DRUG INTERACTIONS

DRUG INTERACTIONS

a source book of adverse interactions, their mechanisms, clinical importance and management

IVAN H. STOCKLEY

B Pharm, PhD (Nott), MRPharm S (Lond), CBiol, MIBiol,
University of Nottingham Medical School,
Nottingham, England

SECOND EDITION

OXFORD

BLACKWELL SCIENTIFIC PUBLICATIONS

LONDON EDINBURGH BOSTON

MELBOURNE PARIS BERLIN VIENNA

© 1981, 1991 Ivan Stockley

Published by
Blackwell Scientific Publications
Editorial Offices:
Osney Mead, Oxford OX2 0EL
25 John Street, London WC1N 2BL
23 Ainslie Place, Edinburgh EH3 6AJ
3 Cambridge Center, Cambridge
  Massachusetts 02142, USA
54 University Street, Carlton
  Victoria 3053, Australia

Other Editorial Offices:
Librairie Arnette SA
2, rue Casimir-Delavigne
75006 Paris
France

Blackwell Wissenschafts-Verlag
Meinekestraße 4
D–1000 Berlin 15
Germany

Blackwell MZV
Feldgasse 13
A–1238 Wien
Austria

First published 1981
Second edition 1991
Reissued in paperback 1992

Typeset by Electronic Village Ltd,
Richmond, Surrey
Printed and bound in Great Britain
at The University Press, Cambridge

DISTRIBUTORS

Marston Book Services Ltd
PO Box 87
Oxford OX2 0DT
(*Orders*: Tel. 0865 791155
        Fax: 0865 791927
        Telex: 837515)

USA
  Blackwell Scientific Publications, Inc.
  3 Cambridge Center
  Cambridge, MA 02142
  (*Orders*: Tel: 800 759–6102
          617 225–0401)

Canada
  Times Mirror Professional Publishing, Ltd
  5240 Finch Avenue East
  Scarborough, Ontario M1S 5A2
  (*Orders*: Tel: 800 268–4178
          416 298–1588)

Australia
  Blackwell Scientific Publications
  (Australia) Pty Ltd
  54 University Street
  Carlton, Victoria 3053
  (*Orders*: Tel: 03 347–0300)

British Library
Cataloguing in Publication Data

Stockley, Ivan H.
  Drug interactions.–2nd. ed.
1. Drugs. Interactions
I. Title
615.7045

ISBN 0-632-03499-8

Praise the LORD, O my soul;
  all my inmost being, praise his holy
  name.
Praise the LORD, O my soul;
  and forget not all his benefits—
who forgives all your sins
  and heals all your diseases.
who redeems your life from the pit
  and crowns you with love and
  compassion,
who satisfies your desires with good
  things
  so that your youth is renewed like
  the eagle's.

For as high as the heavens are above
  the earth,
so great is his love for those who
  fear him,
as far as the east is from the west
  so far has he removed our
  transgressions from us.
As a father has compassion on his
  children,
so the LORD has compassion on
  those who fear him.

          Psalm 103 vv 1–5, 11–13 (NIV)

CONTENTS

PREFACE TO THE SECOND EDITION

This book, its previous edition and its predecessor were all written for doctors, pharmacists, surgeons, nurses and associated health professionals who want to know what happens if drugs are given together, and who do not have either the time or the facilities to make their own searches through the world's medical literature.

My aim has been to answer for them a number of practical everyday questions: What, if anything, happens if the drugs in question are given together? Does it affect everybody? Why does it happen? How can it be managed, and if not what can be used instead which is safer?

To answer these and other questions comprehensively but concisely I have, as before, subdivided the book into a series of synopses, each of which deals with particular interactions between pairs of drugs or groups of drugs. These are categorized into 24 chapters under the drugs which are affected. The synopses have a common format but some of them are condensed where information is sparse. The length of the reference list gives a very fair idea of how much is known about any particular interaction. All of the 650 synopses in the first edition have been reviewed and updated, and an almost equal number of new ones has been added.

Most of what is written in this book is derived from original case reports and clinical studies in man which have been published in medical and related journals worldwide, but some of it also comes from unpublished work on the files of drug companies. I am particularly grateful to numerous people (far too many to name individually here) who work in the information and medical departments of the international drug companies in the UK and elsewhere who have sent me company reports, shared their expert opinions with me, offered constructive suggestions and criticisms, and drawn my attention to obscure reports I might otherwise have missed.

My thanks are also due to many other people, but particularly the staff in the University of Nottingham Medical School library for their ever-willing help, and Dr Alison Ramsey who has provided the computer expertise I lack and given invaluable help in obtaining and filing the thousands of papers used in writing this book.

This book is written to stand alone, but it is also intended to complement the multi-language *Drug Interaction Alert* ready-reference chart, published and distributed worldwide by Boehringer Ingelheim International, whose generous support of my studies and whose permission to reproduce the *Alert* on the jacket of this book I gratefully acknowledge here. The book similarly complements the *Drug Interaction Automatic Alerting System* which is currently in use on the Richardson Pharmacy Computer systems in the UK.

The maintenance of the Drug Interaction Database which underpins this book is like the legendary painting of the Forth Bridge, a never-ending task. If you have informed and constructive comments to make or any additional information which would increase the breadth and accuracy of the database and future editions of this book, I should be pleased to hear from you.

Ivan H. Stockley
University of Nottingham
Medical School

PREFACE TO THE
FIRST EDITION

Plans for this book were drawn up as long ago as 1971, but they were shelved in favour of writing a series of articles on interactions for *The Pharmaceutical Journal* at the invitation of the editor. Later in 1974 these articles were reprinted in facsimile form, with an index, and published under the title *Drug Interactions and their Mechanisms*, so there seemed little point at that time in writing another book on the same subject. A supplement on oral contraceptives was added to the 1978 reprint, but eventually it became clear that a complete rewrite was necessary, incorporating the old material as well as the mass of new data published since the articles were first written. This book is therefore the up-dated successor to the familiar yellow-backed reprinted series of articles.

My aim, as before, has been to present to the practising doctor, pharmacist, surgeon or nurse, or anyone else who has neither the time nor the facilities to carry out detailed literature searches of their own, what is known about the hundreds of drug interactions now on record. I have attempted not only to answer the question of what is likely to happen if two drugs are given concurrently, but also the important associated questions such as these: Is it a genuine, reported, interaction or is it still only theoretical? Has it been described many times or only once? Is the interaction, when it occurs, serious or not? Are all patients affected or only a few? Is it best to avoid the concurrent use of the drugs altogether, or can the interaction be accommodated in some way? And what alternative drugs can be used which do not interact?

So that these questions can be answered succinctly, the material has been organized into a series of individual drug–drug or drug–food synopses—600 or so in all—and categorized into 20 chapters. A very brief outline of the most common mechanisms of interaction has been included at the beginning of the book and a few chapters also include a very short pharmacological introduction for the benefit of those whose pharmacology is not as fresh as it might be. The synopses have a common format with a summary for rapid reading, but very extensive bibliographies are included for those who wish to study the original literature in depth. The synopses are assembled into chapters according to the drugs whose activity is changed, although where the same drug is the affecting or interacting agent, it is usually categorized elsewhere. For this reason the index *must* be used to ensure that the whole range of interactions can be identified.

Through the generosity of the Leverhulme Trust in particular, and a number of Pharmaceutical Companies—Boots, Geistlich, Glaxo, Janssen, Lepetit, Leo, Ortho, Pfizer, Roche, Upjohn and Warner-Lambert—I was able to accumulate sufficient funds for my University to pay a temporary replacement member of staff to undertake my teaching duties for a year, thus enabling me to take sabbatical leave to write this book. I am indebted to all of those, within and without the university, who in one way or another gave me the support I needed.

I also owe a debt of gratitude to many other people: the library staff of the Science and Medical Libraries in the University of Nottingham; the staff of the drug information and medical departments of many of the pharmaceutical companies in the UK; numerous individuals who have drawn my attention to obscure papers and articles which I might otherwise have missed; Dr J. S. B. Stuart for some of the documentation of chapter 12; Böhringer Ingelheim for allowing me to reproduce the

Drug Interaction Alert chart on the jacket of this book; Mr Per Saugman and his staff at Blackwell Scientific Publications, in particular John Robson and Dominic Vaughan; and my wife Bridget, and children Alex, Rosalind, Ben and Beth who with such good grace put up with my acquisition of an intended playroom for a study, and a house strewn, seemingly for ever, with papers.

Ivan H. Stockley
University of Nottingham

BEFORE USING THIS BOOK...

...it is important to realize the extent and the limitations of our knowledge of interactions so that the data summarized here can be properly used.

What we know about interactions comes from a range of sources of widely varying quality and reliability. The best information comes from clinical studies carried out with large numbers of patients where the conditions are scrupulously controlled and the results well analysed. From data of this kind a very good idea of the importance and the incidence of the interaction can be deduced.

However, what is known about very many interactions comes from much less reliable sources: from observations on only one or two patients, possibly in uncontrolled situations where it would be undesirable or unethical to re-challenge the patients with both drugs to confirm the interaction. It may be confined to the results of animal experiments or even based solely on theoretical considerations. Not that this kind of data is to be despised. Quite the contrary. Many of the now very well-confirmed interactions were initially detected in only one patient or even in laboratory animals, but such observations need careful confirmation before their clinical importance can be assessed, and a clear distinction must be drawn between these possible interactions and those which are now well-established.

It also needs to be remembered that patients are not like selected batches of laboratory animals, of the same age, weight, sex and strain which can be expected to respond to drugs with some degree of uniformity. Every ward, surgery, office or clinic contains a mixture of individuals who are very unlikely to respond uniformly to one or more drugs because their genetic make-up, sex, renal and hepatic functions, disease and nutritional states, ages and other parameters are all different. By the same token, the drug dosages, their form, route, duration and order of administration can have a vital bearing on the way a patient responds, and on whether an interaction develops or not.

The sum of all these variables is that while it is possible to say what has already been seen to occur when drugs are given together, the outcome of giving the same drugs to other patients is never totally predictable because when a patient is given one or more drugs for the first time, a new and unique 'experiment' is being undertaken. Despite this element of uncertainty, some idea of the probable outcome of using pairs of drugs in patients can be based on the clinical experience already available—the more extensive the data, the firmer the predictions. The 'importance and management' sections of the synopses are therefore intended to be broad assessments of the incidence and clinical importance of the interactions, with suggestions about how they can be managed. Readers should modify and refine what is written in these sections with the data they have about their own patients so that the measures taken can be individually tailored to fit their patient's needs.

1

GENERAL CONSIDERATIONS AND AN OUTLINE SURVEY OF SOME BASIC INTERACTION MECHANISMS

1. What is a drug interaction?

An interaction is said to occur when the effects of one drug are changed by the presence of another drug, food, drink or by some environmental chemical agent. The outcome may be harmful if the interaction causes an increase in the efficacy or toxicity of the drug. For example, patients already taking warfarin may begin to bleed if given azapropazone or phenylbutazone unless the warfarin dosage is reduced appropriately. Patients taking monoamine oxidase inhibitor anti-depressants may experience an acute and life-threatening hypertensive crisis if they eat tyramine-rich foods. A reduction in efficacy as a result of an interaction may also be harmful. Thus patients on warfarin given rifampicin will need an increase in the dosage of warfarin to maintain adequate anti-coagulation, and patients taking tetracycline anti-biotics should avoid antacids and milky foods because the antibacterial effects can be drastically reduced.

These unwanted and unsought-for interactions are one kind of adverse drug reaction but there are other interactions which can be beneficial rather than adverse. Antihypertensive drugs and diuretics are commonly given together for the treatment of hypertension, and sulphamethoxazole is given with trimethoprim (as co-trimoxazole) because the combined effects are greater than either drug alone. The mechanisms of both types of inter-action, adverse or beneficial, are very similar, but only the adverse interactions form the subject of this book.

Sometimes the term 'drug interaction' is used for the physico-chemical reactions which can occur if drugs are mixed in intravenous fluids, causing precipitation or inactivation. It is also often used for the interference which drugs may have on the biochemical and other assays carried out on body fluids which can invalidate the results. A long-established and less ambiguous term for the former is 'pharmaceutical incompatibilities'. There is no brief and widely accepted term for the drug-biochemical test interactions, but the simple term 'drug interactions' is possibly best reserved for the reactions which go on within, rather than outside, the body.

2. What is the incidence of drug interactions?

The more drugs a patient takes the greater the likelihood that an adverse reaction will occur. One hospital study found that the rate was 7% in those taking 6–10 drugs but 40% in those taking 16–20 drugs which represents a disproportionate increase.[1] A possible explanation is that the drugs were interacting together.

Some of the early studies on the frequency of interactions uncritically compared drugs prescribed with the lists of possible drug interactions, without appreciating that many interactions may be clinically trivial or totally theoretical. As a result an unrealistically high incidence was suggested. Most of the later studies have avoided this error by considering only potentially clinically important interactions and incidences of 4.7%,[2] 6.3%[3] and 8.8%[6] have been found. Even so not all of these studies took into account the distinction which must be made between the incidence of potential interactions and the incidence of those where clinical problems actually arise. That is to say, some patients experience serious reactions while others appear not to react at all.

1

For example a screening of 2422 patients over a total of 25,005 days revealed that 113 (4.7%) were taking combinations of drugs which could interact, but evidence of interactions was observed in only seven patients, representing 0.3%.[2] In another hospital study of 44 patients over a 5-day period taking 10–17 drugs, 77 potential drug interactions were identified, but only one probable and four possible adverse reactions (6.4%) were detected.[5] These figures are low compared with those of a hospital survey which monitored 927 patients who had had 1004 potentially interacting drug combinations. Changes in drug dosage were made in 44% of these cases.[4]

These discordant figures need to be put into the context of under-reporting of adverse reactions of any kind by doctors, for reasons which include pressure of work, indifference, indolence or the fear of litigation. Both doctors and patients may not recognize adverse reactions and interactions, and many outpatients simply stop taking their drugs without saying why. None of these studies gives a clear answer to the question of how frequently drug interactions occur, but even if the incidence is as low as some of the studies suggest, it still represents a very considerable number of patients who appear to be at risk when one remembers the large numbers of drugs administered and prescriptions handled every day by many doctors and pharmacists.

3. How seriously should interactions be regarded and handled?

It would be very easy to conclude after leafing through this book that it is extremely risky to treat patients with more than one drug at a time, but this would be an over-reaction. The figures quoted in the previous section illustrate that many drugs which are known to interact in some patients simply fail to do so in others. This partially explains why some quite important drug interactions remained virtually un-noticed for many years, a good example of this being the effect which quinidine has on serum digoxin levels (see Fig 1.1). Examples of this kind suggest that patients apparently tolerate adverse interactions remarkably well and that many experienced physicians accommodate the effects (such as rises or falls in serum drug levels) without consciously recognizing that

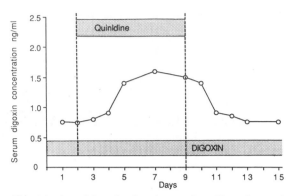

Fig. 1.1 A multi-mechanism interaction. The effects of quinidine (1 mg daily) on the serum digoxin levels of five subjects taking constant doses of digoxin (after Doering W, N Eng J Med (1979) 301, 400, with permission). The mechanisms involved include changes in renal and non-renal clearance, and possibly absorption and tissue-binding.

what they are seeing is the result of an interaction. One of the reasons it is often difficult to detect an interaction is that, as already mentioned, patient variability is very considerable. We now know many of the predisposing and protective factors which determine whether an interaction occurs or not, but in practice it is still very difficult to predict what will happen when an individual patient is given two potentially interacting drugs. An easy solution to this practical problem is to choose a non-interacting alternative. But if none is available it is frequently possible to give known interacting drugs provided appropriate precautions are taken. If the effects are well monitored and the dosages well adjusted, the effects of the interaction can often be allowed for. The reasons this can be done are that many interactions are dose related so that if the dosage is reduced the effects will be reduced accordingly. For example, isoniazid causes the levels of phenytoin to rise, particularly in those individuals who are slow acetylators of isoniazid, and levels may climb into the toxic range. If the serum phenytoin levels are monitored and its dosage reduced appropriately, the concentrations can be kept within the therapeutic range. The dosage of the interacting drug may also be critical. Thus a small dosage of cimetidine may fail to inhibit the metabolism of warfarin, whereas a larger dose may have profound clinical effects.

Some interactions can be accommodated by using another member of the same group of drugs. For example, the serum levels of doxycycline can fall to subtherapeutic concentrations if phenytoin, barbiturates or carbamazepine are given, but other tetracyclines do not seem to be affected. Cimetidine causes serum warfarin levels to rise because it inhibits its metabolism, but not those of phenprocoumon because these two anticoagulants are metabolized in different ways. It is therefore clearly important not to extrapolate uncritically the interactions seen with one drug to all members of the same group.

The variability in patient response has lead to some extreme responses among prescribers. Some clinicians have become over-anxious about interactions so that their patients are denied useful drugs which they might reasonably be given if appropriate precautions are taken. This attitude is exacerbated by some of the more alarmist lists and charts of interactions which fail to make a distinction between interactions which are very well documented and well established, and those which have only been encountered in a single patient and which in the final analysis are probably totally idiosyncratic. 'One swallow does not make a summer', nor does a serious reaction in a single patient mean that the drugs in question should never again be administered to anyone else. At the other extreme there are a some clinicians who have personally encountered few interactions and therefore virtually disregard their existence so that some of their patients are potentially put at risk. The responsible position lies between these two extremes because a very substantial number of interacting drugs can be given together safely if the appropriate precautions are taken, whereas there are relatively few pairs of drugs which should always be avoided.

4. Mechanisms of drug interaction

Some drugs interact together in totally unique ways but, as the many examples in this book amply illustrate, there are certain mechanisms of interaction which are encountered time and time again. Some of these common mechanisms are discussed here in greater detail than space will allow in the individual synopses so that only the briefest reference need be made within the synopses.

Mechanisms which are unusual or peculiar to particular pairs of drugs are detailed within the synopses. Very many drugs which interact do so, not by a single mechanism, but often by two or more mechanisms acting in concert, although for clarity most of the mechanisms are dealt with here as though they occur in isolation. For convenience the mechanisms of interactions can be subdivided into those which involve the pharmacokinetics of a drug and those which are pharmacodynamic.

4.1 Pharmacokinetic interactions

Pharmacokinetic interactions are those which can affect the processes by which drugs are absorbed, distributed, metabolized and excreted (the so-called ADME interactions).

4.1.1 Drug absorption interactions

Most drugs are given orally for absorption through the mucous membranes of the gastrointestinal tract, and most of the interactions which go on within the gut result in reduced rather than increased absorption. A clear distinction must be made between those which decrease the *rate* of absorption and those which alter the *total* amount absorbed. For drugs which are given chronically on a multiple dose regimen (e.g. the oral anticoagulants) the rate of absorption is usually unimportant, provided the total amount of drug absorbed is not markedly altered. On the other hand for drugs which are given as single doses intended to be absorbed rapidly (e.g. hypnotics or analgesics) where a rapidly achieved high concentration is needed, a reduction in the rate of absorption may result in failure to achieve adequate serum levels. Table 1.1 lists some of the drug interactions which result from changes in absorption.

4.1.1.1 Effects of changes in gastrointestinal pH The ability of drugs to pass through mucous membranes by simple passive diffusion depends upon the extent to which they exist in the non-ionized lipid-soluble form. Absorption is therefore governed by the pKa of the drug, its lipid-solubility, the pH of the contents of gut and various other parameters relating to the pharmaceutical formulation of the drug. Thus the absorption of salicylic acid by the stomach is much higher at low pH than at high. On theoretical grounds it might be expected therefore that alterations in gastric pH caused by drugs such as antacids would have a marked effect on absorption,

Table 1.1 Some drug absorption interactions

Drug affected	Interacting drugs	Effect of interaction
Tetracyclines	Antacids containing Al^{3+}, Ca^{2+}, Mg^{2+}, Bi^{2+}, milk, Zn^{2+}, Fe^{2+}	Formation of poorly soluble chelates resulting in reduced antibiotic absorption (see Fig 1.2)
Digoxin Thyroxine Warfarin	Cholestyramine	Reduced absorption of digoxin, thyroxine, warfarin due to binding/complexation with cholestyramine
Penicillamine	Al^{3+} and Mg^{2+} containing antacids, food, iron preparations	Formation of less soluble penicillamine chelates resulting in reduced absorption of penicillamine
Digoxin	Metoclopramide Propantheline	Reduced digoxin absorption and increased digoxin absorption due to changes in gut motility
Penicillin	Neomycin	Neomycin-induced malabsorption state

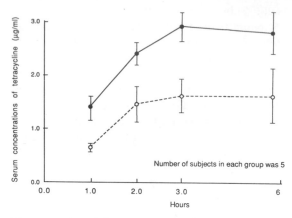

Fig. 1.2 A drug chelation interaction. Tetracycline forms a less-soluble chelate with iron if the two drugs are allowed to mix within the gut. This reduces the absorption and depresses the serum levels and the antibacterial effects (after Neuvonen PJ, Br Med J (1970) 4, 532, with permission). The same interaction can occur with other ions such as Al^{3+}, Ca^{2+}, Mg^{2+}, Bi^{2+} and Zn^{2+}.

but in practice the outcome is often uncertain because a number of other mechanisms may also come into play such as chelation, adsorption and changes in gut motility which can considerably affect what actually happens.

4.1.1.2 Adsorption, chelation and other complexing mechanisms Activated charcoal is intended to act as an adsorbing agent within the gut for the treatment of drug overdosage or to remove other toxic materials, but inevitably it can affect the absorption of drugs given in therapeutic doses. Antacids can also adsorb a very considerable number of drugs but often other mechanisms of interaction are also involved. For example the tetracycline antibiotics can chelate with a number of di- and trivalent metallic ions such as calcium, aluminium, bismuth and iron to form complexes which not only are poorly absorbed but have reduced antibacterial effects (see Figure 1.2).

These metallic ions are found in dairy products

and antacids. Separating the dosages by 2–3 h goes some way towards reducing the effects of this type of interaction. The marked reduction in the bioavailability of penicillamine by some antacids seems also to be due to chelation, although adsorption may have some part to play. Cholestyramine, an anionic exchange resin intended to bind bile acids and cholesterol metabolites in the gut, binds to a considerable number of drugs if co-administered (e.g. digoxin, warfarin, thyroxine) thereby reducing their absorption. Table 1.1 lists these drugs which chelate or complex or adsorb other drugs thereby reducing their absorption.

4.1.1.3 Changes in gastrointestinal motility Since most drugs are largely absorbed in the upper part of the small intestine, drugs which alter the rate at which the stomach empties its contents can affect absorption. Propantheline, for example, delays gastric emptying and reduces paracetamol (acetaminophen) absorption whereas metoclopramide has the opposite effect, however the total amount of drug absorbed remains unaltered. These two drugs have quite the opposite effect on the absorption of hydrochlorothiazide and slowly dissolving brands of digoxin. Anticholinergic drugs decrease the motility of the gut, thus the tricyclic antidepressants can increase the absorption of dicoumarol probably because they increase the time available for dissolution and absorption, but in the case of levodopa they reduce the absorption possibly because the exposure time to intestinal mucosal metabolism is increased. The same reduced levodopa absorption has also been seen with homatropine. On the other hand benzhexol (another anticholinergic) reduces the absorption of chlorpromazine. Other examples of changes in motility which affect absorption include the reduced absorption caused by pethidine and diamorphine. These examples illustrate that what actually happens is sometimes unpredictable because the final outcome may be the result of several different mechanisms.

4.1.1.4 Malabsorption caused by drugs Neomycin causes a malabsorption syndrome which is similar to that seen with non-tropical sprue. The effect is to impair the absorption of a number of drugs including digoxin and penicillin V.

4.1.2 Drug displacement (protein-binding) interactions

Following absorption, drugs are rapidly distributed around the body by the circulation. Some drugs are totally dissolved in the plasma water, but many others are transported with some proportion of their molecules in solution and the rest bound to plasma proteins, particularly the albumins. The extent of this binding varies enormously but some drugs are extremely highly bound. For example, dicoumarol has only four out of every 1000 molecules remaining unbound at serum concentrations of 0.5 mg%. Drugs can also become bound to albumin in the interstitial fluid, and some such as digoxin can bind to the heart muscle tissue.

The binding of drugs to the plasma proteins is reversible, an equilibrium being established between those molecules which are bound and those which are not. Only the unbound molecules remain free and pharmacologically active, while those which are bound form a circulating but pharmacologically inactive reservoir which, in the case of 'restrictive' drugs, is temporarily protected from metabolism and excretion. As the free molecules become metabolized, so some of the bound molecules become unbound and pass into solution to exert their normal pharmacological actions, before they, in their turn are metabolized and excreted.

Depending on the concentrations and their relative affinities for the binding sites, one drug may suc-

cessfully compete with another and displace it from the sites it is already occupying. The displaced (and now active) drug molecules pour into plasma water where their concentration rapidly rises. So for example, a drug which reduces the binding from (say) 99 to 95% would thereby increase the unbound concentration of free and active drug from 1 to 4% (a fourfold increase). This displacement is only likely to raise the number of free and active molecules significantly if the majority of the drug is within the plasma rather than the tissues, so that only drugs with a low apparent volume of distribution (V_d) will be affected. Such drugs include the sulphonylureas such as tolbutamide (96% bound, V_d 10 l), oral anticoagulants such as warfarin (99% bound, V_d 9 l) and phenytoin (90% bound, V_d 35 l). Other highly bound drugs include diazoxide, ethacrynic acid, methotrexate, nalidixic acid, phenylbutazone and the sulphonamides.

Displacement of this kind happens when patients stabilized on warfarin are given chloral hydrate because its major metabolite, trichloroacetic acid, is a highly bound compound which successfully displaces warfarin, thereby increasing its anticoagulant effects. This effect is only very short-lived because the now free and active warfarin molecules become exposed to metabolism as the blood flows through the liver and the total amount of drug rapidly falls. A small but transient increase in the anticoagulant effects can be seen and the warfarin requirements fall briefly by about a third, but within about five days a new equilibrium becomes established with the same concentration of unbound warfarin, even though the free fraction has increased. Normally no change in the warfarin dosage is needed.[7]

In vitro many commonly used drugs are capable of being displaced by others, but in the body the effects seem almost always to be buffered so effectively that the outcome is normally clinically unimportant, and it would seem that the importance of this interaction mechanism has been grossly overemphasized, despite statements made to the contrary in numerous papers, reviews and drug data sheets. It is difficult to find an example of a clinically important interaction due to this mechanism alone. One possible example is the marked diuresis which was seen in patients with nephrotic syndrome when they were given clofibrate.[8] Usually this mechanism has a minor part to play compared with other mechanisms which are going on at the same time. However it may need to be taken into account in some circumstances.

Suppose, for example, an epileptic patient has a total serum phenytoin concentration of 50 μmol/l of which 45 μmol/l is bound and 5 μmol/l free (i.e. 10% free). If now another drug is given which displaces a further 10%, more of the phenytoin thereby becomes exposed to metabolism and excretion so that the total serum phenytoin concentration is halved (to 25 μmol/ l) with a free concentration of 20% but which still remains at 5 μmol/l. From the patient's point of view the effective amount of phenytoin stays the same, even though the total amount of phenytoin in circulation has halved. Under these circumstances there would be no need to change the phenytoin dosage, and to do so in order to accommodate the change in total levels might lead to overdosage.

Basic drugs as well as acidic drugs can be highly protein bound, but clinically important displacement interactions do not seem to have been described. The reasons seem to be that the binding sites within the plasma are different from those occupied by acidic drugs (alpha-1-acid glycoprotein rather than albumin) and, in addition, basic drugs have a large V_d with only a small proportion of the total amount of drug being within the plasma.

4.1.3 Drug metabolism (biotransformation) interactions

Although some drugs are lost from the body simply by being excreted unchanged in the urine, a very large number are chemically altered within the body to less lipid-soluble compounds which are more easily excreted by the kidneys. If this were not so, many drugs would remain in the body for extended periods of time and continue to exert their effects. This chemical change is called metabolism, biotransformation, biochemical degradation or sometimes detoxification. Some drug metabolism goes on in the serum, the kidneys, the skin and the intestines, but by far the greatest proportion is carried out by enzymes which are found in the membranes of the endoplasmic reticulum of the liver cells. If liver is homogenized and then centrifuged, the reticulum breaks up into small sacs called microsomes which carry the enzymes, and it is for this reason that the metabolizing enzymes of the liver are frequently referred to as the

'liver microsomal enzymes'.

4.1.3.1 *Enzyme induction* A phenomenon familiar to prescribers is the 'tolerance' which develops to some drugs. For example, when barbiturates were widely used as hypnotics it was found necessary to keep on increasing the dosage as time went by to achieve the same hypnotic effect, the reason being that the barbiturates increase the activity of the microsomal enzymes so that pace of metabolism and excretion increases. This phenomenon of enzyme stimulation or 'induction' not only accounts for the tolerance, but if another drug is present as well which is metabolized by the same range of enzymes (an oral anticoagulant for example), its enzymic metabolism is similarly increased and larger doses are needed to maintain the same therapeutic effect. Figure 1.3 shows the effects of an enzyme inducing agent, dichloralphenazone, on the metabolism and anticoagulant effects of warfarin. Figures 1.4 and 1.5 show the effects of another enzyme inducing agent, rifampicin (rifampin) on the serum levels of ketoconazole and cyclosporin. Table 1.2 lists some of the interactions due to enzyme induction and Table 1.3 contains some of the potent enzyme-inducing drugs.

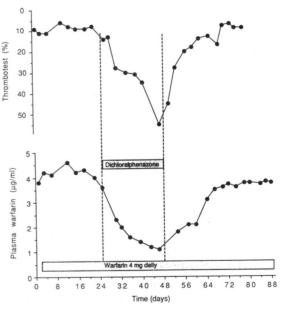

Fig. 1.3 *An enzyme induction interaction.* In this patient the hypnotic dichloralpenazone (*Welldorm*) increased the metabolism of the warfarin, thereby reducing its serum levels and its effects (thrombotest percentages) (after Breckenridge A et al., Clin Sci (1971) 40, 351, with permission).

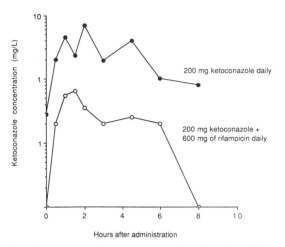

Fig. 1.4 *An enzyme induction interaction.* Rifampicin (600 mg daily plus isoniazid) increased the metabolism of the ketoconazole in this patient, thereby reducing the serum levels (after Brass C, Antimicrob Ag Chemother (1982) 21, 151, with permission).

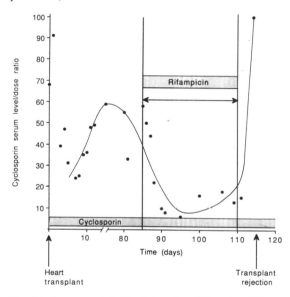

Fig. 1.5 *An enzyme induction interaction.* Rifampicin (600 mg daily) increased the metabolism of cyclosporin in this patient, thereby reducing the trough serum levels. He subsequently died because his heart transplant was rejected (after Van Buren D et al., Transplant Proc (1984) 16, 1642, with permission).

A metabolic pathway which is commonly affected is Phase I oxidation, this term covering a number of metabolic biotransformations, all of which require the presence of NADPH and the haem-containing protein cytochrome P450. When enzyme induction occurs the amount of endoplasmic reticulum within the liver cells increases and the cytochrome P450

Table 1.2 Interactions due to enzyme induction

Drug affected	Inducing agent(s)	Effect of interaction
Anticoagulants (oral)	Aminoglutethimide Barbiturates Carbamazepine Dichloralphenazone Glutethimide Phenazone Rifampicin (rifampin)	Anticoagulant effects reduced (see Fig. 1.3)
Contraceptives (oral)	Barbiturates Carbamazepine Phenytoin Primidone Rifampicin	Break-through bleeding. Contraceptive failures.
Corticosteroids	Aminoglutethimide Barbiturates Carbamazepine Phenytoin Primidone Rifampicin	Corticosteroid effects reduced
Haloperidol	Tobacco smoke	Haloperidol effects reduced
Phenytoin	Rifampicin	Phenytoin effects reduced. Seizure-risk increased
Theophylline	Barbiturates Rifampicin Tobacco smoke	Theophylline effects reduced

Table 1.3 Enzyme inducing drugs

Aminoglutethimide
Barbiturates
Carbamazepine
Dichloralphenazone
Glutethimide
Phenazone
Phenytoin
Primidone
Rifampicin (rifampin)
Tobacco smoke

levels also rise. The extent of the enzyme induction depends on the drug and its dosage, but its development may take days or weeks, and persist for a similar length of time after withdrawal of the inducing agent so that enzyme induction interactions are delayed in both starting and stopping. Enzyme induction is an extremely common mechanism of interaction and is not confined to drugs but is also caused by the chlorinated hydrocarbon insecticides such as dicophane and lindane, and after smoking tobacco.

It is possible to accommodate this kind of interaction by increasing the dose of the drug which is being affected, but the effects require thorough monitoring and there are obvious dangers if the inducing drug is withdrawn without reducing the dosage of the other drug. The raised drug dosage will be an overdose when the drug metabolism has returned to normal.

4.1.3.2 Enzyme inhibition Just as some drugs can stimulate the activity of the microsomal enzymes, so there are others which have the opposite effect and act as inhibitors. The normal pace of drug metabolism is slackened so that the metabolism of other drugs given concurrently is also reduced and they begin to accumulate within the body, the effect being essentially the same as when the dosage is increased. Figure 1.6 shows what happened when an epileptic patient on phenytoin was given chloramphenicol. The accumulating phenytoin was not detected until it reached levels at which the patient began to manifest toxicity. Figure 1.7 illustrates the sharp and potentially hazardous rise in blood pressure which can occur if the normally protective monoamine oxidase within the gut wall and liver is inhibited by the presence of an MAO-inhibitory drug (tranylcypromine). Other mechanisms of interaction are also involved. Table 1.4 lists some other interactions due to the inhibition of microsomal and other enzymes, and Table 1.5 is a list of enzyme-inhibiting drugs. Numerous other examples are to be found throughout this book. The clinical significance of many enzyme inhibition interactions depends on the extent to which the serum levels of the drug rise. If the serum levels remain within the therapeutic range the interaction may be advantageous. If not, the interaction becomes adverse as the serum levels climb into the toxic range.

4.1.3.3 Changes in blood flow through the liver After absorption in the intestine, the portal circulation takes drugs directly to the liver before they are distributed by the blood flow around the rest of the body. A number of highly lipid-soluble drugs undergo substantial biotransformation during this 'first pass' through the gut wall and liver and there is evidence that some concurrently administered drugs can have a marked effect on the extent of first pass metabolism. Cimetidine (but not ranitidine) decreases hepatic blood flow and thereby increases

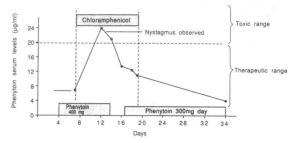

Fig. 1.6 *An enzyme inhibition interaction.* The chloramphenicol inhibited the metabolism of the phenytoin in this patient so that the serum levels climbed into the toxic range and intoxication developed (indicated by nystagmus). The problem was solved by stopping the phenytoin and later re-starting at a lower dosage (after Ballek RE et al., Lancet (1973) i, 150, with permission).

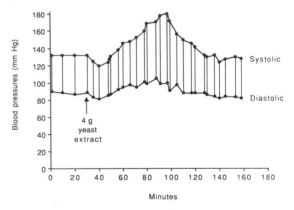

Fig. 1.7 *An enzyme inhibition interaction.* The effect of 4 g *Marmite* (a tyramine-rich yeast extract) on the diastolic and systolic blood pressures of a patient taking a Monoamine Oxidase Inhibitor (tranylcypromine) (after Blackwell B, Br J Psychiat (1967) 113, 349, with permission).

the bioavailability of propranolol. Propranolol also reduces both its own clearance and that of other drugs such as lignocaine (lidocaine). A number of other drugs have the opposite effect and increase the flow of blood through the liver so that their metabolism is increased.

4.1.4 Interactions due to changes in excretion

With the exception of the inhalation anaesthetics, most drugs are excreted either in the bile or in the urine. Blood entering the kidneys along the renal arteries is, first of all, delivered to the glomeruli of the tubules where molecules small enough to pass through the pores of the glomerular membrane (e.g. water, salts, some drugs) are filtered through into the lumen of the tubules. Larger molecules,

Table 1.4 Interactions due to enzyme inhibition

Drug affected	Inhibiting agent(s)	Clinical outcome
Alcohol	Chlorpropamide Disulfiram Latamoxef	Disulfiram-reaction due to a rise in blood acetaldehyde levels
Anticoagulants (oral)	Metronidazole Phenylbutazone Sulphinpyrazone	Anticoagulant effects increased. Bleeding possible
Azathioprine Mercaptopurine	Allopurinol	Azathioprine/ mercaptopurine effects increased; toxicity
Caffeine	Idrocilamide	Caffeine effects increased. Intoxication possible
Corticosteroids	Erythromycin Triacetyloleandomycin	Corticosteroid effects increased. Toxicity possible.
Phenytoin	Chloramphenicol Isoniazid	Phenytoin effects increased. Intoxication possible (see Fig. 1.6)
Suxamethonium	Ecothiophate	Neuromuscular blockade increased. Prolonged apnoea possible.
Tolbutamide Chloramphenicol	Azapropazone Phenylbutazone	Tolbutamide effects increased. Hypoglycaemia possible.
Tyramine-containing food-stuffs	Monoamine oxidase inhibitors	Tyramine-induced hypertensive crisis (other mechanisms also involved) see Fig. 1.7

Table 1.5 Some Enzyme inhibitors

Allopurinol
Azapropazone
Chloramphenicol
Ciprofloxacin
Cimetidine
Disulfiram
Enoxacin
Erythromycin
Idrocilamide
Isoniazid
Ketoconazole
Phenylbutazone
Sulphinpyrazone
Triacetyloleandomycin

such as plasma proteins, and blood cells are retained. The blood flow then passes to the remaining parts of the kidney tubules where active energy-using transport systems are able to remove drugs and their metabolites from the blood and secrete them into the tubular filtrate. The tubule cells additionally possess active and passive transport systems for the reabsorption of drugs. Interference by drugs with kidney tubule fluid pH, with active transport systems and with blood flow to the kidney can alter the excretion of other drugs.

4.1.4.1 Changes in urinary pH As with drug absorption in the gut, passive reabsorption of drugs depends upon the extent to which the drug exists in the non-ionized lipid-soluble form which in its turn depends on its pKa and the pH of the urine. Only the un-ionized form is lipid-soluble and able to diffuse back through the lipid membranes of the tubule cells. Thus at high pH values (alkaline), weakly acid drugs (pKa 3.0–7.5) largely exist as ionized lipid-insoluble molecules which are unable to diffuse into the tubule cells and will therefore be lost in the urine. The converse will be true for weak organic bases with pKa values of 7.5–10.5. Thus pH changes which increase the amount in the un-ionized form (alkaline urine for acidic drugs, acid for bases) increase the loss of the drug, whereas moving the pH in the opposite directions will increase their retention. Figure 1.8 illustrates the situation with a weakly acidic drug.

The clinical significance of this interaction mechanism is small because although a very large number of drugs are either weak acids or bases, almost all are largely metabolized by the liver to inactive compounds and few are excreted in the urine unchanged. In practice therefore only a handful of drugs seem to be affected by changes in urinary pH (the exceptions include changes in the excretion of quinidine and salicylate due to alterations in urinary pH caused by antacids). In cases of overdosage, deliberate urinary pH changes have been used to increase the loss of drugs such as phenobarbitone and salicylates.

4.1.4.2 Changes in active kidney tubule excretion Drugs which use the same active transport systems in the kidney tubules can compete with one another for excretion. For example, probenecid reduces the excretion of penicillin and other drugs by successfully

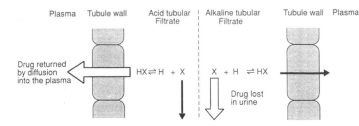

Plasma | Tubule wall | Acid tubular Filtrate | Alkaline tubular Filtrate | Tubule wall | Plasma

Drug returned by diffusion into the plasma

$HX \rightleftharpoons H + X$ $X + H \rightleftharpoons HX$

Drug lost in urine

Fig. 1.8 *An excretion interaction.* If the tubular filtrate is acidified, most of the molecules of weakly acid drugs (HX) exist in an un-ionized lipid-soluble form and are able to return through the lipid membranes of the tubule cells by simple diffusion. Thus they are retained. In alkaline urine most of the drug molecules exist in an ionized non-lipid souble form (X). In this form the molecules are unable to diffuse freely through these membranes and are therefore lost in the urine.

competing for an excretory mechanism, thus the 'loser' (penicillin) is retained. But even the 'winner' (probenecid) is also later retained because it is passively reabsorbed further along the kidney tubule. See Figure 1.9. Table 1.6 contains some examples of drugs which interact in this way.

4.1.4.3 Changes in kidney blood flow The flow of blood through the kidney is partially controlled by the production of renal vasodilatory prostaglandins. If the synthesis of these prostaglandins is inhibited (e.g. by indomethacin), the renal excretion of lithium is reduced and its serum levels rise as a result.

4.1.4.4 Biliary excretion and the entero-hepatic shunt A number of drugs are excreted in the bile, either unchanged or conjugated (e.g. as the glucuronide) to make them more water soluble. Some of the conjugates are metabolized to the parent compound by the gut flora which are then reabsorbed. This recycling process prolongs the stay of the drug within the body, but if activity of the gut flora is decimated by the presence of an antibiotic, the drug is not recycled and is lost more quickly. This may possibly explain the rare failure of the oral contraceptives which can be brought about by the concurrent use of penicillins or tetracyclines.

4.2 Pharmacodynamic interactions

Pharmacodynamic interactions are those where the effects of one drug are changed by the presence of another drug at its site of action. Sometimes the drugs directly compete for particular receptors (e.g. beta-2 agonists such as salbutamol and beta-antagonists) but often the reaction is more indirect and involves the interference with physiological mechanisms. These interactions are much less easy to classify neatly than those which are pharmacokinetic.

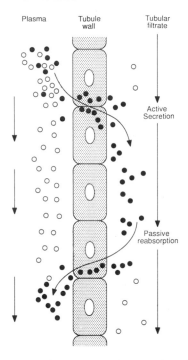

Plasma | Tubule wall | Tubular filtrate

Active Secretion

Passive reabsorption

Fig. 1.9 *Competitive interaction between drugs for active tubular secretion.* Probenecid (●) is able successfully to compete with some of the other drugs (○) for active secretory mechanisms in the kidney tubules which reduces their loss in the urine and raises serum levels. The probenecid is later passively reabsorbed.

4.2.1 Additive or synergistic interactions and combined toxicity

If two drugs which have the same pharmacological effect are given together, the effects can be additive. For example, alcohol depresses the central nervous system and, if taken in moderate amounts with normal therapeutic doses of any of a large number of drugs (e.g. hypnosedatives, tranquillizers, etc.), the result may be excessive drowsiness. Strictly speaking these are not interactions within the definition given at the beginning of this chapter, nevertheless it is

Table 1.6 Interactions due to changes in renal transport

Drug affected	Interacting drug	Result of interaction
Cephalosporins Dapsone Indomethacin Nalidixic acid Penicillin PAS (amino-salicylic acid)	Probenecid	Serum levels of affected raised; possibility of toxicity with some drugs. See Fig. 1.8
Methotrexate	Salicylates and some other NSAID's	Methotrexate serum levels raised. Serious methotrexate toxicity possible
Acetohexamide Glibenclamide Tolbutamide	Phenylbutazone	Hypoglycaemic effects increased and pro-longed due to reduced renal excretion

Table 1.7 Additive, synergistic or summation interactions

Drugs	Result of interaction
Anticholinergics + anticholinergics (anti-parkinsonian agents, butyrophenones phenothiazines, tricyclic antidepressants, etc.)	Increased anticholinergic effects; heat stroke in hot and humid conditions; adynamic ileus; toxic psychoses
Antihypertensives + drugs causing hypotension (anti-anginals, vasodilators, phenothiazines)	Increased antihypertensive effects; orthostasis
CNS depressants + CNS depressants (alcohol, anti-emetics, antihistamines hypnosedatives, tranquillizers etc)	Impaired psychomotor skills, reduced alertness, drowsiness, stupor, respiratory depression, coma, death
Methotrexate + co-trimoxazole	Bone marrow megaloblastosis due to folic acid antagonism
Nephrotoxic drugs + nephrotoxic drugs (gentamicin or tobramycin with cephalothin)	Increased nephrotoxicity
Neuromuscular blockers + drugs with neuromuscular blocking effects (e.g. aminoglycoside antibiotics)	Increased neuromuscular blockade; prolonged apnoea
Potassium supplements + potassium-sparing diuretics (triamterene)	Marked hyperkalaemia

Table 1.8 Opposing or antagonistic interactions

Drug affected	Interacting drug	Results of interaction
Anticoagulants	Vitamin K	Anticoagulant effects opposed
Carbenoxolone	Spironolactone	Ulcer-healing effects opposed
Hypoglycaemic agents	Glucocorticoids	Hypoglycaemic effects opposed
Hypnotic drugs	Caffeine	Hypnosis prevented
Levodopa	Antipsychotics (those with Parkinson side effects)	Antiparkinsonian opposed

convenient to consider them within the broad context of the clinical outcome of giving two drugs together. Additive effects can occur with both the main effects of the drugs as well as their side-effects, thus an additive 'interaction' can occur with anticholinergic antiparkinson drugs (main effect) or butyrophenones (side effect) which can result in serious anticholinergic toxicity. Sometimes the additive effects are solely toxic (e.g. additive ototoxicity, nephrotoxicity or bone marrow depression). Examples of these reactions are listed in Table 1.7. It is common to use the terms 'additive', 'summation', 'synergy' or 'potentiation' to describe what happens if two or more drugs behave like this. These words have precise pharmacological definitions but they are often used rather loosely as synonyms because in practice in man it is often very difficult to know the extent of the increased activity, that is to say whether the effects are greater or smaller than the sum of the individual effects.

4.2.2 Antagonistic or opposing interactions

In contrast to additive interactions, there are some pairs of drugs with activities which are opposed to one another. For example the oral anticoagulants can prolong the blood clotting time by com-petitively inhibiting the effects of dietary vitamin K. If the intake of vitamin K is increased the effects of the oral anticoagulant are antagonized and the prothrombin time can return to normal thereby cancelling out the therapeutic benefits of anti-coagulant treatment. Other examples of this type of interaction are listed in Table 1.8.

4.2.3 Interactions due to changes in drug transport mechanisms

A number of drugs whose actions occur at adrenergic neurones can be prevented from reaching those sites of action by the presence of other drugs.

Table 1.9 Interactions due to changes in drug transport mechanisms

Drug affected	Interacting drug	Results of interaction
Clonidine	Tricyclic anti-depressants	Antidepressant effects opposed, possibly due to interference in CNS with clonidine uptake.
Guanethidine like antihypertensives (debrisoquine, guanoclor, etc.)	Tricyclic anti-depressants Chlorpromazine Haloperidol Thiothixene Indirectly-acting sympathomimetics	Antihypertensive effects opposed, due to inhibition of uptake into adrenergic neurones. See Fig. 1.10
Noradrenaline (norepinephrine)	Tricyclic anti-depressants	Pressor effects increased due to inhibition of nor-adrenaline uptake into adrenergic neurones.

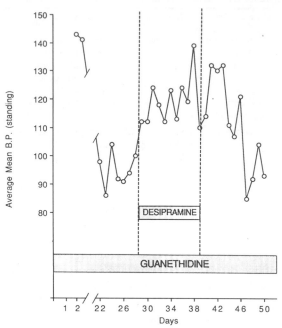

Fig. 1.10 *A pharmacodynamic interaction.* The desipramine (75–100 mg daily) inhibited the uptake of guanethidine (150 mg daily) into adrenergic neurones of the sympathetic nervous system thereby stopping its antihypertensive effects. As a result the blood pressure in this patient rose once again (after Oates JA et al., Ann NY Acad Sci (1971) 179, 302, with permission).

Thus the uptake of guanethidine and related drugs (guanoclor, bethanidine, debrisoquine, etc.) is blocked by chlorpromazine, haloperidol, thiothix-ene, a number of indirectly-acting sympathomimetic amines and the tricyclic antidepressants so that the antihypertensive effect is prevented. This is il-lustrated in Figure 1.10. The tricyclic antidepressants also prevent the re-uptake of noradrenaline into peripheral adrenergic neurones so that its pressor effects are increased. The antihypertensive effects of clonidine are also prevented by the tricyclic anti-depressants, one possible reason being that the up-take of clonidine within the CNS is blocked. Some of these interactions at adrenergic neurones are il-lustrated in Figure 1.11. See also Table 1.9.

4.2.4 Interactions due to disturbances in fluid and electrolyte balance

An increase in the sensitivity of the myocardium to the digitalis glycosides, and resultant toxicity, can result from a fall in plasma potassium concentrations brought about by potassium-depleting diuretics such as frusemide. Plasma lithium levels can rise if thiazide diuretics are used because the clearance of the lithium by the kidney is changed, probably as a result of the changes in sodium excretion which can accompany the use of these diuretics. Table 1.10 lists some examples.

Table 1.10 Interactions due to disturbances in fluid and electrolyte balance

Drug affected	Interacting drug	Results of interaction
Digitalis	Potassium-depleting diuretics	Digitalis toxicity related to changes in ionic balance at the myocardium
Lithium chloride	Dietary salt restriction	Increased serum lithium levels; intoxication possible
	Increased salt intake	Reduced serum lithium levels
		Both changes related to changes in sodium excretion
Lithium chloride	Thiazide and related diuretics	Increased serum lithium levels. Intoxication possible
Guanethidine Chlorothiazide	Kebuzone Phenylbutazone	Antihypertensive effects opposed due to salt and water retention

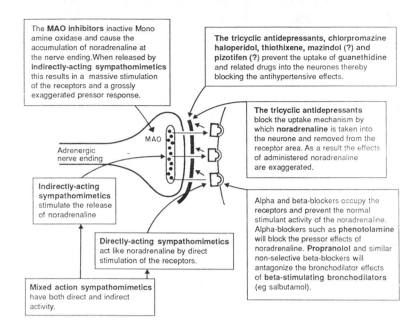

The **MAO inhibitors** inactive Mono amine oxidase and cause the accumulation of noradrenaline at the nerve ending. When released by **indirectly-acting sympathomimetics** this results in a massive stimulation of the receptors and a grossly exaggerated pressor response.

The tricyclic antidepressants, chlorpromazine **haloperidol, thiothixene, mazindol (?)** and **pizotifen (?)** prevent the uptake of guanethidine and related drugs into the neurones thereby blocking the antihypertensive effects.

MAO

The tricyclic antidepressants block the uptake mechanism by which **noradrenaline** is taken into the neurone and removed from the receptor area. As a result the effects of administered noradrenaline are exaggerated.

Adrenergic nerve ending

Indirectly-acting sympathomimetics stimulate the release of noradrenaline

Directly-acting sympathomimetics act like noradrenaline by direct stimulation of the receptors.

Alpha and beta-blockers occupy the receptors and prevent the normal stimulant activity of the noradrenaline. Alpha-blockers such as **phenotolamine** will block the pressor effects of noradrenaline. **Propranolol** and similar non-selective beta-blockers will antagonize the bronchodilator effects of **beta-stimulating bronchodilators** (eg salbutamol).

Mixed action sympathomimetics have both direct and indirect activity.

Fig. 1.11 *Interactions at adrenergic neurones.* A highly simplified composite diagram of an adrenergic neurone (molecules of noradrenaline (norepinephrine) indicated as (●) contained in single vesicle at the nerve-ending) to illustrate in outline some of the different sites where drugs can interact. More details of these interactions are to be found in individual synopses.

5. Conclusions

It is quite impossible to remember all the known clinically important interactions and how they occur, which is why this reference book has been written, but there are some broad general principles which need little memorizing. Be on the alert with any drugs which have a narrow therapeutic window or where it is necessary to keep serum levels at or above a suitable level (anticoagulants, anticonvulsants, cytotoxics, antihypertensives, antiinfectives, digitalis glycosides, hypoglycaemic agents, immunosuppressants, etc.). Remember those drugs which are enzyme inducing agents (phenytoin, barbiturates) and enzyme inhibitors (cimetidine), and keep in mind that the elderly are most at risk because of reduced liver and kidney function on which drug clearance depends. And think about the basic pharmacology of the drugs under consideration so that obvious problems (additive CNS depression for example) are not overlooked.

References

1   Smith JW, Seidl LG and Cluff LE. Studies on the epidemiology of adverse drug reactions. V. Clinical factors influencing susceptibility. Ann Intern Med (1969) 65, 629.
2   Puckett WH and Visconti JA. An epidemiological study of the clinical significance of drug-drug interaction in a private community hospital. Amer J Hosp Pharm (1971) 28, 247.
3   Shinn AF, Shrewsbury RP and Anderson KW. Development of a computerized drug interaction database (Medicom) for use in a patient specific environment. Drug Inform (1983) 17, 205.
4   Haumschild MJ, Ward ES, Bishop JM and Haumschild MS. Pharmacy-based computer system for monitoring and reporting drug interactions. Am J Hosp Pharm (1987) 44, 345.
5   Schuster BG, Fleckenstein L, Wilson JP and Peck CC. Low incidence of adverse reactions due to drug-drug interaction in a potentially high risk population of medical inpatients. Clin Res (1982) 30, 258A.
6   Ishikura C and Ishizuka H. Evaluation of a computerized drug interaction checking system. Int J Bio-Medical Computing (1983) 14, 311.
7   Boston Collaborative Drug Surveillance Program. Interaction between chloral hydrate and warfarin. N Eng J Med (1972) 286, 53.
8   Bridgeman JF, Rosem SM and Thorp JM. Complications during clofibrate treatment of nephrotic syndrome hyperlipoproteinaemia. Lancet (1972) ii, 506.

2
ALCOHOL INTERACTIONS

For social and historical reasons we normally buy alcohol in a bar instead of in a Pharmacy because it is considered to be a drink and not a drug, but pharmacologically speaking it has much in common with medicinal drugs which depress the central nervous system. Objective tests show that as blood-alcohol levels rise, the ability to perform a number of skills gradually deteriorates because of the progessive disorganization of the brain. The myth that alcohol is a stimulant has arisen because at parties and social occasions it helps people to lose some of their inhibitions and allows them to relax and unwind. Professor JH Gaddum put it amusingly and succinctly when, describing the early effects of moderate amounts of alcohol, he wrote that '...logical thought is difficult but after dinner speeches easy...' The expansiveness and locquaciousness which are socially acceptable lead on, with increasing amounts of alcohol, to unrestrained behaviour in normally well-controlled individuals, through drunkeness, unconsciousness and finally death from respiratory failure. These effects are all a reflection of the progressive and deepening depression of the CNS. Since alcohol impairs the skills needed to drive a car safely, almost all national and state authorities have imposed maximum legal blood-alcohol limits. In the UK and a number of other countries this is currently 80 mg%, but impairment is clearly detectable at lower concentrations and because of this some countries have imposed much lower legal limits.

Table 2.1 gives an indication in very broad terms of the reactions of men and women to different amounts and concentrations of alcohol. On the whole women are smaller than men and their body fluids also represent a smaller proportion of their total body mass, so that after taking the same drink the blood-alcohol level of a woman is likely to be higher than that of a man. The values given assume that the drinkers regularly drink, have had a meal and weigh between 9 and 11 stones (55–70 kg). Higher blood alcohol levels would occur if drunk on an empty stomach and lower values in much heavier individuals. The liver metabolizes about one unit per hour so that the values will fall with time.

Probably the most common drug interaction of all occurs if alcohol is drunk while taking other drugs which have CNS depressant activity. This can occur with some antihistamines, analgesics, antidepressants, hypno-sedatives, tranquillizers, travel-sickness remedies and others (see Alcohol & CNS depressants). This chapter contains a number of synopses which describe the results of formal studies on recognized CNS depressants (see the index), but there are large numbers of other drugs which still await study of this kind and which undoubtedly represent a real hazard.

A less serious but not uncommon interaction between alcohol and some other drugs and chemical agents is the flushing (Antabuse) reaction which is exploited in the case of disulfiram. See the Index.

Table 2.1 Reactions to different concentrations of alcohol

Amounts of alcohol drunk		Blood-alcohol concentrations mg %	Reactions to different % of alcohol in the blood
Man 11 stones (70 kg)	**Woman** 9 stones (55 kg)		
2 units	1 unit	25–30 mg%	Sense of well-being enhanced. Reaction times reduced.
4 units	2 units	50–60 mg%	Mild loss of inhibition, judgement impaired, increased risk of accidents at home, at work and on the road; no overt signs of drunkeness.
5 units	3 units	75–80 mg%	Physical co-ordination reduced, marked loss of inhibition; noticeably under the influence; at the legal limit for driving in the UK.
7 units	4 units	100+ mg%	Clumsiness, loss of physical control, tendency to extreme responses; definite intoxication.
10 units	6 units	150 mg%	Slurred speech, possible loss of memory the following day, probably drunk and disorderly.
24 units	14 units	360 mg%	Dead drunk, sleepiness, possible loss of consciousness.
33 units	20 units	500 mg %	Coma and possibly death.

1 unit   = half pint (300 ml) medium strength beer (3–4%)   = glass wine (100 ml)   = single sherry or martini (a third of a gill (50 ml))   = single spirit one-sixth gill (25 ml)

3–4% alcohol (8° proof)   11% alcohol (20° proof)   17–20% alcohol (30–5° proof)   37–40% alcohol (65–70° proof)

After *Which?* October 1984, page 447 and others.

Alcohol + Anticholinergics

Abstract/Summary

A marked impairment of attention occurs if alcohol is taken in the presence of atropine or glycopyrrhonium. This may make driving more hazardous.

Clinical evidence, mechanism, importance and management

A study in healthy subjects of the effects of 0.5 mg atropine or 1.0 mg glycopyrrhonium, in combination with alcohol (0.5 mg/kg) showed that while reaction times and co-ordination were unaffected or even improved, there was a marked impairment of attention which was large enough to make driving more hazardous.[1] Patients should be warned.

Reference

1 Linnoila M. Drug effects of psychomotor skills related to driving: interaction of atropine, glycopyrrhonium and alcohol. Eur J clin Pharmacol (1973) 6, 107.

Alcohol + Antihistamines

Abstract/Summary

Some antihistamines cause drowsiness which can be increased by alcohol. The detrimental effects of alcohol on driving skills are considerably increased by the use of the older more sedative antihistamines (promethazine, chlorpheniramine, diphenhydramine, etc.), but are much less marked with other antihistamines (clemastine, clemizole, cyclizine, cyprohepatadine, pheniramine, tripelennamine, triprolidine, etc.) and appears to be minimal or absent with some of the newer antihistamines (acrivastine, astemizole, loratadine, terfenadine).

Clinical evidence

(a) Alcohol + the most sedative antihistamines (chlorpheniramine, diphenhydramine, promethazine)

A double blind study on the effects of alcohol (0.75 g/kg) and dexchlorpheniramine (4 mg/70 kg) on 13 subjects showed that together they significantly impaired the performance of a number of tests (standing steadiness, reaction time, manual dexterity, perception, etc.).[7] A significant impairment in psychomotor performance was also seen in another study in subjects given 12 mg chlorpheniramine with alcohol (0.5 mg/kg body weight).[19] Other studies also describe this interaction.[3] Diphenhydramine in doses of 25 or 50 mg was shown to increase the detrimental effects of alcohol on the performance of choice reaction and co-ordination tests by subjects who had taken 0.5 g/kg alcohol, and its interaction in doses of 50, 75 or 100 mg has been confirmed in other reports.[1,4,9,10,11] A marked interaction can also occur with promethazine,[8] and I am aware of a double motor fatality attributed to the overwhelming sedative effects of promethazine taken with alcohol and chlordiazepoxide.

(b) Alcohol + less sedative antihistamines (clemastine, clemizole, cyclizine, cyproheptadine, mebhydrolin, pheniramine, tripelennamine, triprolidine)

An investigation on 16 normal subjects examined the effects of alcohol (blood levels about 50 mg%) and antihistamines, alone or together, on the performance of tests designed to assess mental and motor performance. Clemizole (40 mg), tripelennamine (50 mg) did not significantly affect the performance under the stress of delayed auditory feedback. Clemastine in 3 mg doses also affected co-ordination, whereas 1.5 mg and 1 mg did not.[2,4,5] A study[12] on five subjects showed that the detrimental effects of 100 ml whiskey on the performance of driving tests on a racing car simulator (blood alcohol estimated as less than 80 mg%) were not increased by 50 mg cyclizine. However three of the subjects experienced drowsiness after cyclizine, and other studies[13] have shown that cyclizine alone causes drowsiness in the majority. A study in 20 subjects of the effects of alcohol and mebhydrolin (0.71 mg/kg) showed that the performance of a number of tests on perceptual, cognitive and motor functions was impaired to some extent.[14] No interaction was detected in one study of the combined effects of 4 mg pheniramine or 4 mg cyproheptadine and alcohol (0.7 g/kg),[6] however triprolidine (10 mg) further impairs the deterioration in driving caused by alcohol.[17]

(c) Alcohol + least sedative antihistamines (acrivastine, astemizole, loratadine, terfenadine)

A double blind study showed that terfenadine alone (60–240 mg) did not affect psychomotor skills, nor did it affect the adverse effects of alcohol.[9] Two other studies have shown that astemizole (10–30 mg daily) does not interact with alcohol[15,16,19] and another showed that neither terfenadine (60 mg) nor loratadine (10–20 mg) interact with alcohol.[17] Acrivastine (4 and 8 mg) with and without alcohol was found in another study to behave like terfenadine.[18]

Mechanism

When an interaction occurs it appears to be due to the combined or additive central nervous depressant effects of both the alcohol and the antihistamine.

Importance and management

An adverse interaction between alcohol and the more sedative antihistamines (diphenydramine, chlorpheniramine, promethazine) is well established and clinically important. These antihistamines can cause marked drowsiness when taken alone, and the addition of even quite small amounts of alcohol can make activities such as driving or handling other potentially dangerous machinery much more hazardous. Patients should certainly be warned. Remember also that a number of the more sedative antihistamines appear 'in disguise' as antiemetics, sedatives and as components of cough/cold and influenza remedies which can be bought over the counter. The situation with a number of other antihistamines (clemastine, clemizole, cyclizine, cyproheptadine, mebhydrolin, pheniramine, tripelannamine and triprolidine) is less clear cut. These antihistamines are much less sedative and tests with some of them failed to detect an interaction with normal doses and moderate amounts of alcohol, nevertheless it would seem prudent to issue some cautionary warning, particularly if the patient is likely to drive. The newest antihistamines (acrivastine, astemizole, loratadine, terfenadine) seem to cause little or no drowsiness in most patients and the risk appears to be minimal or absent.

References

1   Hughes FW and Forney RB. Comparative effect of three antihistamines and ethanol on mental and motor performance. Clin Pharmacol Ther (1961) 5, 414.
2   Linnoila M. Effects of drugs on psychomotor skills related to driving: antihistamines, chlormezanone and alcohol. Europ J Clin Pharmacol (1973) 5, 87.
3   Smith RB, Rossie GV and Orzechowski RF. Interactions of chlorpheniramine-ethanol combinations: acute toxicity and antihistamine activity. Toxicol Appl Pharmacol (1974) 28, 240.
4   Tang PC and Rosenstein R. Influence of alcohol and dramamine alone and in combination on psychomotor performance. Aerospace Med (1967) 38, 818.
5   Franks HM, Hensley VR, Hensley WJ, Starmer GA and Teo RKC. The interaction between ethanol and antihistamines. 2. Clemastine. Med J Aust (1979) 1, 185.
6   Landauer AA and Milner G. Antihistamines alone and together with alcohol in relation to driving safety. J Forens Med (1971) 18, 127.
7   Franks HM, Hensley VR, Hensley WJ, Starmer GA and Teo RKC. The interaction between ethanol and antihistamines. 1: Dexchlorpheniramine. Med J Aust (1978) 1, 449.
8   Hedges A, Hills M and Maclay WP. Some drug and peripheral effects of meclastine, a new antihistamine drug in man. J Clin Pharmacol (1971) 11, 112.
9   Moser L, Huther KJ, Koch-Weser J and Lundt PV. Effects of terfenadine and diphenhydramine alone or in combination with diazepam or alcohol on psychomotor performance and subjective feelings. Europ J Clin Pharmacol (1978) 14, 417.
10 Baugh R and Calvert RT. The effects of diphenhydramine alone and in combination with ethanol on histamine skin response and mental performance. Europ J Clin Pharmacol (1977) 12, 201.
11 Burns M and Moskowitz H. Effects of diphenhydramine and alcohol on skills performance. Europ J Clin Pharmacol (1980) 17, 259.
12 Hughes DTD, Cramer F and Knight GJ. Use of a racing car simulator for medical research. The effects of marzine and alcohol on driving performances. Med Sci Law (1967) October, 200.
13 Brand JJ, Colquhoun WP, Gould AH and Perry WLM. (-)Hyoscine and cyclizine as motion sickness remedies. Br J Pharmac Chemother (1967) 30, 463.
14 Franks HM, Lawrie M, Schabinsky VV, Starmer GA and Teo RKC. Interaction of alcohol and antihistamines: 3. Mebhydrolin. Med J Aust (1981) 2, 447–9.
15 Bateman DN, Chapman PH and Rawlins MD. Lack of effect of astemizole on ethanol dynamics or kinetics. Eur J Clin Pharmacol (1983) 25, 567–8.
16 Moser L, Plum H and Bruckmann M. Interaktionen eines neuen Antihistaminikums mit Diazepam und Alkohol. Med Welt (1984) 35, 296–9.
17 Riedel WJ, Schoenmakers EAJM and O'Hanlon JF. The effects of loratadine alone and in combination with alcohol on actual driving performance. Institute for Drugs, Safety and Behaviour, University of Limburg, Maastricht, The Netherlands, August 1987.
18 Cohen AF, Hamilton MJ and Peck AW. The effects of acrivastine (BW825C), diphenhydramine and terfenadine in combination with alcohol on human CNS preformance. Eur J Clin Pharmacol (1987) 32, 279–88.
19 Hindmarch I and Bhatti JZ. Psychomotor effects of astemizole and chlorpheniramine, alone and in combination with alcohol. Int Clin Psychopharmacol (1987) 2, 117–19.

Alcohol + Aspirin and Salicylates

Abstract/Summary

A small increase in the gastrointestinal blood loss caused by aspirin occurs in patients if they drink, but any increased damage to the lining of the stomach is small and appears usually to be of minimal importance in normal individuals. Buffered aspirin, paracetamol and diflunisal do not interact in this way.

Clinical evidence

(a) Alcohol + unbuffered aspirin

A study in 13 men showed that their mean daily blood loss from the gut was 0.4 ml while taking no medication, 3.2 ml while taking 2100 mg of soluble unbuffered aspirin (*Disprin*) and 5.3 ml while also taking 180 ml Australian whiskey (31.8% w/v ethanol). Alcohol alone did not cause gastrointestinal bleeding.[1]

A not dissimilar study showed that the daily blood loss increased from 2.15 to 5.32 ml when, in addition to 2400 mg aspirin daily, the subjects drank 140 ml vodka (40% alcohol) and 200 ml table wine.[5] An epidemiological study of patients admitted to hospital with gastrointestinal haemorrhage showed a statistical association between bleeding and the ingestion of aspirin with or without alcohol.[2] Endoscopic examination has shown that aspirin and alcohol have additive damaging effects on the gastric mucosa (not on the duodenum) but the extent is small.[7]

(b) Alcohol + buffered aspirin

A study in 22 normal men who were given three double whiskeys (equivalent to 142 ml 40% ethanol) and 728 g sodium acetylsalicylate showed that no increase in gastrointestinal bleeding took place.[3]

Mechanism

Both aspirin and alcohol can damage the normal mucosal lining of the stomach, one measure of the injury being a fall in the gastric potential difference. An additive fall has been seen with unbuffered aspirin and alcohol, whereas an increase occurs with buffered aspirin.[4] Once the protective mucosal barrier is breached, exfoliation of the cells occurs and damage to the capillaries follows. Aspirin causes a marked prolongation in bleeding times, and this can be increased by alcohol.[6] The total picture is complex.

Importance and management

An established interaction but of limited importance. Aspirin ingestion causes some blood loss in most people, 3 g daily for a period of 3–5 days inducing an average blood loss of about 5 ml or so. Some increased loss undoubtedly occurs with alcohol, but it seems to be quite small and there is no evidence to suggest that it is usually of much importance in most normal individuals using moderate doses. In one study alcohol was described as being a mild damaging agent or a mild potentiating agent for other damaging drugs.[7] Buffered aspirin, paracetamol (acetaminophen) or diflunisal[5] are preferable because they do not interact with alcohol. Only a small interaction occurs with ibuprofen. On the other hand it should be remembered that chronic and/or gross overuse of salicylates and alcohol may result in gastric ulceration.

References

1 Goulston K and Cooke AR. Alcohol, Aspirin and gastrointestinal bleeding. Brit Med J (1968) 4, 644.
2 Needham CD, Kyle J, Jones PF, Johnstone SJ and Kerridge DF. Aspirin and alcohol in gastrointestinal haemorrhage. Gut (1971) 12, 819.
3 Bouchier JAD and Williams HS. Determination of faecal blood-loss after combined alcohol and sodium acetylsalicylate intake. Lancet (1969) i, 178.
4 Murray HS, Strottman MP and Cooke AR. Effect of several drugs on gastric potential differences in man. Brit Med J (1974) 1, 19.
5 De Schepper PJ, Tjandramaga TB, De Roo M, Verhaest L, Daurio C, Steelman SL and Tempero KF. Gastrointestinal blood loss after diflunisal and after aspirin. Clin Pharmacol Ther (1978) 23, 669.
6 Rosove MH and Harwig SSL. Confirmation that ethanol potentiates aspirin-induced prolongation of the bleeding time. Thromb Res (1983) 31, 525–7.
7 Lanza FL, Royer GL, Nelson RS, Rack MF and Seckman CC. Ethanol, aspirin, ibuprofen, and the gastroduodenal mucosa: an endoscopic assessment. Gastroenterology (1985) 80, 767–9.

Alcohol + Barbiturates

Abstract/Summary

Alcohol and the barbiturates are CNS depressants which if taken together can have additive (possibly more than additive effects). Any activity requiring alertness and good co-ordination, particularly driving a car or handling other potentially dangerous machinery, will be made more difficult and more hazardous.

Clinical evidence

A study in man of the effects of alcohol (0.5 mg/kg), taken the morning after using 100 mg amylobarbitone as a hypnotic the night before, showed that the performance of co-ordination skills was much more impaired than with either drug alone.[1]

Increased CNS depression has been described in a number of other clinical studies,[2-4] and has featured very many times in coroners' reports of fatal accidents and suicides. A study of the fatalities due to this interaction indicated that with some barbiturates the CNS depressant effects are more than additive.[9]

In addition there is some evidence that blood alcohol levels may be reduced in the presence of a barbiturate.[3,5,7]

Mechanisms

Both alcohol and the barbiturates are CNS depressants, and simple additive CNS depression provides part of the explanation. The Ferguson principle may account for the more than

additive effects.[10] Acute alcohol ingestion may inhibit the liver enzymes concerned with the metabolism of the barbiturates.[4,8]

Importance and management

The effects of concurrent use (particularly the fatal effects) are very well recognized, but not many formal studies of this interaction in normal clinical situations have been made. Nevertheless it is clearly potentially serious and of practical importance. The most obvious hazards are increased drowsiness, lack of alertness and impaired co-ordination which make the handling of potentially dangerous machinery (e.g. car driving) more difficult and dangerous, but it has also been rightly pointed out that other risks are increased: '...many old people may have a whiskey nightcap with their barbiturate sleeping pill. They then have to get out of bed in the middle of the night to empty their bladder; they are unsteady, they fall, they are found in the morning with a fractured femur or in a hypothermic state. No figures are available to give a reliable idea of the scale of this problem...'[6] The hangover effects of some hypnotics are still present next morning and can continue to interact significantly with alcohol. Patients should be warned.

References

1 Saario I and Linnoila M. Effect of subacute treatment with hypnotics alone or in combination with alcohol, on psychomotor skills relating to driving. Acta pharmacol et toxicol (1976) 38, 382.
2 Kielholz P, Goldberg L, Obersteg JI, Poldinger W, Ramseyer A and Schmid P. Fahrversuche zur Frage der Beeintrachtigung der Verkehrstuchtigkeit durch Alkohol, Tranquilizer und Hypnotika. Dtsch Med Wsch (1969) 94, 301.
3 Morrelli PL, Veneroni E, Zaccala M and Bizzi A. Further observations on the interaction betwen ethanol and psychotropic drugs. Arzneim-Forsch (Drug Res) (1971) 21, 20.
4 Wegener H and Kotter L. Analgetica und Verkehrstuchtigkeit Wirkung einer Kombination von 5-Allyl-5-isobutyl-saure. Dimethylamino-phenazon und Coffeine nach einmaliger under wiederholter Applika-tion. Arzneim-Forsch (Drug Res) (1971) 21, 47.
5 Mould GP, Curry SH and Binns TB. Interaction of glutethimide and phenobarbitone with ethanol in man. J Pharm Pharmac (1972) 24, 894.
6 Wilkes E. Are you still prescribing those outdated drugs ? MIMS Magazine (1976) 27, 84.
7 Mezey E and Robles EA. Effects of phenobarbital administration on rates of ethanol clearance and on ethanol-oxidising enzymes in man. Gastroenterology (1974) 66, 248.
8 Rubin E and Lieber CS. Inhibition of drug metabolism by acute ethanol intoxication. A hepatic microsomal mechanism. Am J Med (1970) 49, 801.
9 Stead AH and Moffat AC. Quantification of the interaction between barbiturates and alcohol and interpretation of fatal blood concentra-tions. Human Toxicol (1983) 2, 5–14.
10 King LA. Thermodynamic interpretation of synergism in bar-biturate/ethanol poisoning. Human Toxicol (1985) 4, 633-5.

Alcohol + Benzodiazepines

Abstract/Summary

The concurrent use of the benzodiazepines tranquillizers increases the CNS depressant effects of alcohol to some extent, but usually not as much as other more obviously sedative drugs. The risks of car driving and handling other potentially dangerous machinery are increased, particularly because the patient may be unaware of being affected. Some hypnotic benzodiazepines used at night are still present in appreciable amounts next day and may interact with alcoholic drinks taken during the morning.

Clinical evidence

It is very difficult to assess and compare the results of the very many studies of this interaction because of the differences between the tests, their duration, the dosages of the benzodiazepines and alcohol, whether given chronically or acutely, and a number of other variables. However the overall picture seems to be that diazepam[6,8–13,16,21,26,27,37] has a more marked effect than chlordiazepoxide,[1–7] medazepam,[17] or oxazepam,[16] but possibly the same as triazolam.[29,31] The effects of lormetazepam may be greater than diazepam.[38] The potencies of bromazepam,[14] clobazam,[15] lorazepam,[25,30,37] oxazolam,[39] metaclazepam,[40] potassium clorazepate[23] and triazolam[29] are unclear, but brotizolam seems to have a small effect.[36] Those on lorazepam and triazolam may be unaware of the extent of the impairment which occurs[25,29] and the anxiolytic effects of lorazepam may be opposed by alcohol.[30]

The hypnotic benzodiazepines flurazepam,[18,33,34] nitrazepam,[10,19] temazepam[33] and flunitrazepam[24,25,35] when taken the night before can interact with alcohol the next morning, but midazolam[28] appears not to do so. Loprazolam may mitigate the effects of alcohol and may possibly have less of a hangover effect.[32]

Mechanism

It would appear that the CNS depressant actions of the benzodiazepines and alcohol are additive. Alcohol also increases the absorption and raises the serum levels of some benzodiazepines.[15,20,22]

Importance and management

Very extensively studied interactions. The overall picture is that benzodiazepine tranquillizers worsen the detrimental effects of alcohol. Up to a 20–30% increase has been suggested.[29] The extent will depend on the particular benzodiazepine (see 'Clinical evidence' above), its dosage and the amounts of alcohol but diazepam appears to be high on the list and, with alcohol, is commonly found in the blood of car drivers involved in traffic accidents.[41] With small amounts of alcohol the importance of the interaction may be quite small, but patients should be warned that their usual response to alcohol may be greater than expected, and their ability to drive a car or carry out other tasks requiring alertness may be impaired. They may also be unaware of the deterioration. The same warning applies to the hypnotic benzodiazepines taken the night before because the body may still contain significant amounts the next morning.

References

1 Reggiani G, Hurlimann A and Theiss E. Some aspects of the experimental and clinical toxicology of chlordiazepoxide. Acta pharmacol et toxicol (1979) 45, 257.

2 Hughers FW, Forney RB and Richards AB. Comparative effect in human subjects of chlordiazepoxide, diazepam and placebo on mental and physical performance. Clin Pharmacol Ther (1965) 6, 139.

3 Linnoila M. Effects of diazepam, chlordiazepoxide, thioridazine, haloperidol, flupenthixol and alcohol on psychomotor skills related to driving. Ann Med Exp Biol Fenn (1973) 51, 125.

4 Linnoila M, Saario I, Olkoniemi J, Liljequist R, Himberg JJ and Maki M. Effect of two weeks' treatment with chlordiazepoxide or flupenthixol alone or in combination with alcohol on psychomotor skills related to driving. Arzneim Forsch/Drug Res (1975) 25, 1088.

5 Hoffer A. Lack of potentiation by chlordiazepoxide (Librium) of depression of excitation due to alcohol. Canad Med Ass J (1962) 87, 920.

6 Dundee JW and Isaac M. Interaction of alcohol with sedatives and tranquillizers (a study of blood levels at loss of consciousness following rapid infusion). Med Sci Law (1970) 10, 220.

7 Kielholz P, Goldberg L, Obersteg JI, Poldinger W, Ramseyer A and Schmid P. Fahrversuche zur Frage der Beeintrachtigung der Verkehrsuchtigkeit durch Alkohol Tranquilizer und Hypnotika. Dtsch Med Wsch (1969) 94, 301.

8 Morselli PL, Veneroni E, Zaccala M and Bizzi A. Further observations on the interaction between ethanol and psychotropic drugs. Arzneim-Forsch/Drug Res (1971) 21, 20.

9 Linnoila M and Hakkinen S. Effects of diazepam and codeine, alone and in combination with alcohol, on simulated driving. Clin Pharmacol Ther (1974) 15, 368.

10 Linnoila M. Drug interaction on psychomotor skills related to driving: hypnotics and alcohol. Ann Med Exp Biol Fenn (1973) 51, 118.

11 Missen AW, Cleary W, Eng L and McMillan S. Diazepam, alcohol and drivers. NZ Med J (1978) 87, 275.

12 Laisu U, Linnoil M, Seppala T, Himberg JJ and Mattila MJ. Pharmacokinetic and pharmacodynamic interactions of diazepam with different alcoholic beverages. Eur J clin Pharmacol (1979) 16, 263.

13 Palva ES, Linnoila M, Saario I, Mattila MJ. Acute and subacute effects of diazepam on psychomotor skills: interaction with alcohol. Acta pharmacol et toxicol (1979) 45, 257.

14 Seppala T, Saario I and Mattila MJ. Two weeks' treatment with chlorpromazine, thioridazine, sulpiride or bromazepam: actions and interactions with alcohol on psychomotor skills relating to driving. Mod Probl Pharmacopsych (1976) 11, 85.

15 Tauber K, Badian M, Brettell HF, Royen Th, Rupp K, Sitting W and Uihlein M. Kinetic and dynamic interaction of clobazam and alcohol. Br J clin Pharmacol (1979) 7, 91S.

16 Molander L and Durhok C. Acute effects of oxazepam, diazepam and methylperone, alone and in combination with alcohol on sedation, coordination and mood. Acta pharmacol et toxicol (1976) 38, 145.

17 Landauer AA, Pocock DA and Prott FW. The effect of medazepam and alcohol on cognitive and motor skills used in car driving. Psychopharmacologia (1974) 37, 159.

18 Saario I and Mattila M. Effect of subacute treatment with hypnotics alone or in combination with alcohol on psychomotor skills related to driving. Acta pharmacol et toxicol (1976) 38, 382.

19 Saario I, Linnoila M and Maki M. Interaction of drugs with alcohol on human psychomotor skills related to driving: effect of sleep deprivation or two weeks' treatment with hypnotics. J Clin Pharmacol (1975) 15, 52.

20 MacLeod SM, Giles HG, Patzalek G, Thiessen JJ and Sellers EM. Diazepam actions and plasma concentrations following ethanol ingestion. Eur J clin Pharmacol (1977) 11, 345.

21 Curry SH and Smith CM. Diazepam-ethanol interaction in humans: addition or potentiation? Comm Psychopharmacol (1979) 3, 101.

22 Laisi U, Linnoila M, Seppala T, Himberg J-J and Mattila MJ. Pharmacokinetic and pharmacodynamic interactions of diazepam with different alcoholic beverages. Eur J Clin Pharmacol (1979) 16, 263.

23 Staak M, Raff G and Nusser W. Pharmacopsychological investigations concerning the combined effects of dipotassium clorazepate and ethanol. Int J Clin Pharmacol Biopharm (1979) 17, 205.

24 Linnoila M, Erwin CW, Brendle A and Logue P. Effects of alcohol and flunitrazepam on mood and performance in healthy young men. J Clin Pharmacol (1981) 21, 430–5.

25 Sappala T, Aranko K, Mattila MJ and Shrotriya RC. Effects of alcohol on buspirone and lorazepam actions. Clin Pharmacol Ther (1982) 32, 201–7.

26 Smiley A and Moskowitz H. Effects of long-term administration of buspirone and diazepam on driver steering control. Am J Med (1986) 80 (Suppl 3B) 22–9.

27 Erwin CW, Linnoila M, Hartwell J, Erwin A and Guthrie S. Effects of buspirone and diazepam, alone and in combination with alcohol, on skilled performance and evoked potentials. J Clin Psychopharmacol (1986) 6, 199.

28 Hindmarch I and Subhanz Z. The effects of midazolam in conjunction with alcohol on sleep, psychomotor performance and car driving ability. Int J Clin Pharm Res (1983) III, 323–9.

29 Dorian P, Sellers EM, Kaplan HL, Hamilton C, Greenblatt DJ and Abernethy D. Triazolam and ethanol interaction: kinetic and dynamic consequences. Clin Pharmacol Ther (1985) 37, 558–62.

30 Lister RG and File SE. Performance impairment and increased anxiety resulting from the combination of alcohol and lorazepam. J Clin Psychopharmacol (1983) 3, 66–71.

31 Ochs HR, Greenblatt DJ, Arendt RM, Hubbel W and Shader RI. Pharmacokinetic noninteraction of triazolam and ethanol. J Clin Psychopharmacol (1984) 4, 106–7.

32 McManus IC, Ankier SI, Norfolk J, Phillips M and Priest RG. Effects of psychological performance of the benzodiazepine loprazolam alone and with alcohol. Br J clin Pharmac (1983) 16, 291–300.

33 Betts TA and Birtle J. Effect of two hypnotic drugs on actual driving performance next morning. Br Med J (1982) 285, 852.

34 Hindmarch I and Gudgeon AC. Loprazolam (HR158) and flurazepam with ethanol compared on tests of psychomotor ability. Eur J Clin Pharmacol (1982) 23, 509–12.

35 Seppala T, Nuotto E and Dreyfus JF. Drug-alcohol interactions on psychomotor skills: zopiclone and flunitrazepam. Pharmacology (1983) 27, Suppl 2, 127–35.

36 Scavone JM, Greenblatt DJ, Harmatz JS and Shader RI. Kinetic and dynamic interaction of brotizolam and ethanol. Br J clin Pharmac (1986) 21, 197–204.

37 Aranko K, Seppala T, Pellinen J and Mattila MJ. Interaction of diazepam or lorazepam with alcohol. Psychomotor effects and bioassayed serum levels after single and repeated doses. Eur J Clin Pharmacol (1985) 28, 559–65.

38 Willumeit H-P, Ott H, Neubert W, Hemmerling K-G, Schratzer K and Fichte K. Alcohol interaction of lormetazepam, mepindol sulphate and diazepam measured by performance on the driving simulator. Pharmacopsychiat (1984) 17, 36–43.

39 Hopes H and Debus G. Untersuchungen zu Kombinationseffekten von Oxazolam und Alkohol auf Leistung und Befinden bei gesunden Probanden. Arzneim-Forsch/Drug Res (1984) 34, 921–6.

40 Schmidt V. Experimentelle Untersuchunger zur Wechselwirkung zwischen Alkohol und Metaclazepam. Beitr Gerichtl Med (1983) 41, 413–7.

41 Chan AWK. Effects of combined alcohol and benzodiazepine: a review. Drug and Alcohol Dependence (1984) 13, 315–41.

Alcohol + Bromvaletone or Ethinamate

Abstract/Summary

The detrimental effects of alcohol on the skills related to driving are made worse by bromvaletone, but the interaction with ethinamate is mild. Both showed hangover effects and can interact with alcohol next morning.

Clinical evidence, mechanism, importance and management

A study on a very large number of subjects given 1 g ethinamate or 0.6 g bromvaletone, either alone or with 0.5 g/kg alcohol, showed that the performance of a number of psychomotor skills related to driving was slightly impaired by ethinamate, but strongly impaired by bromvaletone. There was sufficient hangover for both drugs to interact with alcohol next morning after being used as hypnotics the night

before.[1] The CNS depressant effects of these hypnotics and alcohol would seem to be additive. Patients should be warned.

Reference

1 Linnoila M. Drug interaction on psychomotor skills related to driving: hypnotics and alcohol. Ann Med Exp Biol Fenn (1973) 51, 118.

Alcohol + Buspirone

Abstract/Summary

Buspirone does not appear to interact with alcohol directly, but it can cause drowsiness and weakness which may make driving more hazardous.

Clinical evidence, mechanism, importance and management

Studies in 12 normal subjects showed that 10 or 20 mg buspirone did not appear to interact with alcohol (i.e. worsen the performance of certain psychomotor tests) but it did make them feel drowsy and weak. The tentative conclusion was drawn that patients might therefore be more aware of feeling 'under par' than with some other drugs (e.g. the benzodiazepines) and less likely to take risks.[1,2] Nevertheless it would seem prudent to warn patients of the potential hazards of driving or handling other potentially dangerous machinery.

References

1 Mattila MJ, Aranko K and Sappala T. Acute effects of buspirone and alcohol on psychomotor skills. J Clin Psychiatry (1982) 43, 56–60.
2 Seppala T, Aranko K, Mattila MJ and Shrotriya RC. Effects of alcohol on buspirone and lorazepam actions. Clin Pharmacol Ther (1982) 32, 201–7.

Alcohol + Butyraldoxime

Abstract/Summary

A disulfiram-like reaction can occur in those exposed to N-butyraldoxime if they drink alcohol.

Clinical evidence, mechanism, importance and management

Workers in a printing company complained of flushing of the face, shortness of breath, tachycardia and drowsiness very shortly after drinking quite small quantities of alcohol (one and a half ounces of whiskey). It was found that the printing ink contained N-butyraldoxime as an anti-oxidant. Increased blood levels of acetaldehyde were found in the workers exposed to N-butyraldoxime when given alcohol.[1] The reason for the reaction seems to be that N-butyraldoxime, like disulfiram, can inhibit the metabolism of alcohol so that acetaldehyde accumulates (see 'Alcohol + Disulfiram').

This reaction would seem to be more unpleasant and socially disagreeable than serious. No treatment seems necessary.

Reference

1 Lewis W and Schwartz L. An occupational agent (N-butyraldoxime) causing reaction to alcohol. Med Ann DC (1956) 25, 485–90.

Alcohol + Caffeine

Abstract/Summary

Despite popular belief, objective tests show that caffeine does not counteract the effects of alcohol. It does not sober up those who have drunk too much and may even make them more accident-prone.

Clinical evidence, mechanism, importance and management

A study on a large number of subjects given 300 mg caffeine, either alone or with alcohol (0.75 mg/kg), showed that the caffeine did not antagonize the deleterious effect of alcohol on the performance of psychomotor skill tests. Only reaction times were reversed.[1] In another investigation on eight subjects it was found that, contrary to expectations, caffeine increased the frequency of errors in the performance of a serial reaction task.[2] Yet another double-blind study clearly showed that caffeine does not antagonize the effects of alcohol.[3] A further study found no evidence that caffeine opposes the actions of alcohol, instead it appeared that it increases the detrimental effects.[4] The reasons for this are not understood. These investigations show that despite the time-hallowed belief in the value of strong black coffee in sobering up those who have drunk too much, it is not effective. It not only does not make it safe for them to drive or handle dangerous machinery, it may even make them more accident-prone.

References

1 Franks HM, Hagedorn H and Hensley VR. The effect of caffeine on human performance, alone and in combination with alcohol. Pyschopharmacology (1975) 45, 177.
2 Lee DJ and Lowe G. Interaction of alcohol and caffeine in a perceptual-motor task. IRCS Med Sci: Libr Compend (1980) 8, 420.
3 Nuotto E, Mattila MJ, Sappala T and Konno K. Caffeine and coffee and alcohol effects on psychomotor function. Clin Pharmacol Ther (1982) 31, 68–76.
4 Osborne DJ and Rogers Y. Interactions of alcohol and caffeine on human reaction time. Aviat Space Environ Med (1983) 54, 528–34.

Alcohol + Calcium channel blockers

Abstract/Summary

Blood alcohol levels can possibly be raised by verapamil and may remain elevated for a much longer period of time.

Clinical evidence

10 normal subjects were given 80 mg verapamil three times daily for six days and on day 6 they were additionally given 0.8 mg/kg alcohol. Peak serum alcohol levels were found to be raised by 16.7% (from 106.45 to 124.24 mg/dl) and the AUC (area under the concentration-time curve) was raised by almost 30%. The time that serum alcohol levels exceeded 100 mg/dl was prolonged from 0.2 to 1.3 h.[1]

Mechanism

Not understood. It seems possible that the verapamil inhibits the metabolism of the alcohol by the liver, thereby reducing its loss from the body.

Importance and management

Information seems to be limited to this report and it needs confirmation, but patients on verapamil should be warned that the effects of alcohol may possibly be increased. A rise of almost 17% is small but it could be enough to lift legal blood levels to illegal levels if driving. Moreover the intoxicant effects of alcohol may persist for a much longer period of time. There seems to be nothing documented about any of the other calcium channel blockers and alcohol. More study is needed.

Reference

1 Schumock G, Bauer LA, Horn J and Opheim K. Verapamil inhibits ethanol elimination. Pharmacotherapy (1989) 9, 184–5.

Alcohol + Cephalosporin antibiotics

Abstract/Summary

Disulfiram-like reactions can occur in those taking latamoxef (moxalactam), cephamandole, cefoperazone, cefmenoxime and cefotetan after drinking alcohol or following an injection of alcohol. This is not a general reaction of the commonly used cephalosporins but is confined to those with a particular chemical structure.

Clinical evidence

A young man with cystic fibrosis was given 2 g latamoxef (moxalactam) intravenously every 8 h for pneumonia. After three days' treatment he drank, as was his custom, a can of beer with lunch. He rapidly became flushed with a florid macular eruption over his face and chest. This faded over the next 30 min but he complained of severe nausea and headache. A woman patient also on latamoxef became flushed, diaphoretic and nauseated after drinking a cocktail of vodka and tomato juice.[1]

This reaction has been described in at least five other subjects who drank alcohol while receiving latamoxef.[6–8] The symptoms experienced have included flushing of the face, arms and neck, shortness of breath, headache, tachycardia, dizziness, hyper- and hypotension, and vomiting. Similar reactions have been described in patients on cephamandole,[2,5] cefoperazone,[3,12,14,17–20] cefmenoxime[15] and cefotetan[23] after drinking wine, beer, or other alcoholic drinks,[4,11,13] and after the ingestion of an 8% alcoholic elixir.[15] It has also been seen following the injection of alcohol into the para-aortic space for celiac plexus block.[18]

Mechanism

These reactions appear to have the same pharmacological basis as the disulfiram-alcohol reaction (see appropriate synopsis). Studies in rats have shown that three of these antibiotics (latamoxef, cephamandole and cefoperazone) can raise blood acetaldehyde levels when alcohol is given, but to a lesser extent than disulfiram.[6,11] It appears that the reaction is confined to those cephalosporins which possess a methyltetrazolethiol group in the 3-position on the cephalosporin molecule.[21]

Importance and management

An established interaction. The incidence appears to vary. One report[1] says that one out of 30 on latamoxef showed this reaction, and in another study only two out of 10 did so.[8] The incidence is possibly slightly higher with cefoperazone and it occurred in five out of eight subjects in a study of cefotetan.[23] It is usually more embarrassing or unpleasant and possibly frightening than serious, with the symptoms subsiding spontaneously after a few hours. There is evidence that the severity varies (cefoperazone > latamoxef > cefmetazole.[22]) Treatment is not usually needed but there are two reports[2,7] of two elderly patients who needed treatment for hypotension which was life-threatening in one case;[7] plasma expanders and dopamine have been used as treatment.[2,7]

Since the reaction is unpredictable, all patients on the antibiotics known to interact should be warned that it can occur during and up to three days after the course of treatment is over. Advise them to avoid alcohol. Those with kidney or liver disease in whom the drug clearance is prolonged should wait a week. It should not be forgotten that some foods and pharmaceuticals contain substantial amounts of alcohol, and a reaction with some topically applied products cannot be excluded (see 'Alcohol + Disulfiram').

This disulfiram-like reaction is not a general reaction of all the cephalosporins. There are no reports of reactions in patients taking cephalothin, cephradine, cefoxitin, cephazolin, or cefsulodin.[16] Ceftizoxime and cefonicid do not interact with alcohol in man.[9,24] A number of less widely used cephalosporins and others which are still the subject of investigation are possible candidates for this reaction because they possess the methyltetrazolethiol group in the 3-position. These include cefazaflur,[11] cefotiam, ceforanide, cefpiramide (SM-1652, Yamanouchi), 7-methoxy cefazaflur (SKF 73678), SKF 80000, T-1982 (Toyoma), P-75123 (Pierrel), SQ 14359 and SQ 67590(Squibb).[15,21]

References

1 Neu HC and Prince AS. Interaction between moxalactam and alcohol. Lancet (1980), i, 1422.
2 Portier H, Chalopin JM, Freysz M and Tanter Y. Interaction between cephalosporins and alcohol. Lancet (1980), ii, 263.
3 Foster TS, Raehl CL and Wilson HD. Disulfiram-like reaction associated with parenteral cephalosporin. Amer J Hosp Pharm (1980) 37, 858.
4 Reeves DS and Davies AJ. Alcohol-cephalosporin interaction. Lancet (1980) ii, 540.
5 Drummer S, Hauser WE and Remington JS. Antabuse-like effect of beta-lactam antibiotics. N Eng J Med (1980) 303, 1417.
6 Beuning MK, Wold JS, Isreal KS and Kammer RB. Disulfiram-like reaction to beta-lactams. J Amer Med Ass (1981) 245, 2027.
7 Brown KR, Guglielmo BJ, Pons VG and Jacobs RA. Theophylline elixir, moxalactam and a disulfiram-like reaction. Ann Int Med (1982), 97, 621–2.
8 Elenbaas RM, Ryan JL, Robinson WA. Singsank MJ, Harvey MJ and Klaasen CD. Investigation of the disulfiram-like activity of moxalactam. Clin Pharmacol Ther (1982) 32, 347–55.
9 McMahon FG and Noveck RJ. Lack of disulfiram-like reactions with ceftizoxime. J Antimicrob Chemother (1982) Suppl C, 129–33.
10 Beuning MK and Wolds JS. Ethanol-moxalactam interactions in vivo. Rev Inf Dis (1982) 4, Suppl Nov/Dec S555–63.
11 Yanagihara M, Okada K, Nozaki M, Tsurumi K and Fujimura H. Cepheim antibiotics and alcohol metabolism. Disulfiram-like reaction resulting from intravenous administration of cepheim antibiotics. Fol Pharmacol Japon (1982) 79, 55–60.
12 Allaz AF, Dayer P, Fabre J, Rudhardt M and Balant L. Pharmacocinetique d'une novelle cephalosporine, la cefoperazone. Schweiz Med Wsch (1979), 109, 1999–2005.
13 McMahon FG. Disulfiram-like reaction to cephalosporin. J Amer Med Ass (1980), 243, 2397.
14 Kemmerich B and Lode H. Cefoperazone—another cephalosporin associated with a disufiram type alcohol incompatibility. Infection (1981) 9, 110.
15 Uri JV and Parks DB. Disulfiram-like reaction to certain cephalosporins. Ther Drug Monit (1983) 5, 219–24.
16 McMahon FG. Quoted in 15 as personal communication.
17 Kannangara DW, Gallaagher K and Lefrock JL. Disulfiram-like reactions with newer cephalosporins: cefmenoxime. Amer J Med Sci (1984) 287, 45–7.
18 Umeda S and Arai T. Disufiram-like reaction to moxalactam after celiac plexus block. Anesth Analg (1985) 65, 377.
19 Bailey RR, Peddie B, Blake E, Bishop V and Reddy J. Cefoperazone in the treatment of severe or complicated infections. Drugs (1981) 22 (Suppl 1), 76–86.
20 Ellis-Pegler RB and Lang SDR. Cefoperazone in Klebsiella Meningitis: A case report. Drugs (1981) 22 (Suppl 1), 69–71.
21 Norrby SR. Adverse reactions and interactions with newer cephalosporin and cephamycin antibiotics. Med Toxicol (1986) 1, 32–46.
22 Nakamura K, Nakagawa A and Tanaka M. Effects of cephem antibiotics on ethanol metabolism. Fol Pharmacol Jap (1984) 83, 183–91.
23 Kline SS, Mauro VF, Forney RB, Freimer EH and Somani P. Cefotetan-induced disulfiram-type reactions and hypoprothrombinaemia. Antimicrob Ag Chemother (1987) 31, 1328–31.
24 McMahon FG, Ryan JR, Jain AK, LaCorte W and Ginzler F. Absence of disulfiram-type reactions to single and multiple doses of cefonicid: a placebo-controlled study. J Antimicrol Chemother (1987) 20, 913–8.

Alcohol + Chloral hydrate

Abstract/Summary

Both alcohol and chloral are CNS depressants and their effects may be additive, possibly even more than additive. Some patients may experience a disulfiram-like flushing reaction if they drink after taking chloral for several days.

Clinical evidence

Studies in five subjects given chloral (15 mg/kg) and alcohol (0.5 mg/kg) showed that both drugs given alone impaired their ability to carry out complex motor tasks. When taken together, the effects were additive, and possibly even more than additive. After taking chloral for seven days, one of the subjects experienced a disulfiram-like reaction (bright red-purple flushing of the face, tachycardia, hypotension, anxiety and persistent headache) after drinking alcohol.[1,2]

The disulfiram-like reaction has been described in other reports.[3,4] One of these was published more than a century ago in 1872 and describes two patients on chloral who experienced this reaction after drinking only half a bottle of beer.[3]

Mechanism

Alcohol, chloral and trichloroethanol (to which chloral is metabolized) are all CNS depressants. During concurrent use, the metabolic pathways used for their elimination are mutually inhibited: blood-alcohol levels rise because the trichloroethanol competitively depresses the oxidation of alcohol to acetaldehyde, while trichloroethanol levels also rise because its production from chloral is increased and its further conversion and clearance as the glucuronide is inhibited. As a result the rises in the blood levels of alcohol and trichloroethanol are exaggerated, and their effects are accordingly greater.[1,2,5,6] Blood levels of acetaldehyde are raised by only 50% during the use of chloral, so that the flushing reaction, despite its resemblance to the disulfiram reaction, may possibly have a partially different basis.[2]

Importance and management

A well-documented and established interaction. Only a few references are given here. A comprehensive bibliography is to found in references 1 and 2. Patients given chloral should be warned about the extensive CNS depression which can occur if they drink, and of the disulfiram-like reaction which may occur after taking chloral for a period of time. Its incidence is uncertain. There seems to be little clinical evidence to support the idea of the legendary 'Mickey Finn', concocted of chloral and alcohol, which is reputed to be so potent that deep sleep can be induced in the unsuspecting victim within minutes of ingestion—at least in normal therapeutic doses of 0.3–2.0 g. Larger doses may cause serious and potentially life-threatening CNS depression.

It seems likely that chloral betaine, triclofos and other compounds closely related to chloral hydrate will interact with alcohol in a similar manner, but this requires confirmation.

References

1 Sellers EM, Carr G, Bernstein JG, Sellers S and Koch-Weser J. Interaction of chloral hydrate and ethanol in man. II. Hemodynamic and performance. Clin Pharmacol Ther (1972) 13, 50.
2 Sellers EM, Lang M, Koch-Weser J, LeBlanc E and Kalant H. Interaction of chloral hydrate and ethanol in man. I. Metabolism. Clin Pharmacol Ther (1972) 13, 37.
3 Bjorstrom F. On the effect of alcoholic beverages and simultaneous use of chloral. Uppsala Lakareforenings Forhandlingar (1872) 8, 114.
4 Bardodej Z. Intolerance alkohlu po chloralhydratu. Ceskolov farm (1965) 14, 478.
5 Owens AH, Marshall EK and Brown GO. A comparative evaluation of the hypnotic potency of chloral hydrate and trichloroethanol. Bull Johns Hopkins Hosp (1955) 96, 71.
6 Wong LK and Biemann K. A study of drug interaction by gas chromatography–mass spectrometry. Synergism of chloral hydrate and ethanol. Biochem Pharmacol (1978) 27, 1019.

Alcohol + Cimetidine, Famotidine or Ranitidine

Abstract/Summary

Some studies have shown that blood alcohol levels can be raised to some extent in those taking H_2-blockers, whereas others report that no significant interaction occurs.

Clinical Evidence

(a) Evidence of an interaction

A double-blind study on six volunteers showed that after taking 1200 mg cimetidine daily for seven days, their peak blood alcohol levels following the ingestion of 0.8 g/kg alcohol were raised about 12% (from 146 to 163 mg%). The area under the time/concentration curve was increased about 7% (from 717 to 771 mg/100 ml/h). The subjects assessed themselves as being more intoxicated while taking cimetidine and alcohol than with alcohol alone.[1]

In an essentially similar study[2,12] other workers found that the blood alcohol levels were raised 17% (from 73 to 86 mg%) by cimetidine but not by ranitidine. A later study in six normal subjects found that after taking 800 mg cimetidine daily for a week the AUC following a single 0.15 mg/kg oral dose of alcohol was approximately doubled (from 0.89 to 1.64 mM.h) and peak levels were raised about 33%. No changes were seen when the alcohol was given intravenously.[13] Another study[3] in subjects given cimetidine or ranitidine for only two days showed that peak blood alcohol levels were raised by 17 and 27% respectively, and the time for which blood levels remained above the 80 mg% mark (the legal driving limit in the UK and some other countries) was prolonged by about one-third.

(b) Evidence of no interaction

The makers of cimetidine (SKF) have on file three unpublished studies which failed to find any evidence that cimetidine or ranitidine significantly increased the blood levels of alcohol. One study was on six normal subjects given single 400 mg doses of cimetidine, another on six normal subjects given 1 g cimetidine daily for 14 days, and the last on 10 normal subjects given either 1 g cimetidine daily or 300 mg ranitidine daily.[7] Six other studies also failed to demonstrate significant interactions involving either cimetidine, ranitidine or famotidine and a number of different alcoholic drinks.[5,6,8–11]

Mechanism

Uncertain. The rate of elimination of alcohol from the body is not altered by cimetidine[2,3] or ranitidine[3] so it seems possible that, if any interaction occurs, these drugs act by enhancing the rate of alcohol absorption from the gut. This would seem to be confirmed by studies which showed no interaction with cimetidine when the alcohol was given intravenously.[4,13]

Importance and management

A controversial interaction which is not established. The weight of evidence suggests that neither cimetidine, famotidine nor ranitidine usually cause a significant rise in the blood levels of alcohol: eight studies found no evidence of an interaction and three found only a relatively small rise. Only one found a substantial rise (AUC doubled, peak levels+33%).[13] The authors of the first report describing this interaction (peak levels+12%) concluded that it is 'unlikely to result in socially significant consequences'[1] yet they also say that the subjects in this study said that the intoxicant effects of alcohol were perceptibly increased by cimetidine.[1] Another study failed to confirm that this was so.[6] With so many questions remaining unanswered this interaction certainly cannot be dimissed entirely, but it seems not to be of major importance. The ultracautious may wish to warn patients that an increase in the effects of alcohol may sometimes occur. More study is needed.

References

1 Feeley J and Wood AJJ. Effects of cimetidine on the elimination and actions of alcohol. J Amer Med Ass (1982) 247, 2819–21.
2 Seitz HK, Bosche J, Czygan P, Veith S, Simon B and Kommerell B. Increased blood ethanol levels following cimetidine but not ranitidine. Lancet (1983) i, 760.
3 Webster LK, Jones DB and Smallwood RA. Influence of cimetidine and ranitidine on ethanol pharmacokinetics. Aust NZ J Med (1985) 15, 359–60.
4 Couzigou P, Fleury B, Bourjac M, Betbeder A-M, Vincon G, Richard-Molard B, Albin H, Amouretti M and Beraud C. Pharmacocinetique de l'alcool apres perfusion intraveineuse de trois heures avec et sans cimetidine chez dix sujets sains non alcooliques. Gastroenterol Clin Biol (1984) 8, 103–8.
5 Dobrilla G, de Pretis G, Piazzi L, Chilovi F, Comberlato M, Valentini M, Pastorino A and Vallaperta P. Is ethanol metabolism affected by oral administration of cimetidine and ranitidine in therapeutic doses? Hepato-gastroenterol (1984) 31, 35–7.
6 Johnston KI, Fenzl E and Hein B. Einfluss von Cimetidine auf den Abbau und die Wirkung des Alkohols. Arzneim-Forsch/Drug Res (1984) 34, 734–6.
7 Robson AS (Smith Kline and French). Personal communication (1989).
8. Tanaka E and Nakamura K. Effects of H2-receptor antagonists on ethanol metabolism in Japanese volunteers. Br J clin Pharmac (1988) 26, 96–9.
9 Tan OT, Stafford TJ, Sarkany I, Gaylarde PM, Tilsey C and Payne JP. Suppression of alcohol-induced flushing by a combination of H1 and H2 histamine antagonists. Br J Dermatol (1982) 107, 647–52.
10 Holtmann G and Singer MV. Histamine H2-receptor antagonists and
blood alcohol levels. Dig Dis Sci (1988) 33, 767–8.
11 Holtmann G, Singer MV, Knop D, Becker S and Goebell H. Effect of histamine H2-receptor antagonists on blood alcohol levels. Gastroenterology (1988) 94, A190.
12 Seitz HK, Veith S, Czygan P, Bosche J, Simon B, Gugler R and Kommerell B. In vivo interactions between H2-receptor antagonists and ethanol metabolism in man and in rats. Hepatology (1984) 4, 1231–4.
13 Caballeria J, Baraona E, Rodamilans M and Lieber CS. Effects of cimetidine on gastric alcohol dehydrogenase activity and blood alcohol levels. Gastroenterology (1989) 96, 388–92.

Alcohol + CNS depressants

Abstract/Summary

The concurrent use of small or moderate amounts of alcohol and therapeutic doses of drugs which are CNS depressants can increase drowsiness and reduce alertness. These drugs include analgesics, anticonvulsants, antidepressants, antihistamines, antinauseants, neuroleptics, tranquillizers, hypno-sedatives and others. This increases the risk of accident when driving or handling other potentially dangerous machinery and may make the performance of everyday tasks more difficult and hazardous.

Clinical evidence, mechanism, importance and management

Alcohol is a CNS depressant (see the introduction to this chapter). With only small or moderate amounts of alcohol and blood alcohol levels well within legal driving limits, it may be quite unsafe to drive if another CNS depressant is being taken concurrently. The details of drugs which have been tested are set out in the synopses in this chapter (see the Index), but there are others which nobody seems to have tested formally. The Abstract/Summary above lists some of those which commonly cause drowsiness. Quite apart from driving, almost everyone meets potentially dangerous situations every day at home, in the garden, in the street and at work. Crossing a busy street or even walking downstairs can become much more risky under the influence of drugs and drink. A cause for concern is that the patient may be partially or totally unware of the extent of the deterioration in his skills. Patients should be warned.

Alcohol + Codeine

Abstract/Summary

Codeine in 50 mg doses, both alone and with alcohol, impairs the ability to drive safely but no interaction of importance would be expected with the relatively small amounts of codeine in most compound analgesic preparations.

Clinical evidence, mechanism, importance and management

Double blind studies on a very large number of professional army drivers showed that 50 mg of codeine and alcohol

(0.5 mg/kg), both alone and together, impaired their ability to drive safely on a static driving simulator. The number of 'collisions', neglected instructions and the times they 'drove off the road' were increased.[1,2] Codeine dosages of this order are given in the form of Codeine Phosphate Syrup (BPC 1973) and in Tablets of Codeine Phosphate BP so that these preparations, particularly with alcohol, could make drivers more accident-prone, but the increased hazard is difficult to quantify. Doses of 15, 25 or 30 mg codeine phosphate occur in some elixirs and linctuses, but only relatively small amounts of codeine (5–8 mg) are found in most proprietary compound analgesic tablets. Alcohol appears not to affect the pharmacokinetics of codeine.[3]

References

1 Linnoila M and Hakkinen S. Effects of diazepam and codeine, alone and in combination with alcohol, on simulated driving. Clin Pharmacol Ther (1974) 15, 368.
2 Linnoila M and Mattila MJ. Interaction of alcohol and drugs on psychomotor skills as demonstrated by a driving simulator. Br J Pharmac (1973) 47, 671P.
3 Bodd E, Beylich KM. Christopherson AS and Morland J. Oral administration of codeine in the presence of ethanol: a pharmacokinetic study in man. Pharmacol Toxicol (1987) 61, 297–300.

Alcohol + Dextropropoxyphene

Abstract/Summary

The central nervous depressant effects of alcohol are increased to some extent by dextropropoxyphene in normal therapeutic doses, but the effect appears to be small and of limited clinical importance. In deliberate suicidal overdosage the CNS depressant effects appear to be additive and can be fatal.

Clinical evidence

A study in eight volunteers of the effects of dextropropoxyphene on motor co-ordination, mental performance and stability of stance showed that alcohol alone (blood levels of 50 mg%) impaired the performance of the tests to a greater degree than 65 mg dextropropoxyphene given alone. When given together there was some evidence that the effects were greater than with either alone, but in some instances the impairment was no greater than with just alcohol. The effect of alcohol clearly predominated.[1]

Another study[2] showed that the effects of alcohol (95 mg) on the performance of two psychomotor tests were not altered in subjects who had been given two tablets of *Distalgesic* (dextropropoxyphene 32.5 mg + paracetamol 325 mg in each tablet).

Mechanism

Not understood. Both drugs are CNS depressants and in overdosage the fatal dose of dextropropoxyphene is reduced by the presence of alcohol. Their effects seem to be additive.[4,5] Neither affects the serum levels of the other.[3]

Importance and management

Numerous reports describe the severe and often fatal respiratory depression which can follow alcohol/dextropropoxyphene overdosage, but information about the combined effects of moderate social drinking and therapeutic doses of dextropropoxyphene is limited. The objective evidence indicates that the interaction with moderate doses of both is quite small. Even so it would seem prudent (at the risk of being overcautious) to warn patients that dextropropoxyphene can cause drowsiness and this may be exaggerated to some extent by alcohol. They should be warned that driving or handling potentially hazardous machinery may be more risky.

References

1 Kiplinger GF, Sokol G and Rodda BE. Effects of combined alcohol and propoxyphene on human performance. Arch int Pharmacodyn (1974) 212, 175.
2 Edwards C, Gard PR, Handley SL, Hunter M and Whittington RM. Distalgesic and ethanol-impaired function. Lancet (1982) ii, 384.
3 Sellers EM, Hamilton CA, Kaplan HL, Degani NC and Foltz RL. Pharmacokinetic interaction of propoxyphene and alcohol. Br J clin Pharmac (1985) 19, 398–401.
4 Carson DJL and Carson ED. Fatal dextropropoxyphene poisoning in Northern Ireland. Review of 30 cases. Lancet (1977) i, 894–7.
5 Whittington RM and Barclay AD. The epidemiology of dextropropoxyphene (Distalgesic) overdose fatalities in Birmingham and the West Midlands. J Clin Hosp Pharm (1981) 6, 251–7.

Alcohol + Dimethylformamide

Abstract/Summary

A disulfiram-like reaction can occur in about 20% of those who drink alcohol after being exposed to dimethylformamide (DMF) vapour.

Clinical evidence

A three-year study in a chemical plant where dimethylformamide (DMF) was used showed that about 20% (19 out of 102 men) exposed to the vapour developed this reaction after drinking alcohol.[3] Flushing of the face, and often of the neck, arms, hands and chest occurred after drinking alcohol, and sometimes dizziness, nausea and tightness of the chest. A single glass of beer was enough to induce a flush lasting 2 h. The majority of the men experienced the reaction within 24 h of exposure to DMF, but it could occur even after four days.

Three further cases of this interaction are described in other reports.[1,2]

Mechanism

Men exposed to DMF vapour develop substantial amounts of DMF and its metabolite (N-methylformamide) in their blood and urine.[3] This latter compound in particular has been shown in rats[4] given alcohol to raise their blood acetaldehyde levels by a factor of 5, so it would seem probable that the N-methylformamide is responsible for this disulfiram-like reaction (see 'Alcohol+Disulfiram').

Importance and management

An established interaction, the incidence being about 20%.[3] Those who come into contact with DMF, even in very low concentrations, should be warned of this possible interaction with alcohol. It would appear to be more unpleasant than serious in most instances, and normally requires no treatment.

References

1 Chivers CP. Disulfiram effect from inhalation of dimethylformamide. Lancet (1978) i, 331.
2 Reinl W and Urba HJ. Erkrankungen durch dimethylformamid. Int Arch Gewerbepath Gewerbehyg (1965) 21, 333.
3 Lyle WH, Spence TWM, McKinneley WM and Duckers K. Dimethyl-formamide and alcohol intolerance. Brit J Ind Med (1979) 36, 63.
4 Hanasono GK, Fuller RW, Broddle WD and Gibson WR. Studies on the effects of N,N-dimethylformamide on ethanol disposition and monoamine oxidase activity in rats. Toxicol Appl Pharmacol (1977) 39, 461.

Alcohol + Disulfiram

Abstract/Summary

The ingestion of alcohol while taking disulfiram will result in flushing and fullness of the face and neck, tachycardia, breathlessness, giddiness and hypotension, nausea and vomiting. This is also called the Antabuse reaction. It is used to deter alcoholic patients from drinking. A mild skin flush reaction may possibly occur in particularly sensitive individuals if alcohol is applied to the skin or if the vapour is inhaled.

Clinical evidence

This toxic interaction was first observed in 1937 by Dr EE Williams amongst workers in the rubber industry who were handling tetraethylthiuram disulphide:

'Beer will cause a flushing of the face and hands, with rapid pulse, and some of the men describe palpitations and a terrible fullness of the face, eyes and head. After a glass of beer (six ounces) the blood pressure falls about 10 points, the pulse is slightly accelerated and the skin becomes flushed in the face and wrists. In 15 min the blood pressure falls another 10 points, the heart is more rapid, and the patient complains of fullness in the head'.[1]

The later observation[2] by Hald and his colleagues of the same reaction with the ethyl congener (disulfiram) led to its introduction as a drink deterrent. Some patients also experience giddiness, sweating, nausea, vomiting, difficulty in breathing and headache. The severity of the reaction can depend upon the amount of alcohol ingested but some individuals are extremely sensitive. Respiratory depression, cardiovascular collapse, cardiac arrhythmias, unconsciousness and convulsions may occur. There have been fatalities.[4,5]

A mild disulfiram reaction is said to occur in some patients who apply alcohol to the skin. This has been reported after using after-shave lotion,[7] tar gel (33% alcohol)[6] and a beer-containing shampoo (3% alcohol).[8] The reaction has also been described in a patient who inhaled vapour from paint in a poorly ventilated area and from the inhalation of 'mineral spirits'.[11] A woman on disulfiram reported vaginal stinging and soreness during sexual intercourse, and similar discomfort to her husband's penis, which seemed to be related to the disulfiram dosage and how intoxicated her husband was.[13]

Mechanism

Largely, but not totally understood. Normally alcohol is rapidly metabolized within the body, firstly to acetaldehyde and then by a series of biochemical steps to water and carbon dioxide. Disulfiram inhibits the enzyme (acetaldehyde dehydrogenase) which is concerned with the metabolism of acetaldehyde and, as a result, the acetaldehyde accumulates in the body. But not all the symptoms of the reaction can be reproduced by injecting acetaldehyde, so that some other biochemical mechanism must also be involved. For example, it is thought that the inhibition of dopamine-beta-hydroxy-lase may have some part to play. It has been suggested that the mild skin flush which can occur if alcohol is applied to the skin is not a true disulfiram reaction.[12]

Importance and management

An extremely well-documented and important interaction exploited therapeutically to deter alcoholics from drinking. Initial treatment should be given under close supervision because an extremely intense reaction can occur in some patients with even quite small doses of alcohol. Apart from the usual warnings about drinking, patients should also be warned about the unwitting ingestion of alcohol in some pharmaceutical preparations. The alcohol-content of nearly 500 American products has been published which is too extensive to be reproduced here.[10] The risk of a reaction is real. It has been seen following a single dose of an alcohol-containing cough mixture,[3] whereas the ingestion of small amounts of communion wine and the absorption of alcohol from a bronchial nebulizer spray is said not to result in any reaction.[9]

References

1 Williams EE. Effects of alcohol on workers with carbon disulfide. J Amer med Ass (1937) 109, 1472.
2 Hald J, Jacobssen E and Larsen V. The sensitizing effects of tetra-ethylthiuram disulphide (Antabuse) to ethyl alcohol. Acta Pharmacol (1948) 4, 285.
3 Koff RS, Popadimas I and Honig E. Alcohol in cough medicines: hazards to the disulfiram user. J Amer med Ass (1971) 215, 1988.
4 Garber RS and Bennett RE. Unusual reaction to antabuse: report of three cases. J Med Soc NJ (1950) 47, 168.
5 Kwentus J and Major LF. Disulfiram in the treatment of alcoholism. A review. J Stud Alc (1979) 40, 428.
6 Ellis CN, Mitchell AJ and Beardsley GR. Tar gel interaction with disulfiram. Arch Dermatol (1979) 115, 1367.
7 Mercurio F. Antabuse-alcohol reaction following the use of after-shave lotion. J Amer med Ass (1952) 149, 82.
8 Stoll D and King LE. Disulfiram-alcohol skin reaction to beer-containing shampoo. J Amer med Ass (1980) 244, 2045.

9 Rothstein E. Use of disulfiram (Antabuse) in alcoholism. N Eng J Med (1970) 283, 936.
10 Parker WA. Alcohol-containing pharmaceuticals. Am J Drug Alcohol Abuse (1982–3) 9, 195–209.
11 Scott GE and Little FW. Disulfiram reaction to organic solvents other than ethanol. N Eng J Med (1985) 312, 790.
12 Haddock NF and Wilkin JK. Cutaneous reactions to lower aliphatic alcohols before and during disulfiram therapy. Arch Dermatol (1982) 118, 157–9.
13 Chick JD. Disulfiram reaction during sexual intercourse. Br J Psychiatry (1988) 152, 438.

Alcohol + Edible fungi

Abstract/Summary

A disulfiram-like reaction can occur if alcohol if taken after eating the smooth ink(y) caps fungus (Coprinus atramentarius), Boletus luridus *and certain other edible fungi.*

Clinical evidence

A man who drank three pints of beer, 2 h after eating a meal of freshly picked and fried inky caps, developed facial flushing and a blotchy red rash over the upper half of his body. His face and hands swelled and he became breathless, sweated profusely, and vomited during the 3 h when the reaction was most severe. On admission to hospital he demonstrated tachycardia and some cardiac arrhythmia. The man's wife who ate the same fungi but without alcohol did not show the reaction.[1]

This reaction has been described on many occasions in medical and pharmacological reports[9,11,13] and in books devoted to descriptions of edible and poisonous fungi.[10] Only a few are listed here. Mild hypotension and '...alarming orthostatic features...'[2,3] are said to be common symptoms but arrhythmia seen in the case cited here[1] appears to be rare. Recovery from this interaction is usually spontaneous and uncomplicated. A similar reaction has been described after eating *Boletus luridus*,[14] and other fungi including *Coprinus micaceus, Clitocybe claviceps* and certain morels.[14]

Mechanism

An early and attractive idea was that this reaction was due to disulfiram (one group of workers actually claimed to have isolated it from the fungus[4]), but this was not confirmed by later work[5,12] and it now appears that the active ingredient is coprine (N-5-(1-hydroxycyclopropyl)-glutamine).[6,7] This is metabolized in the body to 1-aminocyclopropanol which appears, like disulfiram, to inhibit aldehyde dehydrogenase (see 'Alcohol + Disulfiram'). The active ingredients in the other fungi are unknown.

Importance and management

An established and well documented interaction. It is said to occur up to 24 h after eating the fungi. The intensity depends upon the quantities of fungus and alcohol consumed, and the time interval between them.[1,2] Despite the widespread consumption of edible fungi in Europe (and many people drink with a meal), reports of this reaction are few and far between, suggesting that while it can certainly be very unpleasant and frightening, the outcome is usually uncomplicated. Treatment appears normally not to be necessary.

The related fungus *Coprinus comatus* (the 'shaggy ink cap' or 'Lawyers wig') is said not to interact with alcohol,[3,8] nor is there anything to suggest that it ever occurs with the common field mushroom (*Agaricus campestris*) or the cultivated variety (*Agaricus bisporis*).[8]

References

1 Caley MJ and Clarke RA. Cardiac arrhythmias after mushroom ingestion. Brit Med J (1977) 2, 1633.
2 Buck RW. Mushroom toxins—brief review of literature. N Engl J Med (1961) 265, 681.
3 Broadhurst-Zingrich L. Ink caps and alcohol. Brit Med J (1978) 1, 511.
4 Simandl J and Franc J. Isolation of tetraethylthiuram disulfide from Coprinus atramentarius. Chem Listy (1956) 50, 1862.
5 Vanhaelen M, Vanhaelen-Fastre R, Hoyois J and Mardens Y. Reinvestigation of disulfiram-like activity of Coprinus atramentarius (Bull.ex Fr) Fr. extracts. J Pharm Sci (1976) 65, 1774.
6 Hatfield GM and Schaumberg IP. Isolation and structural studies of coprine, the disulfiram-like constituent of Coprinus atramentarius. Lloydia (1975) 38, 489.
7 Lindberg P, Bergman R and Wickberg B. Isolation and structure of coprine, a novel physiologically active cyclopropane derivative from Coprinus atramentarius and its synthesis via 1-amino-cyclo-propanol. J Chem Soc Chem Commun (1975) 946.
8 Radford AP. Ink caps and mushrooms. Brit Med J (1978) 1, 112.
9 Reynold WA and Lowe FH. Mushrooms and a toxic reaction to alcohol. Report of four cases. N Engl J Med (1965) 189, 630.
10 Ramsbottom J. Mushrooms and Toadstools. Collins, London (1953) p 55.
11 Wildervanck LS. Alcohol en de kale inktzwam. Ned T Geneesk (1978) 122, 913.
12 Wier JK and Tyler VE. An investigation of Coprinus atramentarius for the presence of disulfiram. J Am Pharm Ass (1960) 49, 427.
13 Tottmar O, Marchner H and Lindberg P., in 'Alcohol and Aldehyde Metabolising Systems', ed Thuram RG, Williamson JR, Drott HR and Chance B. vol 2. Academic Press, NY. (1977) pp. 203–12.
14 Budmiger H and Kocher F. Hexenrohrling (Boletus luridus) mit alkohol. Ein Kasuistischer Beitrag. Schweiz med Wsch (1982) 112, 1179–81.

Alcohol + Fluoxetine and Femoxetine

Abstract/Summary

Neither fluoxetine nor femoxetine in therapeutic doses appear to interact with alcohol.

Clinical evidence, mechanism, importance and management

A study in normal subjects showed that neither fluoxetine (30–60 mg) nor alcohol (4 oz whiskey) affected the pharmacokinetics of the other, and no changes in psychomotor activity was seen (stability of stance, motor performance, manual co-ordination).[1] A study in 12 subjects demonstrated that blood alcohol levels of 80 mg% (80 mg/dl) impaired the performance of a number of psychomotor tests but the addition of 40 mg fluoxetine daily taken for six days had little further effect.[3] Another study also found no change in the performance of a number of psychophysiological tests when fluoxetine was combined with alcohol.[4] No significant interaction was seen in another study with femoxetine (200–600 mg) and alcohol (1 g/kg).[2]

References

1 Lemberger L, Rowe H, Bergstrom RF, Farid KZ and Enas GG. Effect of fluoxetine on psychomotor performance, physiologic response, and kinetics of ethanol. Clin Pharmacol Ther (1985) 37, 658–64.
2 Stromberg C and Mattila MJ. Acute and subacute effects on psychomotor performance of femoxetine alone and with alcohol. Eur J Clin Pharmacol (1985) 28, 641–7.
3 Allen D, Lader M, Curran HV. A comparative study of the interactions of alcohol with amitriptyline, fluoxetine and placebo in normal subjects. Prog Neuro-Psychopharmacol and Biol Psychiat (1988) 12, 63–80.
4 Schaffler K. Study on performance and alcohol interaction with the antidepressant fluoxetine. Int Clin Psychopharmacol (1989)

Alcohol + Fluvoxamine or Clovoxamine

Abstract/Summary

There is some evidence that the sedative effects of alcohol and fluvoxamine may be additive, but clovoxamine appears not to interact.

Clinical evidence, mechanism, importance and management

A study in normal subjects given 100 mg fluvoxamine found that it tended to enhance night-time sedation and cause some difficulty in alertness next morning.[1] Another study found that 150 mg fluvoxamine daily with alcohol (0.5%) impaired alertness and attention more than alcohol alone.[3] Concurrent use may therefore make driving and handling other potentially dangerous machinery more hazardous. No sedation was seen in a study with 150 mg clovoxamine daily.[1] Another study in 12 subjects found no evidence that single doses of 50, 100 or 150 mg clovoxamine increased the effects of alcohol (0.8 g/kg) as measured by a number of psychomotor tests.[2]

References

1 Ochs HR, Greenblatt DJ, Verburg-Ochs B, Labedski L. Chronic treatment with fluvoxamine, clovoxamine and placebo: interaction with digoxin and effects on sleep and alertness. J Clin Pharmacol (1989) 29, 91–5.
2 Stromberg C, Mattila MJ. Acute comparison of clovoxamine and mianserin, alone and in combination with ethanol, on human psychomotor performance. Pharmacol Toxicol (1987) 60, 374–9.
3 Herberg K-W, Menke H. Study of the effects of the antidepressant fluvoxamine on driving skills and its interaction with alcohol. Duphar Laboratories. Data on file 1981.

Alcohol + Glutethimide

Abstract/Summary

The sedative effects of glutethimide are increased by alcohol and the performance of psychomotor skills is impaired. Driving or handling other potentially dangerous machinery is made more hazardous.

Clinical evidence, mechanism, importance and management

A double-blind study on normal subjects given 250 mg glutethimide, either alone or with alcohol (0.5 mg/kg), showed that concurrent use subjectively and objectively impaired the performance of a number of psychomotor skill tests related to driving (choice reaction, coordination, divided attention).[1] Both are CNS depressants and their effects would appear to be additive. It has also been reported that blood alcohol levels can be raised 11–30% by glutethimide and blood glutethimide levels are reduced,[2] but a later study was unable to confirm this.[1] It was also claimed that effects of alcohol and glutethimide were antagonistic rather than additive.[2]

The information is limited and somewhat contradictory, nevertheless patients should be warned about the probable results of taking glutethimide and alcohol together. Driving a car, handling dangerous machinery or undertaking any task needing alertness and full coordination is likely to be made more difficult and hazardous. There is no evidence of a hangover effect which could result in an interaction with alcohol the next day.[1]

References

1 Saario I and Linnoila M. Effect of subacute treatment with hypnotics, alone or in combination with alcohol, on psychomotor skills related to driving. Acta pharmacol et toxicol (1976) 38, 382.
2 Mould GP, Curry SH and Binns TB. Interactions of glutethimide and phenobarbitone with ethanol in man. J Pharm Pharmac (1972) 24, 894.

Alcohol + Glyceryl trinitrate

Abstract/Summary

Patients who take glyceryl trinitrate (nitroglycerin) while drinking may feel faint and dizzy.

Clinical evidence, mechanism, importance and management

The results of studies[1,5] on the combined haemodynamic effects of alcohol and glyceryl trinitrate give support to claims made in 1965 and 1980 that concurrent use increases the risk of exaggerated hypotension and fainting.[2,3] Their vasodilatory effects[4] would appear to be additive. The greatest effect was seen when the glyceryl trinitrate was taken 1 h after starting to drink.[1] It is suggested that this increased susceptibility to postural hypotension should not be allowed to stop patients from using glyceryl trinitrate if they drink, but they should be warned and told what to do if they feel faint and dizzy.[1]

References

1   Kupari M, Heikkila J and Ylikahri R. Does alcohol intensify the hemodynamic effects of nitroglycerin? Clin Cardiol (1984) 7, 382–6.
2   Shafer N. Hypotension due to nitroglycerin combined with alcohol. N Engl J Med (1965) 272, 1169.
3   Opi.e. LH. Drugs and the heart. Nitrates. Lancet (1980) i, 750–2.
4   Allison RD, Kraner JC and Roth GM. Effects of alcohol and nitroglycerin on vascular responses in man. Angiology (1971) 22, 211–222.
5   Abrams J, Schroeder K, Raizada V and Gibbs D. Potentially adverse effects of sublingual nitroglycerin during consumption of alcohol. J Amer Coll Cardiol (1990) 15, 226A.

Alcohol + Griseofulvin

Abstract/Summary

An increase in the intoxicant effects of alcohol has been reported to occur in a very small number of patients. A flushing reaction has also been described in one patient.

Clinical evidence, mechanism, importance and management

The descriptions of this interaction are very brief. One of them describes a man who had '. . .decreased tolerance to alcohol and emotional instability manifested by crying and nervousness so severe that the drug was stopped.'[1] Another states that '. . .a possible potentiation of the effects of alcohol has been noted in a very small number of patients.'[2] I am also personally aware of a man who experienced a marked increase in the intoxicant effects of alcohol while taking griseofulvin. A single case of flushing and tachycardia attributed to concurrent use has also been described.[2]

The documentation is extremely sparse which would seem to suggest that interactions between alcohol and griseofulvin are uncommon. Normally concurrent use need not be avoided.

References

1   Drowns BV, Fuhrman DL and Dennie CC. Use, abuse and limitations of griseofulvin. Missouri Med (1960) 57, 1473.
2   Simon HJ and Rantz LA. Reactions to antimicrobial agents. Ann Rev Med (1961) 12, 119.

Alcohol + Hydromorphone

Abstract/Summary

A single case report describes a fatality due to the combined CNS depressant effects of hydromorphone and alcohol.

Clinical evidence, mechanism, importance and management

A young man died from the combined cardiovascular and respiratory depressant effects of hydromorphone (*Dilaudid*) and alcohol.[1] He fell into a sleep, the serious nature of which was not recognized by those around him. Post mortem analysis revealed alcohol and hydromorphone concentrations of 900 mg/l and 0.1 mg/l, neither of which is particularly excessive. This case emphasizes the importance of warning patients about the potentially hazardous consequences of drinking while taking potent CNS depressants of this kind.

Reference

1   Levine B, Saady J, Fierro M and Valentour J. A hydromophone and ethanol fatality. J Forensic Sci (1984) 29, 655–9.

Alcohol + Indomethacin or Phenylbutazone

Abstract/Summary

The skills related to driving are impaired by indomethacin and phenylbutazone. Further impairment occurs if patients drink while taking phenylbutazone, but this does not appear to occur with indomethacin.

Clinical evidence, mechanism, importance and management

A study on a large number of normal subjects showed that the performance of various psychomotor skills related to driving (choice reaction, coordination, divided attention tests) were impaired by 50 mg indomethacin or 200 mg phenylbutazone. The concurrent ingestion of alcohol (0.5 mg/kg) made things worse in those taking phenylbutazone, but the performance of those taking indomethacin was improved to some extent.[1] The reasons are not understood. The study showed that the subjects were subjectively unaware of the adverse effects of phenylbutazone. Information is very limited, but patients should be warned if they intend to drive.

Reference

1   Linnoila M, Seppala T and Mattila MJ. Acute effect of antipyretic analgesics, alone or in combination with alcohol, on human psychomotor skills related to driving. Br J clin Pharmac (1974) 1, 477.

Alcohol + Isoniazid

Abstract/Summary

Isoniazid increases the hazards of driving after drinking alcohol.

Clinical evidence, mechanism, importance and management

The effects of 750 mg isoniazid with 0.5 g/kg alcohol were examined in 100 volunteers given various psychomotor tests and using a driving simulator. No major interaction was seen in the psychomotor tests, but the number of drivers who 'drove off the road' on the simulator was increased.[1,2] There would therefore appear to be some extra risks for patients on isoniazid who drink and drive, but the effect does not appear to be large. Patients should nevertheless be warned.

References

1 Linnoila M and Matilla MJ. Effects of isoniazid on psychomotor skills related to driving. J clin Pharmacol (1973) 13, 343.
2 Linnoila M and Matilla MJ. Interaction of alcohol and drugs on psychomotor skills as demonstrated by a driving simulator. Br J Pharmacol (1973) 47, 671 P.

Alcohol + Ketoconazole

Abstract/Summary

Disulfiram-like reactions have been seen in a few patients taking ketoconazole after drinking alcohol.

Clinical evidence

One patient out of group of 12 taking 200 mg ketoconazole daily experienced a disulfiram-like reaction (nausea, vomiting, facial flushing) after drinking.[1] No further details are given and the report does not say whether any of the others drank alcohol. A woman on 200 mg ketoconazole daily developed a disulfiram-like reaction when she drank.[3] Another report describes a transient 'sunburn-like' rash or flush on the face, upper chest and back of a patient taking 200 mg ketoconazole daily when she drank modest quantities of wine or beer.[2] The reasons are not known but it seems possible that ketoconazole may act like disulfiram and inhibit the activity of acetaldehyde dehydrogenase (see 'Alcohol + Disulfiram').

The incidence of this reaction appears to be low (these appear to be the only reports) and its importance is probably small, but patients should be warned. Reactions of this kind are usually more unpleasant than serious, disulfiram itself being the possible exception.

References

1 Fazio RA, Wickremesinghe PC and Arsura EL. Ketoconazole therapy of candida esophagitis—a prospective study of 12 cases. Am J Gastroenterol (1983) 79, 261–4
2 Magnasco AJ and Magnasco LD. Interaction of ketoconazole and ethanol. Clin Pharm (1986) 5, 522–3.
3 Meyboom RHB and Pater BW. Overgevoeligheid voor alcoholische dranken tijdens behandeling met ketoconazol. Ned Tijdsch Geneeskd (1989) 133, 1463–4.

Alcohol + Lithium carbonate

Abstract/Summary

Some limited evidence suggests that lithium carbonate alone or combined with alcohol may make car driving more hazardous.

Clinical evidence, mechanism, importance and management

A study on 20 normal subjects given lithium carbonate to achieve blood levels of 0.75 meq/l and 0.5 g/kg alcohol, and who were subjected to various tests (choice reaction, coordination, attention) to assess any impairment of psychomotor skills related to driving, indicated that lithium alone and with alcohol may increase the risk of accident.[1] Information is very limited but patients should be warned.

Reference

1 Linnoila M, Saario I and Maki M. Effects of treatment with diazepam or lithium and alcohol on psychomotor skills related to driving. Eur J clin Pharmacol (1974) 7, 337.

Alcohol + Maprotiline

Abstract/Summary

The sedative effects of maprotiline and alcohol combined can make car driving or handling dangerous machinery more hazardous.

Clinical evidence, mechanism, importance and management

A double blind cross-over trial in 12 normal subjects found that single 75 mg oral doses of maprotiline subjectively caused drowsiness which was increased by alcohol (1 g/kg) and worsened the performance of a number of tests.[1] Patients should be warned of the hazards, particularly if they drive.

Reference

1 Stromberg C, Seppala T and Mattila MJ. Acute effects of maprotiline, doxepin and zimeldine with alcohol in healthy volunteers. Arch Int Pharmacodyn (1988) 291, 217–228.

Alcohol + Meprobamate

Abstract/Summary

The intoxicant effects of alcohol can be considerably increased by the presence of normal daily doses of meprobamate. Driving or handling other potentially dangerous machinery is made much more hazardous.

Clinical evidence

A study on 24 subjects, given 2.4 mg meprobamate daily for a week, showed that with blood alcohol levels of 50 mg% their performance of a number of co-ordination and judgement tests was much more impaired than with either drug alone. Some of the subjects were quite obviously drunk while taking both and showed '...marked muscular inco-ordination and little or no concern for the social proprieties....Two could not walk without assistance....Nothing approaching this was seen with alcohol alone.'[1]

Other studies confirm this interaction, although the effects appeared to be less pronounced.[2–7]

Mechanism

Both meprobamate and alcohol are CNS depressants which appear to have additive effects. There is also evidence that alcohol may inhibit or increase meprobamate metabolism, depending on whether it is taken acutely or chronically, but the contribution of this to the enhanced CNS depression is uncertain.[8,9]

Importance and management

A well-documented and potentially serious interaction. Normal daily dosages of meprobamate in association with relatively moderate blood-alcohol concentrations, well within the UK legal limit for driving, can result in obviously hazardous intoxication. Patients should be warned.

References

1 Zirkle GA, McAtee OB, King PD and Van Dyke R. Meprobamate and small amounts of alcohol. Effects on human ability, coordination and judgement. J Amer Med Ass (1960) 173, 1823.
2 Reisby N and Theilgaard A. The interaction of alcohol and meprobamate in man. Acta Psychiatr Scand (1969) Suppl 208, 192.
3 Forney RB and Hughes FW. Meprobamate, ethanol or meprobamate-ethanol combinations on performance of human subjects under delayed audiofeedback (DAF). J Psychol (1964) 57, 431.
4 Goldberg L. Behavioural and physiological effects of alcohol on man. Psychosom Med (1966) 28, 570.
5 Ashford JR and Cobby JM. Drug interactions. The effects of alcohol and meprobamate applied singly and jointly in human subjects. IV. J Stud Alc (1975) Suppl 7, 140.
6 Cobby JM and Ashford JR. Drug interactions. The effects of alcohol and meprobamate applied singly and jointly in human subjects. V. J Stud Alc (1975) Suppl 7, 162.
7 Ashford JR and Carpenter JA. Drug interactions. The effects of alcohol and meprobamate applied singly and jointly in human subjects. VI. J Stud Alc (1975) Suppl 7, 177.
8 Misra PS, Lefevre A, Ishi H, Rubin E and Lieber CS. Increase of ethanol, meprobamate and pentobarbital metabolism after chronic ethanol administration in man and in rats. Am J Med (1971) 51, 346.
9 Rubin E, Gang H, Misra PS and Lieber CS. Inhibition of drug metabolism by acute ethanol intoxication. A hepatic microsomal mechanism. Am J Med (1970) 49, 801.

Alcohol + Methaqualone or *Mandrax* (methaqualone + diphenhydramine)

Abstract/Summary

*The CNS depressant effects of alcohol and its detrimental effects on the skills relating to driving or handling other potentially dangerous machinery are increased by the concurrent use of methaqualone or **Mandrax**.*

Clinical evidence

(a) Alcohol + methaqualone

A retrospective study of drivers arrested for driving under the influence of drugs and/or drink showed that, generally speaking, those with blood-methaqualone levels of 1.0 mg/l or less showed no symptoms of sedation, whereas those above 2.0 mg/l demonstrated serious deterioration (staggering gait, drowsiness, incoherence and slurred speech). These effects were increased if the drivers had also been drinking. The authors write that '...the levels (of methaqualone) necessary for driving impairment are considerably lowered (by alcohol)...', but no precise measure of this is presented in the paper. A similar effect was seen in drivers taking methaqualone and diazepam.[3]

(b) Alcohol + Mandrax (methaqualone 250 mg + diphenhydramine 25 mg)

A double-blind study on 12 subjects given two *Mandrax* tablets showed that both mental and physical sedation and a reduction in cognitive skills were enhanced by alcohol (0.5 mg/kg). Residual amounts of *Mandrax* continued to interact as long as 72 h after a single dose. Methaqualone blood levels are also raised by regular moderate amounts of alcohol.[1]

Enhanced effects were also seen in another study.[2]

Mechanism

Alcohol, methaqualone and diphenhydramine are all CNS depressants, the effects of which are additive. The diphenhydramine–alcohol interaction is discussed under 'Alcohol + Antihistamines'. A hangover can occur because the elimination half-life of methaqualone is long (10–40 h).

Importance and management

An established interaction of importance. Those taking either methaqualone or *Mandrax* should be warned that handling machinery, driving a car, or any other task requiring alertness and full co-ordination, will be made more difficult and hazardous if they drink. Doses of alcohol below the legal driving limit with normal amounts of methaqualone may cause considerable intoxication. Patients should also be told that a significant interaction may possibly occur the following day because methaqualone taken on the previous day can have a hangover effect.

References

1 Roden S, Harvey P and Mitchard M. The effect of ethanol on residual plasma concentrations and behaviour in volunteers who have taken Mandrax. Br J clin Pharmac (1977) 4, 245.

2 Saario I and Linnoila M. Effect of subacute treatment with hypnotics, alone or in combination with alcohol, on psychomotor skills related to driving. Acta pharmacol et toxicol (1976) 38, 3382.

3 McCurdy HH, Solomons ET and Holbrook JM. Incidence of methaqualone in driving-under-the-influence (DUI) cases in the State of Georgia. J Anal Toxicol (1981) 5, 270–4.

Alcohol + Metoclopramide

Abstract/Summary

There is some as yet unconfirmed evidence that metoclopramide can increase the sedative effects of alcohol.

Clinical evidence, mechanism, importance and management

A study in seven normal subjects found that 10 mg metoclopramide given intravenously accelerated the rate of absorption of alcohol (70 mg/kg) given orally and increased its peak levels but not to a statistically significant extent. Blood alcohol levels remained below 12 mg%. More importantly the sedative effects of the alcohol were found to be increased.[1] The mechanisms of these interactions are not understood. Nobody else seems to have examined this interaction so that its clinical importance is uncertain but some care would seem appropriate if patients on metoclopramide take alcohol. More study is needed.

Reference

1 Bateman D, Kahn C, Mashiter K and Davies DS. Pharmacokinetic and concentration-effect studies with IV metoclopramide. Br J clin Pharmac (1978) 6, 401–5.

Alcohol + Metronidazole

Abstract/Summary

A disulfiram-like reaction can occur in patients taking metronidazole who drink alcohol. It also occurred in a woman while using a vaginal insert containing metronidazole. The existence of this interaction is disputed in some reports.

Clinical evidence

A man who had been in a drunken stupor for three days was given two metronidazole tablets (total of 500 mg) 1 h apart by his wife in the belief that they might sober him up. 20 min after the first tablet he was awake and complaining that he had been given disulfiram (which he had experienced some months before). Immediately after the second tablet he took another drink and developed a classic disulfiram-like reaction with flushing of the face and neck, nausea and epigastric discomfort.[1]

All of 10 alcoholic patients who took part in a test of the value of metronidazole (250 mg twice daily) as a possible drink-deterrent experienced some disulfiram-like reactions of varying intensity (facial flushing, headaches, sensation of heat, fall in blood pressure, vomiting).[4] Another report on 60 patients, given 250–750 mg daily, stated that all of them developed mild to moderate disulfiram-like reactions.[5] Other reports describe the same reaction, but the incidence is said to be lower: 24%,[6] 10%[7] and 2%.[2] A disulfiram-like reaction has been seen in a patient treated intravenously with metronidazole and a trimethoprim-sulphamethoxazole preparation containing 10% alcohol as a diluent.[11] Another report describes a reaction when metronidazole was used as a vaginal insert.[12] It has also been reported that alcohol tastes badly[1,4] or is less pleasurable[2] while taking metronidazole. Some drug abusers apparently exploit the reaction for 'kicks'.[10] In contrast, there are other reports which claim that metronidazole has no disulfiram-like effects whatsoever.[8,9]

Mechanism

Metronidazole, like disulfiram, can inhibit the activity of acetaldehyde dehydrogenase.[3] The accumulation of acetaldehyde is responsible for most of the symptoms (see 'Alcohol+Disulfiram'). It also appears that enough can be absorbed from the vagina for a reaction to occur.[12]

Importance and management

Numerous studies have been made of this interaction, but it remains a controversial issue, the incidence being variously reported as 100%, and at the other extreme 0%. Despite this patients given metronidazole by mouth should be warned what may happen if they drink. If and when it occurs, it seems normally to be more unpleasant and possibly frightening than serious, and usually requires no treatment. The risk of a reaction with metronidazole used intravaginally seems to be small because the absorption is low (about 20% compared with about 100% orally) but evidently it can happen. Patients should be warned.

References

1 Taylor JAT. Metronidazole—a new agent for combined somatic and psychic therapy for alcoholism. Bull Los Angeles Neurol Soc (1964) 29, 158.

2 Penick SB, Carrier RN and Sheldon JR. Metronidazole in the treatment of alcoholism. Amer J Psychiat (1969) 125, 1063.

3 Fried R and Fried L. The effect of Flagyl on xanthine oxidase and alcohol dehydrogenase. Biochem Pharmacol (1966) 15, 1890.

4 Ban TA, Lehmann HE and Roy P. Preliminary report on the therapeutic effect of FLAGYL in alcoholism. L'Union Medicale du Canada (1966) 95, 147.

5 Sansoy OM and Vegas L. Evaluation of metronidazole in the treatment of alcoholism. J Ind Med Ass (1970) 55, 29.

6 de Mattos H. Relationship between alcoholism and the digestive system. Hospital (1968) 74, 281.

7 Channabasavanna SM, Kaliaperumal VG and Mathew G. Metronidazole in the treatment of alcoholism: a controlled trial. Ind J
   Psychiat (1979) 21, 90.
8 Goodwin DW. Metronidazole in the treatment of alcoholism. Amer J
   Psychiat (1968) 123, 1276–8.
9 Gelder MG and Edwards G. Metronidazole in the treatment of alcohol
   addiction. A controlled trial. Br J Psychiat (1968) 114, 473–5.
10 Giannini AJ and DeFrance DT. Metronidazole and alcohol—potential
   for combinative abuse. J Toxicol.-Clin Toxicol (1983) 20, 509–15.
11 Edwards DL, Fink PC and Van Dyke PO. Disulfiram-like reaction
   associated with intravenous trimethoprim-sulphamethoxazole and
   metronidazole. Clin Pharm (1986) 5, 999–1000.
12 Plosker GL. Possible interaction between ethanol and vaginally administered metronidazole. Clin Pharm (1987) 6, 189–93.

Alcohol + Milk

Abstract/Summary

*Blood levels of alcohol and its intoxicant effects are reduced
if milk has been drunk.*

Clinical evidence, mechanism, importance and management

10 subjects were given 25 ml alcohol (equivalent to a double
whiskey) after drinking a pint and a half of water or milk
during the previous 90 min. Blood alcohol levels measured
90 min later were reduced about 40% by the presence of the
milk, and about 25% half an hour later. The intoxicant effects
of the alcohol were also obviously reduced.[1] The reasons are
not understood, but a possible reason is that the absorption
of the alcohol by the gut is reduced by the milk. These findings appear to confirm a long and widely-held belief among
drinkers, but whether this interaction can be regarded as advantageous or undesirable is a moot point.

Reference

1 Miller DS, Stirling JL and Yudkin J. Effect of ingestion of milk on concentrations of blood alcohol. Nature (1966) 212, 1051.

Alcohol + Monosulfiram

Abstract/Summary

*Disulfiram-like reactions have been seen in two men who drank
alcohol after using a solution of monosulfiram on the skin for
the treatment of scabies.*

Clinical evidence, mechanism, importance and management

A man who used undiluted *Tetmosol* (a solution of monosulfiram) for three days on the skin all over his body
developed a disulfiram-like reaction (flushing, sweating, skin
swelling, severe tachycardia and nausea) on the third day
after drinking three double whiskeys. The same thing happened on two subsequent evenings after drinking.[1] A

similar reaction has been described in another patient when
he drank after using *Tetmosol* for five days.[2] Monosulfiram
(tetraethylthiuram monosulphide) is closely related to
disulfiram (tetraethylthiuram disulphide) and it seems probable that the pharmacological basis of the reaction is similar
to the disulfiram reaction (see 'Alcohol + Disulfiram').

The manufacturers advise abstention from alcohol before and
for at least 48 h after applying *Tetmosol*, but this may not
always be necessary. The writer of a letter, commenting on
the first case cited, wrote that he had never encountered this
reaction when using a diluted solution of *Tetmosol* on patients
at the Dreadnought Seamen's Hospital in London who
'. . . are not necessarily abstemious,'[3] which suggests that the
reaction is uncommon and unlikely to occur if the solution
is diluted correctly, usually with 2–3 parts of water. This
would reduce the amount absorbed through the skin. Nevertheless patients should be warned that this reaction can occur
sometimes.

References

1 Gold S. A skinful of alcohol. Lancet (1966) ii, 1417.
2 Dantas W. Monosulfiram como causa de sindrome do acetaldeido. Arq
   Cat Med (1980) 9, 29–30.
3 Erskine D. A skinful of alcohol. Lancet (1967) i, 54.

Alcohol + Nitrofurantoin

Abstract/Summary, Clinical evidence, mechanism, import- ance and management

*An extensive literature survey[1] failed to find any experimental
or clinical evidence for an alleged disulfiram-like reaction between alcohol and nitrofurantoin. It is concluded that this 'interaction' is erroneous.*

Reference

1 Rowles B and Worthen DB. Clinical drug information: a case of misin-
   formation. New Eng J Med (1982) 306, 113–4.

Alcohol + Nitroimidazoles

Abstract/Summary

*It is alleged that benznidazole, nimorazole, ornidazole and
tinidazole can cause a disulfiram-like reaction with alcohol.*

Clinical evidence, mechanism, importance and management

It has been claimed that all of the nitroimidazoles (benznidazole, metronidazole, nimorazole, ornidazole, tinidazole) can
cause a disulfiram-like reaction with alcohol (flushing of the
face and neck, palpitations, dizziness, nausea, etc.)[1,2] but so
far I have been unable to find direct evidence confirming

this interaction except with metronidazole (see 'Alcohol + Metronidazole'). Roche, the manufacturers of benznidazole, also say they have no record of this interaction on their drug database.[3] If and when this reaction occurs it is usually more unpleasant and frightening than serious, and requires no treatment.

References

1 Bodino JAJ, Lopez EL. Schistosomiasis drugs. In 'Antimicrobial therapy in infants and children' edited by Koren G, Prober CG, Gold R, published by Marcel Dekker, NY (1988) pp 687–727.
2 Ralph ED. Nitroimidazoles. In 'Antimicrobial therapy in infants and children' edited by Koren G, Prober CG, Gold R, published by Marcel Dekker, NY (1988) pp 729–745.
3 Roche UK. Personal communication (1989).

Alcohol + Paraldehyde

Abstract/Summary

Both alcohol and paraldehyde have CNS depressant effects which can be additive. Their concurrent use in the treatment of acute intoxication has had a fatal outcome.

Clinical evidence, mechanism, importance and management

A report describes eight patients who died suddenly and unexpectedly after treatment for acute intoxication with 30–60 ml paraldehyde (normal dose range 3–30 ml; fatal dose 120 ml or more).[1] Both are CNS depressants and may therefore be expected to have additive effects at any dosage, although an animal study suggested that it may be less than additive.[2]

References

1 Kaye S and Haag HB. Study of death due to combined action of alcohol and paraldehyde in man. Toxicol Appl Pharmacol (1964) 6, 316.
2 Gessner PK and Shakarjian MP. Interactions of paraldehyde with ethanol and chloral hydrate. J Pharmacol Exp Ther (1985) 235, 32–6.

Alcohol + Phenothiazines, Butyrophenones and other psychotropic drugs

Abstract/Summary

The detrimental effects of alcohol on the skills related to driving are made worse by thioridazine and flupenthixol. Any interaction with sulpiride, tiapride or haloperidol seems to be milder. There is evidence that drinking can precipitate the emergence of extrapyramidal side-effects in patients taking neuroleptics.

Clinical evidence

(a) Effect on driving skills

A double-blind study in subjects given 0.5 mg flupenthixol, three times a day for two weeks, showed that when combined with 0.5 mg/kg alcohol their performance of a number of tests (choice reaction, coordination, attention) was impaired to such an extent that driving or handling other potentially dangerous machinery could be hazardous.[1,2] No interaction of any importance was seen with single 0.5 mg doses of haloperidol.[1,2] Subjects given 150 mg sulpiride daily for two weeks demonstrated only a mild interaction with alcohol, whereas when given 30–60 mg thioridazine daily for two weeks some additive effects with alcohol were seen, with a moderately deleterious effect on attention.[2,3] A study in nine alcoholics given 400–600 mg tiapride daily showed that wakefulness was not impaired when combined with alcohol (0.5 mg/kg) and in fact appeared to be improved, but the effect on driving skills was not studied.[7]

(b) Precipitation of extra-pyramidal side-effects

A report[4] describes in detail seven patients who developed acute extrapyramidal side-effects (akathisia, dystonia) while taking trifluoperazine, fluphenazine and chlorpromazine when they drank alcohol. The author stated that these were examples of numerous such alcohol-induced neuroleptic toxicity reactions observed by him over an 18-year period involving phenothiazines and butyrophenones. Elsewhere he describes the emergence of drug-induced parkinsonism in a woman taking perphenazine and amitriptyline when she began to drink.[5] 18 cases of haloperidol-induced extrapyramidal reactions among young drug abusers, in most instances associated with the ingestion of alcohol, have also been described.[6]

Mechanisms

Uncertain. (a) Additive CNS depressant effects are one explanation of this interaction. (b) One suggestion to account for the emergence of the drug side-effects is that alcohol lowers the threshold of resistance to the neurotoxicity of these drugs. In addition is seems possible that alcohol impairs the activity of tyrosine hydroxylase so that the dopamine/acetylcholine balance within the corpus striatum is upset.[5]

Importance and management

The documentation is limited. Patients should be warned that if they drink while taking thioridazine or flupenthixol (probably other related drugs as well) they may become very drowsy, and should not drive or handle other potentially dangerous machinery. The effects of alcohol with haloperidol, sulpiride and tiapride appear to be minimal. The author of the reports describing the emergence of serious neuroleptic side-effects in those who drink, considers that patients should routinely be advised to abstain from alcohol during neuroleptic treatment.

References

1 Linnoila M. Effects of diazepam, chlordiazepoxide, thioridazine, haloperidol, flupenthixol and alcohol on psychomotor skills related to driving. Ann Med Exp Biol Fenn (1973) 51, 125.
2 Linnoila M, Saario I, Olkonieme J, Liljequist R, Himberg JJ and Maki M. Effect of two weeks treatment with chlordiazepoxide or flupenthixol, alone or in combination with alcohol, on psychomotor skills related to driving. Arzneim-Forsch (Drug Res) (1975) 25, 1088.
3 Seppala T, Saario I and Matilla MJ. Two weeks' treatment with chlorpromazine, thioridazine, sulpiride or bromazepam: actions and interactions with alcohol on psychomotor skills related to driving. Mod Probl Pharmacopsych (1976) 11, 85.
4 Lutz EG. Neuroleptic-induced akathisia and dystonia triggered by alcohol. J Amer Med Ass (1977) 236, 2422.
5 Lutz EG. Neuroleptic-induced parkinsonism facilitated by alcohol. J Med Soc NJ (1978) 75, 473–5.
6 Kenyon-David D. Haloperidol intoxication. NZ Med J (1981) 92, 165.
7 Vandel B, Bonim B, Vandel S, Blum D, Rey E and Volmat R. Etude de l'interaction entre le tiapride et l'alcool chez l'homme. Sem Hop Paris (1984) 60, 175–7.

Alcohol + Procarbazine

Abstract/Summary

A flushing reaction has been seen in patients on procarbazine after drinking alcohol.

Clinical evidence, mechanism, importance and management

A report describes five patients taking procarbazine whose faces became very red and hot when they drank wine.[1] Another report states that flushing occurred in three patients on procarbazine after drinking beer.[2] A third report says that two out of 40 patients complained of flushing of the face after taking a small alcoholic drink, and another patient thought that the effects of alcohol were markedly increased.[3] Whether this flushing reaction is related to the alcohol–disulfiram reaction (see 'Alcohol+Disulfiram') is not known. The evidence is very limited, but clearly this reaction is a possibility in patients on procarbazine who drink. It seems to be more embarrassing, possibly frightening, than serious, and if it occurs it is unlikely to require treatment. Patients should be warned.

References

1 Mathe G, Berumen L, Schweisguth O, Brule G, Schneider M, Cattan A, Amiel JL and Schwarzenberg L. Methyl-hydrazine in the treatment of Hodgkin's disease and various forms of haematosarcoma and leukaemia. Lancet (1963) ii, 1077.
2 Dawson WB. Ibenzmethyzin in the management of late Hodgkin's disease. In 'Natulan, Ibenzmethyzin'. Report of the proceedings of a symposium, Downing College, Cambridge, June 1965. Edited by Jelliffe AM and Marks J. John Wright, Bristol (1965) p 31.
3 Todd IDH. Natulan in the management of late Hodgkin's disease, other lymphoreticular neoplasms, and malignant melanoma. Br Med J (1965) 1, 326–7.

Alcohol + Sodium cromoglycate

Abstract/Summary

No adverse interaction occurs between sodium cromoglycate and alcohol.

Clinical evidence, mechanism. importance and management

A double-blind cross over trial on 17 subjects showed that 40 mg sodium cromoglycate had little or no effect on the performance of a number of tests on human perceptual, cognitive and motor skills, whether taken alone or with alcohol (0.75 g/kg). Nor did it affect blood alcohol levels.[1] This is in line with the common experience of patients, and no special precautions seem to be necessary.

Reference

1 Crawford WA, Frank HM, Hensley VR, Hensley WJ, Starmer GA and Teo RCK. The effect of sodium cromoglycate on human performance alone and in combination with ethanol. Med J Aust (1976) 2, 997.

Alcohol + Tetracyclic antidepressants

Abstract/Summary

Mianserin can cause drowsiness and impair the ability to drive or handle other dangerous machinery, particularly during the first few days of treatment. This impairment is increased by alcohol. Pirlindole appears not to interact with alcohol.

Clinical evidence

(a) Mianserin

A double-blind cross-over study in 13 normal subjects given 20–60 mg mianserin daily for eight days, with and without alcohol (1 g/kg), showed that their performance of a number of psychomotor tests (choice reaction, coordination, critical flicker frequency) were impaired by concurrent use. The subjects were aware of feeling drowsy and muzzy, and less able to carry out the tests.[1]

These results confirm the findings of other studies.[2,3,5]

(b) Pirlindole

A study in subjects given pirlindole indicated that it did not affect the performance of a number of psychomotor tests, with or without alcohol.[4]

Mechanism

The CNS depressant effects of mianserin appear to be additive with those of alcohol.

Importance and management

Drowsiness is a frequently reported side-effect of mianserin, particularly during the first few days of treatment. Patients should be warned that driving or handling dangerous machinery will be made more hazardous if they drink. Pirlindole appears not to interact.

References

1 Seppala T, Stromberg C and Bergman I. Effect of zimelidine, mianserin and amitriptyline on psychomotor skills and their interaction with alcohol. A placebo controlled study. Eur J Clin Pharmacol (1984) 27, 181–9.
2 Matilla MJ, Liljequist R and Seppala T. Effects of amitriptyline and mianserin on psychomotor skills and memory in man. Br J clin Pharmac (1978) 5, 53S.
3 Seppala T. Psychomotor skills during acute and two-week treatment with mianserin (Org GB 94) and amitriptyline and their combined effects with alcohol. Ann Clin Res (1977) 9, 66.
4 Ehlers T and Ritter M. Effects of the tetracyclic antidepressant pirlindole on sensorimotor performance and subjective condition in comparison to imipramine and during interaction with alcohol. Neuropsychobiology (1984) 12, 48–54.
5 Stromberg C and Mattila MJ. Acute comparison of clovoxamine and mianserin, alone and in combination with ethanol, on human psychomotor performance. Pharmacol Toxicol (1987) 60, 374–9.

Alcohol + Tolazoline

Abstract/Summary

A disulfiram-like reaction may occur in patients on tolazoline if they drink.

Clinical evidence, mechanism, importance and management

Seven normal subjects were given 500 mg tolazoline daily for four days. Within 15 and 90 min of drinking 90 ml port wine (18.2% alcohol) six of the seven experienced tingling over the head, and four developed warmth and fullness of the head. The reasons are not understood, but this reaction is not unlike a mild disulfiram reaction and may possibly have a similar mechanism (see 'Alcohol+Disulfiram'). Patients given tolazoline should be warned about this reaction if they drink and advised to limit their consumption. Reactions of this kind with drugs other than disulfiram are usually more frightening than serious and treatment is rarely needed.

Reference

1 Boyd EM. A search for drugs with disulfiram-like activity. QJ Stud Alcohol (1960) 21, 23–5.

Alcohol + Trazodone

Abstract/Summary

Trazodone makes driving or handling other dangerous machinery more hazardous, and further impairment may occur with alcohol.

Clinical evidence, mechanism, importance and management

In a study in six normal subjects which compared the effects of amitriptyline (50 mg) and trazodone (100 mg) it was found that both drugs impaired the performance of a number of psychomotor tests, causing drowsiness and reducing 'clear-headedness' to approximately the same extent. Only manual dexterity was further impaired when the subjects on trazodone were given sufficient alcohol to give blood levels of about 40 mg%.[1] Patients given trazodone should be warned that their ability to drive, handle dangerous machinery or to do other tasks needing complex psychomotor skills may be impaired.

Reference

1 Warrington SJ, Ankier SI and Turner P. Evaluation of possible interactions between ethanol and trazodone or amitriptyline. Neuropschobiology (1986) 15 (Suppl 1) 31–7.

Alcohol + Trichloroethylene

Abstract/Summary

A flushing skin reaction similar to a mild disulfiram reaction can occur in those exposed to trichloroethylene when they drink alcohol.

Clinical evidence

An engineer from a factory where trichloroethylene was being used as a degreasing agent, developed facial flushing, a sensation of increased pressure in the head, lacrymation, tachypnoea and blurred vision within 12 min of drinking 3 oz bourbon whiskey. The reaction did not develop when he was no longer exposed to the trichloroethylene. Other workers in the same plant reported the same experience.[1]

Vivid red blotches in a symmetrical pattern on the face, neck, shoulders and back were seen in other workers exposed for a few hours each day to 20–220 ppm trichloroethylene when they drank only half a pint (300 ml) of beer,[3] and it has also been reported elsewhere.[2] It has been described as the 'degreasers flush'. There is also some evidence that long-term exposure may possibly reduce mental capacity.[4]

Mechanism

Uncertain. One suggested mechanism is a disulfiram-like inhibition of acetaldehyde metabolism by trichloroethylene (see 'Alcohol+Disulfiram').

Importance and management

An established interaction. It would seem to be more unpleasant and socially disagreeable than serious, and normally requires no treatment. The whole question of whether long-term exposure to trichloroethylene is desirable does not seem to have been answered.

References

1 Pardys S and Brotman M. Trichloroethylene and alcohol: a straight flush. J Amer Med Ass (1974) 229, 521.
2 Smith GF. Trichloroethylene. A review. Brit J Industr Med (1966) 23, 249.
3 Stewart RD, Hake CL and Peterson JE. 'Degreasers Flush', dermal response to trichloroethylene and ethanol. Arch Environm Hlth (1974) 29, 1.
4 Windemuller FJB and Ettema JH. Effects of combined exposure to trichloroethylene and alcohol on mental capacity. Int Arch Occup Environ Hlth (1978) 41, 77.

Alcohol + Tricyclic antidepressants

Abstract/Summary

The ability to drive, to handle dangerous machinery or to do other tasks requiring complex psychomotor skills may be impaired by amitriptyline and to a lesser extent by doxepin, particularly during the first few days of treatment. This impairment is increased by alcohol. Nortriptyline, clomipramine, desipramine and amoxapine appear to interact with alcohol only minimally. Information about other tricyclic antidepressants appears to be lacking.

Clinical evidence

(a) Alcohol + amitriptyline

A study in 21 normal subjects showed that blood alcohol levels of about 80 mg% impaired the performance of three motor skills tests related to driving, and after additionally taking 0.8 mg/kg amitriptyline the performance was even further impaired.[1]

Similar results have been very clearly demonstrated in considerable numbers of subjects using a variety of psychomotor skill tests,[1-7] the interaction being most marked during the first few days of treatment, but tending to wane as treatment continued.[5] There is also some limited evidence from animal studies that amitriptyline may possibly enhance the fatty changes induced in the liver by alcohol,[8] but this still needs confirmation from human studies. Unexplained blackouts lasting a few hours have also been described in three women after drinking only modest amounts;[9] they had been taking amitriptyline or imipramine for only a month.

(b) Alcohol + doxepin

A double-blind cross-over trial on 21 subjects given various combinations of alcohol and either doxepin or a placebo showed that with blood-alcohol levels of 40–50 mg% choice reaction test times were prolonged and the number of mistakes increased. Coordination was obviously impaired after seven days treatment with doxepin, but not after 14 days.[3]

In an earlier study doxepin appeared to cancel out the deleterious effects of alcohol on the performance of a simulated driving test.[10]

(c) Alcohol + amoxapine, clomipramine, desipramine, nortriptyline

Studies in subjects with blood-alcohol levels of 40–50 mg% showed that clomipramine and nortriptyline had only slight or no effects on various choice reaction, coordination, memory and learning tests.[3,11,12] The amoxapine–alcohol interaction was found to be slight,[14] but two patients have been described who experienced reversible extrapyramidal symptoms (parkinsonism, akathisia) while taking amoxapine, apparently caused by drinking.[16] Tests in subjects given 100 mg desipramine indicated that no significant interaction occurred with alcohol.[15]

Mechanisms

Part of the explanation is that both alcohol and some of the tricyclics, particularly amitriptyline, cause drowsiness and other CNS depressant effects which can be additive with the effects of alcohol.[6] The sedative effects in descending order are said in one review to be as follows: amitriptyline, doxepin, imipramine, nortriptyline, desipramine, protriptyline.[13] In addition, alcohol causes marked increases (+100–200%) in the plasma concentrations of amitriptyline, probably by inhibiting its metabolism during its first pass through the liver.[4]

Importance and management

The amitriptyline–alcohol interaction is very well documented. Patients should be warned that driving or handling dangerous machinery may be made more hazardous if they drink, particularly during the first few days, but the effects of the interaction diminish during prolonged treatment. The alcohol–doxepin interaction is less well documented and the information is conflicting, but to be on the safe side a similar warning should be given. Nortriptyline, clomipramine, desipramine and amoxapine appear to interact only minimally with alcohol. Direct information about other tricyclics seems to be lacking, but there appear to be no particular reasons for avoiding concurrent use. However prescribers may feel it appropriate to offer some precautionary advice because during the first 1–2 weeks of treatment many tricyclics (without alcohol) may temporarily impair the skills related to driving.[14]

References

1 Landauer AA, Milner G and Patman J. Alcohol and amitriptyline effects on skills related to driving behaviour. Science (1969) 163, 1467.
2 Seppala T. Psychomotor skills during acute and two-week treatment with mianserin (ORG GB 94) and amitriptyline and their combined effects with alcohol. Ann Clin Res (1977) 9, 66.
3 Seppala T, Linnoila M, Elonen E, Matilla MJ and Maki M. Effect of tricyclic antidepressants and alcohol on psychomotor skills related to driving. Clin Pharmacol Ther (1975) 17, 515.

4 Dorian P, Sellers EM, Reed KL, Warsh JJ, Hamilton C, Kaplan HL and Fan T. Amitriptyline and ethanol: pharmacokinetic and pharmacodynamic interaction. Eur J Clin Pharmacol (1983) 25, 325–331.

5 Seppala T, Stromberg C and Bergman I. Effects of zimelidine, mianserin and amitriptyline on psychomotor skills and their interaction with ethanol. A placebo controlled cross-over study. Eur J Clin Pharmacol (1984) 27, 181–9.

6 Scott DB, Fagan D and Tiplady B. Effects of amitriptyline and zimelidine in combination with alcohol. Psychopharmacology (1982) 76, 209–11.

7 Matilla M, Liljequist R and Seppala T. Effects of amitriptyline and mianserin on psychomotor skills and memory in man. Br J Clin Pharmacol (1978) 5, 53S.

8 Milner G and Kakulas K. The potentiation by amitriptyline of liver changes induced by ethanol in mice. Pathology (1969) 1, 113.

9 Hudson CJ. Tricyclic antidepressants and alcoholic blackouts. J Nerv Ment Dis (1981) 169, 381.

10 Milner G and Landauer AA. The effects of doxepin, alone and together with alcohol in relation to driving safety. Med J Aust (1978) 1, 837.

11 Hughes FW and Forney RB. Delayed audiofeedback (DAF) for induction of anxiety. Effect of nortriptyline, ethanol or nortriptyline-ethanol combinations on performance with DAF. J Amer Med Ass (1963) 185, 556.

12 Liljequist R, Linnoila M and Matilla M. Effect of two weeks' treatment with chlorimipramine and nortriptyline, alone or in combination with alcohol on learning and memory. Psychopharmacology (1974) 39, 181.

13 Marco LA and Randels RM. Drug interactions in alcoholic patients. Hillside J Clin Psychiatry (1981) 3, 27–44.

14 Linnoila M and Seppala T. Antidepressants and driving. Accid Anal and Prev (1985) 17, 297–301.

15 Linnoila M, Johnson J, Dubyoski K, Buchsbaum MS, Schneinin M and Kilts C. Effects of antidepressants on skilled performance. Br J clin Pharmac (1984) 18, 109–120S.

16 Shen WW. Alcohol, amoxapine and akathisia. Biol Psychiatry (1984) 19, 929–30.

Alcohol + Viqualine (Ivoqualine)

Abstract/Summary

No adverse interaction occurs if alcohol and viqualine are taken together.

Clinical evidence, mechanism, importance and management

A controlled study in 16 normal subjects found that alcohol (serum levels 17–22 mmol/l) had no effect on the steady-state serum levels of ivoqualine (75 mg twice daily for three days), nor was there any evidence of a disulfiram-like reaction. The deleterious effects of alcohol on a number of skills (word recall, manual tracking, body sway) and self-ratings of intoxication, sedation and performance were not altered by the ivoqualine.[1] On the basis of this study there would seem to be no good reason for those taking ivoqualine to avoid alcoholic drinks.

Reference

1 Sullivan JT, Naranjo CA, Shaw CA, Kaplan HL, Kadlec KE and Sellers EM. Kinetic and dynamic interactions of oral viqualine and ethanol in man. Eur J Clin Pharmacol (1989) 36, 93–6.

Alcohol + Xylene

Abstract/Summary

Some individuals exposed to xylene vapour who subsequently drink alcohol may experience dizziness and nausea. A flushing skin reaction has also been seen.

Clinical evidence, mechanism, importance and management

Studies[1] in volunteers exposed to m-xylene vapour at concentrations of 140 or 250 ppm for 4 h who were then given alcohol to drink (0.8 g/kg) showed that about 10% experienced dizziness and nausea. One subject exposed to 300 ppm developed a conspicuous dermal flush on his face, neck, chest and back. He also showed some erythema on alcohol alone. The reasons for these reactions are not understood.

Reference

1 Riilimaki V, Laine A, Savolainene K and Sippel H. Acute solvent-ethanol interactions with special reference to xylene. Scand j work environ hlth (1982) 8, 77–9.

3

ANALGESIC AND NON-STEROIDAL ANTI-INFLAMMATORY DRUG INTERACTIONS

The drugs dealt with in this chapter are listed in Table 3.1 with their proprietary names. In addition the list also contains other analgesic and non-steroidal anti-inflammatory drugs which act as interacting agents and are dealt with in other chapters. The Index should be consulted for the full listing.

Table 3.1 Analgesics and Non-steroidal Anti-inflammatory Drugs (NSAID'S)

Non-proprietary names	Proprietary names
Analgesics (Non-narcotic)	
Alclofenac	*Allopydin, Argun, Darkeyfenac, Desiflam, Epinal, Mervan, Prinalgin, Vanadian, Zumaril*
Azapropazone	*Cinnamin, Pentosol, Prolixan, Rheumox, Tolyprin*
Clometacin	*Duperan*
Diclofenac	*Aflamin, Blesin, Delphimix, Dichronic, Diclo Attritin,-Phlogont,-Spondyril, Dicloreum, Dolobasan, Dolotren, Duravolten, Effekton, Flogofenac, Forgenac, Inflamac, Monoflam, Myogit, Neriodin, Novapirina, Panamor, Rheumavincin, Rhumalgan, Seecoren, Sofarin, Toryxil, Tsudohmin, Voltarol, Voltarene,*
Diflunisal	*Adomal, Algobid, Antadar, Artrodol, Diflonid, Difludol, Diflunil, Diflusan, Dolisal, Dolobid, Dolobis, Donobid, Dopanone, Dorbid, Flulisin, Fluniget, Fluodonil, Flustar, Ilacen, Reuflos, Unisal*
Fenoprofen	*Fenopron, Fepron, Nalfon, Nalgesic, Progesic*
Feprazone	*Analud, Brotazona, Cocresol, Danfenona, Grisona, Impremial, Methrazone, Naloven, Nessazona, Nilatin, Prenakes, Prenazon, Rangozona, Represil, Tabien,*
Floctafenine	*Idalon, Idarac,*
Flufenamic acid	*Alfenamin, Ansatin, Arlef, Meralen, Sastridex, Surika*
Flurbiprofen	*Ansaid, Cebutid, Flugalin, Flurofen, Froben, Ocufen*
Glafenine	*Exidol, Glifan, Osodent, Privadol*
Ibuprofen	*Advul, Algofen, Anco, Artrene, Brufen, Cuprofen, Emodin, Fenbid, Ibucasen, Inflam, Lidifen, Liptan, Migrafen, Motrin, Neobrufen, Novaprin, Novoprofen, Nurofen, Pacifene, Reclofen, Suspren, Uniprofen, Vesicum (incomplete list).*
Indobufen	*Ibustrin*
Indomethacin	*Agilex, Amuno, Arthrexin, Atracin, Boutycin, Confortid, Flexin, Indocid, Imbrilon, Inacid, Indomet, Indotard, Infrocin, Metindol, Sadeorum, Tannex, Vonum*
Isoxicam	*Maxicam, Pacyl, Vectren*
Kebuzone	*Chebutan, Chepirol, Chetopir, Gammachetone, Neo-panagyl, Neufenil*
Ketoprofen	*Alrheumat, Anaus, Arcental, Capisten, Fastum, Flexen, Ketalgin, Ketoartril, Ketoprosil, Meprofen, Orudis, Oruvail, Profenid, Reuprofen, Salient, Tafirol, Wasserprofen*
Meclofenamic acid	*Meclomen, Movens*
Mefenamic acid	*Bafameritin-m, Bonabol, Citronamic, Coslan, Lysalgo, Mefalgic, Mefedolo, Parkemed, Ponalar, Ponstan, Ponstil, Pontal*

Table 3.1 *(continued)*

Non-proprietary names	Proprietary names
Mofebutazone	*Chemiartrol, Monazone, Monbutina, Monoprine, Rheumatox*
Nabumetone	*Relifex, Relifen*
Naproxen	*Alganil, Anaprox, Denaxpren, Floginax, Laraflex, Madaprox, Naprium, Naprorex, Naprosyn, Naproval, Piproxen, Proxen, Proxine, Rofanten, Xenar*
Nefopam	*Acupan, Dolitrone, Lenipan, Nefadol, Nefam, Oxadol, Sinalgico*
Oxametacin	*Dinulcid, Flogar, Restid*
Oxyphenbutazone	*Artroflog, Artzone, Butofen, Flogitolo, Oxibutol, Piraflogin, Rheumapax, Tandacote, Tandearil, Tanderil, Validil*
Paracetamol (acetaminophen)	
Penicillamine	*Artamin, Atamir, Cuprenil, Cuprimine, Depamine, Depen, Distamine, Mercatyl, Pendramine, Rhumantin, Sufortan, Trolovol, Vistamin*
Phenazone (antipyrine)	
Phenylbutazone	*Algoverine, Artrizin, Butacote, Butazolidin, Butalan, Butazina, Butoz, Ditrone, Denilbutina, Intra-butazone, Megazone, Panazone, Rheumaphen, Sinobutina,*
Piroxicam	*Antiflog, Baxo, Dexicam, Doblexan, Feldene, Flogobene, Improntal, Larapram, Polipirox, Remoxicam, Reumagil, Roxene, Roxiden, Vitaxicam, Zamcam*
Salicylates	
Aspirin	
Aloxiprin	*Lyman tabs, Palaprin, Paloxin, Rumatral, Supperpyrin, Tiatral*
Benorylate	*Benoral, Benorile, Benortan, Benotamol, Bentum, Doline, Duvium, Salipran, Vetedol, Winolate*
Choline salicylate	
Sodium salicylate	
Sulindac	*Aflodac, Algocetil, Arthrocine, Citireuma, Clinoril, Clisundac, Lyndac, Reumofil, Sudac, Sulartrene, Sulen, Sulic, Sulindal, Sulindol,*
Tiaprofenoic acid	*Surgam(amyl), Surgamic, Tioprofen*
Tolfenamic acid	*Clotam*
Tolmetin	*Benetazon*
Analgesics (Narcotic and Related)	
Alfentanil	*Alfenta, Rapifen*
Codeine	
(Dextro)propoxyphene	*Abalgin, Algafen, Antalvic, Daraphen, Depronal, Dolene, Dolocap, Dolorphen, Dolotard, Doloxene, Liberen, Novoproxyn, Proxagesic. Also contained in Cosalgesic, Distalgesic, Darvon Co*
Dextromoramide	*Jetrium, Palfium,*
Diamorphine (heroin)	
Dihydrocodeine	*DF118*
Fentanyl	*Fentanest, Leptanal, Sublimaze, Thalamonal*
Hydromorphone	*Dilaudid*
Methadone	*Physeptone, Dolophine, Westalone, L-Polamidon*
Morphine	
Oxymorphone	*Numorphan*
Papaveretum	*Escopon, Omnopon*
Pentazocine	*Fortagesic, Fortral, Sosegon, Talwin, Fortal*
Pethidine (meperidine)	*Demerol,*
Phenoperidine	

Alfentanil + Erythromycin

Abstract/Summary

Some patients may experience prolonged and increased alfentanil effects if they are treated with erythromycin.

Clinical evidence, mechanism, importance and management

A study in six subjects showed that after taking 1 g erythromycin daily for seven days the mean half-life of alfentanil was increased by 56% (from 84 to 131 min) and the clearance was decreased from 3.9 to 2.9 ml/kg/min. Some of the subjects were much more sensitive than others: two showed marked changes; two showed little changes, and the other two showed intermediate effects. The two most sensitive subjects demonstrated considerable changes within a day of taking only 500 mg erythromycin. Inhibition of the metabolism of the alfentanil by the erythromycin seems to be the mechanism of this interaction.[1]

Direct evidence appears to be limited to this report but it indicates that the outcome of concurrent use is unpredictable. Some patients may experience prolonged alfentanil effects and respiratory depression. The authors of the report suggest that alfentanil should be given in reduced amounts or avoided in patients who have recently had erythromycin.

Reference

1 Bartkowski RR, Goldberg ME, Larijani GE and Boerner T. Inhibition of alfentanil metabolism by erythromycin. Clin Pharmacol Ther (1989) 46, 99–102.

Antirheumatic agents + Mazindol

Abstract/Summary

Mazindol is reported not to interact adversely with indomethacin, salicylates and other analgesics and anti-inflammatory drugs.

Clinical evidence, mechanism, importance and management

A double-blind study of mazindol and a placebo was carried out on 26 obese arthritics, 15 of whom were on salicylates, 11 on indomethacin and one on dextropropoxyphene with paracetamol. Additional drugs used were ibuprofen (four patients), phenylbutazone (one patient), dextropropoxyphene (seven patients), paracetamol (three patients) and prednisone (nine patients). No adverse interactions were seen.[1]

Reference

1 Thorpe PC, Isaac PF and Rodgers JA. A controlled trial of mazindol (Sanjorex, Teronac) in the management of obese rheumatic patients. Curr Ther Res (1975) 17, 149.

Aspirin and Salicylates + Antacids

Abstract/Summary

The serum salicylate concentrations of patients taking large doses of aspirin as an anti-inflammatory agent can be reduced to sub-therapeutic levels by the concurrent use of some antacids.

Clinical evidence

A child with rheumatic fever taking 0.6 g aspirin five times daily with 30 ml *Maalox* (aluminium and magnesium hydroxide suspension) had a serum salicylate concentration of between 8.2 and 11.8 mg/100 ml. When the *Maalox* was withdrawn, the urinary pH fell from a range of 7–8 to 5.0–6.4, whereupon the serum salicylate level rose to about 38 mg/100 ml, calling for a reduction in dosage.[1] An associated study in 13 normal subjects taking 4 g aspirin daily for a week showed that the concurrent use of 4 g sodium bicarbonate daily reduced serum salicylate levels from 27 to 15 mg/100 ml. This reflected a rise in the urinary pH from a range of 5.6–6.1 to 6.2–6.9.[1]

Similar changes have been reported in other studies.[3,5,6]

Mechanism

Aspirin and other salicylates are acidic compounds which are excreted by the kidney tubules and are ionized in solution. In alkaline solution, much of the drug exists in the ionized form which is not readily reabsorbed and therefore is lost in the urine. If the urine is made more acidic, much more of the drug exists in the un-ionized form which is readily reabsorbed so that less is lost in the urine and the drug is retained in the body. Magnesium oxide also strongly adsorbs aspirin and sodium salicylate.[4]

Importance and management

A well-established and clinically important interaction for those on chronic treatment with large doses of salicylates because the serum salicylate may be reduced to sub-therapeutic levels. This interaction can occur with both 'systemic' antacids (e.g. sodium bicarbonate) as well as some 'non-systemic' antacids (e.g. magnesium-aluminium hydroxides), although some evidence suggests that some aluminium-containing antacids (*Amphojel*—aluminium hydroxide, and *Robalate*—aluminium aminoacetate) may have minimal effects on urinary pH.[1,2] Care should be taken to monitor serum salicylate levels if any antacid is started or stopped in patients where the control of salicylate levels is critical. No important interaction would be expected in those taking occasional doses of aspirin for analgesia.

References

1 Levy C. Interactions of salicylates with antacids. Clinical implications with respect to gastrointestinal bleeding and anti-inflammatory activity. Frontiers of Internal Medicine 1974, 12th Int Congr Intern Med, Tel Aviv, 1974, p 404, Karger, Basel (1975).

2 Muirden KR and Barraclough DRE. Drug interaction in the management of rheumatoid arthritis. Aust NZ J Med (1976) 6 (Suppl 1) 14.

3 Levy G, Lampman T, Kamath BL and Garrettson LK. Decreased serum salicylate concentration in children with rheumatic fever treated with antacid. N Engl J Med (1975) 293, 323.

4 Naggar VF, Khalil SA and Daabis NA. The in-vitro adsorption of some anti-rheumatics on antacids. Pharmazie (1976) 31, 461.

5 Hansten PD and Hayton WL. Effect of antacid and ascorbic acid on serum salicylate concentration. J Clin Pharmacol (1980) 24, 326.

6 Shastri RA. Effect of antacids on salicylate kinetics. Int J Clin Pharmacol ther Tox (1985) 23, 480–4.

Aspirin and Salicylates + Carbonic anhydrase inhibitors

Abstract/Summary

Severe and even life-threatening salicylate intoxication can occur in those on high dose salicylate treatment concurrently treated with carbonic anhydrase inhibitors (acetazolamide, dichlorphenamide) unless the salicylate dosage is reduced appropriately.

Clinical evidence

A boy of eight with chronic juvenile arthritis, well controlled on prednisolone, indomethacin and aloxiprin, was admitted to hospital with drowsiness, vomiting and hyperventilation (diagnosed as metabolic acidosis) within a month of increasing the aloxiprin dosage from 3 to 3.5 g daily and adding 75 mg dichlorphenamide daily for glaucoma.[1]

Other cases of salicylate toxicity (metabolic acidosis) occurred in a 22-year-old woman on salsalate when additionally given 1000 mg acetazolamide daily,[1] and in two elderly women on large doses of aspirin when they were given acetazolamide or dichlorphenamide.[2] Coma developed in an 85-year-old taking 3.9 g aspirin daily when the dosage of acetazolamide was increased from 0.5 to 1 g,[3] and toxicity in another very old man given both drugs.[5] Salicylate poisoning developed in a man on dichlorphenamide within 10 days of starting to take 3.9 g aspirin daily.[4]

Mechanism

One suggestion is that carbonic anhydrase inhibitors (acetazolamide, dichlorphenamide) lower the plasma pH so that more of the salicylate exists in the non-ionized (lipid-soluble) form which can enter the CNS and other tissues more easily, leading to salicylate intoxication.[2] Another idea is that it is due to changes in plasma protein binding and in the excretion of the carbonic anhydrase inhibitor by the kidney.[5] Animal studies confirm that carbonic anhydrase inhibitors increase the lethality of aspirin.

Importance and management

There are few clinical cases on record, but the interaction is established (well confirmed by animal studies) and potentially serious. Carbonic anhydrase inhibitors should probably be avoided in those on high dose salicylate treatment. If they are used, since the interaction may develop slowly, the patient should be monitored for any evidence of toxicity (confusion, lethargy, hyperventilation, tinnitus) and the salicylate dosage reduced accordingly.[2] In this context other non-steroidal anti-inflammatory drugs may be safer. Naproxen proved to be a satisfactory substitute in one case.[1]

References

1 Cowan RA, Hartnell GG, Lowdell CP, McLean BI and Leak AM. Metabolic acidosis induced by carbonic anhydrase inhibitors and salicylates in patients with normal renal function. Brit Med J (1984) 289, 347–8.

2 Anderson CJ, Kaufman PL and Sturm RJ. Toxicity of combined therapy with carbonic anhydrase inhibitors and aspirin. Am J Ophthalmol (1978) 86, 516–19.

3 Chapron DJ, Brandt JL, Sweeny KR and Olesen-Zammett L. Interaction between acetazolamide and aspirin—A possible unrecognized cause of drug-induced coma. J Am Geriat Soc (1984) 32, S18.

4 Hurwitz GA, Wingfield W, Cowart TD and Jollow DJ. Toxic interaction between salicylates and a carbonic anhydrase inhibitor: the role of cerebral edema. Vet Hum Toxicol (1980) 22 (Suppl) 42–4.

5 Sweeney KR, Chapron DJ, Brandt JL, Gomolin IH, Feig PU and Kramer PA. Toxic interaction between acetazolamide and salicylate: case reports and a pharmacokinetic explanation. Clin Pharmacol Ther (1986) 40, 518–24.

Aspirin and Salicylates + Cimetidine or Ranitidine

Abstract/Summary

Cimetidine causes a slight increase in serum salicylate levels if taken with aspirin, but this is probably of little or no clinical importance. Ranitidine does not interact.

Clinical evidence, mechanism, importance and management

A study with six subjects given 1200 mg aspirin 1 h after 300 mg cimetidine showed that a modest increase occurred in the serum salicylate levels of three of them.[1] In another study in 13 patients with rheumatoid arthritis, given enteric-coated aspirin, it was found that after taking 1200 mg cimetidine daily for seven days the total amount of aspirin absorbed was unaltered, but serum levels were slightly raised (from 161 to 180 μg/ml).[2] Six normal subjects showed little change in the pharmacokinetics of a single 1 g dose of aspirin after being given 150 mg ranitidine twice daily for a week.[3]

There seems to be no evidence suggesting that concurrent use should be avoided.

References

1 Khoury W, Geraci K, Askari A and Johnson M. The effect of cimetidine on aspirin absorption. Gastroenterology (1979) 76, 1169.

2 Willoughby JS, Paton TW, Walker SE and Little AH. The effect of cimetidine on enteric-coated ASA disposition. Clin Pharmacol Ther (1983) 33, 268.

3 Corrocher R, Bambara LM, Caramaschi P, Testi R, Girelli M, Pellegatti M and Lomeo A. Effect of ranitidine on the absorption of aspirin. Digestion (1987) 37, 178–83.

Aspirin and Salicylates + Corticosteroids

Abstract/Summary

Concurrent use is very common but the incidence of gastro-intestinal bleeding and ulceration may be increased. Serum salicylate levels are reduced by corticosteroids and can rise, possibly to toxic concentrations, if the corticosteroid is withdrawn without reducing the salicylate dosage.

Clinical evidence

A 4-year-old boy chronically treated with at least 20 mg prednisone daily was additionally given 3.6 g choline salicylate daily, the prednisone gradually being tapered off to 2 mg daily over a three-month period. Severe salicylate intoxication developed and, in a retrospective investigation of the cause using frozen serum samples drawn for other purposes, it was found that the serum salicylate levels had climbed from about 10 to 90 mg% during the withdrawal of the prednisone.[1] Later studies in three other patients on choline salicylate or aspirin and either prednisone or another unnamed corticosteroid, demonstrated similar but less spectacular rises (about threefold) during corticosteroid withdrawal.[1]

A serum salicylate rise of similar proportions has been described in a patient on aloxiprin when prednisolone was withdrawn.[2] Other studies in considerable numbers of both adults and children show that prednisone, methylprednisolone, betamethasone and ACTH reduce serum salicylate levels.[4,5,8] Another study in patients also showed that intra-articular doses of steroids (dexamethasone, methylprednisolone, triamcinolone) reduced serum salicylate levels when given as enteric-coated aspirin.[6]

Mechanism

Uncertain. One idea is that the presence of the corticosteroid increases the glomerular filtration rate resulting in an increase in the clearance of the salicylate. When the corticosteroid is withdrawn, the clearance returns to normal and the salicylate accumulates. Another suggestion is that the corticosteroids increase the metabolism of the salicylate.[4] Studies in mice have shown that cortisone protects them from the development of salicylism.[3]

Importance and management

A well-established interaction. Concurrent use is very common but patients should be monitored to ensure that salicylate levels remain adequate when corticosteroids are added[5] and do not become excessive if they are withdrawn. It should also be remembered that concurrent use may increase the incidence of gastrointestinal bleeding[7] and ulceration.

References

1 Klinenberg JR and Miller F. Effect of corticosteroids on blood salicylate concentration. J Amer Med Ass (1965) 194, 601.

2 Muirden KD and Barraclough DRE. Drug interactions in the management of rheumatoid arthritis. Aust NZ J Med (1976) 6 (Suppl 1) 14.

3 Montuori E. Accion de la cortisone sobre le toxicidad del salicilato di sodio. Rev Soc Argent Biol (1954) 30, 44.

4 Graham GG, Champion GD, Day RO and Paull PD. Patterns of plasma concentrations and urinary excretion of salicylate in rheumatoid arthritis. Clin Pharmacol Ther (1977) 22, 410–20.

5 Bardare M, Cislaghi GU, Mandelli M and Sereni F. Value of monitoring plasma salicylate levels in treating juvenile rheumatoid arthritis. Arch Dis Child (1978) 53, 381–5.

6 Edelman J, Potter JM and Hackett LP. The effect of intra-articular steroids on plasma salicylate concentrations. Br J clin Pharmac (1986) 21, 301–7.

7 Carson JL, Strom BL, Schinnar R, Sim E, Maislin G and Morse ML. Do corticosteroids really cause upper GI bleeding? Clin Res (1987) 35, 340A.

8 Koren G, Roifman C, Gelfand E, Lavi S, Suria D and Stein L. Corticosteroids-salicylate interaction in a case of juvenile rheumatoid arthritis. Ther Drug Monit (1987) 9, 177–9.

Aspirin and Salicylates + Food

Abstract/Summary

Avoid food if rapid analgesia is needed because it delays the absorption of aspirin.

Clinical evidence, mechanism, importance and management

A study in 25 subjects given 650 mg aspirin in five different aspirin preparations showed that food roughly halved their serum salicylate levels when measured 10 and 20 min later, compared with those seen when the same dose was taken while fasting.[1] Similar results were found in another study in subjects given 1500 mg calcium aspirin.[2] In yet another study on eight subjects who were given 900 mg effervescent aspirin, their serum salicylate levels were roughly halved by food at 15 min, but were almost the same after an hour.[3] A possible reason for the reduced absorption is that the aspirin becomes adsorbed onto the food. Food also delays gastric emptying. So if rapid analgesia is needed, aspirin should be taken without food.

References

1 Wood JH. Effect of food on aspirin absorption. Lancet (1967) ii, 212.

2 Spiers ASD and Malone HF. Effect of food on aspirin absorption. Lancet (1967) i, 440.

3 Volans GN. Effects of food and exercise on the absorption of effervescent aspirin. Br J clin Pharmac (1974) 1, 137–41.

Aspirin and Salicylates + Levamisole

Abstract/Summary

A rise in serum salicylate levels in a patient on aspirin when given levamisole was not confirmed in subsequent controlled studies.

Clinical evidence, mechanism, importance and management

A preliminary report of a patient who showed an increase in serum salicylate levels when levamisole was given with aspirin[1] prompted a study of this possible interaction. Nine normal subjects were given 3.9 g of sustained-release aspirin daily in two divided doses over a period of three weeks. During this period they were also given 50 mg levamisole three times a day for a week, each subject acting as his own control. No significant changes in serum salicylate levels were found.[2]

References

1 Laidlaw DA. Rheumatoid arthritis improved by treatment with levamisole and L-histidine. Med J Aust (1976) 2, 382.
2 Rumble RH, Brooks PM and Roberts MS. Interaction between levamisole and aspirin. Br J clin Pharmac (1979) 7, 631.

Aspirin and Salicylates + Misoprostol

Abstract/Summary

Aspirin and misoprostol appear not to interact.

Clinical evidence, mechanism, importance and management

18 normal subjects were given 200 μg misoprostol or 975 mg aspirin or both drugs together. The pharmacokinetics of neither was significantly changed by concurrent use.

Reference

1 Karim A, Rozek LF and Leese PT. Absorption of misoprostol (Cytotec), an antiulcer prostaglandin, or aspirin is not affected when given concomitantly to healthy human subjects. Gastroenterology (1987) 92, 1742.

Aspirin and Salicylates + Phenylbutazone

Abstract/Summary

Phenylbutazone reduces the uricosuric effects of aspirin.

Clinical evidence

The observation that several patients given both drugs developed elevated serum urate levels, prompted a study on four patients without gout. This showed that 2 g aspirin daily had little effect on the excretion of uric acid in the urine, but marked uricosuria occurred with 5 g daily. When phenylbutazone was additionally given (200, 400 and then 600 mg daily over three days) the uricosuria was abolished. Serum uric acid levels rose from an average of 4 to 6 mg%. The inter-

action was confirmed in a patient with tophaceous gout. Retention of uric acid also occurred if the phenylbutazone was given first.[1]

Mechanism

Not understood. It seems likely that some interference occurs within the kidney tubules.

Importance and management

An established but sparsely documented interaction. If serum urate measurements are taken for diagnostic purposes, full account should be taken of this interaction. The potential problems arising from this interaction should also be recognized in patients given both drugs.

Reference

1 Oyer JH, Wagner SL and Schmid FR. Suppression of salicylate-induced uricosuria by phenylbutazone. Am J Med Sci (1966) 225, 40–5.

Aspirin and Salicylates + Probenecid

Abstract/Summary

The uricosuric effects of aspirin or other salicylates and probenecid are not additive as might be expected but are mutually antagonistic.

Clinical evidence

A study showed that the urinary uric acid excretion in mg/average 24 h was found to be 673 mg with a single 3 g daily dose of probenecid, 909 mg with a 6 g daily dose of sodium salicylate, but only 114 mg when both drugs were used concurrently.[1]

Similar antagonism has been seen in other studies in patients given 2.6–5.2 g aspirin daily.[2-4] No antagonism is seen until serum salicylate levels of 5–10 mg/100 ml are reached.[4]

Mechanism

Not understood. The interference probably occurs at the site of renal tubular secretion, but it also seems that both drugs can occupy the same site on plasma albumins.

Importance and management

A well-established and clinically important interaction. Regular dosing with substantial amounts of salicylates should be avoided if this antagonism is to be avoided, but small occasional analgesic doses do not matter. Serum salicylate levels of 5–10 mg/100 ml are necessary before this interaction occurs.

References

1 Seegmiller JE and Grayzel AI. Use of the newer uricosuric agents in the management of gout. J Amer Med Ass (1960) 173, 1076.
2 Pascale LR, Dubin A and Hoffman WS. Therapeutic value of probenecid (Benemid) in gout. J Amer Med Ass (1952) 149, 1188.
3 Gutman AB and Yu TF. Benemid (p-di-n-propylsulfamyl-benzoic acid) as uricosuric agent in chronic gout arthritis. Trans Ass Amer Phys (1951) 64, 279.
4 Pascale LR, Dubin A, Bronsky D and Hoffman WS. Inhibition of the uricosuric action of Benemid by salicylate. J Lab Clin Med (1955) 45, 771–7.

Aspirin and Salicylates + Sulphinpyrazone

Abstract/Summary

The uricosuric effects of the salicylates and sulphinpyrazone are not additive as might be expected but are mutually antagonistic.

Clinical evidence

6 g sodium salicylate with 600 mg sulphinpyrazone daily caused a urinary uric acid excretion in a patient of only 30 mg/average 24 h, whereas when each drug was used by itself in the same doses the excretion was 281 and 527 mg/av 24 h respectively.[1] A later study on five gouty men infused with sulphinpyrazone (300 mg to prime followed by 10 mg/min) for about an hour showed that the additional infusion with sodium salicylate (3 g to prime followed by 10–20 mg/min) virtually abolished the uricosuria. When the drugs were given in the reverse order to three other patients the same result was seen.[2]

The uricosuria caused by 400 mg sulphinpyrazone was shown in another study to be completely abolished by 3.5 g aspirin.[3]

Mechanism

Not fully understood. Sulphinpyrazone competes successfully with salicylate for excretion by the kidney tubules so that salicylate excretion is reduced, but the salicylate blocks the inhibitory effect of sulphinpyrazone on the tubular reabsorption of uric acid so that the uric acid accumulates within the body.[2]

Importance and management

An established and clinically important interaction. Concurrent use for uricosuria should be avoided. Doses of aspirin as low as 700 mg can cause an appreciable fall in uric acid excretion[3] but the effects of the occasional small dose are probably of little practical importance.

References

1 Seegmiller JE and Grayzel AI. Use of the newer uricosuric agents in the management of gout. J Amer Med Ass (1960) 173, 1076.

2 Yu TF, Dayton PG and Gutman AB. Mutual suppression of the uricosuric effects of sulphinpyrazone and salicylate: a study in interaction between drugs. J Clin Invest (1963) 42, 1330.
3 Kersley GD, Cook ER and Tovey DCJ. Value of uricosuric agents and in particular of G 28315 in gout. Ann Rheum Dis (1958) 17, 326–33.

Azapropazone + Miscellaneous drugs

Abstract/Summary

The serum levels of azapropazone are not significantly changed by the concurrent use of chloroquine, dihydroxy-aluminium sodium carbonate, magnesium aluminium silicate, bisacodyl or anthraquinone laxatives.

Clinical evidence, mechanism, importance and management

A study in 12 subjects given 300 mg azapropazone three times a day showed that the serum levels of azapropazone, measured at 4 h, were not affected by the concurrent use of chloroquine, 250 mg daily for seven days.[1] Another study in 15 patients taking the same dosage of azapropazone found that the concurrent use of dihydroxy-aluminium sodium carbonate, magnesium aluminium silicate, bisacodyl or anthraquinone laxatives only caused a minor (5–6%) reduction in azapropazone serum levels.[2] No special precautions would seem to be needed if these drugs are given together.

References

1 Faust-Tinnefeldt G and Geissler HE. Azapropazon und rheumatologische Basistherapie mit Chloroquin unter dem Aspekt der Arzneimittelinteraktion. Arzneim-Forsch/Drug Res (1977) 27, 2170.
2 Faust-Tinnefeldt G, Geissler HE and Mutschler E. Azapropazon-Plasmaspiegel unter Begleitmedikation mit einem Antacidum oder Laxans. Arzneim-Forsch/Drug Res (1977) 27, 2411.

Buprenorphine + Amitriptyline

Abstract/Summary

No marked increase in the CNS and respiratory depressant effects of buprenorphine occurs if amitriptyline is given concurrently.

Clinical evidence, mechanism, importance and management

A study in 12 normal subjects found that both 0.4 mg buprenorphine given sublingually and 50 mg amitriptyline given orally impaired the performance of a number of psychomotor tests (digit symbol substitution, flicker fusion, Maddox wing, hand-to-eye coordination, reactive skills) and the subjects felt drowsy, feeble, mentally slow and muzzy. When given together the effects were only moderately increased and the increase in the respiratory depressant effects of the buprenorphine was only mild.[1] There seems to be no good reason for avoiding concurrent use.

Reference

1 Saarialho-Kere U, Mattila MJ, Paloheimo M and Seppala T. Psychomotor, respiratory and neuroendocrinological effects of buprenorphine
and amitriptyline in healthy volunteers. Eur J Clin Pharmacol (1987)
33, 139–46.

Dextromoramide + Triacetyloleandomycin

Abstract/Summary

*An isolated report describes a marked increase in the effects of
dextromoramide and coma in a man when he was treated with
triacetyloleandomycin.*

Clinical evidence, mechanism, importance and management

A man on dextromoramide developed signs of overdosage
(a morphine-like coma, mydriasis and depressed respiration)
three days after starting treatment with triacetylolandomycin
for a dental infection. He recovered when treated with naloxone. A possible explanation is that the triacetyloleandomycin
reduced the metabolism of the dextromoramide, thereby
reducing its loss from the body and increasing its serum
levels and effects.[1] The general importance of this interaction is uncertain but concurrent use should be well
monitored.

Reference

1 Carry PV, Ducluzeau R, Jourdan C, Bourrat Ch, Vigneau C and
Descotes J. De nouvelles interactions avec les macrolides? Lyon Med
(1982) 248, 189–90.

Dextropropoxyphene + Food

Abstract/Summary

*Food can delay the absorption of dextropropoxyphene, but the
total amount absorbed may be slightly increased.*

Clinical evidence, mechanism, importance and management

A study in normal subjects showed that, while fasting, peak
serum dextropropoxyphene levels were reached after about
2 h. High fat and high carbohydrate meals delayed peak
serum levels to about 3 h, and high protein to about 4 h.
Both the protein and carbohydrate meals caused a small increase in the total amount of dextropropoxyphene absorbed.[1] Likely reasons for the delay in absorption are that
food delays gastric emptying and possibly also physically
prevents the dextropropoxyphene from coming into contact
with the absorbing surface of the gut. Avoid food if rapid
analgesic effects are needed.

Reference

1 Musa MN and Lyons LL. Effect of food and liquid on the pharmacokinetics of propoxyphene. Curr Ther Res (1976) 19, 669.

Dextropropoxyphene + Orphenadrine

Abstract/Summary

*An alleged adverse interaction between dextropropoxyphene and
orphenadrine which is said to cause mental confusion, anxiety,
and tremors seems to be very rare, if indeed it ever occurs.*

Clinical evidence

Riker, the manufacturers of orphenadrine, used to state in
their package insert that 'mental confusion, anxiety and
tremors have been reported in patients receiving orphenadrine and dextropropoxyphene (propoxyphene) concurrently.' Eli Lilley, the manufacturers of propoxyphene,
issued a similar warning. However in correspondence with
both manufacturers, two investigators of this interaction
(Pearson and Salter[1]) were told that the basis of these
statements consisted of either anecdotal reports from clinicians or cases where patients had received twice the recommended dose of orphenadrine, in all a total of 13 cases. In
every case the adverse reactions seen were similar to those
reported with either drug alone. A brief study on five
patients given both drugs to investigate this alleged interaction failed to reveal an adverse interaction.[2]

Importance and management

The documentation is sparse (to say the least) and no case
of interaction has been firmly established. The investigators
cited[1] calculated that the two drugs were probably being
used together on three million prescriptions a year, and at
that time (1970) a maximum of 13 doubtful cases had been
reported. There seems therefore little reason for avoiding concurrent use, although prescribers should know that the advisability of using the two drugs together has been the
subject of some debate.

References

1 Pearson RE and Salter FJ. Drug interaction?—Orphenadrine with propoxyphene. N Engl J Med (1970) 282, 1215.
2 Puckett WH and Visconti JA. Orphenadrine and propoxyphene (cont.)
N Engl J Med (1970) 283, 544.

Dextropropoxyphene + Tobacco smoking

Abstract/Summary

*Dextropropoxyphene is less effective as an analgesic in those
who smoke than in those who do not.*

Clinical evidence

A study on 835 patients who were given dextropropoxy-phene hydrochloride for mild or moderate pain or headache showed that its efficacy as an analgesic was decreased by smoking. The drug was rated as ineffective by the physicians in 10.1% of 335 non-smokers, 15% of 347 patients who smoked up to 20 cigarettes daily, and 20.3% of 153 patients who smoked more than 20 cigarettes daily.[1]

Mechanism

It is thought that tobacco smoke contains chemical compounds which increase the activity of the liver enzymes concerned with the metabolism of dextropropoxyphene, thereby increasing its loss from the body and diminishing its effectiveness as an analgesic.[1]

Importance and management

The interaction appears to be well established. Prescribers should be aware that dextropropoxyphene is twice as likely to be ineffective (1 in 5) in those who smoke 20 cigarettes a day as in those who do not smoke (1 in 10).

Reference

1 Boston Collaborative Drug Surveillance Program. Decreased clinical efficacy of propoxyphene in cigarette smokers. Clin Pharmacol Ther (1973) 14, 259.

Diclofenac + Miscellaneous drugs

Abstract/Summary

Aluminium hydroxide, digitoxin, doxycycline and cefadroxil do not interact with diclofenac.

Clinical evidence, mechanism, importance and management

A study in nine normal subjects showed that two teaspoons of a 5.8% suspension of aluminium hydroxide had no effect on the bioavailability of a single 50 mg dose of diclofenac. The concurrent use of 0.1 mg digitoxin also had no effect on the serum levels of diclofenac (50 mg twice daily) of eight normal subjects.[1] In another study neither 2 g cefadroxil (eight patients) nor 200 mg doxycycline (seven patients) when taken daily for a week had any effect on the pharmacokinetics of 100 mg diclofenac.[2]

References

1 Schumacher A, Faust-Tinnefeldt G, Geissler HE, Gilfrich HJ and Mutschler E. Untersuchungen potentieller Interaktionen von Diclofenac-Natrium (Voltaren) mit einem Antazidum und mit Digitoxin. Therapiewoche (1983) 33, 2619–25.
2 Schumacher A, Geissler HE, Mutschler E and Osterburg M. Untersuchungen potentieller Interaktionen von Diclofenac-Natrium (Voltaren) mit Antibiotika. Z Rheumatol (1983) 42, 25–7.

Diflunisal + Antacids

Abstract/Summary

Aluminium and magnesium containing antacids can reduce the absorption of diflunisal by up to 40%, but no important interaction occurs if food is taken at the same time.

Clinical evidence, mechanism, importance and management

A study on four normal subjects showed that when given three 15 ml doses of *Aludrox* (aluminium hydroxide), 2 h before, together with and 2 h after a single 500 mg oral dose of diflunisal, the absorption was reduced about 40%.[1] Another study[2] showed that the absorption of a single 500 mg dose of difunisal was reduced 13% when given with 30 ml *Maalox* (aluminium-magnesium hydroxides), 21% when given 1 h later, and 32% when the antacid was given on a four-times-a-day schedule. Yet another study demonstrated a 26% reduction in absorption by 15 ml aluminium hydroxide gel.[3] However the bioavailability of diflunisal was not significantly altered in those taking aluminium-magnesium hydroxides if also taken with food.[4] Just how these antacids cause a reduced absorption is not clear but adsorption has been suggested.[4] The clinical importance of this interaction is uncertain.

References

1 Verbeeck R, Tjandramaga TB, Mullie TB, Verbesselt R and De Schepper PJ. Effect of aluminium hydroxide on diflunisal absorption. Br J clin Pharmac (1979) 7, 519.
2 Holmes GI, Irvin JD, Schrogie JJ, Lavies RO, Breault GO, Rogers JL, Huber PB and Zinny MA. Effects of Maalox on the bioavailability of diflunisal. Clin Pharmacol Ther (1979) 25, 228.
3 Tobert JA, De Schepper P, Tjandramaga TB, Mullie A, Meisinger MAP, Buntinx AP, Huber PB and Yeh KC. The effect of antacids on the bioavailability of diflunisal. Clin Pharmacol Ther (1979) 25, 251.
4 Tobert JA, De Schepper P, Tjandramaga TB, Mullie A, Buntinx AP, Meisinger MAP, Huber PB, Hall TIP and Yeh KC. Effect of antacids on the bioavailability of diflunisal in the fasting and prostprandial states. Clin Pharmacol Ther (1981) 30, 385.

Diflunisal + Non-steroidal anti-inflammatory agents (NSAID's) and Analgesics

Abstract/Summary

Aspirin can reduce serum diflunisal levels. Diflunisal raises serum indomethacin levels 2–3-fold and concurrent use should be avoided. Paracetamol levels are increased by diflunisal but not those of naproxen.

Clinical evidence, mechanism, importance and management

(a) Diflunisal + aspirin

The concurrent use of aspirin (600 mg four times daily) has been shown to cause a 15% fall in plasma diflunisal levels after two 250 mg doses daily over three days.[2] This would seem to be clinically unimportant.

(b) Diflunisal + indomethacin

A study in 16 normal subjects showed that diflunisal (500 mg twice daily) raised the steady-state serum levels and the AUC (area under the curve) of indomethacin (50 mg twice daily) two- to threefold. The reason appears to be that the diflunisal inhibits the glucuronidation of the indomethacin. The diflunisal appeared to have no clear effect on the blood loss in the faeces.[8] In another study it was found that two 250 mg doses of diflunisal daily with 75 mg indomethacin increased plasma indomethacin levels by 30–35%.[3] Despite evidence that diflunisal protects the human gastric mucosa against the damaging effects of indomethacin,[6] fatal gastrointestinal haemorrhage has occurred in three patients concurrently treated with diflunisal and indomethacin, and the manufacturers advise avoidance.[5]

(c) Diflunisal + paracetamol and naproxen

Diflunisal raises serum paracetamol (acetaminophen) levels by 50% but the total bioavailability is unchanged.[7] Diflunisal has been found to have no effect on serum naproxen levels in daily doses of 500 mg.[4]

References

1 Tempero KF, Cirillo VJ and Stellman SL. Diflunisal: a review of pharmacokinetic and pharmacodynamic properties, drug interactions and special tolerability studies in humans. Br J clin Pharmac (1977) 4, 315.
2 Perrier CV. Unpublished observations quoted in ref.1.
3 De Schepper P. Unpublished observations quoted in ref.1.
4 Dresse A, Gerard MA, Quiraux N, Fischer P and Gerardy J. Effect of diflunisal on human plasma levels and on the urinary excretion of naproxen. Arch Int Pharmacodyn (1978) 236, 276.
5 Edwards IR. Medicines Adverse Reactions Committee: eighteenth annual report. NZ Med J (1984) 97, 729–32.
6 Cohen MM. Diflunisal protects human gastric mucosa against damage by indomethacin. Dig Dis Sci (1983) 28, 1070–77.
7 Diggins JB, (Merck Sharp Dohme). Personal communication (1988)
8 Van Hecken A, Verbesselt R, Tjandra-Maga TB and De Schepper PJ. Pharmacokinetic interaction between indomethacin and diflunisal. Eur J Clin Pharmacol (1989) 36, 507–12.

Flufenamic, Mefenamic and Tolfenamic acids, Oxyphenbutazone or Phenylbutazone + Antacids

Abstract/Summary

The absorption of the fenamates is markedly accelerated by magnesium hydroxide but retarded by aluminium hydroxide. Sodium bicarbonate appears not to interact, and in vitro studies suggest that oxyphenbutazone and phenylbutazone are little affected.

Clinical evidence

Studies in six normal subjects given single 500 mg doses of mefenamic acid or 400 mg tolfenamic acid showed that magnesium hydroxide accelerated the absorption of both drugs (the mefanamic acid AUC after 1 h was increased threefold and of tolfenamic acid sevenfold) but the total bioavailability was only slightly increased. Sodium bicarbonate had no significant effect, but aluminium hydroxide markedly retarded the rate of absorption but no marked change in the total amount absorbed was seen.[2]

The table below summarizes some *in vitro* adsorption and elution studies undertaken with a number of antacids, designed to mimic the conditions which occur as drugs are moved through the intestinal tract.[1]

Mechanisms

A partially or totally reversible adsorption can occur with some of these antacids. It is not understood why the absorption of both mefenamic and tolfenamic acids is increased by magnesium hydroxide.

Importance and management

Information is very limited but it would appear that if rapid analgesia is needed with either mefenamic or tolfenamic acid, magnesium hydroxide can be given concurrently but aluminium hydroxide should be avoided. Aluminium hydroxide markedly retards the speed of absorption but only reduces the total absorption by about 20%. Sodium bicarbonate does not interact. The data in the table suggest that flufenamic acid is possibly similarly affected but whether the other antacids listed interact significantly is not known. There appears to be little problem with oxyphenbutazone or

Table 3.2 These figures represent the percent antirheumatic drug adsorbed per gram of adsorbent. The figures in brackets are the percent eluted using either 0.01 N.HCl (first figure) or 0.014 N.NaHCO3 (second figure).

	Magnesium trisilicate	Magnesium oxide	Aluminium hydroxide	Bismuth oxycarbonate	Calcium carbonate	Kaolin
Flufenamic acid	0	90 (26.-)	10	79	37	44
Mefenamic acid	0	95 (40.-)	69	26	2	90
Oxyphenbutazone	0	24 (100.-)	27	0	0	0
Phenylbutazone	0	12 (100.100)	0	0	0	0

phenylbutazone, however the full significance of the data in the table needs to be evaluated clinically.

References

1 Naggar VF, Khalil SA and Daabis NA. The *in vitro* adsorption of some antirheumatics on antacids. Pharmazie (1976) 31, 461.
2 Neuvonen PJ and Kivisto KT. Effect of magnesium hydroxide on the absorption of tolfenamic and mefenamic acids. Eur J Clin Pharmacol (1988) 35, 495–502.

Flufenamic or Mefenamic acid + Cholestyramine

Abstract/Summary

The absorption of both flufenamic and mefenamic acid is markedly reduced in animals by the concurrent use of cholestyramine, but whether this is an important interaction in man is uncertain.

Clinical evidence, mechanism, importance and management

In vitro studies with physiological concentrations of bile salt anions have shown that chlolestyramine binds to both flufenamic and mefenamic acid, while in studies in rats a 60–70% reduction in the gastrointestinal absorption of both acids has been seen in the presence of cholestyramine.[1] The same interaction seems likely in man, but so far nobody appears to have carried out a clinical study.

Reference

1 Rosenberg HA and Bates TR. Inhibitory effect of cholestyramine on the absorption of flufenamic and mefenamic acids in rats. Proc Soc Exp Biol Med (1974) 145, 93.

Ibuprofen + Antacids

Abstract/Summary

No clinically important interaction has been seen when ibuprofen is taken with an antacid (aluminium-magnesium hydroxide).

Clinical evidence, mechanism, importance and management

A study in eight normal subjects showed that doses of an antacid (aluminium and magnesium hydroxide) given before, with and after a single 400 mg dose of ibuprofen did not alter its pharmacokinetics.[1] There would seem to be no good reason for avoiding concurrent use.

Reference

1 Gontarz N, Small RE, Comstock TJ, Stalker DJ, Johnson SM and Willis HE. Effect of antacid suspension on the pharmacokinetics of ibuprofen. Clin Pharm (1987) 6, 413–16.

Ibuprofen or Flurbiprofen + Cimetidine, Nizatidine or Ranitidine

Abstract/Summary

Cimetidine causes a small increase in the serum levels of ibuprofen and flurbiprofen, but this is unlikely to be of clinical importance. Neither nizatidine nor ranitidine appear to interact.

Clinical evidence

(a) Ibuprofen

A controlled study in 13 normal subjects showed that while taking 1200 mg cimetidine daily, their peak serum ibuprofen levels after taking single 600 mg doses were raised 14% (from 56 to 64 μg/ml) and their AUC's by 6%. While taking 300 mg ranitidine daily no changes were seen.[1] No changes were seen in two other single dose studies with ibuprofen and cimetidine,[2,4] one of which also found no interaction between ibuprofen and nizatidine.[4]

(b) Flurbiprofen

A study in which 30 patients with rheumatoid arthritis were given 150–300 mg flurbiprofen daily for two weeks found that the concurrent use of 300 mg cimetidine three times a day increased the maximal serum level of flurbiprofen, but not when given 150 mg ranitidine twice daily. The efficacy of the flurbiprofen (assessed by Ritchie score, 50' walking time, grip strength) was not altered.[1]

Another study in normal subjects taking single 200 mg doses of flurbiprofen found that serum flurbiprofen serum levels were very slightly raised by cimetidine and the AUC was raised 11%, but no significant interaction occurred with ranitidine.[3]

Mechanism

Not understood.

Importance and management

The effects of cimetidine on serum ibuprofen and flurbiprofen levels would seem to be established but they are unlikely to be clinically important.

References

1 Ochs HR, Greenblatt DJ, Matlis R and Weinbrenner J. Interaction of ibuprofen with the H$_2$ receptor antagonists ranitidine and cimetidine. Clin Pharmacol Ther (1985) 38, 648–51.
2 Conrad KA, Mayersohn M and Bliss M. Cimetidine does not alter

ibuprofen kinetics after a single dose. Br J clin Pharmac (1984) 18, 624–6.

3 Sullivan KM, Small RE, Rock WL, Cox SR and Willis HE. Effects of cimetidine or ranitidine on the pharmacokinetics of flurbiprofen. Clin Pharm (1986) 5, 586–9.

4 Forsyth DR, Jayasinghe KSA and Roberts CJC. Do nizatidine and cimetidine interact with ibuprofen? Eur J Clin Pharmacol (1988) 35, 85–8.

5 Kreeft JH, Bellamy N, Freeman D. Do H2-antagonists alter the kinetics and effects of chronically administered flurbiprofen in rheumatoid arthritis? Clin Invest Med (1987) 10 (four Suppl B) B58.

Indomethacin + Allopurinol

Abstract/Summary

Allopurinol does not affect serum indomethacin levels.

Clinical evidence, mechanism, importance and management

Eight patients were treated for five days with 300 mg allopurinol and 50 mg indomethacin eight-hourly. The allopurinol had no significant effect on the AUC of indomethacin and the amounts of indomethacin excreted in the urine were not significantly altered.[1,2] There seems to be no reason for avoiding concurrent use.

References

1 Pullar T, Myall O, Dixon JS, Haigh JRM, Lowe JR and Bird HA. Allopurinol has no effect on steady-state concentrations of indomethacin. Br J clin Pharmac (1988) 23, 672P.

2 Pullar T, Myall O, Haigh JRM, Lowe JR, Dixon JS, Bird HA. The effect of allopurinol on the steady-state pharmacokinetics of indomethacin. Br J clin Pharmac (1988) 25, 755–7.

Indomethacin + Antacids

Abstract/Summary

The irritation of the gut caused by indomethacin can be relieved by the concurrent use of antacids, but serum indomethacin levels may be reduced to some extent as a result. This appears not to be clinically important.

Clinical evidence

A study in 12 normal subjects showed that the absorption of a single 50 mg dose of indomethacin was reduced by 35% when taken with 80% *Mergel* (an antacid formulation of aluminium hydroxide, magnesium carbonate and hydroxide).[1]

In another study in normal subjects 700 mg aluminium hydroxide suspension caused a marked fall in peak indomethacin serum levels,[2] whereas in yet another study 30 ml magnesium-aluminium hydroxide caused only slight changes in the absorption of a 50 mg dose of indomethacin.[3]

Mechanism

In vitro studies[4] have shown that indomethacin can be adsorbed by various antacids (magnesium trisilicate, magnesium oxide, magnesium hydroxide, bismuth oxycarbonate, calcium carbonate). This may explain some of the reduction in gastrointestinal absorption, but other mechanisms may also be involved.

Importance and management

Adequately but not extensively documented. Some reduction in serum levels is possible. Despite this the manufacturers of indomethacin recommend that it is taken with food, milk or an antacid to minimize gastrointestinal disturbances. Check that the indomethacin remains effective.

References

1 Galeazzi RL. The effect of an antacid on the bioavailability of indomethacin. Europ J clin Pharmacol (1977) 12, 65–8.

2 Garnham JC, Kaspi T, Kaye CM and Oh VMS. Different effects of sodium bicarbonate and aluminium hydroxide on the absorption of indomethacin in man. Postgrad Med J (1977) 53, 126–9.

3 Emori HW, Paulus H, Bluestone R, Champion GD and Pearson C. Indomethacin serum concentrations in man. Effects of dosage, food and antacid. Ann Rheum Dis (1976) 35, 333–8.

4 Naggar VF, Khalil SA and Daabis NA. The in-vitro adsorption of some antirheumatics on antacids. Pharmazie (1976) 31, 461.

Indomethacin + Aspirin and Salicylates

Abstract/Summary

Aspirin is reported to increase, decrease or have no effect on serum indomethacin levels, but none of these changes has been clearly shown to be of significant clinical importance.

Clinical evidence

The overall picture is confusing and contradictory. Some studies report that aspirin reduces serum indomethacin levels.[1-3,10] Others claim that no interaction occurs[4-6,11] and no changes in clinical effectiveness take place.[6,7] Yet other studies using buffered aspirin claim that it increases the absorption of indomethacin and is associated with an increase in side-effects.[8,9]

Mechanism

Not resolved. Changes in the rates of absorption and renal clearance have been proposed.

Importance and management

Although extensively studied, there seems to be no clear evidence, one way or the other, that there are either advantages or disadvantages in using both drugs concurrently. It might be prudent to check on the effects on the gastrointestinal tract since both can cause irritation and bleeding.

References

1 Rubin A, Rodda BE, Warrack P, Gruber CM and Ridolfo AS. Interactions of aspirin with nonsteroidal antiinflammatory drugs in man. Arth Rheum (1973) 16, 635.

2 Kaldestad E, Hansen T and Brath HK. Interaction of indomethacin and acetylsalicylic acid as shown by the serum concentrations of indomethacin and salicylate. Eur J clin Pharmacol (1975) 9, 199.

3 Jeremy R and Towson J. Interaction between aspirin and indomethacin in the treatment of rheumatoid arthritis. Med J Aust (1970) 1, 127.

4 Champion D, Mongan E, Paulus H, Sarkissian E, Okun R and Pearson C. Effect of concurrent aspirin (ASA) administration on serum concentrations of indomethacin (I) Arth Rheum (1971) 14, 375.

5 Lindquist B, Jensen KM, Johansson H and Hansen T. Effect of concurrent administration of aspirin and indomethacin on serum concentrations. Clin Pharmacol Ther (1974) 15, 247.

6 Brooks PM, Walker JJ, Bell MA, Buchanan WW and Rhymer AR. Indomethacin-aspirin interaction: a clinical appraisal. Br Med J (1975) 2, 69.

7 The Cooperating Clinical Committee of the American Rheumatism Association. A three-month trial of indomethacin in rheumatoid arthritis with special reference to analysis and inference. Clin Pharmacol Ther (1967) 8, 11.

8 Turner P and Garnham JC. Indomethacin-aspirin interaction. Br Med J (1975) 2, 368.

9 Garnham JC, Raymond K, Shotton E and Turner P. The effect of buffered aspirin on plasma indomethacin. Eur J clin Pharmacol (1975) 8, 107.

10 Lei BW, Kwan KC, Duggan DE, Breault GO and Davis RL. The influence of aspirin on the absorption and disposition of indomethacin. Clin Pharmacol Ther (1976) 19, 110.

11 Barraclough DRE, Muirden KD and Laby B. Salicylate therapy and drug interaction in rheumatoid arthritis. Aust NZ J Med (1975) 5, 518–23.

Indomethacin + Cimetidine

Abstract/Summary

Cimetidine can cause a small reduction in the serum levels of indomethacin but its anti-inflammatory effects do not seem to be significantly altered.

Clinical evidence, mechanism, importance and management

10 patients with rheumatoid arthritis who had been taking 100–200 mg indomethacin daily for over a year were additionally given 1 g cimetidine daily for a fortnight. Their serum indomethacin levels fell by an average of 18% (from 1.64 to 1.34 ng/ml) but there was no significant change in the clinical effectiveness of the anti-inflammatory treatment (as measured by articular index, pain, grip strength and ESR). The fall in indomethacin levels is thought to be due to some alteration in the absorption from the gut.[1] No special precautions would seem to be necessary during concurrent use.

Reference

1 Howes CA, Pullar T, Sourindhrin I, Mistra PC, Capel H, Lawson DH and Tilstone WJ. Reduced steady-state plasma concentrations of chlorpromazine and indomethacin in patients receiving cimetidine. Eur J Clin Pharmacol (1983) 24, 99–102.

Indomethacin + Food

Abstract/Summary

Gastric upset caused by indomethacin can be minimized by taking it with food or milk. Any interaction seems to be of minimal importance.

Clinical evidence, mechanism, importance and management

Studies in patients and normal subjects, given single or multiple oral doses of indomethacin, have shown that food causes marked and complex changes in the immediate serum indomethacin levels (peak levels are delayed and altered), but fluctuations in levels are somewhat ironed out.[1] However another study comparing indomethacin concentrations in serum and synovial fluids found that they were about the same 5–9 h after taking the indomethacin.[2] So it seems that the fluctuations and alterations which go on during the first 5 h are probably much less important than overall serum levels. The likelihood of an undesirable interaction seems to be small, whereas the advantages of taking the indomethacin at meal times to avoid gastric upset (a manufacturer's recommendation) are considerable.

References

1 Emori HW, Paulus H, Bluestone R, Champion GD and Pearson C. Indomethacin serum concentrations in man. Effects of dosage, food and antacid. Ann Rheum Dis (1976) 35, 333–8.

2 Emori HW, Champion GD, Bluestone R and Paulus HE. The simultaneous pharmacokinetics of indomethacin in serum and synovial fluid. Ann Rheum Dis (1973) 32, 433.

Indomethacin + Probenecid

Abstract/Summary

Serum indomethacin levels can be doubled by the concurrent use of probenecid. This can result in clinical improvement in patients with arthritic diseases, but indomethacin toxicity may also occur, particularly in those whose kidney function is impaired. The uricosuric effects of probenecid are not affected.

Clinical evidence

A study on 28 patients with osteoarthritis, taking 50–150 mg indomethacin daily, showed that 0.5–1.0 g probenecid daily roughly doubled their indomethacin serum levels and this paralleled the increased effectiveness (relief of morning stiffness, joint tenderness and raised grip strength indices). But four patients demonstrated indomethacin toxicity.[1]

Other studies have also demonstrated the marked rise in serum indomethacin levels caused by probenecid.[2-4] Clear signs of indomethacin toxicity (nausea, headache, tinnitus, confusion and a rise in blood urea) occurred in a woman with stable mild renal impairment when given probenecid.[5] The uricosuric effects of probenecid are not altered.[2]

Mechanism

Uncertain. It seems possible that the indomethacin and probenecid compete for the same kidney tubule secretory mechanisms, which leads to a decrease in the loss of the indomethacin.[2] There may also be some reduction in biliary excretion of indomethacin as well.[6]

Importance and management

An established and adequately documented interaction. Concurrent use should be very well monitored because, while clinical improvement can undoubtedly occur, some patients may develop indomethacin toxicity (headache, dizziness, light-headedness, nausea, etc.). This is particularly likely in those with some impaired kidney function. Reduce the indomethacin dosage as necessary.

References

1 Brooks PM, Bell MA, Sturrock RD, Famaey JP and Dick WC. The clinical significance of indomethacin-probenecid interaction. Br J clin Pharmac (1974) 1, 287.
2 Skeith MD, Simkin PA and Healey LA. The renal excretion of indomethacin and its inhibition by probenecid. Clin Pharmacol Ther (1968) 9, 89.
3 Emori W, Paulus HE, Bluestone R and Pearson CM. The pharmacokinetics of indomethacin in serum. Clin Pharmacol Ther (1973) 14, 134.
4 Baber N, Halliday L, Littler T, Orme ML'E and Sibeon R. Clinical studies of the interaction between indomethacin and probenecid. Br J Clin Pharmac (1978) 5, 364P.
5 Sinclair H and Gibson T. Interaction between probenecid and indomethacin. Brit J Rheumatol (1986) 25, 316–17.
6 Duggan DE, Hooke KF, White JD, Noll RM and Stevenson CR. The effects of probenecid upon the individual components of indomethacin elimination. J Pharmac Exp Ther (1977) 201, 463.

Indomethacin + Vaccines

Abstract/Summary

Some very limited evidence suggests that the response of the body to immunization with live vaccines may be more severe than usual in the presence of indomethacin.

Clinical evidence

A man with ankylosing spondylitis, taking 25 mg indomethacin three times a day, had a strong primary type reaction 12 days after smallpox vaccination. He experienced three days of severe malaise, headache and nausea, as well as enlarged lymph nodes. The scab which formed was unusually large (3 cm diameter) but he suffered no long term ill-effects.[1]

Mechanism

Uncertain. The suggestion is that the indomethacin alters the response of the body to viral infections, whether originating from vaccines or not.[1] For example, a child taking indomethacin who developed haemorrhagic chickenpox during a ward outbreak of the disease suffered severe scarring.[2] The manufacturers (MSD) of indomethacin state that indomethacin may mask the signs and symptoms of infection.

Importance and management

Information is very sparse and the interaction is not adequately established, but be aware that a more severe reaction may possibly occur if live vaccines (e.g. rubella, measles, etc.) are used in patients using indomethacin.

References

1 Maddock AC. Indomethacin and vaccination. Lancet (1973) ii, 210–11.
2 Rodriguez RS and Barbabosa E. Haemorrhagic chicken pox after indomethacin. N Engl J Med (1971) 235, 690.

Isoxicam + Miscellaneous drugs

Abstract/Summary

Aspirin may possibly causes changes in the serum levels of isoxicam but the importance of this is uncertain. Blood loss is increased. Isoxicam is reported not to be affected by either cimetidine or phenytoin.

Clinical evidence, mechanism, importance and management

A study in normal subjects found that the concurrent daily use of 200–300 mg isoxicam and 1800 mg aspirin for 14 days caused small rises in the serum levels of both drugs. Gastrointestinal blood loss was significantly increased.[1] In contrast another study found that 3.9 g aspirin daily approximately halved the serum levels of isoxicam.[2] Reduced serum isoxicam levels were seen in another study.[3] Whether any of these changes has any important effect on the clinical efficacy of isoxicam is uncertain but the possible increase in gastrointestinal blood loss should not be overlooked.

Other studies found that 1200 mg cimetidine daily had no effect on the rate and extent of absorption of isoxicam,[1] and phenytoin is also reported not to change the pharmacokinetics of isoxicam.[4]

References

1 DJ Farnham. Studies of isoxicam in combination with aspirin, warfarin sodium and cimetidine. Sem Arth Rheum (1982) 12 (Suppl 2), 179–183.
2 Grace EM, Mewa AAM, Sweeney GD, Rosenfeld JM, Darke AC and Buchanan WW. Lowering of plasma isoxicam concentrations with acetylsalicylic acid. J Rheumatol (1986) 13, 1119–21.
3 Esquivel M, Cussenot F, Ogilvie RI, East DS, Shaw DH. Interaction of isoxicam with acetylsalicylic acid. Br J clin Pharmac (1984) 18, 576–81.
4 Caille A. The effect of the administration of phenytoin on the pharmacokinetics of isoxicam. In preparation. Quoted by Downie WW, Gluckman MI, Ziehmer BA, Boyle JA. Clin Rheum Dis (1984) 10, 385–99.

Ketoprofen + Probenecid

Abstract/Summary

Probenecid can reduce the loss of ketoprofen from the body and increase its serum levels. Increased toxicity is a possibility.

Clinical evidence, mechanism, importance and management

A study in six normal subjects given 50 mg doses of ketoprofen six-hourly found that the concurrent use of 500 mg probenecid six-hourly reduced the ketoprofen clearance by 67%.[1] The reason is not understood but the probenecid possibly inhibits the metabolism (conjugation) of the ketoprofen by the liver. The clinical importance of this interaction is uncertain but be alert for any evidence of adverse effects caused by excessive ketoprofen serum levels. The authors of the report suggest that the ketoprofen dosage could be markedly reduced.

Reference

1 Upton RA, Williams RL, Buskin JN and Jones RM. Effects of probenecid on ketoprofen kinetics. Clin Pharmacol Ther (1982) 31, 705–12.

Meclofenamic acid + Aspirin

Abstract/Summary

Aspirin can cause a small and probably clinically unimportant reduction in serum meclofenamate levels, but intestinal bleeding is increased by concurrent use.

Clinical evidence, mechanism, importance and management

10 normal subjects given 1.8 g aspirin daily and 300 mg sodium meclofenamate daily for 14 days showed no significant reductions in serum salicylate levels, but serum meclofenamate levels were depressed to some extent. The clinical significance of this is uncertain, but it is probably limited. The gastrointestinal blood loss was approximately doubled compared with either drug alone.[1]

Reference

1 Baragar FD and Smith TC. Drug interaction studies with sodium meclofenamate (Meclomen). Curr Ther Res (1978) 23, April Suppl. S51.

Methadone + Anticonvulsants

Abstract/Summary

Serum methadone levels can be reduced by the concurrent use of carbamazepine, phenobarbitone or phenytoin. An increase in the methadone dosage may be needed.

Clinical evidence

(a) Carbamazepine

A study in 37 patients on methadone maintenance showed that only those on enzyme-inducing drugs (10 patients) had low trough methadone levels (less than 100 ng/ml). One was taking carbamazepine and he complained of daily withdrawal symptoms. He had signs of opioid abstinence.[1] The other nine were taking phenobarbitone (five patients) or phenytoin (four patients).[1]

(b) Phenobarbitone

In the study cited above, five patients on methadone maintenance who were on phenobarbitone had low trough serum methadone levels.[1]

(c) Phenytoin

Five patients on methadone began to experience methadone-withdrawal symptoms within 3–4 days of starting to take 300–500 mg phenytoin daily for five days. Methadone serum levels were depressed about 60%. The symptoms disappeared within 2–3 days of stopping the phenytoin and the serum methadone levels rapidly climbed to their former values.[2]

Reduced serum methadone levels have been described in other patients taking phenytoin.[1,3] See (a) above.

Mechanism

Not fully established but all of these anticonvulsants are recognized enzyme-inducing agents which can increase the metabolism of other drugs by the liver, thereby hastening their loss from the body. In one of the studies it was found that while taking phenytoin the excretion into the urine of the main metabolite of methadone was increased.[2]

Importance and management

Information is limited but the interaction appears to be established and of clinical importance. Anticipate the need to increase the methadone dosage in patients taking any of these anticonvulsants. It may be necessary to give methadone twice daily to prevent withdrawal symptoms appearing towards the end of the day.

References

1 Bell J, Seves V, Bowren P, Lewis J and Batey R. The use of serum methadone levels in patients receiving methadone maintenance. Clin Pharmacol Ther (1988) 43, 623–9.
2 Tong TG, Pond SM, Kreek MJ, Jaffery NF and Benowitz NL. Phenytoin-induced methadone withdrawal. Ann Intern Med (1981) 94, 349.
3 Finelli PF. Phenytoin and methadone tolerance. N Engl J Med (1976) 294, 227.

Methadone + Cimetidine

Abstract/Summary

Two elderly patients taking methadone developed apnoea when additionally treated with cimetidine.

Clinical evidence, mechanism, importance and management

An elderly patient taking 25 mg methadone daily developed apnoea two days after starting to take 1200 mg cimetidine daily.[1] Another elderly patient on methadone and morphine also developed apnoea (two breaths per minute) after taking 1200 mg cimetidine daily for six days.[2] This was controlled with naloxone. The probable reason is that the cimetidine (a well-recognized enzyme-inhibiting agent) depresses the activity of the liver enzymes concerned with the N-demethylation of the methadone (demonstrated in studies with liver microsomes taken from rats[1]) so that it accumulates in the body. So the effects seen were apparently due to the respiratory depressant effects of too much methadone. Liver impairment might possibly have contributed to the development of this interaction since both of the patients were elderly.

Information seems to be limited to these two observations, but it would seem reasonable to monitor the effects of concurrent use closely in any patient to make sure that the serum methadone levels do not rise too high. The outcome of this interaction could possibly be life-threatening. If the suggested mechanism of interaction is true, then ranitidine may prove to be a non-interacting alternative to cimetidine because it does not cause enzyme inhibition.

References

1 Dawson GW and Vestal RE. Cimetidine inhibits the *in vitro* N-demethylation of methadone. Res Comm Chem Pathol Pharmacol (1984) 46, 301–4.
2 Sorkin EM and Ogawa GS. Cimetidine potentiation of narcotic action. Drug Intell Clin Pharm (1983) 17, 60–1.

Methadone + Disulfiram

Abstract/Summary

No adverse interaction has been seen in patients treated concurrently with methadone and disulfiram.

Clinical evidence, mechanism, importance and management

Seven opiate addicts, without chronic alcoholism or liver disease, and who were on methadone-maintenance treatment (45–65 mg daily) showed an increase in the urinary excretion of the major pyrrolidine metabolite of methadone (an indicator of increased N-demethylation) when given 500 mg disulfiram daily for seven days, but there was no effect on the degree of opiate intoxication nor were withdrawal symp-

toms experienced.[1] No special precautions would seem to be necessary.

References

1 Tong TG, Benowitz NL and Kreek MJ. Methadone-disulfiram interaction during methadone maintenance. J Clin Pharmacol (1980) 20, 507.

Methadone + Rifampicin (Rifampin)

Abstract/Summary

Serum methadone levels can be markedly reduced by rifampicin. A dosage increase may be needed both for narcotic-dependent patients to prevent the development of withdrawal-symptoms, and for patients given methadone as an analgesic.

Clinical evidence

Following the observation that former heroin addicts complained of withdrawal symptoms when given rifampicin, a study was made on 30 patients on methadone. 21 developed withdrawal symptoms within 1–33 days of starting 600–900 mg rifampicin and 300 mg isoniazid daily. Seven of the most severely affected developed symptoms within a week and their serum methadone concentrations fell by 33–68%. None of 56 other patients on methadone and other anti-tubercular treatment (which included isoniazid but not rifampicin) showed withdrawal symptoms.[1–3]

Other cases of this interaction have been reported.[4–5] One patient needed a 50% increase in the dosage of methadone.[5] Another needed an increase from 45 to 140 mg daily.[5]

Mechanism

Rifampicin is a potent enzyme-inducing agent which increases the activity of the liver enzymes concerned with the metabolism of methadone, as a result of which its clearance from the body is markedly increased. In the study cited the urinary excretion of the major metabolite of methadone rose by 250%.[1]

Importance and management

An established interaction of clinical importance. The incidence is high. Two-thirds (21) of the narcotic-dependent patients in the study cited[1] developed this interaction, 14 of whom were able with the support of counselling to tolerate the relatively mild symptoms. Withdrawal symptoms may develop within 24 h. The analgesic effects of methadone would also be expected to be reduced. Concurrent use need not be avoided, but the effects should be monitored and appropriate dosage increases made where necessary.

References

1 Kreek MJ, Garfield JN, Gutjah CL and Giusti LM. Rifampicin-induced methadone withdrawal. N Eng J Med (1976) 294, 1104–6.
2 Garfield JW, Kreek MJ and Giusti L. Rifampin-methadone relationship.

1. The clinical effects of rifampin-methadone interaction. Am Rev Resp Dis (1975) 111, 262.
3 Kreek MJ, Garfield JW, Gutjah CL, Bowen D, Field F and Rothschild M. Rifampin-methadone relationship. 2. Rifampin effects on plasma concentration, metabolism and excretion of methadone. Am Rev Resp Dis (1975) 111, 926–7.
4 Bending MR and Skacel PO. Rifampicin and methadone withdrawal. Lancet (1977) i, 1211.
5 Van Leeuwen DJ. Rifampicine leidt tot onthoudingsverschijnselen bij methadonegebruikers. Ned Tijdsch Geneeskd (1986) 130, 548–50.

Methadone + Urinary acidifiers or alkalinizers

Abstract/Summary

The loss of methadone from the body in the urine is increased if the urine is made acid and reduced if it is made alkaline. There can be a two- to threefold difference.

Clinical evidence, mechanism, importance and management

Although methadone is metabolized to a considerable extent by the liver, about half of it is excreted unchanged in the urine.[2,3] Since is it a weak base (pKa 8.4) its renal clearance is pH-dependent. A study in patients on methadone showed that the urinary clearance of those with urinary pH's of less than 6 was three times greater than those with higher urinary pH's.[1] In one subject it was shown that when his urinary pH was lowered from 6.2 to 5.5, the loss of unchanged methadone in the urine was doubled.[3] The reason is that in acid urine little of the drug is in the un-ionized form, so that little can be reabsorbed by simple passive diffusion, whereas in alkaline solution most of the drug is in the un-ionized form which is readily reabsorbed by the kidney tubules and little is lost in the urine. Changes in the urinary pH brought about by drugs such as acetazolamide or sodium bicarbonate (alkalinization), or ammonium chloride (acidification), would be expected to have an influence on the response to methadone, but the clinical importance of this interaction has not been established. Some antacids and foods can also alter the urinary pH.

References

1 Bellward GD, Warren DM, Howald W, Axelson JE and Abbott FS. Methadone maintenance; effect of urinary pH on renal clearance in chronic high and low doses. Clin Pharmacol Ther (1977) 22, 92–9.
2 Baselt RC and Casarett LJ. Urinary excretion of methadone in man. Clin Pharmacol Ther (1972) 13, 64.
3 Inturrisi CE and Verebeley K. Disposition of methadone in man after a single oral dose. Clin Pharmacol Ther (1972) 13, 923.

Morphine + Cimetidine or Ranitidine

Abstract/Summary

The pharmacokinetics of morphine are unchanged by cimetidine but a slight and clinically unimportant increase in the respiratory depression can occur. Ranitidine also normally seems not to interact significantly. However an isolated report describes apnoea, confusion, agitation and muscular twitching in an acutely ill patient given morphine or papaveretum and cimetidine. Another isolated report describes disorientation, confusion and agitation in a patient given morphine and ranitidine.

Clinical evidence

(a) Cimetidine

Cimetidine (1200 mg for four days) given to seven normal subjects had no effect on the pharmacokinetics of morphine and the extent and duration of the pupillary miosis caused by morphine was unchanged.[2] In another study in normal subjects it was found that premedication with 600 mg cimetidine 1 h before 10 mg morphine (IM) prolonged the respiratory depression due to morphine, but the extent was small and clinically insignificant.[3]

An acutely ill patient with grand mal epilepsy, gastrointestinal bleeding and an intertrochanteric fracture who was undergoing haemodialysis three times a week, was being treated with 900 mg cimetidine daily. After being given the sixth dose of morphine (15 mg four-hourly) he became apnoeic (three respirations per minute) which was controlled with naloxone. He remained confused and agitated for the next 80 h with muscular twitching and further periods of apnoea controlled with naloxone. He had had nine 10 mg doses of morphine on a previous occasion in the absence of cimetidine without problems. About a month later he experienced the same adverse reactions when given papaveretum while still taking cimetidine.[1]

(b) Ranitidine

A man with terminal cancer on 150 mg ranitidine IV eight-hourly became confused, disorientated and agitated when given the ranitidine after an IV infusion of morphine (50 mg daily) was started. When the ranitidine was stopped his mental state improved but worsened when he was given ranitidine again 8 and 16 h later. He improved when the ranitidine was stopped.[5]

Another report describes hallucinations in a patient given sustained-release morphine and ranitidine, but the author discounted the possibility of an interaction.[6]

Mechanism

Studies with human liver microsomal enzymes have shown that the metabolism of morphine is not affected by cimetidine or ranitidine.[4] The isolated cases of interaction remain unexplained.[1,5] It would seem that unidentified factors conspired to cause these reactions.

Importance and management

The absence of an important morphine–cimetidine interaction is adequately documented. Concurrent use causes only a slight and unimportant prolongation of the respiratory depression due to morphine. Whether this might possibly have some importance in patients with pre-existing breathing disorders is uncertain. The available *in vitro* evidence[4] also suggests that ranitidine is unlikely to interact with morphine significantly, however the unexplained reports of adverse interactions which are cited here emphasize the importance of monitoring the concurrent use of morphine or papaveretum and these H_2-blockers.

References

1 Fine A and Churchill DN. Potential lethal interaction of cimetidine and morphine. Can Med Ass J (1981) 124, 1434.
2 Mojaverian P, Fedder IL, Vlasses PH, Rotmensch HH, Rocci ML, Swanson BN and Ferguson RK. Cimetidine does not alter morphine disposition. Br J clin Pharmac (1982) 14, 809–13.
3 Lam AM and Clement JL. Effect of cimetidine premedication on morphine-induced ventilatory depression. Can Anaesth Soc J (1984) 31, 36–43.
4 Knodell RG, Holtzman JL, Crankshaw DL, Steele NM and Stanley LN. Drug metabolism by rat and human hepatic microsomes in response to interaction with H_2-receptor antagonists. Gastroenterology (1982) 82, 84–7.
5 Martinez-Abad M, Gomis FD and Ferrer JM. Ranitidine-induced confusion with concomitant morphine. Drug Intell Clin Pharm (1988) 22, 914.
6 Jellema JG. Hallucinations during sustained-release morphine and methadone administration. Lancet (1987) ii, 392.

Morphine + Contraceptives (oral)

Abstract/Summary

The clearance of morphine is approximately doubled by the concurrent use of the oral contraceptives.

Clinical evidence, mechanism, importance and management

A controlled study in six young women showed that, while taking an oral contraceptive, the clearance of morphine given intravenously (1 mg) was increased by 75%, and given orally (10 mg) by 120%.[1] The suggested reason is that the oestrogen component of the contraceptive increases the activity of the liver enzymes (glucuronyl transferase) concerned with the metabolism of the morphine. This implies that the dosage of morphine would need to be virtually doubled to achieve the same degree of analgesia. Whether this is so in practice requires confirmation.

Reference

1 Watson KJR, Ghabrial H, Mashford ML, Harman PJ, Breen KJ and Desmond PV. The oral contraceptive pill increases morphine clearance but does not increase hepatic blood flow. Gastroenterol (1986) 90, 1779.

Morphine + Food

Abstract/Summary

Food increases the bioavailability of oral morphine and raises the serum levels.

Clinical evidence, mechanism, importance and management

12 patients with chronic pain were given 50 mg morphine hydrochloride by mouth in 200 ml water either while fasting or after a high fat breakfast (fried eggs and bacon, toast with butter, and milk). The maximum blood morphine concentrations and the time to achieve these concentrations were unaltered by the presence of the food, but the AUC (area under the concentration-time curve) was increased by 34% and blood morphine levels were maintained at higher levels over the period from 4 to 10 h after being given the morphine. The reasons are not understood. The inference to be drawn is that pain relief is likely to be increased if the morphine is given with food. This appears to be an advantageous interaction. More confirmatory study is needed.

Reference

1 Gourlay GK, Plummer JL, Cherry DA, Foate JA and Cousins MJ. Influence of a high-fat meal on the absorption of morphine from oral solutions. Clin Pharmacol Ther (1989) 46, 463–8.

Morphine + Metoclopramide

Abstract/Summary

Metoclopramide increases the rate of absorption of oral morphine and increases its sedative effects.

Clinical evidence

A study in 20 patients undergoing surgery showed that 10 mg metoclopramide orally markedly increased the extent and the speed of sedation due to a 20 mg oral dose of morphine (*MST-Continus Tablets*—Napp Laboratories) over a period of 3–4 h. Peak serum morphine levels and the total absorption remained unaltered.[1]

Mechanism

Metoclopramide increases the rate of gastric emptying so that the rate of morphine absorption from the small intestine is increased. An alternative idea is that both drugs act additively on opiate receptors to increase sedation.[1]

Importance and management

An established interaction which can be usefully exploited in anaesthetic practice, but the increased sedation may also represent a problem if the morphine is being given long-term.

Reference

1 Manara AR, Shelley MP, Quinn K and Park GR. The effect of metoclopramide on the absorption of oral controlled release morphine. Br J clin Pharmac (1988) 25, 518–21.

Morphine + Tricyclic antidepressants

Abstract/Summary

The bioavailability and the degree of analgesia of oral morphine is increased by the concurrent use of clomipramine or amitriptyline. This is a useful interaction, but it also seems possible that the toxicity of morphine may be increased.

Clinical evidence, mechanism, importance and management

A study in 24 patients being treated with oral morphine for the control of cancer pain showed that clomipramine or amitriptyline in daily doses of 20 or 50 mg increased the AUC of morphine (area under the concentration/time curve) by amounts ranging from 28 to 111%. The half-life of morphine was also prolonged.[1] The reasons are not understood. The increased analgesia may not only be due to the increased serum levels of morphine, but may possibly involve an analgesic effect of the antidepressant. This is a useful interaction, but the possibility of increased morphine toxicity should also be borne in mind. Whether other tricyclic antidepressants behave similarly is uncertain.

Reference

1 Ventafridda V, Ripamonti C, De Conno F, Bianchi M, Pazzuconi F and Panerai AE. Antidepressants increase bioavailability of morphine in cancer patients. Lancet (1987) i, 1204.

Nabumetone + Miscellaneous drugs

Abstract/Summary

Nabumetone does not interact with warfarin and appears not to interact with antihypertensive drugs. It is not affected by aluminium hydroxide, paracetamol or aspirin but its absorption is increased by food and milk.

Clinical evidence, mechanism, importance and management

A study in normal volunteers found that nabumetone had no significant effect on the anticoagulant effects of warfarin.[1] Other single dose studies have shown that the absorption of nabumetone is also not significantly altered by aluminium hydroxide, aspirin or paracetamol but it is increased by food and milk.[2] No significant changes in blood pressure were seen in large numbers of hypertensive patients when given nabumetone.[3] Because the active metabolite of nabumetone is highly protein bound and can displace other highly protein bound drugs the manufacturers of nabumetone say that the effects of hydantoin anticonvulsants (phenytoin) and the sulphonylureas may possibly be increased, but the risk seems to be more theoretical than real.[3]

References

1 Fitzgerald DE. Double blind study to establish whether there is any interaction between nabumetone and warfarin in healthy adult male volunteers. Roy Soc Med Int Congr Symp (1985) Series 69, 47–53.
2 Von Schrader HW, Buscher G, Dierdorf D, Mugge H and Wolf D. Nabumetone—a novel anti-inflammatory drug: the influence of food, milk, antacids, and analgesics on bioavailability of single oral doses. Int J Clin Pharmacol Ther Tox (1983) 21, 311–21.
3 Reliflex Product Booklet. Bencard (1987).

Naproxen + Antacids

Abstract/Summary

There is evidence that the absorption of naproxen can be altered (increased or decreased) by some antacids, but the clinical importance of this is uncertain.

Clinical evidence, mechanism, importance and management

A study in 14 normal subjects given single 300 mg doses of naproxen showed that 700 or 1400 mg sodium bicarbonate increased the rate and extent of absorption whereas 700 mg magnesium oxide or magnesium hydroxide reduced both. On the other hand when 15 or 60 ml *Maalox* were given, the rate and extent of absorption were slightly increased.[1] The reasons are not fully understood, but naproxen becomes more soluble as the pH rises which may account for the increased absorption with sodium bicarbonate, whereas magnesium and aluminium may form less soluble complexes.[2] The clinical importance of these observations is uncertain because single dose, short term studies (these studies only extended over 3 h) do not reliably predict what may happen when multiple doses are taken. Concurrent use need not be avoided but the effectiveness of the naproxen should be monitored.

References

1 Segre EJ, Sevelius H and Varady J. Effects of antacids on naproxen absorption. N Engl J Med (1974) 291, 582.
2 Segre EJ. Drug interactions with naproxen. Eur J Rheumatol Inflamm (1979) 2, 12.

Naproxen + Aspirin and Salicylates

Abstract/Summary

Serum naproxen levels can be reduced by salicylates but this does not appear to worsen the clinical effectiveness of combined use and it has even been claimed that it is increased.

Clinical evidence, mechanism, importance and management

A study in six normal subjects given 1200 mg naproxen showed that the serum levels were slighly depressed by the use of aspirin. The AUC (area under the curve) was depressed by 16%.[1,2] Another study in patients with rheumatoid arthritis found that choline magnesium trisilicate increased the clearance of naproxen by 56% and decreased its serum levels by 26%. It was concluded that increases in clinical efficacy were minimal compared with full doses of either drug alone.[4] However the authors of another study claimed that concurrent treatment was more effective in the treatment of rheumatoid arthritis than aspirin alone.[3] The value of concurrent use is therefore debatable but there would seem to be little reason for avoiding the use of both drugs, however the gastric irritant effects of both drugs should be borne in mind.

References

1 Segre EJ, Chaplin M, Forchielli E, Runkel R and Sevelius H. Naproxen-aspirin interactions in man. Clin Pharmacol Ther (1974) 15, 374.
2 Segre E, Sevelius H, Chaplin M, Forchielli E, Runkel R and Rooks W. Interaction of naproxen and aspirin in the rat and in man. Scand J Rheumatol (1973) Suppl 2, 37.
3 Williken RF and Segre EJ. Combination therapy with naproxen and aspirin in rheumatoid arthritis. Arth Rheum (1976) 19, 677.
4 Furst DE, Sarkissian E, Blocka K, Cassell S, Dromgoole S, Harris ER, Hirschberg JM, Josephson N and Paulus HE. Arth Rheum (1987) 30, 1157–61.

Naproxen + Cholestyramine

Abstract/Summary

Cholestyramine delays but does not reduce the absorption of naproxen.

Clinical evidence, mechanism, importance and management

A study in eight normal subjects showed the absorption of naproxen (a single 250 mg dose) was delayed but not reduced when given with cholestyramine (4 g in 100 ml orange juice). The amount absorbed after 2 h was reduced from 96 to 51%, but was complete after 5 h.[1] Since naproxen is given chronically, this delay is probably not important. This needs confirmation.

Reference

1 Calvo MV and Dominguez-Gil A. Interaction of naproxen with cholestyramine. Biopharm Drug Dis (1984) 5, 33–42.

Naproxen + Cimetidine

Abstract/Summary, clinical evidence, mechanism, importance and management

Naproxen and cimetidine do not interact together nor does naproxen alter the beneficial effects of cimetidine on gastric acid secretion.[1]

Reference

1 Holford NHG, Riegelman S, Buskin JN and Upton RA. Pharmacokinetic and pharmacodynamic study of cimetidine administered with naproxen. Clin Pharmacol Ther (1981) 29, 251.

Naproxen + Probenecid

Abstract/Summary

Serum naproxen levels are raised 50% by the concurrent use of probenecid. The clinical importance of this is uncertain, but probably minimal.

Clinical evidence, importance and management

A study carried out on six normal subjects who were taking 250 mg naproxen twice daily showed that the concurrent use of probenecid, 500 mg twice daily, increased the serum naproxen levels by 50%.[1] Probenecid apparently inhibits the loss of unchanged naproxen in the urine (half-life prolonged from 14 to 37 h) and also alters its metabolism by the liver.[2,3]

There seem to be no reports of adverse effects due to this interaction, but prescribers should be aware that naproxen serum levels will be raised during concurrent use.

References

1 Runkel R, Mroszcak E, Chaplin M, Sevelius H and Segre E. Naproxen-probenecid interaction. Clin Pharmacol Ther (1978) 24, 706.
2 Runkel R, Forschielli E, Boost G, Chaplin M, Hill R, Sevelius H, Thompson G and Segre E. Naproxen metabolism, excretion and comparative pharmacokinetics, Scand J Rheumatol (1973) 2, 29.
3 Runkel R, Chaplin MD, Sevelius H, Ortega E and Segre E. Pharmacokinetics of naproxen overdoses. Clin Pharmacol Ther (1976) 20, 269.

Naproxen + Sulglycotide

Abstract/Summary

Sulglycotide does not affect the absorption of naproxen.

Clinical evidence, mechanism, importance and management

A study in 12 normal subjects showed that 200 mg sulglycotide had no significant effects on the· pharmacokinetics of single 500 mg doses of naproxen.[1] Sulglycotide may therefore be used to protect the gastric mucosa from possible injury by naproxen without altering its absorption.

Reference

1 Berte F, Feletti F, De Barnardi di Valserra M, Nazzari M, Cenedese A and Cornelli U. Lack of influence of suglycotide on naproxen bioavailability in healthy volunteers. Int J Clin Pharmacol Ther Tox (1988) 26, 125–8.

Narcotic analgesics + Benzodiazepines

Abstract/Summary

The respiratory depressant effects of opiates such as diamorphine and phenoperidine appear to be opposed by the presence of benzodiazepines. Patients on methadone who are given diazepam may experience increased drowsiness.

Clinical evidence, mechanism, importance and management

A 14-year-old boy with staphylococcal pneumonia secondary to influenza developed adult respiratory distress syndrome. It was decided to suppress his voluntary breathing with opiates and use assisted ventilation, so he was given phenoperidine and diazepam for 11 days, and later diamorphine with lorazepam. Despite very high doses (19.2 g diamorphine in 24 h) his respiratory drive was not suppressed. On day 17 with serum morphine and lorazepam levels of 320 and 5.3 μg/ml respectively he remained conscious and his pupils were not constricted.[1] Later animal studies confirmed that lorazepam opposed the respiratory depressant effects of morphine.[1] In this situation this was an unwanted interaction, but under some circumstances it might be used to advantage. The effects on analgesia were not measured.

Four addicts, maintained on methadone for at least six months, were given 0.3 mg/kg diazepam for nine days. The pharmacokinetics were unaltered (confirmed in other studies[3,4]) and the opiate effects of the methadone remained unchanged, but all four were sedated.[2] The CNS depressant effects of both drugs would seem to be additive. Concurrent use need not be avoided but patients given both drugs are likely to experience increased drowsiness.

References

1 McDonald CF, Thomson SA, Scott NC, Scott W, Grant IWB and Crompton GK. Benzodiazepine-opiate antagonism—a problem in intensive care therapy. Intensive Care Med (1986) 12, 39–42.
2 Pond SM, Benowitz NL, Jacob P and Rigod J. Lack of effect of diazepam on methadone metabolism in methadone-maintained addicts. Clin Pharmacol Ther (1982) 31, 139–43.
3 Preston KL, Griffiths RR, Stitzer ML, Bigelow GE and Liebson IA. Diazepam and methadone interactions in methadone maintenance. Clin Pharmacol Ther (1984) 36, 534–41.
4 Preston KL, Griffiths RR, Cone EJ, Darwin WD and Gorodetzky CW. Diazepam and methadone blood levels following concurrent administration of diazepam and methadone. Drug Alc Dep (1986) 18, 195–202.

Narcotic analgesics + Promethazine

Abstract/Summary

Although promethazine can be used to reduce the dosage of many narcotic analgesics, it has potent sedative effects which would be expected to be additive with CNS depressant effects of the narcotics

Clinical evidence

A study in more than 300 patients treated with a number of different narcotic analgesics (morphine, pethidine, oxymorphone, hydromorphone, fentanyl, pentazocine) showed that their analgesic requirements were reduced 28–44% when they were given promethazine, 50 mg/70 kg body weight.[1] This possible advantageous interaction would be expected to be accompanied by increased sedation since promethazine is a potent CNS depressant which would be additive with the CNS depressant effects of the narcotics. See also 'Pethidine (Meperidine) + Chlorpromazine and other Phenothiazines'.

Reference

1 Keeri-Szanto M. The mode of action of promethazine in potentiation of narcotic drugs. Br J Anaesth (1974) 46, 918–24.

Nefopam + Miscellaneous drugs

Abstract/Summary

Nefopam should not be given to patients taking anticonvulsants or the MAOI. Be cautious with tricyclic antidepressants, anticholinergics and sympathomimetics. The intensity and incidence of side-effects are somewhat increased when nefopam is given with codeine, pentazocine or dextropropoxyphene.

Clinical evidence, mechanism, importance and management

Detailed information about adverse interactions between nefopam and other drugs seems not to be available, but convulsions have been seen in a few patients and the manufacturers say that nefopam is contraindicated in patients with a history of convulsive disorders. Caution should be exercised with the tricyclic antidepressants and other drugs with anticholinergic side-effects because the convulsive threshold may be lowered and the side-effects may be additive. The CSM has a number of reports of urinary retention caused by nefopam which would be expected to be worsened by drugs with anticholinergic activity.[3] Nefopam appears to have sympathomimetic activity and the makers say it should not be given with the MAOI. A controlled trial in 45 normal subjects divided into nine groups of five, each given 60 mg nefopam daily for three days with either 650 mg aspirin, 5 mg diazepam, 60 mg phenobarbitone, 65 mg dextropropoxyphene, 60 mg codeine, 50 mg pentazocine, 25 mg indomethacin or 50 mg hydroxyzine pamoate found that the only changes were possibly an additive increase in the intensity and incidence of side-effects with nefopam and codeine, pentazocine or dextropropoxyphene.[1] The incidence of sedation with nefopam is 20–30% which, depending on the circumstances, may present a problem if given with other sedative drugs.[2]

References

1 Lasseter KC, Cohen A and Back EL. Neofam HCl interaction study with eight other drugs. J Int Med Res (1976) 4, 195.
2 Heel RC, Brogden RN, Pakes GE, Speight TM and Avery GS. Nefopam: a review of its pharmacological properties and therapeutic efficacy. Drugs (1980) 19, 249–57.
3 Committee on the Safety of Medicines (CSM). Nefopam hydrochloride (Acupan). Current Problems no 24, January 1989.

Non-steroidal anti-inflammatory agents (NSAID's) + Antacids

Abstract/Summary

The absorption of suprofen, tolmetin and zomepirac are not significantly affected by the concurrent use of magnesium-aluminium hydroxide but a small reduction can occur with ketoprofen.

Clinical evidence, mechanism, importance and management

24 normal subjects were given 200 mg suprofen with either 8 oz water or 30 ml *Maalox* in water after an overnight fast. The bioavailability of the suprofen was not significantly affected by the antacid.[1] Neither single dose nor longer-term administration of 20 ml doses of *Maalox* affects the absorption or the plasma elimination half-life of 100 mg doses of zomepirac.[3] A detailed pharmacokinetic study on 24 subjects similarly showed that *Maalox*, given as single 20 ml doses four times a day over a three-day period, had no significant effect on the absorption from the gut of tolmetin given as single 400 mg doses.[4] Five normal subjects showed a 22% reduction in the absorption of 50 mg ketoprofen (as measured by the amount excreted in the urine) when given 1 g aluminium hydroxide, largely as a result of the adsorption of the ketoprofen by the antacid.[2]

No particular precautions are needed if these antacids are given with suprofen, tolmetin or zomepirac, and it seems doubtful if the effects of ketoprofen will be reduced to any great extent.

References

1 Abrams LS, Marriott TB and Van Horn A. The effect of Maalox on the bioavailability of suprofen. Clin Res (1983) 31, 626A.
2 Ismail FA, Khalafallah N and Khalil SA. Adsorption of ketoprofen and bumadizone calcium on aluminium-containing antacids and its effect on ketoprofen bioavailability in man. Int J Pharmaceut (1987) 34, 189–96.
3 Nayak RK, Ng KT and Gottlieb S. Effect of chronic and acute antacid

administration on zomepirac pharmacokinetics. Clin Pharmacol Ther (1980) 27, 275.
4 Ayres JW, Weidler DJ, Mackichan J, Sakmar E, Hallmark MB, Lemanowicz EF and Wagner JG. Pharmacokinetics of tolmetin with and without concomitant administration of antacid in man. Eur J Clin Pharmacol (1977) 12, 421.

Non-steroidal anti-inflammatory drugs (NSAID's) + Sucralfate

Abstract/Summary

Sucralfate appears not to interact adversely with aspirin, ibuprofen, indomethacin, ketoprofen or naproxen, and may also possibly protect the gastric mucosa from damage.

Clinical evidence

Six normal subjects were given 2 g sucralfate half an hour before taking single doses of either 50 mg ketoprofen, 50 mg indomethacin or 500 mg naproxen. Some changes were seen (reduced maximal serum concentrations of ketoprofen, reduced rate of absorption of naproxen and indomethacin, increased time to achieve maximal serum concentrations with indomethacin) but no alterations in bioavailability occurred.[1] A delay, but no reduction in the total absorption of naproxen is described by the same authors in another report. They say that it is unlikely that its clinical efficacy will be reduced.[5] 2 g sucralfate daily for two days was found not to decrease the rate of absorption of single 400 mg doses of ibuprofen[2] nor of 650 mg doses of aspirin.[3] In another study 5 g sucralfate in divided doses did not significantly alter the absorption of single 600 mg doses of ibuprofen.[4] Sucralfate can protect human gastric mucosa from damage by aspirin.[6]

Mechanism

The protective effects of sucralfate may possibly be related to stimulation of prostaglandin production.

Importance and management

Single dose studies are not necessarily reliable predictors of what will happen when patients take drugs regularly, but the evidence available suggests that the sucralfate is unlikely to have an adverse effect on treatment with aspirin, ibuprofen, indomethacin, ketoprofen or naproxen, and may possibly have some protective effect on the gastric mucosa.

References

1 Caille G, Du Souich P, Gervais P, Besner J-G. Single dose pharmacokinetics of ketoprofen, indomethacin and naproxen taken alone or with sucralfate. Biopharm Drug Disp (1987) 8, 173–83.
2 Anaya AL, Mayersohn M, Conrad KA and Dimmitt DC. The influence of sucralfate on ibuprofen absorption in healthy adult males. Biopharm Drug Disp (1986) 7, 443–51.
3 Lau A, Chang C-W and Schlesinger P. Evaluation of a potential drug interaction between sucralfate and aspirin. Gastroenterology (1985) 88, 1465.
4 Pugh MC, Small RE, Garnett WR, Townsend RJ and Willis HE. Effect

of sucralfate on ibuprofen absorption in normal volunteers. Clin Pharm (1984) 3, 630–3.

5 Caille G, du Souich P, Gervais P, Besner JG and Vezina M. Effects of concurrent sucralfate administration on pharmacokinetics of naproxen. Am J Med (1987) 83 (Suppl 3B) 67–73.

6 Stern AI, Ward F and Hartley G. Protective effect of sucralfate against aspirin-induced damage to human gastric mucosa. Am J Med (1987) 83 (Suppl 3B) 83–5.

Oxyphenbutazone and Phenyl-butazone + Anabolic steroids

Abstract/Summary

Serum oxyphenbutazone levels are raised 40% by the use of methandrostenolone. Phenylbutazone appears to be unaffected.

Clinical evidence

A study in six subjects taking 300–400 mg oxyphenbutazone daily for 2–5 weeks showed that oxyphenbutazone levels were raised 43% (range 5–100%) by 5 or 10 mg/kg methandrostenolone. Neither 5 mg prednisone nor 1.5 mg dexamethasone daily were found to affect oxyphenbutazone levels.[1]

Two other studies confirm this interaction with oxyphenbutazone.[2,3] One of them found no interaction with phenylbutazone.[2]

Mechanism

Uncertain. One idea is that the anabolic steroids alter the distribution of oxyphenbutazone between the tissues and plasma so that more remains in circulation. There may also possibly be some changes in metabolism. Phenylbutazone possibly does not interact because it displaces oxyphenbut-azone (its normal metabolite) from the plasma binding sites, thereby raising the levels of unbound oxyphenbutazone and obliterating the effect of the steroid.

Importance and management

The interaction is established but its importance is uncertain. There seem to be no reports of toxicity arising from concurrent use but the possibility should be borne in mind.

References

1 Weiner M, Siddiqui AA, Shahani RT and Dayton PG. Effect of steroids on disposition of oxyphenbutazone in man. Proc Soc Exp Biol Med (1976) 124, 1170.

2 Hvidberg E, Dayton PG, Read JM and Wilson CH. Studies of the inter-action of phenylbutazone, oxyphenbutazone and methandrostenolone in man. Proc Soc Exp Biol Med (1968) 129, 438.

3 Weiner M, Siddiqui AA, Bostanci N and Dayton PG. Drug inter-actions. The effect of combined administration on the half-life of coumarin and pyrazolone drugs in man. Fed Proc (1965) 24, 153.

Paracetamol (Acetaminophen) + Alcohol

Abstract/Summary

Severe liver damage, fatal in some instances, can occur in alcoholics and persistent heavy drinkers who take only moderate doses of paracetamol. Moderate drinkers do not seem to be at risk.

Clinical evidence

Three chronic alcoholic patients developed severe liver damage after taking only slightly above recommended doses of paracetamol (acetaminophen). They demonstrated SGOT levels of 5000–10,000 iu. Two of them had taken only 10 g paracetamol over the two days prior to admission (normal dosage is up to 4 g daily). One of them died in hepatic coma and a post mortem revealed typical paracetamol toxicity. Two of them also developed renal failure.[1]

There are numerous other reports of liver toxicity in a total of about 30 alcoholics attributed to the concurrent use of alcohol and paracetamol. About a third had been taking daily doses within the recommended daily maximum (4 g daily), and a third had had doses within the range 4–8 g daily.[2–17]

Mechanism

Paracetamol is normally predominantly metabolized by the liver to non-toxic sulphate and glucuronide conjugates. Per-sistent heavy drinking stimulates a normally minor biochemical pathway, the cytochrome P-450 dependent mixed function oxidase system, which allows the production of unusually large amounts of highly hepatotoxic metabolites. Unless sufficient glutathione is present to detoxify these metabolites (alcoholics often have an inadequate intake of protein), they become covalently bound to liver macro-molecules and damage results. Other factors may also have some part to play. Acute ingestion of alcohol by non-alcoholics on the other hand appears to protect against damage because the damaging biochemical pathway is in-hibited rather than stimulated.

Importance and management

An established and clinically important interaction. The in-cidence is uncertain but possibly small bearing in mind the very wide-spread use of paracetamol and alcohol. However damage, when it occurs, can be serious and therefore alcoholics and those who persistently drink heavily should be advised to avoid paracetamol or limit their intake con-siderably. The normal daily recommended maximum of 4 g is almost certainly too high in some individuals. The risk for non-alcoholics, moderate drinkers and those who very occa-sionally drink a lot appears to be low.

References

1 McClain CJ, Kromhout JP, Peterson FJ and Holtzman JL. Potentiation of acetaminophen hepatotoxicity by alcohol. J Amer Med Ass (1980) 244, 251.

2 Emby DJ and Fraser BN. Hepatotoxicity of paracetamol enhanced by ingestion of alcohol. S Afr Med J (1977) 51, 208.

3 Goldfinger R, Ahmed KS, Pichumoni CS and Weseley SA. Concomitant alcohol and drug abuse enhancing acetaminophen toxicity. Am J Gastroenterol (1978) 70, 385.

4 Barker JD, de Carle DJ and Anuras S. Chronic excessive acetaminophen use and liver damage. Ann Intern Med (1977) 87, 299.

5 O'dell JR, Zetterman RK and Burnett DA. Centrilobular hepatic fibrosis following acetaminophen-induced necrosis in an alcoholic. J Amer Med Ass (1986) 255, 2636–7.

6 McJunkin B, Barwick KW, Little WC and Winfield JB. Fatal massive hepatic necrosis following acetaminophen overdosage. J Amer Med Ass (1976) 236, 1874–5.

7 LaBrecque DT and Mitros FA. Increased hepatotoxicity of acetaminophen in the alcoholic. Gastroenterology (1980) 78, 1310.

8 Johnson MW, Friedman PA and Mitch WE. Alcoholism, nonprescription drugs and hepatotoxicity. The risk of unknown acetaminophen ingestion. Am J Gastroenterol (1981) 76, 530–3.

9 Licht H, Seeff LB and Zimmerman HJ. Apparent potentiation of acetaminophen toxicity by alcohol. Ann Intern Med (1980) 92, 511.

10 Black M, Cornell JF, Rabin L and Schachter N. Late presentation of acetaminophen toxicity. Dig Dis Sci (1982) 27, 370–4.

11 Fleckenstein JL. Nyquil and acute hepatic necrosis. N Engl J Med (1985) 313, 48.

12 Gerber MA, Kaufmann H, Klion F and Alpert LI. Acetaminophen associated hepatic injury: report of two cases showing an unusual portal tract reaction. Human Pathol (1980) 11, 37–42.

13 Leist MH, Giuskin LE and Payne JA. Enhanced toxicity of acetaminophen in alcoholics. Report of three cases. J Clin Gastroenterol (1985) 7, 55–9.

14 Himmelstein DU, Woolandler SJ and Adler RD. Elevated SGOT/SGPT ratio in patients with acetaminophen hepatotoxicity. Am J Gastroenterol (1984) 79, 718–20.

15 Levinson M. Ulcer, back pain and jaundice in an alcoholic. Hosp Prac (1983) 18, 48N, 48S.

16 Seeff LB, Cuccherini BA, Zimmerman HJ, Adler E and Benjamin SB. Acetaminophen hepatotoxicity in alcoholics. Ann Intern Med (1986) 104, 399–404.

17 Floren C-H, Thesleff P and Nilsson A. Severe liver damaged caused by therapeutic doses of acetaminophen. Acta Med Scand (1987) 222, 285–8.

Paracetamol (Acetaminophen) + Anticholinergic agents

Abstract/Summary

Anticholinergic drugs can delay gastric emptying so that the onset of analgesia with paracetamol may be delayed.

Clinical evidence

A study in six convalescent patients given 1.5 g paracetamol showed that the concurrent use of propantheline (30 mg IV) delayed the peak serum levels from about 1 h to 3 h, and peak concentrations were lowered by about a third. The total amount of paracetamol absorbed was unchanged.[1]

Mechanism

Propantheline is an anticholinergic drug which slows the rate at which the stomach empties so that the rate of absorption in the gut is reduced.

Importance and management

Information is very limited but this interaction would seem to be established. Rapid pain relief with paracetamol would be expected to be delayed and reduced by any drug with anticholinergic activity (e.g. some antiparkinson drugs, tricyclic antidepressants, some phenothiazines and antihistamines, etc.) but this needs clinical confirmation. Nobody seems to have studied any of these drugs except propantheline. If the paracetamol is being taken in repeated doses over extended periods it seems unlikely to be an important interaction because the total amount absorbed is unchanged.

Reference

1 Nimmo J, Heading RC, Tothill P and Prescott LF. Pharmacological modification of gastric emptying: effects of propantheline and metoclopramide on paracetamol absorption. Br Med J (1973) 1, 587.

Paracetamol (Acetaminophen) + Barbiturates

Abstract/Summary

Hepatotoxicity developed in a woman on phenobarbitone while taking paracetamol.

Clinical evidence, mechanism, importance and management

An epileptic woman on 100 mg phenobarbitone daily developed hepatitis after taking 1 g paracetamol daily for three months for headaches. Within two weeks of stopping the paracetamol her serum transaminase levels fell within the normal range which implied that her hepatitis was due to drug-induced liver damage.[1] It could be that the liver enzyme induction caused by the phenobarbitone resulted in an increase in the production of the hepatotoxic metabolites of paracetamol which exceeded the normal glutathione binding capacity. The author of the report suggests that other patients taking normal low doses of paracetamol with phenobarbitone may also run the risk of liver toxicity. So far this isolated report remains unconfirmed.

Reference

1 Pirotte JH. Apparent potentiation by phenobarbital of hepatotoxicity from small doses of acetaminophen. Ann Intern Med (1984) 101, 403.

Paracetamol (Acetaminophen) + Cholestyramine

Abstract/Summary

The absorption of paracetamol may possibly be reduced if cholestyramine is given at the same time, but if the cholestyramine is given an hour later the reduction in absorption is small.

Clinical evidence

A study in four normal subjects given 12 g cholestyramine and 2 g paracetamol together showed that the absorption of the paracetamol was reduced by 60% (range 30—98%) at 2 h but the results were said not to be statistically significant. When the cholestyramine was given 1 h after the paracetamol, the absorption was reduced by only 16%.

Mechanism

Cholestyramine reduces the absorption, presumably because it binds with the paracetamol in the gut. Separating the dosages prevents mixing in the gut.

Importance and management

An established interaction. The cholestyramine should not be given within 1 h of the paracetamol if maximal analgesia is to be achieved.

Reference

1 Dorboni B, Willson RA, Thompson RPH and Williams R. Reduced absorption of paracetamol by activated charcoal and cholestyramine. Br Med J (1973) 3, 86.

Paracetamol (Acetaminophen) + Cimetidine

Abstract/Summary, clinical evidence, mechanism, importance and management

No clinically important interaction has been seen when used concurrently.[1]

Reference

1 Chen MM and Lee CS. Cimetidine-acetaminophen interaction in humans. J Clin Pharmacol (1985) 25, 227–9.

Paracetamol (Acetaminophen) and Other drugs + Opiate analgesics

Abstract/Summary

Morphine and diamorphine delay gastric emptying so that the rate of absorption of other drugs given orally may be reduced.

Clinical evidence, mechanism, importance and management

A study in eight normal subjects showed that the absorption of a single 20 mg/kg dose of paracetamol was markedly delayed and reduced 30 m after an IM injection of either pethidine (150 mg) or diamorphine (10 mg). Peak plasma paracetamol levels were reduced from 20 to 13.8 and 5.2μg/ml

respectively, and delayed from 22 to 114 and 142 min respectively.[1] This interaction was also observed by the same workers in women in labour who had been given opiate analgesics.[2] The underlying mechanism of interaction is that these opiate analgesics delay gastric emptying so that the rate of absorption of the paracetamol is reduced, but the total amount of paracetamol absorbed is not affected. In the study cited the paracetamol was principally being used as a model drug to identify the way in which these analgesics affect drug absorption, but it seems probable that other oral drugs intended to have a rapid effect may be affected similarly. One example is mexiletine (see 'Mexiletine + Morphine').

References

1 Nimmo WS, Heading RC, Wilson J, Tothill P and Prescott LF. Inhibition of gastric emptying and drug absorption by narcotic analgesics. Br J clin Pharmac (1975) 2, 509–13.
2 Nimmo WS, Wilson J and Prescott LF. Narcotic analgesics and delayed gastric emptying during labour. Lancet (1975) i, 890–3.

Paracetamol (Acetaminophen) + Oral contraceptives

Abstract/Summary

Paracetamol (acetaminophen) is cleared from the body more quickly in women taking oral contraceptives and the analgesic effects are expected to be reduced. An increase in the dosage may be necessary. Paracetamol also increases the absorption of ethinyloestradiol from the gut by about 20%.

Clinical evidence

(a) Effect of oral contraceptives on paracetamol

A controlled study[1] in seven women showed that while taking oral contraceptives the plasma clearance of paracetamol, following a single 1.5 g dose, was increased by 63% (from 287 to 470 ml/min) and the elimination half-life decreased by 43% (from 2.40 to 1.67 h) when compared with women not taking oral contraceptives.

Other studies found increases in paracetamol clearance of 86%, 49% and 30%, and corresponding half-life decreases in women on oral contraceptives.[2–4]

(b) Effect of paracetamol on oral contraceptives

A single dose study in six normal women showed that 1 g paracetamol increased the AUC (area under time/concentration curve) of ethinyloestradiol by 21.6%.[5,6]

Mechanism

The evidence suggests that the oral contraceptives increase the metabolism (both oxidation and glucuronidation) by the liver of the paracetamol so that it is cleared from the body more quickly.[3] The increased absorption of the ethinyloestradiol is probably because the paracetamol reduces its metabolism by the gut wall during absorption.[5,6]

Importance and management

The effect of the oral contraceptives on paracetamol is well-established. Its clinical importance has not been directly studied, but it seems likely that an increase in the dosage of paracetamol (acetaminophen) will be needed to achieve optimal analgesic effects in women on the pill. The clinical importance of the increased ethinyloestradiol absorption is uncertain.

References

1   Mitchell MC, Hanew T, Meredith CG and Schenker S. Effects of oral contraceptive steroids on acetaminophen metabolism and elimination. Clin Pharmacol Ther (1983) 34, 48–53.
2   Abernethy DR, Divoll M, Ochs HR, Ameer B and Greenblatt DJ. Increased metabolic clearance of acetaminophen with oral contraceptive use. Obst Gynecol (1982) 60, 338–41.
3   Miners JO, Attwood J and Birkett DJ. Influence of sex and oral contraceptive steroids on paracetamol metabolism. Br J Clin Pharmacol (1983) 16, 503–9.
4   Mucklow JC, Fraser HS, Bulpitt CJ, Kahn C, Mould G and Dollery CT. Environmental factors affecting paracetamol metabolism in London factory and office workers. Br J Clin Pharmacol (1980) 10, 67–74.
5   Rogers SM, Back DJ, Stevenson P, Grimmer SFM and Orme ML'E. Paracetamol interaction with oral contraceptive steroids. Br J Clin Pharmacol (1987) 23, 615 P.
6   Rogers SM, Back DJ, Stevenson P, Grimmer SFM and Orme ML'E. Paracetamol interaction with oral contraceptive steroids: increased plasma concentration of ethinyloestradiol. Br J clin Pharmac (1987) 23, 721–5.

Penicillamine + Antacids

Abstract/Summary

The absorption of pencillamine from the gut can be reduced by 30–40% if antacids containing aluminium and magnesium hydroxides are taken concurrently.

Clinical evidence

A study in six normal subjects showed that the concurrent use of 30 ml *Maalox-plus* (aluminium hydroxide, magnesium hydroxide, simethicone) reduced the absorption of a single 500 mg dose of penicillamine by a third.[1] In another study it was found that 30 ml *Aludrox* (aluminium and magnesium hydroxides) reduced the absorption by almost 40%.[2]

Mechanism

The most likely explanation is that the penicillamine forms less soluble chelates with magnesium and aluminium ions in the gut which reduces its absorption.[2] Another idea is that the penicillamine is possibly less stable at the higher pH caused by the antacid.[1]

Importance and management

An established interaction. If maximal absorption is needed the administration of the two drugs should be separated to avoid mixing in the gut. Two hours or so has been found enough for most other drugs which interact similarly. There seems to be nothing documented about other antacids.

References

1   Osman MA, Patel RB, Schuna A, Sundstrom WR and Welling PG. Reduction in oral penicillamine absorption by food, antacid and ferrous sulphate. Clin Pharmacol Ther (1983) 33, 465–70.
2   Ifan A and Welling PG. Pharmacokinetics of oral 500-mg penicillamine: effect of antacids on absorption. Biopharm Drug Disp (1986) 7, 401–5.

Penicillamine + Food

Abstract/Summary

Food can reduce the absorption of penicillamine by as much as a half.

Clinical evidence

A study in normal subjects given 500 mg penicillamine showed that the presence of food reduced the serum penicillamine levels by about 50% (from 3.05 to 1.52 μg/ml). The total amount absorbed was reduced similarly (AUC_{0-12h} reduced from 14.7 to 7.16 $h^{-1}ml^{-1}$).[1,3]

These figures are in good agreement with previous findings.[2]

Mechanism

Uncertain. One suggestion is that food delays stomach emptying so that the penicillamine is exposed to more prolonged degradation in the stomach.[2] Another idea is that the protein in food increases the oxidation of the penicillamine to disulphides which are less easily absorbed.[2]

Importance and management

An established interaction. If maximal effects are required the penicillamine should not be taken with food.

References

1   Schuna A, Osman MA, Patel RB, Welling PG and Sundstrom WR. Reduction in oral penicillamine absorption by food, antacid and ferrous sulphate. J Rheumatol (1983) 10, 95–7.
2   Bergstrom RF, Kay DR, Harcom TM and Wagner JG. Penicillamine kinetics in normal subjects. Clin Pharmacol Ther (1981) 30, 404–13.
3   Osman MA, Patel RB, Schuna A, Sundstrom WR and Welling PG. Reduction in oral penicillamine absorption by food, antacid and ferrous sulphate. Clin Pharmacol Ther (1983) 33, 465–70.

Penicillamine + Iron preparations

Abstract/Summary

The absorption of penicillamine can be reduced as much as two-thirds by the concurrent use of iron preparations.

Clinical evidence

A study in five normal subjects given 250 mg penicillamine showed that when they were also given 90 mg ferrous iron (*Fersamal*) the absorption of the penicillamine was reduced by about two-thirds (using the cupiuretic effects of penicillamine as a measure).[1]

A two-thirds reduction in absorption has been described in another study in subjects given 500 mg penicillamine and 300 mg ferrous sulphate.[5] Other studies confirm this interaction.[2,3] There is also evidence that withdrawal of iron from patients stabilized on penicillamine without a reduction in the dosage can lead to the development of toxicity (nephropathy).[4]

Mechanism

It is believed that the iron and penicillamine form a chemical complex or chelate in the gut which is less easily absorbed.

Importance and management

An established and clinically important interaction. If maximal absorption of the penicillamine is required the iron should be given at least 2 h after the penicillamine to prevent, as far as possible, their admixture in the gut.[1] Care should be taken not to withdraw iron suddenly from patients stabilized on penicillamine because the marked increase in absorption which follows may precipitate penicillamine toxicity. The toxic effects of penicillamine seem to be dependent on the size of the dose and possibly also related to the rate at which the dosage is increased.[4]

References

1 Lyle WH. Penicillamine and iron. Lancet (1976) ii, 240.
2 Lyle WH, Pearcy DF and Hui M. Inhibition of penicillamine-induced cupiuresis by oral iron. Proc Roy Soc Med (1977) (Suppl 3) 48–9.
3 Hall ND, Blake DR, Alexander GJM, Vaisey C and Bacon PA. Serum SH reactivity: a simple assessment of D-penicillamine absorption Rheumatol Int (1981) 1, 39–41.
4 Harkness JAL and Blake DR. Penicillamine nephropathy and iron. Lancet (1982) ii, 1368–9.
5 Osman MA, Patel RB, Schuna A, Sundstrom WR and Welling PG. Reduction in oral penicillamine absorption by food, antacid and ferrous sulphate. Clin Pharmacol Ther (1983) 33, 465–70.

Pentazocine + Tobacco smoking and Environmental pollution

Abstract/Summary

Those who smoke or who live in urban areas where the air is heavily polluted may need about 50% more pentazocine to achieve satisfactory analgesia than those who do not smoke or who live where the air is clean.

Clinical evidence, mechanism, importance and management

A study in which pentazocine was used to supplement nitrous oxide relaxant anaesthesia showed that patients who came from an urban environment needed about 50% more pentazocine than those who lived in the country (3.6 compared with 2.4 µg/kg/min). Roughly the same difference was seen between those who smoked and those who did not (3.8 compared with 2.5 µg/kg/min).[1] In another study it was found that those who smoked metabolized 40% more pentazocine than those who did not smoke.[2] The likely reason for these differences is that tobacco smoke and polluted city air contains chemical compounds which act as enzyme inducing agents which increase the rate at which the liver metabolizes pentazocine (and probably other drugs as well). Smokers and urban dwellers from polluted areas may need about 40–50% more pentazocine than country dwellers and non-smokers to achieve the equivalent amount of analgesia.

References

1 Keeri-Szanto M and Pomeroy JR. Atmospheric pollution and pentazocine metabolism. Lancet (1971) i, 947–9.
2 Vaughan DP, Beckett AH and Robbie DS. The influence of smoking on the intersubject variation in pentazocine elimination. Br J clin Pharmac (1976) 3, 279–83.

Pethidine (Meperidine) + Acyclovir

Abstract/Summary

An isolated report describes pethidine toxicity associated with the concurrent use of high dose acyclovir.

Clinical evidence, mechanism, importance and management

A man with Hodgkin's disease was treated with high dose acyclovir for localized herpes zoster, and with pethidine, methadone and carbidopa-levodopa for pain. On the second day he experienced nausea, vomiting and confusion, and later dysarthria, lethargy and ataxia. Despite vigorous treatment he later died. It was concluded that some of the adverse effects were due to pethidine toxicity arising from norpethidine accumulation associated with renal impairment due to the acyclovir.[1]

Reference

1 Johnson R, Douglas J, Corey L and Krasney H. Adverse effects with acyclovir and meperidine. Ann Intern Med (1985) 103, 962–3.

Pethidine (Meperidine) + Barbiturates

Abstract/Summary

A single case report describes greatly increased sedation with severe CNS toxicity in a woman given pethidine after receiving phenobarbitone for a fortnight.

Clinical evidence

A woman whose pain had been satisfactorily controlled with pethidine without particular CNS depression, showed prolonged sedation with severe CNS toxicity when later given pethidine after being treated with 120 mg phenobarbitone daily for a fortnight as anticonvulsant therapy.[1]

Mechanism

Studies in the patient cited, four other patients and two normal subjects revealed that phenobarbitone stimulates the liver enzymes concerned with the metabolism—N-demethylation—of pethidine so that the production of its more toxic metabolite (norpethidine, normeperidine) is increased. The toxicity seen appears to be the combined effects of this compound and the directly sedative effects of the barbiturate.[1,2]

Importance and management

There is only one report of toxicity but the metabolic changes described under 'Mechanism' were seen in other patients and subjects. The general clinical importance is uncertain but concurrent use should be undertaken with care. Since the metabolic product of pethidine is a less effective analgesic than the parent compound, the depth of analgesia may be reduced. It has also been suggested that if the pethidine is continued but the barbiturate suddenly withdrawn, the toxic concentrations of norpethidine might lead to convulsions in the absence of the anticonvulsant. Whether other barbiturates behave similarly is not clear, but it is possible. More study is needed to confirm these possibilities.

References

1 Stambaugh JE, Wainer IW, Hemphill DM and Schwartz I. A potentially toxic drug interaction between pethidine (meperidine) and phenobarbitone. Lancet (1977) i, 398.
2 Stambaugh JE, Wainer IW, and Schwartz I. The effect of phenobarbital on the metabolism of meperidine in normal volunteers. J Clin Pharmacol (1978) 18, 482.

Pethidine (Meperidine) + Chlorpromazine and other Phenothiazines

Abstract/Summary

Pethidine (meperidine) and chlorpromazine can be used together for increased analgesia and for premedication before anaesthesia, but increased respiratory depression, sedation, CNS toxicity and hypotension can also occur. Other phenothiazines such as promethazine, prochlorperazine, propiomazine and thioridazine may also interact to cause some of these effects.

Clinical evidence

A study in six normal subjects showed that pethidine alone (100 mg/70 mg body weight) caused respiratory depression whereas chlorpromazine alone (25 mg/70 mg body weight) had no consistent effects. But together the respiratory depressant effects were greater than with pethidine alone. One subject showed marked respiratory depression, beginning about half an hour after receiving both drugs and lasting 2 h.[1]

A single dose study in normal subjects showed no change in the pharmacokinetics of pethidine, but the excretion of the metabolites of pethidine were increased. The symptoms of lightheadedness, dry mouth and lethargy were significantly increased and four subjects experienced such marked debilitation that they required assistance to continue the study. Systolic and diastolic blood pressures were also depressed.[2]

A patient on chronic thioridazine treatment (100 mg daily) given premedication with pethidine, diphenhydramine and glycopyrrolate was very lethargic after surgery and stopped breathing. He responded to naloxone.[7] Studies with other phenothiazines have shown that promethazine increases the analgesic effects of pethidine,[3] and propiomazine can increase its respiratory depressant effects,[5] but the effects of prochlorperazine[4] on respiration were not statistically significant.

Mechanism

There is evidence that chlorpromazine can increase the activity of the liver microsomal enzymes so that the metabolism of pethidine to normeperidine and normeperidinic acid are increased. These are toxic and probably account for the lethargy and hypotension seen in one study.[2] The effects of the phenothiazines on pethidine-induced respiratory depression may be related.

Importance and management

Lower doses of pethidine can be used if chlorpromazine is given,[6] but concurrent use is clearly not without its problems. A marked increase in respiratory depression can occur in some susceptible individuals.[1] The authors of one study offer the opinion that '...the debilitation observed after meperidine-chlorpromazine combinations again raises the question as to whether the clinical use of this combination is justified. The risks of increased CNS toxicity and hypotension outweigh the uncertain advantages, and the use of the combination as an analgesic should probably be discontinued.'[2]

Information about other adverse pethidine–phenothiazine interactions seems to be very limited. The pethidine–thioridazine interaction cited here seems to be the only one recorded.[7] Increased analgesia may occur but it may be accompanied by increased respiratory depression[3,5] which is undesirable in patients with existing respiratory insufficiency.

One manufacturer of pethidine (Roche) advises that severe hypotension may take place with phenothiazines, but particular drugs are not named.

References

1 Lambertsen CJ, Wendel H and Longenhagen JB. The separate and combined respiratory effects of chlorpromazine and meperidine in normal men controlled at 46 mm Hg alveolar pCO_2. J Pharm Exptl Ther (1961) 131, 381–93.
2 Stambaugh JE and Wainer IW. Drug interaction: meperidine and chlorpromazine, a toxic combination. J Clin Pharmacol (1981) 21, 140.
3 Keeri-Szanto M. The mode of action of promethazine in potentiating narcotic drugs. Br J Anaesth (1974) 46, 918–24.
4 Steen SN and Yates M. The effects of benzquinamide and prochlorperazine separately and combined on the human respiratory centre. Anesthesiology (1972) 36, 519–20.
5 Hoffman JC and Smith TC. The respiratory effects of meperidine and propiomazine in man. Anesthesiology (1970) 32, 325–31.
6 Sadove MS, Levin MJ, Rose RF, Schwartz L and Witt FW. Chlorpromazine and narcotics in the management of pain of malignant lesions. J Amer Med Ass (1954) 155, 626–8.
7 Ereshefsky L, Jann MW and Fidone GS. Clinical implication of the neuroleptic-opioid interaction. Drug Intell Clin Pharm (1986) 20, 75–7.

Pethidine + Cimetidine or Ranitidine

Abstract/Summary

Cimetidine reduces the loss of pethidine from the body, but the extent to which this increases its analgesic and toxic effects is uncertain. It is probably not large. Ranitidine does not interact.

Clinical evidence, mechanism, importance and management

A study in eight normal subjects showed that after taking 1200 mg cimetidine daily for a week, the total body clearance of a single 70 mg intravenous dose of pethidine was decreased by 22%.[1] The probable reason is that the cimetidine inhibits the liver microsomal enzymes concerned with metabolism of the pethidine because it was found that the production of the normal metabolite of pethidine, norpethidine, was reduced by 23%.[1] This is supported by other studies with both animal and human liver microsomes.[2] The clinical importance of this interaction has not been assessed, but it is probably not great. However since the effects of the pethidine, both analgesic and toxic, would be expected to be increased to some extent, concurrent use should be monitored. Direct clinical information about this interaction seems to be limited to the study cited.[1] An alternative would be to use ranitidine which has been shown not to interact.[3]

References

1 Guay DRP, Meatherall RC, Chalmers JL and Grahame GR. Cimetidine alters pethidine disposition in man. Br J clin Pharmac (1984) 18, 907–14.
2 Knodell RG, Holtzman JL, Crankshaw DL, Steele NM and Stanley LN. Drug metabolism by rat and human hepatic microsomes in response to interaction with H_2-receptor antagonists. Gastroenterology (1982) 82, 84–8.

3 Guay DRP, Meatherall RC, Chalmers JL, Grahame GR and Hudson RJ. Ranitidine does not alter pethidine disposition in man. Br J clin Pharmac (1985) 20, 55–9.

Pethidine (Meperidine) + Furazolidine

Abstract/Summary

On the basis of animal experiments it has been suggested that a serious hyperpyrexic reaction may occur similar to that seen with the antidepressant MAOI if pethidine and furazolidone are used concurrently in man. This has yet to be confirmed.

Clinical evidence, mechanism, importance and management

Studies in rabbits have shown that fatal hyperpyrexia follows the injection of pethidine into animals who have taken furazolidone by mouth for four days.[1] On the basis of this reaction, the known MAO-inhibitory properties of furazolidone in man,[2] and the well-documented MAOI-pethidine interaction in man, there would seem to be the possibility of some risk if these two drugs are used together. More study is needed.

References

1 Eltayeb IB and Osman OH. Furazolidine–pethidine interactions in rabbits. Br J Pharmac (1975) 55, 497.
2 Pettinger WA, Soyangio FG and Oates JA. Monoamine oxidase inhibition by furazolidine in man. Clin Res (1966) 14, 258.

Pethidine (Meperidine) + Monoamine oxidase inhibitors (MAOI)

Abstract/Summary

The concurrent use of pethidine (meperidine) and MAOI has resulted in a serious and potentially life-threatening reaction in a few patients. Excitement, muscle rigidity, hyperpyrexia, flushing, sweating and unconsciousness occur very rapidly. Respiratory depression and hypotension are also seen. Pethidine should not be used in patients on MAOI unless a lack of sensitivity has been confirmed.

Clinical evidence

Severe, rapid and potentially fatal toxic reactions, both excitatory and depressant can occur.

A woman on iproniazid, 100 mg daily, was given 100 mg pethidine to treat acute precordial pain. She became restless and incoherent almost immediately and was comatose within 20 min. Within an hour she was flushed, sweating and showed Cheyne-Stokes respiration. Her pupils were dilated and unreactive. Deep reflexes could not be initiated and plantar reflexes were extensor. Her pulse rate was 82 and blood pressure 156/110 mm Hg. She was rousable within 10 min of receiving an intravenous injection of 25 mg prednisolone hemi-succinate.[1]

A woman who, unknown to her doctor, was taking tranylcypromine, was given 100 mg pethidine. Within minutes she became unconscious, noisy and restless, having to be held down by three people. Her breathing was stertorus and the pulse impalpable. Generalized tonic spasm developed with ankle clonus, extensor plantar reflexes, shallow respiration and cyanosis. On admission to hospital she had a pulse rate of 160, a blood pressure of 90/60 mm Hg and was sweating profusely (temperature 38°C). Her condition gradually improved and 4 h after admission she was conscious but drowsy. Recovery was complete the next day.[10]

This interaction has been seen in other patients treated with iproniazid,[1,3-5] pargyline,[2] phenelzine,[6-9] tranylcypromine[10] and mebanazine.[11] Fatalities have occurred.[6,11]

Mechanism

Not understood, despite the extensive studies undertaken.[15-17] There is some evidence that the reactions may be due to an increase in levels of 5-HT within the brain, and that a critically high level must be reached before the toxicity manifests itself.

Importance and management

A well-documented, serious and potentially fatal interaction first observed in the mid 1950s. The incidence is not known, but it is probably quite low. A study of this interaction on 15 patients given various MAOI failed to demonstrate it.[12] Nevertheless, patients on MAOI should not be given pethidine (meperidine) unless they are known not to be sensitive.

Churchill-Davidson has suggested[15] that sensitivity can be checked by giving a test dose of 5 mg pethidine, after which all the vital signs (pulse, respiration, blood pressure) are checked at 5 min intervals for 20 min, and then at 10 min intervals for the rest of the hour. If no obvious change has occurred, the whole check is repeated over the next hour with 10 mg pethidine, then with 20 mg, and after 3 h with 40 mg. It is not thought necessary to carry on further because by this stage any sensitivity should have revealed itself. Churchill-Davidson quotes the case of a patient who demonstrated sensitivity after 5 mg pethidine with a systolic blood pressure fall of 30 mm Hg, a pulse rate rise of 20 beats/min, and drowsiness.

The interaction has been successfully treated with prednisolone hemisuccinate, 25 mg[1] or chlorpromazine.[4] Acidification of the urine would also effectively increase the rate of clearance.[14]

References

1 Shee JC. Dangerous potentiation of pethidine by iproniazid, and its treatment. Br Med J (1960) 2, 507.
2 Vigran IM. Dangerous potentiation of meperidine hydrochloride by pargyline hydrochloride. J Amer Med Ass (1964) 187, 953.
3 Clement AJ and Benazon D. Reactions to other drugs in patients taking monoamine oxidase inhibitors. Lancet (1962) ii, 197.
4 Papp C and Benaim S. Toxic effects of iproniazid in a patient with angina. Br Med J (1958) 2, 1070.
5 Mitchell RS. Fatal toxic encephalitis occurring during iproniazid therapy in pulmonary tuberculosis. An Inter Med (1955) 42, 417.
6 Palmer H. Potentiation of pethidine. Br Med J (1960) 2, 944.
7 Taylor DC. Alarming reaction to pethidine in patients on phenelzine. Lancet (1962) ii, 409.
8 Cocks DP and Passemore Rowe A. Dangers of monoamine oxidase inhibitors. Br Med J (1962) 2, 1545.
9 Reid NCRW and Jones D. Pethidine and phenelzine. Br Med J (1962) 1, 408.
10 Denton PH, Borrelli VM and Edwards NV. Dangers of monoamine oxidase inhibitors. Br Med J (1962) 2, 1752.
11 Anon. Death from drugs combination. Pharm J (1965) 195, 341.
12 Prosser Evans CDG. The use of pethidine and morphine in the presence of monoamine oxidase inhibitors. Br J Anest (1968) 40, 279.
13 Churchill-Davidson HC. Anaesthesia and monoamine oxidase inhibitors. Br Med J (1962) 1, 520.
14 London DR and Milne MD. Dangers of monoamine oxidase inhibitors. Br Med J (1962) 2, 1752.
15 Leander JD, Batten J and Hargis GW. Pethidine interaction with clorgyline, pargyline or 5-hydroxytryptophan: lack of enhanced pethidine lethality or hyperpyrexia in mice. J Pharm Pharmac (1978) 30, 396.
16 Rogers KJ and Thornton JA. The interaction between monoamine oxidase inhibitors and narcotic analgesics in mice. Br J Pharmacol (1969) 36, 470.
17 Gessher PK and Soble AG. A study of the tranylcypromine-meperidine interaction: effects of p-chlorophenylalanine and 1-5-hydroxy-tryptophan. J Pharmacol Exp Ther (1973) 186, 276.

Pethidine (Meperidine) + Phenytoin

Abstract/Summary

Phenytoin can reduce the serum levels of pethidine and increase the levels of its toxic metabolite, but whether this is of clinical importance is uncertain.

Clinical evidence, mechanism, importance and management

Studies[1,2] in four normal subjects showed that 300 mg phenytoin daily for nine days decreased the elimination half-life of pethidine (100 mg orally and 50 mg IV) from 6.4 to 4.3 h, and the systemic clearance increased from 14.3 to 18.2 mo/min/kg. The production of normeperidine, the metabolic product of pethidine, was increased which suggests that the phenytoin (a known enzyme-inducing agent) had increased the metabolism (N-demethylation) of the pethidine by the liver. It is uncertain whether in practice this means that the analgesic effects of pethidine are reduced by phenytoin, or that the toxic effects of normeperidine are increased, but this should be considered if both drugs are used concurrently. There seem to be no reports confirming that this is an interaction of clinical importance.

References

1 Pond SM and Kretzschmar KM. Decreased bioavailability and increased clearance of meperidine during phenytoin administration. Clin Pharmacol Ther (1981) 29, 273.

2 Pond SM and Kretzschmar KM. Effect of phenytoin on meperidine clearance and normeperidine formation. Clin Pharmacol Ther (1981) 30, 680.

Phenazone (Antipyrine) + Miscellaneous drugs

Abstract/Summary

Changes in the half-life of phenazone (reduced by many liver enzyme-inducers, prolonged by many liver enzyme-inhibitors) are used to detect the effects of drugs on liver enzyme activity.

Clinical evidence, mechanism, importance and management

Phenazone is metabolized by mixed function oxidase enzymes in the liver, for which reason it is extensively used as a model drug for studying whether other drugs stimulate (induce) or inhibit liver enzymes. For example, barbiturates reduce the half-life of phenazone. In one study amylobarbitone caused a 42% reduction thereby demonstrating that the liver enzymes were being stimulated by the barbiturate to metabolize the phenazone more rapidly.[1] In contrast, those drugs which are enzyme inhibitors cause the half-life of phenazone to be prolonged which shows that the activity of the metabolizing enzymes is reduced. Thus phenazone often features in reports of drug interaction studies, but phenazone itself has only a minor role to play as an analgesic and antipyretic.

Reference

1 Vesell ES and Page JG. Genetic control of the phenobarbital-induced shortening of plasma antipyrine half-lives in man. J Clin Invest (1969) 48, 220.

Phenoperidine + Antacids

Abstract/Summary

An antacid has been shown to increase the serum levels of phenoperidine given intravenously.

Clinical evidence, mechanism, importance and management

A study in six normal subjects showed that when given an antacid (*Andursil*—aluminium and magnesium hydroxides, magnesium carbonate, dimethicone) the serum levels of phenoperidine over the 20 min period following a 15 μ/kg IV dose were considerably raised. The peak level rose 60% (from 9.1 to 14.7 ng/ml) but fell after 20 min to about the same

levels. The AUC (area under the plasma concentration-time curve) over this period was increased by 47%. The secondary peaks in the plasma concentrations were also ironed out. A possible reason is that changes in gastric pH may alter the secretion of phenoperidine in the stomach (this also occurs with pethidine). The clinical significance of this study is uncertain, but it seems possible that in the presence of antacids there may be an increase in both the analgesic and respiratory depressant effects of phenoperidine. More study is needed.

Reference

1 Calvey TN, Milne LA, Williams NE, Chan K and Murray GR. Effect of antacids on the plasma concentration of phenoperidine. Br J Anesth (1983) 55, 535–9.

Phenoperidine + Beta-blockers

Abstract/Summary

An isolated report describes a patient with tetanus who showed a very marked fall in blood pressure when given phenoperidine following a dose of propranolol.

Clinical evidence, mechanism, importance and management

A patient with tetanus was treated uneventfully with 2 mg phenoperidine on five occasions over 24 h. Later 2 mg propranolol IV was used to reduce the heart rate from 150 to 120 beats per minute, without any fall in blood pressure. When 2 mg phenoperidine was subsequently given, the systolic blood pressure fell to 30 mm Hg (heart rate 100–120 bpm) and this persisted for 5–10 min until reversed by naloxone.[1] The reasons for this marked hypotensive response are not understood. The general importance of this is uncertain because this incident occurred in the context of tetanus.

Reference

1 Woods KL. Hypotensive effect of propranolol and phenoperidine in tetanus. Br Med J (1978) 2, 1164.

Phenylbutazone + Allopurinol

Abstract/Summary

Allopurinol appears not to interact significantly with phenylbutazone.

Clinical evidence, mechanism, importance and management

The daily administration of 300 mg allopurinol to six normal subjects for a month had no effect on the elimination of a 200 mg daily dose of phenylbutazone, and no effect on the steady-state serum levels of phenylbutazone in three patients taking 200 or 300 mg daily.[1] In another study on six patients with acute gouty arthritis it was found that 300 mg allopurinol produced small but clinically unimportant effects on the half-life of phenylbutazone (6 mg/kg).[2] No special precautions would seem necessary if both drugs are given.

References

1 Rawlins MD and Smith SE. Influence of allopurinol on drug metabolism in man. Br J Pharmac (1973) 48, 693.
2 Horwitz D, Thorgeirsson SS and Mitchell JR. The influence of allopurinol and size of dose on the metabolism of phenylbutazone in patients with gout. Eur J Clin Pharmacol (1977) 12, 133.

Phenylbutazone + Barbiturates

Abstract/Summary

Some reduction in the serum levels of phenylbutazone may be expected if phenobarbitone is given concurrently, but the practical importance of this is uncertain.

Clinical evidence, mechanism, importance and management

Studies in man have shown that the half-life of phenylbutazone is reduced (from 78 to 57 h) by the concurrent use of 90 mg phenobarbitone daily,[1] and other studies confirm that it increases the loss of phenylbutazone from the body.[2,3] It is thought that this is because phenobarbitone is a potent liver enzyme inducing agent which increases the metabolism of phenylbutazone by the liver, thereby hastening its clearance. Whether this is important or not seems not to have been studied. Concurrent use need not be avoided but be alert for any evidence of a deterioration in the response to phenylbutazone treatment if phenobarbitone is added to established treatment. The same precautions would be appropriate with any barbiturate because they are all potent liver enzyme inducing agents.

References

1 Levi AJ, Sherlock S and Walker D. Phenylbutazone and isoniazid metabolism in patients with liver disease in relation to previous drug therapy. Lancet (1968) i, 1275.
2 Whittaker JA and Price Evans DA. Genetic control of phenylbutazone metabolism in man. Br Med J (1970) 3, 323.
3 Anderson KE, Peterson CM, Alvares AP and Kappas A. Oxidative drug metabolism and inducibility by phenobarbital in sickle cell anaemia. Clin Pharmacol Ther (1977) 22, 580.

Phenylbutazone + Indomethacin

Abstract/Summary, clinical evidence, mechanism, importance and management

An isolated report describes transient deterioration in renal

function in a patient during recovery from phenylbutazone-induced renal failure when given 25 mg indomethacin three times a day.[1] A possible reason is that the indomethacin displaced the residual phenylbutazone from its plasma protein binding sites.[1]

References

1 Kimberly R and Brandstetter RD. Exacerbation of phenylbutazone-related renal failure by indomethacin. Arch Intern Med (1978) 138, 1711.
2 Solomon HM, Schrogie JJ and Williams D. The displacement of phenylbutazone-^{14}C and warfarin-^{14}C from human albumin by various drugs and fatty acids. Biochem Pharmacol (1968) 17, 143.

Phenylbutazone + Methylphenidate

Abstract/Summary

Serum phenylbutazone levels are raised by methylphenidate.

Clinical evidence, mechanism, importance and management

Single dose and chronic studies in man using normal daily doses of phenylbutazone (200–400 mg) and methylphenidate showed that serum phenylbutazone levels were significantly increased in five out of six subjects, due, it is suggested to inhibition of liver metabolizing enzymes.[1] The clinical importance of this is uncertain.

Reference

1 Dayton PG, Perel JM, Israili ZH, Faraj BA, Rodewig K, Black N and Goldberg LI. Studies with methylphenidate: drug interactions and metabolism. Int Symp Alc Drug Addiction. Toronto, Ontario, October 1973. (Ed Sellers, EM) Clinical Pharmacology of Psychoactive Drugs, Addiction Res Foundation. ISBN-0–88868–007–4, pages 183–202.

Phenylbutazone + Pesticides

Abstract/Summary

Chronic exposure to lindane and other chlorinated pesticides can increase the rate of metabolism of phenylbutazone.

Clinical evidence, mechanism, importance and management

A study showed that the plasma half-life of phenylbutazone in a group of men who regularly used chlorinated insecticide sprays—mainly lindane—as part of their work, was shorter (51 h) than in a control group (64 h) due, it is believed, to the enzyme-inducing effects of the insecticides.[1] This is of doubtful direct clinical importance, but it illustrates the changed metabolism which can occur in those exposed to environmental chemical agents.

Reference

1 Kolomodin-Hedman B. Decreased plasma half-life of phenylbutazone in workers exposed to chlorinated pesticides. Eur J clin Pharmacol (1973) 5, 195.

Phenylbutazone + Tobacco smoking

Abstract/Summary

The loss of phenylbutazone from the body is greater in smokers than in non-smokers.

Clinical evidence, mechanism, importance and management

A comparative study showed that the half-life of a single dose of phenylbutazone was 37 h in a group of smokers (10 or more cigarettes daily for two years) compared with 64 h in a group of non-smokers. The metabolic clearance was approximately doubled.[1] The conclusion to be drawn is that those who smoke may possibly need larger or more frequent doses of phenylbutazone to achieve the same therapeutic response, but this needs confirmation.

Reference

1 Garg SK and Kiran TNR. Effect of smoking on phenylbutazone disposition. Int J Clin Pharmacol Ther Toxicol (1983) 20, 289–90.

Phenylbutazone or Oxyphenbutazone + Tricyclic antidepressants

Abstract/Summary

The tricyclic antidepressants can delay the absorption of phenylbutazone and oxyphenbutazone from the gut, but their antirheumatic effects are probably not affected.

Clinical evidence, mechanism, importance and management

A study in four depressed women showed that when treated with 75 mg desipramine daily the absorption of phenylbutazone was considerably delayed, but the total amount absorbed (measured by the urinary excretion of oxyphenbutazone) remained unchanged.[1] In another five depressed women it was shown that the half-life of oxyphenbutazone was unaltered by 75 mg desipramine or nortriptyline daily.[2] Animal studies have confirmed that the absorption of phenylbutazone and oxyphenbutazone are delayed by the tricyclic antidepressants, probably because of their anticholinergic effects which reduce the motility of the gut,[3,4] but there seems to be no direct clinical evidence that the antirheumatic effects of either drug are reduced by this interaction. No particular precautions appear to be needed.

References

1 Consolo S, Morselli M, Zaccala M and Garattini S. Delayed absorption of phenylbutazone caused by desmethylimipramine in humans. Eur J Pharmacol (1970) 10, 239.
2 Hammer W, Martens S and Sjoqvist F. A comparative study of the metabolism of desmethylimipramine, nortriptyline and oxyphenbutazone in man. Clin Pharmacol Ther (1969) 10, 44.
3 Consolo S. An interaction between desipramine and phenylbutazone. J Pharm Pharmac (1968) 20, 574.
4 Consolo S and Garattini S. Effect of desipramine on intestinal absorption of phenylbutazone and other drugs. Eur J Pharmacol (1969) 6, 322.

Piroxicam and Tenoxicam + Cholestyramine

Abstract/Summary

Cholestyramine increases the loss of both piroxicam and tenoxicam from the body and their therapeutic effects would be expected to be reduced accordingly.

Clinical evidence

A study in eight normal subjects showed that when given 4 g cholestyramine three times a day, the clearances of 20 mg oral doses of piroxicam and 20 mg IV doses of tenoxicam were increased by 52% and 105% respectively, and their half-lives reduced by 40 and 52% respectively. The cholestyramine was not given until after the piroxicam had been absorbed.

Mechanism

Cholestyramine binds with other drugs in the gut. Since the cholestyramine was not given until the piroxicam had been absorbed and the tenoxicam was given intravenously, it would seem probable that the cholestyramine binds with these drugs following their excretion in the bile, thereby preventing their reabsorption and increasing their loss.

Importance and management

Direct information appears to be limited to this study. Unlike the situation with a number of other drugs, this interaction can be reduced but not avoided by separating the dosages. Monitor the effects of concurrent use and increase the dosage of the piroxicam or tenoxicam as necessary. Alternatively use other NSAID's or hypolipidaemic drugs.

Reference

1 Guentert TS, Defoin R and Mosberg H. Accelerated elimination of tenoxicam and piroxicam by cholestyramine. Clin Pharmacol Ther (1988) 43, 179.

Piroxicam + Cimetidine

Abstract/Summary

Cimetidine does not interact significantly with piroxicam.

Clinical evidence, mechanism, importance and management

A study in 10 normal subjects showed that after taking 1200 mg cimetidine daily for seven days the half-life and the AUC of a single dose of piroxicam were slightly increased (by 7 and 16% respectively) but these changes are unlikely to be clinically important.[1]

Reference

1 Mailhot C, Dahl SL and Ward JR. The effect of cimetidine on serum concentrations of piroxicam. Pharmacotherapy (1986) 6, 112–17.

Sulindac + Dimethylsulfoxide (DMSO)

Abstract/Summary

A single case report describes a patient on sulindac who developed a serious peripheral neuropathy when he applied DMSO to his skin.

Clinical evidence, mechanism, importance and management

A man with a long history of degenerative arthritis was treated uneventfully with 400 mg sulindac daily for six months until, without his doctor's knowledge, he began regularly to apply a topical preparation containing 90% DMSO to his upper and lower extremities. Soon afterwards he began to experience pain, weakness in all his extremities, and difficulty in standing or walking. He was found to have both segmental demyelination and axonal neuropathy. He made a partial recovery but was unable to walk without an artificial aid.[1] The reason for this reaction is not known, but studies in rats have shown that DMSO can inhibit a reductase enzyme by which sulindac is metabolized,[2] and it may be that the high concentrations of unmetabolized sulindac increased the neurotoxic activity of the DMSO. Although there is only this case on record, its seriousness suggests that patients should not use sulindac and DMSO-containing preparations concurrently.

References

1 Reinstein L, Mahon R and Russo GL. Peripheral neuropathy after concomitant dimethylsulfoxide use and sulindac therapy. Arch Phys Med Rehabil (1982) 63, 581–4.
2 Swanson BN, Mojaverian P, Boppana VK and Dudash M. Dimethyl sulfoxide (DMSO) interaction with sulindac (SO). Pharmacologist (1981) 23, 196.

4

ANTIARRHYTHMIC
DRUG INTERACTIONS

This chapter is concerned with the Class I anti-arrhythmic agents which possess some local anaesthetic properties, and with Class III drugs. Antiarrhythmic agents which fall into other classes are dealt with in the chapters devoted to specific groups of drugs (Beta-blockers, Digitalis Glyco-sides, Calcium channel blockers). Interactions in which the antiarrhythmic drug is the affecting agent, rather than the drug whose activity is alter-ed, are dealt with in other chapters. Consult the Index for a full listing.

Table 4.1. Antiarrhythmic agents

Non-proprietary names	Proprietary names
Ajmaline	*Aritmina, Cardiorhythmine, Gilurytmal, Nororytmina*
Amiodarone	*Atlansil, Coronovo, Cordarone (X), Trangorex*
Aprindine	*Amidonal, Fibocil, Fiboran*
Bretylium	*Bretylate, Bretylol*
Disopyramide	*Dicorynan, Dirythmin SA, Durbis, Norpace, Norpaso, Rhythmodan, Ritmodan, Ritmoforine, Rythmodul*
Encainide	-
Flecainide	-
Lignocaine (lidocaine)	-
Lorcainide	*Remivox*
Mexiletine	*Mexitil*
Moricizine (ethmo(z/s)ine)	
Pirmenol	-
Procainimide	*Bicoryl, Novacamid, Procamide, Procainamid Duriles, Procainamide Durettes, Procan SR, Procapan, Pronestyl*
Propafenone	-
Quinidine	*Biquin, Cardioquin(e), Chinidin-Duriles, Cin-Quin, Duraquin, Galactoquin, Galatturil-Chinidina, Gluquine, Kiditard, Kinichron, Kinidine Durettes, Kinidin Duriles, Kinilentin, Longachin, Longacor, Naticardina, Natisedina, Natisedine, Neochinidin, Prosedyl, Optochinidin retard, Quinaglute, Quinate, Quincardina, Quinicardine, Quinidex, Quinidoxin, Quini Durules, Quinidurile, Quinobarb, Quinora, Ritmocor, Sedoquin, Systodin*
Tocainide	*Tonocard*

Ajmaline + Lignocaine (Lidocaine) or Quinidine

Abstract/Summary

An isolated report describes cardiac failure in a patient given ajmaline and lignocaine concurrently. Quinidine causes a very considerable increase in the serum levels of ajmaline.

Clinical evidence, mechanism, importance and management

A woman of 67 showed marked aggravation of cardiac failure when treated with ajmaline orally and lignocaine intravenously for repeated ventricular tachycardias.[1] A study in four normal subjects showed that if a single 200 mg oral dose of quinidine was given with a single 50 mg oral dose of ajmaline, the AUC (area under the time-concentration curve) of ajmaline was increased 10- to 30-fold and the maximal serum concentrations increased from 0.018 to 0.141 μg/ml. The reason is not known.[2] The clinical importance of these interactions is uncertain but concurrent use should be well monitored.

References

1 Bleifeld W. Side effects of antiarrhythmics. Naunyn Schmiedbergs Arch Pharmakol (1971) 269, 282–97.
2 Hori R, Okumura K, Inui K-I, Yasuhara M, Yamada K, Sakurai T and Kawai C. Quinidine-induced rise in ajmaline plasma concentration. J Pharm Pharmacol (1984) 36, 205–7.

Amiodarone + Anaesthetics

Abstract/Summary

There is evidence that the presence of amiodarone possibly increases the risk of complications and death during general anaesthesia.

Clinical evidence, mechanism, importance and management

One study reported that there is no increased risk if patients on amiodarone undergo general anaesthesia[1] whereas three others suggest that severe intra-operative complications may occur.[2–4] A comparative retrospective review of patients undergoing cardio-pulmonary bypass surgery (16 patients with and 30 without amiodarone) showed that the incidence of slow nodal rhythm, complete heart block or pacemaker dependency rose from 17 to 66%, intra-aortic balloon pump augmentation was 7% compared with 50%, and low SVR and high cardiac output rose from 0 to 13%. Mortality was 19% in the amiodarone group and 0% in the control group. Fentanyl and diazepam were used for most of the patients, but other anaesthetics included isoflurane, enflurane and halothane. Another study of 37 patients found no problems with eight non-cardiac surgery patients, but 29 cardiac surgery patients had dysrhythmic complications (52%),

sometimes necessitating a pacemaker (24%). One patient had fatal vasoplegia after cardio-pulmonary bypass.[5] The authors of this report note that amiodarone persists in the body for many weeks which complicates any decision to withdraw the drug since there may be risks in delaying surgery. More study is needed.

References

1 Elliott PL, Schauble JF, Rogers MC and Reid PR. Risk of decompensation during anesthesia in the presence of amiodarone. Circulation (1983) 68, Suppl III-280.
2 Gallagher JD, Lieberman RW, Meranze J, Spielman SR and Ellison N. Amiodarone-induced complications during coronary artery surgery. Anesthesiology (1981) 55, 186–8.
3 MacKinnon G, Landymore R and Marble A. Should oral amiodarone be used for sustained ventricular tachycardia in patients requiring open-heart surgery? Can J Surg (1983) 26, 355–7.
4 Liberman BA and Teasdale SJ. Anesthesia and amiodarone. Can Anaesth Soc J (1985) 32, 629–38.
5 Van Dyck M, Baele Ph, Rennotte M Th, Matta A, Dion R and Kestens-Servaye Y. Should amiodarone by discontinued before cardiac surgery? Acta Anaesth Belg (1988) 39, 5–10.

Amiodarone + Beta-blockers

Abstract/Summary

Bradycardia, ventricular fibrillation and asystole have been seen in a few patients on amiodarone when additionally given propranolol or metoprolol.

Clinical evidence

A woman of 64 was treated for hypertrophic cardiomyopathy with amiodarone (1200 mg daily) and atenolol (50 mg daily). Five days later the atenolol was replaced by metoprolol (100 mg daily). Within 3 h she complained of dizziness, weakness and blurred vision. On examination she was found to be pale and sweating with a pulse rate of 20. Her systolic pressure was 60 mmHg. She responded to atropine and isoprenaline (isoproterenol).[1] Another report describes two cases of cardiac arrest in patients on amiodarone shortly after starting to take propranolol.[2] One developed ventricular fibrillation and the other asystole.

Mechanism

Not understood. The clinical picture is that of excessive beta-blockade. A possible explanation is that the amiodarone reduces the metabolism of some beta-blockers (propranolol, metoprolol) thereby markedly increasing their bradycardial effects which are additive with those of amiodarone. The effects of atenolol perhaps remained unaltered because it is largely cleared in the urine unchanged. Other pharmacodynamic effects may also come into play. Increased bradycardia and EEG changes have been seen with amiodarone and practolol.[3]

Importance and management

Concurrent use is not uncommon and may be therapeutically useful but the reports of adverse reactions cited here (they seem to be the only ones so far documented) emphasize the need for caution. Beta-blockers which are extensively metabolized by the liver (e.g. propranolol, metoprolol) may possibly be more risky than those which are not.

References

1 Leor J, Levartowsky D, Sharon C and Farvel Z. Amiodarone and beta-adrenergic blockers: an interaction with metoprolol but not with atenolol. Amer Heart J (1988) 116, 206–7.
2 Derrida JP, Ollagnier J, Benaim R, Haiat R and Chiche P. Amiodarone et propranolol; une association dangereuse? Nouv Presse Med (1979) 8, 1429.
3 Antonelli G, Cristallo E, Cesario S and Calabrese P. Modificazioni elet-trocardiografiche indotte dalla somminstrazione di amiodarone associato a practololo. Boll Soc Ital Cardiol (1973) 18, 236.

Amiodarone + Calcium channel blockers

Abstract/Summary

Sinus arrest and serious hypotension occurred in a woman on diltiazem when given amiodarone.

Clinical evidence, mechanism, importance and management

A woman with compensated congestive heart failure, paroxysmal atrial fibrillation and ventricular arrhythmias was treated with frusemide and 90 mg diltiazem six-hourly. Four days after starting additional treatment with amiodarone, 600 mg 12-hourly, she developed sinus arrest and a life-threatening low cardiac output state (systolic pressure 80 mm Hg) with oliguria. Both drugs were stopped and she was treated with pressor drugs and ventricular pacing. She had previously had no problems on diltiazem or verapamil alone, and later she did well on 400 mg amiodarone daily without diltiazem. The reason for this reaction is thought to be the additive effects of both drugs on myocardial contractility, and on sinus and atrioventricular nodal function.[1] Before this isolated case report was published, another author predicted this interaction on theoretical grounds and warned of the risks if dysfunction of the sinus node such as bradycardia or sick sinus syndrome is suspected, or if partial AV block exists.[2]

References

1 Lee TH, Friedman PL, Goldman L, Stone PH and Antman EM. Sinus arrest and hypotension with combined amiodarone-diltiazem. Am Heart J (1985) 109, 163–4.
2 Marcus FI. Drug interactions with amiodarone. Am Heart J (1983) 106, 924–30.

Amiodarone + Cholestyramine

Abstract/Summary

Cholestyramine binds with amiodarone within the gut and reduces its absorption.

Clinical evidence, mechanism, importance and management

A study on 11 patients showed that when 4 g cholestyramine were given 1.5 h after a single 400 mg dose of amiodarone, the serum amiodarone levels 7 h later were depressed by about 50%. The probable reason is that the cholestyramine binds with the amiodarone in the gut, thereby reducing its absorption.[1] A reduced response to the amiodarone would be expected. It is uncertain whether separating the dosages to avoid mixing the gut is an effective way of preventing this interaction because amiodarone is extensively secreted in the bile.

Reference

1 Nitsch J and Luderitz B. Beschleunigte Elimination von Amiodaron durch Colestyramin. Dtsch med Wochesch (1986) 111, 1241–4.

Amiodarone + Cimetidine

Abstract/Summary

Cimetidine causes a rise in the serum levels of amiodarone.

Clinical evidence

The amiodarone serum levels of 12 patients on long-term treatment (200 mg daily) rose by an average of 38% (from 1.4 to 1.93 μg/ml) when given 1200 mg cimetidine daily for a week. Only 8 of the 12 showed this effect.[1]

Mechanism

Not understood. Cimetidine is a well-recognized enzyme inhibitor which reduces the metabolism of many drugs (and possibly amiodarone) so that they are cleared more slowly.

Importance and management

Information seems to be limited to this study. It would appear to be of clinical importance. Monitor the serum amiodarone levels if cimetidine is started, anticipating a rise. Not all patients appear to be affected. Remember that amiodarone is lost from the body very slowly (half-life 25–100 days) so that the results of the one week study cited here may possibly not adequately reflect the magnitude of this interaction. More study is needed.

Reference

1 Landau S, Tepper D and Somberg J. Cimetidine-amiodarone interaction. J Clin Pharmacol (1988) 28, 909.

Amiodarone + Disopyramide, Propafenone or Mexiletine

Abstract/Summary

The risk of atypical ventricular tachycardia or torsades de pointes seems to be increased if amiodarone is used with these antiarrhythmics.

Clinical evidence, mechanism, importance and management

A very brief report describes the concurrent use of amiodarone and disopyramide, propafenone or mexiletine in four patients, three of whom developed atypical ventricular contractions (AVT or torsades de pointes). Their QT intervals become markedly prolonged (more than 0.50 sec).[1] In another study five patients given amiodarone and disopyramide all had QT intervals of 0.60 sec immediately before developing torsades de pointes.[4] It has been suggested that, in general, class I antiarrhythmics should be avoided or used with caution if amiodarone is also used because of their additive effects in delaying conduction.[1,2] Concurrent use should be very well monitored. Prolongation of the QT interval rather than QT_c or QRS widening is thought to be a warning sign that the treatment needs modification.[4] The successful use of amiodarone (100–600 mg daily) with mexiletine (600 mg daily)[3,5] or disopyramide (300–500 mg daily)[6] has been described.

References

1 Tartini R, Kappenberger L, Steinbrunn W and Meyer UA. Dangerous interaction between amiodarone and quinidine. Lancet (1982) i, 1327–9.
2 Tartini R, Kappenberger L and Steinbrunn W. Gefährliche interaktionen zwischen amiodaron und antiarrhythmika der klass I. Schweiz Med Wsch (1982)
3 Waleffe A, Mary-Rabine L, Legrand V, Demoulin JC and Kulbertus HE. Combined mexiletine and amiodarone treatment of refractory recurrent ventricular tachycardia. Am Heart J (1980) 100, 788–93.
4 Keren A, Tzivoni D, Gavish D, Levi J, Gottlieb S, Benhorin J and Stern S. Etiology, warning signs and therapy of Torsade de Pointes. Circulation (1981) 64, 1167–74.
5 Hoffman A, Follath F and Burckhardt D. Safe treatment of resistant ventricular arrhythmias with combination of amiodarone and quinidine or mexiletine. Lancet (1983) i, 704
6 James MA, Papouchado M and Vann Jones J. Combined therapy with disopyramide and amiodarone: a report of 11 cases. Int J Cardiol (1986) 13, 248–52.

Aprindine + Amiodarone

Abstract/Summary

Serum aprindine levels can be increased by the concurrent use of amiodarone. Toxicity may occur.

Clinical evidence, mechanism, importance and management

Two patients experienced a rise in serum aprindine levels accompanied by signs of toxicity (nausea, ataxia, etc.) when additionally treated with amiodarone. One of them on 100 mg aprindine daily showed a progressive rise in trough serum levels from 2.3 to 3.5 mg/l over a five-week period when given 1200 mg and later 600 mg amiodarone daily. Even when the aprindine dosage was reduced, serum levels remained higher than before beginning the amiodarone.[1] The authors say that those given both drugs need less aprindine than those on aprindine alone. The mechanism of this interaction is not understood. Monitor the effects of concurrent use and reduce the dosage if necessary.

Reference

1 Southworthy W, Friday KJ and Ruffy R. Possible amiodarone-aprindine interaction. Amer Heart J (1982) 104, 323.

Disopyramide or Procainamide + Antacids

Abstract/Summary

There is some inconclusive evidence that aluminium-containing antacids may possibly cause a small reduction in the absorption of these antiarrhythmic agents.

Clinical evidence, mechanism, importance and management

A study in 10 patients showed that an aluminium phosphate antacid had no statistically significant effect on the pharmacokinetics of a single 200 mg oral dose of disopyramide, but did affect the pharmacokinetics of a single 750 mg oral dose of procainamide. However the antacid appeared to reduce the absorption of both antiarrhythmic agents to a some extent in individual subjects.[1] An aluminium hydroxide antacid but not magnesium oxide has also been shown to reduce maximal procainamide serum levels in animals.[2] The clinical importance of these interactions is uncertain but probably small.

References

1 Albin H, Vincon G, Bertolaso D and Dangoumau J. Influence du phosphate d'aluminium sur la biodisponibilie de la procainamide et du disopyramide. Therapie (1981) 36, 541–6.
2 Remon JP, Belpaire F, Van Severen R and Braeckman P. Interaction of antacids with antiarrhythmics.V. Effect of aluminium hydroxide and magnesium oxide on the bioavailability of quinidine, procainamide and propranolol in dogs. Arzneimittel Forsch (1983) 33, 117–120.

Disopyramide + Anticholinergic agents

Abstract/Summary

The anticholinergic effects of disopyramide may be expected to be additive with other drugs possessing anticholinergic activity.

Clinical evidence, mechanism, importance and management

Disopyramide has anticholinergic side-effects. One study on 24 patients reported that eight complained of dry mouth, one of dysuria and one of disturbed accommodation.[1] In another study on 17 patients, four experienced dry mouth and one had difficulty in urinating.[2] Be alert for an increased incidence of anticholinergic side-effects if disopyramide is used with other drugs possessing this activity (e.g. antiparkinson agents, tricyclic antidepressants, antihistamines, anti-emetics, phenothiazines, butyrophenones, thioxanthenes, etc.). See 'Anticholinergics + Anticholinergics'.

References

1 Hartel G, Louhija A and Konttinen A. Disopyramide in the prevention of recurrence of atrial fibrillation after electroconversion. Clin Pharmacol Ther (1974) 15, 551.
2 Vismara LA, Mason DT and Amsterdam EA. Disopyramide phosphate. Clinical efficacy of a new oral anti-arrhythmic agent. Clin Pharmacol Ther (1974) 16, 330.

Disopyramide + Beta-blockers

Abstract/Summary

Four patients treated for supraventricular tachycardia with intravenous disopyramide and practolol or pindolol developed severe bradycardia. One of them died. Other studies on patients and normal subjects suggest that adverse interactions between these drugs may be uncommon.

Clinical evidence

Two patients with supraventricular tachycardia (180 beat/min) were treated firstly with intravenous practolol (20 and 10 mg respectively) and shortly afterwards with disopyramide (150 and 80 mg respectively). The first patient rapidly developed sinus bradycardia of 25 beats/min, lost consciousness and became profoundly hypotensive. He failed to respond to 0.6 mg atropine but later his heart rate increased to 60 while a temporary pacemaker was being inserted.[1] Another patient similarly treated also developed severe bradycardia and asystole, despite the use of atropine. He was resuscitated with adrenaline but later died.[1]

Two other patients have been reported who developed severe bradycardia when treated for supraventricular tachycardia with either practolol[2] or pindolol[3] and disopyramide.

In contrast, studies in healthy subjects have shown that no adverse effects on left ventricular function occur if propranolol and disopyramide are used concurrently,[6,7] nor are the pharmacokinetics of either drug affected.[5] Atenolol (100 mg daily) has been shown to increase the serum disopyramide steady-state levels from 3.46 to 4.25 μg/ml and reduce the clearance of disopyramide in healthy subjects and patients with ischaemic heart disease by 16% (from 1.9 to 1.59 ml/kg/min).[4] None of the subjects developed any adverse reactions or symptoms of heart failure, apart from one of the volunteers who showed transient first degree heart block.[4]

Mechanism

Not understood. Both drugs can depress the contractility and conductivity of the heart muscle.

Importance and management

The general clinical importance of this interaction is uncertain. The only clear risk seems to be in patients who are treated for supraventricular tachycardia with disopyramide and either practolol or pindolol given intravenously. Considerable caution should be exercised in these patients. More study is needed to find out the factors which contribute to the development of this potentially serious interaction.

References

1 Cumming AD and Robertson C. Interaction between disopyramide and practolol. Br Med J (1979) 2, 1264.
2 Gelipter D and Hazell M. Interaction between disopyramide and practolol. Br Med J (1980) 1, 52.
3 Pedersen C, Josephsen P and Lindvig K. Interaktion mellem disopyramide og pindolol efter oral indgift. Ugskr Laeg (1983) 145, 3266–7.
4 Bonde J, Bodtker S, Angelo HR, Svendsen TL and Kampmann JP. Atenolol inhibits the elimination of disopyramide. Eur J Clin Pharmacol (1986) 28, 41–3.
5 Karim A, Nissen C and Azarnoff DL. Clinical pharmacokinetics of disopyramide. J Pharmacokinet Biopharm (1982) 10, 465–94.
6 Cathcart-Rake WF, Coker JE, Atkins FL, Huffman DF, Hassanein KM, Shen DD and Azarnoff DL. The effect of concurrent oral administration of propranolol and disopyramide on cardiac function in healthy men. Circulation (1980) 61, 938–45.
7 Cathcart-Rake WF, Coker JE, Shen D, Huffman D and Azarnoff DL. The pharmacodynamics of concurrent disopyramide and propranolol. Clin Pharmacol Ther (1979) 25, 217.

Disopyramide + Erythromycin

Abstract/Summary

Two patients taking disopyramide developed cardiac arrhythmias when given erythromycin. Disopyramide serum levels were raised.

Clinical evidence

A woman with ventricular ectopy on disopyramide (300 mg alternating with 150 mg six-hourly) developed new arrhythmias (ventricular asystoles and later polymorphic ventricular tachycardia) within 36 h of starting 1 g erythromycin lactobionate IV 6-hourly and cephamandole. Her serum disopyramide level was found to be 16 μmol/l. The problem resolved when the disopyramide was stopped and bretylium given, but it returned when the disopyramide was restarted. It resolved again when the erythromycin was stopped.[1]

Another patient with ventricular tachycardia, well controlled over five years with 200 mg disopyramide four times daily, showed ventricular tachycardia within a few days of starting 500 mg erythromycin base four times daily. His serum disopyramide levels were found to be elevated (30 μmol/l). The problem resolved when both drugs were withdrawn.[1]

Mechanism

Unknown. Erythromycin possibly inhibits the metabolism of the disopyramide by the liver, thereby reducing its loss from the body and increasing its serum levels. Both patients developed high serum disopyramide levels.

Importance and management

Information seems to be limited to these two cases. The effects of concurrent use should be well monitored if erythromycin is added to disopyramide. Be alert for the development of raised serum disopyramide levels. More study is needed.

Reference

1 Ragosta M, Weihl AC and Rosenfeld LE. Potentially fatal interaction between erythromycin and disopyramide. Amer J Med (1989) 86, 465–6.

Disopyramide + Phenobarbitone

Abstract/Summary

Serum disopyramide levels are reduced by the concurrent use of phenobarbitone.

Clinical evidence, mechanism, importance and management

A study in 16 normal subjects showed that after taking 100 mg phenobarbitone daily for 21 days the half-life and AUC (area under the time-concentration curve) of a single 200 mg dose of disopyramide were reduced about 35%. No significant differences were seen between those who smoked and those who did not.[1] It seems that the phenobarbitone (a known enzyme inducing agent) increases the metabolism of disopyramide by the liver, and thereby increases its loss from the body. The extent to which this reduces the control of arrhythmias by disopyramide in patients is unknown but monitor the effects and the serum levels of disopyramide if phenobarbitone is added or withdrawn. Other barbiturates would be expected to interact similarly.

Reference

1 Kapil RP, Axelson JE, Mansfield IL, Edwards DJ, McErlane B, Mason MA, Lalka D and Kerr CR. Disopyramide pharmacokinetics and metabolism: effect of inducers. Br J clin Pharmac (1987) 24, 781–91.

Disopyramide + Phenytoin

Abstract/Summary

Serum disopyramide levels are reduced by the concurrent use of phenytoin and may fall below therapeutic concentrations. Loss of arrhythmic control may occur.

Clinical evidence.

Eight patients with ventricular tachycardia treated with disopyramide (600–2000 mg daily) showed a 54% fall in their serum disopyramide levels (from a mean of 3.99 to 1.82 μg/ml) when concurrently treated with phenytoin (200–600 mg daily) for a week. Two of the patients who were monitored showed a 53- and 2000-fold increase in ventricular premature beat frequency as a result of this interaction.[1]

Falls in serum disopyramide levels (about 30%) which, in some instances, were then below the therapeutic range, have been described in other reports.[2,3,5] A marked fall in serum disopyramide levels (75% in one case) was seen in two patients after taking phenytoin (300–700 mg daily) for up to two weeks.[4] A pharmacokinetic study in normal subjects confirms this interaction.[5]

Mechanism

Phenytoin, which is a known enzyme-inducing agent, increases the metabolism of the disopyramide by the liver. The major metabolite (N-dealkyldisopyramide) also possesses antiarrhythmic activity neverthless the net effect is a reduction in arrhythmic control.[1]

Importance and management

An established interaction of clinical importance. Some loss of arrhythmic control can occur during concurrent use. Serum disopyramide levels and the antiarrhythmic response should be well monitored. An increase in the dosage of disopyramide may be necessary. Serum disopyramide levels return to normal within two weeks of withdrawing the phenytoin.

References

1 Matos JA, Fisher JD and Kim SG. Disopyramide-phenytoin interaction. Clin Res (1982) 29, 655A.
2 Aitio M-L and Vuorenmaa T. Enhanced metabolism and diminished efficacy of disopyramide by enzyme induction. Br J clin Pharmacol (1980) 9, 149–152.
3 Aitio M-L, Mansury L, Tala E, Haataja M and Aitio A. The effect of enzyme induction on the metabolism of disopyramide in man. Br J clin Pharmacol (1981) 279–85.
4 Kessler JM, Keys PW and Stafford RW. Disopyramide and phenytoin interaction. Clin Pharm (1982) 1, 263–4.

5 Nightingale J and Nappi JM. Effect of phenytoin on serum disopyramide concentrations. Clin Pharm (1987) 6, 46–50.

Reference

1 Aito M-L, Mansury L, Tala E, Haataja M and Aitio A. The effect of
enzyme induction on the metabolism of disopyramide in man. Br J clin
Pharmac (1981) 11, 279–85.

Disopyramide + Quinidine

Abstract/Summary

*Disospyramide serum levels may be slightly raised by
quinidine.*

Clinical evidence, mechanism, importance and management

A study in 16 normal subjects showed that in the presence
of quinidine the peak serum levels of disopyramide given as
single 150 mg doses were raised by 20% (from 2.68 to
3.23 µg/ml) and by 14% when given chronically as 150 mg
four times a day. Serum quinidine levels were decreased
26%. The frequency of adverse effects such as dry mouth,
blurred vision, urine retention and nausea were also
somewhat increased. The mechanism of this interaction is not
understood. Concurrent use would generally appear to be
safe except in those whose disopyramide levels are already
in the near-toxic range. The anticholinergic side-effects of
disopyramide may be increased.

Reference

1 Baker BJ, Gammill J, Massengill J, Schubert E, Karin A and Doherty
JE. Concurrent use of quinidine and disopyramide: evaluation of serum
concentrations and electrocardiographic effects. Am Heart J (1983) 105,
12–15.

Disopyramide + Rifampicin

Abstract/Summary

*The serum levels of disopyramide can be markedly reduced by
the concurrent use of rifampicin.*

Clinical evidence, mechanism, importance and management

A study in 12 patients with tuberculosis showed that after
taking rifampicin for 14 days their plasma levels of disopyramide following single 200 or 300 mg doses were approximately halved (AUC's before and after were 20.3 and 8.22 µg
ml^{-1} h respectively; half-life reduced from 5.9 to 3.25 h).[1]
The most probable explanation is that rifampicin markedly
increases the metabolism of the disopyramide by the liver.

Information seems to be limited to this study, but what is
known suggests that the dosage of disopyramide will need
to be increased in patients taking rifampicin. So far there
appear to be no clinical reports of adverse reactions.

Encainide + Diltiazem

Abstract/Summary

*Diltiazem causes a marked increase in the serum levels of en-
cainide but the levels of its active metabolites are only slightly
increased.*

Clinical evidence

A study in six normal subjects (extensive metabolizers) given
25 mg encainide eight-hourly for seven days showed that the
concurrent use of 90 mg diltiazem eight-hourly for seven
days increased the encainide AUC (area under the concentration-time curve) 2–3-fold (from 130 to 333 ng.h/ml), but
the active metabolites of encainide were only slightly increased (+8–10%).[1]

Mechanism

Diltiazem appears to inhibit the metabolism of encainide by
the liver, thereby increasing its serum levels.

Importance and management

Information is very limited. The active metabolites of encainide are largely responsible for its antiarrhythmic effects
and these were little unaffected by this interaction, nevertheless the response should be monitored if diltiazem is
started or stopped. More study is needed. Nifedipine is
reported not to interact.[2] There seems to be no information
about other calcium channel blocking drugs.

References

1 Bottorff MB, Hoon TJ, Lalone RL, Kazierad DJ and Mirvis DM. Effects
of diltiazem on the disposition of encainide and its active metabolites.
Clin Pharmacol Ther (1988) 43, 195.
2 Quart BD, Gallo DG, Sami MH and Wood AJJ. Drug interaction
studies and encainide use in renal and hepatic impairment. Am J Cardiol (1986) 58, 104–113C.

Encainide + Miscellaneous drugs

Abstract/Summary

*No clinically significant interactions have been seen to occur
between encainide and warfarin, acenocoumarol, sulphonylureas, insulin, beta-blockers, nifedipine, diuretics, antipsychotics or amiodarone but the effects of cimetidine should
be monitored.*

Clinical evidence, mechanism, importance and management

A study in 13 normal subjects showed that the concurrent use of 1200 mg cimetidine daily for seven days while taking 75 mg encainide daily increased the AUC (area under the curve) of encainide by 32%, and of two metabolites of encainide (O-demethyl encainide and 3-methoxy-O-demethyl encainide) by 43 and 36% respectively. Although a retrospective evaluation of 33 patients who had had both drugs revealed no evidence of any clinically significant interaction, the authors suggest that if cimetidine is added the effects should be monitored.[1] Retrospective analyses of large numbers of patients taking encainide and warfarin or nicoumalone (78 patients), oral sulphonylureas or insulin (40 patients), beta-blockers (88 patients), nifedipine (24 patients), un-named diuretics (229), and amiodarone and other anti-arrhythmics (118) and un-named antipsychotics (23 patients) revealed no clinically significant interactions.[1] See also 'Encainide + Quinidine'.

Reference

1 Quart BD, Gallo DG, Sami MH and Wood AJJ. Drug interaction studies and encainide use in renal and hepatic impairment. Am J Cardiol (1986) 58, 104–113C.

Encainide + Quinidine

Abstract/Summary

Quinidine causes a marked reduction in the clearance of encainide in those who are extensive metabolizers of encainide.

Clinical evidence

Seven normal subjects who were extensive metabolizers of encainide were given 60 mg encainide orally and 4.5 mg encainide C^{14} intravenously before and after taking 50 mg quinidine six-hourly for five days. The quinidine decreased the systemic clearance from 935 to 190 ml/min and the non-renal clearance from 782 to 95 ml/min. Serum encainide levels were markedly increased and the levels of the active metabolites of encainide were reduced. These changes were reflected to some extent in the ECG measurements made. A parallel study showed that no interaction occurred in four poor metabolizers of encainide.[1]

Mechanism

Quinidine causes a marked reduction in the metabolism of encainide by the liver in extensive metabolizers.

Importance and management

An established interaction and expected to occur in most patients (most people are extensive metabolizers) but its clinical importance is uncertain. Monitor the encainide effects if quinidine is given concurrently, or withdrawn.

Reference

1 Funck-Bretano C, Turgeon J, Woosely RL and Rogen DM. Effect of low dose quinidine on encainide pharmacokinetics and pharmacodynamics. Influence of genetic polymorphism. J Pharmacol Exp Ther (1989) 249, 134–42.

Flecainide + Amiodarone

Abstract/Summary

Serum flecainide levels are increased by the concurrent use of amiodarone. The flecainide dosage should be reduced by a third.

Clinical evidence

Seven patients on oral flecainide (200–500 mg daily) were given reduced doses when amiodarone was added (1200 mg loading doses, later reduced to 600 mg daily) because it was observed that the trough plasma levels of flecainide were increased. The flecainide dosage was reduced by a third (averaging a reduction from 325 to 225 mg daily) to keep the flecainide levels under control. Observations on two patients suggest that the interaction begins soon after the amiodarone is added, and it takes about two weeks to develop fully. Other reports confirm this interaction.[2,3] The authors of these two reports reduced the flecainide dosage by a half, but did not measure plasma levels.

Mechanism

Not understood

Importance and management

An established interaction, but the documentation is limited. A reduction in the flecainide dosage is necessary if the adverse effects of flecainide overdosage are to be avoided. A one third reduction has proved to be satisfactory.[1] Remember that amiodarone is cleared from the body exceptionally slowly so that this interaction may persist for some time after it has been withdrawn.

References

1 Shea P, Roop L, Kim SS, Schechtman K and Ruffy R. Flecainide and amiodarone interaction. J Am Coll Cardiol (1986) 7, 1127–30.
2 Leclerq JF and Coumel P. La flecainide: un nouvel anti-arythmique. Arch Mal Coeur (1983) 76, 1218–30.
3 Fontaine G, Frank R and Tonet JL. Association amiodarone-flecainide dans le traitement des troubles du rythme ventriculaires graves. Arch Mal Coeur (1984) 77, 1421–2.

Flecainide + Cholestyramine

Abstract/Summary

An isolated report describes reduced serum flecainide levels in a patient given cholestyramine. Studies in other subjects failed to demonstrate any interaction.

Clinical evidence, mechanism, importance and management

A patient on 100 mg flecainide twice daily had unusually low trough serum levels (100 ng/ml). When he stopped taking cholestyramine (4 g three times daily) his plasma flecainide levels rose. However a later study on three normal subjects given 100 mg flecainide and 4 g cholestyramine three times daily, found little or no evidence of an interaction (steady-state flecainide levels of 63.1 and 59.1 ng/ml without and with cholestyramine). *In vitro* studies also failed to demonstrate any binding between flecainide and cholestyramine which might result in reduced absorption from the gut.

Information seems to be limited to this report. Its general importance seems to be small, nevertheless the outcome of concurrent use should be monitored so that unusual cases like this can be identified.

Reference

1 Stein H and Hoppe U. Is there an interaction between flecainide and cholestyramine? Naunyn-Schmiedbergs Arch Pharmakol (1989) 339 (Suppl) R114.

Flecainide + Cimetidine

Abstract/Summary

Some preliminary evidence indicates that cimetidine can increase flecainide serum levels.

Clinical evidence, mechanism, importance and management

A study in eight normal subjects given single 200 mg oral doses of flecainide showed that after taking 1 g cimetidine daily for a week the flecainide serum levels were raised 28% and clearance was reduced 27%. The results suggested that the cimetidine reduced both the renal clearance and the metabolism of the flecainide by the liver.[1-3] The clinical importance of these findings is uncertain but be alert for the need to reduce the flecainide dosage if cimetidine is added. More study is needed.

Reference

1 Tjandra Maga TB, Verbesselt R, Van Hecken A, Van Melle P and De Schepper PJ. Oral flecainide elimination kinetics: effects of cimetidine. Circulation (1983) 68, Supp III-416.
2 Tjandra Maga TB, Van Hecken A, Van Melle P, Verbesselt R and De

Schepper PJ. Altered pharmacokinetics of oral flecainide by cimetidine. Br J clin Pharmac (1986) 22, 108–110.
3 Verbesselt R, Tjandra Maga TB, Van Hecken A, Van Melle P and De Schepper PJ. Effects of cimetidine on the elimination of oral flecainide. Eur Heart J (1984) 5, 136.

Flecainide + Food or Antacids

Abstract/Summary

The absorption of flecainide is not significantly altered if taken with food or an aluminium hydroxide antacid in adults, but it may possibly be reduced by milk in infants.

Clinical evidence, mechanism, importance and management

Studies in normal adult subjects showed that the neither food nor 15 ml of *Aludrox* (280 mg aluminium hydroxide per 5 ml) had any significant effect on the absorption of a single 200 mg dose of flecainide.[1] No special precautions seem necessary if taken together. However a premature baby being treated for refractory atrio-ventricular tachycardia with high doses of flecainide (40 mg/kg daily or 25 mg six-hourly) developed flecainide toxicity (seen as ventricular tachycardia) when his milk feed was replaced by 5% dextrose. His serum flecainide levels approximately doubled, the conclusion being drawn that the milk had reduced the absorption.[2] Milk-fed infants on high doses may therefore possibly need a reduced flecainide dosage if milk is reduced of stopped. Monitor the effects.

Reference

1 Tjandra-Maga TB, Verbesselt R, Van Hecken A, Mullie A and De Schepper PJ. Flecainide: single and multiple oral dose kinetics, absolute bioavailability and effect of food and antacid in man. Br J clin Pharmac (1986) 22, 309–16.

Flecainide + Quinine

Abstract/Summary

Quinine reduces the metabolism of flecainide.

Clinical evidence, mechanism, importance and management

A study in four subjects showed that a single 500 mg dose of quinine increased the AUC (area under the concentration/time curve) of a single 150 mg IV dose of flecainide by 23% (from 189 to 232 mg.min/l) and reduced the systemic clearance by 19% (from 793 to 646 ml/min). Renal clearance remained unchanged.[1] It would seem that quinine reduces the metabolism of flecainide. The clinical importance of this interaction is uncertain. More study is needed.

Reference

1 Munafo A, Reymond G and Borgeat J. Influence of quinine administration on flecainide kinetics. Clin Res (1988) 36, 368A.

Flecainide + Tobacco smoking

Abstract/Summary

Tobacco smokers need larger doses of flecainide than non-smokers to achieve the same therapeutic effects.

Clinical evidence

Prompted by the chance observation that smokers appeared to have a reduced pharmacodynamic response to flecainide than non-smokers, a large-scale analysis (described as meta-analysis) was undertaken of the findings of seven pharmacokinetic studies[2-4] and five multicentre efficacy trials[5] in which flecainide had been studied and in which the smoking habits of the subjects had been also been recorded: a total of 338 smokers and 288 non-smokers. This meta-analysis confirmed that smokers needed higher doses of flecainide to achieve the same steady-state serum levels. Trough serum plasma concentrations (ng/ml/mg dose) were 1.74 for the smokers and 2.18 for the non-smokers.[1]

Mechanism

The probable reason is that some components of the tobacco smoke stimulate the cytochrome P-450s in the liver concerned with the O-dealkylation of flecainide so that it is cleared from the body more quickly.

Importance and management

An established interaction. Anticipate the need to give smokers higher doses of flecainide than non-smokers to achieve the required therapeutic response.

References

1 Holtzman JL, Weeks CE, Kvam DC, Berry DA, Mottonen L, Ekholm BP, Chang SF and Conard GJ. Identification of drug interactions by meta-analysis of premarketing trials: The effect of smoking on the pharmacokinetic and dosage requirements of flecainide acetate. Clin Pharmacol Ther (1989) 46, 1–8.
2 Holtzman JL, Kvam DC, Berry DA, Borrell G, Harrison LI and Conard GJ. The pharmacodynamic and pharmacokinetic interaction of flecainide acetate with propranolol: effects on cardiac function and drug clearance. Eur J Clin Pharmacol (1987) 33, 97–9.
3 Conard GJ and Ober RE. Metabolism of flecainide. Am J Cardiol (1984) 53, 41–51B.
4 Holtzman JL, Finley D, Mottonen L, Berry DA, Ekholm BP, Kvam DC, McQuinn RL and Miller AM. The pharmacodynamic and pharmacokinetic interaction between single doses of flecainide acetate and verapamil: effects on cardiac function and drug clearance. Clin Pharmacol Ther (1989) 46, 26–32.
5 Morganroth J, Anderson JL and Gentzkow GD. Classification by type of ventricular arrhythmia predicts frequency of adverse cardiac events from flecainide. J Am Coll Cardiol (1986) 8, 607–15.

Lignocaine (Lidocaine) + Barbiturates

Abstract/Summary

Serum lignocaine levels following intravenous infusion may be lower in those who are taking barbiturates.

Clinical evidence

Two tests were carried out on seven epileptic patients: firstly while taking their usual anti-epileptic drugs and/sedatives (phenytoin, barbiturates, phenothiazines, benzodiazepines) and the other after taking only 300 mg phenobarbitone daily for four weeks. It was found that the phenobarbitone treatment caused a small increase (10–25%) in serum lignocaine levels given by infusion (2 mg/kg) but all of the levels were up to 40% lower at 30 and 60 min than in the six control subjects who had not received any drugs.[1]

In a study in *dogs*, four out of six given lignocaine in therapeutic doses died from respiratory arrest when concurrently given a 30 mg/kg pentobarbitone infusion over 1 min. The other two showed apnoea.[2]

Mechanism

Not fully understood. One suggestion is that the barbiturates increase the activity of the liver microsomal enzymes, thereby increasing the rate of metabolism of the lignocaine.[1] The death of the dogs appeared to result from the additive depressant effects of the two drugs on the respiratory centre.

Importance and management

Direct information is very limited but the interaction in man appears to be established. It may be necessary to increase the dosage of lignocaine to achieve the desired therapeutic response in patients on phenobarbitone or other barbiturates. The clinical importance of the serious interaction seen in dogs is uncertain.

References

1 Heinonen J, Takki S and Jarho L. Plasma lidocaine levels in patients treated with potential inducers of microsomal enzymes. Acta anaesth Scandinav (1970) 14, 89–95.
2 LeLorier J. Lidocaine and pentobarbital: a potentially lethal drug-drug interaction. Toxicol Appl Pharmacol (1978) 44, 657.

Lignocaine (Lidocaine) + Beta-blockers

Abstract/Summary

The serum levels of lignocaine can be increased by the concurrent use of propranolol. Two cases of toxicity attributed to this interaction have been reported. Nadolol possibly interacts similarly, but there is uncertainty about metoprolol. Atenolol and pindolol appear not to interact but an increased loading dosage of lignocaine in the presence of penbutolol has been suggested.

Clinical evidence

(a) Lignocaine + atenolol, penbutolol, pindolol

Studies with atenolol (50 mg daily),[5] pindolol and penbutolol[6] found that these beta-blockers appear not to affect the clearance of lignocaine, but the volume of distribution of penbutolol was altered so that it is possible that a higher loading dose of lignocaine may be needed.[6]

(b) Lignocaine + metoprolol

A single dose study in normal subjects given 100 mg metoprolol twice daily for two days showed that it did not affect the pharmacokinetics of lignocaine,[7] and another study in seven normal subjects failed to find any changes in the pharmacokinetics of lignocaine after one week's treatment with metoprolol (100 mg 12-hourly).[5] In contrast another study found that lignocaine clearance was reduced 31% by metoprolol.[9]

(c) Lignocaine + nadolol

A study in six normal subjects receiving 30-h infusions of lignocaine (2 mg/min) showed that three days' pretreatment with 160 mg nadolol daily raised the steady-state serum lignocaine levels by 28% (from 2.1 to 2.7 μg/ml) and reduced the plasma clearance by 17% (from 1030 to 850 ml/min).[1]

(d) Lignocaine + propranolol

A study on six normal subjects receiving 30-h infusions of lignocaine (2 mg/min) showed that three days' pretreatment with propranolol (80 mg eight-hourly) raised the steady-state serum lignocaine levels by 19% (from 2.1 to 2.5 μg/ml) and reduced the plasma clearance by 15% (1030 to 866 ml/min).[1] Other studies found a 30%[8] and a 22.5%[2] increase in steady-state serum lignocaine levels and a 46%[9] fall in plasma clearance due to the concurrent use of propranolol. Two cases of lignocaine toxicity attributed to lignocaine–propranolol interaction occur in the FDA adverse drug reaction file.[10]

(e) Lignocaine + un-named beta-blockers

A matched study in 50 patients showed that concurrent use of lignocaine and beta-blockers decreased arrhythmias and increased lignocaine toxicity, the mean serum lignocaine levels being raised by 39% (from 3.6 to 5.0 μg/ml).[3]

Mechanism

Not fully agreed. There is some debate about whether the increased serum lignocaine levels largely occurs because of the decreased cardiac output caused by the beta-blockers which decreases the flow of blood through the liver thereby reducing the metabolism of the lignocaine,[1] or because of direct liver enzyme inhibition.[4]

Importance and management

The lignocaine–propranolol interaction is established and of clinical importance. Monitor the effects of concurrent use and reduce the lignocaine dosage if necessary to avoid toxicity. The situation with other beta-blockers is less clear. Nadolol appears to interact like propranolol, but it is uncertain whether metoprolol interacts or not. Atenolol, penbutolol and pindolol are reported not to interact, although it has been suggested that a higher loading dose (but not a higher maintenance dose) of lignocaine may be needed if penbutolol is used.[6] The suggestion has been made that a significant interaction is only likely to occur with non-selective beta-blockers without intrinsic sympathomimetic activity.[4] Until the situation is better defined it would seem prudent to monitor the effects of concurrent use with any beta-blocker.

References

1 Schneck DW, Luderer JR, Davis D and Vary J. Effects of nadolol and propranolol on plasma lidocaine clearance. Clin Pharmacol Ther (1984) 36, 584–7.
2 Svendsen TL, Tango M, Waldorff S, Steiness E and Trap-Jensen J. Effects of propranolol and pindolol on plasma lignocaine clearance. Br J clin Pharmac (1982) 13, 223–6S.
3 Wyse DG, Kellen J, Tam Y and Rademaker AW. Increased efficacy and toxicity of lidocaine in patients on beta-blockers. Circulation (1986) 74, II-43.
4 Bax NDS, Tucker GT, Lennard MS and Woods HF. The impairment of lignocaine clearance by propranolol—major contribution from enzyme inhibition. Br J clin Pharmac (1985) 19, 597–603.
5 Miners JO, Wing LMH, Lillywhite KJ and Smith KJ. Failure of 'therapeutic' doses of beta-adrenoceptor antagonists to alter the disposition of tolbutamide and lignocaine. Br J clin Pharmac (1984) 18, 853–60.
6 Ochs HR, Skanderra D, Abernethy DR and Greenblatt DJ. Effect of penbutolol on lidocaine kinetics. Arzneim-Forsch/Drug Res (1983) 33, 1680–1.
7 Jordo L, Johnsson G, Lundborg P and Regardh C-G. Pharmacokinetics of lidocaine in healthy individuals pretreated with multiple dose of metoprolol. Int J Clin Pharmacol Ther Tox (1984) 22, 312–15.
8 Ochs HR, Carstens G and Greenblatt DJ. Reduction of lidocaine clearance during continuous infusion and by co-administration of propranolol. N Engl J Med (1980) 303, 373.
9 Conrad KA, Byers JM, Finley PR and Burnham L. Lidocaine elimination: effects of metoprolol and of propranolol. Clin Pharmacol Ther (1983) 33, 133–8.
10 Graham CM, Turner WM and Jones JK. Lidocaine-propranolol interactions. N Engl J Med (1981) 304, 1301.

Lignocaine (Lidocaine) + Cimetidine

Abstract/Summary

Cimetidine reduces the clearance of lignocaine and raises serum levels in some patients. Lignocaine toxicity may occur if the dosage is not reduced. Ranitidine appears to interact minimally.

Clinical evidence

(a) Studies with cimetidine in patients

15 patients were given 1 mg/kg lignocaine IV followed by a constant infusion of 2 or 3 mg/min until steady-state serum levels were established. 6 h later they were started on cimetidine (initial dose 300 mg IV, then 300 mg six-hourly by mouth). After 12 h the lignocaine serum levels of 14 of the 15 had risen by an average of 75% (to 5.6 μg/ml) but only a 30% increase when compared with the control group (4.3 μg/ml). Six patients developed toxic serum levels (+ 5 μg/ml) and two experienced lethargy and confusion attributable to toxicity which disappeared when the lignocaine was stopped.[1]

A study in patients with suspected myocardial infarction given two 300 mg oral doses of cimetidine 4 h apart, starting 11–20 h after a 2 mg/min infusion of lignocaine began, showed that total lignocaine serum levels had risen by 28% after 24 h and unbound levels by 18%. In three of these patients whose diagnosis was subsequently confirmed, rises in total and unbound lignocaine serum levels of 24% and 9% occurred by 24 h.[3] In contrast, a study in six patients with suspected myocardial infarction given lignocaine infusions, followed later by a cimetidine infusion, failed to find a significant increase in the plasma accumulation of lignocaine.[6]

(b) Studies with cimetidine in normal subjects

A rise in peak serum lignocaine levels of 50% was seen in a study in six normal subjects given 300 mg cimetidine six-hourly for a day. Systemic clearance fell by 35% (from 766 to 576 ml/min) and five of the six experienced toxicity.[2] 18 normal subjects taking 1 g cimetidine daily for three days showed a 21% fall in lignocaine clearance.[4] A 30% fall in lignocaine clearance was described in another study in seven normal subjects.[5] In another study on six normal subjects the lignocaine clearance under steady-state conditions was reduced 34%.[7]

(c) Studies with ranitidine in normal subjects

A study in 10 normal subjects given 150 mg ranitidine twice daily for five days showed that it increased the systemic clearance of lignocaine (given orally or intravenously) by 9%.[8] Another study in six normal subjects given the same dose of ranitidine for one day found no change in the clearance of lignocaine given intravenously.[9]

Mechanism

Not established. It seems possible that the metabolism of the lignocaine is reduced both by a fall in blood flow to the liver and by direct inhibition of the activity of the liver microsomal enzymes. As a result its clearance is reduced and its serum levels rise.

Importance and management

The lignocaine–cimetidine interaction is well studied but controversial. It is confused by the differences between the studies (healthy subjects, patients with different diseases, different modes of drug administration, etc.). A fall in the clearance of lignocaine (35% or more) and a resultant rise in the serum levels should be looked for if cimetidine is used, but a clinically significant alteration may not occur in every patient. It may possibly be of less importance in patients following a myocardial infarction because of the increased amounts of alpha-1-acid glycoprotein which alters the levels of bound and free lignocaine.[3] Monitor all patients closely for evidence of toxicity and check serum lignocaine levels regularly. A reduced infusion rate may be needed. Ranitidine would appear to be a suitable alternative for cimetidine.

References

1 Knapp AB, Maguire W, Keren G, Karmen A, Levitt B, Miura DS and Somberg JC. The cimetidine-lidocaine interaction. Ann Intern Med (1983) 98, 174–7.
2 Feeley J, Wilkinson GR, McAllister CB and Wood AJJ. Increased toxicity and reduced clearance of lidocaine by cimetidine. Ann Intern Med (1982) 96, 592–4.
3 Berk SI, Gal P, Bauman JL, Douglas JB, McCue JD and Powell JR. The effect of oral cimetidine on total and unbound serum lignocaine concentrations in patients with suspected myocardial infarction. Int J Cardiol (1987) 14, 91–4.
4 Wing LMH. Miners JO, Birkett DJ, Foenander T, Lillywhite K and Wanwimolruk S. Lidocaine disposition—sex differences and effects of cimetidine. Clin Pharmacol Ther (1984) 35, 695–701.
5 Bauer LA, Edwards WAD, Randolph FP and Blouin RA. Cimetidine-induced decrease in lidocaine metabolism. Am Heart J (1984) 108, 413–15.
6 Patterson JH, Foster J, Powell JR, Cross R, Wargin W and Clark JL. Influence of a continuous cimetidine infusion on lidocaine plasma concentrations in patients. J Clin Pharmacol (1985) 25, 607–9.
7 Powell JR, Foster J, Patterson JH, Cross R and Wargin W. Effect of duration of lidocaine infusion and route of cimetidine administration on lignocaine pharmacokinetics. Clin Pharm (1986) 5, 993–8.
8 Robson RA, Wing LMH, Miners JO, Lilleywhite KJ and Birkett DJ. The effect of ranitidine on the disposition of lignocaine. Br J clin Pharmac (1985) 20, 170–3.
9 Feeley J and Guy E. Lack of effect of ranitidine on the disposition of lignocaine. Br J clin Pharmac (1983) 15, 378–9.

Lignocaine (Lidocaine) + Disopyramide

Abstract/Summary

Laboratory studies show that disopyramide can increase the levels of unbound lignocaine, but whether in practice their combined effects have a clinically important depressant effect on the heart is not known.

Clinical evidence

An *in vitro* study using serum taken from nine patients receiving lignocaine for severe ventricular arrhythmias showed that there was an average 20% increase in its free (unbound) fraction when disopyramide in a concentration of 14.7 μmol/l was added.

Mechanism

Disopyramide can displace lignocaine from its binding sites on plasma proteins (alpha-1-acid glycoprotein).

Importance and management

The importance of this displacement interaction in clinical practice uncertain. The suggestion made by the authors of the study is that a transient 20% increase in levels of free and active lignocaine plus the negative inotropic effects of the disopyramide might possibly be hazardous in patients with reduced heart function. More study is needed.

Reference

1 Bonde J, Jensen NM, Burgaard P, Angelo HR, Graudal N, Kampmann JP and Pedersen LE. Displacement of lidocaine from human plasma proteins by disopyramide. Pharmacol Toxicol (1987) 60, 151–5.

Lignocaine (Lidocaine) + Morphine

Abstract/Summary

Morphine given as an intravenous bolus does not alter lignocaine serum levels given as a continuous intravenous infusion.

Clinical evidence, mechanism, importance and management

A controlled study in 10 subjects who were receiving continuous lignocaine infusions during suspected myocardial infarction found that a 10 mg IV morphine sulphate bolus did not significantly alter the steady-state serum levels of lignocaine (about 2.45 μg/ml).[1]

Reference

1 Vacek JL, Wilson DB, Hurwitz A, Gollub SB and Dunn MI. The effect of morphine sulphate on serum lidocaine levels. Clin Res (1988) 36, 325A.

Lignocaine (Lidocaine) + Phenytoin

Abstract/Summary

The incidence of central toxic side-effects may be increased following the concurrent intravenous infusion of lignocaine and phenytoin. Sinoatrial arrest has been reported in one patient. In patients taking phenytoin as an anticonvulsant, serum lignocaine levels are slightly reduced when given intravenously, but markedly reduced if given orally.

Clinical evidence

(a) Cardiac depression and increased side-effects

A study in five patients given 0.5–3.0 mg/min lignocaine intravenously for at least 24 h, followed by additional intravenous infusions of phenytoin, showed that serum levels of both drugs remained normal and unchanged but the incidence of side-effects (vertigo, nausea, nystagmus, diplopia, impaired hearing) were unusually high.[4]

Sinoatrial arrest occurred in a man following a suspected myocardial infarction with heart block, after receiving 1 mg/kg lignocaine infused intravenously in 1 min, followed 3 min later by 250 mg phenytoin over 5 min. The patient lost consciousness and his blood pressure could not be measured, but he responded to 200 μg isoprenaline.[1]

(b) Reduced serum lignocaine levels

A study found that the clearance of intravenous lignocaine is slightly greater in patients taking anticonvulsants than in normal subjects (0.85 compared with 0.77 l/min) but this difference was not statistically significant.[2] Other studies in epileptic patients and normal subjects showed that when taking phenytoin the bioavailability of lignocaine (lidocaine) given *orally* was halved.[2,3]

Mechanisms

(a) Phenytoin and lignocaine appear to have additive depressant actions on the heart. (b) The reduced lignocaine serum levels is possibly due to liver enzyme induction; when given orally the marked reduction results from the stimulation of hepatic first-pass metabolism phenytoin.[2,3]

Importance and management

Information is limited and the importance of the interactions is not well established. (a) The case of sinoatrial arrest emphasizes the need to exercise caution when giving two drugs which have depressant actions on the heart. (b) The reduction in serum lignocaine levels given intravenously to patients taking anticonvulsants, including phenytoin, is small and appears not to be of any clinical significance. Since lignocaine is not usually given orally, the practical importance of the marked reduction in bioavailability would also seem to be small.

References

1 Wood RA. Sinoatrial arrest: an interaction between phenytoin and lignocaine. Br Med J (1971) 645.
2 Perucca E and Richens A. Reduction of oral bioavailability of lignocaine by induction of first pass metabolism in epileptic patients. Br J clin Pharmac (1979) 8, 21–31.
3 Perucca E, Hedges A, Makki KA and Richens A. A comparative study of antipyrine and ligocaine disposition in normal subjects and in patients treated with enzyme-inducing drugs. Br J clin Pharmac (1980) 10, 491–7.
4 Karlsson E, Collste P and Rawlins ML. Plasma levels of lidocaine during combined treatment with phenytoin and procainamide. Europ J clin Pharmacol (1974) 7, 455

Lignocaine (Lidocaine) + Procainamide

Abstract/Summary

An isolated case of delerium has been described in a patient given lignocaine and procainamide.

Clinical evidence, mechanism, importance and management

A man with paroxysmal tachycardia, under treatment with oral procainamide and increasing doses of lignocaine by intravenous infusion, became restless, noisy and delerious when given a further intravenous dose of procainamide.[1] The reason is not understood but the symptoms suggest that the neurotoxic effects of the two drugs might be additive. Other studies in patients have shown that lignocaine plasma levels are unaffected by procainamide.[2]

References

1 Ilyas M, Owens D and Kvasnicka G. Delerium induced by a combination of anti-arrhythmic drugs. Lancet (1969) ii, 1368.
2 Karlsson E, Collste P and Rawlins MD. Plasma levels of lidocaine during combined treatment with phenytoin and procainamide. Eur J clin Pharmacol (1974) 7, 455.

Lignocaine (Lidocaine) + Tocainide

Abstract/Summary

An isolated report describes a tonic-clonic seizure in a man which occurred during the period when his treatment for arrhythmia with lignocaine was being changed for tocainide.

Clinical evidence, mechanism, importance and management

An elderly man treated with frusemide and co-trimoxazole experienced a tonic-clonic seizure while his treatment with lignocaine was being changed to tocainide, although the serum levels of both antiarrhythmics remained within their therapeutic ranges. The patient became progressively agitated and disorientated about 2 h after taking the second of two 600 mg (six-hourly) oral doses of tocainide while still receiving 2 mg/min lignocaine IV, and about 1 h later he had the seizure. The patient subsequently tolerated each drug separately at concentrations similar to those which preceded the seizure without problems.[1] The reason for this reaction is not understood.

Reference

1 Forrence E, Covinsky JO and Mullen C. A seizure induced by concurrent lidocaine-tocainide therapy—Is it just a case of additive toxicity? Drug Intell Clin Pharm (1986) 20, 56–9.

Lorcainide + Rifampicin

Abstract/Summary

A report describes a marked reduction in serum lorcainide concentrations and failure to control ventricular tachycardia in a man treated with rifampicin.

Clinical evidence, mechanism, importance and management

A 62-year-old on 600 mg rifampicin daily for tuberculosis had his treatment for ventricular tachycardia changed from lignocaine to lorcainide. It was found necessary to given him three times the normal dosage (800–900 mg daily instead of 200–300 mg) to control his condition and to achieve satisfactory serum levels (0.29 μg/ml). The likely reason is that the rifampicin (a known, potent enzyme inducing agent) increased the metabolism of the lorcainide by the liver, thereby hastening its loss from the body and reducing the serum levels.[1] This seems to be the first and only report of this interaction, but be alert for it in any patient receiving these drugs and anticipate the need to increase the lorcainide dosage.

Reference

1 Mauro VF, Somani P and Temesy-Armos PN. Drug interaction between lorcainide and rifampicin. Eur J Clin Pharmacol (1987) 31, 737–8.

Mexiletine + Antacids, Urinary acidifiers and Alkalinizers

Abstract/Summary

Changes in urinary pH caused by the concurrent use of acidifying or alkalinizing drugs do not normally have a marked effect on the plasma levels of mexiletine, but a few patients may be affected. The absorption is unaltered by the concurrent use of Gelusil.

Clinical evidence, mechanism, importance and management

Mexiletine is normally largely cleared from the body by liver metabolism[1] and only about 10% is excreted unchanged in the urine. Although changes in urinary pH can affect the amounts lost in the urine,[2,3,5] alterations brought about by diet or the concurrent use of alkalinizers or acidifiers (antacids, acetazolamide, etc.) would not be expected to have a marked effect on the plasma concentrations of mexiletine in most patients. There appear to be no reports of adverse interactions but concurrent use should be monitored. A single dose study showed that the bioavailability of mexiletine was unchanged by *Gelusil*.[4]

References

1 Beckett AH and Chidomere EC. The distribution, metabolism and excretion of mexiletine in man. Postgrad Med J (1977) 53 (Suppl 1) 60–6.
2 Kiddie MA, Kaye CM and Turner P. The influence of urinary pH on the elimination of mexiletine. Br J clin Pharmac (1974) 1, 229–32.
3 Johnston A, Burgess CD, Warrington SJ, Wadsworth J and Hamer NAJ. The effect of spontaneous changes in urinary pH on mexiletine plasma concentrations and excretion during chronic administration to healthy volunteers. Br J clin Pharmac (1979) 8, 349–52.
4 Herzog P, Holtermuller KH, Kasper W, Meinertz T, Trenk D and Jahnchen E. Absorption of mexiletine after treatment with gastric antacids. Br J clin Pharmac (1982) 14, 746–7.

5   Mitchell BG, Clements JA, Pottage A and Prescott LF. Mexiletine
    disposition: individual variation in response to urine acidification and
    alkalinization. Br J clin Pharmac (1983) 16, 281–4.

Mexiletine + Antiarrhythmic drugs

Abstract/Summary

*The concurrent use of mexiletine and either propranolol or
quinidine is reported to be beneficial, and side-effects may be
reduced. The same is possibly also true for amiodarone.*

Clinical evidence, mechanism, importance and management

A study in patients showed that a combination of mexiletine
and propranolol (240 mg daily) was more effective in blocking ventricular premature depolarizations (VPD) and ventricular tachycardia, without significant side effects, than
mexiletine alone.[1] A statistical decrease in VPDs in a considerable number of patients given combined treatment is
described elsewhere.[2] Mexiletine and quinidine given concurrently are reported to be more effective than quinidine
alone, and the incidence of side-effects is reduced.[3]

References

1   Leahey EB, Heissenbuttel RH, Giardina EGV and Bigger JT. Combined
    mexiletine and propranolol treatment of refractory ventricular tachycar-
    dia. Br Med J (1980) 281, 357.
2   Quoted as unpublished data by Bigger JT. The interaction of mexiletine
    with other cardiovascular drugs. Am Heart J (1984) 107, 1079–85.
3   Duff HJ, Roden D, Primm RK, Oates JA and Woosley RL. Mexiletine
    in the treatment of resistant ventricular arrhythmias: enhancement of
    efficacy and reduction of dose-related side effects by combination with
    quinidine. Circulation (1983) 67, 1124.

Mexiletine + Cimetidine or Ranitidine

Abstract/Summary

*No adverse interaction occurs if mexiletine and cimetidine or
ranitidine are given concurrently. Cimetidine can reduce the
gastric side-effects of mexiletine.*

Clinical evidence, mechanism, importance and management

A study in 11 patients showed that their peak and trough
serum mexiletine levels were unaltered when given
cimetidine, 1 g daily for a week, and the frequency and
severity of the ventricular arrhythmias for which they were
receiving treatment remained unchanged. Moreover the
gastric side effects of mexiletine were reduced in half of the
patients.[1] This study in patients confirms two other single-
dose studies[2,3] using cimetidine and ranitidine in normal
subjects. There would seem to be no problems with giving
these drugs concurrently, and some advantages.

References

1   Klein AL and Sami MH. Usefulness and safety of cimetidine in
    patients receiving mexiletine for ventricular arrhythmia. Am Heart
    J (1985) 109, 1281.
2   Klein A, Sami M and Selinger K. Mexiletine kinetics in healthy sub-
    jects taking cimetidine. Clin Pharmacol Ther (1985) 37, 669–73.
3   Brockmeyer NH, Breithaupt H, Hattingberg MV and Ohnhaus EE.
    Metabolism of mexiletine alone and in combination with cimetidine
    and ranitidine *in vivo* and *in vitro*. Br J clin Pharmac (1987) 39, 246P.

Mexiletine + Diamorphine or Morphine

Abstract/Summary

*The absorption of mexiletine is depressed in patients follow-
ing a myocardial infarction, and very markedly depressed and
delayed if diamorphine or morphine are used concurrently. This
can limit its value as an antiarrhythmic agent during the first
few hours following an infarction.*

Clinical evidence

A pharmacokinetic study in patients and normal subjects
showed that the serum levels of mexiletine (400 mg orally
followed by 200 mg 2 h later) in patients who had had a
myocardial infarction and who had been given diamorphine
(5–10 mg) or morphine (10–15 mg) were reduced as
follows: at 2 h to 33%; 3 h 40%; 4 h 53%; 6 h 70% and 8 h
80%. The peak concentrations in the subjects and the patients
occurred at 3 and 6 h respectively.[1,2]

Mechanism

The reduced absorption of mexiletine would seem to result
from inhibition by the narcotics of gastric emptying. Other
mechanisms probably contribute to its delayed clearance.

Importance and management

An established interaction although information is limited.
The delay and reduction in the absorption would seem to
limit the value of oral mexiletine during the first few hours
after a myocardial infarction, particularly if these narcotic
analgesics are used.

References

1   Prescott LF, Pottage A and Clements JA. Absorption, distribution and
    elimination of mexiletine. Postgrad Med J (1977) 53 (Suppl 1) 50–5.
2   Pottage A, Campbell RWF, Achuff SC, Murray A, Julian DC and
    Prescott LF. The absorption of oral mexiletine in coronary care patients.
    Eur J clin Pharmac (1978) 13, 393–9.

Mexiletine + Phenytoin

Abstract/Summary

Serum mexiletine levels are reduced by the concurrent use of phenytoin. An increase in the dosage may be necessary.

Clinical evidence

The observation of three patients who had unusually low serum mexiletine levels while taking phenytoin, prompted a pharmacokinetic study in six normal subjects. After taking 300 mg phenytoin daily for a week, the mean area under the mexiletine plasma concentration/time curve and its half-life following single 400 mg doses were reduced by an average of about 50% (AUC reduced from 17.7 to 8.0 μg/ml/h; half-life reduced from 17.2 to 8.4 h).[1]

Mechanism

The most likely explanation is that phenytoin, a potent liver enzyme-inducing agent, increases the metabolism and clearance of mexiletine from the body.

Importance and management

Information seems to be limited to this report,[1] but the interaction appears to be established. It seems possible that the fall in mexiletine levels will be clinically important in some individuals. Monitor the serum mexiletine levels and raise the dosage if necessary.

Reference

1 Begg EJ, Chinwah PM, Day RO and Wade DN. Enhanced metabolism of mexiletine after phenytoin administration. Br J clin Pharmac (1982) 14, 219–23.

Mexiletine + Rifampicin (Rifampin)

Abstract/Summary

The clearance of mexiletine from the body is increased by the concurrent use of rifampicin. An increase in the dosage of mexiletine may be necessary.

Clinical evidence, mechanism, importance and management

A pharmacokinetic study on eight normal subjects showed that after taking 600 mg rifampicin daily for 10 days, the half-life of a single 400 mg dose of mexiletine was reduced by 40% (from 8.5 to 5 h).[1,2] The probable reason is that the rifampicin (a known, potent enzyme-inducing agent) increases the metabolism and clearance of the mexiletine from the body. It seems likely that the mexiletine dosage will need to be increased during concurrent use, but by how much is uncertain. More study is needed to confirm the clinical importance of this interaction.

References

1 Pentikainen PJ, Koivula IH and Hiltunen HA. Effect of enzyme induction on pharmacokinetics of mexiletine. Clin Pharmacol Ther (1982) 31, 260.
2 Pentikainen PJ, Koivula IH and Hiltunen HA. Effect of rifampicin treatment on the kinetics of mexiletine. Eur J Clin Pharmacol (1982) 23, 261–6.

Moricizine (Ethomozine) + Cimetidine

Abstract/Summary

Cimetidine increases the serum levels of moricizine.

Clinical evidence, mechanism, importance and management

A study in eight normal subjects showed that seven days' treatment with 300 mg cimetidine four times daily halved the clearance of a single 500 mg dose of moricizine (from 38.2 to 19.7 ml/kg/min) and increased both its half-life (from 3.3 to 4.6 h) and the AUC (from 5.6 to 7.8 μg.ml/h). Despite the increase in serum moricizine levels, the PR and QRS intervals were not further prolonged. It is believed that the moricizine serum levels rise because the cimetidine reduces its metabolism by the liver.[1] Concurrent use should be well monitored to ensure that the increased serum moricizine levels do not result in toxicity. Reduce the dosage as necessary.

Reference

1 Biollaz J, Shaheen O and Wood AJJ. Cimetidine inhibition of moricizine metabolism. Clin Pharmacol Ther (1985) 37, 665–8.

Pirmenol + Rifampicin (Rifampin)

Abstract/Summary

Rifampicin markedly increases the loss of pirmenol from the body. A reduction in its antiarrhythmic effects is likely to occur.

Clinical evidence

A study in 12 normal subjects showed that 14 days' treatment with 600 mg rifampicin daily markedly affected the pharmacokinetics of a single 150 mg dose of pirmenol. The apparent plasma clearance increased sevenfold (from 12.8 to 88.2 l/h) and the AUC (area under the curve) decreased 83% (from 13.34 to 2.28 mg/h/l).[1,2]

Mechanism

The probable reason is that the rifampicin (a well-recognized enzyme inducer) increases the metabolism of the pirmenol by the liver, thereby increasing its loss from the body.

Importance and management

Direct information seems to be limited to this study but what occurred is consistent with the way rifampicin interacts with other drugs. Anticipate the need to increase the dosage of pirmenol if rifampicin is used concurrently.

References

1 Stringer KA, Thomas RW, Cetnarowski AB and Goldfarb AL. Effect of rifampin on the disposition of pirmenol. J Clin Pharmacol (1987) 27, 709.
2 Stringer KA, Cetnarowski AB, Goldfarb AB, Lebsack ME, Chang TS and Allen J. Enhanced pirmenol elimination by rifampin. J Clin Pharmacol (1988) 28, 1094–7.

Procainamide + Amiodarone

Abstract/Summary

Serum procainamide levels are increased by about 60% and of N-acetylprocainamide by about 30% if amiodarone is given concurrently. Reduce the dosage of procainamide to avoid toxicity.

Clinical evidence

A study in 12 patients stabilized on procainamide (2–6 g daily, or about 900 mg six-hourly) showed that when concurrently treated with amiodarone (600 mg loading dose 12-hourly for 5–7 days, then 600 mg daily) their mean serum procainamide levels rose by 57% (from 6.8 to 10.6 μg/ml) and their serum N-acetylprocainamide (NAPA) levels rose by 32% (from 6.9 to 9.1 μg/ml). Procainamide levels increased by more than 3.0 μg/ml in six patients. The increases usually occurred within 24 h, but in other patients as late as four or five days. Toxicity was seen in two patients. Despite lowering the procainamide dosages by 20%, serum procainamide levels were still higher (at 7.7 μg/ml) than before the amiodarone was started.[1]

An increase of 35% in trough serum procainimide level was seen in four other patients after four days treatment with amiodarone, 6–15 μg/kg.[2]

Mechanism

Not understood.

Importance and management

Information appears to be limited to these studies, but the interaction would seem to be established and clinically important. Its incidence is high (11 out of 12 in the report cited[1]), and it develops rapidly. The dosage of procainamide may need to be reduced 30–50% if amiodarone is given. Serum levels should be monitored and patients observed for side effects.[1]

References

1 Saal AK, Werner JA, Greene HL, Sears GK and Graham EL. Effect of amiodarone on serum quinidine and procainamide levels. Am J Cardiol (1984) 53, 1265–7.
2 Windle JR, Prystowsky EN, Miles WM, Zipes DP and Heger JJ. Pharmacokinetic and pharmacodynamic interaction of amiodarone and procainamide. J Am Coll Cardiol (1985) 5, 481.

Procainamide + Beta-blockers

Abstract/Summary

The pharmacokinetics of procainamide are little changed by either propranolol or metoprolol.

Clinical evidence, mechanism, importance and management

One study in six normal subjects found that long-term treatment with propranolol (period and dosage not stated) increased the procainamide half-life from 1.71 to 2.66 h and reduced the plasma clearance by 16%.[1] However a later study in eight normal subjects showed that the pharmacokinetics of a single 500 mg dose of procainamide hydrochloride were only slightly altered by the concurrent use of either 80 mg propranolol three times daily or 100 mg metoprolol twice daily. The procainamide half-life increased from 1.9 to 2.2 h with propranolol and to 2.3 h with metoprolol, but no significant changes in total clearance occurred. No changes in the AUC of N-acetyl procainamide were seen.[2] It seems unlikely that a clinically important adverse interaction normally occurs between these drugs. There seems to be no information about other beta-blockers.

References

1 Weidler DJ, Gang DC, Jalad NS and McFarland MA. The effect of long-term propranolol on the pharmacokinetics of procainamide in humans. Clin Pharmacol Ther (1981) 29, 289.
2 Ochs HR, Carstens G, Roberts G-M and Greenblatt DJ. Metoprolol or propranolol does not alter the kinetics of procainamide. J Cardiovasc Pharmacol (1983) 5, 392–5.

Procainamide + Cimetidine or Ranitidine

Abstract/Summary

Serum procainimide levels can be increased if cimetidine is given concurrently and toxicity may develop particularly in those who have a reduced renal clearance such as the elderly. Ranitidine appears not to interact significantly.

Clinical evidence

(a) Cimetidine

An elderly man developed procainamide toxicity when given 1200 mg cimetidine daily and it was necessary roughly to halve the procainamide dosage (from 937 to 500 mg daily) to bring the serum levels of procainamide and N-acetylprocainamide into the accepted therapeutic range.[2]

A study in six normal subjects showed that after taking 1 g cimetidine for a day the AUC (area under the curve) of a 1 g oral dose of procainamide was increased by 35% (from 27 to 36.5 μg/ml/h) and the elimination half-life was prolonged from 2.9 to 3.8 h.[1,3] Another study in normal subjects also found that cimetidine inhibited the loss of procainamide through the kidneys by 35%.[4] A study in six normal subjects found a steady-state serum level increase of 45% when given 1200 mg cimetidine daily.[6]

(b) Ranitidine

A study using ranitidine showed that ranitidine reduced the absorption of procainamide from the gut and reduced the kidney excretion,[5] whereas no change in the pharmacokinetics of procainamide by ranitidine was found in another study.[6]

Mechanism

Procainamide levels in the body are increased because the cimetidine virtually halves its excretion by the kidney[1] but the precise mechanism is uncertain. One suggestion is that it interferes with the active secretion of procainamide by the kidney tubules.[3,4]

Importance and management

The procainamide–cimetidine interaction is established. Concurrent use should be undertaken with care because the safety margin of procainamide is low. Reduce the dosage as necessary. This is particularly important in the elderly because they have a reduced ability to clear both drugs. Ranitidine appears not to interact significantly.

References

1 Somogyi A and Heinzow B. Cimetidine reduces procainamide elimination. N Engl J Med (1982) 307, 1080.
2 Higbee MD, Wood JS and Mead RA. Case report. Procainamide-cimetidine interaction. A potential toxic interaction in the elderly. J Am Geriatr Soc (1984) 32, 162–4.
3 Somogyi A, McLean A and Heinzow B. Cimetidine-procainamide pharmacokinetic interaction in man: evidence of competition for tubular secretion of basic drugs. Eur J Clin Pharmacol (1983) 25, 339–45.
4 Christian CD, Meredith CG and Speeg KV. Cimetidine inhibits renal procainamide clearance. Clin Pharmacol Ther (1984) 36, 221–7.
5 Somogyi A and Bochner F. Dose and concentration dependent effect of ranitidine on procainamide disposition and renal clearance in man. Br J clin Pharmac (1984) 18, 175–81.
6 Paloucek F, Rodvold K, Jang D and Gallestegui J. The effects of cimetidine and ranitidine on steady-state pharmacokinetics of procainamide. J Clin Pharmacol (1986) 26, 557.

Procainamide + Para-aminobenzoic acid (PABA)

Abstract/Summary

A single case report shows that para-aminobenzoic acid can reduce the metabolism of procainamide, increase its serum levels and reduce the production of N-acetylprocainamide.

Clinical evidence, mechanism, importance and management

A 61-year-old man, treated with procainamide for sustained ventricular tachycardia, was found to be a rapid acetylator of procainamide so that the serum levels of the procainamide metabolite (N-acetylprocainamide) were particularly high and he experienced some N-acetylprocainamide toxicity (this metabolite has some anti-arrhythmic properties but can also be toxic). When he was additionally given 1.5 g PABA six-hourly for 30 h to suppress the production of this metabolite, the control of his arrhythmia improved.[1]

In this instance the interaction was exploited for the patient's benefit as part of an experimental study, but it draws attention to the possibility of increased procainamide levels in other patients concurrently treated with PABA. The importance of this is uncertain but the outcome should be monitored if PABA is added or withdrawn.

Reference

1 Nylen ES, Cohen AI, Wish MH, Lima JL and Finkelstein JD. Reduced acetylation of procainamide by para-aminobenzoic acid. J Amer Coll Cardiol (1986) 7, 185–7.

Procainamide + Quinidine

Abstract/Summary

A single case report describes a marked increase in the serum procainamide levels of a patient when concurrently treated with quinidine.

Clinical evidence, mechanism, importance and management

A man with sustained ventricular tachycardia on high dose intravenous procainamide (2 g eight-hourly) showed a 70% increase (a rise from 9.1 to 15.4 ng/ml) in his steady-state serum procainamide levels when concurrently treated with 324 mg quinidine gluconate eight-hourly. The procainamide half-life increased from 3.7 to 7.2 h and its clearance fell from 27 to 16 l/h. The mechanism of interaction suggested by the authors of the report is that the quinidine interferes with one or more of renal pathways by which procainamide is cleared from the body.[1] Information so far seems to be limited to this report but it would seem prudent to monitor the effects if high-dose procainamide is given with quinidine. More study is needed to find out the general importance of this interaction.

Reference

1   Hughes B, Dyer JE and Schwartz AB. Increased procainamide plasma concentrations caused by quinidine: a new drug interaction. Am Heart J (1987) 114, 908–9.

Procainamide + Trimethoprim

Abstract/Summary

Trimethoprim causes a marked increase in the serum levels of procainamide and its active metabolite, N-acetyl procainamide.

Clinical evidence

A study in eight normal subjects given 500 mg procainamide six-hourly for three days showed that the concurrent use of 200 mg trimethoprim daily increased the AUC (area under the time/concentration curve from 0 to 12 h) of procainamide by 63% and of its active metabolite, N-acetyl procainamide, by 51%. Another study found that 200 mg daily reduced the renal clearance of procainamide by 45% and of N-acetyl procainamide by 26%.[2]

Mechanism

The reason would appear to be that the trimethoprim decreases losses in the urine of both procainamide and its active metabolite by successfully competing for active secretion. It may also cause a small decrease in the metabolism of the procainamide.[1]

Importance and management

An established interaction but its documentation is limited. The need to reduce the procainamide dosage should be anticipated if trimethoprim is given to patients already controlled on procainamide. The daily dosage of trimethoprim in co-trimoxazole (trimethoprim 160 mg + sulphamethoxazole 800 mg) may equal or exceed the dosages used in the study cited.

References

1   Kosoglou T, Rocci ML and Vlasses PH. Evaluation of trimethoprim/procainamide interaction at steady-state in normal volunteers. Clin Pharmacol Ther (1988) 43, 131.
2   Vlasses PH, Kosoglou T, Chase SL, Greenspon AJ, Lottes S, Andress E, Ferguson RK and Rocci ML. Trimethoprim inhibition of the renal clearance of procainamide and N-acetylprocainamide. Arch Intern Med (1989) 149, 1350–3.

Propafenone + Cimetidine

Abstract/Summary

Cimetidine appears not to interact adversely with propafenone.

Clinical evidence, mechanism, importance and management

A study in 12 normal subjects given 225 mg propafenone eight-hourly showed that the concurrent use of 400 mg cimetidine eight-hourly caused some changes in the pharmacokinetics and pharmacodynamics of the propafenone. Raised peak and steady-state serum levels were seen but these were not statistically significant. A slight increase in the QRS duration also occurred.[1] None of the changes seems likely to be clinically important.

Reference

1   Pritchett ELC, Smith WM and Kirsten EB. Pharmacokinetic and pharmacodynamic interactions of propafenone and cimetidine. J Clin Pharmacol (1988) 28, 619–24.

Propafenone + Miscellaneous drugs

Abstract/Summary

Propafenone can oppose the effects of anticholinesterases used for myasthenia gravis and have anticholinergic effects which may possibly be additive with other anticholinergic drugs. Shortness of breath and a worsening of the control of asthma have also been reported.

Clinical evidence, mechanism, importance and management

Propafenone is reported to aggravate myasthenia gravis, possibly due to its anticholinergic effects on nicotinic receptors on skeletal muscle. This was seen in a patient well controlled on pyridostigmine. Improvement occurred when the propafenone was withdrawn. Other cases have also been described. Avoidance of concurrent use has been advised.[1] Propafenone also has other anticholinergic effects (constipation, dry mouth, blurred vision)[1] which may possibly be additive with other drugs possessing anticholinergic effects (e.g. tricyclic antidepressants). Shortness of breath and a worsening of asthma have also been reported in a handful of cases, attributed to the beta-blocking effects of propafenone. Caution is advised in those with chronic airways disease,[1] but see also 'Beta-blockers + Propafenone'.

Reference

1   Committee on the Safety of Medicines (CSM) Current Problems Series, No 29, August (1990).

Propafenone + Quinidine

Abstract/Summary

Quinidine doubles the serum levels of propafenone and halves the levels of its active metabolite in 'extensive' metabolizers, but the antiarrhythmic effects remain unaffected.

Clinical evidence

Nine patients on propafenone for frequent isolated ventricular ectopic beats firstly had their dosage reduced to 150 mg eight-hourly and then four days later 50 mg quinidine daily was added.

Four days later the steady-state serum propafenone levels in seven patients ('extensive' metabolizers) had more than doubled (from 408 to 1096 ng/ml) but the ECG intervals and arrhythmia frequency were unaltered. The steady-state serum propafenone levels remained unchanged in the other two patients ('poor' metabolizers).[1]

Mechanism

Quinidine inhibits the metabolism (cytochrome P450-dependent 5-hydroxylation) of propafenone by the liver in those who are 'extensive' metabolizers so that it is cleared more slowly. Its serum levels are doubled as a result, but the overall antiarrhythmic effects remain effectively unchanged because the production of its active antiarrhythmic metabolite (5-hydroxypropafenone) is simultaneously halved.[1] Whether one is an 'extensive' or a 'poor' metabolizer is genetically predetermined.

Importance and management

An established interaction but apparently of little clinical importance, however until these results have been confirmed concurrent use should be well monitored. The patients described had their propafenone dosage approximately halved before the study began. The metabolic status of patients seems in this instance not to be important.

Reference

1 Funck-Bretano C, Kroemer HK, Pavlou H, Woosley RL and Roden DM. Genetically determined interaction between propafenone and low dose quinidine: role of active metabolites in modulating net drug effect. Br J clin Pharmac (1989) 27, 435–44.

Quinidine + Amiodarone

Abstract/Summary

Serum quinidine levels can be approximately doubled by the concurrent use of amiodarone. Reduce the quinidine dosage appropriately to avoid quinidine toxicity and the risk of atypical ventricular tachycardia (AVT or torasades de pointes).

Clinical evidence

A study in 11 patients stabilized on quinidine (daily doses of 4200–1200 mg) showed that when concurrently treated with amiodarone (600 mg loading dose 12-hourly for 5–7 days, then 600 mg daily) their mean serum quinidine levels rose by an average of 32% (from 4.4 to 5.8 μg/ml). Three of the patients showed a substantial increase (+2.0 μg/ml). Signs of toxicity (diarrhoea, nausea, vomiting, hypotension, etc.)

were seen in some patients and the quinidine dosage was reduced in 9 of the 11 by an average of 37%. Even so, the quinidine serum levels were still higher (at 5.2 μg/ml) than before the amiodarone was started.

A test on a normal subject showed that when 600 mg amiodarone was added to a daily quinidine dosage of 1200 mg, the serum quinidine levels doubled within three days and the QT interval was prolonged from 1.0 (no drugs) to 1.2 (on quinidine alone) to 1.4 (on quinidine and amiodarone).[2] This report describes two patients with minor heart arrhythmias which developed into atypical ventricular tachycardia (AVT or 'torsades de pointes') when given both drugs.[2]

Mechanism

Not understood.

Importance and management

An established and clinically important interaction. It appears to occur in most patients, and to develop rapidly. It has been recommended that the dosage of quinidine should be reduced 30–50% if amiodarone is given, the serum levels should be monitored and patients observed closely for side-effects.[1] It has also been suggested that the ECG should be monitored for evidence of a prolongation of the QT interval.[2] An uncorrected QT interval greater than 0.60 sec may be an indication that the patient runs the risk of developing atypical ventricular tachycardia.[3] Successful and uneventful concurrent use is described in a report of patients on quinidine (dose not stated) and 200 mg amiodarone five times weekly.[4]

References

1 Saal AK, Werner JA, Greene HL, Sears GK and Graham EL. Effect of amiodarone on serum quinidine and procainamide levels. Am J Cardiol (1984) 53, 1265–7.

2 Tartini R, Kappenberger L, Steinbrunn W and Meyer UA. Dangerous interaction between amiodarone and quinidine. Lancet (1982) i, 1327–9.

3 Keren A, Tzivoni D, Gavish D, Levi J, Gottlieb S, Benhorin J and Stern S. Etiology, warning signs and therapy of Torsade de Pointes. Circulation (1981) 64, 1167–74.

4 Hoffman A, Follath F and Burckhardt D. Safe treatment of resistant ventricular arrhythmias with a combination of amiodarone and quinidine or mexiletine. Lancet (1983) i, 704.

Quinidine + Anticonvulsants

Abstract/Summary

Serum quinidine levels can be reduced by the concurrent use of phenytoin, phenobarbitone or primidone. Loss of arrhythmia control is possible if the quinidine dosage is not increased.

Clinical evidence

When two patients appeared to have an increased quinidine clearance when given phenytoin and primidone, further study was made in four normal subjects. After two weeks treatment with either phenytoin or phenobarbitone (in dosages adjusted to give 10–20 μg/ml) the elimination half-life of a single 300 mg dose of quinidine was reduced by about 50% and the total area under the time-concentration curve by about 60%.[1]

Similar results were found in another study in three normal subjects.[2] This interaction was observed in a patient with recurrent ventricular tachycardia.[3] Changes in quinidine levels due to pentobarbitone have been described in another report.[4] An estimated 70% reduction in the half-life of quinidine as a result of adding phenytoin to concurrent treatment with phenobarbitone is described in a three-year-old child.[5] Difficulty in achieving adequate serum quinidine levels has been reported in a woman on phenytoin and primidone. Her quinidine half-life was approximately halved.[6]

Mechanism

The evidence suggests that phenytoin, primidone or phenobarbitone (all known enzyme-inducing agents) increase the metabolism by the liver of the quinidine and increase its loss from the body.

Importance and management

An established interaction of clinical importance although the documentation is not great. The concurrent use of phenytoin, primidone, phenobarbitone or any other barbiturate need not be avoided but be alert for the need to increase the quinidine dosage. If the anticonvulsants are withdrawn the quinidine dosage may need to be reduced to avoid quinidine intoxication. Quinidine serum levels should be monitored.

References

1   Data JL, Wilkinson GR and Nies AS. Interaction of quinidine with anticonvulsant drugs. N Engl J Med (1976) 294, 699.
2   Russo ME, Russo J, Smith RA and Pershing LK. The effect of phenytoin on quinidine pharmacokinetics. Drug Intell Clin Pharm (1982) 16, 480.
3   Urbano AM. Phenytoin-quinidine interaction in a patient with recurrent ventricular tachyarrhythmias. N Engl J Med (1983) 308, 225.
4   Chapron DJ, Mumford D and Pitegoff GJ. Apparent quinidine-induced digoxin toxicity after withdrawal of pentobarbital. A case of sequential drug interactions. Arch Intern Med (1979) 139, 363.
5   Rodgers GC and Blackman MS. Quinidine interaction with anticonvulsants. Drug Intell Clin Pharm (1983) 17, 819–20.
6   Kroboth FJ, Kroboth PD and Logan T. Phenytoin-theophylline-quinidine interaction. N Engl J Med (1983) 308, 725.

Quinidine + Aspirin

Abstract/Summary

A patient and two normal subjects given quinidine and aspirin showed a two- to threefold increase in bleeding times. The patient bled.

Clinical evidence, mechanism, importance and management

A patient with a prolonged history of paroxysmal atrial tachycardia was given quinidine (800 mg daily) and aspirin (325 mg twice daily). After a week he showed generalized petechiae and blood in his faeces. His prothrombin and partial prothrombin times were normal but the template bleeding time was more than 35 min (normal 2–10 min). Further study in two normal subjects showed that quinidine alone (975 mg daily for five days) and aspirin alone (650 mg three times a day for five days) prolonged bleeding times by 125% and 163% respectively; given together the bleeding times were prolonged by 288%.[1] The underlying mechanism is not totally understood but it is believed to be the outcome of the additive effects of two drugs, both of which can reduce blood platelet aggregation.

This seems to be the only study of this adverse interaction, but what is known from other studies about the effects of both drugs on platelet function when given alone supports this report. Concurrent use in other patients should be well monitored to check that bleeding does not occur.

Reference

1   Lawson D, Mehta J, Mehta P, Lipman BC and Imperi GA. Culmulative effects of quinidine and aspirin on bleeding time and platelet alpha-2-adrenoceptors: potential mechanism of bleeding diathesis in patients receiving this combination. J Lab Clin Med (1986) 108, 581–6.

Quinidine + Beta-blockers

Abstract/Summary

Normally an advantageous interaction. Relatively modest doses of quinidine and propranolol can control atrial fibrillation in patients resistant to high doses of quinidine. Propranolol serum levels are raised. An isolated report describes a patient on quinidine who developed marked bradycardia (36 beats/min) when using timolol eye drops. Another describes orthostatic hypotension with quinidine and propranolol.

Clinical evidence

(a) Advantageous interactions

A man with atrial fibrillation of 10 year's duration which was totally resistant to large doses of quinidine, returned to sinus rhythm after treatment with 80 mg propranolol daily for 10 days, to which was then added 0.2 g quinidine three times a day. He was later maintained on the same dose of quinidine with only 20 mg propranolol.[1]

Similar successes with combined treatment are described elsewhere: 9 out of 10 responded favourably in one study,[2] 34 out of 48 in another,[3] and 13 out of 17 in yet another.[4]

A pharmacokinetic study showed that concurrent use can double the AUC (area under the concentration-time curve) and the peak serum levels of propranolol. Maximum heart rates during exercise were significantly more suppressed.[5] Peak serum quinidine levels were found in one study to be raised by over 50% and its clearance reduced by almost 40% by the presence of propranolol,[6] but this was not confirmed in two other studies.[7,8]

(b) Adverse interactions

An elderly man who for six months had been uneventfully taking 500 mg quinidine three times a day for atrial premature beats, was hospitalized with dizziness after starting to use 0.5% timolol eye drops for open-angle glaucoma. He was found to have a sinus bradycardia of 36 beats/min. The symptoms abated when the drugs were withdrawn and normal sinus rhythm returned after 24 h. The same symptoms developed within 30 h of re-starting concurrent use, but disappeared when the quinidine was withdrawn.[7] In another report a man on quinidine and propranolol is described who felt dizzy and faint when standing, which worsened with exercise but disappeared when sitting or lying down.[10]

Mechanism

Both propranolol and quinidine increase the refractory period and reduce the conduction velocity of heart muscle. Together they appear to be better than quinidine alone in the control of arrhythmias. Just why quinidine increases propranolol serum levels is not understood. The adverse quinidine–timolol interaction possibly arose because the negative chronotropic effects of the quinidine and the timolol-induced reduction in sinus rates were additive.[9] Other unidentified factors may also have had a part to play.

Importance and management

The propranolol-quinidine is normally an advantageous interaction. Combined use can be exploited in the treatment of atrial fibrillation. Prescribers who intend to use quinidine and timolol eye drops concurrently should be aware of the adverse interaction report cited above, and of the possibility of orthostatic hypotension.

References

1 Stern S. Synergistic action of propranolol with quinidine. Am Heart J (1962) 72, 569.
2 Stern S and Borman JB. Early conversion of atrial fibrillation after open-heart surgery by combined propranolol and quinidine treatment. Isr J med Sci (1969) 5, 102.
3 Fors WJ, Vanderark CR and Reynolds JW. Evaluation of propranolol and quinidine in the treatment of quinidine-resistant arrhythmias. Amer J Cardiol (1971) 27, 190.
4 Stern S. Conversion of chronic atrial fibrillation to sinus rhythm witha combined propranolol and quinidine treatment. Amer Heart J (1967) 74, 170.
5 Sakurai T, Kawai C, Yasuhara M, Okumura K and Hori R. Increased plasma concentration of propranolol by a pharmacokinetic interaction with quinidine. Jap Circ J (1983) 47, 872.
6 Kessler KM, Humphries WC, Black M and Spann JF. Quinidine pharmacokinetics in patients with cirrhosis or receiving propranolol. Amer Heart J (1978) 96, 627–35.
7 Kates RE and Blandford MF. Disposition kinetics of oral quinidine when administered concurrently with propranolol. J Clin Pharmacol (1979) 19, 378.
8 Fenster P, Perrier D, Mayersohn M and Marcus FI. Kinetic evaluation of the propranolol-quinidine combination. Clin Pharmacol Ther (1980) 27, 450–3.
9 Dinai Y, Sharir M, Naveh (Floman) N and Halkin H. Bradycardia induced by interaction between quinidine and ophthalmic timolol. Ann Intern Med (1985) 103, 890–1.
10 Loon NR, Wilcox CS and Folger W. Orthostatic hypotension due to quinidine and propranolol. Am J Med (1986) 81, 1101–4.

Quinidine + Calcium channel blockers

Abstract/Summary

Four patients have been described whose quinidine serum levels were depressed when concurrently treated with nifedipine, and which doubled when the nifedipine was withdrawn. In contrast, verapamil reduces the clearance of quinidine and in one patient the serum quinidine levels doubled. He experienced quinidine toxicity. Acute hypotension has also been seen in three patients on quinidine when given verapamil intravenously. Diltiazem appears not to interact.

Clinical evidence

(a) Diltiazem

A study in 10 normal subjects given 0.6 mg quinidine twice daily and 120 mg diltiazem daily for seven days showed that the pharmacokinetics of neither drug was affected by the presence of the other.[4]

(b) Nifedipine

Two patients taking 300–400 mg quinidine six-hourly and 10 mg nifedipine six or eight-hourly showed a doubling of their serum quinidine levels (from 2–2.5 to 4.6 μg/ml and from 1.8–1.6 to 3.5 μg/ml respectively) when the nifedipine was withdrawn. The increased serum quinidine levels were reflected in a prolongation of the QT_c interval. Four other patients failed to demonstrate this interaction.[1]

Two other reports describe the same response:[2,3] the quinidine serum level doubled in one patient when the nifedipine was stopped,[2] and in the other it was found difficult to achieve adequate serum quinidine levels during concurrent use, even when the quinidine dosage was increased threefold. When the nifedipine was withdrawn, the quinidine levels rose once again.[3] A study in 12 patients found that no significant change occurred in serum quinidine levels in the group as a whole when given nifedipine, but one patient showed a 41% decrease.[8]

(c) Verapamil

A cross-over study in six normal subjects showed that after taking 80 mg verapamil daily for three days the clearance of a single 400 mg dose of quinidine was decreased by 32% (from 17 to 11.69 l/h) and the half-life was increased by 35% (from 6.87 to 9.29 h).[5]

A patient given 648 mg quinidine bisulphate six-hourly showed an increase in serum levels from 2.3 to 5.6 μg/ml when given 80 mg verapamil eight-hourly for a week. He became dizzy and had blurred vision. In a subsequent study in this patient it was found that the verapamil halved the quinidine clearance and almost doubled the serum half-life.[6] Three other patients given quinidine orally showed marked hypotension (falls in systolic pressures to 80 and 60 mm Hg were seen in two patients, and in the other patient a systolic/diastolic pressure fall from 130/70 to 80/50 mm Hg) when given verapamil intravenously.[7]

Mechanism

Not understood. One suggestion is that the quinidine-nifedipine interaction is due to changes in cardiovascular haemodynamics.[1] The quinidine–verapamil interaction is possibly due to an inhibitory effect of verapamil on the metabolism of quinidine. The marked hypotension[7] observed may be related to the antagonistic effects of the two drugs on catecholamine-induced alpha-receptor induced vasoconstriction.

Importance and management

The quinidine–nifedipine interaction is established and clinically important but its incidence seems to be small. Concurrent use should be well monitored. An increase in the dosage of quinidine may be needed. What is known about the quinidine–verapamil interaction suggests that a reduction in the dosage of the quinidine may be needed to avoid toxicity. If the verapamil is given intravenously, be alert for evidence of acute hypotension. Monitor the effects of concurrent use closely. No interaction apparently occurs between quinidine and diltiazem.

References

1 Farringer JA, Green JA, O'Rourke RA, Linn WA and Clementi WA. Nifedipine-induced alterations in serum quinidine concentrations. Am Heart J (1984) 108, 1570–2.
2 Van Lith RM and Appleby DH. Quinidine-nifedipine interaction. Drug Intell Clin Pharm (1985) 19, 829–30.
3 Green JA, Clementi WA, Porter C and Stigelman W. Nifedipine-quinidine interaction. Clin Pharm (1983) 2, 461–5.
4 Matera MG, De Santis D, Vacca C, Fici F, Romano AR, Marrazzo R and Marmo E. Quinidine-diltiazem: pharmacokinetic interaction in humans. Curr Ther Res (1986) 40, 653–6.
5 Lavoie R, Blevins RD, Rubenfire M and Edwards DJ. The effect of verapamil on quinidine pharmacokinetics in man. Drug Intell Clin Pharm (1986) 20, 457.
6 Trohman RG, Estes DM, Castellanos A, Palomo AR, Myerburg RJ and Kessler KM. Increased plasma concentrations during administration of verapamil; a new quinidine-verapamil interaction. Am J Cardiol (1986) 57, 706–7.
7 Maisel AS, Motulsky HJ and Insel PA. Hypotension after quinidine plus verapamil. Possible additive competition at alpha-adrenergic receptors. N Engl J Med (1985) 312, 167–70.
8 Munger MA, Jarvis RC, Nair R, Kasmer RJ, Nara AR, Urbanic A and Green JA. Elucidation of the nifedipine–quinidine interaction. Clin Pharmacol Ther (1989) 45, 411–16.

Quinidine + Cimetidine and Ranitidine

Abstract/Summary

Quinidine serum levels can rise and intoxication may develop in some patients when concurrently treated with cimetidine. An isolated case of ventricular bigeminy occurred in a patient on quinidine and ranitidine.

Clinical evidence

A study in six normal subjects showed that 1200 mg cimetidine for seven days prolonged the elimination half-life of a single dose of quinidine by 55% (from 5.8 to 9.0 h). Peak serum levels were raised by 21%. These changes were reflected in ECG changes (+50% and +28% respectively in the mean areas under the Q-T and $Q-T_c$ time curves), but these were said not to be statistically significant.[1]

A later study, prompted by the observation of two patients who developed toxic quinidine levels when given cimetidine, found essentially the same. The AUC and half-life of quinidine were increased by 14.5 and 22.6% respectively, and the clearance was decreased by 25%.[2] A study in four normal subjects found that 1200 mg cimetidine daily for five days prolonged the elimination half-life of quinidine by 54% and decreased the body clearance by 36%. Cimetidine prolonged the QT by 30% above quinidine's effect alone.[5,6] Another single case report describes marked increases in both quinidine and digoxin concentrations in a woman when given cimetidine.[3] Ventricular bigeminy occurred in a man on quinidine when given ranitidine. His serum quinidine levels remained unchanged.[4]

Mechanism

It is believed[2] that the cimetidine depresses the metabolism of the quinidine by the liver so that it is cleared more slowly, as a result its effects are increased.

Importance and management

This interaction is established and of clinical importance. The incidence is unknown. Be alert for changes in the response to quinidine if cimetidine is started or stopped. Ideally the quinidine serum levels should be monitored and the dosage reduced as necessary. Reductions of 25% (oral) and 35% (intravenous) have been recommended.[6] Those at greatest risk are likely to be patients with impaired liver function, the elderly and those with serum quinidine levels already at the top end of the range.[2] The situation with ranitidine is uncertain.

References

1 Hardy BG, Zador IT, Golden L, Lalka D and Schentag JJ. Effect of cimetidine on the pharmacokinetics and pharmacodynamics of quinidine. Amer J Cardiol (1983) 52, 172–5.
2 Kolb KW, Garnett WR, Small RE, Vetrovec GW, Kline BJ and Fox T. Effect of cimetidine on quinidine clearance. Ther Drug Monitor (1984) 6, 306–12.
3 Polish LB, Branch RA and Fitzgerald GA. Digitoxin-quinidine inter-

action: potentiation during administration of cimetidine. South Med J (1981) 74, 633–4.

4 Iliopoulou A, Kontogiannis D, Tsoutsos D and Moulopoulos S. Quinidine-ranitidine adverse reaction. Eur Heart J (1986) 7, 360.

5 Boudoulas H, MacKichan JJ and Schall SF. Effect of cimetidine on quinidine pharmacokinetics and pharmacodynamics. Clin Res (1987) 35, 874A.

6 MacKichan JJ, Boudoulas H and Schaal SF. Effect of cimetidine on quinidine bioavailability. Biopharm Drug Dis (1989) 10, 121–5.

Quinidine + Kaolin-pectin

Abstract/Summary

There is some evidence that kaolin-pectin can reduce the absorption of quinidine and lower serum levels.

Clinical evidence, mechanism, importance and management

A study in four normal subjects showed that when given 30 ml of *Kaopectate* (kaolin + pectin) the maximal salivary quinidine concentration after a single 100 mg oral dose was reduced by 54% and the AUC (area under the curve) by 58%.[1] There is a correlation between salivary and serum concentrations after a single dose of the drug.[2] This is consistent with an *in vitro* study in which 40 ml of a 40 mg/100 ml solution were mixed with 1 g kaolin. The amount of quinidine adsorbed onto 1 g kaolin rose from 3.54 to 5.81 mg over the pH range 2 to 5.5–7.5 (i.e. those occurring within the gut).[1] Quinidine is also bound by pectin. More study is needed to confirm these two studies but be alert for the need to increase the quinidine dosage if kaolin-pectin is used concurrently.

References

1 Moustafa MA, Al-Shora HI, Gaber M and Gouda MW. Decreased bioavailability of quinidine sulphate due to interactions with adsorbent antacids and antidiarrhoeal mixtures. Int J Pharmaceutics (1987) 34, 207–11.

2 Narang PK, Carliner NH, Fisher ML and Crouthamel WG. Quinidine saliva concentrations; absence of correlation with serum concentrations at steady-state. Clin Pharmacol Ther (1983) 34, 695–702.

3 Bucci AJ, Myre SA, Tan HSI and Shenouda LS. In vitro interaction of quinidine with kaolin and pectin. J Pharm Sci (1981) 70, 999–1002.

Quinidine + Ketoconazole

Abstract/Summary

An isolated report describes a marked increase in serum quinidine levels in man when additionally treated with ketoconazole.

Clinical evidence, mechanism, importance and management

An elderly man with chronic atrial fibrillation, treated with 300 mg quinidine four times daily, was additionally given 200 mg ketoconazole daily for candidal oesophagitis. Within seven days his serum quinidine levels had risen from a range of 1.4–2.7 mg/l to 6.9 mg/l but he showed no evidence of toxicity. The elimination half-life of quinidine was found to be 25 h (normal values in healthy subjects 6.7 h). The quinidine dosage was reduced to 200 mg twice daily but it needed to be increased to its former value by the end of a month. The reasons for this reaction are not understood.[1]

This is an isolated case so that its general importance is uncertain, but it draws attention to the need to monitor serum quinidine levels in any patient if ketoconazole is added.

Reference

1 McNulty RM, Lazor JA and Sketch M. Transient increase in plasma quinidine concentrations during ketoconazole-quinidine therapy. Clin Pharm (1989) 8, 222–5.

Quinidine + Laxatives

Abstract/Summary

Quinidine serum levels can be reduced by the concurrent use of an anthraquinone-containing laxative.

Clinical evidence, mechanism, importance and management

Studies on patients with heart arrhythmias taking 500 mg quinidine bisulphate 12-hourly showed that concurrent use of an anthraquinone-containing laxative (*Liquedepur*, Fa.Natterman, Cologne) reduced serum quinidine levels measured 12 h after the last dose of quinidine by about 25%.[1] This might be of clinical importance in patients whose serum levels are barely adequate to control their arrhythmia.

Reference

1 Guckenbiehl W, Gilfrich HJ and Just H. Einfluss von Laxantien und Metoclopramid auf die Chindin-Plasmakonzentration wahrend Langzeittherapie bei Patienten mit Herzrhythmusstorungen. Med Welt (1976) 27, 1273.

Quinidine + Lignocaine (Lidocaine)

Abstract/Summary

A single case report describes a man on quinidine who had sinoatrial arrest when he was given lignocaine.

Clinical evidence, mechanism, importance and management

A man with Parkinson's disease was given 300 mg quinidine six-hourly for the control of ventricular ectopic beats. After receiving 600 mg he was given lignocaine as well, initially a bolus of 80 mg, followed by an infusion of 4 mg/min because persistent premature ventricular beats developed. Within 2.5 h the patient complained of dizziness and weakness, and was found to have sinus bradycardia, SA arrest and atrioventricular escape rhythm. Normal sinus rhythm resumed when the lignocaine was stopped. The reasons for this reaction are not understood.[1]

Reference

1 Jerestay RM, Kahn AH and Landry AB. Sinoatrial arrest due to lidocaine in a patient receiving quinidine. Chest (1972) 61, 683.

Quinidine + Metoclopramide

Abstract/Summary

Metoclopramide can reduce the absorption of quinidine from a sustained-release formulation but may increase the absorption with other preparations.

Clinical evidence

A study of this interaction was prompted by the case of a patient on sustained-release quinidine (*Quinidex*) whose arrhythmia failed to be controlled when metoclopramide was added. Five normal subjects were given 10 mg metoclopramide six-hourly 24 h before and 48 h after a single oral dose of 600 mg or 900 mg quinidine. Five others received the quinidine but not the metoclopramide. It was found that the metoclopramide caused a mean decrease in the quinidine absorption of 10%, but two subjects had decreases of 22.5 and 28.1%.[1] Another study in patients taking 500 mg quinidine 12-hourly found that 30 mg daily doses of metoclopramide increased the mean serum levels measured 3.5 h after the last dose of quinidine by almost 20% (from 1.6 to 1.9 μg/ml) and at 12 h by about 16% (from 2.4 to 2.8 μg/ml).[2]

Mechanism

Not understood. Metoclopramide alters both the gastric emptying time and gastrointestinal motility which can affect absorption.

Importance and management

Direct information seems to be limited to these studies using different quinidine preparations. Since the outcome of concurrent use is uncertain, the effects should be well monitored. More study is needed.

References

1 Yuen GJ, Hansten PD and Collins J. Effect of metoclopramide on the adsorption of an oral sustained-release product. Clin Pharm (1987) 6, 722–5.
2 Guckenbiehl W, Gilfrich HJ and Just H. Einfluss von Laxantien und Metoclopramid auf die Chindin-Plasmakonzentration wahrend Langzeittherapie bei Patienten mit Herzrhythmusstorugen. Med Welt (1976) 27, 1273.

Quinidine + Rifampicin (Rifampin)

Abstract/Summary

The serum levels of quinidine and its therapeutic effects can be markedly reduced by the concurrent use of rifampicin.

Clinical evidence

It was noted that control of ventricular dysrhythmia with quinidine was lost in a patient when he was given rifampicin. Further study in normal subjects showed that concurrent treatment with 600 mg rifampicin daily reduced the mean half-life of the quinidine by almost 60% (from 6.1 to 2.3 h), and the AUC (area under the plasma-concentration time curve) fell from 20.1 to 3.4 μg/ml/h.[1,2]

Another report described a patient taking 800–1200 mg quinidine daily who showed a reduction in serum levels from 4 to 0.5 μg/ml within a fortnight of starting 600 mg rifampicin daily.[3] Yet another patient failed to achieve adequate serum quinidine levels despite large daily doses of quinidine (3200 mg) while taking rifampicin. When the rifampicin was stopped, the quinidine dosage was reduced 44% (to 1800 mg daily) but the serum levels rose 43% (from 1.4 to 2 μg/ml).[4] A 'double interaction' was seen in a patient on quinidine and digoxin when given rifampicin: the quinidine levels fell resulting in a fall in digoxin levels.[5]

Mechanism

Rifampicin is a potent enzyme-inducing agent which increases the metabolism of the quinidine by the liver 3–4-fold, thereby increasing its loss from the body and reducing its effects. It has been suggested that two of the quinidine metabolites (3-hydroxquinidine and 2-oxoquinidinone) may be as potent as quinidine itself which might offset to some extent the effects of this interaction.[6]

Importance and management

An established and clinically important interaction. The dosage of quinidine will need to be increased if rifampicin is given concurrently. Monitor the serum levels. Doubling the dose may not be enough.[2,5] An equivalent dosage reduction will be needed if the rifampicin is stopped.

References

1 Twum-Barima Y and Carruthers SG. Evaluation of rifampicin-quinidine interaction. Clin Pharmacol Ther (1980) 27, 290.
2 Twum-Barima Y and Carruthers SG. Quinidine-rifampicin interaction. N Engl J Med (1981) 304, 1466.
3 Ahmad D, Mathur P, Ahunjma S, Henerson R and Carruthers G. Rifampicin-quinidine interaction. Br J dis Chest (1979) 73, 409.
4 Schwartz A and Brown JR. Quinidine-rifampin interaction. Am Heart J (1984) 107, 789–90.
5 Bussey HI, Merritt GJ and Hill EG. The influence of rifampin on quinidine and digoxin. Arch Intern Med (1984) 144, 1021–3.
6 Bussey HI, Farringer J, and Merritt GJ. Influence of rifampin on quinidine and digoxin. Drug Intell Clin Pharm (1983) 17, 436.

Quinidine + Urinary alkalinizers and Antacids

Abstract/Summary

Large rises in urinary pH due to the concurrent use of some antacids, diuretics or alkaline salts can cause the retention of quinidine which may lead to quinidine intoxication. The outcome of using many antacids with quinidine is uncertain.

Clinical evidence

The urinary excretion of quinidine in four normal subjects taking 200 mg six-hourly by mouth was reduced by an average of 50% (from 53 to 26 ml/min) when their urine was made alkaline (i.e. changed from pH 6–7 to pH 7–8) with sodium bicarbonate and acetazolamide (0.5 g every 12 h). Below pH 6 their serum quinidine excretion averaged 115 mg/l, whereas when urinary pH values rose above 7.5 their average excretion fell to 13 mg/l. The quinidine excretion rate decreased from 103 to 31 μg/min. In six other subjects the rise in serum quinidine levels was reflected in a prolongation of the Q-T interval. Raising the urinary pH from about 6 to 7.5 in one individual increased serum quinidine levels from about 1.6 to 2.6 μg/ml.[1]

A patient on quinidine who took about eight *Mylanta* tablets daily (aluminium hydroxide gel 200 mg, magnesium hydroxide 200 mg) for a week and large amounts of citrus fruit juice developed quinidine intoxication.[2]

Mechanism

In acid urine much of the quinidine excreted by the kidney tubules is in the ionized (lipid-insoluble) form which is unable to diffuse freely back into the cells and so is lost in the urine. In alkaline urine more of the quinidine is in the un-ionized (lipid-soluble) form which freely diffuses back into the cells and is retained. In this way the pH of the urine determines how much quinidine is lost or retained and thereby governs the serum levels. Changes in pH and adsorbtion effects within the gut due to antacids may also possibly affect the absorption of quinidine.[4,5]

Importance and management

An established interaction. Monitor the effects if drugs which can markedly change urinary pH are started or stopped. Reduce the quinidine dosage accordingly. Acetazolamide and sodium bicarbonate can both raise the urinary pH significantly, depending on the dosages used.[1] Other urinary alkalinizers are expected to behave similarly.

The effects of those antacids which are known to raise the urinary pH is less certain because there is some indirect evidence that the interaction is possibly offset by reductions in absorption from the gut.[4,5] There is a single case report of quinidine intoxication due to *Mylanta* (aluminium-magnesium hydroxide),[2] and *Maalox* can raise the pH by 1.0 and may possibly interact similarly.[3] *Milk of magnesia* (magnesium hydroxide) and *Titralac* (calcium carbonate-glycine) in normal doses raise the pH by 0.5 so that a smaller effect is likely.[3]

Amphogel (aluminium hydroxide) and *Robalate* (dihydrox-aluminium glycinate) are reported to have no effect on urinary pH.[3] In those instances where the antacids do not affect urinary pH at all but reduce the quinidine absorption from the gut (magnesium trisilicate?[5]), an increase in the quinidine dosage may possibly be needed. More study is needed to find out which, if any, of these antacids normally interacts significantly, and by how much. Until more is known, monitor the effects of concurrent use.

References

1 Gerhardt RE, Knouss RF, Thyrium PT, Luchi RJ and Morris JJ. Quinidine excretion in aciduria and alkaluria. Ann Intern Med (1969) 71, 927.

2 Zinn MB. Quinidine intoxication from alkali ingestion. Texas med (1970) 66, 64.

3 Gibaldi M. Effect of antacids on pH of urine. Clin Pharmacol Ther (1974) 16, 520.

4 Remon JP, Van Severen R and Braeckman P. Interaction entre anti-arrythmiques, antiacides et antidiarrheques. III. Influence d'antacides et d'antidiarrheques sur la reabsorption *in vitro* de sels de quinidine. Pharm Acta Helv (1979) 54, 19.

5 Moustafa MA, Al-Sora HI, Gaber M and Gouda MW. Decreased bioavailability of quinidine sulphate due to interactions with adsorbent antacids and antidiarrhoeal mixtures. Int J Pharmaceutics (1987) 34, 207–11.

Tocainide + Antacids or Urinary alkalinizers

Abstract/Summary

Raising the pH of the urine can reduce the loss of tocainide in the urine.

Clinical evidence

When five normal subjects took 30 ml of an un-named antacid four times a day for 48 h before and 58 h after a single 600 mg dose of tocainide, the urinary pH rose from 5.9 to 6.9. The total clearance fell by 28% (from 2.55 to 1.85 ml/kg/min). Peak serum levels rose by 24% (from 4.2 to 3.4 μg/ml), the half-life and AUC (area under the time-concentration curve) rose from 13.2 to 15.4 h and from 51.7 to 68.5 μg.h/ml respectively.[1]

Mechanism

Tocainide is a weak base so that its loss in the urine will be affected by the pH of the urine. Alkalinization of the urine increases the number of un-ionized molecules available for passive reabsorption, thereby reducing the urinary loss and raising the serum levels.

Importance and management

Information is limited and the clinical importance uncertain, but the outcome of concurrent use should be well monitored. More study is needed. Be alert for any evidence of increased tocainide effects and possible toxicity if other drugs are given which can alter urinary pH. Reduce the tocainide dosage if necessary. Aluminium-magnesium hydroxide (*Mylanta*) and *Maalox* can raise urinary pH by 1.0 whereas *Milk of magnesia* (magnesium hydroxide) and *Titralac* (calcium carbonate-glycine) in normal doses raise the pH by only 0.5.[2] *Amphogel* (aluminium hydroxide) and *Robalate* (dihydroxy aluminium glycinate) are reported to have no effect on urinary pH.[2]

References

1 Meneilly GP, Scavone JM, Meneilly GS and Wei JY. Tocainide: pharmacokinetic alterations during antacid-induced urinary alkalinization. Clin Pharmacol Ther (1987) 41, 178.
2 Gibaldi M. Effect of antacids on pH of urine. Clin Pharmacol Ther (1974) 16, 520.

Tocainide + Cimetidine

Abstract/Summary

There is some evidence that cimetidine can reduce the bioavailability and serum levels of tocainide but ranitidine appears not to interact.

Clinical evidence, mechanism, importance and management

A study in 11 normal subjects showed that treatment with cimetidine (dosage not stated) for four days had an effect on the pharmacokinetics of 500 mg tocainide given intravenously over 15 min (half-life increased, clearance decreased), but too small to be clinically important.[1] However another study in seven normal subjects found that 1200 mg cimetidine daily for two days reduced the AUC (area under the time-concentration curve) of a single 400 mg oral dose of tocainide by about a third (from 31.6 to 23.1 μg/ml) and reduced peak serum levels from 2.4 to 1.7 μg/ml, but no changes in the half-life or renal clearance occurred.[2] The reasons for this and its clinical importance are uncertain, but be alert for evidence of a reduced response to tocainide in the presence of cimetidine. 150 mg ranitidine twice daily was found not to interact.[2]

References

1 Holmes GI, Antonello J, Yeh KC, Demstriades J, Irvin JD and McMahon FG. Intravenous tocainide maintains safe therapeutic levels when administered concomitantly with cimetidine. Clin Pharmacol Ther (1987), 41, 237.
2 Lalonde RL, North DS, Mattern AL and Kapil RP. Tocainide pharmacokinetic after H-2 antagonists. Clin Pharmacol Ther (1987) 41, 241.

Tocainide + Rifampicin (Rifampin)

Abstract/Summary

The loss of tocainide from the body is increased by the concurrent use of rifampicin.

Clinical evidence

Eight normal subjects were given 300 mg rifampicin twice daily for five days. The AUC (area under the concentration-time curve) of a single 600 mg oral dose of tocainide was reduced by almost 30% (from 76.8 to 55 mg/h/l) and the half-life was also reduced about 30% (from 13.2 to 9.4 h).[1]

Mechanism

These findings are consistent with the well-recognized enzyme inducing effects of rifampicin which increase the metabolism of drugs by the liver, thereby increasing their loss from the body and reducing their serum levels.

Importance and management

Information is limited to this single dose study in normal subjects but the interaction would seem to be established. It seems probable that it is of clinical importance. Monitor patients who are additionally given rifampicin for evidence of reduced tocainide serum levels and reduced effects. Increase the dosage as necessary. Reduce the tocainide dosage if the rifampicin is withdrawn. More study is needed.

Reference

1 Rice TL, Patterson JH, Celestin C, Foster JR, Powell JR. Influence of rifampin on tocainide pharmacokinetics in humans. Clin Pharm (1989) 8, 200.

5

ANTIBIOTIC AND ANTI-INFECTIVE DRUG INTERACTIONS

'Most physicians...have the vague feeling that if one anti-microbial drug is good, two should be better, and three should cure almost everybody of almost every ailment.'

This 'vague feeling' has proved to be valid in a number of instances, but there is also good evidence that sometimes the very opposite is true. This situation has fuelled a keen debate about the desirability or otherwise of combining antimicrobial agents which has gone on for many years, and various schemes have been published which try to provide a logical framework for predicting the likely outcome. One of the serious difficulties is the often poor correlation between *in vitro* and *in vivo* studies so that it is difficult to get a thoroughly reliable indication of how antimicrobial agents will behave together in clinical practice. Some of the synopses in this chapter illustrate these difficulties very clearly.

Some of the arguments in favour of combining antimicrobial agents are as follows. Where the infections are acute and undiagnosed the presence of more than one drug increases the chance that at least one effective antimicrobial is present. This may be especially important if the patient is infected by more than one organism. The possibility of the emergence of resistant organisms is decreased by the use of more than one drug, and in some cases two drugs acting at different sites may be more effective than one drug alone. It may

also be that two drugs administered below their toxic thresholds may be as effective and less toxic than one drug at a higher concentration.

In contrast there are other arguments against using antimicrobials together. One serious objection is that two drugs may actually be less effective than one on its own. In theory this could arise if a bactericidal drug, which requires actively dividing cells for it to be effective, were used with a bacteriostatic drug. However in practice this seems to be less important than might be supposed and there are relatively few well-authenticated clinical examples. Another objection is that some broad-spectrum drugs may be suboptimal for particular organisms and may inadequately control the infection. Toxic side-effects may possibly also be increased by the use of more than one drug.

An indiscriminate and 'blunderbuss' approach to the treatment of infections is no longer in favour, the general consensus of informed opinion being that the advantages of combined antimicrobial treatment are balanced by a number of clear disadvantages, and that usually one drug alone, properly chosen, is likely to be equally effective.

Some of the synopses in this chapter are concerned with the adverse effects of combining antimicrobials together but most of them deal with the interactions caused by non-infective agents. Interactions where the antimicrobials are the affecting or interacting agent are dealt with in other chapters. A complete listing is to be found in the Index.

Table 5.1 Antibiotics

Aminoglycosides	Cephalosporins		Penicillins	Polypeptides
Amikacin	Cefacetrile	Cephaloridine	Amoxycillin	Bacitracin
Dibekacin	Cefaclor	Cephradine	Ampicillin	Colistin
Dihydrostreptomycin	Cefadroxil	Cephaloglycin	Azlocillin	Polymyxin B
Framycetin	Cefamandole	Cephalothin	Bacampicillin	Vancomycin
Gentamicin	Cefazaflur	Cephamandole	Benzylpenicillin	
Kanamycin	Cefmetazole	Cephapirin	Carbenicillin	Quinolones
Neomycin	Ceforanide	Cephazolin	Ciclacillin	Ciprofloxacin
Netilmicin	Cefotaxime	Chloramphenicol	Cloxacillin	Enoxacin
Paromomycin	Cefotetan	Clindamycin	Dicloxacillin	Nalidixic acid
Ribostamycin	Cefotiam	Fusidic acid	Flucloxacillin	Norfloxacin
Sissomycin	Cefoxitin	Lincomycin	Methicillin	Ofloxacin
Streptomycin	Cefpiramide		Mezlocillin	Pefloxacin
Tobramycin	Cefsulodin	Macrolides	Nafcillin	
	Cefuroxime	Erythromycin	Oxacillin	Rifampicin (rifampin)
Antifungals	Ceftazidine	Josamycin	Phenethicillin	
Amphotericin B	Ceftizoxime	Midecamycin	Piperacillin	Tetracyclines
Fluconazole	Ceftriaxone	Miocamycin	Pivampicillin	Chlortetracyline
Griseofulvin	Cephalexin	Spiramycin	Ticarcillin	Demeclocycline
Ketoconazole	Cephaloglycin	Triacetyloleandomycin	Phenoxymethyl-	Doxycycline
Miconazole	Cephacetrile		penicillin	Methacycline
			(penicillin V)	Minocycline
				Oxytetracycline
				Rolitetracycline
				Tetracycline

Table 5.2 Non-antibiotic anti-infectives

Antimalarials	Antiprotozoals	Antituberculars and antileprotics	Antivirals	Sulphonamides
Chloroquine	Metronidazole		Acyclovir	Co-trimoxazole
Hydroxychloroquine		Aminosalicylic acid	Interferon	Sulphadiazine
Mepacrine Pamaquine	Anthelmintics	(PAS)	Vidarabine	Sulphamethoxine
Primaquine	Levamisole	Clofazimine	Zidovudine	Sulphadimidine
Proguanil	Metriphonate	Cycloserine		(-methazine,
Pyrimethamine	Piperazine	Dapsone	Furazolidone	-merazine)
	Praziquantel	Ethambutol	Hexamine	Sulphafurazole
		Isoniazid	(methenamine)	(sulfisoxazole)
		Prothionamide	Nitrofurantoin	Sulphamerazine
		Pyrazinamide	Sulphasalazine	Sulphamethizole
				Sulphamethoxazole
				Sulphamethoxypyri-
				dazine
				Sulphametopyridazine
				Sulphaphenazole
				Sulphasomidine
				Sulphathiazole

Aminoglycoside antibiotics + Amphotericin

Abstract/Summary

Nephrotoxicity attributed to the concurrent use of gentamicin and amphotericin has been described in four patients.

Clinical evidence, mechanism, importance and management

Four patients given moderate doses of gentamicin showed renal deterioration when additionally given amphotericin. Both antibiotics in sufficiently high doses are known to be nephrotoxic and it is suggested, on the basis of what was seen, that low doses of each may have additive nephrotoxic effects.[1] The documentation seems to be limited to this report. Until more is known it would be prudent to monitor renal function carefully if these two antibiotics are used.

Reference

1 Churchill DN and Seeley J. Nephrotoxicity associated with combined gentamicin-amphotericin B. Nephron (1977) 19, 176.

Aminoglycoside antibiotics + Cephalosporins

Abstract/Summary

The nephrotoxic effects of gentamicin and tobramycin can be increased by the concurrent use of cephalothin. This may possibly be true for other aminoglycosides.

Clinical evidence

A randomized double-blind trial in patients with sepsis showed the following incidence of definite nephrotoxicity: gentamicin + cephalothin 30% (seven of 23); tobramycin + cephalothin 21% (five of 24); gentamicin + methicillin 10% (two of 20); tobramycin + methicillin 4% (one of 23).[1]

A very considerable number of studies and case reports confirm this increase in the incidence of nephrotoxicity when gentamicin[2–12] or tobramycin[13,14] are used with cephalothin. However the opposite conclusion has been reached by a few others.[15–17] Cefuroxime[18] and cefotaxime[19] are reported not to increase the nephrotoxic effects of tobramycin. Hypokalaemia has also been described in patients taking cytotoxic drugs for leukaemia when they were given gentamicin and cephalexin.[20]

Mechanism

Uncertain. The nephrotoxic effects of gentamicin and tobramycin are well documented and it appears that these effects can be additive with cephalothin in some patients. Doses which are well tolerated separately can be nephrotoxic when given together.[12]

Importance and management

The weight of evidence is that this is a potentially serious interaction. The gentamicin–cephalothin interaction is very well documented, but there is less information about tobramycin with cephalothin. The risk of nephrotoxicity is probably greatest if high doses are used in those with some existing renal impairment. Concurrent use is not totally contraindicated (see the report cited above[1]) but renal function should be very closely monitored and dosages kept to a minimum. This drug combination is probably best avoided in high risk patients wherever possible. Possible alternatives with a much reduced risk of nephrotoxicity are gentamicin or tobramycin with methicillin,[1] or tobramycin with cefuroxime and cefotaxime.[18,19] Whether other aminoglycosides interact similarly is uncertain, but the possibility should be borne in mind.

References

1 Wade JC, Smith CR, Petty BG, Lipsky JJ, Conrad G, Ellner J and Lietman PS. Cephalothin plus an aminoglycoside is more nephrotoxic than methicillin plus an aminoglycoside. Lancet (1978) ii, 604.
2 Opitz A, Herrman I, von Harrath D and Schaefer K. Akute niereninsuffizienz nach Gentamicin-cephalosporin-Kombinatic.nstherapie. Med Welt (1971) 22, 434.
3 Plager JE. Association of renal injury with con ined cephalothin-gentamicin therapy among patients severely il . ith malignant disease. Cancer (1976) 37, 1937.
4 Burck HC and Sorgel G. Nephrotoxicity of the combined application of cephalothin and gentamicin, in, Proceedings of 6th International Congress of Nephrology. Int Congr Nephrology, Florence, Italy. (1975) Abstract 700.
5 EORTC International Antimicrobial Therapy Project Group. The antibiotic regimens in the treatment of infection in febrile granulocytopenic patients with cancer. J Infect Dis (1978) 137, 14.
6 Kleinknecht D, Ganeval D and Droz D. Acute renal failure after high doses of gentamicin and cephalothin. Lancet (1973) i, 1129.
7 Noone P, Pattison JR and Shafi MS. Renal failure in combined gentamicin and cephalothin therapy. Br Med J (1973) 2, 777.
8 Bobrow SN, Jaffe E and Young RC. Anuria and acute tubular necrosis associated with gentamicin and cephalothin. J Amer Med Ass (1972) 222, 1546.
9 Fillastre JP, Laumonier R, Humbert G, Dubois D, Metayer J, Delpech A, Leroy J and Robert M. Acute renal failure associated with combined gentamicin and cephalothin therapy. Br Med J (1973) 2, 396.
10 Zazgornik J, Schmidt P, Lugscheider R and Kopsa H. Akutes Nierenversagen bei kombinierter Cephaloridin-Gentamycin-Therapie. Wien Klin Wsch (1973) 85, 839.
11 Cabanillas F, Burgos RC, Rodriguez RC and Baldizon C. Nephrotoxicity of combined cephalothin-gentamicin regimen. Arch Intern Med (1975) 135, 850.
12 Tvedgaard E. Interaction between gentamicin and cephalothin as cause of acute renal failure. Lancet (1976) ii, 581.
13 Tobias JS, Whitehouse JM and Wrigley PF. Severe renal dysfunction after tobramycin/cephalothin therapy. Lancet (1976) i, 425.
14 Klastersky J, Hensgens C and Debusscher L. Empiric therapy for cancer patients: comparative study of ticarcillin-tobramycin, ticarcillin-cephalothin, and cephalothin-tobramycin. Antimicrob Ag Chemother (1975) 7, 640.
15 Fanning WL, Gump D and Jick H. Gentamicin- and cephalothin-associated rises in blood urea nitrogen. Antimicrob Ag Chemother (1976) 10, 80.
16 Stille W and Arndt I. Argumente gegen eine Nephrotoxizitat von Cephalothin und Gentamcyin. Med Welt (1972) 23, 1603
17 Wellwood JM, Simpson PM, Tighe JR and Thompson EE. Evidence of gentamicin nephrotoxicity in patients with renal allografts. Br Med J (1975) 3, 278.
18 Trollford B, Alestig K, Rodjer S, Sandberg T and Westin J. Renal function in patients treated with tobramycin-cefuroxime or tobramycin-penicillin G. J Antimicrob Chemother (1983) 12, 641–5.

19 Kuhlmann J, Seidl G, Richter E and Grotsch H. Tobramycin nephrotoxicity: failure of cefotaxime to potentiate injury in patient. Naunyn Schmied Arch Pharmakol (1981) 316, R80.
20 Young GP, Sullivan J and Hurley A. Hypokalaemia due to gentamicin/cephalexin in leukaemia. Lancet (1973) ii, 855.

Aminoglycosides + Clindamycin

Abstract/Summary

Three cases of acute renal failure have been tentatively attributed to the concurrent use of gentamicin and clindamycin

Clinical evidence, mechanism, importance and management

Three patients with normal renal function developed acute renal failure when they were concurrently treated with gentamicin (4–5 mg/kg/day for 13–18 days) and clindamycin (0.9–1.8 mg/kg/day for 7–13 days). They recovered within 3–5 days of discontinuing the antibiotics.[1] The reasons for the renal failure are not known, but clindamycin has been shown to produce lysosomal changes in the kidney cells of rats which are similar to those produced by gentamicin.[2] Until more is known it would be prudent to monitor renal function carefully if these antibiotics are used together. Tobramycin with clindamycin is reported not to be nephrotoxic.[3]

References

1 Butkus DE, de Torrente A and Terman. Renal failure following gentamicin in combination with clindamycin. Gentamicin nephrotoxicity. Nephron (1976) 17, 307.
2 Gray JE, Purmalis A, Purmalis B and Mathews J. Ultrastructural studies of the hepatic changes brought about by clindamycin in animals. Toxical Appl Pharmacol (1971) 19, 217.
3 Gillett P, Wise R, Melkian V and Falk R. Tobramycin/cepholothin nephrotoxicity. Lancet (1976) i, 547.

Aminoglycosides + Dimenhydrinate

Abstract/Summary

The manufacturers of dimenhydrinate (diphenhydramine) suggest that it may possibly undesirably mask the ototoxic effects of streptomycin and other aminoglycoside antibiotics.

Clinical evidence, mechanism, importance and management

Dimenhydrinate can block the dizziness, nausea and vomiting which can occur during treatment with streptomycin.[1,2] However Searle, the manufacturers of dimenhydrinate, warn that '...caution should be used when *Dramamine* (dimenhydrinate) is given in conjunction with certain antibiotics which may cause ototoxicity, since *Dramamine* is capable of masking ototoxic symptoms and an irreversible

state may be reached.'[1,3] There seems to be no direct clinical evidence to confirm this, but there would seem to be an obvious hazard in not taking sufficient notice of the warning signs of developing ototoxicity with streptomycin or any other aminoglycoside.

References

1 Titche LL and Nady A. Control of vestibular toxic effects of streptomycin by Dramamine. Dis Chest (1950) 18, 386.
2 Cohen AC and Glinsky GC. Hypersensitivity to streptomycin. J Allergy (1951) 22, 63.
3 Physicians Desk Reference (1972), p 1246. Medical Economics Inc., USA.

Aminoglycosides + Ethacrynic acid

Abstract/Summary

The concurrent use of aminoglycoside antibiotics and ethacrynic acid should be avoided because their damaging actions on the ear can be additive. Intravenous administration and renal impairment are additional causative factors. Even sequential administration may not be safe.

Clinical evidence

Four patients with some renal impairment became permanently deaf after treatment with 1.0–1.5 g kanamycin and 50–150 mg ethacrynic acid. One of the patients was given the drugs 2 h apart and was deaf within 30 min. Another showed deafness which took almost a fortnight to develop. He was given kanamycin on the first and fifth days of treatment and ethacrynic acid on the second.[1]

There are other reports describing temporary, partial or total permanent deafness in man as a result of giving ethacrynic acid with gentamicin,[5] kanamycin,[3,5,7] streptomycin,[1,2,6] or neomycin.[2,8] This interaction has been very extensively demonstrated in animals.

Mechanism

Both the aminoglycosides and ethacrynic acid given singly can damage the ear and cause deafness, the site of action of the aminoglycosides being the hair cell and that of ethacrynic acid the stria vascularis. Studies in animals have shown that neomycin can cause a marked increase (fivefold) in the concentration of ethacrynate in cochlear tissues, and it may be that the aminoglycoside has some effect on the tissues which allows the ethacrynic acid to penetrate more easily.[4]

Importance and management

A well-established and well-documented interaction. Concurrent and sequential use should be avoided because permanent deafness may result. Patients with renal impairment seem to be particularly at risk, probably because the drugs are less rapidly cleared. Most of the reports describe deafness after intravenous administration but it has also been seen when given orally. If it is deemed absolutely necessary to use both drugs, minimal doses should be used and the effects on hearing should be monitored continuously. Not every aminoglycoside has been implicated, but their ototoxicity is clearly established and they may be expected to interact in a similar way.

References

1 Johnson AH and Hamilton CA. Kanamycin ototoxicity—possible potentiation by other drugs. S Med J (1970) 63, 511.
2 Mathog RH and Klein WJ. Ototoxicity of ethacrynic acid and aminoglycoside antibiotics in uremia. N Engl J Med (1969) 280, 1223.
3 Ng PS, Conley CE and Ing TS. Deafness after ethacrynic acid. Lancet (1969) i, 673.
4 Orsulakova A and Schacht J. A biochemical mechanism of the ototoxic interaction between neomycin and ethacrynic acid. Acta Otolaryngol (1981) 93, 43–8.
5 Meriwether WD, Mangi RJ and Serpick AA. Deafness following standard intravenous dose of ethacrynic acid. J Amer Med Ass (1971) 216, 795–8.
6 Schneider WJ and Becker EL. Acute transient hearing loss after ethacrynic acid therapy. Arch Intern Med (1966) 117, 715–17.
7 Slone D, Jick H, Lewis GP, Shapiro S and Miettinen OS. Intravenously given ethacrynic acid and gastrointestinal bleeding. J Amer Med Ass (1969) 209, 1668–71.
8 Matz GJ, Beal DDC and Krames L. Ototoxicity of ethacrynic acid. Demonstrated in a human temporal bone. Arch Otolaryngol (1969) 90, 152–5.

Aminoglycosides + Extended spectrum penicillins

Abstract/Summary

Gentamicin, netilmicin, tobramycin and sisomicin are chemically inactivated if mixed in intravenous fluids with carbenicillin, ticarcillin, azlocillin, piperacillin or mezlocillin. Some inactivation can occur if both drugs are given to patients with severe renal impairment or those undergoing haemodialysis, but no interaction of importance appears to occur in those with normal renal function.

Clinical evidence

(a) Aminoglycosides + penicillins in vitro

In vitro studies with solutions of gentamicin, 5 μg/ml, and carbenicillin, 200 μg/ml, showed that the gentamicin became inactivated. These studies were undertaken to check on clinical observations of suspected inactivation.[1]

Inactivation has also been described in other reports involving carbenicillin with gentamicin,[2–6] netilmicin,[12] tobramycin[5] or sisomicin;[5] ticarcillin with gentamicin,[5,6] tobramycin[5] or sisomicin;[5] azlocillin with gentamicin, tobramycin and netilmicin;[12] mezlocillin with gentamicin, tobramycin and netilmicin;[12] and piperacillin with amikacin, gentamicin and tobramycin.[20]

(b) Aminoglycosides + penicillins in patients with renal impairment

A study in six patients with severe renal failure who were receiving carbenicillin (1.5–15 g daily) administered in divided doses 3–6 times daily by intravenous infusion, showed that the presence of the penicillin prevented the achievement of serum gentamicin levels above 4 μg/ml even though large doses were given.[7] A similar interaction was seen with carbenicillin and tobramycin.[7]

Other reports similarly describe the adverse interaction of gentamicin with carbenicillin[2,6,11], ticarcillin,[6] and piperacillin;[19] and tobramycin with ticarcillin.[16] A reduction in the half-life of gentamicin to about a half or a third has been described as well.[6,9]

(c) Aminoglycosides + penicillins in patients undergoing haemodialysis

A study in six chronic haemodialysis patients showed that when given 4 g piperacillin 12-hourly the pharmacokinetics of netilmicin (2 mg/kg) were unchanged whereas the clearance of tobramycin (2 mg/kg) was more than doubled (from 3.6 to 8.3 ml/min) and the half-life reduced from 73 to 22 h.[21]

(d) Aminoglycosides + penicillins in patients with normal renal function

A patient with normal renal function was given 80 mg gentamicin intravenously, with and without 4 g carbenicillin. The serum gentamicin concentration profiles in both cases were very similar, with only a fraction of depression due to the carbenicillin.[2]

No interaction was seen in 10 patients with normal renal function given tobramycin and piperacillin.[18]

Mechanism

These penicillins interact chemically with the aminoglycoside antibiotics to form biologically inactive amides by a reaction between the amino groups on the aminoglycosides and the beta-lactam ring on the penicillins.[8] Thus both antibiotics are inactivated.

Importance and management

These interactions are well documented and of clinical importance. Gentamicin, netilmicin, tobramycin and sisomicin should not be mixed with carbenicillin, ticarcillin, azlocillin, piperacillin or mezocillin in infusion fluids before administration because inactivation occurs. Inactivation can also occur in patients with renal failure. Where concurrent use is thought necessary, it has been recommended that the dosage of the penicillin should be adjusted to renal function and the serum levels of both antibiotics closely monitored.[7] There is some *in vitro* evidence that minimal inactivation occurs in serum between amikacin and ticarcillin or carbenicillin,[5] and the authors of another study suggest using amikacin with piperacillin, keeping the latter at concentrations of 250 μg/ml or lower.[15] However this requires confirmation and it would be prudent to monitor concurrent use very closely. Piperacillin appears to affect tobramycin in patients on haemodialysis, but not netilmicin.

There would seem to be no reason for avoiding concurrent use in patients with normal renal function because no significant *in vivo* inactivation appears to occur. Moreover there is good clinical evidence that concurrent use is valuable in the treatment of *Pseudomonas* infections.[2,10]

It has been shown that significant inactivation of tobramycin in particular, and gentamicin and amikacin to a lesser extent, by carbenicillin, ticarcillin, penicillin and ampicillin can occur in samples of serum taken for laboratory assay if left at room temperature (losses up to 25% after 12 h) or even frozen (losses up to 20% after 24 h).[13,14,17] It has been suggested that samples which cannot be assayed at once should have 50 mega units per litre of penicillinase added.[13]

References

1 McLaughlin JE and Reeves DS. Clinical and laboratory evidence for the inactivation of gentamicin by carbenicillin. Lancet (1971) i, 261.

2 Eykyn S, Phillips I and Ridley M. Gentamicin plus carbenicillin. Lancet (1971) i, 545.

3 Levison ME and Kaye D. Carbenicillin plus gentamicin. Lancet (1971) ii, 45.

4 Lynn B. Carbenicillin plus gentamicin. Lancet (1971) i, 653.

5 Holt HA, Broughall JM, McCarthy M and Reeves DS. Interactions between aminoglycoside antibiotics and carbenicillin or ticarcillin. Infection (1976) 4, 109.

6 Davies M, Morgan JR and Anand C. Interactions of carbenicillin and ticarcillin with gentamicin. Antimicrob Ag Chemother (1975) 7, 431.

7 Weibert R, Keane W and Shapiro F. Carbenicillin inactivation of aminoglycosides in patients with severe renal failure. Trans Amer Soc Artif Int Organs (1976) 22, 439.

8 Perenyi T, Graber H and Arr M. Uber die Wechselwirkung der Penizilline und Aminoglykosid-Antibiotika. Int J Clin Pharmacol Ther Toxicol (1974) 10, 50.

9 Riff LJ and Jackson GG. Laboratory and clinical conditions for gentamicin activation by carbenicillin. Arch Intern Med (1972) 130, 887.

10 Kluge RM, Standiford HC, Tatem B, Young VM, Schimpff SC, Greene WH, Calia FM and Hornick RB. The carbenicillin-gentamicin combination against pseudomonas aeruginosa. Correlation of effect with gentamicin sensitivity. An Intern Med (1974) 81, 584.

11 Weibert RT and Keanse WF. Carbenicillin-gentamicin interaction in acute renal failure. Am J Hosp Pharm (1977) 43, 1137.

12 Henderson JL, Polk RE and Kline BJ. In vitro inactivation of gentamicin, tobramycin and netilmicin by carbenicillin, azlocillin or mezlocillin. Amer J Hosp Pharm (1981) 38, 1167.

13 Edwards DJ and Schentag JJ. In vitro interactions between beta-lactam antibiotics and tobramycin. Clin Chem (1981) 27, 341.

14 Polk RE and Kline BJ. Mall order tobramycin serum levels: low values caused by ticarcillin. Amer J Hosp Pharm (1980) 37, 920.

15 Hale DC, Jenkins R and Matsen JM. In vitro inactivation of aminoglycoside antibiotics by piperacillin and carbenicillin. Amer J Clin Pathol (1980) 74, 316.

16 Chow MSS, Quintiliani R and Nightingale CH. In vivo inactivation of tobramycin by ticarcillin. A case report. J Amer Med Ass (1982) 247, 658–65.

17 Tindula RJ, Ambrose PJ and Harralson AF. Aminoglycoside inactivation by penicillins and cephalosporins and its impact on drug level monitoring. Drug Intell Clin Pharm (1983) 17, 906–8.

18 Lau A, Lee M, Flascha S, Prasad R and Sharifi R. Effect of piperacillin on tobramycin pharmacokinetics in patients with normal renal function. Antimicrob Ag Chemother (1983) 24, 533–7.

19 Thompson MIB, Russo ME, Saxon BJ, Atkin-Thor E and Matsen JM. Gentamicin inactivation by piperacillin or carbenicillin in patients with end-stage renal disease. Antimicrob Ag Chemother (1982) 21, 268–73.

20 Hale DC, Jenkins R and Matsen JM. In vitro inactivation of aminoglycoside anibiotics by piperacillin and carbenicillin. Am J Clin Pathol (1980) 74, 316–19.

21 Halstenson CE, Heim KL, Abraham PA and Keane WF. Netilmicin disposition is not altered by concomitant piperacillin administration. Clin Pharmacol Ther (1985) 41, 210.

Aminoglycosides + Frusemide (Furosemide) or Bumetanide

Abstract/Summary

Although some patients have developed nephrotoxicity and/or ototoxicity while taking both drugs, it has not been established that the damage resulted from an interaction. Nevertheless concurrent use should be well monitored.

Clinical evidence

An analysis of three prospective, controlled, randomized and double blind trials showed that the concurrent use of aminoglycosides (gentamicin, tobramycin, amikacin) and frusemide did not increase either aminoglycoside-induced nephrotoxicity or ototoxicity. Nephrotoxicity developed in 20% (10 of 50 patients) given frusemide and 17.1% (38 of 222) not given frusemide. Auditory toxicity developed in 21.7% (five of 23) given frusemide and 23.5% (28 of 119) not given frusemide.[1]

A clinical study evaluating a possible interaction found that frusemide increased the aminoglycoside-induced renal damage, whereas two other clinical studies found no interaction.[2-4] There are clinical reports claiming that concurrent use results in ototoxicity, but usually only small numbers of patients were involved and control groups were not included.[5-8] A patient has been described[1] on gentamicin who rapidly developed deafness only when frusemide was replaced by ethacrynic acid. There seem to be no clinical reports of an aminoglycoside–bumetanide interaction, but it has been described in animals.[12,13]

Mechanism

Normally none, although both the aminoglycosides and frusemide given singly are associated with ototoxicity. Studies in patients and normal subjects have shown that frusemide reduces the renal clearance of gentamicin and can cause both a rise in serum gentamicin[9,10] and tobramycin levels.[11]

Importance and management

Although there is ample evidence of an adverse interaction in animals, the weight of evidence suggests that frusemide does not normally increase either the nephrotoxicity or ototoxicity of the aminoglycosides in man. Nevertheless as there is still a little uncertainty about the safety of concurrent use it would be prudent to monitor for any evidence of changes in aminoglycoside serum levels or of kidney or ear damage. The authors of the major study cited[1] caution that an interaction may possibly exist if high dose infusions of frusemide are used. See also 'Mechanism' above. The same precautions would also be appropriate with bumetanide.

References

1 Smith CR and Lietman PS. Effect of furosemide on aminoglycoside-induced nephrotoxicity and auditory toxicity in humans. Antimicrob Ag Chemother (1983) 23, 133–7.

2 Bygbjerg IC and Moller R. Gentamicin-induced nephropathy. Scand J Infect Dis (1976) 8, 203–8.

3 Prince RA, Ling MH, Hepler CD, Rainville EC, Kealey GP, Doivta ST, LeFrock JL and Kowalsky SF. Factors associated with creatinine clearance changes following gentamicin therapy. Am J Hosp Pharm (1980) 37, 1489–95.

4 Smith CR, Maxwell RR, Edward CQ, Rogers JF and Lietman PS. Nephrotoxicity induced by gentamicin and amikacin. Johns Hopkins MJ (1978) 142, 85–90.

5 Gallagher KL and Jones JK. Furosemide-induced ototoxicity. Ann Intern Med (1979) 91, 744–5.

6 Noel P and Levy V-G. Toxicite renale de l'association gentamicine-furosemide. Une observation. Nouv Presse Med (1978) 7, 351.

7 Brown CB, Ogg CS, Cameron JS and Bewick M. High dose frusemide in acute reversible intrinsic renal failure. Scot med J (1974) 19, 35.

8 Thomsen J, Bech P and Szpirt W. Otological symptoms in chronic renal failure. The possible role of aminoglycoside-furosemide interaction. Arch Oto-Rhino-Laryng (1976) 214, 71.

9 Lawson DH, Tilstone WJ and Semple PF. Furosemide interactions: studies in normal volunteers. Clin Res (1976) 24, 3.

10 Lawson DH, Tilstone WJ, Gray JMB and Srivastava PK. Effect of furosemide on the pharmacokinetics of gentamicin in patients. J Clin Pharmacol (1982) 22, 254–8.

11 Kak JS, Lyman C and Kilarski DJ. Tobramycin-furosemide interaction. Drug Intell Clin Pharm (1984) 18, 235–8.

12 Ohtani I, Ohtsuki K, Omata T, Ouchi J and Saito T. Interaction of bumetanide and kanamycin. Oto-Rhino-Laryngol (1978) 40, 216.

13 Brummett RE, Bendrick T and Himes D. Comparative ototoxicity of bumetanide and furosemide when used in combination with kanamycin. J Clin Pharmacol (1981) 21, 628–36.

Importance and management

Information seems to be limited to these studies[1,2] although supporting evidence comes from the fact that indomethacin also causes the retention of digoxin in premature babies. The authors of the second study[2] suggest that the different results may be because their own aminoglycoside serum levels were lower before the indomethacin was given and because they measured the new steady-state levels after 40–60 h instead of 24 h. Whatever the explanation, concurrent use should be very closely monitored because toxicity is associated with raised aminoglycoside serum levels. The authors of the first study[1] suggest that the aminoglycoside dosage should be reduced before giving indomethacin and the serum levels and kidney function well monitored during concurrent use. Other aminoglycosides possibly behave similarly. This interaction does not seem to have been studied in adults.

References

1 Zarfin Y, Koren G, Maresky D, Perlman M and MacLeod S. Possible indomethacin-aminoglycoside interaction in pre-term infants. J Pediatr (1985) 106, 511–13.

2 Jerome M and Davis JC. The effects of indomethacin on gentamicin serum levels. Proc West Pharmacol Soc (1987) 30, 85–7.

Aminoglycosides + Indomethacin

Abstract/Summary

Conflicting reports claim that serum gentamicin and amikacin levels are or are not raised in premature babies when given indomethacin to close patent ductus arteriosis.

Clinical evidence

(a) Aminoglycoside serum levels increased

A study in 22 preterm (premature) infants with gestational ages ranging from 25 to 34 weeks, showed that the use of indomethacin (0.2 mg/kg) caused a rise in the serum levels of either gentamicin or amikacin which they were being given concurrently. Trough and peak levels of gentamicin were raised 48 and 32% respectively, and of amikacin 28 and 17%.[1]

(b) Aminoglycoside serum levels unchanged

Eight out of 13 infants showed no increase in serum gentamicin levels when given 0.2–0.25 mg/kg indomethacin, four showed slight to moderate rises and one had a substantial rise.[2]

Mechanism

Indomethacin reduces the filtration rate of the kidney tubules. Since the aminoglycosides are lost from the body by kidney filtration, the effect of the indomethacin is possibly to cause the retention of the antibiotic in the body.

Aminoglycosides + Magnesium salts

Abstract/Summary

Respiratory arrest occurred in a baby with elevated serum magnesium levels when given gentamicin.

Clinical evidence

A baby girl born to a woman whose pre-eclampsia had been treated with magnesium sulphate was found to have muscle weakness and a serum magnesium concentration of 4.3 mg/dl. When 12 h old the baby was given ampicillin, 100 mg/kg IV and gentamicin 2.5 mg/kg IM every 12 h. Soon after the second dose of gentamicin she stopped breathing and needed intubation. The gentamicin was stopped and the baby improved.[1]

Animal studies confirm this interaction.[1]

Mechanism

Magnesium ions and the aminoglycoside antibiotics have neuromuscular blocking acitivity which can be additive (see also 'Neuromuscular blockers + Magnesium salts and Neuromuscular blockers' and/ or 'Anaesthetics + Aminoglycoside antibiotics'). In this case it was enough to block the actions of the respiratory muscles.

Importance and management

Direct information about this interaction is very limited but it is well supported by the well-recognized pharmacological actions of magnesium and the aminoglycosides, and their interactions with conventional neuromuscular blockers. The aminoglycosides as a group should be avoided in hypermagnesemic infants needing antimicrobial treatment. If this is not possible, the effects on their respiration should be closely monitored.

Reference

1 L'Hommedieu CS, Nicholas D, Armes DA, Jones P, Nelson T and Pickering LK. Potentiation of magnesium sulfate-induced neuromuscular weakness by gentamicin, tobramycin and amikacin. J Pediatr (1983) 102, 629–31.

Aminoglycosides + Miconazole

Abstract/Summary

A report describes a reduction in serum tobramycin levels due to miconazole.

Clinical evidence, mechanism, importance and management

A study in nine patients undergoing bone marrow transplantation showed that intravenous miconazole significantly lowered their peak serum tobramycin levels (from 9.1 to 6.7μg/ml) and six of them needed dosage adjustments.[1] The reasons are not understood. Concurrent use should be monitored. More study is needed.

Reference

1 Hatfield SM, Crane LR, Duman K, Karanes C and Kiel RJ. Miconazole-induced alteration in tobramycin pharmacokinetics. Clin Pharm (1986) 5, 415–19.

Aminoglycosides + Penicillin V

Abstract/Summary

The serum levels of penicillin V (phenoxymethylpenicillin) when given orally can be halved by the concurrent use of neomycin.

Clinical evidence, mechanism, importance and management

The serum concentrations of penicillin V in five normal subjects, given 250 mg oral doses, were reduced by 50% while also taking 12 g neomycin daily, a return to normal not being achieved until six days after the neomycin was withdrawn.[1] The probable reason is that neomycin causes a reversible malabsorption syndrome which affects the absorption of several drugs. It seems possible that kanamycin and paromomycin might do the same, but this needs confirmation. Parenteral administration of the penicillin or an increase in the oral dosage would seem to be logical answers to this

problem, but whether these are effective seems not to have been documented. This study appears to be the only direct evidence of this interaction.

Reference

1 Cheng SH and White A. Effect of orally administered neomycin on the absorption of penicillin V. N Engl J Med (1962) 267, 1296.

Aminoglycosides + Vancomycin

Abstract/Summary

There is some evidence that the nephrotoxicity of the aminoglycosides and vancomycin may be additive.

Clinical evidence, mechanism, importance and management

Although the combination of an aminoglycoside and vancomycin may possibly be valuable in the treatment of resistant staphylococcal infections, a retrospective study has shown that the incidence of nephrotoxicity in patients given both drugs was high (35%) compared with that for either drug given alone (2–10%).[1,2] Additive nephrotoxicity has also been clearly demonstrated in rats.[3] On the basis of this evidence it would be prudent to monitor concurrent use carefully both for nephrotoxicity and possibly also for ototoxicity.

References

1 Farber B and Moellering R. Retrospective study of the toxicity of preparations of vancomycin from 1974–1981. Antimicrob Ag Chemother (1981) 23, 138–41.
2 Hewitt W. Gentamicin toxicity in perspective. Postgrad Med J (1974) 50 (Suppl 7) 55–9.
3 Wold J and Turnipseed A. Toxicity of vancomycin in laboratory animals. Rev Infect Dis (1981) three (Suppl) 224–9.

Aminosalicylic acid (PAS) + Alcohol

Abstract/Summary

Alcohol can completely nullify the blood-lipid-lowering effects of PAS

Clinical evidence, mechanism, importance and management

A study was made in a group of 65 patients of the effectiveness of PAS-C (purified PAS recrystallized in vitamin C) and diet on the treatment of hyperlipidaemia types IIa and IIb. When three of them drank unstated amounts of beer, the effects of the PAS-C on lowering serum cholesterol, triglyceride and LDL-cholesterol levels were completely abolished.[1] The reasons are not understood. Patients given PAS to reduce blood-lipid levels should avoid alcohol. There seems to be no evidence that alcohol affects the treatment of tuberculosis with PAS.

Reference

1 Kuo PT, Fan WC, Kostis JB and Hayase K. Combined para-aminosalicylic acid and dietary therapy in long term control of hypercholesterolemia and hypertriglyceridemia (types IIa and IIb hyperlipoproteinaemia). Circulation (1976) 53, 338–41.

Aminosalicylic acid (PAS) + Aspirin and Salicylates

Abstract/Summary

Additive gastrointestinal irritation is possible with these drugs, but whether other adverse interactions occur is uncertain.

Clinical evidence, mechanism, importance and management

There seems to be little or no direct evidence of adverse interactions between these drugs although Martindale's Extra Pharmacopoeia states that the adverse effects of aminosalicylic acid and the salicylates may be additive. No clinical details or references are given. However since a common problem with both aminosalicylic acid and aspirin is gastrointestinal irritation and even gastric bleeding, it might be prudent to avoid regular concurrent use. Occasional use probably does not matter.

Reference

1 Reynolds JEF (ed). Martindale. The Extra Pharmacopoeia. 29th Edtn. Pharm Press, London (1989) p 554.

Aminosalicylic acid (PAS) + Diphenhydramine

Abstract/Summary

Diphenhydramine can cause a small reduction in the absorption of aminosalicylic acid from the gut, but the clinical importance of this is uncertain.

Clinical evidence, mechanism, importance and management

A study in nine subjects (and in rats) showed that when 50 mg diphenhydramine was injected intramuscularly 10 min before giving 2 g aminosalicylic acid by mouth, the mean peak serum aminosalicylic acid levels were reduced about 15%, and the total amount absorbed over 2 h was reduced about 10%.[1] The possible reason is that the diphenhydramine reduces peristalsis in the gut which in some way reduces aminosalicylic acid absorption. The extent to which diphenhydramine or any other anticholinergic drug

diminishes the therapeutic response to long-term treatment with aminosalicylic acid is uncertain, but it should be borne in mind.

Reference

1 Lavigne J-G and Marchand C. Inhibition of the gastrointestinal absorption of p-aminosalicylate (PAS) in rats and humans by diphenhydramine. Clin Pharmacol Ther (1973) 14, 404–12.

Aminosalicylic acid (PAS) + Probenecid

Abstract/Summary

The serum levels of aminosalicylic acid can be raised two- to fourfold by the concurrent use of probenecid.

Clinical evidence, mechanism, importance and management

A study in man showed that when 0.5 g probenecid was administered six-hourly, the serum levels of aminosalicylic acid following single 4 g doses were increased two- to fourfold.[1] Similar results are described in another report.[2] The reasons are uncertain but it seems probable that the probenecid successfully competes with the aminosalicylic acid for active excretion by the kidney tubules, resulting in its retention and accumulation in the body.

The documentation is limited but the interaction appears to be established. Such large increases in serum aminosalicylic acid levels would be expected to lead to toxicity and it also seems probable that the dosage of aminosalicylic acid could be reduced without losing the required therapeutic response. This needs confirmation. Concurrent use should be undertaken with caution.

References

1 Boger WP and Pitts FW. Influence of p-(di-N-propylsulfamyl)-benzoic acid, 'Benemid' on para-aminosalicylic (PAS) plasma concentrations. Amer Rev Tuberc (1950) 61, 682.
2 Carr DT, Karlson AG and Bridge EV. Concentration of PAS and tuberculostatic potency of serum after administration of PAS with and without Benemid. Proc Staff Meet Mayo Clin (1952) 27, 209.

Amphotericin + Corticosteroids

Abstract/Summary

Amphotericin and the corticosteroids can cause potassium loss as well as salt and water retention which can have adverse effects on cardiac function.

Clinical evidence

Four patients treated with amphotericin and 25–40 mg hydrocortisone daily developed cardiac enlargement and congestive heart failure. The cardiac size decreased and the failure disappeared within two weeks of stopping the hydrocortisone. The amphotericin was continued successfully with the addition of potassium supplements.[1]

Mechanism

Amphotericin causes potassium to be lost in the urine. Hydrocortisone can cause potassium to be lost and salt and water to be retained. Working in concert these could account for the hypokalaemic cardiopathy and the circulatory overload which was seen.

Importance and management

Information is limited but the interaction would seem to be established. Monitor the electrolyte and fluid balance and the cardiac function during concurrent use. The elderly would seem to be particularly at risk. Corticosteroids can be used to control the immediate side-effects of amphotericin (fever, chills, headache, nausea, vomiting) but bear in mind that the corticosteroids can also reduce the resistance to infection.

Reference

1 Chung D-K and Koenig MG. Reversible cardiac enlargement during treatment with amphotericin B and hydrocortisone. Report of three cases. Am Rev Resp Dis (1971) 103, 831–41.

Amphotericin + Low salt diet

Abstract/Summary, clinical evidence, mechanism, importance and management

The renal toxicity of amphotericin B can be associated with sodium depletion. When the sodium is replaced the renal function improves.[1,2]

References

1 Feeley J, Heidemann H, Gerkens J, Roberts LJ and Branch RA. Sodium depletion enhances nephrotoxicity of amphotericin B. Lancet (1981) i, 1422–3.
2 Heidemann HT, Gerkens JF, Spickard WA, Jackson EK and Branch RA. Amphotericin B nephrotoxicity in humans decreased by salt repletion. Am J Med (1983) 75, 476–81.

Amphotericin + Miconazole or Ketoconazole

Abstract/Summary

There is evidence that amphotericin with either miconazole or ketoconazole may possibly be less effective than amphotericin alone.

Clinical evidence, mechanism, importance and management

Studies in a few patients and *in vitro* experiments[1,4] suggest that the antifungal effects of amphotericin and miconazole used together may be antagonistic, and not additive as might be expected. In another study four out of six patients who failed to respond to amphotericin treatment were concurrently receiving ketoconazole, whereas it was successful in 5/6 others who stopped taking either miconazole or ketoconazole.[3] Other *in vitro* studies similarly suggest that amphotericin and ketoconazole may be less effective than amphotericin alone,[2] whereas in contrast yet another *in vitro* study indicates that the antifungal effects may be increased.[5] The reasons are not understood. Until more is known it might be better to avoid concurrent use, or at least the outcome should be very well monitored.

References

1 Schachter LP, Owellen RJ, Rathbun HK and Buchanan B. Antagonism between miconazole and amphotericin B. Lancet (1976) ii, 318.
2 Sud IJ and Feingold DS. Effect of ketoconazole on the fungicidal action of amphotericin B in Candida albicans. Antimicrob Ag Chemother (1983) 23, 185–7.
3 Meunier-Carpentier F, Cruciani M and Klastersky J. Oral prophylaxis with miconazole or ketoconazole of invasive fungal disease in neutropenic cancer patients. Eur J Cancer Clin Oncol (1983) 19, 43–8.
4 Cosgrove RF, Beezer AE and Miles RJ. *In vitro* studies of amphotericin B in combination with the imidazole antifungal compounds clotrimazole and miconazole. J Infect Dis (1979) 138, 681–5.
5 Odds FC. Interactions among amphotericin B, 5-fluorocytosine, ketoconazole, and miconazole against pathogenic fungi *in vitro*. Antimicrob Ag Chemother (1982) 22, 763–70.

Ampicillin or Amoxycillin + Allopurinol

Abstract/Summary

The incidence of skin rashes among those taking either ampicillin or amoxycillin is increased by the concurrent use of allopurinol.

Clinical evidence

A retrospective search through the records of 1324 patients, 67 of whom were taking allopurinol and ampicillin, showed that 15 of them (22%) developed a skin rash compared with 94 (7.5%) of the rest not taking allopurinol.[1] The types of rash were not defined.

Another study[2] showed similar results: 35 out of 252 patients (13.9%) compared with 251 out of 4434 (5.9%). A parallel study revealed that 8 out of 36 patients (22%) on amoxycillin and allopurinol developed a rash, whereas only 52 out of 887 (5.9%) did so on amoxycillin alone.[2]

Mechanism

Not understood. One suggestion is that the allopurinol itself was responsible.[1] Another is that hyperuricaemic individuals may possibly have an altered immunological reactivity.[3]

Importance and management

An established interaction of limited importance. There would seem to be no strong reason for avoiding concurrent use, but prescribers should recognize that the development of a rash is by no means unusual. Whether this also occurs with penicillins other than ampicillin or amoxycillin is uncertain. It appears not to have been reported.

References

1 Boston Collaborative Drug Surveillance Programme. Excess of ampicillin rashes associated with allopurinol or hyperuricaemia. N Engl J Med (1972) 286, 505.
2 Jick H and Porter JB. Potentiation of ampicillin skin reactions by allopurinol or hyperuricaemia. J Clin Pharmacol (1981) 21, 456.
3 Fessel WJ. Immunological reactivity in hyperuricaemic patients. N Engl J Med (1972) 286, 1218.

Antibiotics + Alcohol

Abstract/Summary

No adverse interaction normally occurs between alcohol and most antibiotics, with the exception of some cephalosporins, griseofulvin and possibly doxycycline.

Clinical evidence, mechanism, importance and management

A long-standing and very common belief among members of the general public (presumably derived from advice given by doctors and pharmacists) is that alcohol should be strictly avoided while taking any antibiotic. This belief was expressed in 1965 by Dr W Kitto of Chicago who, in answer to a question posed in the Journal of the American Medical Association, claimed that alcohol increases the degradation of penicillin in the gut and reduces the amount available for absorption.[2] However a much later study in 1987 showed that the pharmacokinetics of phenoxymethylpenicillin were unaffected by alcoholic drinks.[1] Another study found that alcohol delayed the absorption of amoxicillin but did not affect the total amount absorbed.[3]

It is difficult to know how this clinical folklore arose because there is little to support it for most antibiotics. The few exceptions include latamoxef, cephamandole, cefoperazone, cefmenoxime, a few other uncommon cephalosporins, and griseofulvin, all of which sometimes cause an unpleasant disulfiram-like reaction with alcohol. This does not happen with most of the commonly prescribed cephalosporins. It is also recognized that serum doxycycline levels may be significantly reduced by alcohol in alcoholics, but not in normal subjects. Details of these interactions are to be found in the appropriate synopses.

References

1 Lindberg RLP, Huupponen RK, Viljanen S and Pihlajamaki KK. Ethanol and the absorption of oral penicillin in man. Int J Clin Pharmacol Ther Toxicol (1987) 25, 536–8.

2 Kitto W. Antibiotics and alcohol ingestion. J Amer Med Ass (1965) 193, 411.
3 Morasso MI, Hip A, Marquez M, Gonzalez C and Arancibia A. Amoxicillin kinetics and ethanol ingestion. Int J Clin Pharmacol Ther Toxicol (1988) 26, 428–31.

Anti-infective agents + Cimetidine

Abstract/Summary, clinical evidence, mechanism, importance and management

Human studies show that cimetidine does not adversely affect the bioavailability of ampicillin or co-trimoxazole.[1] The bioavailability of benzylpenicillin may even be increased.[2]

References

1 Rogers HJ, James CA, Morrison PJ and Bradbrook ID. Effect of cimetidine on oral absorption of ampicillin and co-trimoxazole. J Antimicrob Chemother (1980) 6, 297.
2 Fairfax AJ, Adam J and Pagan FS. Effect of cimetidine on absorption of oral benzylpenicillin. Br Med J (1977) 2, 820.

Antimalarials + Antacids, Antidiarrhoeals

Abstract/Summary

The absorption of chloroquine can be reduced about 20% by the concurrent use of magnesium trisilicate, and about 30% by kaolin. In vitro studies suggest that pyrimethamine may possibly be similarly affected.

Clinical evidence

Six normal subjects were given 1 g chloroquine with either 1 g magnesium trisilicate or 1 g kaolin after an overnight fast. The magnesium trisilicate reduced the AUC (area under the concentration/time curve) of the chloroquine by 18.2% and the kaolin reduced it by 28.6%.[1]

Related in vitro studies by the same authors using segments of everted rat intestine showed that the absorption of chloroquine and pyrimethamine respectively were decreased as follows: magnesium trisilicate (-31.3 and -37.5%), kaolin (-46.5 and -49.9%), calcium carbonate (-52.8 and -31.5%), and gerdiga (-36.1 and -38.0%). Gerdiga is a clay containing hydrated silicates with sodium and potassium carbonates and bicarbonates. It is used in rural areas of the Sudan as an antacid and is similar to attapulgite.[2]

Mechanism

These antacid and antidiarrhoeal compounds adsorb chloroquine thereby reducing the amount available for absorption by the gut. Pyrimethamine appears to be similarly affected.

Importance and management

The chloroquine/magnesium trisilicate and chloroquine/kaolin interactions are established. Whether the therapeutic effects of the chloroquine are significantly reduced is uncertain, nevertheless it would seem prudent to separate the doses as much as possible to reduce admixture in the gut. Nobody seems to have checked if other antacids interact similarly. There does not seem to be any direct evidence from clinical studies that the effects of pyrimethamine are significantly reduced by antacids and antidiarrhoeals, however it should be pointed out that its *in vitro* absorption pattern in animal studies is similar to chloroquine.[2]

References

1 McElnay JC, Mukhtar HA, D'Arcy PF, Temple DJ and Collier PS. The effect of magnesium trisicate and kaolin on the *in vivo* absorption of chloroquine. J Trop Med Hyg (1982) 85, 159–63.
2 McElnay JC, Mukhtar HA, D'Arcy PF and Temple DJ. In vitro experiments on chloroquine and pyrimethamine absorption in the presence of antacid constituents of kaolin. J Trop Med Hyg (1982) 85, 153–8.

Cephalosporins + Cholestyramine

Abstract/Summary

Cholestyramine binds with cefadroxil and cephalexin in the gut which delays their absorption. The importance of this is uncertain but probably small.

Clinical evidence

A cross-over study in four normal subjects showed that peak serum levels of cefadroxil (after a 500 mg oral dose) were reduced and delayed if the antibiotic was taken with 10 g cholestyramine, but the total amount absorbed was not affected.[1]

Similar results were found in a study involving cephalexin and cholestyramine.[2]

Mechanism

Cholestyramine is an ion-exchange resin which binds with these two cephalosporins in the gut. This prevents the early and rapid absorption of the antibiotic, but as the cholestyramine-cephalosporin complex passes along the gastro-intestinal tract, the antibiotic is progressively released and eventually virtually all of it becomes available for absorption.[1]

Importance and management

Direct information seems to be limited to the studies cited. The clinical significance is uncertain, but as the total amount of antibiotic absorbed is not reduced it is probably of little importance. This needs confirmation. Information about other cephalosporins seems to be lacking.

References

1 Marino EL, Vicente MT and Dominguez-Gil A. Influence of cholestyramine on the pharmacokinetic parameters of cefadroxil after simultaneous administration. Int J Pharmaceutics (1983) 16, 23–30.
2 Parson RL, Paddock GM and Hossack GM. Cholestyramine-induced antibiotic malabsorption. Chemotherapy 4. In Williams JD and Geddes AM. (eds) Pharmacology of Antibiotics. Plenum Press, New York, London (1975) pp 191–8.

Cephalosporins + Frusemide (Furosemide)

Abstract/Summary

The nephrotoxic effects of cephaloridine appear to be increased by the concurrent use of frusemide. Whether cephalothin and cephacetrile are similarly affected is as yet uncertain. Cephradine levels in the brain are reduced by frusemide.

Clinical evidence

Nine out of 36 patients who developed acute renal failure while taking cephaloridine had also been treated with a diuretic, frusemide being used in seven cases. Other factors such as age and dosage may also have been involved. The authors of this report related their observations to previous animal studies which showed that potent diuretics such as frusemide and ethacrynic acid enhanced the incidence and extent of tubular necrosis.[1,2]

Several other reports describe nephrotoxicity in patients given both drugs.[3,4,6] Brain concentrations of cephradine are markedly reduced by frusemide.[13]

Mechanism

Cephaloridine alone is nephrotoxic, but why this should be increased by frusemide is not understood. The clearance of cephaloridine is reduced by frusemide.[7,12] One clinical study showed that frusemide (80 mg) increased the serum half-life of cephaloridine by 25%,[8] but whether this has any bearing on the matter is uncertain.

Importance and management

The cephaloridine-frusemide interaction is not well-established, but there is enough evidence to suggest that concurrent use should be undertaken with caution. Age and/or renal impairment may possibly be predisposing factors. Renal function should be checked frequently. A pharmacokinetic study suggests that the development of this adverse interaction may possibly depend on the time relationship of drug administration, and it has been recommended that frusemide should be avoided 3 or 4 h before the cephaloridine.[11]

Most other cephalosporins appear not to interact with frusemide with a few possible exceptions: There is a question mark hanging over cephalothin and cephacetrile because animal studies have demonstrated increased nephrotoxicity,[9,10] and nephrotoxicity has been seen in a patient on cephalothin and frusemide.[3] Frusemide is also reported markedly to reduce brain concentrations of cephradine.[12] On the other hand studies in man have shown that cefoxitin seems to be relatively free of nephrotoxicity alone or combined with frusemide.[5] Ceftriaxone does not interfere with the diuretic effects of frusemide.[14]

References

1 Foord RD. Cephaloridine and the kidney. Proc VIth Int Cong Chemother, Tokyo (1969) 1, 597.
2 Dodds MG and Foord RD. Enhancement by potent diuretics of renal tubular necrosis induced by cephaloridine. Br J Pharmacol (1970) 40, 227.
3 Simpson IJ. Nephrotoxicity and acute renal failure associated with cephalothin and cephaloridine. NZ Med J (1971) 74, 312.
4 Kleinknecht D, Jungers P and Fillastre J-P. Nephrotoxicity of cephaloridine. Ann Intern Med (1974) 80, 421.
5 Trolifors B. Effects on renal function of treatment with cefoxitin alone or in combination with furosemide. Scand J Inf Dis (1978) (Suppl) 13, 73.
6 Lawson DH, Macadam RF, Singh H, Gavras H and Linton AL. The nephrotoxicity of cephaloridine. Postgrad Med J (1970) 46 (Suppl) 36.
7 Lawson DH, Tilstone WJ and Semple PF. Furosemide interactions: studies in normal volunteers. Clin Res (1976) 24, 3.
8 Norrby R, Stenqvist K and Elgefors B. Interaction between cephaloridine and furosemide in man. Scand J Inf Dis (1976) 8, 209.
9 Lawson DH, Macadam RF, Singh H, Gavras H, Hartz S, Turnbull D and Linton A. Effect of furosemide on antibiotic induced renal damage in rats. J Inf Dis (1972) 126, 593.
10 Luscombe DK and Nichols PJ. Possible interaction between cephacetrile and frusemide in rabbits and rats. J Antimicrob Chemother (1972) 1, 67.
11 Kosmsidis J, Polyzos A and Daikos GK. Pharmacokinetic interactions between cephalosporins and furosemide are influenced by administration time relationships. Curr Chemother Infect Dis. PISF Int Cong Chemother 11th (1979 and 1980) p 673.
12 Tilstone WJ, Semple PF, Lawson DH and Boyle JA. Effects of furosemide on glomerular filtration rate and clearance of practolol, digoxin, cephaloridine and gentamicin. Clin Pharmacol Ther (1976) 22, 389.
13 Adam D, Jacoby W and Raff WK. Beeinflusung der Antibiotika-Konzentration im Gewebe durch ein Saluretikum. Klin Wsch (1978) 56, 247.
14 Korn H, Eichler HG and Gasic S. A drug interaction study of ceftriaxone and frusemine in healthy volunteers. Int J Clin Pharmacol Ther Tox (1986) 24, 262–4.

Cephalosporins + Penicillins

Abstract/Summary

Mezlocillin reduces the loss of cefotaxime from the body.

Clinical evidence, mechanism, importance and management

A study in eight normal subjects showed that when cefotaxime (30 mg/kg) and mezlocillin (50 mg/kg) were infused together over 30 min, the kinetics of the mezlocillin were unchanged but the clearance of the cefotaxime was reduced by 40%. The clinical significance of this is uncertain.[1]

Reference

1 Flaherty J, Barriere S and Gambertoglio J. Interaction between cefotaxime and mezlocillin. Clin Pharmacol Ther (1985) 41, 196.

Cephalosporins + Probenecid

Abstract/Summary

The serum levels of many but not all cephalosporins are raised by the concurrent use of probenecid. This can be exploited in the treatment of some conditions, but it may also increase the risk of nephrotoxicity with cephaloridine and possibly cephalothin.

Clinical evidence

A study in 10 normal subjects given single 500 mg oral doses of cephradine or cefaclor showed that the concurrent use of probenecid (500 mg doses taken 25, 13 and 2 h before the antibiotic) markedly raised the serum concentrations of both antibiotics. Peak serum levels were very roughly doubled.[1]

Probenecid also raises the serum levels and prolongs the half-life of cefmetazole,[15] cephaloridine,[2] cephazolin,[3] cephacetrile,[4] cephradine,[5] cephaloglycin,[6] cephalothin,[7] cephamandole,[8] cefoxitin,[9,11] ceftizoxime[12] and cephalexin.[10] However probenecid is reported to lack any effect on the pharmacokinetics of ceftriaxone[13] and ceforanide.[14]

Mechanism

Probenecid inhibits the excretion of the cephalosporins by the kidney tubules by successfully competing for the excretory mechanisms (a fuller explanation of this mechanism is set out in the introductory chapter). Thus the cephalosporin is retained in the body and its serum levels rise. The extent of the rise cannot be fully accounted for by this mechanism alone and it is suggested that some change in tissue distribution may also have a part to play.[1]

Importance and management

An extremely well-documented interaction, only a few representative references being listed here. Serum levels of many cephalosporins will be higher if probenecid is used concurrently, but no special precautions are normally needed. This interaction has been exploited in the treatment of gonorrhoea. However elevated serum levels of some cephalosporins, in particular cephaloridine and cephalothin, carry the risk of increased nephrotoxicity.

References

1 Welling PG, Dean S, Selen A, Kendall MJ and Wise R. Probenecid: an unexplained effect on cephalosporin pharmacology. Br J clin Pharmac (1979) 8, 491.
2 Kaplan KS, Reisberg BE and Weinstein L. Cephaloridine: antimicrobial activity and pharmacologic behaviour. Amer J Med Sci (1967) 253, 667.
3 Duncan WC. Treatment of gonorrhoea with cefazolin plus probenecid. J Infect Dis (1974) 120, 398.

4 Wise R and Reeves DS. Pharmacological studies on cephacetrile in human volunteers. Curr Med Res Opin (1974) 2, 249.

5 Mischler TW, Sugerman AA, Willard SA, Bannick LJ and Neiss ES. Influence of probenecid and food on the bioavailability of cephradine in normal male subjects. J Clin Pharmacol (1974) 14, 604.

6 Applestein JM, Crosby EB, Johnson WD and Kaye D. In-vitro antimicrobial activity and human pharmacology of cephaloglycin. Appl Microbiol (1968) 16, 1006.

7 Tuano SB, Brodie JL and Kirby WMM. Cephaloridine versus cephalothin: relation of the kidney to blood level differences after parenteral administration. Antimicrob Ag Chemother (1966) 101.

8 Griffith RS, Black HR, Brier GL and Wolney JD. Effect of probenecid on the blood levels and urinary excretion of cefamandole. Antimicrob Ag Chemother (1977) 11, 809.

9 Bint AJ, Reeves DS and Holt HA. Effect of probenecid on serum cefoxitin concentrations. J Antimicrob Chemother (1977) 3, 627.

10 Taylor WA and Holloway WJ. Cephalexin in the treatment of gonorrhoea. Int J Clin Pharmacol (1972) 6, 7.

11 Reeves DS, Bullock DW, Bywater MJ, Holt HA, White LO and Thornhill DP. The effect of probenecid on the pharmacokinetics and distribution of cefoxitin in healthy volunteers. Br J clin Pharmac (1981) 11, 353.

12 LeBel M, Paone RP and Lewis GP. Effect of probenecid on the pharmacokinetics of ceftizoxime. J Antimicrob Chemother (1983) 12, 147–55.

13 Stockel K, McNamara PJ, Brandt R and Ziegler WH. The influence of protein binding on the pharmacokinetics of 'Rocephin' Roche. 12th Int Congr Chemother, Florence. (1981) 987.

14 Jovanovich JF, Saravolatz LD, Burch K and Pohlod DJ. Failure of probenecid to alter the pharmacokinetics of ceforanide. Antimicrob Ag Chemother (1981) 20, 530–2.

15 Ko H, Cathcart KS, Griffith DL, Peters GR and Adams WJ. Pharmacokinetics of intravenously administered cefmetazole and cefoxitin and effects of probenecid on cefmetazole elimination. Antimicrob Ag Chemother (1989) 33, 356–61.

Cephalothin + Colistin sulphomethate sodium

Abstract/Summary

Renal failure has been attributed to the concurrent use of cephalothin and colistin sulphomethate sodium (colistimethate sodium).

Clinical evidence, mechanism, importance and management

Four patients developed acute renal failure during treatment with colistin sulphomethate sodium. Three were given cephalothin concurrently and the fourth had previously been treated with this antibiotic.[1] An increase in renal toxicity associated with concurrent use has been described in another report.[2] The reason for this reaction is not known. What is know suggests that renal function should be closely monitored if these antibiotics are given concurrently or sequentially.

References

1 Adler S and Segal DP. Nonoliguric renal failure secondary to sodium colistimethate. A report of four cases. Amer J Med Sci (1971) 262, 109.

2 Koch-Weser J, Sidel VW, Federman EB, Karnarek F, Finer DC and Eaton AE. Adverse effects of sodium colistimethate. Manifestations and specific reaction rates during 317 courses of therapy. Ann Intern Med (1970) 72, 857.

Chloramphenicol + Paracetamol (Acetaminophen)

Abstract/Summary

Paracetamol is reported to increase, decrease or to have no effect on chloramphenicol serum levels. The outcome of concurrent use is therefore uncertain.

Clinical evidence, mechanism, importance and management

Following an initial observation that the half-life of chloramphenicol in children with kwashiorkor was prolonged by paracetamol, a study on six adults showed that the half-life of chloramphenicol (1 g intravenously) was increased from 3.25 to 15 h by 100 mg paracetamol (given intravenously 2 h later). The reason is not understood.[1] Later studies in 26 child patients[2] and eight normal adults[3] failed to confirm the existence of this interaction. Another study[4] in five child patients found that the clearance of chloramphenicol was *increased* and its half-life *reduced* from 3 to 1.2 h in five child patients.

These contradictory reports make the whole situation very confusing indeed. The outcome of concurrent use is uncertain, but it would clearly be prudent to monitor serum chloramphenicol levels closely. A reversible form of bone marrow depression which is dose-related can take place when chloramphenicol concentrations reach the 25–35 μg/ ml range. More study is needed.

References

1 Buchanan N and Moodley GP. Interaction between chloramphenicol and paracetamol. Br Med J (1979) 2, 307.

2 Kearns GL, Bocchini JA, Brown RD, Cotter DL and Wilson JT. Absence of a pharmacokinetic interaction between chloramphenicol and acetaminophen in children. J Pediatr (1985) 107, 134–9.

3 Rajpurohit R and Krishnaswamy K. Lack of effect of paracetamol on the pharmacokinetics of chloramphenicol in adult human subjects. Ind J Pharmac (1984) 124–8.

4 Spika JS, Davis DJ, Martin SR, Beharry K, Rex J and Aranda JV. Interaction between chloramphenicol and acetaminophen. Arch Dis Child (1986) 61, 1121–4.

Chloramphenicol + Penicillins, Streptomycin or Cephalosporins

Abstract/Summary

Antagonism between chloramphenicol and other antibiotics has been described in a case of staphylococcal endocarditis, in bacterial meningitis in a large group of patients and in an infant, and in experimental Pneumococcal meningitis in dogs. In contrast, no antagonism and even additive antibiotic effects have been described in other infections.

Clinical evidence

(a) Antibiotic antagonism

A study on 264 patients (adults and children of more than two months) with acute bacterial meningitis showed that on ampicillin alone the case-fatality ratio was 4.3% compared with 10.5% on a combination of ampicillin, chloramphenicol and streptomycin. The neurological sequelae (hemiparesis, deafness, cranial nerve palsies) were also markedly increased by the use of the combined drugs.[6]

A man with acute *Staphylococcus aureus* endocarditis showed clinical deterioration and positive blood culture when chloramphenicol was added to methicillin. The patient's serum inhibited the infecting organism at a dilution of 1 in 64, but was not bactericidal even at 1 in 2. After withdrawal of the chloramphenicol, methicillin alone was successful. The patient's serum was then still inhibitory at 1 in 64 but had become bactericidal at 1 in 32.[4]

Antagonism has also been described in an infant of two-and-a-half months with meningitis due to *Salmonella enteritidis* treated with chloramphenicol and ceftazidime,[7] and in experimental pneumococcal meningitis in dogs treated with chloramphenicol and penicillin.[1]

(b) Lack of antagonism and increased antibiotic effects

A report claims that no antagonism was seen in 65 of 66 patients given chloramphenicol and benzylpenicillin for bronchitis or bronchopneumonia.[2] Ampicillin with chloramphenicol is more effective than chloramphenicol alone in the treatment of typhoid,[3] and benzyl procaine penicillin with chloramphenicol is more effective than chloramphenicol alone in the treatment of gonorrhoea (failure rates of 1.8 compared with 8.5%).[8] In a study on premature, newborn children and infants it was found that the presence of pencillin markedly raised the serum concentrations of concurrently administered chloramphenicol.[5]

Mechanism

By no means fully understood. Chloramphenicol inhibits bacterial protein synthesis and can change an actively growing bacterial colony into a static one. Thus the effects of a bactericide, such as penicillin, which interferes with cell wall synthesis, are blunted, and the death of the organism occurs more slowly. This would seem to explain the antagonism seen with some organisms.

Importance and management

Proven cases of antibiotic antagonism in patients seem to be few in number (although *in vitro* evidence is available). Some practitioners totally avoid concurrent use, but there is certainly insufficient evidence to impose a general prohibition because (depending on the organism) they have sometimes been used together with clear advantage.[3,8] The authors of one report[1] point out that, where the diagnosis of the meningitis is still not clear, and when chloramphenicol is thought to be necessary because the condition could be due to *H. influenzae* or one of the enterobacteriaceae, it would seem reasonable to use the pencillin or other bactericide first of all, withholding treatment with the bacteriostat for at least an hour.

References

1 Wallace JF, Smith RH, Garcia M and Petersdorf RG. Studies on the pathogenesis of meningitis. VI. Antagonism between penicillin and chloramphenicol in experimental pneumococcal meningitis. J Lab Clin Med (1967) 70, 408.

2 Ardalan P. Zur frage des Antagonismus von Penicillin und Chloramphenicolus Klinischer sicht. Prax Pneumol (1969) 23, 722.

3 De Ritis R, Giammanco G and Manzillo G. Chloramphenicol combined with ampicillin in the treatment of typhoid. Br Med J (1972) 4, 17.

4 Percival A. In Antibiotic Interactions. Williams JD (ed) (1979) Academic Press.

5 Windorfer A and Pringsheim W. Studies on the concentrations of chloramphenicol in the serum and cerebrospinal fluid of neonates, infants and small children. Europ J Pediatr (1977) 124, 129–38.

6 Mathies AW, Leedom JM, Ivler D, Wehrle PF and Portnoy B. Antibiotic antagonism in bacterial meningitis. Antimicrob Ag Chemother (1967) 218–24.

7 French GL, Ling TKW, Davies DP and Leung DTY. Antagonism of ceftazidime by chloramphenicol *in vitro* and *in vivo* during treatment of Gram negative meningitis. Br Med J (1985) 291, 636–7.

8 Gjessing HC and Odegaard K. Oral chloramphenicol alone and with intramuscular procaine penicillin in the treatment of gonorrhoea. Br J Ven Dis (1967) 43, 133–6.

Chloramphenicol + Phenobarbitone

Abstract/Summary

Studies in children show that phenobarbitone can markedly depress serum chloramphenicol levels. There is a single report of markedly increased serum phenobarbitone levels in a man caused by the use of chloramphenicol.

Clinical evidence

(a) Decreased serum chloramphenicol concentrations

Two children of three and seven months treated for *H. influenzae* meningitis with 100 mg/kg/day chloramphenicol, initially intravenously but later orally, failed to achieve the expected peak serum levels of 15–25 mg/l while concurrently receiving phenobarbitone (10 mg/kg/day) to prevent convulsions. One child had serum chloramphenicol levels of only 5 mg/l or less until the chloramphenicol dosage was doubled, when they rose to 7–11 mg/l.[1]

This interaction has been described in another single case report of a child who was also being treated with phenytoin.[6] Other studies in neonates (20 patients) confirm that this interaction can occur, but no statistically significant effect was confirmed in infants (40 patients).[7]

(b) Decreased serum phenobarbitone concentrations

A man admitted to hospital on numerous occasions for pulmonary complications associated with cystic fibrosis, had average serum phenobarbitone concentrations of 35 mg/l while taking 200 mg phenobarbitone daily and chloramphenicol. When the antibiotic was withdrawn, his serum phenobarbitone levels fell by a third (to 24 mg/l) even though the phenobarbitone dosage was increased from 200 to 300 mg daily.[4]

Mechanism

Phenobarbitone is a potent liver enzyme inducing agent which can increase the metabolism and clearance of chloramphenicol (clearly demonstrated in rats[2]) so that its serum levels fall and its effects are reduced. Chloramphenicol has the opposite effect and inhibits the metabolism of the phenobarbitone (also demonstrated in animals[5]) so that the effects of the barbiturate are increased.

Importance and management

The documentation of these interactions is limited. Their incidence is not known. Concurrent use should be well monitored to ensure that chloramphenicol serum levels are adequate, and that phenobarbitone levels do not become too high. Make appropriate dosage adjustments as necessary. Other barbiturates also act like phenobarbitone and may be expected to interact similarly. Sodium valproate has little or no enzyme-inducing activity and may be a suitable anticonvulsant alternative for phenobarbitone.[3]

References

1 Bloxham RA, Durbin GM, Johnson T and Winterborn MH. Chloramphenicol and phenobarbitone—a drug interaction. Arch Dis Child (1979) 54, 76.
2 Bella DD, Ferrari V, Marca G and Bonanomi L. Chloramphenicol metabolism in the phenobarbital-induced liver. Comparison with thiamphenicol. Biochem Pharmacol (1968) 17, 2381.
3 Oxley J, Hedges A, Makki KA, Monks A and Richens A. Lack of hepatic enzyme-inducing effect of sodium valproate. Br J clin Pharmac (1979) 8, 189.
4 Koup JR, Gibaldi M, McNamara P, Hilligoss DM, Colburn W and Bruck E. Interaction of chloramphenicol with phenytoin and phenobarbital. Case report. Clin Pharmacol Ther (1978) 24, 571.
5 Adams HR. Prolonged barbiturate anaesthesia by chloramphenicol in animals. J Amer Vet Med Assoc (1970) 157, 1908.
6 Powell DA, Nahala MC, Durrell DC, Glazer JP and Hilty MJ. Interactions among chloramphenicol, phenytoin and phenobarbitone in a pediatric patient. J Pediatr (1981) 98, 1001.
7 Windorfer A and Pringsheim W. Studies on the concentrations of chloramphenicol in the serum and cerebrospinal fluid of neonates, infants and small children. Eur J Pediat (1977) 124, 129–38.

Chloramphenicol + Rifampicin (Rifampin)

Abstract/Summary

The chloramphenicol serum levels of two children were markedly lowered when additionally treated with rifampicin.

Clinical evidence

Two children aged two and five, under treatment for meningitis due to *Haemophilus influenzae*, were given 100 mg/kg/day chloramphenicol in four divided doses by slow infusion. Within three days of starting additional treatment with rifampicin (20 mg/kg/day) their peak serum chloramphenicol levels were markedly depressed (by 85 and 64% respectively) and only returned into the therapeutic range after the dosage of chloramphenicol was increased to 125 mg/kg/day.[1]

Mechanism

It is thought that rifampicin, a potent enzyme inducing agent, markedly increased the metabolism of the chloramphenicol by the liver, thereby lowering its serum levels.[1]

Importance and management

Even though so far only these two cases have been reported, the evidence is sufficiently strong for this interaction to be taken seriously. There is a risk that the serum chloramphenicol will fall to sub-therapeutic levels unless the dosage is increased appropriately.

Reference

1 Prober CG. Effect of rifampin on chloramphenicol levels. N Engl J Med (1985) 312, 788–9.

Chloroquine + Cimetidine or Ranitidine

Abstract/Summary

Cimetidine reduces the metabolism and the loss of chloroquine from the body. The clinical importance of this is still uncertain. Ranitidine appears not to interact.

Clinical evidence, mechanism, importance and management

A study in 10 normal subjects found that 400 mg cimetidine daily for four days approximately halved (from 0.49 to 0.23 l/d/kg) the clearance of a single dose of chloroquine (600 mg base). The elimination half-life was prolonged from 3.11 to 4.62 days.[1] The suggested reason is that the cimetidine inhibits the metabolism of the chloroquine by the liver, thereby reducing its loss from the body. The clinical importance of this interaction is uncertain, but since the main metabolite of chloroquine has pharmacological activity it would seem prudent to be alert for any signs of chloroquine toxicity during concurrent use. A similar study by the same authors found that ranitidine does not interact with chloroquine.[2]

References

1 Ette EI, Brown-Awala EA and Essien EE. Chloroquine elimination in humans: effect of low-dose cimetidine. J Clin Pharmacol (1987) 27, 813–16.
2 Ette EI, Brown-Awala EA and Essien EE. Effect of ranitidine on chloroquine disposition. Drug Intell Clin Pharm (1987) 21, 732–4.

Co-trimoxazole + Folic acid

Abstract/Summary

The effects of folic acid used to treat megaloblastic anaemia can be reduced or abolished by co-trimoxazole.

Clinical evidence

Four patients failed to respond to their treatment for megaloblastic anaemia while concurrently taking co-trimoxazole. The expected reticulocyte response failed to occur in three of the patients and the fourth showed no clinical improvement until the co-trimoxazole was withdrawn.[1]

This interaction has been described in other reports.[2,3]

Mechanism

Not understood. In theory neither sulphamethoxazole nor trimethoprim should disturb folate metabolism in man. Along with other mammmals we rely on folate in the diet rather than on an ability to synthesize it from PABA. Moreover mammalian dihydrofolate reductase is about 50,000 times less sensitive to trimethoprim than the bacterial enzyme. But in practice haematological changes can occur in man.

Importance and management

An established interaction. The 'antifolate' effects of co-trimoxazole are well documented. In normal individuals the effects are usually mild and relatively unimportant, but in patients with megaloblastic anaemia the effects are much more serious and co-trimoxazole should therefore be avoided.

References

1 Chanarin I and England JM. Toxicity of trimethoprim-sulphamethoxazole in patients with megaloblastic anaemia. Br Med J (1972) 1, 651.
2 Rooney PJ and Housley E. Trimethoprim-sulphamethoxazole in folic acid deficiency. Br Med J (1972) 2, 656.
3 Hill AVL and Kerr DNS. Toxicity of co-trimoxazole in nutritional haematinic deficiency. Postgrad Med J (1973) 49, 596.

Co-trimoxazole + Kaolin-pectin

Abstract/Summary

Kaolin-pectin can cause a small but probably clinically unimportant reduction in serum co-trimoxazole levels.

Clinical evidence

Eight normal subjects were given 20 ml co-trimoxazole suspension (160 mg trimethoprim + 800 mg sulphamethoxazole, *Septran* paediatric) with and without 20 ml kaolin-pectin suspension. The kaolin-pectin reduced the AUC of the trimethoprim by 12% and of the sulphamethoxazole by 9.5%. The maximal serum levels were reduced by 20% and 7.6% respectively.[1]

Mechanism

The probable reason is that the drugs are adsorbed onto the the kaolin-pectin which reduces their bioavailability.

Importance and management

These reductions are small and unlikely to be clinically relevant, but this needs confirmation.

Reference

1 Gupta KC, Desai NK, Satoskar RS, Gupta C and Goswami SN. Effect of pectin and kaolin on bioavailability of co-trimoxazole suspension. Int J Clin Pharmacol Ther Tox (1987) 25, 320–1.

Co-trimoxazole + Prilocaine-lignocaine (Lidocaine) cream

Abstract/Summary

Methaemoglobinaemia developed in a baby treated with co-trimoxazole when a prilocaine-lignocaine cream was applied to his skin.

Clinical evidence, mechanism, importance and management

A twelve-week-old child on co-trimoxazole (sulphamethoxazole+trimethoprim) for two months for pyelitis was treated with 5 g of EMLA cream (25 mg prilocaine and 25 mg lidocaine per gram) applied to the back of his hands and in the cubital regions. This cream allows pain-free venipuncture. 5 h later just before an operation began his skin was noted to be pale and his lips had a brownish cyanotic colour. This was found to be due to the presence of 28% methaemoglobin. The authors of the report suggest that the prilocaine together with the sulphamethoxazole (both known to be able to cause methaemoglobin formation) suppressed the activity of two enzymes (NADH-dehydrogenase and NADP-diaphorase) which normally keep blood levels of methaemoglobin to a minimum. The authors advise caution in using EMLA cream on infants because they appear to be predisposed to methaemoglobin formation with prilocaine.[1]

Reference

1 Jakobson B and Nilsson A. Methemoglobinemia associated with a prilocaine-lidocaine cream and trimetoprim-sulphamethoxazole. A case report. Acta Anaesthesiol Scand (1985) 29, 453–55.

Cycloserine + Alcohol, Isoniazid, Phenytoin

Abstract/Summary

Cycloserine is reported to increase the effects of alcohol and phenytoin. Its CNS side-effects are increased by isoniazid.

Clinical evidence, mechanism, importance and management

A brief report describes an enhancement of the actions of alcohol in two patients on cycloserine.[1] Patients should be warned. In a report about the concurrent use of cycloserine and isoniazid, both increased and decreased serum cycloserine levels were seen but the mean values were not significantly changed. Only one out of 11 on cycloserine alone developed CNS effects (drowsiness, dizziness, unstable gait), but when given in conjunction with isoniazid, nine of the 11 developed these effects.[2] Lilley who market cycloserine also say that it reduces the metabolism of phenytoin so that the risk of phenytoin intoxication is increased but the documentation for this is uncertain.

References

1 Glass F, Mallach HJ and Simsch A. Beobachtungen und Unter-suchungen uber die gemeinsame wirkung von Alkohol und D-Cycloserin. Arzneim-Forsch (Drug Res) (1965) 15, 684.
2 Mattila MJ, Nieminen E and Tiitinen H. Serum levels, urinary excre-tion, and side-effects of cycloserine in the presence of isoniazid and p-aminosalicylic acid. Scand J Resp Dis (1969) 50, 291–300.

Dapsone + Clofazimine

Abstract/Summary

Dapsone can reduce the anti-inflammatory effects of clofazimine.

Clinical evidence, mechanism, importance and management

14 out of 16 patients with severe recurrent erythema nodosum leprosum (ENL) failed to respond adequately when given dapsone and clofazimine and needed additional therapy with corticosteroids. When the dapsone was stopped the patients responded to clofazimine alone and in some in-stances they were controlled on smaller doses.[1] Further evidence of this interaction comes from a laboratory study which suggests that the actions of clofazimine may be related to its ability to inhibit neutrophil migration (resulting in decreased numbers of neutrophils in areas of inflammation), whereas dapsone can have the opposite effect.[1] Clofazimine does not affect the pharmacokinetics of dapsone.[2] Although the information is very limited, it would seem prudent to avoid concurrent use in the treatment of ENL. The authors of the report cited[1] are at great pains to emphasize that what they describe only relates to the effects of dapsone on the anti-inflammatory effects of clofazimine, and not to the beneficial effects of combined use when treating drug-resistant *Mycobacterium leprae*.

References

1 Imkamp FMJH, Anderson R and Gatner EMS. Possible incompatibility of dapsone with clofazimine in the treatment of patients with erythema nodosum leprosum. Lepr Rev (1982) 53, 148–53.
2 Venkatesan K, Mathur A, Girdhar BK and Bharadwaj VP. The effect of clofazimine on the pharmacokinetics of rifampicin and dapsone in leprosy. J Antimicrob Chemother (1986) 18, 715–18.

Dapsone + Probenecid

Abstract/Summary

The serum levels of dapsone can be markedly raised by the concurrent use of probenecid.

Clinical evidence

A study in 12 men given 500 mg dapsone with 300 mg pro-benecid, and 3 h later another 500 mg dapsone, showed that the dapsone serum levels were raised about 50% when measured at 4 h. The urinary excretion of dapsone and its metabolites were found to be reduced.[1]

Mechanism

Not fully examined. It seems probable that the probenecid inhibits the renal excretion of dapsone by the kidney.

Importance and management

The documentation is very limited, but it seems to be an established interaction. It is likely that the probenecid will raise the serum levels of dapsone given chronically. The im-portance of this is uncertain, but the extent of the rise and the evidence that the haematological toxicity of dapsone may be dose-related[2] suggests that it may well have some clinical importance. This needs confirmation.

References

1 Goodwin CS and Sparell G. Inhibition of dapsone excretion by pro-benecid. Lancet (1969) ii, 884.
2 Ellard GA. Dapsone acetylation in dermatitis herpetiformis. Br J Derm (1974) 90, 441.

Dapsone + Rifampicin (Rifampin)

Abstract/Summary

Rifampicin increases the excretion of dapsone and lowers its serum levels.

Clinical evidence, mechanism, importance and management

A study in seven patients with leprosy given single doses of dapsone (100 mg) and rifampicin (600 mg), alone or together, showed that while the pharmacokinetics of rifampicin were not significantly changed by dapsone, the half-life of the dapsone was halved and the AUC was reduced by about 20%.[1] This confirms previous studies in patients given both drugs for several days who had reduced dapsone serum levels and an increased urinary excretion.[2,3]

Mechanism

It seems probable that the rifampicin, well recognized as a potent liver-enzyme inducing agent, increases the metabolism and loss of dapsone from the body.

Importance and management

This interaction is established, but its clinical importance is uncertain. Concurrent use should be well monitored to confirm that treatment is effective. It may be necessary to raise the dosage of dapsone.

References

1 Krishna DR, Appa Rao AVN, Ramanakar TV and Prabhakar MC. Pharmacokinetic interaction between dapsone and rifampicin (rifampin) in leprosy patients. Drug Dev Ind Pharmacy (1986) 12, 443–9.
2 Balakrishnan S and Seshadri PS. Drug interactions, the influence of rifampicin (rifampin) and clofazimine on the urinary excretion of DDS. Lepr India (1970) 53, 17–22.
3 Peters JH, Murray JF, Gordon GR, Gelber RH, Levy L, Laing ABG and Waters MFR. Tissue levels of dapsone in mice, rats and man. Int J Lepr (1976) 44, 545.

Erythromycin + Antacids

Abstract/Summary

Mylanta *can prolong the absorption of erythromycin but the clinical importance of this is uncertain.*

Clinical evidence, mechanism, importance and management

A study in eight normal subjects found that 30 ml *Mylanta* (aluminium hydroxide, magnesium hydroxide, dimethicone) given with 500 mg erythromycin stearate had no significant effect on the AUC, peak serum concentration, or time to peak serum concentration of the erythromycin, but the mean elimination rate constant was 0.44 compared with 0.2 h^{-1}. Thus the total amount of erythromycin absorbed remained unaltered but its absorption appeared to be prolonged.[1] The reason for this is not clear nor is its clinical importance known.

Reference

1 Yamreudeewong W, Scavone JM, Paone RP and Lewis GP. Effect of antacid co-administration on the bioavailability of erythromycin stearate. Clin Pharmacy (1989) 8, 352–4.

Erythromycin + Other antibiotics

Abstract/Summary

There is evidence that the effectiveness of concurrent treatment with erythromycin and other antibiotics (e.g. penicillin, ampicillin, lincomycin) may sometimes be more, and sometimes less, effective than with only one antibiotic.

Clinical evidence, mechanism, importance and management

The penicillins and erythromycin have a similar range of antibacterial activity so that so that it is fairly unusual to use them them together and not much is known about the effectiveness of concurrent use. A large scale clinical study of uncomplicated scarlatina showed that penicillin was more effective than erythromycin, while the two antibiotics together were slightly less effective, as judged by the duration of the fever and the disappearance of the haemolytic streptococci.[1] This antagonism was seen in an *in vitro* study.[2] It has been suggested that combined treatment may possibly be more effective in the case of double infections with penicillinase-producing staphylococci.[1] There is also evidence that erythromycin with ampicillin is effective in pulmonary nocardiosis.[3] *In vitro* antagonism has been seen when a strain of staphylococci (resistant to erythromycin but sensitive to lincomycin) was exposed to both antibiotics together.[4] Whether this is likely to occur *in vivo* is uncertain. The general points for and against concurrent treatment with antibiotics and anti-infective agents are outlined in the introduction to this chapter.

References

1 Strom J. Penicillin and erythromycin singly and in combination in scarlatina therapy and the interference between them. Antibiot Chemotherap (1961) 11, 694.
2 Manten A. Synergism and antagonism between antibiotic mixtures containing erythromycin. Antibiot Chemotherap (1954) 4, 1228.
3 Bach MC, Monaco AP and Finland M. Pulmonary nocardiosis: therapy with minocycline and with erythromycin plus ampicillin. J Amer Med Ass (1973) 224, 1378.
4 Griffint LJ, Ostrande WE, Mullins CG and Beswick DE. Drug antagonism between lincomycin and erythromycin. Science (1964) 147, 746.

Erythromycin + Urinary acidifiers or Alkalinizers

Abstract/Summary

In the treatment of urinary tract infections, the antibacterial activity of erythromycin is maximal in alkaline urine and minimal in acid urine.

Clinical evidence

Urine taken from seven volunteers taking 1 g erythromycin, four times a day, was tested against five genera of Gram-negative bacilli (*Escherichia coli, Klebsiella pneumoniae, P. mirabilis, Ps. aeruginosa* and *Serrata sp.*) both before and after treatment with acetazolamide or sodium bicarbonate. A direct correlation was found between the activity of the antibiotic and the pH of the urine. Normally acid urine had little or no antibacterial activity, whereas alkalinized urine had activity.[1]

Clinical studies have confirmed the increased antibacterial effectiveness of erythromycin in the treatment of bacteriuria when the urine is made alkaline.[2,3]

Mechanism

The pH of the urine does not apparently affect the way the kidney handles the antibiotic (most of it is excreted actively rather than passively) but it does have a direct influence on the way the antibiotic affects the micro-organisms. Mechanisms suggested include effects of bacterial cell receptors, induction of active transport mechanisms on bacterial cells walls, and changes in ionization of the antibiotic which enables it to enter the bacterial cell more effectively.

Importance and management

An established interaction which can be exploited. The effectiveness of the antibiotic in treating urinary tract infections can be maximized by making the urine alkaline (for example with acetazolamide or sodium bicarbonate). Treatment with urinary acidifiers will minimize the activity of the erythromycin and should be avoided.

References

1 Sabath LD, Gerstein DA, Loder PB and Finland M. Excretion of erythromycin and its enhanced activity in urine against gram-negative bacilli with alkalinization. J Lab Clin Med (1968) 72, 916.
2 Zinner SH, Sabath LD, Casey JI and Finland M. Erythromycin and alkalinization of the urine in the treatment of urinary tract infections due to gram-negative bacilli. Lancet (1971) i, 1267.
3 Zinner SH, Sabath LD, Casey JI and Finland M. Evythromycin plus alkalization in the treatment of urinary infection Antimicrob Ag Chemother (1969) 9, 413

Ethambutol + Antacids

Abstract/Summary

Aluminium hydroxide can cause a small, and probably clinically unimportant, reduction in the absorption of ethambutol in some patients.

Clinical evidence, mechanism, importance and management

A study in 13 patients with tuberculosis, given single 50 mg/kg doses of ethambutol, showed that when they were also given 1.5 g aluminium hydroxide at the same time and repeated 15 and 30 min later, their serum ethambutol levels were delayed and reduced. The average urinary excretion of ethambutol over a 10 h period was reduced about 15%. There were marked variations. Some showed no interaction and others and increased absorption. No interaction was in six normal subjects similarly treated.[1] Just why this interaction occurs is not understood, but aluminium hydroxide can affect gastric emptying. The reduction in absorption is generally small and variable, and it seems doubtful if it will have a significant effect on the treatment of tuberculosis.

Reference

1 Mattila MJ, Linnoila M, Seppala T and Koskinen R. Effect of aluminium hydroxide and glycpyrrhonium on the absorption of ethambutol and alcohol in man. Br J clin Pharmacol (1978) 5, 161.

Ethionamide + Miscellaneous drugs

Abstract/Summary

Ethionamide has been associated in a few cases with mental depression, psychiatric disturbances, hypoglycaemia, hypothyroidism and alcohol-related psychotoxicity.

Clinical evidence, mechanism, importance and management

Ethionamide can cause depression, mental disturbances and hypoglycaemia.[1,4,5] Caution has been advised in patients under treatment for these psychiatric conditions, epilepsy and diabetes mellitus.[1] Hypothyroidism and thyroid enlargement have also been reported in a few patients treated with ethionamide and particular care may therefore be necessary in patients under treatment for thyroid malfunction.[2] A psychotoxic reaction has also been seen in a patient on ethionamide attributed to the heavy consumption of alcohol.[3] The incidence and importance of all of these reactions is uncertain, but prescribers should take them into account if ethionamide is prescribed with other drugs.

References

1 Martindale. The Extra Pharmacopoeia, edition 28 (1982).
2 Moulding T and Fraser R. Hypothyroidism related to ethionamide. Amer Rev Resp Dis (1970) 101, 90.

3 Lansdown FS, Beran M and Litwak T. Psychotoxic reaction during ethionamide therapy. Am Rev Resp Dis (1967) 95, 1053.
4 Narang RK. Acute psychotic reaction probably caused by ethionamide. Tubercle (1972) 53, 137.
5 Sharma GS, Gupta PK, Jain NK, Shanker A and Nanawati V. Toxic psychosis to isoniazid and ethionamide in a patient with pulmonary tuberculosis. Tubercle (1979) 60, 171.

Flucytosine + Cytarabine

Abstract/Summary

Some very limited evidence suggests that cytarabine may oppose the activity of 5-flucytosine.

Clinical evidence, mechanism, importance and management

A man with Hodgkin's disease treated for cryptococcal meningitis with 100 mg/kg 5-flucytosine daily showed a fall in his serum and CSF levels from 30–40 mg/l to undetectable levels when given cytarabine intravenously. *In vitro* tests showed that 1 mg/l cytarabine completely abolished the activity of up to 50 mg/l 5-flucytosine against the patient's strain of cryptococcus, whereas procarbazine did not. When the cytarabine was replaced by procarbazine in the patient, his body fluid levels of 5-flucytosine returned to their former values.[1] In another study in a patient with myeloid leukaemia it was found that the predose and postdose 5-flucytosine levels fell from 65 and 80 mg/l to 42 and 53 mg/l respectively while concurrently receiving cytarabine and daunorubicin.[2] This was attributed to an improvement in renal function rather than antagonism between the two drugs.[2] No changes in the activity of 5-flucytosine against 14 out of 16 wild isolates of cryptococcus in the presence of cytarabine was seen in an *in vitro* study, although an increase was seen in one and a decrease in the other.[2]

The evidence for this interaction is very limited indeed and its general clinical importance remains uncertain, but the manufacturers warn against concurrent use. It has been suggested that if both drugs are used, the flucytosine should be given 3 h or more after the cytarabine when the serum levels will have fallen.[3]

References

1 Holt RJ. Clinical problems with 5-flucytosine. Mykosen (1978) 21, 363–9.
2 Wingfield HJ. Absence of fungistatic antagonism between flucytosine and cytarabine *in vitro* and *in vivo*. J Antimicrob Chemother (1987) 20, 523–7.
3 Scoffield RE (Pfizer). Personal communication (1988).

Flucytosine + Miscellaneous drugs

Abstract/Summary

The interactions of flucytosine with amphotericin B and aluminium hydroxide–magnesium hydroxide do not appear to be of clinical importance.

Clinical evidence, mechanism, importance and management

The combined use of flucytosine and amphotericin B is more effective than flucytosine alone in the treatment of cryptococcal meningitis, but the amphotericin causes some deterioration in kidney function which can result in raised flucytosine blood levels and some increase in toxicity. Nevertheless combined use is thought to be useful.[1] Aluminium hydroxide–magnesium hydroxide delays the absorption of flucytosine from the gut, but the total amount absorbed remains unaffected.[2]

References

1 Bennett JE, Dismukes WE, Duma RJ, Medoff G, Sande MA, Gallis A, Leonard J, Fields BT, Bradshaw M, Haywood H, McGee ZA, Cate TR, Cobbs CG, Warner JF and Alling DW. A comparison of amphotericin B alone and combined with flucytosine in the treatment of cryptococcal meningitis. N Engl J Med (1979) 301, 126–31.
2 Cutler RE, Blair AD and Kelly MR. Flucytosine kinetics in subjects with normal and impaired renal function. Clin Pharmacol Ther (1978) 24, 333–42.

Griseofulvin + Phenobarbitone

Abstract/Summary

The antifungal effects of griseofulvin can be reduced or even abolished by the the concurrent use of phenobarbitone (phenobarbital).

Clinical evidence

Two epileptic children of seven and eight, taking 40 mg phenobarbitone daily, failed to respond to long-term treatment for tinea capitis with griseofulvin, 400 mg daily, until the barbiturate was withdrawn.[7]

Two other patients have been reported who similarly failed to respond to griseofulvin while taking phenobarbitone.[3,6] Two studies, one in six and the other in eight normal subjects, showed that while taking 90 mg phenobarbitone daily the absorption of griseofulvin given orally was reduced by 45% and 33% respectively. The peak serum levels after 8 h were reduced 33% (from 1.35 to 0.9 μg/ml) in the latter study.[1,2]

Mechanism

Not fully understood. Initially it was thought[4] that the phenobarbitone increased the metabolism and clearance of the griseofulvin but it now seems that it reduces the absorption of griseofulvin from the gut.[2] One idea is that the phenobarbitone increases peristalsis so that the opportunity for absorption is diminished.[2] Another suggestion is that the phenobarbitone forms a complex with the griseofulvin which makes an already poorly soluble drug even less soluble, and therefore less readily absorbed.[5]

Importance and management

An established interaction of clinical importance, although the evidence seems to be limited to the reports cited. If the barbiturate must be given, it has been suggested that the griseofulvin should be given in divided doses three times a day to give it a better chance of being absorbed.[2] The effect of increasing the dosage of griseofulvin appears not to have been studied. An alternative is to exchange the phenobarbitone for a non-interacting anticonvulsant such as sodium valproate. This proved to be successful in one of the cases cited.[7]

References

1 Busfield D, Child KJ, Atkinson RM and Tomich EG. An effect of phenobarbitone on blood levels of griseofulvin in man. Lancet (1963) ii, 1042.
2 Riegleman S, Rowland M and Epstein WL. Griseofulvin-phenobarbital interaction in man. J Amer Med Ass (1970) 213, 426.
3 Lorenc E. A new factor in griseofulvin treatment failures. Missouri Med (1967) 64, 32.
4 Busfield D, Child KJ and Tomich EG. An effect of phenobarbitone on griseofulvin metabolism in the rat. Brit J Pharmacol (1964) 22, 137.
5 Abougela IKA, Bigford DJ, McCorquodale K and Grant DJW. Complex formation and other physico-chemical interactions between griseofulvin and phenobarbitone. J Pharm Pharmac (1976) 28, 44P.
6 Stepanova Zh V and Sheklahova AA. Liuminal kak prichina neudachi griseoful'vinoterapii bol'nogo mikrospoviei. (Luminal as a cause of failure of griseofulvin therapy of a patient with microsporosis). Vestn Dermatol Venereol (1975) 12, 63–5.
7 Beurey J, Weber M and Vignaud J-M. Traitment des teignes microsporiques. Interference metabolique entre phenobarbital et griseofulvine. Ann Dermatol Venereol (Paris) (1982) 109, 567–70.

Hexamine compounds + Urinary acidifiers or Alkalinizers and Sulphonamides

Abstract/Summary

Urinary alkalinizers (e.g. potassium citrate) and those antacids which can raise the urinary pH above 5 should not be used during treatment with hexamine compounds (methenamine). If some of the older less-soluble sulphonamides are also used there is the risk of kidney damage due to crystalluria at low urinary pH values.

Clinical evidence, mechanism, importance and management

(a) Hexamine + urinary acidifiers or alkalinizers

Hexamine (methenamine) and hexamine mandelate are only effective as urinary antiseptics if the pH is about 5 or lower when formaldehyde is released. This is normally achieved by giving urinary acidifiers such as ammonium chloride or sodium acid phosphate. In the case of hexamine hippurate, the acidification of the urine is achieved by the presence of hippuric acid. The concurrent use of compounds which raise the urinary pH such as acetazolamide, sodium bicarbonate, potassium citrate, etc. is clearly contraindicated.[1] Potassium citrate mixture BPC at normal therapeutic doses has been shown to raise the pH by more than 1 thereby making the urine sufficiently alkaline to interfere with the activation of methenamine to formaldehyde.[2] Concurrent use should therefore be avoided. Some antacids can also cause a very significant rise in the pH of the urine.[1]

(b) Hexamine + urinary acidifiers + sulphonamides

At pH values of 5 and below at which hexamine is effective many of the older sulphonamides (sulphapyridine, sulphadiazine, sulphamethizole, etc.) are insoluble and can crystallize out in the kidney tubules causing physical damage.[1] Although this is much less likely to occur with the newer, more soluble sulphonamides, it would seem preferable to avoid the problem by using some other form of treatment.

References

1 Levy C. Interactions of salicylates with antacids. Clinical implications with respect to gastrointestinal bleeding and anti-inflammatory activity. Frontiers of Internal Medicine 1974, 12th Int Congr Intern Med, Tel Aviv 1974. Karger, Basel (1975) p 404.
2 Lipton JH. Incompatibility between sulfamethizole and methenamine mandelate. N Engl J Med (1963) 268, 92.

8-Hydroxyquinoline + Zinc oxide

Abstract/Summary

The presence of zinc oxide inhibits the therapeutic effects of 8-hydroxyquinoline in ointments.

Incompatibility

The observation that a patient had an allergic reaction to 8-hydroxyquinoline in ointments with a paraffin base, but not a zinc oxide base, prompted further study of a possible incompatibility. A study in 13 patients confirmed that zinc oxide reduces the eczematogenic (allergic) properties of the 8-hydroxyquinoline, but it also inhibits its antibacterial and antimycotic effects as well, and appears to stimulate the growth of *Candida albicans*.[1]

Mechanism

It seems almost certain that the zinc ions form chelates with 8-hydroxyquinoline which have little or no antibacterial properties.[1,2]

Importance and management

The documentation is limited but the reaction appears to be established. There is no point in using zinc oxide to reduce the allergic properties of the 8-hydroxyquinoline if, at the same time, the therapeutic effects disappear.

References

1 Fischer T. On 8-hydroxyquinoline-zinc oxide incompatibility. Dermatologica (1974) 149, 129.
2 Alberta A, Rubbo SD, Goldacre RJ and Balfour BJ. The influence of chemical constitution on antibacterial activity III. A study of 8-hydroxyquinoline (oxine) and related compounds. Brit J exp Path (1974) 28, 69.

Imipenem + Aminoglycosides

Abstract/Summary

It has been suggested that the nephrotoxic effects of imipenem and the aminoglycosides may possibly be additive.

Clinical evidence, mechanism, importance and management

When animal studies showed that imipenem caused renal toxicity, cilastin was added to the imipenem to prevent its renal metabolism. This raises the question of the possible additive nephrotoxic effects of other drugs (such as the aminoglycosides) when given concurrently. Monitoring of combined use has been advised but so far there is no direct evidence that their use should be avoided.[1] More study is needed.

Reference

1 Albrecht LM and Rybak MJ. Combination imipenem-aminoglycoside therapy. Drug Intell Clin Pharm (1986) 20, 506.

Influenza vaccine + Paracetamol (Acetaminophen), Alprazolam and Lorazepam

Abstract/Summary

These drugs are not affected by influenza vaccine.

Clinical evidence, mechanism, importance and management

A study in normal healthy subjects showed that the pharmacokinetics of single doses of 650 mg paracetamol (acetaminophen) given IV, alprazolam 1 mg orally or lorazepam 2 mg IV remained unaffected when measured 7 and 14 days after 0.5 ml influenza vaccine given intramuscularly.[1] No special precautions seem necessary.

Reference

1 Scavone JM, Blyden GT, LeDuc BW and Greenblatt DJ. Effect of influenza vaccine on acetaminophen, alprazolam, antipyrine and lorazepam pharmacokinetics. J Clin Pharmacol (1986) 26, 556.

Interferon + Aspirin, Paracetamol or Prednisone

Abstract/Summary

Aspirin and paracetamol (acetaminophen) appear neither to reduce the effects of interferon nor its side-effects. Prednisone also does not reduce its side-effects but it may possibly reduce its biological activity.

Clinical evidence

Studies were made in eight normal subjects given a single IM dose of 18×10^6 U interferon (rHuIFN alpha 2a*) alone or after 24 h of an eight-day course of either aspirin (650 mg four-hourly), paracetamol (acetaminophen) (650 mg four-hourly) or prednisone (40 mg daily). None of these additional drugs reduced the interferon side-effects (fever or chills, headache or myalgia) nor was the activity of the interferon affected as measured by a virus yield inhibition assay with vesicular stomatitis virus. However the prednisone reduced the AUC of 2'-5'-oligoadenylate synthetase activity (a measure of the activity of the interferon) by almost 40%.[1]

Mechanism

Not understood.

Importance and management

Information seems to be limited to this study, on the basis of which there would seem to be no point in using either aspirin or paracetamol to reduce the side effects of interferon but apparently no adverse interaction occurs. In the case of prednisone (and possibly other corticosteroids) the reduction in the biological activity of the interferon would seem to be a disadvantage but more confirmatory study of this is needed.

Reference

1 Witter FR, Woods AS, Griffin MD, Smith CR, Nadler P, Lietman PS. Effects of prednisone, aspirin and acetaminophen on an *in vivo* biologic response to interferon in humans. Clin Pharmacol Ther (1988) 44, 239–43.

Isoniazid + Aminosalicylic acid (PAS)

Abstract/Summary

Isoniazid serum levels are raised by the concurrent use of aminosalicylic acid. A generally advantageous interaction.

Clinical evidence, mechanism, importance and management

A study in man showed that the concurrent administration of aminosalicylic acid significantly increased the serum levels and half-lives of isoniazid due, it is suggested, to the inhibition of the isoniazid metabolism by the aminosalicylic acid. The effect was most marked among the 'fast' acetylators of isoniazid.[1] No precise figures were stated. There seem to be no reports of isoniazid toxicity arising from this interaction and it would appear to be an advantageous interaction.

Reference

1 Boman G, Borga O, Hanngren A, Malmborg A-S and Sjoqvist F. Pharmacokinetic interactions between the tuberculostatics rifampicin (rifampin), para-aminosalicylic acid and isoniazid. Acta Pharmac Toxicol (1970) 28 (suppl 1) 15.

Isoniazid + Antacids

Abstract/Summary

The absorption of isoniazid from the gut is reduced by the concurrent use of aluminium hydroxide. The isoniazid should be given at least an hour before the antacid to minimize the effects of this interaction.

Clinical evidence

10 patients with tuberculosis were given 45 ml aluminium hydroxide (*Amphojel*) at 6, 7 and 8 am, followed immediately by isoniazid and any other medication they were receiving. 1 h serum isoniazid levels and the AUC (drug concentration time curves) were depressed, and peak serum concentrations occurring between 1 and 2 h after ingestion were reduced about 16%, or expressed in $\mu g/ml/mg$ or isoniazid/kg body weight to allow for different dosages, by 25%.[1] The effect of magaldrate (hydrated magnesium aluminate) was less.

Mechanism

Aluminium hydroxide delays gastric emptying (demonstrated in man and rats[2,3]), causing retention of the isoniazid in the stomach. Since isoniazid is largely absorbed from the intestine, the decrease in serum isoniazid concentrations is explained. It also appears to inhibit absorption as well.

Importance and management

This interaction appears to be established, although information is limited. Its clinical importance is uncertain, but as single high doses of isoniazid are more effective in arresting tuberculosis than the same amount of drug in divided doses[4,5] it would seem wise to avoid this interaction by following the recommendations made in the study cited, namely to give the isoniazid at least an hour before the aluminium hydroxide.[1] There seems to be no information about the effects of other antacids.

References

1 Hurwitz A and Schlozman DL. Effects of antacids on gastrointestinal absorption of isoniazid in rat and man. Amer Rev Resp Dis (1974) 109, 41.
2 Hava M and Hurwitz A. The relaxing effect of aluminium hydroxide on rat and human gastric smooth muscle *in vitro*. Europ J Pharmac (1973) 7, 156.
3 Vats TS, Hurwitz A, Robinson RG and Herrin W. Effects of antacids on gastric emptying in children. Pediatr Res (1973) 22, 340.
4 Fox W. General considerations in intermittent drug therapy of pulmonary tuberculosis. Postgrad med J (1971) 47, 729.
5 Hudson LD and Sharbara JA. Twice weekly tuberculosis chemotherapy. J Amer Med Ass (1973) 223, 139.

Isoniazid + Cheese or Fish

Abstract/Summary

Patients taking isoniazid who eat histamine-rich foods (e.g. cheese, certain tropical fish such as tuna) may experience a flushing reaction with headache, difficulty in breathing, nausea and tachycardia.

Clinical evidence

Three months after starting to take 300 mg isoniazid daily, a woman experienced a series of unpleasant reactions 10–30 min after eating cheese. These reactions included chills, headache (sometimes severe), itching of the face and scalp, slight diarrhoea, flushing of the face and on one occasion the whole body, variable and mild tachycardia and a bursting sensation in the head. Blood pressure measurements showed only a modest rise (from 95/65 to 110/80 mm Hg). No physical or biochemical abnormalities were found.[1]

Headache, dizziness, blurred vision, tachycardia, flushing of the skin and redness of the eyes, burning sensation of the body, difficulty in breathing, abdominal colic, diarrhoea, vomiting, sweating and wheezing have all been described in other patients on isoniazid after eating cheese[3,5,9] and certain tropical fish including tuna (skipjack or bonito—*Katsuwanus pelamis*),[4,6,7,11] *Sardinella (Amblygaster) sirm*,[8] *Rastrigella kanagurta*[2] and others.[10] There are well over 300 cases of this reaction on record.

Mechanism

The most likely explanation is these samples of food contained unusually large amounts of histamine produced by the decarboxylating activity of certain bacteria on the amino acid histidine. Normally this is inactivated by histaminase in the body, but in the presence of isoniazid which is a potent inhibitor of this enzyme, it can be absorbed largely unchanged and histamine intoxication develops. Histamine survives all but very prolonged cooking. Tuna fish contains 180–500 mg histamine per 100 g.[11]

Importance and management

An established and well-documented interaction. The incidence appears to be small. With the exception of one patient who appeared to have had a cerebrovascular accident,[7] the reactions experienced by the others were unpleasant and alarming but not serious or life-threatening, and required little or no treatment. Two reports say that treatment with antihistamines was effective.[10,11] Isoniazid has been in use since 1956 and there would seem little need now to introduce any general dietary restrictions, but if any of these reactions is experienced, it would be worthwhile examining the patient's diet and advising the avoidance of probable offending foodstuffs. Very mature cheese and fish which is not fresh are to be treated with suspicion, but there is no way one can guess the likely histamine content of food without undertaking a detailed analysis.

References

1 Smith CK and Durack DT. Isoniazid and cheese reaction. Ann Intern Med (1978) 88, 520.
2 Uragoda CG. Histamine intoxication with isoniazid and a species of fish. Ceylon Med J (1978) 23, 109–10.
3 Uragoda CG and Lodha SC. Histamine intoxication in a tuberculous patient after ingestion of cheese. Tubercle (1979) 60, 59.
4 Uragoda CG and Kottegoda SR. Adverse reactions to isoniazid on ingestion of fish with a high histamine content. Tubercle (1977) 58, 83.
5 Lejonc JL, Gusmini D and Brochard P. Isoniazid and reaction to cheese. Ann Intern Med (1979) 91, 793.
6 Uragoda CG. Histamine poisoning in tuberculous patients after ingestion of tuna fish. Amer Rev Resp Dis (1980) 121, 157.
7 Senanayake N, Vyravanthan S and Kanagasuriyama S. Cerebrovascular accident after a 'skipjack' reaction in a patient taking isoniazid. Brit Med J (1978) 2, 1127.
8 Uragoda CG. Histamine poisoning in tuberculous patients on ingestion of tropical fish. J Trop Med Hyg (1978) 81, 243.
9 Hauser MJ and Baier H. Interactions of isoniazid with foods. Drug Intell Clin Pharm (1982) 16, 617–8.
10 Diao Y et al. Histamine like reaction in tuberculosis patients taking fishes containing much of histamine under treatment with isoniazid in 277 cases. Chin J Tubercul Resp Dis (Chung Hua Chieh Ho Ho Hu Hsi Hsi Chi Ping Tsa Chih) (1986) 9, 267–9, 317–18.
11 Senanayake N and Vryavanthan S. Histamine reactions due to ingestion of tuna fish (Thunnus argentivittatus) in patients on antituberculous therapy. Toxicon (1982) 19, 184–5.

Isoniazid + Cimetidine or Ranitidine

Abstract/Summary

Pharmacokinetic evidence suggests that neither cimetidine nor ranitidine interact with isoniazid.

Clinical evidence, mechanism, importance and management

A pharmacokinetic study in 12 normal subjects showed that 400 mg cimetidine or 300 mg ranitidine, three times a day, for three days had no effect on the pharmacokinetics of single 10 mg/kg doses of isoniazid. Neither the absorption nor the metabolism of isoniazid were changed.[1] The absence of an interaction indicated by this study needs clinical confirmation.

Reference

1 Paulsen O, Hoglund P, Nilsson L-G and Gredeby H. No interaction between H₂ blockers and isoniazid. Eur J Respir Dis (1986) 68, 286–90.

Isoniazid + Disulfiram

Abstract/Summary

Seven patients on isoniazid have been described who experienced difficulties in co-ordination and changes in affect and behaviour after taking disulfiram concurrently. Four others became drowsy.

Clinical evidence

Seven patients with tuberculosis who had been taking 0.6–1.0 g isoniazid daily for not less than 30 days, without problems, experienced adverse reactions within 2–8 days of starting to take 0.5 g disulfiram daily. Among the symptoms seen were dizziness, disorientation, a staggering gait, insomnia, irritable and querulous behaviour, listlessness and lethargy. One patient showed hypomania. Most of them were also taking chlordiazepoxide and other drugs including PAS, streptomycin and phenobarbitone. The adverse reactions decreased or disappeared when the disulifiram was either reduced to 0.25–0.125 g daily, or withdrawn. These seven patients represented less than a third of those who received both drugs. Four other patients given only isoniazid and disulfiram also showed drowsiness and depression.[1]

Mechanism

Not understood. One idea is that some kind of synergy occurred between the two drugs because both can produce not dissimilar side effects if given in high doses. The authors of the report[1] speculate that isoniazid and disulfiram together inhibit two of three biochemical pathways concerned with the metabolism of dopamine. One of these metabolizes dopamine by dopamine beta-hydroxylase to noradrenaline, and then by MAO to 3,4-dihydroxyphenyl acetic acid. This leaves a third pathway open, catalyzed by COMT, which produces a number of methylated products of dopamine. These may possibly have been responsible for the mental and physical reactions seen.

Importance and management

Information about this interaction appears to be limited to the report cited[1] and one other.[2] Its incidence is uncertain, but two-thirds of the group failed to show this interaction and no interaction occurred in another patient taking both drugs and rifampicin (rifampin).[2] If concurrent use is undertaken, the response should be closely monitored and where necessary the dosage of disulfiram should be reduced, or withdrawn.

References

1 Whittington HG and Grey L. Possible interaction between disulfiram and isoniazid. Amer J Psychiat (1969) 125, 1725.
2 Rothstein E. Rifampin with disulfiram. J Amer Med Ass (1972) 219, 1216.

Isoniazid + Ethambutol

Abstract/Summary

There is experimental evidence that ethambutol does not affect serum isoniazid levels but there is also some evidence which suggests that the optic neuropathy of ethambutol may be increased by the concurrent use of isoniazid.

Clinical evidence, mechanism, importance and management

A study in 10 patients with tuberculosis showed that the mean serum levels of isoniazid after taking a single 300 mg dose were not significantly changed when they were also given a single 20 mg/kg dose of ethambutol.[1] The possible effects of concurrent use over a period of time were not studied. However there is some evidence that the optic neuropathy of ethambutol may be increased by the concurrent use of isoniazid.[1-4]

References

1 Singhai KC, Varshney DP, Rathi R, Kishore K and Varshney SC. Serum concentration of isoniazid administered with and without ethambutol in pulmonary tuberculosis patients. Indian J Med Res (1986) 83, 360–2.
2 Renard G and Morax PV. Nevrite optique au cours des traitements anti-tuberculeux. Ann Oculist (Paris) (1977) 210, 53–61.
3 Karmon G, Savir H, Zevin D and Levi J. Bilateral optic atrophy due to combined ethambutol and isoniazid treatment. Ann Ophthalmol (1979) 11, 1013–17.
4 Garret CR. Optic neuritis in a patient on ethambutol and isoniazid evaluated by visual evoked potentials. Case report. Mil Med (1985) 150, 43–6.
5 Jumenez-Lucho VE, Del Busto R and Odel J. Isoniazid and ethambutol as a cause of optic neuropathy. Eur J Respir Dis (1987) 71, 42–5.

Isoniazid + Food

Abstract/Summary

The absorption of isoniazid is markedly reduced if taken with food. (See also 'Isoniazid+Cheese or Fish'.)

Clinical evidence

A study in nine normal subjects given 10 mg/kg body weight isoniazid showed that when taken with breakfast, rather than when fasting, the mean peak isoniazid serum concentrations were delayed and reduced to 30%, and the AUC (area under the time-concentration curve) was reduced to 57%.[1]

Similar results were found in another study.[4]

Mechanism

Uncertain. The presence of food delays the gastric emptying so that the absorption further along the gut is also delayed, but the reduced absorption is not understood.

Importance and management

Information is limited but the interaction seems to be established. As single high doses of isoniazid are more effective in arresting tuberculosis than the same amount of drug in divided doses[2,4] it seems probable that this interaction is clinically important. For maximal absorption isoniazid should be taken without food. See also 'Isoniazid+Cheese or Fish'.

References

1 Melander A, Danielson F, Hanson A, Jansson L, Rerup C, Schersten B, Thulin T and Wahlin E. Reduction of isoniazid bioavailability in normal men by concomitant intake of food. Acta Med Scand (1976) 200, 93–7.
2 Fox W. General considerations in intermittent drug therapy of pulmonary tuberculosis. Postgrad med J (1971) 47, 727.
3 Hudson LD and Sharbara JA. Twice weekly tuberculosis chemotherapy. J Amer Med Ass (1973) 223, 139.
4 Mannisto P, Mantyla R and Klinge R. Influence of various diets on the bioavailability of isoniazid. J Antimicrob Chemother (1982) 10, 427–34.

Isoniazid + Levodopa

Abstract/Summary

An isolated case report describes hypertension, tachycardia, flushing and tremor in a patient attributed to the concurrent use of isoniazid and levodopa.

Clinical evidence, mechanism, importance and management

A patient being treated with levodopa developed hypertension, agitation, tachycardia, flushing and severe non-parkinsonian tremor after starting to take isoniazid. He recovered when the isoniazid was stopped.[1] The reasons are not understood. The author suggested that it might be related in some way to the MAOI–levodopa interaction, but the MAO-inhibitory properties of isoniazid are small. Some of the symptoms seen were not dissimilar to those experienced by patients on isoniazid who ate cheese or fish (see 'Isoniazid+Cheese or Fish'). Concurrent use should be monitored.

Reference

1 Morgan JP. Isoniazid and levodopa. Ann Intern Med (1980) 92, 434.

Isoniazid + Pethidine (Meperidine)

Abstract/Summary

An isolated case report describes hypotension and lethargy in a patient following the concurrent use of isoniazid and pethidine (meperidine).

Clinical evidence, mechanism, importance and management

A patient became lethargic and his blood pressure fell from 124/68 to 84/50 mm Hg within 20 min of being given 75 mg pethidine (meperidine) intramuscularly. An hour before he had been given 30 mg isoniazid. There was no evidence of fever or heart arrhythmias, and his serum electrolytes, glucose levels and blood gases were normal. His blood pressure returned to normal over the next 3 h. He had previously had both pethidine and isoniazid separately without incident. He was subsequently treated with morphine sulphate, 4 mg every 2–4 h intravenously, uneventfully.[1] The authors of the report atttribute this reaction to the MAO-inhibitory properties of the isoniazid and equate it with the severe and potentially fatal MAOI–pethidine interaction. But in fact this reaction was mild and lacked many of the characteristics of the more serious reaction. Moreover isoniazid possesses little MAO-inhibitory properties and does not normally interact like the potent antidepressant and antihypertensive MAOI.

There is too little evidence to forbid concurrent use, but clearly it should be undertaken with caution.

Reference

1 Gannon R, Pearsall W and Rowley R. Isoniazid, meperidine and hypotension. Ann Intern Med (1983) 99, 415.

Isoniazid + Propranolol

Abstract/Summary

Propranolol causes a small reduction in the clearance of isoniazid from the body. It seems unlikely to be of much practical importance.

Clinical evidence, mechanism, importance and management

The clearance of single 600 mg intravenous doses of isoniazid was found in six normal subjects to have been reduced by 21% (from 16.4 to 13.0 l/h) after they had been taking 120 mg propranolol daily for three days,[1] a suggested reason being that the propranolol inhibits the metabolism of the isoniazid.[1] However the increase in isoniazid levels is likely to be only modest, and this interaction is probably of little clinical importance.

Reference

1 Santoso B. Impairment of isoniazid clearance by propranolol. Int J Clin Pharmacol Ther Toxicol (1985) 23, 134–6.

Isoniazid + Rifampicin (Rifampin)

Abstract/Summary

Although concurrent use is common and therapeutically valuable, there is evidence that the incidence of isoniazid hepatotoxicity, particularly in slow acetylators, may be increased.

Clinical evidence, mechanism, importance and management

Both drugs used together have a valuable part to play in short-course chemotherapy of tuberculosis. Studies in man have shown that the serum levels and half-lives of both drugs are unaffected,[1] however there is now increasing evidence that the incidence of heptatotoxicity rises if both drugs are used concurrently. Reports from India suggest that the incidence can be as high as 8–10% while much lower figures, 2–3%, are reported in the West.[2] The reasons for the hepatotoxicity are not fully understood but rifampicin alone can cause liver damage by its own toxic action. In addition it is a potent liver enzyme inducing agent which can increase the metabolism of isoniazid, resulting in the formation of hydrazine which is a proven hepatotoxic agent.[2,4] Higher plasma levels of hydrazine are seen in slow acetylators of isoniazid.[2]

Concurrent use need not be avoided, but it would be prudent to be on the watch for signs of liver damage if both drugs are given, and especially in patients also exposed to other potent enzyme inducers such as phenytoin and the barbiturates.[3]

References

1 Boman G. Serum concentration and half-life of rifampicin (rifampin) after simultaneous oral administration of aminosalicylic acid or isoniazid. Europ J clin Pharmacol (1974) 7, 217.
2 Gangadharam PJ. Isoniazid, rifampin and hepatotoxicity. Am Rev Respir Dis (1986) 133, 963–5. (Review).
3 Lenders JWM, Bartelink AKM, van Herwaarden CLA, van Haelst UJGM and van Tongeren JHM. Dodelijke levercelnecrose na kort durende toediening van isoniazide en rifampcin (rifampin)e aan een patient die reeds werd behandeld met anti-epileptika. Ned Tijd Geneeskund (1983) 127, 420–3.
4 Pessayre D, Bentata M, Degott C, Nonel O, Miguet J-P, Rueff B and Nehamour J-P. Isoniazid-rifampicin (rifampin) fulminant hepatitis. A possible consequence of the enhancement of isoniazid hepatotoxicity by enzyme induction. Gastroenterology (1977) 72, 284.

Ketoconazole + Antacids and/or Cimetidine

Abstract/Summary

Antacids and cimetidine which reduce the acidity of the stomach reduce the gastrointestinal absorption of ketoconazole.

Clinical evidence

The observation of a patient who failed to respond to treatment with ketoconazole while taking cimetidine, sodium bicarbonate and aluminium oxide prompted an investigation of this possible interaction. Even when the ketoconazole dosage was raised to 400 mg daily her serum levels remained less than 1 μg/ml (normally 2 μg/ml 2–4 h after a 200 mg dose). A study in three normal subjects showed that when 200 mg ketoconazole was taken 2 h after 400 mg cimetidine, the absorption was considerably reduced (area under the time-concentration curve reduced by 60%). When this was repeated but with 0.5 g sodium bicarbonate as well, the absorption was reduced to about 5%. In contrast, when this was repeated once more but with the ketoconazole in an acidic solution, the absorption was increased by 50%[1].

A study on four patients showed that the concurrent use of *Maalox* reduced the absorption of ketoconazole (AUC reduced by 40%) but the authors of the paper state that it had no statistical significance[2].

Mechanism

Ketoconazole is administered as a poorly soluble base which must be transformed by the acid in the stomach into the soluble hydrochloride salt. Agents which reduce gastric secretion such as cimetidine or antacids (e.g. sodium bicarbonate) raise the pH in the stomach so that the dissolution of the ketoconazole and its absorption are reduced. Conversely, anything which increases the gastric acidity increases the dissolution and the absorption.[2,3]

Importance and management

Direct information seems to be limited to these studies but it appears to be of clinical importance. Advise patients to take antacids and/or cimetidine not less than 2–3 h after the ketoconazole so that absorption can take place before the pH of the gastric contents is changed.[1] Monitor the effects to confirm that the ketoconazole is effective. It seems probable that ranitidine and other H_2-blockers will interact similarly but this needs confirmation. More study is needed.

References

1 Van der Meer JW, Keuning JJ, Scheigrond HW, Heykants J, Van Cutsem J and Brugmans J. The influence of gastric acidity on the bioavailability of ketoconazole. J Antimicrob Chemother (1980) 6, 552-4.
2 Brass C, Galgiani JN, Blaschke TF, Defelice R, O'Reilly RA and Stevens DA. Disposition of ketoconazole, an oral antifungal in humans. Antimicrob Agents Chemother (1982) 21, 151-8.
3 Sutherland CH, Murphy JE and Schlefifer NH. The effects of two gastric acidifying agents on the pharmacokinetics of ketoconazole. 18th Annual Midyear Clinical Meeting of the American Society of Hospital Pharmacists, Atlanta, Georgia, Dec 4-8, 1983, p. 141.

Ketoconazole or Itraconazole + Food

Abstract/Summary

Itraconazole should be taken with or after food to achieve the best results from treatment. The manufacturers also advise taking ketoconazole with food but the background evidence supporting this is confusing and contradictory.

Clinical evidence

(a) Itraconazole

A study in 24 patients with superficial dermatophyte, *Candida albicans* and *pityriasis versicolor* infections given 50 or 100 mg doses of itraconazole daily showed that taking the drug with or after breakfast produced higher serum levels and gave much better treatment results than taking it before.[4]

(b) Ketoconazole

One study found that the AUC (area under the concentration-time curve) and peak serum concentrations of a single 200 mg dose of ketoconazole was reduced by about 40% (from 14.4 to 8.6 mc.h/ml and from 4.1 to 2.3 μg/ml respectively) when taken by 10 normal subjects after a standardized meal.[2] Another study found that high carbohydrate and fat diets tended to reduce the rate and extent of ketoconazole absorption of ketoconazole.[3] This contrasts with another investigation which found that the absorption of single 200 or 800 mg doses of ketoconazole in eight normal subjects was not altered when taken after a standardized breakfast although the peak serum levels were delayed. The absorption of single 400 and 600 mg doses were somewhat increased.[1]

Importance and management

Information about itraconazole is limited but on the basis of the study cited it should be taken with food to get the best results. A confusing and conflicting picture is presented by the studies with ketoconazole, however the manufacturers say that 'absorption of ketoconazole is maximal when taken during a meal, as it depends on stomach acidity' and 'should always be taken with meals'.

References

1 Daneshmend TK, Warnock DW, Ene MD, Johnson EM, Potten MR, Richardson MD and Williamson PJ. Influence of food on the pharmacokinetics of ketoconazole. Antimicrob Ag Chemother (1984) 25, 1–3.
2 Mannisto PT, Mantyla R, Nykanen S, Lamminsivu U and Ottoila P. Impairing effect of food on ketoconazole absorption. Antimicrob Ag Chemother (1982) 21, 730–33.
3 Lelawong P, Barone JA, Colaizzi JL, Hsuan AT, Mechlinski W, Legendre R and Guarnieri J. Effect of food and gastric acidity on absorption of orally administered ketoconazole. Clin Pharmacy (1988) 7, 228–35.
4 Wishart JM. The influence of food on the pharmacokinetics of itraconazole in patients with superficial fungal infection. J Am Acad Dermatol (1987) 17, 220–3.

Ketoconazole + Phenytoin and Phenobarbitone

Abstract/Summary

A report describes a reduction in serum ketoconazole levels and a relapse in the treatment of a fungal infection in a patient when given phenytoin. Another patient developed reduced ketoconazole serum levels when given phenytoin and phenobarbitone.

Clinical evidence, mechanism, importance and management

A man being treated for coccidioidal meningitis with ketoconazole relapsed when he was given 300 mg phenytoin daily. A pharmacokinetic study showed that his peak serum ketoconazole levels and AUC were reduced compared with the values seen before the phenytoin was started (even though the dosage was increased from 400 to 600 mg, and later 1200 mg), and compared with other patients taking half the dose of ketoconazole (400 or 600 mg).[1] Low serum ketoconazole levels were seen in another patient treated with phenytoin and phenobarbitone.[2] The reason is not known for certain but a likely explanation is that the phenytoin, a known potent enzyme-inducing agent, increases the metabolism and clearance of the ketoconazole from the body.

Information appears to be limited to these two reports, but be alert for any signs of a reduced antifungal response during concurrent use in any patient. It may be necessary to increase the dosage of the ketoconazole.

References

1 Brass C, Galgiani JN, Blaschke TF, Deflice R, O'Reilly RA and Stevens DA. Disposition of ketoconazole, an oral antifungal, in humans. Antimicrob Ag Chemother (1982) 21, 151–8.
2 Stockley RJ, Daneshmend TK, Bredow MT, Warnock DW, Richardson MD and Slade RR. Ketoconazole pharmacokinetics during chronic dosing in adults with haematological malignancy. Eur J Clin Microbiol (1986) 5, 513–7.

Ketoconazole + Rifampicin (Rifampin) and Isoniazid

Abstract/Summary

The serum levels of ketoconazole can be markedly reduced (50–90%) by the concurrent use of rifampicin and/ or isoniazid. Serum rifampicin levels can be halved by the concurrent use of ketoconazole, but are unaffected if the drugs are given 12 h apart.

Clinical evidence

(a) Effect on serum ketoconazole levels

The serum ketoconazole levels of a patient taking 200 mg daily were approximately halved (area under the time-concentration curve reduced from 17.33 to 9.19 μg.h/ml) when concurrently treated with 600 mg rifampicin. After five months of concurrent use with rifampicin and 300 mg isoniazid daily, there was a tenfold decrease in peak serum levels (AUC reduced from 17.33 to 2.02 μg.h/ml)[1].

A study in a 3-year-old child who had responded poorly to treatment showed that peak serum ketoconazole levels were reduced 65–80% by the concurrent use of rifampicin and/or isoniazid, and the AUC's were similarly reduced. The interaction also occurred when the dosages were separated by 12 h. When all three drugs were given together the ketoconazole serum levels were undetectable.[3] Other reports confirm this interaction can occur.[2,4–7] One of them found an 80% reduction in the AUC of ketoconazole but no reduction in rifampicin levels.[6]

(b) Effect on serum rifampicin levels

A study in the child cited above showed that rifampicin serum levels were approximately halved by the concurrent use of ketoconazole, but when given 12 h after the ketoconazole, the serum levels remained unaffected.[3]

Mechanisms

It seems probable that rifampicin reduces the serum levels of ketoconazole by increasing its rate of metabolism within the liver, thereby hastening its clearance from the body. Just how isoniazid interacts is uncertain. It is suggested that ketoconazole impairs the absorption of rifampicin from the gut.

Importance and management

The ketoconazole–rifampicin interactions appear to be established and of clinical importance, but there is less information about the ketoconazole–isoniazid interaction. The effects on rifampicin can apparently be avoided by giving the ketoconazole at a different time (12 h apart is known to be effective) but this does not solve the problem of the effects on ketoconazole. The dosage of at least one of the drugs will need to be increased to achieve both good antitubercular and antifungal responses. Concurrent use should be well monitored and dosage increases made if necessary.

References

1 Brass C, Galgiani JN, Blaschke TF, Defelice R, O'Reilly RA and Stevens DA. Disposition of ketoconazole, an oral antifungal, in humans. Antimicrob Ag Chemother (1982) 21, 151–8.
2 Drouhet E and Dupont B. Laboratory and clinical assessment of ketoconazole in deep seated mycoses. Am J Med (1983) 74, (1B) 30–47.
3 Engelhard D, Stutman MR and Marks MI. Interaction of ketoconazole with rifampin and isoniazid. N Engl J Med (1984) 311, 1681–3.
4 Meunier-Carpentier F, Heymans C and Snoeck R. Interaction of rifampin and ketoconazole and Bayer n7133 (Bay) in normal volunteers. Presented at the 23rd Interscience Conference on Antimicrobial Agents and Chemotherapy, Las Vegas, October 24–6, 1983.
5 Doble H, Hykin P, Shaw R and Keal EE. Pulmonary mycobacterium tuberculosis in acquired immune deficiency syndrome. Br Med J (1985) 291, 849–50.
6 Doble H, Shaw R, Rowland-Hill C, Lush M, Warnock DW and Keal EE. Pharmacokinetic study of the interaction between rifampin and ketoconazole. J Antimicrob Chemother (1988) 21, 633–5.
7 Abadie-Kemmerly S, Pankey GA and Dalvisio JR. Failure of ketoconazole treatment of Blastomyces dermatidis due to interaction of isoniazid and rifampin. Ann Intern Med (1988) 109, 844–5.

Lincomycin or Clindamycin + Food or Drinks

Abstract/Summary

The serum levels of lincomycin are markedly depressed (by up to two-thirds) if taken in the presence of food, but clindamycin is not significantly affected. Cyclamate sweeteners can also reduce the absorption of lincomycin.

Clinical evidence

A cross-over study on 10 normal subjects showed that the mean peak serum levels of lincomycin achieved after single 500 mg oral doses were approximately 3 μg/ml when taken 4 h before breakfast, 2 μg/ml when taken 1 h before breakfast, and less than 1 μg/ml when taken after breakfast. The mean total amounts of lincomycin recovered from the urine were respectively 40.4, 23.8 and 8.9 mg. There were considerable individual variations.[1]

Depressed serum lincomycin levels due to the presence of food have been described in other reports,[2,3] but the absorption of clindamycin is not affected.[3,4] Sodium cyclamate used as an artificial sweetener in diet foods, drinks and some pharmaceuticals can also markedly reduce the absorption of lincomycin (reduction in AUC of 75% using 1 Molar equivalent with 500 mg lincomycin).[5]

Mechanism

Not understood.

Importance and management

A well-established interaction of clinical importance. Lincomycin should not be taken with food or within several hours of eating a meal if adequate serum levels are to be achieved. An alternative is clindamycin, a synthetic derivative of lincomycin, which has the same antibacterial spectrum but the absorption of which is not affected by the presence of food. The interaction with sodium cyclamate is an unlikely occurrence because cyclamates have been banned in the UK (and many other countries as well) as a sweetener in foods and drinks, but it is still sometimes found in pharmaceuticals.

References

1 McCall CE, Steigbigel NH and Finland M. Lincomycin: activity *in vitro* and absorption and excretion in normal young men. Amer J Med Sci (1967) 254, 144.

2 Kaplan K, Chew WH and Weinstein L. Microbiological, pharmacological and clinical studies of lincomycin. Amer J Med Sci (1965) 251, 137.

3 McGehee RF, Smith CB, Wilcox C and Finland M. Comparative studies of antibacterial activity *in vitro* and absorption and excretion of lincomycin and clindamycin. Amer J Med Sci (1968) 256, 279.

4 Wagner JG, Novak E, Patel NC, Chidester CG and Lummis WL. Absorption, excretion and half-life of clinimycin in normal adult males. Amer J Med Sci (1968) 256, 25.

5 Wagner JC. Aspects of pharmacokinetics and biopharmaceutics in relation to drug activity. Amer J Pharm (1969) 141, 5.

Lincomycin or Clindamycin + Kaolin

Abstract/Summary

The concurrent use of kaolin-containing anti-diarrhoeal preparations markedly reduces the absorption of lincomycin by the gut. This interaction can be avoided by giving the linocomycin 2 h after the kaolin. Lincomycin-induced diarrhoea is a potential hazard. The rate but not the extent of clindamycin absorption is altered by kaolin-pectin.

Clinical evidence

A four-way crossover study on eight normal subjects showed that when they were given 0.5 g lincomycin and 3 fl oz of *Kaopectate* (kaolin-pectin), the absorption of the antibiotic was reduced about 90%. Administration of the *Kaopectate* 2 h before the antibiotic had little or no effect on its absorption, whereas when given 2 h after, the absorption was reduced about 50%.[1]

This interaction is described in another report.[3] The absorption rate of clindamycin is markedly prolonged by kaolin, but the extent of its absorption remains unaffected.[4]

Mechanism

A probable explanation is that the lincomycin not only becomes adsorbed onto the surface of the kaolin so that the amount available for absorption by the gut is much reduced, but also the kaolin coats the lining of the gut and acts as a physical barrier to absorption.[1,2]

Importance and management

Information appears to be limited to this study, but it appears to be an established interaction of clinical importance. If good absorption and a good antibiotic response are to be achieved the lincomycin should not be allowed to come into contact with the kaolin in the gut. Separate the administration as much as possible, ideally giving the kaolin 2 h before the antibiotic. It should be borne in mind that lincomycin itself can cause diarrhoea in a fairly large proportion of patients which, in some cases, has lead to the the development of fatal pseudomembranous colitis. Marked diarrhoea, according to the manufacturers, is an indication that the lincomycin should be stopped immediately. Clindamycin appears to be a suitable alternative to lincomycin.

References

1 Wagner JG. Design and data analysis of biopharmaceutical studies in man. Can J Pharm Sci (1966) 1, 55.

2 Rowe EL. Quoted in 1 above.

3 Wagner JG. Pharmcokinetics. I. Definitions, modelling and reasons for measuring blood levels and urinary excretion. Drug Intell (1968) 2, 38.

4 Albert KS, De Sante KA, Welch RD and Di Santo AR. Pharmacokinetic evaluation of a drug interaction between kaolin-pectin and clindamycin. J Pharm Sci (1978) 67, 1579.

Mebendazole + Miscellaneous drugs

Abstract/Summary

Cimetidine raises serum mebendazole levels and increases its effectiveness. Phenytoin and carbamazepine, but not sodium valproate, lower serum mebendazole levels.

Clinical evidence, mechanism, importance and management

A study in eight patients (five with peptic ulcers and three with hydatid cysts) taking 1.5 mg mebendazole daily showed that the concurrent use of cimetidine (400 mg three times daily for 30 days) raised the maximum serum mebendazole levels by 48% due, it is believed, to the enzyme inhibitory effects of the cimetidine.[1] The previously unresponsive hepatic hydatid cysts resolved totally. This is a therapeutically valuable interaction, but be alert for any evidence of mebendazole toxicity (allergic reactions, leucopenia, alopecia). A previous study had suggested that the rises in serum mebendazole levels were too small be useful.[2] The same study found that both phenytoin and carbamazepine (but not sodium valproate) lowered serum mebendazole levels, presumably due to their well-recognized enzyme inducing effects which increase the metabolism and loss of mebendazole from the body.[2] It may be necessary to increase the mebendazole dosage in the presence of these two anticonvulsants. This latter interaction is only likely to be important when treating organisms within the tissues which are affected by drug serum levels, rather than when treating infections in the gut.

References

1 Bekhti A and Pirotte J. Cimetidine increases serum mebendazole concentrations. Implications for treatment of hepatic hydatic cysts. Br J clin Pharmac (1987) 24, 390–2.
2 Luder PJ, Siffert B, Witassek F, Meister F and Bircher J. Treatment of hydatid disease with high oral doses of mebendazole. Long-term follow up of plasma mebendazole levels and drug interactions. Eur J clin Pharmac (1986) 31, 443–8.

Metronidazole + Antacid, Kaolin-pectin and Cholestyramine

Abstract/Summary

The absorption of metronidazole from the gut is unaffected by kaolin-pectin, but a small reduction occurs if an aluminium hydroxide antacid or cholestyramine are given concurrently.

Clinical evidence, mechanism, importance and management

A study in five normal subjects showed that the bioavailability of single 1 g doses of metronidazole was not significantly changed by 30 ml of a kaolin-pectin antidiarrhoeal mixture, but 14.5% reduction occurred when given with 30 ml of an aluminium hydroxide and simethicone suspension and a 21.3% reduction with 4 g cholestyramine.[1] The clinical importance of these reductions is uncertain, but probably small, however clinical studies are needed to confirm this. Separating the dosages as much as possible is an effective way of preventing the admixture of drugs within the gut.

Reference

1 Molokhia AM and Al-Rahman S. Effect of concomitant oral administration of some adsorbing drugs on the bioavailability of metronidazole. Drug Dev Ind Pharm (1987) 13, 1229–37.

Metronidazole + Barbiturates

Abstract/Summary

Phenobarbitone increases the loss of metronidazole from the body. Conventional doses of metronidazole failed to clear up a vaginal infection in a woman while she was taking phenobarbitone.

Clinical evidence

A woman patient with vaginal trichomoniasis was given metronidazole on several occasions over the course of a year, but the infection flared up again as soon as it was stopped. Then it was realized that she was also taking 100 mg phenobarbitone daily. A pharmacokinetic study showed that the metronidazole was being cleared from her body much more rapidly than usual (half life 3.5 h compared with the normal 8–9 h). She was therefore treated with twice the normal dose of metronidazole (500 mg three times a day for seven days) and was cured.[1]

A study in six patients with Crohn's disease showed that 120 mg phenobarbitone daily reduced the AUC of metronidazole by about one-third.[2] A further study in seven normal subjects found that 100 mg phenobarbitone daily for seven days increased the clearance of metronidazole 1.5-fold.[3]

Mechanism

Phenobarbitone is a known and potent liver enzyme-inducing agent which increases the metabolism and loss of metronidazole from the body.

Importance and management

An established and clinically important interaction. Monitor the effects of concurrent use and anticipate the need to increase the metronidazole dosage if phenobarbitone or any other barbiturate (all are potent enzyme-inducing agents) is given concurrently.

References

1 Mead PB, Gibson M, Schentag JJ and Ziemniak JA. Possible alteration of metronidazole metabolism by phenobarbital. N Engl J Med (1982) 306, 1490.

2 Eradiri O, Jamali F and Thomson ABR. Interaction of metronidazole with cimetidine and phenobarbital in Crohn's disease. Clin Pharmacol Ther (1987) 41, 235.

3 Loft S, Sonne J, Poulsen HE, Petersen KT, Jorgensen BG and Dossing M. Inhibition and induction of metronidazole and antipyrine metabolism. Eur J Clin Pharmacol (1987) 32, 35–41.

Metronidazole + Chloroquine

Abstract/Summary

An isolated report describes acute dystonia in a patient on metronidazole when given a single dose of chloroquine.

Clinical evidence, mechanism, importance and management

A patient given a seven-day course of metronidazole (400 mg three times daily) and ampicillin, following a laparoscopic investigation, developed acute dystonic reactions (facial grimacing, coarse tremors, etc.) on day six within 10 min of being given a single dose of chloroquine (5 ml of the phosphate, equivalent to 200 mg base, plus 25 mg promethazine IM). She had had chloroquine before without problems. The symptoms subsided within 15 min of being given 5 mg diazepam intravenously. Although extrapyramidal reactions to chloroquine appear to be rare the authors of the report suggest the use of sulphadoxine/pyrimethamine for malarial prophylaxis in patients on metronidazole.[1]

Reference

1 Achumba JI, Ette EI, Thomas WOA and Essien EE. Chloroquine-induced acute dystonic reactions in the presence of metronidazole. Drug Intell Clin Pharm (1988) 22, 308–10.

Metronidazole + Cimetidine

Abstract/Summary

A study found that cimetidine reduces the loss of metronidazole from the body to some extent, but the clinical importance of this is probably small.

Clinical evidence, mechanism, importance and management

A study in six normal subjects found that the half-life of metronidazole (400 mg IV dose) was increased from 6.2 to 7.9 h after taking cimetidine daily for six days. The total plasma clearance was reduced almost 30%.[1] It is believed that this is due to inhibition by cimetidine of the metabolism of the metronidazole by the liver. However in another study in six patients with Crohn's disease cimetidine was found not to affect either the AUC or the half-life of metronidazole,[2] and no evidence of an interaction was found in a further study in six normal subjects.[3]

The effect of this interaction, if and when it occurs, is not large and it seems unlikely that clinical effects will be marked. There appear to be no reports of metronidazole toxicity during concurrent use.

References

1 Gugler R and Jensen JC. Interaction between cimetidine and metronidazole. N Engl J Med (1983) 309, 1518–19.

2 Eradiri O, Jamali F and Thomson ABR. Interaction of metronidazole with cimetidine and phenobarbital in Crohn's disease. Clin Pharmacol Ther (1987) 41, 235.

3 Loft S, Dossing M, Sonne J, Dalhof K, Bjerrum K and Poulsen HE. Lack of effect of cimetidine on the pharmacokinetics and metabolism of a single oral dose of metronidazole. Eur J Clin Pharmacol (1988) 35, 65–8.

Metronidazole + Corticosteroids

Abstract/Summary

Prednisone increases the loss of metronidazole from the body. An increase in the dosage of metronidazole may be needed.

Clinical evidence

A study in six patients with Crohn's disease showed that when given 20 mg prednisone daily for six days, the AUC of metronidazole (250 mg twice daily) was reduced by 31% (from 78.6 to 53.8 mg.h^{-1}).[1]

Mechanism

Prednisone appears to increase the metabolism of metronidazole by enzyme induction, thereby increasing its clearance from the body.[1]

Importance and management

Information appears to be limited to this report, but the interaction would seem to be of moderate clinical importance. Anticipate the need to increase the metronidazole dosage. Information about other corticosteroids is lacking.

Reference

1 Eradiri O, Jamali F and Thomson ABR. Interaction of metronidazole with phenobarbital, cimetidine, prednisone, and sulfasalazine in Crohn's disease. Biopharm Drug Disp (1988) 9, 219–27.

Metronidazole + Disulfiram

Abstract/Summary

Acute psychoses and confusion can result from the concurrent use of metronidazole and disulfiram.

Clinical evidence, mechanism, importance and management

In a double-blind study on 58 hospitalized chronic alcoholics being treated with disulfiram, half of them were given 750 mg metronidazole daily for a month, and then 250 mg daily. Six of the 29 developed acute psychoses or confusion, five had paranoid delusions and three experienced visual and auditory hallucinations. The symptoms increased when the drugs were withdrawn, but disappeared at the end of a fortnight and did not reappear when disulfiram alone was restarted.[1] Similar reactions have been described in two other reports.[2,3]

The reasons for these reactions are not understood but this is an established interaction. The incidence is high. Concurrent use should be avoided.

References

1 Rothstein E and Clancy DD. Toxicity of disulfiram combined with metronidazole. N Engl J Med (1969) 280, 1006.
2 Goodhue WW. Disulfiram-metronidazole (well-identified) toxicity. N Engl J Med (1969) 280, 1482.
3 Scher JM. Psychotic reaction to disulfiram. J Amer Med Ass (1967) 201, 1051.

Nalidixic acid + Nitrofurantoin

Abstract/Summary

In vitro *studies have demonstrated antagonistic antibacterial effects when the two drugs are used together, but whether this also happens in clinical practice is uncertain.*

Clinical evidence, mechanism, importance and management

The antibacterial activity of nalidixic acid can be inhibited by sub-inhibitory concentrations of nitrofurantoin. 44 out of 53 strains of *Escherichia coli*, *Salmonella* and *Proteus* showed antagonism.[1] Another study confirmed these findings.[2] Whether this similarly occurs if both antibacterials are given to patients is uncertain, but the advice[1] that concurrent use should be avoided when treating urinary tract infections seems sound.

References

1 Stille W and Ostner KH. Antagonismus Nitrofurantoin-Nalidixinsaure. Klin Wsch (1966) 44, 155.
2 Piguet D. In vitro inhibitive action of nitrofurantoin on the bacteriostatic activity of nalidixic acid. Ann Inst Pasteur (Paris) (1969) 116, 43.

Nalidixic acid + Probenecid

Abstract/Summary

Serum nalidixic acid levels are markedly increased by the concurrent use of probenecid.

Clinical evidence, mechanism, importance and management

Following the observation of a man who had ingested unknown amounts of several drugs including nalidixic acid and probenecid and who showed grossly elevated nalidixic acid serum levels, the possible interaction between these two drugs was studied. Two volunteers, acting as their own controls, ingested 0.5 g nalidixic acid with and without 0.5 g probenecid. Their peak serum nalidixic acid levels were unaffected at 2 h, but at 8 h the levels were increased threefold by the presence of probenecid.[1] Another study in five women with urinary tract infections treated with nalidixic acid showed that the concurrent use of probenecid increased the maximal serum nalidixic acid concentrations and the AUC (area under the curve) by 43% (from 33 to 48 μg/ml) and 74% (from 82 to 143 μg.h.ml^{-1}) respectively.[2]

Mechanism

The reasons are not well understood but a suggested explanation is that probenecid successfully competes with the nalidixic acid for excretion by the kidney tubules, so that the nalidixic acid is retained in the body.

Importance and management

The importance of this interaction remains uncertain, but be alert for signs of nalidixic acid toxicity if both drugs are used.

References

1 Dash H and Mills J. Severe metabolic acidosis associated with nalidixic acid overdose. Ann Intern Med (1976) 84, 570.
2 Ferry N, Cuisinaud G, Pozet N, Zech PY and Sassard J. Influence du probenecid sur la pharmacocinetique de l'acide nalidixique. Therapie (1982) 37, 645–9.

Nitrofurantoin + Antacids

Abstract/Summary

The antibacterial effectiveness of nitrofurantoin in the treatment of urinary tract infections is possibly reduced by magnesium trisilicate, but aluminium hydroxide is reported not to interact. Whether other antacids interact adversely is uncertain.

Clinical evidence

A cross-over study in six normal subjects showed that 5 g magnesium trisilicate in 150 ml water reduced the absorption of single 100 g oral doses of nitrofurantoin by more than 50%. The time during which the concentration of nitrofurantoin in the urine was at, or above, the minimal antibacterial inhibitory concentration of 32 µg/ml was also reduced.[1] The amounts of nitrofurantoin adsorbed by other antacids in *in vitro* tests were as follows: magnesium trisilicate and charcoal 99%, bismuth oxycarbonate and talc 50–53%, kaolin 31%, magnesium oxide 27%, aluminium hydroxide 2.5% and calcium carbonate 0%.[1]

A cross-over study in six subjects confirmed that aluminium hydroxide gel does not affect the absorption of nitrofurantoin from the gut (as measured by its excretion into the urine).[2]

Mechanism

Antacids can, to a greater or lesser extent, adsorb nitrofurantoin onto their surfaces, as a result less is available for absorption by the gut and for excretion into the urine.

Importance and management

Whether in clinical practice the concurrent use of magnesium trisilicate significantly reduces the antibacterial effectiveness of nitrofurantoin awaits confirmation. The response should be well monitored. It may be necessary to increase the dosage of the nitrofurantoin. The results of the *in vitro* studies suggest that the possible effects of the other antacids are smaller, and aluminium hydroxide is reported not to interact.

References

1 Naggar VF and Khalil SA. Effect of magnesium trisilicate on nitrofurantoin absorption. Clin Pharmacol Ther (1979) 25, 857.
2 Jaffe JM, Hamilton BH and Jeffers S. Nitrofurantoin-antacid interaction. Drug Intell Clin Pharm (1976) 10, 419.

Nitrofurantoin + Anticholinergics and Diphenoxylate

Abstract/Summary

Diphenoxylate and anticholinergic drugs such as propantheline can double the absorption of nitrofurantoin in some patients, but the clinical importance of this is uncertain.

Clinical evidence, mechanism, importance and management

A study[1] in six normal subjects showed that when they were given 100 mg nitrofurantoin with 30 mg propantheline, the absorption of the nitrofurantoin was approximately doubled (as measured by the amounts excreted in the urine). Two out of six men in another study[2] similarly showed a nearly doubled nitrofurantoin absorption when given 200 mg diphenoxylate daily, but the other four showed little effect. The suggested mechanism is that the reduced motility of the gut caused by these drugs allows the nitrofurantoin to dissolve more completely, so that it is absorbed by the gut more easily. Whether this interaction is of any clinical importance is uncertain. It would be expected to be accompanied by an increase in the therapeutic effects of nitrofurantoin and

possibly in the incidence of dose-related adverse reactions. So far there appear to be no reports of any problems arising from concurrent use.

References

1 Jaffe JM. Effect of propantheline on nitrofurantoin absorption. J Pharm Sci (1975) 64, 1729.
2 Callahan M, Bullock FJ, Braun J and Yesair DW. Pharmacodynamics of drug interactions with diphenoxylate. Fed Proc (1974) 33, 513.

Penicillins + Chloroquine

Abstract/Summary

The absorption of ampicillin is reduced by the concurrent use of chloroquine, but bacampicillin is not affected.

Clinical evidence, mechanism, importance and management

A study in seven normal subjects showed that the concurrent use of 1 g chloroquine reduced the absorption of single 1 g doses of ampicillin given orally by about a third (from 29 to 19%) as measured by its excretion in the urine.[1] A likely reason is that the chloroquine irritates the gut so that the ampicillin is moved through more quickly and less time is available for absorption. A reasonable solution to the problem would seem to be to increase the dosage of the ampicillin or possibly to separate the administration of the drugs (not less than 2 h has been suggested[1]). This needs confirmation. An alternative is to use bacampicillin (an ampicillin pro-drug) the bioavailability of which is not affected by chloroquine.[2]

References

1 Ali HM. Reduced ampicillin bioavailability following oral coadministration with chloroquine. J Antimicrob Chemother (1985) 15, 781–4.
2 Ali HM. The effect of Sudanese food and chloroquine on the bioavailability of ampicillin from bacampicillin tablets. Int J Pharmacy (1981) 9, 185–90.

Penicillins + Dietary fibre

Abstract/Summary

Dietary fibre can reduce the absorption of amoxicillin.

Clinical evidence, mechanism, importance and management

The AUC (area under the concentration time curve) of a single 500 mg oral dose of amoxicillin in 10 subjects was found to be 12.17 µg/ml/h while taking a low fibre diet (7.8 g daily) but only 9.65 µg/ml/h while on a high fibre diet (36.2 g daily). Peak serum levels were the same and occurred at 3 h. The subjects used were slum-dwellers in Santiago and the two diets represented the amounts of fibre normally eaten during the winter and summer seasons. A possible reason for the reduced absorption is that the amoxicillin becomes trapped within the fibre. The clinical importance of this interaction is uncertain but it may be necessary to increase the dosage of this antibiotic in those who have a high fibre diet to accommodate the reduced absorption.[1]

Reference

1 Lutz M, Espinoza J, Arancibia A, Araya M, Pacheco I and Brunser O. Effect of structured dietary fibre on bioavailability of amoxicillin. Clin Pharmacol Ther (1987) 42, 220–4.

Penicillins + Miscellaneous drugs

Abstract/Summary

Aspirin, indomethacin, probenecid, phenylbutazone, sulphaphenazole and sulphinpyrazone prolong the half-life of penicillin G significantly, whereas chlorothiazide, sulphamethizole and sulphamethoxypyridazine do not. These interactions do not seem to present any problems in practice. The interaction of probenecid with the penicillins is exploited therapeutically.

Clinical evidence

Studies in patients given the following drugs for 5–7 days showed the following changes in the half-life of penicillin G:

Probenecid also increases the serum concentrations of other penicillins including nafcillin.[2]

Mechanisms

In many cases it seems likely that the interacting drugs successfully compete with penicillin for excretion by the kidney tubules so that the pencillin is retained in the body. This is certainly true for probenecid.

Importance and management

These interactions are not adverse and may be exploited. In the days when penicillin was very expensive, the penicillin–probenecid interaction was used to reduce the loss of the penicillin in the urine. It is still used today to achieve higher and more prolonged plasma concentrations of the penicillins (ampicillin, amoxycillin) in the treatment of gonorrhoea and the prevention of diphtheria and endocarditis. No particular precautions would seem necessary during concurrent use of these drugs and the penicillins.

References

1 Kampmann H, Hansen JM, Siersboek-Nielsen K and Laursen H. Effect of some drugs on penicillin half-life in blood. Clin Pharmacol Ther (1972) 13, 516–19.
2 Waller ES, Sharanevych MA and Yakatan GJ. The effect of probenecid on nafcillin disposition. J Clin Pharmacol (1982) 22, 482–9.

Table 5.3 Changes in half-life of Penicillin G

Drug	Number of patients	Change in half life in minutes		Significance p
		From	To	
Probenecid (2 g)	22	40.4	104.3	<0.001
Phenylbutazone (600 mg)	12	42.8	102.2	<0.01
Sulphinpyrazone (600 mg)	8	42.6	70.3	<0.001
Aspirin (3 g)	11	44.5	72.4	<0.05
Sulphaphenazole (1 g)	7	34.9	50.4	<0.05
Indomethacin (75 mg)	11	42.7	52.2	<0.05
Chlorothiazide (2 g)	6	53.5	62.3	NS
Sulphamethizole (4 g)	5	58.6	70.6	NS
Sulphamethoxypyridazine (500 mg)	6	60.0	50.8	NS

Penicillins + Tetracyclines

Abstract/Summary

Tetracyclines can reduce the effectiveness of penicillin in the treatment of pneumococcal meningitis and probably scarlet fever. It is uncertain whether a similar interaction occurs with other infections. It may possibly only be important with those infections where a rapid kill is essential.

Clinical evidence

A study in patients with pneumococcal meningitis showed that penicillin alone (one million units every 2 h) was more effective than penicillin with chlortetracycline (0.5 g every 6 h). Out of 14 patients given penicillin alone, 70% recovered compared with only 20% in another group of essentially similar patients who had had both antibiotics.[1]

Another report about the treatment of pneumococcal meningitis with penicillin and tetracyclines (chlortetracycline, oxytetracycline, tetracycline) confirmed that the mortality was much less in those given only pencillin.[2] In the treatment of scarlet fever (Group A beta-haemolytic streptococci), no difference was seen in the initial response, but spontaneous reinfection occurred more frequently in those who had had penicillin and chlortetracycline.[3]

Mechanism

The generally accepted explanation is that bactericides such as penicillin which inhibit bacterial cell wall synthesis, require cells to be actively growing and dividing to be maximally effective, a situation which will not occur in the presence of bacteriostatic antibiotics such as the tetracyclines.

Importance and management

An established and important interaction when treating pneumococcal meningitis, and probably scarlet fever as well. The documentation seems to be limited to the reports cited. Concurrent use should be avoided in these infections, but the importance of this interaction with other infections is uncertain. It demonstrably does not occur when treating pneumococcal pneumonia.[4] It has been suggested that antagonism, if it occurs, may only be significant when it is essential to kill bacteria rapidly.[4] The antibiotics implicated in the interaction are penicillin, tetracycline, chlortetracycline and oxytetracycline, but any penicillin and tetracycline would be expected to behave similarly. Among the general rules which should be applied if concurrent use is thought appropriate are: to give the bactericidal penicillin a few hours before the bacteriostatic tetracycline (see 'Mechanism' above), and to ensure that the doses are well above minimally effective levels.

References

1 Lepper MH and Dowling HF. Treatment of pneumococcic meningitis with penicillin compared with penicillin plus aureomycin: studies including observations on an apparent antagonism between penicillin and aureomycin. Arch Intern Med (1951) 88, 489.

2 Olsson RA, Kirby JC and Romansky MJ. Pneumococcal meningitis in the adult. Clinical, therapeutic and prognostic aspects in forty-three patients. Ann Intern Med (1961) 55, 545.

3 Strom J. The question of antagonism between penicillin and chlortetracycline illustrated by therpeutical experiments in Scarlatina. Antibiot Med (1955) 1,6.

4 Ahern JJ and Kirby WMM. Lack of interference of aureomycin in treatment of pneumoccoal pneumonia. Arch Intern Med (1953) 91, 197.

Piperazine + Phenothiazines

Abstract/Summary

An isolated case of convulsions in a child was attributed to the use of chlorpromazine following piperazine.

Clinical evidence, mechanism, importance and management

A child given piperazine for pin worms developed convulsions when treated with chlorpromazine several days later.[1] In a subsequent animal study using 4.5 or 10 mg/kg chlorpromazine, many of the animals died from respiratory arrest after severe clonic convulsions.[1] However a later study failed to confirm these findings[2] so that it is by no means certain whether the adverse reaction was due to an interaction; nevertheless there is enough evidence to warrant some caution if these drugs are used concurrently.

References

1 Boulos BM and Davis LE. Hazard of simultaneous administration of phenothiazine and piperazine. N Engl J Med 91969) 280, 1245.

2 Armbrecht BH. Reaction between piperazine and chlorpromazine. N Engl J Med (1970) 282, 149.

Praziquantel + Corticosteroids

Abstract/Summary

The continuous use of dexamethasone can reduce serum praziquantel levels by 50%.

Clinical evidence

8 patients with parenchymal brain cysticercosis treated with praziquantel (50 mg/kg divided into three doses 8-hourly) showed a 50% reduction in steady-state serum levels (from 3.13 to 1.55 μg/ml) when given 8 mg dexamethasone 8-hourly.

Mechanism

Not understood.

Importance and management

Information is limited to this study but the interaction would appear to be established. It is not known how much it affects the outcome of treatment for cysticercosis because the optimum praziquantel dosage is still uncertain but a reduction in efficacy seems probable. The authors of the report suggest that dexamethasone should not be given continuously with praziquantel but only used transiently for the treatment of the adverse effects arising from the inflammatory response to the dead and dying parasites in the CNS. This interaction is only likely to be important for infections where treatment depends upon the maintenance of adequate serum levels. There seems to be no information about other corticosteroids.

Reference

1 Vazquez ML, Jung H and Sotelo J. Plasma levels of praziquantel decrease when dexamethasone is given simultaneously. Neurology (1987) 37, 1561–2.

Primaquine + Mepacrine (Quinacrine)

Abstract/Summary

Primaquine appears not to interact adversely with mepacrine although theoretically it might be expected to do so.

Clinical evidence, mechanism, importance and management

Patients given pamaquine, the predecessor of primaquine, showed grossly elevated serum levels when concurrently treated with mepacrine.[1,2] The probable reason was that the mepacrine occupies binding sites in the body normally also used by the pamaquine and, as a result, the latter failed to become sequestered at these sites and the serum levels became very high. On theoretical grounds primaquine might be expected to interact with mapacrine similarly, but there seem to be no reports confirming that a clinically important interaction actually takes place.

References

1 Zubrod CG, Kennedy TJ and Shannon JA. Studies on the chemotherapy of the human malarias. VIII. The physiological disposition of pamaquine. J Clin Invest (1948) 27 (Suppl) 114–120.
2 Earle DP, Bigelow FS, Zubrod CG and Kane CA. Studies on the chemotherapy of the human malarias. IX. Effect of pamaquine on the blood cells of man. J Clin Invest (1948) 27, (Suppl) 121–9.

Prothionamide + Rifampicin (Rifampin) and/or Dapsone

Abstract/Summary

Prothionamide appears to be very hepatotoxic, which is possibly increased by the concurrent use of rifampicin or isopiperazinylrifamycin SV. Prothionamide does not affect the pharmacokinetics of either dapsone or rifampicin.

Clinical evidence

39% of 39 patients with leprosy became jaundiced after 24–120 days treatment with dapsone (100 mg daily), prothionamide (300 mg daily) and isopiperazinylrifamycin SV (300–600 mg monthly). Laboratory evidence of liver damage occurred in a total of 56% and despite the withdrawal of the drugs from all the patients, two of them died.[1] All the patients except two had had dapsone before, alone, for 3–227 months without reported problems.[1] 22% of 50 other leprosy patients also showed liver damage after treatment with dapsone (100 mg) and prothionamide (300 mg) daily, with rifampicin (900 mg), prothionamide (500 mg) and clofazimine (300 mg) monthly for 30–50 days. One patient died.[1] Most of the patients recovered within 30–60 days after withdrawing the treatment.

Jaundice, liver damage and deaths have occurred in other leprosy patients given rifampicin and prothionamide or ethionamide.[2–4] Prothionamide does not affect the pharmacokinetics of either dapsone or rifampicin.[5]

Mechanism

Although not certain, it seems probable that the liver damage was primarily caused by the prothionamide, possibly exacerbated by the rifampicin or the isopiperazinylrifamycin SV.

Importance and management

This serious and potentially life-threatening hepatotoxic reaction to prothionamide is established, but the part played by the other drugs, particularly the rifampicin, is uncertain. Strictly speaking this may not be an interaction. If prothionamide is given the liver function should be very closely monitored in order to detect toxicity as soon as possible.

References

1 Baohong J, Jiakun C, Chenmin W and Guang X. Hepatotoxicity of combined therapy with rifampicin and daily prothionamide for leprosy. Lepr Rev (1984) 55, 283–9.
2 Lesobre R, Ruffine J, Teyssier L, Achard F, and Brefort G. Les icterus en cours du traitment par la rifampicine. Rev Tuberc Pneumol (1969) 33, 393–403.
3 Report of the Third Meeting of the Scientific Working Group on Chemotherapy of Leprosy (THELEP) of the UNDP/World Bank/WHO Special Programme for Research and Training in Tropical Diseases. Int J Lepr (1981) 49, 431–6.
4 Cartel JL, Millan J, Guelpa-Lauras CC and Grosset JH. Hepatitis in leprosy patients treated by a daily combination of dapsone, rifampicin and a thioamide. Int J Lepr (1983) 51, 461–5.
5 Mathur A, Venkatesan K, Girdhar BK, Bharadwaj VP, Girdhar A and Bagga AK. A study of drug interactions in leprosy −1. Effect of simultaneous administration of prothionamide on metabolic disposition of rifampicin and dapsone. Lepr Rev (1986) 57, 33–7.

Pyrantel + Piperazine

Abstract/Summary

Piperazine opposes the anthelmintic actions of pyrantel.

Clinical evidence, mechanism, importance and management

Pyrantel acts as an anthelmintic because it depolarizes the neuromuscular junctions of some intestinal nematodes causing the worms to contract. This paralyzes the worms so that they are dislodged by peristalsis and expelled in the faeces. Piperazine also paralyzes nematodes but it does so by causing hyperpolarization of the neuromuscular junctions. These two pharmacological actions oppose one another, as was shown in two *in vitro* pharmacological studies. Strips of whole *Ascaris lumbricoides* which contracted when exposed to pyrantel (1.5 ng/ml) failed to do so when also exposed to piperazine (1 mg/ml).[1] Parallel electrophysiological studies using *Ascaris* cells confirmed that the depolarization due to pyrantel (which causes the paralysis) was opposed by piperazine.[1]

In practical terms this means that piperazine does not add to the anthelmintic effects of pyrantel on *Ascaris* as might be expected, but opposes it. For which reason it is usually recommended that concurrent use should be avoided, but direct clinical evidence confirming that combined use is ineffective seems to be lacking. It seems reasonable to extrapolate the results of these studies on *Ascaris lumbricoides* (roundworm) to the other gastrointestinal parasites for which pyrantel is used, i.e. *Enterobius vermicularis* (threadworm or pinworm), *Ancyclostoma duodenale*, *Necator americanus* (hookworm), *Trichuris trichiura* (whipworm), *Trichostrogylus colubriformis* and *orientalis*, but no one seems to have checked on this directly.

Reference

1 Aubry ML, Cowell P, Davey MJ and Shevde S. Aspects of the pharmacology of a new anthelmintic: pyrantel. Br J Pharmac (1970) 38, 332–44.

Pyrazinamide + Miscellaneous drugs

Abstract/Summary

Pyrazinamide should be used with caution with other potentially hepatotoxic drugs. It may cause hyperuricaemia which is modestly reduced by aminosalicylic acid or probenecid, but more extensively by aspirin. Pyrazinamide may possibly adversely affect the control of diabetes.

Clinical evidence, mechanism, importance and management

Hepatotoxicity is the most common side-effect of pyrazinamide[1,2] and it should therefore be used with caution with other potentially hepatotoxic drugs. It has been used with good effect in the treatment of tuberculosis in combination with other agents such as rifampicin, isoniazid and streptomycin.[1] Pyrazinamide can decrease the urinary output of uric acid by a third to a half, resulting in a rise in the serum levels of urate in the blood (hyperuricaemia).[3,4] This hyperuricaemia is inhibited to some extent by aminosalicyclic acid, but probenecid is no more effective and the response is short-lived.[3,4] On the other hand it is reduced by aspirin (2.4 g daily).[4] Pyrazinamide is contraindicated in patients with existing hyperuricaemia or gouty arthritis.[1] The control of diabetes mellitus is reported to be more difficult in some patients taking pyrazinamide.[1,2]

References

1 Data Sheet Compendium 1985–86, Datapharm Publications 1985. p 942
2 Martindale. The Extra Pharmacopoeia, 28th Edition. Pharmaceutical Press 1982.
3 Cullen JH, LeVine M and Fiore JM. Studies of hyperuricaemia produced by pyrazinamide. Amer J Med (1957) 23, 587–95.
4 Shapiro M and Hyde L. Hyperuricaemia due to pyrazinamide. Amer J Med (1957) 23, 596–9.

Pyrimethamine + Co-trimoxazole or Sulphonamides

Abstract/Summary

Serious pancytopenia and megaloblastic anaemia have been described in patients under treatment with pyrimethamine and either co-trimoxazole or other sulphonamides.

Clinical evidence

A woman taking 50 mg pyrimethamine weekly as malarial prophylaxis, developed petechial haemorrhages and widespread bruising within 10 days of starting to take co-trimoxazole (320 mg trimethoprim + 800 mg sulphamethoxazole daily). She was found to have gross megaloblastic changes and pancytopenia in addition to being obviously pale and ill. After withdrawal of the two drugs she responded rapidly to hydroxycobalamine and folic acid, with chloroquine as malarial prophylaxis.[1]

Similar cases have been described in other patients taking pyrimethamine with co-trimoxazole[2,4–6] or sulphafurazole.[3] Another case has been referred to elsewhere involving a sulphonamide.[7]

Mechanism

Uncertain, but a reasonable surmise can be made. Pyrimethamine and trimethoprim are both 2:4 diaminopyrimidines and both selectively inhibit the actions of the enzyme dihydrofolate reductase which is concerned with the eventual synthesis, amongst other compounds, of the nucleic acids needed for the production of new cells. The sulphonamides inhibit another part of the same synthetic chain. The adverse reactions seen would seem to reflect a gross depression of the normal folate metabolism caused by the combined actions of both drugs. Megaloblastic anaemia and pancytopenia are among the adverse reactions of pyrimethamine and, more rarely, of co-trimoxazole taken alone. In theory this should not occur (see 'Co-trimoxazole + Folic acid') but in practice it clearly does so occasionally.

Importance and management

Information seems to be limited to the reports cited, but the interaction appears to be established. Its incidence is unknown. Concurrent use need not be avoided but the authors of the report cited[1] advise that co-trimoxazole should be prescribed '...with caution and haematological cover...' to patients given pyrimethamine or proguanil for malarial prophylaxis, and '...further caution...' in the tropics because of the folate deficiency associated with pregnancy and malnutrition in children. The manufacturers of co-trimoxazole support this in advising that if the dosage of pyrimethamine is high the blood picture should be monitored regularly.

References

1 Fleming AF, Warrell DA and Dickmeiss H. Co-trimoxazole and the blood. Lancet (1974) ii, 284.
2 Andsell VE, Wright SG and Hutchinson DBA. Megaloblastic anaemia associated with combined pyrimethamine and co-trimoxazole administration. Lancet (1976) ii, 1257.
3 Waxman S and Herbert V. Mechanism of pyrimethamine induced megaloblastosis in human bone marrow. N Engl J Med (1969) 280, 1316.
4 Malfatti S and Piccini A. Anemia megaloblastica pancitopenica in corso di trattemento con pirimetamina, trimethoprim e sulfametossazolo. Haematologica (1976) 61, 349.
5 Borgstein A and Tozer RA. Infectious mononucleosis and megaloblastic anaemia associated with Daraprim and Bactrim. Centr Afr J Med (1974) 20, 185.
6 Whitman EN. Effects in man of prolonged administration of trimethoprim and sulfisoxazole. Postgrad Med J (1969) 45 (Suppl) 46.
7 Weissbach G. Zeitschrift fur Aerzliche Fortbild (1965) 59, 10.

Quinine + Antacids or Urinary acidifiers and Alkalinizers

Abstract/Summary

Urinary alkalinizers can increase the retention of quinine in man, and antacids can reduce the absorption in animals, but neither of these interactions appears to be clinically important.

Clinical evidence, mechanism, importance and management

The excretion of quinine in man is virtually halved (from 17.4 to 8.9%) if the urine is changed from acid to alkaline with agents such as acetazolamide or sodium bicarbonate.[1] The reason is that at alkaline pH values more of the quinine exists in the un-ionized (lipid soluble) form which is more easily reabsorbed by the kidney tubules. However there seem to be no reports of adverse effects arising from the increased serum quinine levels due to this interaction. Magnesium and aluminium hydroxide gel depresses the absorption of quinine from the gut of *rats* and reduces blood quinine levels by 50–70%.[2] The reason appears to be that aluminium hydroxide slows gastric emptying which reduces absorption, and magnesium hydroxide also forms an insoluble precipitate with quinine. There seem to be no clinical reports of a reduction in the therapeutic effectiveness of quinine due to the concurrent use of antacids.

References

1 Haag HB, Larson PS and Schwartz JJ. The effect of urinary pH on the elimination of quinine in man. J Pharmacol Exp Ther (1943) 79, 136.
2 Hurwitz A. The effects of antacids on gastrointestinal drug absorption. II. Effect of sulfadiazine and quinine. J Pharmacol Exp Ther (1971) 179, 485.

Quinine + Cimetidine or Ranitidine

Abstract/Summary

The loss of quinine from the body is reduced by the concurrent use of cimetidine, but not ranitidine. The extent to which this increases the toxicity of quinine has not been determined.

Clinical evidence

A study in six normal subjects showed that after taking 1 g cimetidine daily for a week, the clearance of quinine was reduced by 27% (from 0.182 to 0.133 $l\, h^{-1}\, kg^{-1}$), its half-life was increased by 49% (from 7.6 to 11.3 h) and the AUC was increased by 42% (53.9 to 76.8 $mg\, l^{-1}\, h$). Peak levels were unchanged. No interaction was seen when cimetidine was replaced by ranitidine.[1]

Mechanism

It seems probable that the cimetidine (a recognized enzyme inhibitor) reduces the metabolism of the quinine by the liver so that it is lost from the body more slowly.

Importance and management

The report cited seems to be all that is currently known about this interaction. Its clinical importance is uncertain, but prescribers should be alert for evidence of quinine toxicity during concurrent use (the increase in AUC was 75% in one subject[1]). Ranitidine is apparently a non-interacting alternative.

Reference

1 Wanwimolruk S, Sunbhanich M, Pongmarutai M and Patamasucon P. Effects of cimetidine and ranitidine on the pharmacokinetics of quinine. Br J clin Pharmac (1986) 22, 346–50.

Quinine + Rifampicin (Rifampin)

Abstract/Summary

A single case report describes a reduction in the serum levels and therapeutic effects of quinine in a patient when rifampicin was given.

Clinical evidence

A patient whose myotonia was controlled with quinine reported a worsening of the symptoms within three weeks of starting to take rifampicin for the treatment of tuberculosis. Peak quinine levels were found to be low, but rose again when the rifampicin was stopped. Control of the myotonia was restored after six weeks.[1]

Mechanism

Rifampicin is a potent liver enzyme-inducing agent which increases the metabolism of many drugs by the liver, thereby hastening their clearance from the body and reducing their effects.

Importance and management

Information appears to be limited to this report but it is consistent with the way rifampicin affects a number of other drugs. Monitor the effects of concurrent use and anticipate the need to raise the quinine dosage as necessary. Reduce the dosage when the rifampicin is stopped.

Reference

1 Osborn JE, Pettit MJ, Graham P. Interaction between rifampicin and quinine: case report. Pharm J (1989) 243, 704.

Quinolone antibiotics + Antacids

Abstract/Summary

Serum ciprofloxacin, enoxacin, norfloxacin and pefloxacin (but not ofloxacin) levels can be reduced below therapeutic concentrations by the concurrent use of aluminium and magnesium antacids.

Clinical evidence

10 patients on dialysis (CAPD) because of renal failure were given given 250 mg ciprofloxacin four times daily. The steady-state serum ciprofloxacin levels of three of them concurrently taking aluminium-containing antacids (*Maalox*, *Malinal*) as phosphate binders were reduced by approximately two-thirds (peak serum levels fell from 3.69 to 1.25 μg/ml), whereas the serum levels of three others taking a calcium carbonate containing antacid (*Titralac*) for the same reason were unaffected.[1]

A further study found that peak serum ciprofloxacin levels

and the AUC (area under the curve) were reduced 90% or more by the use of aluminium and magnesium-containing antacids.[2] A later study found that the bioavailability of ciprofloxacin was reduced 77–85% when *Maalox* was given within 2 h before the antibiotic.[11] Reductions in serum levels of 50–98% in serum enoxacin, ciprofloxacin, norfloxacin and pefloxacin levels have been described in other studies and case reports[3,6,7,9] involving aluminium and magnesium-containing antacids. However no clinically important interaction was seen in a study of ofloxacin with a chewing tablet of *Maalox*.[8] Another study found that calcium supplementation with calcium carbonate caused a 40% reduction in ciprofloxacin bioavailability.[10]

Mechanism

It is believed that certain functional groups (3-carbonyl and 4-oxo) on the antibiotics form insoluble chelates with aluminium and magnesium ions in the gut which reduces absorption.[2,6] In addition these chelates appear to be relatively inactive as antibacterials.[4]

Importance and management

The aluminium/magnesium antacid-ciprofloxacin interaction is established and clinically important. Serum antibiotic levels may become subtherapeutic against organisms such as staphylococci and *Pseudomonas aeruginosa*.[5,11] Do not give the antacid and antibiotic at the same time. Separating the dosages as much as possible reduces the effects of this interaction but it is difficult to assess the best time scheduling. Giving the antacid 2–4 h before the antibiotic to avoid mixing in the gut results in reductions in absorption of 30–75%.[6,11] One study suggests that the absorption is reduced 20–40% if the antacid is given 2–4 h after the antibiotic,[6] whereas another suggests that no interaction occurs if given 2 h after the antibiotic.[11] The makers of ciprofloxacin advise avoidance within 4 h of these antacids. Remember also that some antacids can raise the urinary pH. The solubility of ciprofloxacin decreases as the pH rises and excessive urinary alkalinity should be avoided to prevent crystalluria and possible kidney damage.

Much less is known about enoxacin, norfloxacin and pefloxacin but they seem to interact like ciprofloxacin and the same precautions should be followed. An alternative is possibly to use ofloxacin which appears not to interact.

References

1 Fleming LW, Moreland TA, Stewart WK and Scott AC. Ciprofloxacin and antacids. Lancet (1986) ii, 248.
2 Hoffken G, Borner K, Glatzel PD, Koeppa P and Lode H. Reduced enteral absorption of ciprofloxacin in the presence of antacids. Eur J Clin Microbiol (1985) 4, 345.
3 Preheim LC, Cuevas TA, Roccaforte JS, Mellencamp MA and Bittner MJ. Ciprofloxacin and antacids. Lancet (1986) ii, 48.
4 Machka K and Braveny J. Inhibitorische wirkung verschiedener faktoren auf die aktivitat von gyrasehemmern. FAC (1985) 3, 557–62.
5 Rubinstein E and Segev S. Drug interactions with ciprofloxacin and with other non-antibiotics. Am J Med (1987) 82 (Suppl 4A) 119–23.
6 Schentag JJ, Watson WA, Nix DE, Sedman AJ, Frost RW and Letteri J. The dependent interactions between antacids and quinolone antibiotics. Clin Pharmacol Ther (1988) 43, 135.
7 Vinceneux Ph, Weber Ph, Gaudin H and Boussougant Y. Diminution

de l'absorption de la pefloxacin par les pansements gastriques. La Presse Med (1986) 15, 1826.

8 Maesen FPV, Davies BI, Geraedts WH and Shmajow CA. Ofloxacin and antacids. J Antimicrob Chemother (1987) 19, 848–9.
9 Noyes M and Polk RE. Norfloxacin and absorption of magnesium-aluminium. Ann Intern Med (1988) 109, 168–9.
10 Polk RE. Influence of chronic administration of calcium on the bioavailability of oral ciprofloxacin. 29th Int Conf Antimicrob Ag Chemother, Houston, Texas (1989), 211.
11 Nix DE, Watson WA, Lener ME, Frost RW, Krol G, Goldstein H, Letterei J and Schentag JJ. Effects of aluminium and magnesium antacids and ranitidine on the absorption of ciprofloxacin. Clin Pharmacol Ther (1989) 46, 700–5.

Quinolone antibiotics + Cimetidine or Ranitidine

Abstract/Summary

Cimetidine reduces the clearance of pefloxacin from the body, ranitidine reduces the absorption of enoxacin but neither cimetidine nor ranitidine appear to interact with ciprofloxacin.

Clinical evidence, mechanism, importance and management

Neither cimetidine nor ranitidine affect the pharmacokinetics of ciprofloxacin[1,2,5] but a study of the concurrent use of cimetidine and pefloxacin showed that the AUC was increased about 40% (from 49 to 69 μg/h/ml^{-1}), the half-life increased from 10.3 to 15.3 h and the clearance was reduced from 151 to 110 ml/min.[3] The clinical importance of this is uncertain but increased toxicity is a possibility. In contrast 50 mg ranitidine given intravenously 2 h before a single oral dose of enoxacin was found to have reduced the absorption by 26–40%[4,6] which seemed to be related to change in gastric pH caused by the ranitidine.[6] A reduced therapeutic response seems likely. Concurrent use should be monitored. More study is needed.

References

1 Hoffken G, Lode H and Wiley P-D. Pharmacokinetics and interaction in the bioavailability of new quinolones. In: Proc Int Symp on New Quinolones, Geneva 1986, 141.
2 Wingender W, Foerster D and Beerman D. Effect of gastric emptying on rate and extent of the systemic availability of ciprofloxacin. In: Proc 14th Int Congr Chemother, Kyoto, Japan 1986.
3 Soergel F, Koch U, Metz R and Stephan V. Cimetidine inhibits the hepatic metabolism of pefloxacin. In: Proc 26th Interscience Conference on Antimicrobial Agents and Chemotherapy, New Orleans, Louisiana 1986.
4 COMPRECIN (enoxacin) Clinical Information Manual (Parke Davis) April 1989, references 222 and 223: Schentag JJ, Sedman AJ and Wilton DJ. Interaction between enoxacin, ranitidine and antacids. 3rd European Congress of Clinical Microbiology, The Hague (1987). Thomas D, Latts J, Sedman A and Kinkel A. A study to examine potential pharmacokinetic interaction of enoxacin (CI-919) with antacids or ranitidine, (Protocol 919–66), RR-764–00840, 1987.
5 Nix DE, Watson WA, Lener ME, Frost RW, Krol G, Goldstein H, Letterei J and Schentag JJ. Effects of aluminium and magnesium antacids and ranitidine on the absorption of ciprofloxacin. Clin Pharmacol Ther (1989) 46, 700–5.
6 Lebsack M, Nix D, Schentag J, Welage L, Ryerson B, Totthaker R and

Sedman A. Impact of gastric pH on ranitidine-enoxacin drug-drug interaction. J Clin Pharmacol (1988) 28, 939.

Quinolone antibiotics + Iron preparations

Abstract/Summary

Some preliminary evidence shows that iron preparations can reduce the absorption of ciprofloxacin and ofloxacin from the gut. The quinolone-iron complexes formed have reduced antibacterial effects.

Clinical evidence

A cross-over trial in 12 normal subjects given single doses of 500 mg ciprofloxacin or 400 mg ofloxacin showed that the concurrent use of 200 mg iron (in the form of an iron-glycine-sulphate complex) reduced the bioavailability of the ciprofloxacin by 48% and that of ofloxacin by 36%.[1] Another study found that 325 mg ferrous sulphate three times a day reduced the absorption of ciprofloxacin in normal subjects by 65%.[3] Reduced serum levels of ciprofloxacin (peak levels reduced from 5.2 to 0.3–0.5) were recorded in another patient while taking ferrous sulphate.[3]

Mechanism

Uncertain, but the suggestion is that a quinolone-iron complex (chelation between the metal and the 4-oxo- and adjacent carboxyl groups) is formed which is less easily absorbed. An *in vitro* study also showed that antibacterial effects of ciprofloxacin, ofloxacin and norfloxacin are markedly reduced by ferric chloride or ferrous sulphate when tested against *Salmonella typhimurium* and *Shigella sonnei*.[2]

Importance and management

Information is limited but it seems possible that these interactions are of clinical importance. Until more is known, separate the dosages of ciprofloxacin or ofloxacin and iron as much as possible to avoid mixing in the gut, and monitor the effectiveness of the antibiotic treatment. There seems to be no direct information about other quinolones but many of them interact with the metal ions found in a number of antacids and therefore possibly similarly interact with iron.

References

1 Lode H, Stuhlert P, Deppermann KH and Mainz D. Pharmacokinetic interactions between ciprofloxacin/ofloxacin and ferro-salts. 29th Int Conf Antimicrob Ag Chemother, Houston Tex (1989) 213.
2 Smith JT. Oral iron, 4-quinolones and enteric infection. 29th Int Conf Antimicrob Ag Chemother, Houston Tex (1989) 149.
3 Polk RE. Effect of ferrous sulfate and multivitamins with zinc on the absorption of ciprofloxacin in normal volunteers. 29th Int Conf Antimicrob Ag Chemother, Houston Tex (1989) 136.

Quinolone antibiotics + Rifampicin (Rifampin)

Abstract/Summary, Clinical evidence, mechanism, importance and management

Despite evidence that rifampicin can reduce serum ciprofloxacin levels in animals (by enzyme induction), there is some preliminary evidence that no interaction occurs in man.[1]

Reference

1 Rubin J et al, unpublished observations quoted by Polk RE, Drug-drug interactions with ciprofloxacin and other fluoroquinolones. Am J Med (1989) 87 (Suppl 5A) 76–81S.

Quinolone antibiotics + Sucralfate

Abstract/Summary

Sucralfate causes a very marked reduction in the absorption of ciprofloxacin and norfloxacin if taken together, but a smaller reduction occurs if the dosages are separated by 2 h.

Clinical evidence

(a) Ciprofloxacin + sucralfate

A study in 12 normal subjects showed that a 1 g dose of sucralfate 6 and 12 h before a single 750 mg dose of ciprofloxacin, reduced the ciprofloxacin AUC (area under the concentration-time curve) by 30%. Three of the subjects showed little or no changes but a decrease of more than 50% was seen in four others.[2] Another study found that a patient given 1 g sucralfate four times daily had serum ciprofloxacin levels which were 85–90% lower than five other patients who were not taking sucralfate.[3]

(b) Norfloxacin + sucralfate

A study in eight normal subjects showed that while taking sucralfate (1 g four times daily) the bioavailability of single 400 mg doses of norfloxacin as measured by changes in the AUC (area under the time-concentration curve) was markedly reduced: to 1.8% when taken with the sucralfate and to 56.6% when taken 2 h afterwards.[1,4]

Mechanism

Not established, but a likely explanation is that the aluminium hydroxide component of sucralfate (200 mg in each g) forms an insoluble chelate with the quinolone which reduces its absorption. See 'Quinolones and Antacids'.

Importance and management

Information is very limited but this interaction would seem to be established and clinically important. Since it seems possible that serum ciprofloxacin and norfloxacin levels could be reduced to subtherapeutic concentrations if both drugs are taken together, separate the dosages as much as possible (by 2 h or more) giving the quinolone first. More study is needed to confirm both these findings and the effectiveness of separating the dosages. Enoxacin and pefloxacin also interact with antacids containing aluminium hydroxide (see 'Quinolones+Antacids') but ofloxacin appears not to do so.

References

1 Parpia SH, Nix DE, Hejmanowski LG, Wilton JH, Goldstein HR and Schentag JJ. The effect of sucralfate on the oral bioavailability of norfloxacin. Pharmacotherapy (1988) 8, 140.
2 Nix DE, Watson WA, Frost RW and Rescott DL. Decreased ciprofloxacin absorption after pre-treatment with sucralfate. Pharmacotherapy (1989) 9, 190,
3 Yuk JH, Nightingale CN and Quintiliani R. Ciprofloxacin levels when receiving sucralfate. J Amer Med Ass (1989) 262, 901.
4 Parpia SH, Nix DE, Hejmanowski LG, Goldstein HR, Witton JH and Schentag JJ. Sucralfate reduces the gastrointestinal absorption of norfloxacin. Antimicrob Ag Chem (1989) 33, 99–102.

Quinolone antibiotics + Zinc

Abstract/Summary

Zinc can reduce the absorption of ciprofloxacin.

Clinical evidence, mechanism, importance and management

A study in normal subjects found that a multivitamin preparation with zinc (*Stresstabs 600* with zinc, Lederle Labs) reduced the absorption of ciprofloxacin by 24% (range 2–50%).[1] The probable reason is that the zinc forms a less-soluble chelate with the antibiotic (similar to the chelates formed with the metallic ions in antacids and iron preparations). The clinical importance of this awaits assessment but such large reductions in absorption may result in inadequate control of infection. Other quinolones appear to interact similarly with metallic ions and seem likely to interact with zinc as well. More study is needed.

Reference

1 Polk RE. Effect of ferrous sulfate and multivitamins with zinc on the absorption of ciprofloxacin in normal volunteers. 29th Int Conf Antimicrob Ag Chemother, Houston Tex (1989) 8, 140.

Rifampicin + Aminosalicylic acid (PAS)

Abstract/Summary

The serum levels of rifampicin are halved if aminosalicylic acid in granular form containing bentonite is used concurrently. This interaction may be avoided by separating the dosages by 8–12 h or by using an aminosalicylic acid formulation which does not contain bentonite.

Clinical evidence

A study in 30 patients with tuberculosis showed that their serum rifampicin levels (doses 10 mg/kg) were reduced more than 50% (from 6.06 to 2.91 μg/ml) at 2 h by the concurrent use of PAS-Granulate (*Ferrosan*).[1] Subsequent studies by the same workers on six normal subjects showed that this interaction was not due to the aminosalicylic acid itself but to the bentonite which was the main excipient of the granules.[2]

Other studies confirm this marked reduction in serum rifampicin levels in the presence of aminosalicylic acid granules.[3,4]

Mechanism

The bentonite excipient in aminosalicylic acid granules adsorbs the rifampicin so that much less is available for absorption by the gut, resulting in reduced serum levels.

Importance and management

Well-documented and clinically important. Separating the administration of the two drugs by 8–12 h to prevent their mixing in the gut has been suggested as an effective way to prevent this interaction.[1] An alternative is to give aminosalicylic acid preparations which do not contain bentonite or similar substances which can adsorb rifampicin.

References

1 Boman G, Hanngren A, Malmborg A-S, Borga O and Sjoqvist F. Drug Interaction: decreased serum concentrations of rifampicin when given with PAS. Lancet (1971) i, 800.
2 Boman G, Lundgren P and Stjernstrom G. Mechanism of the inhibitory effect of PAS granules on the absorption of rifampicin: absorption of rifampicin by an excipient, bentonite. Eur J clin Pharmacol (1975) 8, 293.
3 Boman G. Serum concentrations and half-life of rifampicin after simultaneous oral administration of aminosalicylic acid or isoniazid. Eur J clin Pharmacol (1974) 7, 217.
4 Boman G, Borga O, Hanngren A, Malmborg A-S and Sjoqvist F. Pharmacokinetic interactions between the tuberculostatics rifampicin, para-aminosalicylic acid and isoniazid. Acta Pharmac Toxicol (1970) 28, (Suppl 1) 15.

Rifampicin (Rifampin) + Antacids

Abstract/Summary

The absorption of rifampicin can be reduced up to 36% by the concurrent use of antacids but the clinical importance of this is uncertain.

Clinical evidence

A study in five normal subjects showed that when single 600 mg doses of rifampicin were taken with different antacids and 200 ml of water the absorption of the rifampicin was reduced as follows (as measured by the fall in the urinary excretion): with 15 or 30 ml aluminium hydroxide gel (20–31% reduction); with 2 or 4 g magnesium trisilicate (32–36% reduction); and with 2 g sodium carbonate (21% reduction).[1]

Mechanism

The rise in the pH within the stomach caused by these antacids reduces the dissolution of the rifampicin thereby inhibiting its absorption. In addition aluminium ions may form less soluble chelates with rifampicin, and magnesium trisilicate can adsorb rifampicin, both of which would also be expected to reduce bioavailability.[1]

Importance and management

Direct information seems to be limited to this report. No one seems to have assessed the effects of a 20–35% reduction in absorption on rifampicin treatment, but if antacids are given it would be prudent to be alert for any evidence that it is less effective than expected.

Reference

1 Khalil SAH, El-Khordagui LK and El-Gholmy ZA. Effect of antacids on oral absorption of rifampicin. Int J Pharmaceut (1984) 20, 99–106.

Rifampicin (Rifampin) + Clofazimine

Abstract/Summary, Clinical evidence, mechanism, importance and management.

The pharmacokinetics of rifampicin are not altered by clofazimine.[1]

Reference

1 Venkatesan K, Mathur A, Girdhar BK and Bharadwaj VP. The effect of clofazimine on the pharmacokinetics of rifampicin and dapsone in leprosy. J Antimicrob Chemother (1986) 18, 715–18.

Rifampicin (Rifampin) + Dipyrone

Abstract/Summary

The pharmacokinetics of rifampicin are not significantly changed by dipyrone.

Clinical evidence, mechanism, importance and management

A study in untreated patients with leprosy showed that the pharmacokinetics of a single 600 mg dose of rifampicin were not statistically significantly changed by 1 g dipyrone, but peak serum rifampicin levels occurred sooner (at 3 instead of 4 h) and were about 50% higher.[1] However it should be emphasized that dipyrone is an unsafe drug because, like the related amidopyrine, it can cause potentially fatal agranulocytosis. It has been stated that it should only be used in serious and life-threatening situations where alternative antipyretics are not available.[2]

References

1 Krishna DR, Ramankar TV and Prabhakar MC. Pharmacokinetics of rifampin in the presence of dipyrone in leprosy patients. Drug Dev Ind Pharm (1984) 10, 101–10.
2 Reynolds JEF (ed). Martindale. The Extra Pharmacopoeia Edition 28, Pharmaceutical Press, London (1982) p 251.

Rifampicin (Rifampin) + Food

Abstract/Summary

Food delays and reduces the absorption of rifampicin from the gut.

Clinical evidence

A study in six normal subjects showed that when a single 10 mg/kg dose of rifampicin was taken with a standard Indian breakfast (125 g wheat, 10 g visible fat, 350 g vegetables) the absorption of the rifampicin was reduced. The AUC (area under the concentration-time curve) after 8 h was reduced by 26%. and the peak serum levels were reduced by 30% (from 11.84 μg/ml at 2 h to 8.35 μg/ml at 4 h).[1]

Mechanism

Not understood.

Importance and management

An established interaction. The recommendation is that rifampicin should be taken on an empty stomach or 30 min before a meal, or 2 h after a meal to ensure rapid and complete absorption.

Reference

1 Polasa K, Krishnaswamy K. Effect of food on bioavailability of rifampicin. J Clin Pharmacol (1983) 23, 433–7.

Rifampicin (Rifampin) + Probenecid

Abstract/Summary

Whether or not the serum levels of rifampicin are increased by the concurrent use of probenecid is unpredictable.

Clinical evidence, mechanism, importance and management

A study in five normal subjects given probenecid before and after taking single 300 mg doses of rifampicin showed that mean peak serum rifampicin levels were raised 86%. At 4, 6 and 9 h the percentage increases were 118, 90 and 102% respectively.[1] However subsequent studies in patients, taking either 600 or 300 mg rifampicin plus 2 g probenecid

taken 30 min before, showed that the latter group achieved serum rifampicin levels which were only about half those achieved by those on 600 g rifampicin.[2] Similar results were found in a study on patients given 450 mg rifampicin.[3] The reasons for these discordant results are not understood.

Rifampicin is effective but expensive, so the idea of giving smaller doses with probenecid to raise serum levels was attractive because costs could hopefully be reduced. But the response of patients is so inconsistent and unpredictable that these drugs cannot be used together routinely for this purpose. It should however be borne in mind that the occasional patient may show elevated rifampicin levels.

References

1 Kenwright S and Levi AJ. Impairment of hepatic uptake of rifamycin antibiotics by probenecid, and its therapeutic implications. Lancet (1973) ii, 1401.
2 Fallon RJ, Lees AE, Allan GW, Smith J and Tyrrell WF. Probenecid and rifampicin serum levels. Lancet (1975) ii, 792.

Rifampicin (Rifampin) + Triacetyloleandomycin

Abstract/Summary

Cholestatic jaundice has been attributed to the concurrent use of these two antibiotics.

Clinical evidence, mechanism, importance and management

Two cases of cholestatic jaundice have been reported in patients treated with both rifampicin and triacetyloleandomycin.[1,2] Both antibiotics are potentially hepatotoxic and it seems possible that their liver damaging effects can be additive. As a general rule the concurrent use of hepatotoxic drugs should be avoided.

References

1 Piette F and Peyrard P. Ictere benin medicamenteux lors d'un traitement associant rifampicin-triacetyloleandomycine. Nouv Presse med (1979) 8, 368.
2 Givaudan JF, Gamby Th and Privat Y. Ictere cholestatique apres association rifampicine-troleandomycin: une nouvelle observation. Nouv Presse med (1979) 8, 2357.

Rifapentine + Other drugs

Abstract/Summary, Clinical evidence, mechanism, importance and management

Rifapentine (MDL 473) is a derivative of rifampicin with a similar antibacterial spectrum, approximately a ten times greater potency and a longer half-life. Like rifampicin it is a potent liver enzyme inducing agent[1] and although so far no

clinically important interactions have been documented, it is
expected to interact with many of the drugs with which rifampicin interacts (see Index).

Reference

1 Durand DV, Hampden C, Boobis AR, Park BK and Davies DS. Induction of mixed function oxidase activity in man by rifapentine (MDL
473), a long-acting rifamycin derivative. Br J clin Pharmac (1986) 21,
1–7.

Sulphasalazine + Antibiotics

Abstract/Summary

*The release in the colon of the active drug (5-aminosalicylic
acid) from sulphasalazine is markedly reduced by the concurrent use of ampicillin and rifampicin which reduce the activity
of the gut bacteria. This interaction seems likely with any other
oral antibiotic which similarly reduces the gut microflora.*

Clinical evidence

(a) Sulphasalazine + ampicillin

A study in five normal subjects given sulphasalazine (2 g
over 72 h) showed that while also taking ampicillin (250 mg
four times a day) the conversion and release by the bacterial
microflora within the gut of the active metabolite of
sulphasalazine(-5-aminosalicylic acid) was reduced by a
third.[1]

(b) Sulphasalazine + rifampicin

A crossover trial on 11 patients with Crohn's disease, on long
term treatment with sulphasalazine, showed that while concurrently taking rifampicin (10 mg/kg/day) and ethambutol
(15 mg/kg/day) their plasma levels of both 5-aminosalicylic
acid and sulphapyridine fell by 60%.[2]

Mechanism

The azo link of sulphasalazine is split by the anaerobic
bacteria in the colon to release sulphapyridine and 5-
aminosalicylic acid, the latter being the active metabolite
which acts locally in the treatment of Crohn's disease. Antibiotics which decimate the gut flora can apparently reduce
this conversion and this is reflected in lower plasma levels.

Importance and management

Information is limited but the interaction appears to be
established. The extent to which these antibiotics reduce the
effectiveness of sulphasalazine in the treatment of Crohn's
disease or ulcerative colitis seems not to have been determined, but it would clearly be prudent to be on the alert for
evidence of a reduced effect if ampicillin, rifampicin or any
other oral antibiotic (demonstrated with neomycin in
animals[3]) is given which affects the activity of the gut
microflora.

References

1 Houston JB, Day J and Walker J. Azo reduction of sulphasalazine in
healthy volunteers. Br J clin Pharmac (1982) 14, 395–8.
2 Shaffer JL and Houston JB. The effect of rifampicin on sulphapyridine
plasma concentrations following sulphasalazine administration. Br J
clin Pharmac (1985) 19, 526–8.
3 Peppercorn MA and Goldman P. The role of intestinal bacteria in the
metabolism of salicylazosulfapyridine. J Pharmacol Exp Ther (1972) 181,
555–62.

Sulphasalazine or Sodium Fusidate + Cholestyramine

Abstract/Summary

*There are animal studies which show that cholestyramine can
bind with these two drugs in the gut, thereby reducing their
activity. Whether this also occurs in man awaits confirmation.*

Clinical evidence, mechanism, importance and management

In vitro and *in vivo* studies with rats show that cholestyramine
binds with sodium fusidate in the gut, thereby reducing the
amount available for absorption.[1] Similarly another study in
rats showed that cholestyramine binds with sulphasalazine
so that the azo-bond is protected against attack by the
bacteria within the gut. As a result the active 5-aminosalicylic
acid is not released and the faecal excretion of intact
sulphasalazine increases 30-fold.[2] It seems possible that both
of these interactions could also occur in man, but confirmation of this is as yet lacking. Separating the dosages to prevent admixture in the gut has proved effective with other
drugs which bind with cholestyramine.

References

1 Johns WE and Bates TR. Drug-cholestyramine interactions. I.
Physicochemical factors affecting *in vitro* binding of sodium fusidate to
cholestyramine. J Pharm Sci (1972) 61, 730.
2 Pieniaszek HJ and Bates TR. Cholestyramine-induced inhibition of
salicylazosulfapyridine (sulfasalazine) metabolism by rat intestinal
microflora. J Pharmacol Exp Ther (1976) 198, 240.

Sulphasalazine + Iron salts

Abstract/Summary

*Sulphasalazine and iron appear to bind together in the gut, but
whether this reduces the therapeutic response to either compound is uncertain.*

Clinical evidence, mechanism, importance and management

A study in five normal subjects given single 50 mg/kg doses
of sulphasalazine, with and without 400 mg ferrous sulphate,
showed that the serum levels of sulphasalazine were reduced

by the iron. At 5 h the serum levels were reduced about 40%. The reasons are not known, but it is suggested that this may be because the sulphasalazine chelates with the iron which interferes with its absorption.[1] The extent to which this suggested chelation affects the ability of the intestinal bacteria to split the sulphasalazine and release its locally active metabolite (5-aminosalicylic acid) and thereby affects the therapeutic response, seems not to have been studied.

Reference

1 Das KM and Eastwood MA. Effect of iron and calcium on salicylazosulphapyridine metabolism. Scott Med J (1973) 18, 45–56.

Sulphasalazine + Metronidazole

Abstract/Summary

Metronidazole appears not to interact adversely with sulphasalazine.

Clinical evidence, mechanism, importance and management

A study in 10 patients (seven with Crohn's disease and five with ulcerative colitis) on long-term sulphasalazine treatment showed that no statistically significant changes in serum sulphapyridine levels occurred while taking 400 mg metronidazole twice daily for 8–14 days.[1] There seems to be no good reason for avoiding concurrent use.

Reference

1 Shaffer JL, Kershaw A and Houston JB. Disposition of metronidazole and its effects on sulphasalazine metabolism in patients with inflammatory bowel disease. Br J clin Pharmac (1986) 21, 431–5.

Sulphonamides + Barbiturates

Abstract/Summary

The anaesthetic effects of thiopentone (-al) are increased but shortened by pretreatment with sulphafurazole (sulfisoxazole). Phenobarbitone appears not to interact signficantly with sulphafurazole or sulphasomidine. There seem to be no reports of any adverse sulphonamide–barbiturate interactions.

Clinical evidence

(a) Thiopentone (-al) + sulphafurazole (sulfisoxazole)

A study in 48 patients showed that the prior intravenous administration of sulphafurazole (sulfisoxazole), 40 mg/kg, reduced the required anaesthetic dosage of thiopentone (thipental) by 40%, but the awakening time was shortened.[1]

This interaction has also been observed in animal experiments.[2]

(b) Sulphafurazole or sulphasomidine + phenobarbitone (-al)

A study in children showed that phenobaritone did not affect the pharmacokinetics of sulphfurazole (sulfisoxazole) or sulphasomidine.[3]

Mechanism

It is suggested that sulphafurazole successfully competes with the thiopentone for the plasma protein binding sites,[4] the result being that more free and active barbiturate molecules remain in circulation to exert their anaesthetic effects and a smaller dose is therefore required.

Importance and management

The evidence for the sulphfurazole–thiopentone interaction is limited, but it appears to be strong. Less thiopentone than usual may be required to achieve adequate anaesthesia, but since the awakening time is shortened repeated doses may be needed. Information about other sulphonamide–barbiturate interactions are also very limited, but none so far reported seems to be of clinical importance.

References

1 Csogor SI and Kerek SF. Enhancement of thiopentone anaesthesia by sulphafurazole. Br J Anaesth (1970) 42, 988.
2 Csogor SI, Palfy B and Feztz G. Influence du sulfathiazol sur l'effet narcotique du thiopental et de l'hexobarbital. Rev Roum Physiol (1971) 8, 81.
3 Krauer B. Comparative investigations of elimination kinetics of two sulphonamides in children with and without phenobarbital administration. Schweiz Med Wsch (1971) 101, 668.
4 Csogor SI and Papp J. Competition between sulphonamides and thiopental for binding sites on plasma proteins. Arzneim-Forsch (1970) 20, 1925.

Sulphonamides + Local anaesthetics

Abstract/Summary

The para-aminobenzoic acid (PABA) derived from certain local anaesthetics can reduce the effects of the sulphonamides and allow the development of local and even generalized infections.

Clinical evidence

Four patients on sulphonamides developed local infections in areas where procaine had been injected prior to diagnostic taps in meningitis, or draining procedures in empyema. Extensive cellulitis of the lumbar region occurred in one case, and the patient died of meningitis despite continued therapy with sulphadiazine.[1]

A study in man[2] demonstrated that the amount of procaine in pleural fluid after anaesthesia for thoracentesis was sufficient to inhibit the antibacterial activity of 5% sulphapyridine against type III pneumococci. Other studies in animals confirm that antagonism can occur both *in vitro*[6] and *in vivo*[3–5] with local anaesthetics which are hydrolyzed to PABA.

Mechanism

The ester type of local anaesthetic is hydrolyzed within the body to produce PABA which antagonizes the effects of the sulphonamides by competitive inhibition. A fuller explanation of the sulphonamide–PABA interaction is given in the 'Sulphonamide + PABA' synopsis.

Importance and management

Clinical examples of this interaction seem to be few but the supporting evidence (human, animal and *in vitro* studies dating back to the mid-1940s) is strong. This would seem to be an interaction of clinical importance. Local anaesthetics of the ester type which are hydrolyzed to PABA (e.g. amethocaine, procaine, benzocaine) should be avoided in patients using sulphonamides, whereas those of the amide type (bupivacaine, cinchocaine [dibucaine], lignocaine [lidocaine], mepivacaine and prilocaine) do not interact adversely.

References

1 Peterson OL and Finland M. Sulfonamide inhibiting action of procaine. Amer J Med Sci (1944) 207, 166.
2 Boroff DA, Cooper A and Bullowa JGM. Inhibition of sulfapyridine by procaine in chest fluids after procaine anaesthesia. Proc Soc Exp Biol Med (1941) 47,182.
3 Pfeiffer CC and Grant CW. The procaine-sulfonamide antagonism: an evaluation of local anesthetics for use with sulfonamide therapy. Anesthesiology (1944) 5, 605.
4 Casten D, Fried JJ and Hallman FA. Inhibitory effect of procaine on bacteriostatic activity of sulfathiazole. Surg Gyn Obst (1943) 76, 726.
5 Powell HM, Krahl ME and Clowes GHA. Inhibition of chemotherapeutic action of sulfapyridine by local anesthetics. J Indiana Med Ass (1942) 35, 62.
6 Walker BS and Derow MA. The antagonism of local anesthetics against the sulfonamides. Amer J Med Sci (1945) 210, 585.

Sulphonamides + Para-aminobenzoic acid (PABA)

Abstract/Summary

The antibacterial effects of the sulphonamides are reduced or abolished by PABA.

Clinical evidence and mechanism

Many micro-organisms can synthesize their own folate if provided with PABA, whereas man needs preformed folate in his diet. The molecular structure of the sulphonamides is sufficiently similar to PABA for micro-organisms to incorporate them into the synthetic biochemical pathways concerned with making folate, but sufficiently dissimilar for the synthesis to fail. Starved of folate in this way, the organism ceases to grow and multiply, and it is in this way that the sulphonamides act as bacteriostatic agents. The term 'competitive antagonist' is used to describe this situation because PABA and the sulphonamide compete with one another to take part in the synthetic reactions, the relative concentrations of each molecule being among the factors which determine the 'winner', hence the clinical importance of achieving adequate concentrations of the sulphonamide and of avoiding the introduction of additional PABA molecules.

Importance and management

The interaction between PABA and the sulphonamides has been very extensively studied and is very well documented. PABA should not be given to patients taking sulphonamides. Although PABA features in both the BP and USP, it is now used largely in topical preparations as a sunscreen agent and it is most unlikely to be absorbed through the skin. Oral administration is probably not common.

Tetracyclines + Alcohol

Abstract/Summary

The serum levels of doxycycline may fall below minimal therapeutic concentrations in alcoholic patients, but tetracycline itself is not affected and it seems likely that the other tetracyclines are also not affected. There is nothing to suggest that moderate amounts of alcohol will significantly affect the serum levels of doxycycline or any other tetracycline in normal non-alcoholic subjects.

Clinical evidence

In a comparative study the half-life of doxycycline was found to be 10.5 h in six alcoholics compared with 14.7 h in six normal healthy volunteers. The serum levels of two of the alcoholic patients fell well below what is generally accepted as the minimum therapeutic concentrations. The half-life of tetracycline was the same in both groups. All of them were given 100 mg doxycycline daily after a 200 mg loading dose, and 500 mg tetracycline twice daily after an initial 750 mg loading dose.[1]

In another study in normal subjects it was found that cheap red wine (but not whiskey) postponed the absorption of doxycycline, probably because of the acetic acid content which slows gastric emptying, but did not affect its total absorption. The authors concluded that '...the acute intake of alcoholic beverages generally does not interfere with the kinetics of doxycycline to an extent which would jeopardise therapeutic levels in tissues.'[4]

Mechanism

Heavy drinkers can metabolize some drugs much more quickly than non-drinkers due to the enzyme-inducing effects of alcohol,[2,3] and this interaction with doxycycline would seem to be due to this effect, possibly associated with some reduction in absorption from the gut.

Importance and management

Information is limited, but the doxycycline–alcohol interaction appears to be established. It seems to be clinically significant in alcoholic subjects but not in normal individuals. One suggested solution to the problem is to dose alcoholic subjects twice daily instead of only once. Alternatively tetracycline could be used because it appears not to be affected. There is nothing to suggest that moderate or even occasional heavy drinking affects any of the tetracylines in normal subjects.

References

1 Neuvonen PJ, Pentilla O, Roos M and Tirkkonen J. Effect of long-term alcohol consumption on the half-life of tetracycline and doxycycline in man.
2 Misra PS, Leferre A, Ishii H, Rubin E and Lieber CS. Increase of ethanol, meprobamate and pentobarbital metabolism after chronic ethanol administration in man and rats. Amer J Med (1971) 571, 346.
3 Neuvonen PJ, Pentilla O, Lehtovaara K and Aho K. Effect of antiepileptic drugs on the elimination of various tetracycline derivatives. Europ J Clin Pharmacol (1975) 9, 147.
4 Mattila MJ, Laisi U, Linnoila M and Salonen R. Effect of alcoholic beverages on the pharmacokinetics of doxycycline in man. Acta pharmacol et toxicol (1982) 50, 370–3.

Tetracyclines + Antacids

Abstract/Summary

The serum levels, and as a consequence the therapeutic effectiveness, of the tetracycline antibiotics can be markedly reduced or even abolished by the concurrent use of antacids containing aluminium, bismuth, calcium or magnesium. Other antacids such as sodium bicarbonate which raise the gastric pH may also reduce the bioavailability of some tetracycline preparations.

Clinical evidence

(a) Aluminium-containing antacids

A study on five patients and six normal subjects given 500 mg chlortetracycline orally every 6 h showed that if they were given two tablespoonfuls of aluminium hydroxide gel (*Amphojel*) at the same time, within 48 h the serum chlortetracycline levels had fallen 80–90%. One patient had a recurrence of her urinary tract infection which only subsided when the antacid was withdrawn.[1] This was confirmed in another study.[2]

Other studies in man showed that 30 ml aluminium hydroxide reduced oxytetracycline serum levels by more than 50%;[3] 20 ml caused a 75% reduction in demeclocycline serum levels;[4] 15 ml caused a 100% reduction in serum doxycycline levels; and 30 ml magnesium-aluminium hydroxide (*Maalox*) caused a 90% reduction in tetracycline serum levels.[6]

(b) Calcium, magnesium or bismuth-containing antacids

Bismuth salicylate markedly reduces the absorption of tetracycline[13] and a 50% reduction in serum doxycycline levels can occur.[14] Bismuth carbonate interacts with the tetracyclines *in vitro*.[9] Magnesium sulphate certainly interacts with tetracycline, but in the clinical study on record[6] the

amount of magnesium was much higher than would normally be found in the usual dose of antacid. Magnesium oxide interacted in an *in vitro* study.[9] There seem to be no direct clinical studies with calcium-containing antacids but a clinically important interaction seems an almost certainty, based on an *in vitro* study with calcium carbonate,[9] studies of calcium in milk (see synopsis on 'Tetracyclines + Milk and Dairy products') and as dicalcium phosphate,[7] and as an excipient in tetracycline capsules.[8]

(c) Sodium-containing antacids

A study in eight subjects showed that when given a 250 mg capsule of tetracycline hydrochloride with 2 g sodium bicarbonate, the mean absorption of the tetracycline was reduced 50%. If however the tetracycline was dissolved before administration, the absorption was unaffected by the sodium bicarbonate.[10]

Another study stated that 2 g sodium bicarbonate had an insignificant effect on tetracycline absorption.[12]

Mechanism

Work in the mid-1950s demonstrated that the tetracyclines bind with aluminium, bismuth, calcium, magnesium and other metallic ions to form compounds (chelates) which are much less soluble and therefore much less readily absorbed by the gut.[11] In addition it has been shown[10] that the solubility of the tetracyclines is a hundred times greater at pH 1–3 than at pH 5–6, so that an antacid which raises the gastric pH above about 4 for 20–30 min could prevent up to 50% of the tetracycline from being fully dissolved in the stomach. Once the undissolved drug is emptied out of the stomach, the pH in the duodenum (5–6) and in the rest of the gut are unfavourable for full dissolution, so that a good proportion of the tetracycline may never dissolve and so it remains unavailable for absorption. This may also explain why sodium bicarbonate interacts with tetracycline. A third reason for the reduced absorption may be because the tetracyclines are adsorbed onto the antacid.[13]

Importance and management

Extremely well-documented, long and well-established interactions. Their clinical importance depends on how much the serum tetracycline levels are lowered, but with normal antacid dosages the reductions cited above (50–100%) are so large that many organisms will not be exposed to minimum inhibitory concentrations (MIC). As a general rule none of the aluminium, bismuth, calcium or magnesium containing antacids, or others such as sodium bicarbonate which can markedly alter gastric pH, should be given at the same time as the tetracycline antibiotics. If they must be used, separate the dosages as much as possible to prevent their admixture in the gut. Sodium bicarbonate and other antacids which only affect the extent of absorption by altering gastric pH will only interact with tetracycline preparations which are not already dissolved before ingestion (e.g. those in capsule form). Patients should be warned about taking any over-the-counter antacids and indigestion preparations.

Instead of using antacids to minimize the gastric irritant ef-

fects of the tetracyclines it is usually recommended that tetracyclines are taken before food, however it is not entirely clear
how much this affects their absorption. One study demonstrated that food reduced the absorption of demeclocycline,[4]
whereas another claimed that it did not.[5]

References

1 Waisbren BA and Hueckel JS. Reduced absorption of Aureomycin
   caused by aluminium hydroxide gel (Amphojel). Proc Soc Exp Biol
   Med NY (1950) 73, 73.
2 Seed JC and Wilson CE. The effect of aluminium hydroxide on serum
   Aureomycin concentrations after simultaneous oral administration. Bull
   Johns Hopkins Hosp (1950) 86, 415.
3 Michel JC, Sayer RJ and Kirby WMM. Effect of food and antacids on
   blood levels of Aureomycin and Terramycin. J Lab Clin Med (1950) 36,
   632.
4 Scheiner J and Altemeier WA. Experimental study of factors inhibiting
   absorption and effective therapeutic levels of declomycin. Surg Gynec
   Obstet (1962) 114, 9.
5 Rosenblatt JE, Barrett JE, Brodie JL and Kirby WMM. Comparison of
   in vitro activity and clinical pharmacology of doxycycline with other
   tetracyclines. Antimicrob Ag Chemother (1966) 134.
6 Harcourt RS and Hamburger M. The effect of magnesium sulphate in
   lowering tetracycline blood levels. J Lab Clin Med (1957) 50, 464.
7 Boger WP and Gavin JJ. An evaluation of tetracycline preparations. N
   Engl J Med (1959) 261, 827.
8 Sweeney WM, Hardy SM, Dornbush AC and Ruegsegger JM. Absorption of tetracycline in human beings as affected by certain excipients.
   Antibiot Med Clin Ther (1957) 4, 642.
9 Christensen EKJ, Kerckhoffs HPM and Huizinga T. De invloed van an-
   tacida op de afgifte in vitro van tetracycline-hydrochloride. Pharm
   Weekblad (1967) 102, 463.
10 Barr WH, Adir J and Garrettson L. Decrease of tetracycline absorption
   in man by sodium bicarbonate. Clin Pharmacol Ther (1971) 12, 779.
11 Albert A and Rees CW. Avidity of the tetracyclines for the cations of
   metals. Nature (1956) 177, 433.
12 Garty M and Hurwitz A. Effect of cimetidine and antacids on
   gastrointestinal absorption of tetracycline. Clin Pharmacol Ther (1980)
   28, 203.
13 Albert KS, Welch RD, De Sante KA and Disanto AR. Decreased tetracycline bioavailability caused by bismuth subsalicylate antidiarrhoeal
   mixture. J Pharm Sci (1979) 68, 586.
14 Ericsson CD, Feldman S, Pickering LK and Cleary TG. Influence of
   subsalicylate bismuth on absorption of doxycycline. J Amer Med Ass
   (1982) 247, 2266.

Tetracyclines + Anticonvulsants

Abstract/Summary

*The serum levels of doxycycline are reduced and may fall below
the accepted therapeutic minimum in patients on long-term
treatment with barbiturates, phenytoin or carbamazepine.
Other tetracyclines appear to be unaffected.*

Clinical evidence

A study in 14 patients taking phenytoin (200–500 mg daily)
and/or carbamazepine (300–1000 mg daily) showed that the
half-life of doxycycline was approximately half that in nine
other patients not taking anticonvulsants (7.1 compared with
15.1 h).[1]

Similar results were found in 16 other patients on anticonvulsant therapy with phenytoin, carbamazepine and
phenobarbitone. The serum doxycycline levels of almost all
of them fell below 0.5 μg/ml during the 12–24 h period
following their last dose of doxycycline (100 mg). Tetracycline, methacycline, oxytetracycline, demeclocycline and
chlortetracycline were not significantly affected by these anticonvulsants.[2] Other studies confirm this interaction between
the anticonvulsant barbiturates (and in one case the hypnotic
amylobarbitone) and doxycycline.[3,4]

Mechanism

Uncertain. These anticonvulsants are known enzyme-
inducing agents and it seems probable that they increase the
metabolism of the doxycycline by the liver, thereby hastening its clearance from the body.

Importance and management

The doxycycline–anticonvulsant interactions are established. The extent to which concurrent use affects treatment
with doxycycline seems not to have been studied, but serum
doxycycline levels below 0.5 μg/ml are less than the accepted
minimum inhibitor concentration (MIC). It seems likely that
the antibiotic will fail to be effective. The suggestion has been
made that the interaction can be accommodated by increasing the doxycycline dosage or by giving it twice daily.[2]
Alternatively, tetracyclines which are reported not to be affected by the anticonvulsants could be used: tetracycline,
methacycline, oxytetracycline, demeclocycline and chlortetracycline.[2]

References

1 Pentilla O, Neuvonen PJ, Aho K and Lehtovaara R. Interaction between doxycycline and some antiepileptic drugs. Br Med J (1974) 2,
   470.
2 Neuvonen PJ, Pentilla O, Lehtovaara R and Aho K. Effect of antiepileptic drugs on the elimination of various tetracycline derivatives.
   Eur J clin Pharmacol (1975) 9, 147.
3 Neuvonen PJ and Pentilla O. Interaction between doxycycline and barbiturates. Br Med J (1974) 1, 535.
4 Alestig K. Studies on the intestinal excretion of doxycycline. Scand J
   Infect Dis (1974) 6, 265.

Tetracyclines + Cimetidine

Abstract/Summary

Cimetidine seems not to affect the serum levels of tetracycline.

Clinical evidence, mechanism, importance and
management

A study in five normal subjects showed that cimetidine
reduced the absorption of a single dose of tetracycline
(500 mg) in capsule form by about 30%, but not when the
tetracyline was given in solution.[1] A similar reduction was
seen in another single dose study,[3] but no interaction was
found in a third single dose study.[2] However when tetracycline in either tablet or suspension form was given to six
subjects with 1 g cimetidine daily for six days, no changes

in the serum levels of tetracycline were seen.[3] So it seems that in practice cimetidine has little or no effect on serum tetracycline levels. No special precautions would seem necessary. Information about other tetracyclines seems to be lacking.

References

1 Cole JJ, Charles BG and Ravenscroft PJ. Interaction of cimetidine with tetracycline absorption. Lancet (1980) ii, 536.
2 Garty M and Hurwitz A. Effect of cimetidine and antacids on gastro-intestinal absorption of tetracycline. Clin Pharmacol Ther (1980) 28, 203.
3 Fisher P, House F, Inns P, Morrison PJ, Rogers HJ and Bradbrook ID. Effect of cimetidine on the absorption of orally administered tetra-cycline. Br J Clin Pharmac (1980) 9, 153–8.

Tetracyclines + Colestipol

Abstract/Summary

Colestipol can markedly reduce the absorption of tetracycline.

Clinical evidence

A study in nine subjects found that 30 g colestipol taken either in 180 ml water or orange juice reduced the absorption of a single 500 mg dose of oral tetracycline hydrochloride by 54–56% (as measured by recovery in the urine).[1]

This confirms a previous study which found a 50–60% reduction in the bioavailability of tetracycline.[2]

Mechanism

Colestipol binds to bile acids in the gut and can also bind with some drugs, thereby reducing their availability for ab-sorption. An *in vitro* study found a 30% binding.[3] The presence of citrate ions in the orange juice which can also bind to colestipol appears not to have a marked effect on the binding of the tetracycline.

Importance and management

Direct information seems to be limited to the reports cited but it is consistent with the way colestipol interacts with other drugs. In practice colestipol is normally given in 15–30 g daily doses, divided into two or four doses, and tetracycline in 250–500 mg doses six-hourly which means that it is dif-ficult to avoid some mixing in the gut. It seems very probable that a clinically important interaction will occur, but by how much the steady-state serum tetracycline levels are affected seems not to have been determined. Tell patients to separate the dosages as much as possible. Monitor the outcome well. It may be necessary to increase the dosage of tetracycline. It also seems likely that other tetracyclines will interact similarly.

References

1 Friedman H, Greenblatt DJ and LeDuc BW. Impaired absorption of tetracycline by colestipol is not reversed by orange juice. J Clin Pharmacol (1989) 29, 748–51.

2 Brown RK. The effect of concomitant administration of colestipol hydrochloride on the bioavailability of orally administered tetracycline hydrochloride. Report on file Upjohn Co (1975).
3 Ko H, Royer ME. *In vitro* binding of drugs to colestipol hydrochloride. J Pharmac Sci (1974) 63, 1914.

Tetracyclines + Diuretics

Abstract/Summary

It has been recommended that the concurrent use of tetra-cyclines and diuretics should be avoided because of their association with rises in blood urea nitrogen levels.

Clinical evidence, mechanism, importance and management

A retrospective study of patient records as part of the Boston Collaborative Drug Surveillance Program showed that a strong association existed between tetracycline administration with diuretics (not named) and rises in blood urea nitrogen (BUN) levels.[1] The suggested reasons are that the tetra-cyclines have anti-anabolic effects, whereas diuretics can decrease the glomerular filtration rate and increase the reab-sorption of filtered urea, both of which can result in rises in BUN levels.[2] The recommendation was made that tetra-cyclines should be avoided in patients on diuretics when alternative antibiotics could be substituted.[1] This would seem to be particularly appropriate for patients with existing renal impairment, however it has been claimed that doxy-cycline may be used in those with renal failure.[2]

References

1 Boston Collaborative Drug Surveillance Program. Tetracycline and drug-attributed rises in blood urea nitrogen. J Amer Med Ass (1972) 220, 377.
2 Alexander MR. Tetracyclines and rises in urea nitrogen. J Amer Med Ass (1972) 221, 713–14.

Tetracyclines + Iron preparations

Abstract/Summary

The absorption from the gut of both the tetracylines and of iron salts is markedly reduced by concurrent use, leading to depressed serum levels. Their therapeutic effectiveness may be reduced or even abolished. If both must be given, their ad-ministration should be separated as much as possible to pre-vent mixing in the gut.

Clinical evidence

(a) Effect of iron on absorption of the tetracyclines

An investigation in 10 normal adults given single oral doses of tetracyclines (200–500 mg) showed that the concurrent use of 200 mg ferrous sulphate decreased the serum antibiotic levels as follows: tetracycline reduced 40–50%; oxytetracycline 50–60%; methacycline and doxycycline 80–90%.[1]

Similar results were found in other studies showing that in some instances the serum levels fell below minimal bacterial inhibitory concentrations (MIC).[2–5] If the iron was given 3 h before or 2 h after the tetracycline the serum levels were not significantly depressed,[2–4] with the exception of doxycycline.[4] Even when the iron was given up to 11 h after the doxycycline, serum concentrations were still lowered 20–45%.[4]

(b) Effect of tetracyclines on the absorption of iron

A study of this interaction showed that when 250 mg ferrous sulphate (equivalent to 50 mg Fe^{2+}) was given with 500 mg tetracycline, the absorption of iron in normal subjects was reduced 37–78%, and in those with depleted iron stores 40–65%.[8,9]

Mechanism

The tetracyclines have a strong affinity for iron and form poorly soluble tetracycline-iron chelates which are much less readily absorbed from the gastrointestinal tract. As a result the serum tetracycline levels achieved are much lower.[6,7] There is also less free iron available for absorption. Separating the administration of the two prevents their admixture,[2,3] but in the case of doxycycline some of the antibiotic is returned into the gut in the bile which tends to thwart any attempt to keep the iron and antibiotic apart.[4] The different extent to which iron salts interact with the tetracyclines appears to be a reflection of their ability to liberate ferrous and ferric ions which are free to combine with the tetracycline.[5]

Importance and management

Well-documented and well-established interactions of clinical importance. Reductions in serum tetracycline levels of the order of 30–90% due to the presence of iron are so large that levels may be reached which are too low to inhibit bacterial growth (MIC).[3] However the extent of the reductions depends on a number of factors. (a) The particular tetracycline used: tetracycline itself in the study cited above was affected the least;[1] (b) the time-interval between the administration of the two drugs: giving iron 3 h before or 2 h after the antibiotic is satisfactory with tetracycline itself[2] but 11 h is inadequate for doxycycline; (c) the particular iron preparation used: with tetracycline the reduction in serum levels with ferrous sulphate was 80–90%, with ferrous fumarate, succinate and gluconate 70–80%; with ferrous tartrate 50%; and with ferrous sodium edetate 30%.[5] The interaction can therefore be accommodated by separating the dosages as much as possible, avoiding the use of doxycycline, and choosing one of the iron preparations causing minimal interference.

One suggestion is a schedule in which 500 mg tetracycline is given 30–60 min before breakfast and dinner (total daily dose 1 g), and 50 mg Fe^{2+} before lunch and 2 h after dinner.[9] This provides the patient with tetracycline serum concentrations of about 3–5 $\mu g/ml$ and a daily iron absorp-

tion of 25 mg, sufficient to allow optimal haemoglobin regeneration values of 0.2–0.3 g%/day.

Only tetracycline, oxytetracycline, methacycline and doxycycline have been shown to interact with iron, but it seems reasonable to expect that the others will behave in a similar way.

References

1 Neuvonen PJ, Gothoni G, Hackman R and Bjorkjsten K. Interference of iron with the absorption of tetracyclines in man. Br Med J (1970) 4, 532.
2 Mattila MJ, Neuvonen PJ, Gothoni G and Hackman CR. Interference of iron preparations and milk with the absorption of tetracyclines. Excerpta Medica Int Congr Series No. 254 (1972). Toxicological problems of drug combinations, 128.
3 Gothoni G, Neuvonen PJ, Mattila M and Hackman R. Iron-tetracycline interaction: effect of time interval between the drugs. Acta Med Scand (1972) 191, 409.
4 Neuvonen PJ and Pentilla O. Effect of oral ferrous sulphate on the half-life of doxycycline in man. Eur J Clin Pharmacol (1974) 7, 361.
5 Neuvonen PJ and Pentilla O. Inhibitory effect of various iron salts on the absorption of tetracycline in man. Eur J clin Pharmacol (1974) 7, 357.
6 Albert A and Rees CW. Avidity of the tetracyclines for the cations of metals. Nature (1956) 177, 433.
7 Albert A and Rees CW. Incompatibility of aluminium hydroxide and certain antibiotics. Br Med J (1955) 2, 1027.
8 Heinrich HC, Oppitz KH and Gabbe EE. Hemmung der Eisenabsorption beim Menschen durch Tetracyclin. Klin Wsch (1974) 52, 493.
9 Heinrich HC and Oppitz KH. Tetracycline inhibits iron absorption in man. Naturwissenschaften (1973) 60, 524.

Tetracyclines + Milk and Dairy products

Abstract/Summary

The absorption of the tetracyclines can be markedly reduced if they are allowed to come into contact in the gut with milk or other dairy products, and as a result their therapeutic effects may be diminished or even abolished. Doxycycline is the least affected.

Clinical evidence

The serum levels of 12 normal subjects given single 300 mg oral doses of demeclocycline were reduced 70–80% when ingested with either 8 oz (a little over a third of a pint) of fresh pasteurized milk, 8 oz buttermilk or 4 oz cottage cheese, when compared with four other subjects given the same amount of antibiotic but with a meal containing no dairy products.[1] A 50% reduction was seen in other subjects given 300–500 mg tetracycline, methacycline or oxytetracycline with 300 ml (about half a pint) of milk. Doxycycline was not affected.[2]

Similar results were found in other studies.[3,4] A 20% reduction in serum doxycycline levels (from 1.79 to 1.45 $\mu g/ml$) were found 2 h after a single 100 mg oral dose with 240 ml milk.[3]

Mechanism

The tetracyclines have a strong affinity for the calcium ions which are found in abundance in milk and dairy products.[5,6] The tetracycline-calcium chelates formed are much less readily absorbed from the gastrointestinal tract, and as a result the serum levels achieved are much lower. It has also been shown *in vitro* that the tetracycline chelates have a very much reduced antibacterial activity.[8] Doxycycline has a lesser tendency to form chelates[7] which explains why its serum levels are reduced to a smaller extent than other tetracyclines.

Importance and management

Well-documented and very well-established interactions of clinical importance. Reductions in serum tetracycline levels of 50–80% are so large that their antibacterial effects may become minimal or even nil. For this reason tetracyclines should not be taken with milk or dairy products such as yoghourt or cheese. Separate the ingestion of these foods and the administration of the tetracycline as much as possible (in the case of iron which interacts by the same mechanism, 2–3 h is enough). The small amounts of milk in tea and coffee probably do not matter very much, but nobody seems to have checked on this. Doxycycline and minocycline[10] are minimally affected by dairy products and in this respect have advantages over other tetracyclines. The manufacturers of tetracycline phosphate (*Tetrex*) claim that the phosphate combines with the calcium leaving more free tetracycline available for absorption. This form also appears to have advantages.[9]

It is common practice to advise patients to take the tetracyclines before food to overcome the gastric irritant effects, but it is not entirely clear whether, or how much, this affects the amount available for absorption. One study with demeclocycline demonstrated that food reduced the absorption,[1] whereas another claimed that it did not.[3]

References

1 Scheiner J and Altemeier WA. Experimental study of factors inhibiting absorption and effective therapeutic levels of declomycin. Surg Gynec Obstet (1962) 114, 9.
2 Neuvonen P, Matilla M, Gothoni H and Hackman R. Interference of iron and milk with absorption of tetracycline. Scand J Clin Lab Invest (1971) 116 (Suppl 27) 76.
3 Rosenblatt JE, Barrett JE, Brodie JL and Kirby WMM. Comparison of *in vitro* activity and clinical pharmacology of doxycycline with other tetracyclines. Antimicrob Ag Chemother (1966) 134.
4 Matilla MJ, Neuvonen PJ, Gothoni G and Hackman CR. Interference of iron preparations and milk with the absorption of tetracyclines. Excerpta Medica Int Congr Series (1971) 254, 128.
5 Albert A and Rees CW. Avidity of the tetracyclines for the cations of metals. Nature (1956) 177, 433.
6 Albert A and Rees CW. Incompatibility of aluminium hydroxide and certain antibiotics. Br Med J (1955) 2, 1027.
7 Schach von Wittenau M. Some pharmacokinetic aspects of doxycycline metabolism in man. Chemotherapy (1968) 13 (Suppl) 41.
8 Weinberg ED. The mutual effects of antimicrobial compounds and metallic ions. Bacteriol Rev (1957) 21, 46.
9 ABPI Data Sheet Compendium 1985–6, Datapharm Publications London (1985) p 266.
10 Ibid p 728.

Tetracyclines + Phenothiazines

Abstract/Summary

An isolated report describes black galactorrhoea in a woman treated with minocycline, perphenazine, amitriptyline and diphenhydramine.

Clinical evidence, mechanism, importance and management

A woman taking 200 mg minocycline daily for four years to control pustulocystic acne, developed irregular darkly pigmented macules in the areas of acne scarring and later began to produce droplets of darkly coloured milk which was found to contain macrophages filled with particles of iron and haemosiderin. The situation resolved when the drugs were withdrawn.[1] Galactorrhoea is a known side-effect of the phenothiazines and is due to an elevation of serum prolactin levels caused by the blockade of dopamine receptors in the hypothalamus. The dark colour appeared to be a side-effect of the minocycline which can cause hemosiderin to be deposited in cells, and in this instance to be scavenged by the macrophages which were then secreted in the milk.

Reference

1 Basler RS and Lynch PJ. Black galactorrhoea as a consequence of minocycline and phenothiazine therapy. Arch Dermatol (1985) 121, 417–18.

Tetracyclines + Rifampicin (Rifampin)

Abstract/summary

Some patients show a marked fall (50%) in serum doxycycline levels if given rifampicin.

Clinical evidence

A pharmacokinetic study in seven patients given 200 mg doxycycline daily showed that the concurrent use of 10 mg/kg rifampicin daily caused a considerable reduction in the serum doxycycline levels. The reduction was very marked in four patients but not significant in the other three. The rifampicin caused a mean fall of 36% (from 14.18 to 9.11 h) in the doxycycline half life in the whole group of seven, a 106% increase in clearance (from 4.7 to 9.67 l/h) and a reduction in the AUC (area under the curve) of 54% (from 54.38 to 24.77 mg.h.l^{-1}).[1]

Mechanism

Uncertain. It seems probable that the rifampicin (a known potent enzyme inducing agent) increases the metabolism of the doxycycline thereby increasing its loss from the body.

Importance and management

Information seems to be limited to this study. This interaction would appear to be clinically important in some patients but not others. More confirmatory study is needed. Monitor the effects of concurrent use and increase the doxycycline dosage as necessary. The study revealed that before the rifampicin was given, the doxycycline half-life in those patients who were affected by this interaction was longer (17.8 h) than in the others (9.2 h). This would seem to be a way of identifying those patients likely to be at risk.

Reference

1 Garraffo R, Dellamonica P, Fournier JP, Lapalaus Ph, Bernard E, Beziau H and Chichmanian RM. Effet de la rifampicine sur la pharmacocinetique de la doxycycline. Path Biol (1987) 35, 746–9.

Tetracyclines + Thiomersal

Abstract/Summary

Patients who are treated with tetracyclines and who use contact lens solutions which contain thiomersal (thimerosal, thiomersalate, mercuriothiolate) may experience an inflammatory ocular reaction.

Clinical evidence, mechanism, importance and management

The observation of two patients who had ocular reactions (red eye, irritation, blepharitis) when they used a 0.004% thiomersal-containing contact-lens solution while taking a tetracycline, prompted further study of this interaction. A questionnaire sent to other patients revealed nine other cases which suddenly began shortly after starting to use a tetracycline, and which cleared when the thiomersal or the tetracycline was stopped. The same reaction was also clearly demonstrated in rabbits.[1] The reasons are not understood.

Reference

1 Crook TG and Freeman JJ. Reactions induced by the concurrent use of thimerosal and tetracycline. Amer J Opt Physiol Optics (1983) 60, 759–61.

Tetracyclines + Zinc sulphate

Abstract/Summary

The absorption of tetracycline can be reduced by as much as 50% if zinc sulphate is taken concurrently. Separating their administration as much as possible minimizes the effects of this interaction. Doxycycline interacts minimally with zinc.

Clinical evidence

Seven subjects given 500 mg tetracycline, either alone or with zinc sulphate (200 mg containing 45 mg Zn^{2+}), had tetracycline serum concentrations which were reduced 30–40% by the presence of the zinc. The areas under the curves were similarly reduced.[1]

A more than 50% reduction was seen in another study,[2] and this interaction was confirmed in yet another.[7] The reduction in serum zinc concentrations was found to be minimal.[2]

Mechanism

Zinc (like iron, calcium, magnesium and aluminium) forms a relatively stable and poorly absorbed chelate with tetracycline within the gut which results in a reduction in the amount of antibiotic available for absorption.[3,4]

Importance and management

An established and moderately well documented interaction of clinical importance. Separate the administration of tetracycline and zinc sulphate as much as possible so that the two come into minimal contact in the gut (in the case of iron which interacts by the same mechanism, 2–3 h is enough.[5]) An alternative is to use doxycycline which has been shown to interact minimally with zinc.[1] Other tetracyclines would be expected to interact like tetracycline itself, but this needs confirmation. The small reduction in serum zinc concentrations is likely to be of little practical importance.[2,6]

References

1 Penttila O, Hurme H and Neuvonen PJ. Effect of zinc sulphate on the absorption of tetracycline and doxycycline in man. Eur J Clin Pharmacol (1975) 9, 131.
2 Andersson K-E, Bratt L, Dencker H, Kamure C and Lanner E. Inhibition of tetracycline absorption by zinc. Eur J Clin Pharmacol (1976) 10, 59.
3 Albert A and Rees CW. Avidity of the tetracyclines for cations of metals. Nature (1956) 177, 433.
4 Doluisio JT and Martin AN. Metal complexation of the tetracycline hydrochlorides. J Med Chem (1963) 16, 16.
5 Gothoni G, Neuvonen PJ, Mattila M and Hackman R. Iron–tetracycline interaction: effect of time interval between drugs. Acta med Scand (1972) 191, 409.
6 Andersson K-E, Bratt L, Dencker H and Lanner E. Some aspects of the intestinal absorption of zinc in man. Eur J Clin Pharmacol (1975) 9, 423.
7 Mapp RK and McCarthy TJ. The effect of zinc sulphate and of bicitropeptide on tetracycline absorption. S Afr Med J (1976) 50, 1829.

Tinidazole + Cimetidine

Abstract/Summary

Cimetidine reduces the loss of tinidazole from the body. The clinical importance of this is uncertain.

Clinical evidence, mechanism, importance and management

A study in six normal subjects showed that after taking 800 mg cimetidine daily for seven days the peak serum levels of tinidazole following a single 600 mg dose were raised by 21% (from 14.1 to 17.1 μg/ml), the 24 h AUC increased by 40% (from 150 to 210 μg/ml^{-1} h) and the half-life increased by 47% (from 7.66 to 11.23 h).[1] The probable reason is that the cimetidine inhibits the metabolism of the tinidazole by the liver, thereby reducing its loss from the body. Some increase in both the therapeutic and the toxic effects of tinidazole would be expected, but the clinical importance of this is uncertain. It appears not to have been studied.

Reference

1 Patel RB, Shah GF, Raval JD, Gandhi TP and Gilbert RN. The effect of cimetidine and rifampicin on tinidazole kinetics in healthy human volunteers. Indian Drugs (1986) 23, 338–41.

Tinidazole + Rifampicin (Rifampin)

Abstract/Summary

Rifampicin increases the loss of tinidazole from the body. The clinical importance of this is uncertain.

Clinical evidence, mechanism, importance and management

A study in six normal subjects showed that after taking 600 mg rifampicin daily for seven days the peak serum levels of tinidazole following a single 600 mg dose were reduced by 21% (from 14.1 to 11.1 μg/ml), the 24h AUC fell by 30% (from 150 to 105 μg/ml^{-1} h) and the half-life fell by 27% (from 7.66 to 5.6 h).[1] The probable reason is that the rifampicin increases the metabolism of the tinidazole by the liver, thereby increasing its loss from the body. Some reduction in the therapeutic effects of tinidazole would be expected, but the clinical importance of this is uncertain. It appears not to have been studied.

Reference

1 Patel RB, Shah GF, Raval JD, Gandhi TP and Gilbert RN. The effect of cimetidine and rifampicin on tinidazole kinetics in healthy human volunteers. Indian Drugs (1986) 23, 338–41.

Trimethoprim + Antacids

Abstract/Summary

Magnesium trisilicate and kaolin-pectin reduce the bioavailability of trimethoprim in rats, but the clinical importance of this is uncertain.

Clinical evidence, mechanism, importance and management

A study in rats showed that magnesium trisilicate and kaolin-pectin reduced the peak serum levels (at 1 hr) of oral trimethoprim by 50 and 30% respectively, and the AUC's (areas under the curve) by 30 and 21%.[1] Whether this interaction affects the clinical effectiveness of trimethoprim in man has not been assessed, but the possibility should be borne in mind.

Reference

1 Babhair SA and Tariq M. Effect of magnesium trisilicate and kaolin-pectin on the bioavailability of trimethoprim. Res Comm Chem Pathol Pharmacol (1983) 40, 165–8.

Trimethoprim + Guar or Food

Abstract/Summary

Guar gum and food can reduce the absorption of trimethoprim from a suspension.

Clinical evidence, mechanism, importance and management

A study over a 24 h period in 12 normal subjects given a single 3 mg/kg oral dose of a trimethoprim suspension showed that mean peak serum levels were depressed 22% and 16% respectively by food and food with guar. Both reduced the AUC (area under the curve) by 22%.[1] The greatest individual reductions were 44% (peak serum levels) and 47% (AUC) with food, and 47% (peak serum levels) and 38% (AUC) with food+guar.[1] The reasons are not understood but it may be due to adsorption of the trimethoprim onto the food and guar.

The clinical importance of this interaction is still uncertain but since a marked reduction in absorption can occur in some individuals it would seem sensible to take trimethoprim suspension between meals. Whether the same interaction occurs with other trimethoprim formulations is not known.

Reference

1 Hoppu K, Tuomisto J, Koskimies O and Simell O. Food and guar decrease absorption of trimethoprim. Eur J Clin Pharmacol (1987) 32, 427–9.

Vidarabine + Allopurinol

Abstract/Summary

There is evidence that if allopurinol and vidarabine (adenine arabinoside) are used concurrently the toxicity of vidarabine may be increased.

Clinical evidence

Two patients with chronic lymphocytic leukaemia, treated with 300 mg allopurinol daily, developed severe neurotoxicity (coarse rhythmic tremors of the extremities and facial muscles, and impaired mentation) four days after starting to take vidarabine for the treatment of viral infections.[1] A computer search to find other patients who had had both drugs for four days revealed a total of 17 patients, five of whom had experienced adverse reactions including tremors, nausea, pain, itching and anaemia.[1]

Mechanism

Uncertain. One suggestion is that the allopurinol allows hypoxanthine arabinoside, the major metabolite of vidarabine, to accumulate. A study with rat liver cytosol showed that allopurinol increased the half-life of this metabolite from 40 min to 4 h.[2]

Importance and management

Information seems to be limited to this study so that the general clinical importance of this possible interaction is uncertain, but it would be prudent to exercise particular care if these drugs are used together. More study is needed.

References

1 Friedman HM and Grasela T. Adenine arabinoside and allopurinol—possible adverse drug interaction. N Engl J Med (1981) 304, 423.
2 Drach JC, Rentea RG and Cowen ME. The metabolic degradation of 9B-D-arabinofuranosyladenine (ara-A) in vitro. Fed Proc (1973) 32, 777.

Zidovudine (Azidothymidine) + Miscellaneous drugs

Abstract/Summary

Paracetamol increases the considerable haematological toxicity of zidovudine (azidothymidine) but acyclovir, aspirin, ketoconazole and co-trimoxazole appear not to do so. Overwhelming fatigue is reported in a patient given zidovudine and acyclovir. Probenecid possibly raises zidovudine serum levels.

Clinical evidence, mechanism, importance and management

A study of zidovudine for the treatment of AIDS in 282 patients showed that haematological abnormalities (anaemia, leukopenia, neutropenia) were very common indeed and 21% needed multiple red cell transfusions. Some of the patients also received acyclovir, aspirin, ketoconazole, co-trimoxazole and paracetamol (acetaminophen) but only the paracetamol increased the haematological toxicity (neutropenia) by an unstated amount. The reason for this increased toxicity is not known but it is suggested that paracetamol may compete with zidovudine for the liver enzymes concerned with metabolism (glucuronidation) of both drugs, resulting in a rise in zidovudine serum levels which increases its toxicity.[1] Probenecid also reduces the kidney tubular excretion of zidovudine and it is suggested that this may possibly have the same effect.[1,3] However successful concurrent use has been described.[4]

On theoretical grounds any drug causing bone marrow suppression might be additive with the effects of zidovudine. A report says that overwhelming fatigue occurred in a patient when given zidovudine and acyclovir on two occasions.[2] The concurrent use of any of these drugs should only be undertaken with great care. More study is needed.

References

1 Richman DD, Fischl MA, Grieco MH, Gottlieb MS, Volberding PA, Laskin OL, Leedom JM, Groopman JE, Mildvan D, Hirsch MS, Jackson GG, Durack DT, Nusinoff-Lehrman S and the AZT Collaborative Working Group. The toxicity of azidothymidine (AZT) in the treatment of patients with AIDS and AIDS-related complex. A double-blind, placebo-controlled trial. N Engl J Med (1987) 317, 192–7.
2 Bach MC. Possible drug interaction during therapy with azidothymidine and acyclovir for AIDS. N Engl J Med (1987) 316, 547.
3 de Miranda P, Good SS and Blum MR et al. The effect of probenecid on the pharmacokinetic disposition of azidothymidine (AZT) Presented at the International Conference on AIDS, Paris (1986). Quoted in reference 1.
4 Duckworth A, Duckworth G, Henderson G and Contreras G. Zidovudine with probenecid. Lancet (1990) 336, 441.

6

ANTICOAGULANT DRUG INTERACTIONS

The blood clotting process

When blood is shed or clotting is initiated in some other way, a highly complex cascade of biochemical reactions is set in motion which ends in the formation of a network or clot of insoluble protein threads enmeshing the blood cells. These threads are produced by the polymerization of the molecules of fibrinogen (a soluble protein present in the plasma) into threads of insoluble fibrin. The penultimate step in the chain of reactions requires the presence of an enzyme, thrombin, which is produced from its precursor prothrombin, already present in the plasma. Figure 6.1 is a highly simplified diagram to illustrate the final stages of this cascade of reactions.

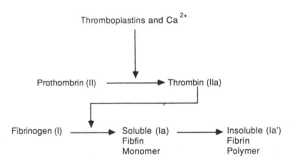

Fig 6.1 A highly simplified flow diagram of the final stages of the blood clotting process.

Mode of action of the anticoagulants

The oral anticoagulants extend the time taken for blood to clot and, it is believed, also inhibit the pathological formation of blood clots within blood vessels by reducing the concentrations within the plasma of a number of components necessary for the cascade to proceed, namely factors VII, IX, X

and II (prothrombin). The parts played by three of these four are not shown in the simplified diagram illustrated but they are essential for the production of the so-called 'thromboplastins'.

The synthesis of normal amounts of these four factors takes place within the liver with vitamin K as one of the essential ingredients, but, in the presence of an oral anticoagulant, the rate of synthesis of all four is retarded. One of the early theories to explain why this happens is based on the observed resemblance between the molecular shapes of vitamin K and the oral anticoagulants. It was suggested that the molecules were sufficiently similar for the anticoagulant actually to take part in the biochemical reactions by which all four are synthesized, but sufficiently dissimilar to prevent the completion of these reactions. The term 'competitive antagonist' is used to describe this situation because vitamin K and the oral anticoagulants compete with one another to take part in the reactions, their relative concentrations being among the factors which determine the 'winner'. This theory is now known to be too simple, but the basic principle of a concentration competition between the two types of molecules remains perfectly valid. A reduction in the concentrations and activity of all four factors is embraced by the portmanteau term 'hypoprothrombinaemia'.

The therapeutic use of the oral anticoagulants

During anticoagulant therapy it is usual to depress the levels of the prothrombin and factors VII, IX and X to those which are believed to give protection against intravascular clotting, without running the risk of excessive depression which leads to bleeding. To achieve this each patient is individually titrated with doses of anticoagulant until the desired response is attained, a procedure which normally takes several days because the oral anticoagulants do not act directly on the blood clotting factors already in circulation, but on the rate of synthesis of new factors by the liver. The 'end point' of the titration is determined by one of a number of different but closely related laboratory *in vitro* tests which measure the extension in the time taken for the blood to clot (e.g. the so-called 'one-stage prothrombin time') although the result of the test may be expressed, not in seconds, but as a ratio or a percentage of normal values.

The normal plasma clotting time, using the Quick one-stage prothrombin time test, is about 12 s, an extension to about 24–30 s or so is usually regarded as adequate in anticoagulant therapy. Other tests include the thrombotest and the prothrombin-proconvertin (P-P) test.

Anticoagulant interactions

Therapeutically desirable prothrombin levels can be upset by a number of factors including diet, disease and the use of other drugs. In the case of drugs, either the addition or the withdrawal may upset the balance in a patient already well stabilized on the anticoagulant. Some drugs increase the activity of the anticoagulants and can cause bleeding if the dosage of the anticoagulant is not reduced appropriately. Others reduce the activity and return the prothrombin time to normal. If one believes in the therapeutic value of the oral anticoagulants, both situations are serious and may be fatal, although excessive hypoprothrombinaemia manifests itself more obviously and immediately as bleeding and is usually regarded as the more serious.

Bleeding and its treatment

When prothrombin times become excessive, bleeding can occur. In order of decreasing frequency the bleeding shows itself as ecchymoses, blood in the urine, uterine bleeding, black faeces, bruising, nose-bleeding, haematoma, gum bleeding, coughing and vomiting blood.

If minor bleeding occurs, the anticoagulant should be stopped at once and 10–20 mg vitamin K1 (phytonadione) given orally. This should return the prothrombin time to normal within about 24 h and the bleeding should cease. If the bleeding is more severe, at least 50 mg vitamin K1 should be given intravenously. If bleeding is not reduced significantly within a few hours, more vitamin K1 should be given and transfusion with fresh whole blood, fresh frozen plasma or plasma concentrates of factors II, IX and V should be undertaken.

This chapter is concerned with those drugs which affect the activity of the anticoagulants. When the anticoagulant is the affecting agent the interaction is dealt with elsewhere in this book. The Index should be consulted.

Table 6.1 Anticoagulants. Not all the anticoagulants listed are in the text

Non-proprietary names	Proprietary names
Oral anticoagulants	
Coumarins	
Cumetharol	*Dicoumoxyl*
Cyclocoumarol	—
Dic(o)umarol (bis-hydroxycoumarin)	*Apekumarol, Baracoumin, Dicumol, Dufalone*
Ethylbiscoum-acetate	*Stabilene, Tromexan(e), Tromexano*
Ethylidene dicoumarin	*Pertromban*
Nicoumalone (acenocoumarol)	*Sint(h)rom(e)*
Phenprocoumon	*Liquamar, Marcoumar, Marcumar*
Tioclomarol	*Apegmone*
Warfarin potassium and sodium	*Aldocumar, Athrombin-K, Coumadan Sodico, Coumadin(e), Marevan, Panwarfin, Sofarin, Warfarin, Warfilone, Warnerin*
Indanediones	
Anisindione	*Miradon, Unidone*
Bromindione	*Fluidane*
Clorindione (chlorphen-indione)	*Indalitan*
Diphenadione	*Dipaxin*
Flurindione	*Previscan*
Phenindione	*Danilone, Dindevan, Emandione, Hedulin, Pindione, Trombantin*
Parenteral anticoagulants	
Heparin	

Anticoagulants + ACE inhibitors

Abstract/Summary

Ramipril appears not to interact with phenprocoumon nor benazepril with either warfarin or nicoumalone (acenocoumarol).

Clinical evidence, mechanism, importance and management

A study in eight normal subjects showed that the concurrent use of 5 mg ramipril daily for seven days had no effect on the pharmacokinetics or anticoagulant effects of phenprocoumon.[1] Another study found that 20 mg benazepril daily did not affect the serum levels of either warfarin or nicoumalone. The anticoagulant activity of nicoumalone was not altered, but the effects of warfarin were slightly reduced but not sufficiently to be clinically important.[2]

References

1 Verho M, Malerczyk V, Grotsch H and Zenbil I. Absence of interaction between ramipril, a new ACE-inhibitor, and phenprocoumon, an anticoagulant agent. Pharmacotherapeutica (1989) 5, 392–9.
2 Van Hecken A, De Lepeleire I, Verbesselt R, Arnout J, Angehrn J, Youngberg C and De Schepper PJ. Effect of benazepril, a converting enzyme inhibitor, on plasma levels and activity of acenocoumarol and warfarin. Int J Clin Pharm Res (1988) VIII, 315–19.

Anticoagulants + Acitretin

Abstract/Summary

Acitretin does not alter the anticoagulant effects of phenprocoumon.

Clinical evidence, mechanism, importance and management

A study in 10 normal subjects on phenprocoumon (1.5–3.0 mg daily) showed that when additionally given 50 mg acitretin daily over 10 days their prothrombin complex activity increased slightly from 22% to 24% (the corresponding INR's were 2.91 and 2.71). There were no important changes in Quick values. There would therefore seem to be no good reason for special precautions if acitretin is given to patients anticoagulated with phenprocoumon, nevertheless the outcome should be monitored. There seems to be no information about other anticoagulants.

Reference

1 Hartmann D, Mosberg H and Weber W. Lack of effect of acitretin on the hypoprothrombinemic action of phenprocoumon in healthy volunteers. Dermatologica (1989) 178, 33–6.

Anticoagulants + Alcohol

Abstract/Summary

The effects of the oral anticoagulants are unlikely to be affected in patients with normal liver function who drink small or moderate amounts of alcohol, but those who drink heavily or who have some liver disease may show considerable fluctuations in their prothrombin times.

Clinical evidence

(a) Patients and subjects free from liver disease

Twenty ounces (one pint or 56.4 g ethanol) of a Californian white table wine a day, given over a three-week period at mealtimes to eight normal subjects anticoagulated with warfarin, were found to have had no significant effects on either the serum warfarin levels or on the anticoagulant response.[8]

Other studies in both patients and normal subjects, anticoagulated with either warfarin or phenprocoumon, have very clearly confirmed the absence of an interaction with alcohol.[1,2,9,10] In one of the studies the subjects were given almost 600 ml of a table wine (12% alcohol) or 300 ml of a fortified wine (20% alcohol).[9,10]

(b) Chronic alcoholics or those with liver disease

In a study[3] in 15 alcoholics, administered a single dose of warfarin, who had been drinking heavily (250 g ethanol or more daily) for at least three months, the results of a previous investigation[4] were confirmed that the half-life of warfarin was reduced from 40.1 to 26.5 h, but, surprisingly, a comparison of their prothrombin times with those of normal subjects showed no differences.

Other reports[2,5] have shown that prothrombin times and warfarin levels of those with liver cirrhosis and other dysfunction can rise markedly after they have been on the binge, but restabilize soon afterwards when the drinking stops.

Mechanism

It seems probable that in man, as in rats,[6] continuous heavy drinking stimulates the hepatic enzymes concerned with the metabolism of warfarin, leading to its more rapid elimination.[3] As a result the half-life shortens. The fluctuations in prothrombin times in those with liver dysfunction[2,5] may possibly occur because sudden large amounts of alcohol exacerbate the general malfunction of the liver and this affects the way it metabolizes warfarin. It may also impair the ability of the liver to synthesize the blood clotting factors.

Importance and management

The absence of an interaction in those free from liver disease is well documented and well established. It appears that it is quite safe for patients on anticoagulants to drink small or moderate amounts of alcohol. Even much less conservative amounts (up to 8 oz/250 ml of spirits[1] or a pint of wine[8]) do not create problems with the anticoagulant control, so that there appears to be a good margin of safety even for the less than abstemious. Only warfarin and phenprocoumon have been investigated, but the other anticoagulants may be expected to behave similarly. Those who drink heavily may possibly need above-average doses of the anticoagulant, while those with liver damage who continue to drink may experience marked fluctuations in their prothrombin times. This typically occurs in alcoholics who go on the binge over the weekend. An attempt to limit their intake of alcohol is desirable from this as well as from other points of view.

References

1   Waris E. Effect of ethyl alcohol on some coagulation factors in man during anticoagulant therapy. Ann Med Exp Biol Fenn (1965) 115, 53.
2   Udall JA. Drug interference with warfarin therapy. Clin Med (1970) 77, 20.
3   Kater RMH, Roggin G, Tobon F, Zieve P and Iber FL. Increased rate of clearance of drugs from the circulation of alcoholics. Amer J Med Sci (1969) 258, 35.
4   Kater RM, Carruli N and Iber FL. Differences in the rate of ethanol metabolism in recently drinking alcoholic and non-alcoholic subjects. Amer J Clin Nutrition (1969) 14, 21.
5   Breckenridge A and Orme M. Clinical implications of enzyme induction. Ann NY Acad Sci (1971) 179, 421.
6   Rubin E, Hutterev F and Lieber CS. Ethanol increases hepatic smooth endoplasmic reticulum and drug metabolising enzymes. Science (1968) 159, 1469.
7   Riedler G. Einfluss des Alkohols auf die Antikoagulantien Therapie. Thromb Diath Haemorr (1966) 16, 613.
8   O'Reilly RA. Warfarin and wine. Clin Res (1978) 26, 145A.
9   O'Reilly RA. Lack of effect of mealtime wine on the hypoprothrombinaemia of oral anticoagulants. Amer J Med Sci (1979) 277, 189.
10 O'Reilly RA. Lack of effect of fortified wine ingested during fasting and anticoagulant therapy. Arch Int Med (1981) 141, 458.

Anticoagulants + Allopurinol

Abstract/Summary

Most patients on oral anticoagulants given allopurinol do not develop an adverse interaction, but since excessive hypoprothombinaemia and bleeding occurs quite unpredictably in a few individuals it is important to monitor the initial anticoagulant response in all patients.

Clinical evidence

In an extensive multi-hospital study of the adverse effects of allopurinol, three patients were observed who developed excessive anticoagulation while concurrently taking warfarin and allopurinol. One of them developed extensive intrapulmonary haemorrhage and had a prothrombin time of 71 s.[6]

A sharp increase in prothrombin times was seen in a very elderly woman on warfarin when given allopurinol,[3] and two patients on long-term treatment with phenprocoumon began to bleed when started on allopurinol.[5] 2.5 mg/kg allopurinol twice daily for 14 days increased the mean half-life of a single dose of dicoumarol in six normal subjects from 51 to 152 h,[1] whereas three other subjects showed an increase from only 13 to 17 h.[4] The disposition of warfarin remained unaltered.[4] No change was seen in the prothrombin ratios of two patients on warfarin who took allopurinol for three weeks,[2] whereas one out of six subjects taking allopurinol for a month demonstrated a 30% reduction in the elimination of warfarin.[2]

Mechanism

It has been suggested that, as in rats, allopurinol inhibits the metabolism of the anticoagulants by the liver, thereby prolonging their effects and half-lives.[1,4] There is a wide individual variability in the effects of allopurinol on drug metabolism in man,[2] so that only a few individuals are affected.

Importance and management

This interaction is established and important. Its incidence is unknown, but it is probably small. It is impossible to predict who is likely to be affected so that prothrombin times should be monitored if allopurinol is added to established anticoagulant treatment. So far the interaction has only been reported with warfarin, phenprocoumon and dicoumarol, but it would be prudent to assume that is it possible with any anticoagulant.

References

1   Vesell ES, Passananti GT and Greene FF. Impairment of drug metabolism in man by allopurinol and nortriptyline. N Eng J Med (1970) 283, 1484.
2   Rawlins MD and Smith SE. Influence of allopurinol on drug metabolism in man. Br J Pharmac (1973) 48, 693.
3   Self TH, Evans WE and Ferguson T. Drug enhancement of warfarin activity. Lancet (1975) ii, 557.
4   Pond SM, Graham GG, Wade DN and Sudlow G. The effect of allopurinol and clofibrate on the elimination of coumarin anticoagulants in man. Aust NZ J Med (1975) 5, 324.
5   Jahnchen E, Meinertz T and Gilfrich MJ. Interaction of allopurinol in man. Klin Wsch (1977) 55, 759.
6   McInnnes GT, Lawson DH and Jick H. Acute adverse reactions attributed to allopurinol in hospitalized patients. Ann Rheum Dis (1981) 40, 245–9.

Anticoagulants + Aminoglutethimide

Abstract/Summary

The anticoagulant effects of warfarin and nicoumalone (acenocoumarol) can be markedly reduced by the concurrent use of aminoglutethimide.

Clinical evidence

Three patients on nicoumalone needed a doubling of their dosage to maintain adequate anticoagulation while taking 250 mg aminoglutethimide four times daily for 3–4 weeks.[1]

Another report describes two patients who needed a 3–4 fold increase in warfarin dosage while taking 250 mg aminoglutethimide four times a day.[2] The increased requirement persisted for two weeks after the aminoglutethimide was stopped, and then declined. Brief mention of the need to take 'much larger doses' of warfarin while on aminoglutethimide is reported elsewhere.[3]

Mechanism

The most probable explanation is that aminoglutethimide, like glutethimide, stimulates the activity of the liver enzymes concerned with the metabolism of the anticoagulants, thereby increasing their loss from the body. This needs confirmation. Some effect on blood steroid levels which might affect coagulation has also been suggested.[2]

Importance and management

Information appears to be limited to the reports cited but the interaction would seem to be established. Monitor the effects if aminoglutethimide is given to patients already taking either warfarin or nicoumalone and increase the anticoagulant dosage as necessary. Reduce the dosage if the aminoglutethimide is withdrawn. Information about other anticoagulants is lacking but it would be prudent to apply the same precautions.

References

1 Bruning PF and Bonfrer JG M. Aminoglutethimide and oral anticoagulant therapy. Lancet (1983) ii, 582.
2 Lonnong PE, Kvinnsland S and Jahren G. Aminoglutethimide and warfarin. A new important drug interaction. Cancer Chemother Pharmacol(1984) 12, 10–12.
3 Murray RML, Pitt P and Jerums G. Medical adrenalectomy with aminoglutethimide in the management of advanced breast cancer. Med J Aust (1981) 1, 179–81.

Anticoagulants + Aminoglycoside antibiotics

Abstract/Summary

If the intake of vitamin K is normal, either no interaction occurs or only a small and clinically unimportant increase in the effects of the oral anticoagulants takes place during concurrent treatment with neomycin, kanamycin or paromomycin. No interaction of any importance is likely with other aminoglycoside antibiotics administered parenterally.

Clinical evidence

Six out of 10 patients on warfarin who were given 2 g neomycin daily over a three-week period showed a gradual increase in their prothrombin times averaging 5.6 seconds.[1] The author of this report also describes another study on 10 patients taking warfarin given 4 g neomycin daily which produced essentially similar results.[2]

A small increase in the effects of an un-named anticoagulant was seen in a study on five patients taking neomycin with bacitracin, three patients on 1 g streptomycin daily, and two patients on 1 g streptomycin with 1 Mu of penicillin daily.[3] No interaction was found in other long-term studies of warfarin with neomycin,[4,5] or dicoumarol with paromomycin.[5]

Mechanism

Not understood. One idea is that these antibiotics increase the anticoagulant effects by decimating the bacterial population in the gut, thereby reducing their production of vitamin K. However this incorrectly supposes that the gut bacteria are normally a necessary and important source of the vitamin.[5] Another suggestion is that these antibiotics decrease the vitamin K absorption as part of a general antibiotic-induced malabsorption syndrome.[6]

Importance and management

A sparsely documented interaction, but common experience seems to confirm that normally no interaction of any significance occurs. Concurrent use need not be avoided. Occasionally vitamin K deficiency and/or spontaneous bleeding[7,8] is seen after the prolonged use of gut-sterilizing antibiotics, a totally inadequate diet, starvation or some other condition in which the intake of vitamin K is very limited. The effects of the oral anticoagulants would be expected to be significantly increased in these circumstances, and appropriate precautions should be taken. Only warfarin and dicoumarol feature in the reports cited, but it seems probable that the other anticoagulants will behave similarly. There is nothing to suggest that an adverse interaction occurs between the oral anticoagulants and aminoglycosides administered parenterally.

References

1 Udall JA. Drug interference with warfarin therapy. Clin Med (1970) 77, 20
2 Udall JA. Human sources and absorption of vitamin K in relation to anticoagulation stability. J Amer Med Ass (1965) 194, 107.
3 Magid E. Tolerance to anticoagulants during antibiotic therapy. Scand J Lab Invest (1962) 14, 565.
4 Schade RWB. A comparative study of the effects of cholestyramine and neomycin in the treatment of type II hyperlipoprotinaemia. Acta Med Scand (1976) 199, 175.
5 Messinger WJ and Samet CM. The effect of bowel sterilizing antibiotic on blood coagulation mechanisms. The anticholesterol effect of paromomycin. Angiology (1965) 16, 29.
6 Faloon WW, Paes IC, Woolfolk D, Nankin H, Wallace K and Haro EN. Effect of neomycin and kanamycin upon intestinal absorption. Ann NY Acad Sci (1966) 132, 879.
7 Haden HT. Vitamin K deficiency associated with prolonged antibiotic administration. Arch Int Med (1957) 100, 986.
8 Frick PG, Riedler G and Brogli H. Dose response and minimal daily requirements for vitamin K in man. J Appl Physiol (1967) 23, 387.

Anticoagulants + Aminosalicylic acid (PAS) and/or Isoniazid

Abstract/Summary

A report attributes a bleeding episode in a patient on warfarin to the concurrent use of isoniazid. Another single report describes a markedly increased anticoagulant response in a patient when given aminosalicylic acid and isoniazid.

Clinical evidence

A man on warfarin and taking 300 mg isoniazid daily began to bleed (haematuria, bleeding gums, etc.) within 10 days of accidentally doubling his dosage of isoniazid. His prothrombin time had increased from 26.3 s to 53.3 s.[1]

Another patient taking digoxin, potassium chloride, dioctyl calcium sulfosuccinate, diazepam and warfarin, was additionally given 12 g aminosalicylic acid, 300 mg isoniazid and 100 mg pyridoxine daily. His prothrombin time increased from 18 to 130 s over 20 days but no signs of haemorrhage were seen.[2] Two patients on isoniazid, aminosalicylic acid and streptomycin (but not taking anticoagulants) developed haemorrhage attributed to the anticoagulant effects of isoniazid.[3]

Mechanism

Not understood. The small depressant effect which aminosalicylic acid has on prothrombin formation in man is unlikely to have been responsible. Isoniazid can increase the anticoagulant effects of dicoumarol in dogs[4] but not of warfarin in rabbits.[5] In dogs the effect is thought to be due to inhibition by the isoniazid of the liver enzymes concerned with the metabolism of the anticoagulant, resulting in a slower clearance from the body.[4]

Importance and management

The interactions of warfarin with isoniazid and aminosalicylic acid are not established. Concurrent use need not be avoided, but prescribers should be aware of these cases and monitor the effects.

References

1 Rosenthal AR, Self TH, Baker ED and Londen RA. Interaction of isoniazid and warfarin. J Amer Med Ass (1977) 238, 2177.
2 Self TH. Interaction of warfarin and aminosalicylic acid. J Amer Med Ass (1973) 223, 1285.
3 Castell FA. Accion anticoagulante de la isoniazide. Enfermedaders de Torax (1969) 69, 153.
4 Eade NR, McLeod PJ and MacLeod SM. Potentiation of bishydroxy-coumarin in dogs by isoniazid and p-aminosalicylic acid. Amer Rev Resp Dis (1971) 103, 792.
5 Kiblawi SS. Influence of isoniazid on the anticoagulant effect of warfarin Clin Ther (1979) 2, 235.

Anticoagulants + Amiodarone

Abstract/Summary

The anticoagulant effects of warfarin, phenprocoumon and nicoumalone (acenocoumarol) are increased by amiodarone and bleeding may occur if the dosage of the anticoagulant is not reduced. A reduction of a third to two-thirds will accommodate this interaction with warfarin and phenprocoumon, a reduction of a third to a quarter with nicoumalone. The onset of this interaction may be slow, but it may also persist long after the amiodarone has been withdrawn.

Clinical evidence

Five out of nine patients well stabilized on warfarin showed signs of bleeding (four had microscopic haematuria and one had diffuse ecchymoses) within 3–4 weeks of starting to take amiodarone (dosage not stated). All nine showed increases in their prothrombin times averaging 21 s. It was necessary to decrease the warfarin dosage by an average of a third (range 16–45%) to return their prothrombin times to the therapeutic range. The effects of amiodarone persisted for 6 to 16 weeks in four of the patients from whom it was withdrawn.[1]

A prolongation in prothrombin times and/or bleeding has been described in other patients on warfarin given 600–800 mg amiodarone daily.[2–4,6,8,10,13,18,20] Amiodarone similarly interacts with phenprocoumon[5] and nicoumalone.[9,11,14–16,21]

Mechanism

Not established. One idea is that the amiodarone inhibits the metabolism of the anticoagulants by the liver, thereby increasing its effects.[3,12,19] Another suggestion is that it may be a result of changes in thyroid function brought about by the amiodarone.

Importance and management

A well documented, established and clinically important interaction. It appears to occur in all patients.[1,6,17,20] The dosage of either warfarin or phenprocoumon should be reduced by a third to two thirds[1,5,12,13,20] to avoid bleeding. One report[13] suggests an average 35% reduction with warfarin in a 70 kg patient on 200 mg amiodarone daily, 50% on 400 mg and 65% on 600 mg and above. The dosage of nicoumalone should be reduced by a quarter to a third.[9,21] These suggested reductions are very broad generalizations and individual patients may need more or less. The interaction develops within two weeks and may persist for weeks after the withdrawal of the amiodarone because up to a third may still be present a month after treatment has ceased.[7] Prothrombin times should be very closely monitored both during and after treatment. One study advises weekly monitoring for the first four weeks.[20] It would seem prudent to assume that other anticoagulants interact similarly, but so far there is no direct evidence that they do so.

References

1 Martinowitz U, Rabinovici J, Goldfarb D, Many A and Bank H. Interaction between warfarin sodium and amiodarone. N Eng J Med (1981) 304, 671.
2 Rees A, Dalal JJ, Reid PG, Henderson AH and Lewis MJ. Dangers of amiodarone and anticoagulant treatment. Br Med J (1981) 282, 1756.
3 Serlin MJ, Sibeon RG and Green GJ. Dangers of amiodarone and anticoagulant treatment. Br Med J (1981) 283, 58.
4 Simpson WT. In 'Amiodarone in Cardiac Arrhythmias'. Simpson WT and Caldwell ADS (eds). Roy Soc Med Int Congr Ser 16. Royal Society of Medicine/Academic Press/Grune and Stratton, London (1979) p 50–2.
5 Broekmans AW and Meyboom RHB. Bijwerkingen van geneesmiddelen. Potentiering van het cumarine-effekt door amiodaron (Cordarone). Ned Tijd Geneesk (1982) 126, 1415.
6 Hamer A, Peter T, Mandel WJ, Scheinman MM and Weiss D. The

potentiation of warfarin anticoagulation by amiodarone. Circulation (1982) 65, 1025–29.

7 Broekhuysen J, Laruel R and Slon R. Recherches dan la serie des benzofuranes. XXXVIII. Etude comparee du transit et du metabolisme de l'amiodarone chez diverses especes d'animales et chez l'homme. Arch Int Pharmacodyn Ther (1969) 177, 340.

8 Ugovern B, Garan H, Kelly E and Ruskin JN. Adverse reactions during treatment with amiodarone. Br Med J (1983) 287. 175–80.

9 Arboix M, Frati ME and Laporte J-R. The potentiation of acenocoumarol anticoagulant effects by amiodarone. Br J clin Pharmac (1984) 18, 355–60.

10 Raeder EA, Podrid PJ and Lown B. Side effects and complications of amiodarone therapy. Am Heart J (1985) 109, 975–83.

11 El Allaf D, Sprynger M and Carlier J. Potentiation of the action of oral anticoagulants by amiodarone. Acta Clin Belg (1984) 39, 306–8.

12 Watt AH, Buss DC, Stephens MR and Routledge PA. Amiodarone reduced plasma warfarin clearance in man. Br J clin Pharmac (1985) 19, 591P.

13 Almog S, Shafran N, Halkin H, Weiss P, Farfel Z, Martinowitz U and Bank H. Mechanism of warfarin potentiation by amiodarone: dose- and concentration-dependent inhibition of warfarin elimination. Eur J Clin Pharmacol(1985) 28, 257–261.

14 Richard C, Riou B, Fournier C, Rimailho A and Auzepy P. Depression of vitamin K-dependent coagulation by amiodarone. Circulation (1983) 68, Suppl III, 278.

15 Richard C, Riou B, Berdeaux A, Forunier C, Khayat D, Rimailho A, Giudicelli JF and Auzepy P. Prospective study of the potentiation of acenocoumarol by amiodarone. Eur J Clin Pharmacol(1985) 28, 625–9.

16 Pini M, Manotti C and Quintavalla R. Interaction between amiodarone and acenocoumarin. Thromb Haem (1985) 54, 549.

17 Kerin N, Blevins R, Goldman L, Faitel K, and Rubenfire M. The amiodarone-warfarin interaction: incidence, time course and clinical significance. JACC (1986) 7, 91A.

18 Watt AH, Stephens MR, Buss DC and Routledge PA. Amiodarone reduces plasma warfarin clearance in man. Br J clin Pharmac (1985) 20, 707–9.

19 O'Reilly RA, Trager WF, Kettie AE and Goulart DA. Interaction of amiodarone with racemic warfarin and its separate enantiomorphs in humans. Clin PharmacolTher (1987) 42, 290–4.

20 Zerin NZ, Blevins RD, Goldman L, Faitel K and Rubenfire M. The incidence, magnitude and time course of the amiodarone-warfarin interaction. Arch InternMed (1988) 148, 1779–81.

21 Fondevila C, Meschengieser S, Lazzari MA. Amiodarone potentiates acenocoumarin. Thromb Res (1988) 52, 203–8.

Anticoagulants + Anabolic steroids and Related sex hormones

Abstract/Summary

The anticoagulant effects of bromindione, dicoumarol, nicoumalone, phenindione, phenprocoumon and warfarin are markedly increased by the concurrent use of danazol, ethyloestrenol, oxymetholone, methandienone (methandrostenolone), methyltestosterone and stanozolol. Bleeding may occur if the anticoagulant dosage is not reduced appropriately.

Clinical evidence

Six patients stabilized on warfarin or phenindione were started on 15 mg oxymetholone daily. One patient developed extensive subcutaneous bleeding and another had haematuria. After 30 days on oxymetholone all six patients had thrombotests of less than 5% which returned to the therapeutic range within a few days of stopping the oxymetholone.[1]

Similarly increased anticoagulant effects and bleeding have been described in studies and case reports of interactions in man taking warfarin with danazol,[13,14] oxymetholone,[4–6] methandienone[2,4,7,8] or stanozolol;[15,17,18] dicoumarol with norethandrolone[2,4] or stanozolol;[12] bromindione with methandienone;[2,4] phenindione with ethyloestrenol;[9] phenprocoumon with methyltestosterone;[10] and nicoumalone with oxymetholone.[11]

One report[6] says that three patients on warfarin given *Sustanon* (containing four combined esters of testosterone) developed no changes in their anticoagulant requirements, whereas another report[16] describes a woman who showed a 78% and a 65% increase in prothrombin times on each of two occasions when using a 2% testosterone propionate vaginal ointment twice daily. A 25% reduction in warfarin dosage was needed.

Mechanism

Not understood. Various theories have been put forward including increased metabolic destruction of the blood clotting factors, or decreased synthesis;[2,3] reduced levels of plasma triglycerides which might reduce vitamin-K availability (though this is disputed);[4,7] and increased concentrations of the anticoagulant at the receptor site or increased receptor affinity.

Importance and management

A well-documented, well-established and clinically important interaction which develops rapidly, possibly within 2–3 days. Most, if not all, patients are affected.[1,3] If concurrent use cannot be avoided, the dosage of the anticoagulant should be appropriately reduced. One recommendation is that the initial dosage should be halved.[14] After withdrawal of the steroid the anticoagulant dosage will need to be increased. It seems probable that all the anticoagulants will interact with any 17-alkyl substituted steroid such as fluoxymesterone and oxandrolone, but as yet there is no direct evidence that they do so. The situation with testosterone and other non 17-alkylated steroids is not clear (see cases cited above).[6,16]

References

1 Longridge RGM, Gilliam PMS and Barton GMG. Decreased anticoagulant tolerance with oxymetholone. Lancet (1971) ii, 90.

2 Pyorala K and Kekki M. Decreased anticoagulant tolerance during methandrostenolone therapy. Scand J Clin Lab Invest (1963) 15, 367.

3 Schrogie JJ and Solomon HM. The anticoagulant response to bishydroxycoumarin. II. The effect of D-thyroxine, clofibrate and norethandrolone. Clin PharmacolTher (1967) 8, 70.

4 Murakami M, Odake K, Matsuda T, Onchi K, Umeda T and Nishuro T. Effects of anabolic steroids on anticoagulant requirements. Jap Circ J (1965) 29, 243.

5 Robinson BHB, Hawkins JB, Ellis JE and Moore-Robinson M. Decreased anticoagulant tolerance with oxymetholone. Lancet (1971) i, 1356.

6 Edwards MS and Curtis JR. Decreased anticoagulant tolerance with oxymetholone. Lancet (1971) ii, 221.

7 Dresdale FC and Hayes JC. Potential dangers in the combined use of methandrostenolone and sodium warfarin. J Med Soc New Jersey (1967) 64, 609.

8 McLaughlin GE, McCarty DJ and Segal BL. Hemarthrosis complicating anticoagulant therapy. A report of three cases. J Amer Med Ass (1966) 196, 1020.

9 Vere DW and Fearnley GR. Suspected interaction between phenindione and ethyloestrenol. Lancet (1968) ii, 281.

10 Husted S, Andreasen F and Foged L. Increased sensitivity to phenprocoumon during methyltestosterone therapy. Europ J clin Pharmacol (1976) 10, 209.

11 De Oyda JC, del Rio A, Noya M and Villeneuva A. Decreased anticoagulant tolerance with oxymetholone in paroxysmal noctural haemoglobinuria. Lancet (1971) ii, 259.

12 Howards CW, Hanson SG and Wahed MA. Anabolic steroids and anticoagulants. Brit Med J (1977) i, 1659.

13 Goulbourne IA and MacLeod DAD. An interaction between danazol and warfarin. Brit J Obst Gyn (1981) 88, 950–1.

14 Small M, Peterkin M, Lowe GDO, McCune G and Thomson JA. Danazol and oral anticoagulants. Scott Med J (1982) 27, 331–2.

15 Acomb C and Shaw PW. A significant interaction between warfarin and stanozolol. Pharm J (1985) 234, 73–4.

16 Lorentz S Mc and Weibert RT. Potentiation of warfarin anticoagulation by topical testosterone ointment. Clin Pharm (1985) 4, 332–4.

17 Cleverly CR. Personal communication (1987).

18 Shaw PW and Smith AM. Possible interaction of warfarin and stanozolol. Clin Pharm (1987) 6, 500–2.

Anticoagulants + Antacids

Abstract/Summary

Aluminium hydroxide does not interact with either warfarin or dicoumarol, and magnesium hydroxide does interact with warfarin. There is some evidence that the absorption of dicoumarol may be increased by magnesium hydroxide and warfarin by magnesium trisilicate, but there is no direct evidence that this is clinically important.

Clinical evidence

(a) Dicoumarol + aluminium or magnesium hydroxide

15 ml of magnesium hydroxide (*Milk of Magnesia*) taken with dicoumarol, and a further dose 3 h later, was found to raise serum dicoumarol levels of six subjects by 75% and the area under the curve by 50%. No interaction occurred with aluminium hydroxide.[2]

(b) Warfarin + aluminium or magnesium hydroxide, or magnesium trisilicate.

30 ml aluminium/magnesium hydroxide (*Maalox*) given with warfarin, and four subsequent doses at 2 h intervals, had no effect on the plasma warfarin levels or on the anticoagulant response of six subjects.[1]

No interaction occurs with warfarin and aluminium hydroxide (*Amphogel*),[2] but an *in vitro* study suggests that the absorption of warfarin may be increased by magnesium trisilicate.[4]

Mechanism

It is suggested that dicoumarol forms a more readily absorbed chelate with magnesium so that its effects are increased.[1,3]

Importance and management

No special precautions need be taken if aluminium or magnesium hydroxide antacids are given to patients on warfarin, or if aluminium hydroxide is given to those on dicoumarol. Choosing these antacids avoids the possibility of an adverse interaction. Despite the evidence from the studies cited, there seems to be no direct clinical evidence of an adverse interaction between any anticoagulant and an antacid.

References

1 Robinson DS, Benjamin DM and McCormack JJ. Interaction of warfarin and nonsystemic gastrointestinal drugs. Clin PharmacolTher (1971) 12, 491.

2 Ambre JJ and Fischer LJ. Effect of coadministration of aluminium and magnesium hydroxides on absorption of anticoagulants in man. Clin PharmacolTher (1973) 12, 231.

3 Akers MA, Lach JL and Fischer LJ. Alterations in the absorption of bishydroxycoumarin by various excipient materials. J Pharm Sci (1973) 62, 391.

4 McElnay JC, Harron DWG, D'Arcy PF and Collier PS. Interaction of warfarin with antacid constituents. Br Med J (1978) 2, 1166.

Anticoagulants + Ascorbic acid (Vitamin C)

Abstract/Summary

Four controlled studies with large numbers of patients failed to demonstrate any interaction, although two isolated cases have been reported in which the effects of warfarin were reduced by ascorbic acid.

Clinical evidence

The prothrombin time of a woman, stabilized on 7.5 mg warfarin daily, who began to take regular amounts of ascorbic acid (dose not stated), fell steadily from 23 s to 19, 17 and then 14 s with no response to an increase in the dosage of warfarin to 10, 15 and finally 20 mg daily. The prothrombin time returned to 28 s within two days of stopping the ascorbic acid.[1]

A woman who had been taking 16 g ascorbic acid daily proved to be unusually resistant to the actions of warfarin and required 25 mg daily before a significant increase in prothrombin times was achieved.[2]

In contrast, no changes in the effects of warfarin were seen in five patients given 1 g ascorbic acid daily for a fortnight,[3] 84 patients given an unstated amount for 10 weeks,[4] 11 patients given up to 4 g daily for two weeks,[10] or 19 patients given up to 5–10 g daily for one or two weeks.[5] In this last study a mean fall of 17.5% in total plasma warfarin concentrations was seen.

Mechanism

Not understood. Some animal studies have demonstrated this interaction[6,7] and others have not,[8,9] but none of them has provided any definite clues about why it ever occurs, and then only rarely. One suggestion is that high doses of ascorbic acid can cause diarrhoea which might prevent adequate absorption of the anticoagulant.

Importance and management

Well-controlled clinical studies in large numbers of patients on warfarin have failed to confirm this interaction, even using very large doses (up to 10 g daily) of ascorbic acid. There is no good reason for avoiding the concurrent use. Information about other anticoagulants is lacking, but it seems likely that they will behave similarly. Check on any patient particularly resistant to the warfarin to confirm that ascorbic acid is not being taken.

References

1 Rosenthal G. Interaction of ascorbic acid and warfarin. J Amer Med Ass (1971) 215, 1671.
2 Smith EC, Skalski RJ, Johnson GC and Rossi GV. Interaction of ascorbic acid with warfarin. J Amer Med Ass (1972) 221, 1166.
3 Hume R, Johnstone JMS and Weyers E. Interaction of ascorbic acid and warfarin. J Amer Med Ass (1972) 219, 1479.
4 Dedichen J. Effect of ascorbic acid given to patients on chronic anti-coagulant therapy. Boll Soc Ital Cardiol (1973) 18, 690.
5 Feetam CL, Leach RH and Meynell MJ. Lack of clinical important interaction between warfarin and ascorbic acid. Toxicol Appl Pharmacol(1975) 31, 544.
6 Sigell LT and Flessa HC. Drug interactions with anticoagulants. J Amer Med Ass (1970) 214, 2035.
7 Sullivan WR, Gangstad EO and Link KP. Studies on the haemorrhagic sweet clover disease. J Biol Chem (1943) 151, 477.
8 Weintraub M and Griner PF. Warfarin and ascorbic acid: lack of evidence for a drug interaction. Toxicol Appl Pharmacol(1974) 28, 53.
9 Deckert FW. Ascorbic acid and warfarin. J Amer Med Ass (1973) 223, 440.
10 Blakely JA. Interaction of warfarin and ascorbic acid. 1st Florence Cnf on Haemostasis and Thrombosis (1977) May. Abstracts p 99.

Anticoagulants + Aspirin and other Salicylates

Abstract/Summary

Aspirin in doses of only 500 mg daily increases the likelihood of bleeding 3–5 times in those taking anticoagulants. Aspirin damages the stomach wall, prolongs bleeding times and in 2–4 g daily doses can increase prothrombin times, but there seems to be no reason for avoiding low-dose aspirin (75 mg daily). Increased warfarin effects have been seen with methyl-salicylate ointment.

Clinical evidence

A study in 534 patients with artificial heart valves showed that three times as many bled (requiring blood transfusion or hospitalization) among those on 500 mg aspirin daily (14%) as among those on warfarin alone (5%).[1] Bleeding was mainly gastrointestinal or cerebral. All of those with intra-cerebral bleeding died.

This finding confirms two other studies[2,3] on a total of 270 patients in whom bleeding was found to be about five times more common in anticoagulated patients taking aspirin (0.5–1.0 g daily) than among those taking only the anticoagulant. Other studies in patients taking dicoumarol, nicoumalone or warfarin found that while also taking 2–4 g aspirin daily the anticoagulant effects were increased and the anticoagulant dosage could be reduced about 30%.[4,5] However another investigator using 3 g aspirin daily failed to find any effect on prothrombin times.[10] Low-dose aspirin (75 mg daily) doubles the normal blood loss from the gastric mucosa but it still remains very small (compared with the 14-fold increase with 2.4 g daily) and warfarin does not increase it.[11] A single case report describes bruising and markedly increased warfarin effects in a woman within two weeks of starting to use methylsalicylate ointment.[12]

Mechanism

Aspirin has a direct irritant effect on the stomach lining and can cause gastrointestinal bleeding. It also decreases platelet aggregation and prolongs bleeding times, all of which would seem to account for the bleeding described.[1–3] In addition, larger doses of aspirin alone are known to have a direct hypoprothrombinaemic effect, like the anticoagulants, which is reversible by vitamin K.[6–9]

Importance and management

The anticoagulant-aspirin interaction is well-documented and clinically important. Patients should avoid aspirin in normal analgesic and anti-inflammatory doses while taking any anticoagulant, although it would appear that only dicoumarol, acenocoumarol and warfarin have been investigated. Low-dose aspirin (75 mg daily) appears not to matter. Warn patients on anticoagulants that many proprietary over-the-counter analgesic and antipyretic preparations contain substantial amounts of aspirin. Paracetamol (acetaminophen) is a safer analgesic substitute. Some of the other salicylates are less irritant and have a smaller effect on platelet function than aspirin so that, on theoretical grounds, the avoidance of concurrent use may be less important. However remember that topical methylsalicylate may cause problems.

References

1 Chesebro JH, Fuster V, Elveback LR, Ugoon DC, Pluth JR, Puga FJ, Wallace RB, Danielson GK, Orszulak TA, Piehler JM and Schaff HV. Trial of combined warfarin plus dipyridamole or aspirin therapy in prosthetic heart valve replacement: danger of aspirin compared with dipyridamole. Amer J Cardiol (1983) 51, 1537–41.
2 Altman R, Boullon F, Rouvier J, Rada R, de la Fuente L and Favaloro R. Aspirin and prophylaxis of thrombo-embolic complications in patients with substitute heart valves. J Thoracic Cardiovasc Surg (1976) 72, 127–9.
3 Dale J, Myhre E, Storstein O, Stormorken H and Efkind L. Prevention of arterial thromboembolism with acetylsalicylic acid: a controlled clinical study in patients with aortic ball valves. Am Heart J (1977) 94, 101–111.
4 Watson RM and Pierson NJ. Effect of anticoagulant therapy upon aspirin-induced gastrointestinal bleeding. Circulation (1961) 24, 613.
5 O'Reilly RA, Sahud MA and Aggeler PM. Impact of aspirin and chlor-

thalidone on the pharmacodynamics of oral anticoagulants drugs in man. Ann NY Acad Sci (1971) 179, 173.

6 Shapiro S. Studies on prothrombin. VI. The effect of synthetic vitamin K on the prothrombinopenia induced by salicylate in man. J Amer Med Ass (1944) 125, 546.

7 Quick AJ and Clesceri L. Influence of acetylsalicylic acid and salicylamide on the coagulation of the blood. J Pharmac Exp Ther (1960) 128, 95.

8 Meyer OO and Howard B. Production of hypoprothrombinaemia and hypocoagulability of the blood with salicylates. J Pharmac Exp Ther (1943) 53, 251.

9 Park BK and Leck JB. On the mechanisms of salicylate-induced hypoprothrombinaemia. J Pharm Pharmacol(1981) 33, 25.

10 Udall JA. Drug interference with warfarin therapy. Amer J Cardiol (1969) 23, 143.

11 Pritchard PJ, Kitchingham GK, Walt RP, Daneshmend TK and Hawkey CJ. Human gastric mucosal bleeding induced by low dose aspirin but not warfarin. Br Med J (1989) 298, 493–6.

12 Chow WH, Cheung KL, Ling HM and See T. Potentiation of warfarin anticoagulation by topical methylsalicylate ointment. J Roy Soc Med (1989) 82, 501–2.

Anticoagulants + Azapropazone

Abstract/Summary

The anticoagulant effects of warfarin are increased by azapropazone and bleeding will occur if the dosage of warfarin is not markedly reduced.

Clinical evidence

A woman taking digoxin, frusemide, spironolactone, allopurinol, and stabilized on warfarin (prothrombin ratio 2.8) developed haematemesis within four days of starting to take 300 mg azapropazone four times a day. On admission to hospital her prothrombin ratio was found to have risen to 15.7 (prothrombin time of 220 s). Subsequent gastroscopic examination revealed a benign ulcer, the presumed site of the bleeding.[1]

Six other patients are reported to have developed this interaction. Three developed bruising within a few days of starting azapropazone,[2] and one had a prothrombin ratio of 10 and developed haematuria.[6] One died.[7] Another patient on warfarin and azapropazone and also taking diclofenac and co-proxamol showed an increase in prothrombin times.[8] The interaction has also been experimentally confirmed in two normal subjects.[3]

Mechanism

Not understood. Azapropazone displaces warfarin from its plasma protein binding sites[3–5] thereby increasing the amount of free and pharmacologically active molecules, but it is almost certain that this on its own does not fully account for the clinical effects reported.

Importance and management

An established interaction of clinical importance, although the documentation is limited. The incidence is uncertain. Concurrent use should be avoided. If it is essential to give azapropazone, the manufacturers recommend that it should only be given to patients if the anticoagulant dosage has been reduced to a very low level, after which daily prothrombin determinations and dosage adjustments should be carried out.

References

1 Powell-Jackson PR. Interaction betwen azapropazone and warfarin. Br Med J (1977) 1, 1193.

2 Green AE, Hort JF, Korn HET and Leach H. Potentiation of warfarin by azapropazone. Br Med J (1977) 1, 1532.

3 McElnay JC and D'Arcy PF. Interaction between azapropazone and warfarin. Br Med J (1977) 2, 773.

4 McElnay JC and D'Arcy PF. The effect of azapropazone on the binding of warfarin to human serum proteins. J Pharm Pharmac (1978) 30 (Suppl) 73P.

5 McElnay JC and D'Arcy PF. Interaction between azapropazone and warfarin. Experientia (1978) 34, 1320.

6 Beeley L. Bulletin of the West Midlands Adverse Drug Reaction Study Group. University of Birmingham, England. January 1980, no 10.

7 Anon. Interactions. Doctors warned on warfarin dangers. Pharm J (1983) 230, 676.

8 Beeley L, Stewart P and Hickey FL. Bull W Midland Centre for Adverse Drug Reaction Reporting (1988) 27, 27.

Anticoagulants + Barbiturates

Abstract/Summary

The effects of the anticoagulants are reduced by the concurrent use of barbiturates and full therapeutic anticoagulation may only be achieved by raising the anticoagulant dosage about 30–60%. If the barbiturate is later withdrawn, the anticoagulant dosage should be reduced to avoid the risk of bleeding.

Clinical evidence

Two examples from many:

A study on 16 patients on long-term warfarin treatment showed that when they were also given 2 g/kg phenobarbitone(-al), their average daily warfarin requirements rose over a four-week period by 25% (from 5.7 to 7.1 mg daily).[1]

An investigation on 12 patients taking either warfarin or phenprocoumon demonstrated that when concurrently given secbutobarbitone sodium (butabarbital), 60 mg daily for the first week and 120 mg daily for the next two weeks, their anticoagulant requirements rose by 35–60%, reaching a maximum after 4–5 weeks.[2]

This interaction has been described in man between warfarin and amylobarbitone(-al),[3,4,23] butobarbitone(-al),[5] heptabarbitone(-al),[6,7] phenobarbitone(-al),[8–12] quinalbarbitone (secobarbital[3,4,12–14,24] and secbutobarbitone (butabarbital);[2] between dicoumarol and aprobarbitone(-al),[15] heptabarbitone(-al),[16,17] phenobarbitone(-al),[18–20] and vinbarbitone (-al);[15] between ethylbiscoumacetate and amylobarbitone (amobarbital),[16,21] pentobarbitone(-al),[22] and phenobarbitone(-al);[21] between phenprocoumon and secbutobarbitone (butabarbital);[2] and between nicoumalone (acenocoumarol) and heptabarbitone(-al).[17]

Mechanism

The evidence from the many studies in man and animals[4,6,8,11,14] clearly shows that the barbiturates are potent liver enzyme inducing agents which increase the metabolism and clearance of the anticoagulants from the body. They may also reduce the absorption of dicoumarol from the gut.[17]

Importance and management

This interaction is clinically important and overwhelmingly well documented. The reduction in the effects of the anticoagulant exposes the patient to the risk of thrombus formation if the dosage is not increased appropriately. A very large number of anticoagulant/barbiturate pairs have been found to interact, and the others may be expected to behave similarly. The only known exception is quinalbarbitone (secbarbital) which in daily doses of 100 mg appears to have little[12] or no[13,14] effect on dicoumarol or warfarin, but in daily doses of 200 mg interacts like the other barbiturates.[13] The barbiturates interact less with R warfarin than S warfarin, but in practice it appears to have little advantage over the usual RS racemic mixture.[25,26]

The reduction in the anticoagulant effects begins within a week, sometimes within 2–4 days, reaching a maximum after about three weeks, and it may still be evident up to six weeks[2] after stopping the barbiturate. Patients' responses can vary considerably. Stable anticoagulant control can be re-established[23] in the presence of the barbiturate by increasing the anticoagulant dosage[1,2,10,20] by about 30–60%. This may be necessary for epileptic patients.[23] Care must be taken not to withdraw the barbiturate without also reducing the anticoagulant dosage, otherwise bleeding will occur.[1,10,23] Alternative non-interacting sedative and hypnotic drugs which are safer and easier to use include nitrazepam, chlordiazepoxide, diazepam, and flurazepam. See 'Anticoagulants + Benzodiazepines'. Information is lacking about anticoagulants other than those cited, but they are expected to interact similarly.

References

1 Robinson DS and McDonald MG. The effect of phenobarbital administration on the control of coagulation achieved during warfarin therapy in man. J PharmacolExp Ther (1966) 153, 250.
2 Antlitz AM, Tolentino M and Kosal MF. Effect of butabarbital on orally administered anticoagulants. Curr Ther Res (1968) 10, 70.
3 Breckenridge A and Orme M. Clinical implications of enzyme induction. Ann NY Acad Sci (1971) 179, 421.
4 Robinson DS and Sylwester D. Interaction of commonly prescribed drugs and warfarin. Ann Int Med (1970) 72, 853.
5 MacGregor AG, Petrie JC and Wood RA. Therapeutic conferences. Drug interaction. Br Med J (1971) 1, 389.
6 Levy G, O'Reilly RA, Aggeler PM and Keech GM. Pharmacokinetic analysis of the effect of barbiturate on the anticoagulant action of warfarin in man. Clin PharmacolTher (1970) 11, 372.
7 O'Reilly RA and Aggeler PM. Effect of barbiturates on oral anticoagulants in man. Clin Res (1969) 17, 153.
8 MacDonald MG, Robinson DS, Sylwester D and Jaffe JJ. The effects of phenobarbital, chloral betaine and glutethimide administration on warfarin plasma levels and hypoprothrombinemic responses in man. Clin PharmacolTher (1969) 10, 80.
9 Seller K and Duckert F. Properties of 3-(1-phenyl-propyl)-4-oxycoumarin (Marcoumar) in the plasma when tested in normal cases and under the influence of drugs. Thromb Diath Haemorrh (1969) 19, 89.
10 MacDonald MG and Robinson DS. Clinical observations of possible barbiturate interference with anticoagulation. J Amer Med Ass (1968) 204, 97.
11 Corn M. Effect of phenobarbital and glutethimide on biological half-life of warfarin. Thromb Diath Haemorrh (1966) 16, 606.
12 Udall JA. Clinical implications of warfarin interactions with five sedatives. Am J Cardiol (1975) 35, 67.
13 Feuer DJ, Wilson WR and Ambre JJ. Duration of effect of secobarbital on the anticoagulant effect and metabolism of warfarin. The Pharmacologist (1971) 3, 195.
14 Breckenridge AM, Orme ML'E, Davies L, Thorgeirsson SS and Davis DS. Dose-dependent enzyme induction. Clin PharmacolTher (1973) 14, 514.
15 Johansson S-A. Apparent resistance to oral anticoagulant therapy and influence of hypnotics on some coagulation factors. Acta Med Scand (1968) 184, 297.
16 Dayton PG, Tarcan Y, Chenkin T and Weiner M. The influence of barbiturates on coumarin plasma levels and prothrombin response. J Clin Invest (1961) 40, 1797.
17 Aggeler PM and O'Reilly RA. Effect of heptabarbital on the response to bishydroxycoumarin in man. J Lab Clin Med (1969) 74, 229.
18 Corn M and Rockett JF. Inhibition of bishydroxycoumarin activity by phenobarbital. Med Ann DC (1965) 34, 578.
19 Cucinell SA, Conney AH, Sansur M and Burns JJ. Drug interactions in man. One lowering effect phenobarbital on plasma levels of bishydroxycoumarin (Dicumarol) and diphenylhydantoin (Dilantin). Clin PharmacolTher (1965) 6, 420.
20 Goss JE and Dickhaus DW. Increased bishydroxycoumarin requirements in patients receiving phenobarbital. N Eng J Med (1965) 273, 1094.
21 Avellaneda M. Interferencia de los barbituricos en la accion del Tromexan. Medicina (1955) 15, 109.
22 Reverchon F and Sapir M. Constatation clinique d'un antagonism entre barbituriques et anticoagulants. La Presse Med (1961) 96, 1570.
23 Williams JRB, Griffin JP and Parkins A. Effect of concomitantly administered drugs on the control of long term anticoagulant therapy. Quart J Med (1976) 45, 63.
24 Cucinell SA, Odessky L, Weiss M and Dayton PG. The effect of chloral hydrate on bishydroxycoumarin metabolism. A fatal outcome. J Amer Med Ass (1966) 197, 360.
25 Orme M and Breckenridge A. Enantiomers of warfarin and phenobarbital. N Eng J Med (1976) 295, 1482.
26 O'Reilly RA, Trager WF, Motley CH and Howald W. Interaction of secobarbital with warfarin pseudoracemates. Clin Pharmacol Ther (1980) 28, 187.

Anticoagulants + Benfluorex

Abstract/Summary

Benfluorex does not alter the anticoagulant effects of phenprocoumon.

Clinical evidence, mechanism, importance and management

25 patients on phenprocoumon showed no significant changes in their prothrombin times while taking 450 mg benfluorex daily for nine weeks when compared with equivalent periods before and after while not taking benfluorex.[1] There seems to be no information about other anticoagulants.

Reference

1 De Witte P and Brems HM. Co-administration of benfluorex with oral anticoagulant therapy. Curr Med Res Opin (1980) 6, 478.

Anticoagulants + Benziodarone

Abstract/Summary

The anticoagulant effects of ethylbiscoumacetate, diphenadione, nicoumalone (acenocoumarol) and warfarin are increased by benziodarone. The dosage of anticoagulant should be reduced appropriately. Chlorindione, dicoumarol and indandione do not interact, but the situation with phenprocoumon is not clear.

Clinical evidence

90 patients on anticoagulants were given 200 mg benziodarone three times a day for two days and 100 mg three times a day thereafter. To maintain constant PP percentages the anticoagulant dosages were reduced as follows: ethylbiscoumacetate 17% (nine patients), diphenadione 42% (eight patients), nicoumalone 25% (seven patients) and warfarin 46% (15 patients). No changes were needed in those taking chlorindione (five patients), dicoumarol (nine patients), phenindione (10 patients) or phenprocoumon (eight patients). A parallel study on 12 normal subjects confirmed the interaction with warfarin.[1]

The absence of an interaction with dicoumarol confirms a previous study,[2] however another study found that 300–600 mg benziodarone daily increased the anticoagulant effects of phenprocoumon in nine out of 29 patients and the ecchymoses observed were more frequent and larger.[3] The metabolism of ethylbiscoumacetate appears to be increased by benziodarone.[3]

Mechanism

Not understood. Benziodarone alone has no definite effect on activity of prothrombin or factors VII, IX or X.

Importance and management

Information appears to be limited to the studies cited, but the interaction would seem to be established. The dosages of the interacting anticoagulants and possibly of phenprocoumon should be reduced appropriately to prevent bleeding. No particular precautions are necessary with the non-interacting anticoagulants.

References

1 Pyorala K, Ikkala E and Siltanen P. Benziodarone (Amplivix) and anticoagulant therapy. Acta Med Scand (1963) 173, 385.
2 Gillot P. Valeur therapeutique du L 2329 dans l'angine de poitrine. Acta Cardiol (1959) 14, 494.
3 Verstraete M, Vermylen J and Claeys H. Dissimilar effect of two antianginal drugs belonging to the benzofuran group on the action of coumarin derivatives. Arch int Pharmacodyn (1968) 176, 33–41.

Anticoagulants + Benzodiazepines

Abstract/Summary

The anticoagulant effects of warfarin are not affected by chlordiazepoxide, diazepam, nitrazepam or flurazepam. The effects of phenprocoumon are not affected by nitrazepam or oxazepam, nor ethylbiscoumacetate by chlordiazepoxide. An interaction between any oral anticoagulant and a benzodiazepine is unlikely, but there are three unexplained and unconfirmed cases attributed to an interaction.

Clinical evidence

A number of studies on a very large number of patients administered anticoagulants and benzodiazepines for extended periods confirm the lack of an interaction between warfarin and chlordiazepoxide,[1–4,7] diazepam,[1,4,7] nitrazepam,[1,4,6] and flurazepam;[5] between ethylbiscoumacetate and chlordiazepoxide;[8] and between phenprocoumon, oxazepam[12] and nitrazepam.[9]

There are three discordant reports: A patient on warfarin showed an increased anticoagulant response when given diazepam.[10] A patient on dicoumarol developed multiple ecchymoses and a prothrombin time of 53 s within a fortnight of starting to take 20 mg diazepam daily.[11] And a patient showed a fall in serum warfarin levels and in the anticoagulant response when given chlordiazepoxide.[6] It is by no means certain that these responses were due to an interaction.

Mechanism

The three discordant reports are not understood. Enzyme induction is a possible explanation in one case[6] because increases in the urinary excretion of 6-beta-hydroxycortisol have been described during chlordiazepoxide use.[1,6]

Importance and management

Well documented and well established. The weight of evidence, including common experience, shows that benzodiazepines can safely be given to patients taking anticoagulants. By no means have all of the anticoagulant/benzodiazepine pairs been examined, but none of them would be expected to interact.

References

1 Orme M, Breckenridge A and Brooks RV. Interactions of benzodiazepines with warfarin. Br Med J (1972) 3, 611.
2 Lackner H and Hunt VE. The effect of Librium on hemostasis. Amer J Med Sci (1986) 256, 368.
3 Robinson DS and Sylwester D. Interaction of commonly prescribed drugs and warfarin. Ann Int Med (1970) 72, 853.
4 Breckenridge A and Orme E. Interaction of benzodiazepines with oral anticoagulants. In 'The Benzodiazepines'. Garattini S, Mussini E and Randall LO (eds) Raven Press, NY. (1973) p 647.
5 Robinson DS and Amidon EI. Interaction of benzodiazepines with warfarin in man. Ibid p 641.
6 Breckenridge A and Orme M. Clinical implications of enzyme induction. Ann NY Acad Sci (1971) 179, 421.
7 Solomon HM, Barakat MJ and Ashley CJ. Mechanisms of drug interaction. J Amer Med Ass (1971) 216, 1997.

8 Van Dam FE and Gribnau-Overkamp MJH. The effect of some
   sedatives (phenobarbital, glutethimide, chlordiazepoxide, chloral
   hydrate) on the rate of disappearance of ethylbiscoumacetate from the
   plasma. Folia Med Neerl (1967) 10, 141.
9 Bieger R, De Jonge H and Loeliger EA. Influence of nitrazepam on oral
   anticoagulation with phenprocoumon. Clin PharmacolTher (1972) 13,
   361.
10 McQueen EG. New Zealand Committee on Adverse Drug Reactions.
   9th Annual Report 1974. NZ Med J (1974) 85, 305.
11 Taylor PJ. Haemorrhage while on anticoagulant therapy precipitated
   by drug interaction. Arizona Med (1967) 24, 697.
12 Schneider J und Kamm G. Beeinflusst Oxazepam (Adumbran) die
   Antikoagulanzientherapie mit Phenprocoumon? Med Klin (1978) 73,
   153.

Anticoagulants + Benzydamine Hydrochloride

Abstract/Summary

Benzydamine does not alter the anticoagulant effects of phenprocoumon.

Clinical evidence, mechanism, importance and management

14 patients on phenprocoumon showed no significant changes in their anticoagulant response while taking 150 mg benzydamine daily for two weeks, although there was some evidence of a fall in blood levels of the anticoagulant.[1] No particular precautions would seem necessary during concurrent use. Information about other anticoagulants is lacking.

Reference

1 Duckert F, Widmer LK and Madar G. Gleichzeitige Behandlung mit
   oraler Antikoagulantien und Benzydamin. Schweiz med Wsch (1974)
   104, 1069.

Anticoagulants + Beta-blockers

Abstract/Summary

The effects of the oral anticoagulants are not normally affected by the concurrent use of beta-blocking drugs.

Clinical evidence, mechanism, importance and management

No clinically important changes in prothrombin times were found in nine patients anticoagulated with nicoumalone (acenocoumarol) or warfarin who were given metoprolol or atenolol.[1] Similarly, no interaction was seen in six subjects on warfarin and propranolol,[2] in 15 patients on phenprocoumon and pindolol,[4] in five patients on warfarin and acebutalol,[8] in eight subjects on warfarin and betaxolol[9] or in 10 men on warfarin and esmolol.[10] Single dose studies in six subjects on warfarin and propranolol, metoprolol or atenolol also demonstrated no significant interaction.[3] A transient in-

crease in phenprocoumon levels was seen in single dose studies in six subjects given metoprolol, but not when given atenolol.[5] In contrast, a patient on warfarin has been reported who showed a marked rise in his British Corrected Ratio when given propranolol.[6] Haemorrhagic tendencies without any changes in Quick time or any other impairment of coagulation have been described in two patients on phenindione and propranolol.[7]

These findings confirm the general clinical experience that the effects of the anticoagulants are not normally affected by the concurrent use of the beta-blockers, but very rarely (and quite unpredictably) some change may be seen.

References

1 Mantero F, Procidano M, Vicariotto MA and Girolami A. Effect of
   atenolol and metoprolol on the anticoagulant activity of
   acenocoumarin. Br J clin Pharmac (1984) 17, 94–6S.
2 Scott AK, Park BK and Breckenridge AM. Interaction between warfarin
   and propranolol. Br J clin Pharmac (1984) 17, 86S.
3 Bax NDS, Lennard MS, Tucker GT, Woods HF, Porter NR, Malia RG
   and Preston FE. The effect of beta-adrenoceptor antagonists on the
   pharmacokinetics and pharmacodynamics of warfarin. Br J clin Pharmac (1984) 17, 85S.
4 Vinazzer H. Effect of the beta-receptor blocking agent Visken on the
   action of coumarin. Int J Clin Pharmacol(1975) 12, 458.
5 Spahn H, Kirch W, Mutschler E, Ohnhaus EE, Kitteringham NR,
   Logering HJ and Paar D. Pharmacokinetic and pharmacodynamic interactions between phenprocoumon and atenolol or metoprolol. Br J clin
   Pharmac (1984) 17, 97–102S.
6 Bax NDS, Lennard MS, Al-Asady S, Deacon CS, Tucker GT and
   Woods HF. Inhibition of drug metabolism by beta-adrenoceptor antagonists. Drugs (1983) 25 (Suppl 2) 121–6.
7 Neilson GH and Seldon WA. Propranolol in angina pectoris. Med J
   Aust (1969) 1, 856.
8 Ryan JR. Clinical pharmacology of acebutolol. Am Heart J (1985) 109,
   1131.
9 Thiercelin JF, Warrington SJ, Thenot JP and Orofiamma B. Lack of
   interaction of betaxolol on warfarin induced hypocoagulability. In Proc
   2nd Eur. Cong Biopharm Pharmacokinet. Vol III: Clinical Pharmacokinetics (published by Imprimerie de l'Universite de Clermont Ferrant,
   1984) edited by Aiache JM and Hirtz J, pp 73–80.
10 Lowenthal DT, Porter RS, Saris SD, Bies CM, Slegowski MB and
   Staudacher A. Clinical pharmacology, pharmacodynamics and interactions of esmolol. Am J Cardiol (1985) 56, 14–17F.

Anticoagulants + 5-Bromo-2'-deoxy-uridine (BUDR)

Abstract/Summary

The anticoagulant effects of warfarin were markedly increased in a patient after receiving a number of courses of BUDR.

Clinical evidence, mechanism, importance and management

A 65-year-old man with grade III anaplastic astrocytoma under treatment with warfarin was given a number of courses of 1400 mg BUDR daily IV as a radiosensitizer. His prothrombin times were unaffected by the first 4-day course of BUDR, but they became more prolonged with successive courses and after the fourth course his prothrombin time climbed to about 45 s which was treated with 10 mg vitamin K. A significant increase also took place when a fifth cycle of 990 mg BUDR was given and the warfarin had to be stopped. The reason for this reaction is not understood. Those using BUDR should be aware that this adverse interaction may occur.

Reference

1 Oster SE and Lawrence HJ. Potentiation of anticoagulant effect of coumadin by 5-bromo-2′-deoxyuridine (BUDR). Cancer Chemother Pharmacol (1988) 22, 181.

Anticoagulants + Calcium channel blockers

Abstract/Summary

Prenylamine does interact adversely with phenprocoumon.

Clinical evidence, mechanism, importance and management

A study in 30 patients with angina treated with phenprocoumon showed that the addition of 60 mg prenylamine three times a day for three weeks had no effect on their prothrombin times.[1] There seems to be no information about other anticoagulants or calcium channel blockers.

Reference

1 Bohm C and Denes G. Untersuchung zur Erfassung eventueller Klinischer Interaktionene zwischen Phenprocoumon und Prenylamin (Ergebnisse einer Multizenterstudie). Acta Ther (1987) 13, 333–43.

Anticoagulants + Carbamazepine

Abstract/Summary

The anticoagulant effects of warfarin can be markedly reduced by carbamazepine. The warfarin dosage may need to be approximately doubled to accommodate this interaction.

Clinical evidence

Two patients on warfarin given carbamazepine (200 mg daily for the first week, 400 mg daily for the second and 600 mg for the third) showed an approximately 50% fall in serum warfarin levels which was reflected in sharp rises in their PP percentages.[1] The half-life of warfarin in three other patients fell by 53, 11 and 60% respectively when similarly treated.[1]

This interaction has been described in five other reports.[2–6]

Mechanism

Uncertain, but the available evidence suggests that carbamazepine increases the metabolism of warfarin by the liver, thereby increasing its loss from the body and reducing its effects.[1,2]

Importance and management

A moderately well-documented, established and clinically important interaction. The incidence is uncertain. Monitor the anticoagulant response if carbamazepine is added to established treatment with warfarin and anticipate the need to double the dosage. Information about other anticoagulants is lacking but it would be prudent to apply the same precautions.

References

1 Hansen JM, Siersbaek-Nielsen K and Skovsted L. Carbamazepine-induced acceleration of diphenylhydantoin and warfarin metabolism in man. Clin Pharmacol Ther (1971) 12, 539.
2 Ross JR and Beeley L. Interaction between carbamazepine and warfarin. Br Med J (1980) 1, 1415.
3 Kendall AG and Boivin M. Warfarin-carbamazepine interaction. Ann InternMed (1981) 94, 280.
4 Massey EW. Effect of carbamazepine on coumarin metabolism. Ann Neurol (1983) 13, 691–2.

Anticoagulants + Carbon tetrachloride

Abstract/Summary

A single case report describes an increase in the anticoagulant effects of dicoumarol in a patient who accidentally drank some carbon tetrachloride.

Clinical evidence, mechanism, importance and management

A patient, well stabilized on dicoumarol, accidentally drank 0.1 ml carbon tetrachloride. Next day his prothrombin time had risen to 41 s (prothrombin activity fall from 18 to 10%). These values were approximately the same next day although the dicoumarol had been withdrawn, and marked hypoprothrombinaemia persisted for another five days.[1]

The probable reason for this reaction is that carbon tetrachloride is very toxic to the liver, the changed anticoagulant response being a manifestation of this. Carbon tetrachloride, once used as an anthelmintic in man, is no longer used in human medicine, but is still employed as an industrial solvent and degreasing agent. On theoretical grounds it would seem possible for anticoagulated patients exposed to substantial amounts of the vapour to experience this interaction but this has not been reported.

Reference

1 Luton EF. Carbon tetrachloride exposure during anticoagulant therapy. Dangerous enhancement of hypoprothrombinemic effect. J Amer Med Ass (1966) 194, 120.

Anticoagulants + Cephalosporins

Abstract/Summary

Cefamandole can increase the anticoagulant effects of warfarin. Hypoprothrombinaemia (without an anticoagulant) and/or bleeding has been seen with cefoperazone, cephazolin, cephalothin and latamoxef (moxalactam). It is suggested that it may also occur with cephaloridine. If these cephalosporins and oral anticoagulants are used together it seems possible that their anticoagulant effects might be additive.

Clinical evidence

(a) Warfarin + cefamandole

A study of a possible interaction was prompted by two patients who developed unusually high prothrombin times (one of them bled) when given both drugs. 60 other patients undergoing heart valve replacement surgery were given antibiotics prophylactically before the chest incision was made, and at six-hourly intervals thereafter for about 72 h. Those given 2 g cefamandole (44 patients) showed a much greater anticoagulant response than those given 500 mg vancomycin (16 patients).[1] A later study by the same workers confirmed these findings.[15] They recommend that those aged over 60 undergoing this kind of surgery, who have a baseline prothrombin time of 14 s or more, should be started on no more than 5 mg warfarin daily if they are to be given cefamandole. Serious bleeding (in the absence of an anticoagulant) following the use of cephamandole has been described in 3 out of 37 patients in another report,[10] and seven other cases are described elsewhere.[11]

(b) Cefoperazone, cephaloridine, cefazolin, cephalothin and latamoxef

It has been claimed that cephaloridine given alone can induce an extension of prothrombin times, but no evidence is given.[2,3] A patient has been described who, 12 days after starting to take 0.5 g cephazolin eight-hourly, was noted to have increased prothrombin and partial thromboplastin times.[4] These returned to normal within 48 h of withdrawing the antibiotic, and recurred 10 days after it was restarted. Increased prothrombin times were found in another study.[15] 17 cases of hypoprothrombinaemia and/or bleeding have been described with latamoxef (moxalactam),[5] and several other cases have been reported with cefoperazone.[6-9,16] Cephalothin has also been implicated.[13]

Mechanism

Not fully understood.[14] One suggestion is that the hypoprothrombinaemia associated with these antibiotics is due to vitamin K deficiency caused by a combination of low vitamin K intake and a suppression of the intestinal bacterial flora which normally act as a supplementary source of vitamin K (cefamandole is secreted in the bile). As a result bleeding occurs because the vitamin K-dependent blood clotting factors fall to very low levels. There is also evidence that these cephalosporins have a direct coumarin-like effect.[16] Latamoxef also inhibits platelet aggregation.[12] The presence of an anticoagulant is an additional factor.

Importance and management

It is well established that bleeding can occur in some patients if these antibiotics are given in the absence of an anticoagulant, but there are few reports of bleeding in patients also taking anticoagulants. Patients most at risk would seem to be those whose intake of vitamin K is restricted (poor diet, malabsorption syndromes, etc.) and those with renal failure. The use of an anticoagulant represents just another factor which may precipitate bleeding. Concurrent use should be well monitored. Excessive hypoprothrombinaemia can be controlled with vitamin K.

References

1 Angaran DM, Dias VC, Arom KV, Northrup WF, Kersten TE, Lindsay WG and Nicoloff DM. The influence of prophylactic antibiotics on the warfarin anticoagulation response in the post-operative prosthetic cardiac valve patient. Ann Surg (1984) 199, 107–111.

2 Council on Drugs. Evaluation of a new antibacterial agent, cephaloridine (Loridine). J Amer Med Ass (1986) 206, 1289.

3 Wade A. Martindales Extra Pharmacopoeia 27th ed. Pharmaceutical Press, London (1977) p 1099.

4 Lerner PI and Lubin A. Coagulopathy with cefazolin in uremia. N Eng J Med (1974) 290, 1324.

5 Beeley L, Beadle R and Lawrence R. Bulletin of the West Midlands Centre for Adverse Drug Reaction Reporting (1984) 19, 15.

6 Meisel S. Hypoprothrombinaemia due to cefoperazone. Drug Intell Clin Pharm (1984) 18, 316.

7 Cristiano P. Hypoprothrombinaemia associated with cefoperazone treatment. Drug Intell Clin Pharm (1984) 18, 314–6.

8 Osborne JC. Hypoprothrombinaemia and bleeding due to cefoperazone. Ann InternMed (1985) 102, 721–2.

9 Freedy HR, Cetnarowski AB, Lumish RM and Schafer FJ. Cefoperazone-induced coagulopathy. Drug Intell Clin Pharm (1986) 20, 281–3.

10 Hooper CA, Haney BB and Stone HH. Gastrointestinal bleeding due to vitamin K deficiency in patients on parenteral cefamandole. Lancet (1980) i, 39–40.

11 Rymer W and Greenlaw CW. Hypoprothrombinaemia associated with cefamandole. Drug Intell Clin Pharm (1980) 14, 780–3.

12 Bang NU, Tessler SS, Heidenreich RO, Marks CA and Mattler LE. Effects of moxalactam on blood coagulation and platelet function. Rev Infect Dis (1982) 4 (Suppl) S546–54.

13 Natelson EA, Brown CH and Bradshaw MW. Influence of cephalosporin antibiotics on blood coagulation and platelet function. Antimicrob Ag Chemother (1976) 9, 91–3.

14 Babiak LM and Rybak MJ. Hematological effects associated with beta-lactam use. Drug Intell Clin Pharm (1986) 20, 833–6.

15 Angaran DM, Dias VD, Arom KV, Northrup WF, Kersten TG, Lindsay WG and Nicoloff DM. The comparative influence of prophylactic antibiotics on the prothrombin response to warfarin in the postoperative prothetic cardiac valve patients. Ann Surg (1987) 206, 155–61.

16 Andrassy K, Kodersich J, Fritz S, Bechtold H and Sonntag H. Alteration of hemostasis associated with cefoperazone treatment. Infection (1986) 14, 27–31.

Anticoagulants + Chloral hydrate

Abstract/Summary

The anticoagulant effects of warfarin are transiently increased by chloral hydrate, but this is of little or no clinical importance. Chloral betaine, petrichloral and triclofos may be expected to have a similar effect.

Clinical evidence

A retrospective study on 32 patients just starting on warfarin showed that while the loading doses of warfarin in the control and chloral-treated groups were the same, the warfarin requirements of the chloral group during the first four days fell by about a third, but rose again to normal by the 5th day.[1]

A study on 10 patients and four normal subjects taking warfarin showed that when given 1 g chloral hydrate each night, there was a minor, clinically unimportant and short-lived increase in the prothrombin times of five of them during the first few days of concurrent treatment, but no change in the overall long-term anticoagulant control.[2]

Similar results have been described in other studies on large numbers of patients taking warfarin and chloral[3–5,8,10,11] or triclofos.[7] Chloral betaine appears to behave similarly.[9] An isolated and by no means fully explained case of fatal hypoprothrombinaemia in a patient on dicoumarol who was given chloral for 10 days, later replaced by secobarbital, has been reported.[6] Another patient on dicoumarol and chloral showed a reduction in prothrombin times.[6]

Mechanism

Chloral hydrate is mainly metabolized to trichloroacetic acid which then successfully competes with warfarin for its binding sites on plasma proteins.[8] As a result, free and active molecules of warfarin flood into plasma water by displacement so that the effects of the warfarin are increased. But this is only short-lived because the warfarin molecules are also exposed to metabolism by the liver, so that the hypoprothrombinaemic effects are reduced once more.

Importance and management

A well-documented and well understood interaction, normally of no clinical importance. There is very good evidence that concurrent use need not be avoided.[1–5,8,10,11] Those who wish to be ultracautious might wish to keep an eye on the anticoagulant response during the first 4–5 days. It is uncertain whether other anticoagulants behave in the same way because the evidence is sparse, indirect and inconclusive,[6,12,13] but what is known suggests that they probably do.

Triclofos[7] and chloral betaine[9] appear to behave like chloral, and petrichloral may also be expected to do so. Dichloralphenazone on the other hand interacts quite differently (see 'Anticoagulants + Dichloralphenazone').

References

1 Boston Collaborative Drug Surveillance Program. Interaction between chloral hydrate and warfarin. N Eng J Med (1972) 286, 53.
2 Udall JA. Warfarin-chloral hydrate interaction. Pharmacological activity and significance. Ann Int Med (1974) 81, 341.
3 Griner PF, Raisz LG, Rickles FR. Wiesner PJ and Odoroff CL. Chloral hydrate and warfarin interaction: clinical significance?
4 Udall JA. Clinical implications of warfarin interactions with five sedatives. Amer J Cardiol (1975) 35, 67.
5 Udall JA. Warfarin interactions with chloral hydrate and glutethimide. Curr Ther Res (1975) 17, 67.
6 Cucinell SA, Odessky K, Weiss M and Dayton PG. The effect of chloral hydrate on bishydroxycoumarin metabolism. A fatal outcome. J Amer Med Ass (1966) 197, 144.
7 Sellers EM, Lang M and Koch-Weser J. Enhancement of warfarin-induced hypoprothrombinaemia by triclofos. Clin PharmacolTher (1972) 13, 911.
8 Sellers EM and Koch-Weser J. Kinetics and clinical importance of displacement of warfarin from albumin by acidic drugs. Ann NY Acad Sci (1971) 179, 213.
9 McDonald MG, Robinson DS, Sylwester D and Jaffe JJ. The effects of phenobarbital, chloral betaine and glutethimide administration on warfarin plasma levels and hypoprothrombinaemic responses in man. Clin PharmacolTher (1969) 10, 80.
10 Breckenridge A, Orme ML'E, Thorgeirsson S, Davies DS and Brooks RV. Drug interactions with warfarin: studies with dichloralphenazone, chloral hydrate and phenazone (antipyrine). Clin Sci (1971) 40, 351.
11 Breckenridge A and Orme M. Clinical implications of enzyme induction. Ann NY Acad Sci (1971) 179, 421.
12 Dayton PG, Tarcam Y, Chenkin Th and Wiener M. The influence of barbiturates on coumarin plasma levels on prothrombin response. J Clin Invest (1961) 40, 1797.
13 Van Dam FE and Gribnau-Overkamp MJH. The effects of some sedatives (phenobarbital, glutethimide, chlordiazepoxide, chloral hydrate) on the rate of disappearance of ethylbiscoumacetate from the plasma. Folis Med Neerl (1967) 10, 141.

Anticoagulants + Chloramphenicol

Abstract/Summary

The anticoagulant effects of dicoumarol and nicoumalone (acenocoumarol) and possibly ethylbiscoumacetate can be increased by the concurrent use of chloramphenicol.

Clinical evidence

A study in four patients showed that the half-life of dicoumarol was increased on average by a factor of three (from 8 to 25 h) when treated with 2 g chloramphenicol daily for 5–8 days.[1]

Three out of nine patients taking an unnamed anticoagulant showed a fall in their Prothrombin-Proconvertin values from a range of 10–30% down to less than 6% when given 1–2 g chloramphenicol daily for 4–6 days.[2] One patient showed a smaller reduction.

There is another report of an increased anticoagulant response involving nicoumalone, and a brief comment implicating, but not confirming, an interaction with dicoumarol and with ethylbiscoumacetate.[3] Hypoprothrombinaemia and bleeding has been described in patients on chloramphenicol in the absence of an anticoagulant.[4,5]

Mechanism

Uncertain. One suggestion is that the chloramphenicol inhibits the liver enzymes concerned with the metabolism of the anticoagulants so that their effects are prolonged and increased.[1] Another is that the antibiotic decimates the gut bacteria thereby decreasing a source of vitamin K, but it is doubtful if these bacteria are an important source of the vitamin except in exceptional cases where dietary levels are very inadequate.[6] A third suggestion is that chloramphenicol blocks production of prothrombin by the liver.[4]

Importance and management

The documentation is very sparse indeed, but what is known suggests that the concurrent use of dicoumarol or nicoumalone and chloramphenicol should be avoided. If concurrent use is undertaken, the anticoagulant dosage should be reduced and the prothrombin time monitored closely. Direct evidence of an interaction with any other anticoagulant is lacking (except possibly ethylbiscoumacetate). It is noteworthy that there is nothing on record about warfarin and chloramphenicol which might imply that no clinically important interaction occurs (?).

References

1 Christensen LK and Skovsted L. Inhibition of drug metabolism by chloramphenicol. Lancet (1969) ii, 1397.
2 Magid E. Tolerance to anticoagulants during antibiotic therapy. Scand J Lab Clin Invest (1962) 14, 565.
3 Johnson R, David A and Chartier Y. Clinical experience with G-23350 (Sintrom). Can Med Ass J (1957) 77, 760.
4 Klippel AP and Pitsinger B. Hypoprothrombinaemia secondary to antibiotic therapy and manifested by massive gastrointestinal haemorrhage. Arch Surg (1968) 96, 266.
5 Matsniotis N, Messaritikas J and Vlachou C. Hypoprothrombinaemia bleeding in infants associated with diarrhoea and antibiotics. Arch Dis Child (1970) 45, 586.
6 Udall JA. Human sources and absorption of vitamin K in relation to anticoagulant stability. J Amer Med Ass (1965), 194, 179.

Anticoagulants + Cholestyramine or Colestipol

Abstract/Summary

The anticoagulant effects of phenprocoumon and warfarin can be reduced by cholestyramine. Separating the dosages as much as possible may help to minimize the effects of this interaction. No important interaction occurs between phenprocoumon or warfarin and colestipol.

Clinical evidence

(a) Phenprocoumon or warfarin + cholestyramine

10 subjects were treated for one-week periods either with warfarin alone or warfarin with 8 g cholestyramine given three times a day. With warfarin alone peak serum levels reached 5.6 μg/ml and prothrombin times were prolonged by 11 s. With cholestyramine given 30 min after the warfarin, peak levels were reduced to 2.7 μg/ml and the prothrombin times were prolonged by 8 s, whereas when the cholestyramine was given 6 h after the warfarin, peak levels reached 4.7 μg/ml and prothrombin times were again prolonged by 11 s.[1]

Comparable results have been found in other studies using single doses of warfarin or phenprocoumon.[2–5,8,12]

(b) Phenprocoumon or warfarin + colestipol

A cross-over study in four normal subjects showed that phenprocoumon serum levels and the prothrombin response were unaffected by the simultaneous administration of 8 g colestipol.[13] No changes in the absorption of single 10 or 40 mg doses of warfarin in the presence of 10 g colestipol were seen in another study.[14]

Mechanism

Cholestyramine binds to bile acids within the gut and to anticoagulants, thereby preventing their absorption.[2,3,5–7] As both warfarin and phenprocoumon undergo entero-hepatic recycling, continuous further contact with the cholestyramine can occur.[4,8] Cholestyramine also reduces the absorption of fat-soluble vitamins such as vitamin K so that it can have some direct hypoprothrombinaemic effects of its own.[10,11] This may offset to some extent the full effects of its interaction with anticoagulants. Colestipol on the other hand appears not to bind to any great extent at the pH values in the gut.[13]

Importance and management

The anticoagulant/cholestyramine interaction is established, but its magnitude and clinical importance is still uncertain. If concurrent use is thought necessary, prothrombin times should be monitored closely and the dosage of the anticoagulant increased appropriately. Giving the cholestyramine 3–6 h after the anticoagulant has been shown to minimize the effects of this interaction.[1,9] Information about other anticoagulants is lacking but as cholestyramine interacts with dicoumarol and ethylbiscoumacetate in animals[7] it would be prudent to assume that they all interact similarly in man.

No special precautions appear necessary if warfarin or phenprocoumon and colestipol are given concurrently. There seems to be no information about other anticoagulants.

References

1 Kventzel WP and Brunk SF. Cholestyramine-warfarin interaction. Clin Res (1970) 18, 594.
2 Robinson DA, Benjamin DM and McCormack JJ. Interaction of warfarin and non-systemic gastrointestinal drugs. Clin Pharmacol Ther (1971) 12, 491.
3 Benjamin D, Robinson DS and McCormack JJ. Cholestyramine binding to warfarin in man and *in vitro*. Clin Res (1970) 18, 336.
4 Jahnchen E, Meinertz T, Gilfrich H-J, Kersting F and Groth U. Enhanced elimination of warfarin during treatment with cholestyramine. Br J clin Pharmac (1978) 5, 437.
5 Hahn KJ, Eiden W, Schettle M, Hahn M, Walter E and Weber E. Effect of cholestyramine on the gastrointestinal absorption of phenprocoumon and acetylsalicylic acid in man. Europ J Clin Pharmacol (1972) 4, 142.
6 Gallo DG, Bailey KK and Sheffner AL. The interaction between cholestyramine and drugs. Proc Soc Exp Biol Med (1965) 120, 60.

7 Tembo AV and Bates TR. Impairment by cholestyramine of dicumarol and tromexan absorption in rats: a potential drug interaction. J Pharmacol Exp Ther. (1974) 191, 53.

8 Meinertz T, Gilfrich H-J, Groth N, Jonen HG and Jahnchen E. Interruption of the enterohepatic circulation of phenprocoumon by cholestyramine. Clin Pharmacol Ther (1977) 147, 166.

9 Cali TJ. Combined therapy with cholestyramine and warfarin. Am J Pharm (1975) 72, 759.

10 Casdorph HR. Safe uses of cholestyramine. Ann Int Med (1970) 72, 759.

11 Gross L and Brotman M. Hypoprothrombinaemia and haemorrhage associated with cholestyramine therapy. Ann Int Med (1970) 72, 95.

12 Meinertz T, Gilfrich H-J, Bork R and Jahnchen E. Treatment of phenprocoumon intoxication with cholestyramine. Br Med J (1977) 2, 439.

13 Harvengt C and Desager JP. Effects of colestipol, a new bile acid sequestrant, on the absorption of phenprocoumon in man. Europ J clin Pharmacol (1973) 6, 19.

14 Hannigan JJ. Colestipol-warfarin drug interaction study. A comparison of plasma warfarin concentrations following oral administration of 10 mg warfarin with and without an ionic exchange resin (colestipol hydrochloride or cholestyramine). On file Upjohn (1975). Quoted by Heel RC, Brogden RN, Pakes GE, Speight TM, Avery GS. Colestipol: a review of its pharmacological properties and therapeutic effects in patients with hypercholesterolaemia. Drugs (1980) 19, 161–80.

Anticoagulants + Cimetidine, Ranitidine or Nizatidine

Abstract/Summary

The anticoagulant effects of warfarin can be increased if cimetidine is given concurrently. Severe bleeding has occurred in a few patients but some show no interaction at all. Nicoumalone (acenocoumarol) and phenindione seem to interact similarly but not phenprocoumon. Ranitidine and nizatidine appear to be non-interacting alternative H_2-blockers.

Clinical evidence

(a) Cimetidine

A very brief report in 1978, published as a letter by the manufacturers of cimetidine, stated that at that time they were aware of 17 cases worldwide indicating that 1 g cimetidine daily could cause a prothrombin time rise of about 20% in those stabilized on warfarin.[1]

A number of studies and case reports have confirmed this interaction with warfarin.[2–5,9–12] Serum warfarin levels are reported to rise (25–80%),[6,11] and prothrombin times can be increased (> 30 s). Severe bleeding (haematuria, internal haemorrhages, etc.) and very prolonged prothrombin times have been seen in handful of patients.[2,4,9,10,12] However one study found that only half of the group of 14 patients studied demonstrated this interaction,[18] and another on 27 patients found that although the AUC of warfarin increased by 21–39% and the clearance fell by 22–28%, prothrombin times only increased by 2–2.6 s.[15] Nicoumalone and phenindione appear to interact like warfarin[3] but not phenprocoumon.[8]

(b) Ranitidine and nizatidine

A study in five subjects given warfarin showed that the concurrent use of 400 mg ranitidine daily for two weeks had no effect on warfarin concentrations or on prothrombin times. In another study[2] with 11 subjects it was found that 300 mg ranitidine daily for three days had no effect on the pharmacodynamics or pharmacokinetics of a single dose of warfarin. In contrast, a third study[16,17] on five subjects reported that 300 mg ranitidine daily for a week reduced the clearance of a single dose of warfarin by almost 30%, but the half-life was not significantly changed and prothrombin times were not measured. 750 mg ranitidine daily given to two subjects was also reported to have reduced the warfarin clearance by more than 50%. A number of aspects of this last study are open to doubt and the validity of the results is questionable. Nizatidine appears to behave like ranitidine.[19]

Mechanism

Cimetidine can inhibit the liver enzymes concerned with the metabolism (phase one hydroxylation) and clearance of warfarin so that its effects are prolonged and increased.[7] This also appears to be true for nicoumalone and phenindione, but not phenprocoumon which is metabolized by different enzymes using another biochemical pathway (phase two glucuronidation).[8] The warfarin–cimetidine interaction has been found to be stereoselective, that is to say the cimetidine interacts with the R(+) isomer but not with the S(−) isomer.[13,14]

Importance and management

The warfarin–cimetidine interaction is well documented and well established. If bleeding is to be avoided, monitor concurrent use closely and anticipate the need to reduce the warfarin dosage. Many patients (probably up to 50%) may not develop this interaction. Nicoumalone and phenindione are reported to interact similarly but the documentation is much more limited. Expect other anticoagulants to behave similarly with the possible exception of phenprocoumon. Ranitidine and nizatidine are non-interacting alternatives to cimetidine.

References

1 Flind AC. Cimetidine and oral anticoagulants. Lancet (1978) ii, 1054.

2 Silver BA and Bell WR. Cimetidine potentiation of the hypoprothrombinaemic effect of warfarin. Ann Intern Med (1979) 90, 348.

3 Serlin MJ, Sibeon RG, Mossman S, Breckenridge AM, Williams JR B, Atwood JL and Willoughby JMT. Cimetidine interaction with oral anticoagulants in man. Lancet (1979) ii, 317.

4 Hetzel D, Birkett D and Miners J. Cimetidine interaction with warfarin. Lancet (1979) ii, 639.

5 Breckenridge AM, Challiner M, Mossman S, Park BK, Serlin MJ, Sibeon RG, Williams JRB and Willoughby JMT. Cimetidine increases the action of warfarin in man. Br J Clin Pharmac (1979) 8, 392 P.

6 Serlin MJ, Sibeon RG and Breckenridge AM. Lack of effect of ranitidine on warfarin action. Br J Clin Pharmac (1981) 12, 791.

7 Henry DA, MacDonald IA, Kitchingman G, Bell GD and Langman MJS. Cimetidine and ranitidine: comparison of effects on hepatic metabolism. Br Med J (1980) 281, 775.

8 Harenberg J, Staiger Ch, de Vries JX, Walter E, Weber E and Zimmerman R. Cimetidine does not increase the anticoagulant effect of phenprocoumon. Br J Clin Pharmac (1982) 14, 292–3.

9 Wallin BA, Jacknowitz A and Raich PC. Cimetidine and effect of warfarin. Ann Inter Med (1979) 90, 993.

10 Kerly B and Ali M. Cimetidine potentiation of warfarin action. Can Med Ass J (1982) 126, 116.

11 O'Reilly RA. Comparative interaction of cimetidine and ranitidine with racemic warfarin in man. Arch Intern Med (1984) 144, 989–91.

12 Davanesen S. Prolongation of prothrombin time with cimetidine. Med J Aust (1981) 1, 537.

13 Choonara IA, Cholerton S, Haynes BP, Breckenridge AM and Park BK. Stereoselective interaction between the R enantiomer of warfarin and cimetidine. Br J Clin Pharmac (1986) 21, 271–77.

14 Toon S, Hopkins KJ, Garstang FM, Diquet B, Gill TS and Rowland M. The warfarin-cimetidine interaction: stereochemical considerations. Br J clin Pharmac (1986) 21, 245–6.

15 Sax MJ, Randolph WC, Peace KE, Chretien S, Frank WO, Braverman AJ, Gray DR, McCree LC, Wyle F, Jackson BJ, Beg MA and Young MD. Effect of two cimetidine regimens on prothrombin time and warfarin pharmacokinetics during long-term warfarin therapy. Clin Pharm (1987) 6, 492–5.

16 Desmond PV, Breen KJ, Harman PJ, Mashford ML and Morphett BJ. Decreased clearance of warfarin after treatment with cimetidine or ranitidine. Aust NZJ Med (1983) 13, 327.

17 Desmond PV, Breen KJ, Harman PJ, Mashford ML and Morphett BJ. Clin Pharmacol Ther (1984) 35, 338–41.

18 Bell WR, Anderson KC, Noe DA and Silver BA. Reduction in the plasma clearance rate of warfarin induced by cimetidine. Arch Intern Med (1986) 146, 2325–8.

19 Callaghan JT and Nyhart EH. Drug interactions between H₂-blockers and theophylline or warfarin. Pharmacologist (1988) 30, A14.

Anticoagulants + Cinchophen

Abstract/Summary

The anticoagulant effects of dicoumarol, ethylbiscoumacetate and phenindione are markedly increased by cinchophen. Bleeding will occur if the anticoagulant dosage is not reduced appropriately.

Clinical evidence

A patient taking an un-named anticoagulant was given a total of 4 g cinchophen over a period of two days, at the end of which his prothrombin levels were found to be less than 5%. The next day he had haematemeses and died. This prompted a study in three patients taking phenindione, ethylbiscoumacetate and dicoumarol. Within two days of starting to take 4 g cinchophen daily, the prothrombin levels of two of them fell sharply from a range of 10–25% to less than 5%. A smaller fall occurred in the third patient.[1]

Mechanism

Cinchophen by itself appears to have a direct effect on the liver, like the oral anticoagulants, which reduces the synthesis of prothrombin.[2] There is a latent period, similar to that of dicoumarol, before the fall in blood prothrombin levels begins, and a short delay after its withdrawal before the prothrombin levels rise again.[1] Its effects can be reversed by the administration of vitamin K.[3] So this interaction seems to result from the additive effects of two anticoagulant drugs.

Importance and management

Direct information about this interaction seems to be limited to the report cited,[1] but what is known suggests that it is of clinical importance. Its incidence is uncertain. Concurrent use should be avoided. Cinchophen should not be given to patients on any anticoagulant unless the prothrombin times can be monitored and the dosage reduced appropriately.

References

1 Jarnum S. Cinchophen and acetylsalicylic acid in anticoagulant treatment. Scand J Lab Invest (1974) 6, 91.

2 Hueper WC. Toxicity and detoxication of cinchophen. Arch Pathol (1946) 41, 592.

3 Rawls A. Prevention of cinchophen toxicity by use of vitamin K. NY State J Med. (1942) 42, 2021.

Anticoagulants + Cisapride

Abstract/Summary

Cisapride causes a small increase in the anticoagulant effects of nicoumalone (acenocoumarol) but appears not to affect warfarin.

Clinical evidence, mechanism, importance and management

22 patients on nicoumalone showed an increase in thrombotest values while taking cisapride (10 mg before meals three times daily for a three-week period) due, it is suggested, to the increase in gastrointestinal motility caused by cisapride which increases nicoumalone absorption. These values fell when the cisapride was stopped. Although the increase was small the prothrombin times should be monitored a week after starting or stopping cisapride so that the anticoagulant dosage can be modified if necessary.[1] Another study in 12 normal subjects on warfarin showed that 10 mg cisapride daily for 25 days had no statistically significant effects on prothrombin times (expressed as international normalized ratios).[2] There seems to be no information about other anticoagulants but monitoring would seem advisable.

References

1 Jonker JJ C. Effect of cisapride on anticoagulant treatment with acenocoumarol. Clinical Research Report, R 51619-NL, August (1985). Janssen unpublished data.

2 Daneshmend TK, Mahida YR, Bhaskar NK and Hawkey CJ. Does cisapride alter the anticoagulant effect of Warfarin? A pharmacodynamic assessment. British Society of Gastroenterology Spring Meeting–12–14 April 1989.

Anticoagulants + Clofibrate, Bezafibrate or Gemfibrozil

Abstract/Summary

The anticoagulant effects of dicoumarol, phenindione and warfarin are increased by clofibrate, and the effects of phenprocoumon are increased by bezafibrate. Bleeding will occur if the anticoagulant dosage is not reduced appropriately. It is uncertain whether gemfibrozil interacts similarly.

Clinical evidence

(a) Anticoagulants + clofibrate

A study in three hospitals of 42 patients taking either pheninidone or warfarin showed that when additionally given either clofibrate or *Atromid* (clofibrate with androsterone) it was necessary to reduce the anticoagulant dosages. 10 out of 15 in Belfast needed a 25% reduction and 5 of them bled. All 9 in Edinburgh needed a 33% reduction, and 14 out of 18 in Johannesburg also needed a reduction.[1]

This interaction has been confirmed in other studies on a considerable number of patients anticoagulated with warfarin,[2–4,7,10,11] phenindione[5,6,8] or dicoumarol.[9] Bleeding has been described frequently, and death due to haemorrhage has occurred in at least two cases.[7,8]

(b) Anticoagulants + bezafibrate

A study on 15 patients with hyperlipidaemia, taking phenprocoumon, showed that while taking 450 mg bezafibrate daily it was necessary to reduce the anticoagulant dosage by 20%, and while taking 600 mg by 33%.[15]

(c) Anticoagulants + gemfibrozil

Gemfibrozil causes haemostatic changes very similar to those seen with clofibrate[16] but there seems to be no direct evidence that it interacts with the oral anticoagulants.

Mechanism

Uncertain. Clofibrate can displace warfarin from its plasma protein binding sites,[12–14] but this does not adequately explain the interaction. Another suggestion is that both clofibrate and bezafibrate increase the affinity of the anticoagulant for the receptor sites.[9,15]

Importance and management

The anticoagulant–clofibrate/bezafibrate interactions are well-documented, established and clinically important. The incidence is reported to be between 20 and 100%,[2,15] but it would be wise to assume that all patients will be affected. If bleeding is to be avoided the anticoagulant dosage should be reduced by about a third. Information about other anticoagulants is lacking, but they may be expected to interact similarly. The manufacturers say that the anticoagulant dosage may need to be reduced if gemfibrozil is given but there seems to be no direct evidence of an interaction.

References

1 Oliver MF, Roberts SD, Hayes D, Pantridge JF, Suzman MM and Bersohn I. Effect of Atromid and ethyl chlorophenoxy-isobutyrate on anticoagulant requirements. Lancet (1963) i, 143.
2 Udall JA. Drug interference with warfarin therapy. Clin Med (1970) 77, 20.
3 Eastham RD. Warfarin dosage, clofibrate and age of patient. Lancet (1973) ii, 554.
4 Roberts SD and Pantridge JF. Effect of Atromid on requirements of warfarin. J Atheroscler Res (1963) 3, 655.
5 Williams GEO and Ferguson JC. Clinical observations on patients

treated with Atromid and anticoagulants. J Atheroscler Res (1963) 3, 671.
6 Rogen AS and Ferguson JC. Clinical observations on patients treated with Atromid and anticoagulants. J Atheroscler Res (1963) 3, 671.
7 Solomon RB and Rosner F. Massive haemorrhage and death during treatment with clofibrate and warfarin. NY State J Med (1973) 73, 2002.
8 Rogen AS and Ferguson JC. Effect of Atromid on anticoagulant requirements. Lancet (1963) i, 272.
9 Schrogie JJ and Solomon HM. The anticoagulant response to bishydroxycoumarin. II. The effect of D-thyroxine, clofibrate and norethandrolone. Clin PharmacolTher (1967) 8, 70.
10 Bjornsson TD, Meffin PJ and Blaschke TF. Interaction of clofibrate with the optical enantiomorphs of warfarin. Pharmacologist (1976) 18, 207.
11 Counihan TB and Keelan P. Atromid in high cholesterol states. J Athersclr Res (1963) 3, 580.
12 Solomon HM, Schrogie JJ and Williams D. The displacement of phenylbutazone-C¹⁴ and warfarin-C¹⁴ from human albumin by various drugs and fatty acids. Biochem Pharmacol(1968) 17, 143.
13 Solomon HM and Schrogie JJ. The effect of various drugs on the binding of warfarin-C¹⁴ to human albumin. Biochem Pharmacol(1967) 16, 1219.
14 Bjornsson TD, Meffin PJ, Swezy S and Blaschke TF. Clofibrate displaces warfarin from plasma proteins in man: an example of a pure displacement interaction. J PharmacolExp Ther (1979) 210, 316.
15 Zimmerman R, Ehlers W, Walter E, Hoffrichter A, Lang PD, Andrassy K and Schlierf G. The effect of bezafibrate on the fibrinolytic system and the drug interaction with phenprocoumon. Atherosclerosis (1978) 29, 477–85.
16 Rasi VPO and Torstila I. The effect of gemfibrozil upon platelet function and blood coagulation. Preliminary report. Proc Roy Soc Med (1976) 69, Suppl 2. 109–11.

Anticoagulants + Contraceptives (oral) and Related sex hormones

Abstract/Summary

The anticoagulant effects of dicoumarol can be increased, and the effects of nicoumalone (acenocoumarol) decreased, by the concurrent use of oral contraceptives. A small dosage adjustment may be necessary.

Clinical evidence

(a) Dicoumarol + oral contraceptives

A study on four healthy subjects given single 150 or 200mg doses of dicoumarol after a 20-day course of *Enovid* (norethynodrel and mestranol) showed that the anticoagulant effects were decreased in three of the four, although the dicoumarol half-life remained unaltered.[1]

(b) Nicoumalone (acenocoumarol) + oral contraceptives

A survey on 12 patients taking nicoumalone showed that, while taking oral contraceptives, over an average of two years their anticoagulant dosage requirements were reduced by about 20%. Even then they were anticoagulated to a higher degree (prothrombin ratio of 1.67 compared with 1.50) than with the anticoagulant alone. The contraceptives used were *Neogynona, Microgynon, Eugynon* (ethinyloestradiol with D-norgestrel) or *Topasel* (IM ampoules of oestradiol enanthate with dihyroxyprogesterone acetophenide).[2] Megestrol is reported to increased bleeding times with anticoagulants (unnamed) in a very brief report on one patient.[4]

Mechanism

Not understood. The oral contraceptives increase plasma levels of some blood clotting factors (particularly factors VII and X) and reduce levels of antithrombin III. They can also inhibit drug metabolism and may possibly affect the oral anticoagulants.

Importance and management

Direct information seems to be limited to these reports. They clearly show that concurrent use need not be avoided, but some modest adjustment in the anticoagulant dosage may be necessary. Information about other anticoagulants is lacking. One study suggests that the progestogen-only contraceptives may not affect the coagulability of the blood as much as the oestrogen/progestogen types, but whether this is reflected in an absence of an interaction with the oral anticoagulants is not documented.[3]

References

1 Schrogie JJ, Solomon HM and Zieve PD. Effect of oral contraceptives on vitamin K dependent clotting activity. Clin PharmacolTher (1967) 8, 670

2 de Teresa E, Vera A, Ortigosa J, Pulpon LA, Arus AP and de Artaza M. Interaction between anticoagulants and contraceptives: an unsuspected finding. Br Med J (1979) 2, 1260.

3 Poller L, Thomson JM, Tabiowo A and Priest CM. Progesterone oral contraception and blood coagulation. Br Med J (1969) 1, 554.

4 Beeley L, Stewart P and Hickey FM. Bull W Midlands Centre for Adverse Drug Reaction Reporting (1988) 27, 24.

Anticoagulants + Corticosteroids or ACTH

Abstract/Summary

Unpredictable but probably small changes (increases or decreases) in the effects of the oral anticoagulants may occur during concurrent treatment with corticosteroids or ACTH.

Clinical evidence

(a) Increased anticoagulant effects

10 out of 14 patients on long-term treatment with either dicoumarol or phenindione showed a small but definite increase in their anticoagulant responses when treated with ACTH for 4–9 days.[1]

A patient controlled on ethylbiscoumacetate began to bleed from the gut and urinary tract within three days of starting treatment with 20 mg ACTH daily.[4]

(b) Decreased anticoagulant effects

A study on 24 patients anticoagulated for several days with dicoumarol showed that 2 h after receiving 10 mg prednisone their silicone coagulation time had decreased from 28 to 24 min, and 2 h later was down to 22 min.[2]

A decrease in the anticoagulant effects of ethyl biscoumacetate is described in two patients given ACTH and cortisone.[3]

Mechanism

Not understood. Corticosteroids can increase the coagulability of the blood in the absence of anticoagulants.[5,6] Increased effects have been described in animals.[4]

Importance and management

Very poorly documented. An interaction is not established. Nothing of any consequence seems to have been reported in the last 20 years or so which suggests that any interaction is usually not very important. The most constructive thing that can be said is that if either ACTH or any corticosteroid is given to patients taking anticoagulants, the effects should be monitored. But it is impossible to predict whether any dosage adjustments will be upward or downward.

References

1 Hellem AJ and Solem JH. The influence of ACTH on prothrombin-proconvertin values in blood during treatment with dicumarol and phenylindandione. Acta Med Scand (1954) 150, 389.

2 Menczel J and Dreyfuss F. Effect of prednisone on blood coagulation time in patients on dicumarol therapy. J Lab Clin Med (1960) 56, 14.

3 Chatterjea JB and Salomon L. Antagonistic effects of ACTH and cortisone on the anticoagulant activity of ethylbiscoumacetate. Br Med J (1954) 2, 790.

4 van Cauwenberge H and Jacques LB. Haemorrhagic effects of ACTH with anticoagulants. Can Med Ass J (1958) 79, 536.

5 Cosgriff SW, Diefenbach AF and Vogt W. Hypercoagulability of the blood associated with ACTH and cortisone therapy. Amer J Med (1950) 9, 752.

6 Ozsoylu S, Strauss HS and Diamond LK. Effects of corticosteroids on coagulation of the blood. Nature (Lond) (1962) 195, 1214

Anticoagulants + Cytotoxic (antineoplastic) agents

Abstract/Summary

A number of single case reports describe an increase in the effects of warfarin, accompanied by bleeding, caused by the concurrent use of cytotoxic drug regimens containing cyclophosphamide, methotrexate, 5-FU, vincristine, vindesine, etoposide, doxorubicin, mustine (methchlorethamine) and procarbazine. A decrease in the effects of warfarin has been seen with regimens of cyclophosphamide, mercaptopurine and mitotane.

Clinical evidence

(a) Anticoagulant effects increased

A woman stabilized on warfarin developed an iliopsoas hematoma three weeks after starting treatment with cyclophosphamide, methotrexate, 5-FU, vincristine and prednisone.[1] The prothrombin times of two women on warfarin approximately doubled, accompanied by bleeding, on day 15 of each cycle of adjuvant treatment with CMF (cyclo-phosphamide, methotrexate and 5-FU).[2] An elderly man showed a marked increase in prothrombin times (prolonga-tion of 8–15 s) on two occasions when given 500 mg etoposide and 5 mg vindesine.[3] The prothrombin times of an elderly man given warfarin increased 50–100% in the middle of three cycles of treatment with *ProMace-Mopp* (cyclophosphamide, doxorubicin, etoposide, methchlor-ethamine, vincristine, procarbazine, methotrexate and pred-nisone), and he developed a subconjunctival haemorrhage during the first cycle.[3]

(b) Anticoagulant effects decreased

A man well stabilized on warfarin showed a marked reduc-tion in his anticoagulant response on two occasions when treated with mercaptopurine,[4] but no changes occured when given busulfan, cyclophosphamide, cytarabine or mephalan. A woman on warfarin showed a marked rise in prothrom-bin times when her treatment with cyclophosphamide was withdrawn.[5] The anticoagulant effects of warfarin were pro-gressively reduced in a woman while receiving mitotane.[8] Later this effect began to reverse.

Mechanisms, importance and management

Just why these responses occurred is not understood. It is not even possible in some cases to identify precisely the drug or drugs responsible. The absence of problems in studies using warfarin as an adjunct to chemotherapy[6,7] and the mere handful of reports describing difficulties suggest that these interactions are uncommon events. Concurrent use need not be avoided but there is clearly a need to monitor the effects of warfarin closely both during and after treatment with these and other cytotoxic agents to ensure that prothrombin times are well controlled.

References

1 Booth BW and Weiss RB. Venous thrombosis during adjuvant chemotherapy. N Engl J Med (1982) 305, 170.
2 Seifter EJ, Brooks BJ and Urbs WJ. Possible interactions between war-farin and antineoplastic drugs. Cancer Treat Rep (1985) 69, 244–5.
3 Ward K and Bitran JD. Warfarin, etoposide and vindesine interactions. Cancer Treat Rep (1984) 68, 817–18.
4 Spiers ASD and Misbashan RS. Increased warfarin requirement during mercaptopurine therapy: a new drug interaction. Lancet (1974) ii, 221.
5 Tashima CK. Cyclophosphamide effect on coumarin anticoagulation. South Med J (1979) 72, 633.
6 Zacharski LR, Henderson WG, Rickles FR, Forman WB, Cornell CJ, Forcier RJ, Edwards RL, Headley E, Kim S-E, O'Donnell JF, O'Dell R, Tornyos K and Kwaan HC. Effect of warfarin anticoagulation on sur-vival in carcinoma of the lung, colon, head and neck, and prostate. Cancer (1984) 53, 2046–52.
7 Ibid. Effect of warfarin on survival in small cell carcinoma of the lung. J Amer Med Ass (1981) 245, 831–5.
8 Cuddy PG and Loftus LS. Influence of mitotane on the hypo-prothrombinemic effect of warfarin. South Med J (1986) 79, 387–8.

Anticoagulants + Dextropropoxyphene

Abstract/Summary

Five patients on warfarin showed a marked increase in prothrombin times and/or bleeding when given Distalgesic *(dextropropoxyphene-paracetamol (acetaminophen)). Other patients on unnamed anticoagulants have been reported not to develop this interaction.*

Clinical evidence

A man on 6 mg warfarin daily showed marked haematuria within six days of starting to take two tablets of *Distalgesic* (dextropropoxyhene 32.5 mg, paracetamol (acetaminophen) 325 mg per tablet) three times a day. His plasma warfarin levels had risen by a third (from 1.8 to 2.4 μg/ml).[1] Another patient controlled for six weeks on warfarin showed gross haematuria within only 5 h of taking six tablets of *Distalgesic* over a 6 h period. Her prothrombin time increased from about 30/40 s to 130 s.[1]

This interaction has been seen in three other patients on war-farin.[2,4,7] The prothrombin time of one of them[4] rose from 28/44 to 80 s within three days of substituting paracetamol (acetaminophen) by two tablets of *Distalgesic* four times a day. Another developed a prothrombin time of more than 50 s after taking 30 tablets of *Darvocet-N* 100 (dextropropoxyphene 100 mg, paracetamol (acetaminophen) 650 mg) and possibly an unknown amount of ibuprofen over a 3-day period.[8] Death due to unknown causes in a patient on warfarin and dextropropoxyphene has also been reported.[3]

In contrast, a double-blind trial on 23 patients anticoagulated with un-named coumarol derivatives and given 450 mg dextropropoxyphene daily for 15 days failed to show any change in prothrombin times.[6]

Mechanism

Not understood. It seem possible that in man, as in animals,[5] dextropropoxyphene inhibits or competes with the liver enzymes concerned with the metabolic clearance of war-farin, thereby prolonging and increasing its effects. There is also the possibility that the paracetamol (acetaminophen) component of the *Distalgesic* and *Darvocet* had some part to play (see 'Anticoagulants + Paracetamol').

Importance and management

Information is very limited but what is known suggests that only a few patients are likely to develop this interaction. Con-current use need not be avoided but it would be prudent to monitor the effects closely, whether using warfarin or any other anticoagulant, because the occasional patient may show a marked interaction.

References

1 Orme M and Breckenridge A. Warfarin and Distalgesic interaction. Br Med J (1976) i, 200.
2 Jones RV. Warfarin and Distalgesic interaction. Br Med J (1976) i, 460.

3 Udall JA. Drug interference with warfarin therapy. Clin Med (1970) 77, 20.

4 Smith R, Pruden D and Hawkes C. Propoxyphene and warfarin interaction. Drug Intell Clin Pharm (1984) 18, 822.

5 Breckenridge A, Orme ML'E, Thorgeirsson S, Davies DS and Brooks RV. Drug interactions with warfarin: studies with dichloralphenazone, chloral hydrate and phenazone (antipyrine). Clin Sci (1971) 40, 351.

6 Franchimont P and Heden G. Comparative studies of ibuprofen and dextropropoxyphene in scapulo-humeral periarthritis following myocardial infarction. XIII Int Cong Rheumatol 30th Sept–6th Oct 1973, Kyoto, Japan.

7 Justice JL and Kline SS. Analgesics and warfarin. A case that brings up questions and cautions. Postgrad Med (1988) 83, 217.

Anticoagulants + Dichloralphenazone

Abstract/Summary

The anticoagulant effects of warfarin are reduced by the concurrent use of dichloralphenazone. It seems likely that other anticoagulants will interact similarly.

Clinical evidence

Five patients on long-term warfarin treatment showed an approximately 50% (20.2–68.5%) reduction in plasma warfarin levels, and a fall in the anticoagulant response, when given 1.3 g doses of dichloralphenazone each night for a fortnight. Another patient given the same doses nightly over a month showed a 70% fall in plasma warfarin levels and a thrombotest percentage rise from 9 to 55%. These values returned to normal when the hypnotic was withdrawn.[2]

Similar results have been described in other reports.[1,3]

Mechanism

The phenazone (antipyrine) component of the hypnotic is a potent liver enzyme inducing agent which increases the metabolism and clearance of the warfarin, thereby reducing its effects.[2,3] The effects of the chloral appear to be minimal, (see 'Anticoagulants + Chloral hydrate').

Importance and management

Information is limited, but it appears to be an established and clinically important interaction. It would seem to affect most patients. The dosage of warfarin will need to be increased to accommodate this interaction. Dichloralphenazone is therefore an inconvenient hypnotic for patients on warfarin and probably any other oral anticoagulant. Non-interacting alternatives for dichloralphenazone may be found among the benzodiazepines (see 'Anticoagulants + Benzodiazepines'). If the dosage of warfarin has been disturbed by using dichloralphenazone, it may take up to a month for it to restabilize.

References

1 Breckenridge A, Orme ML'E, Davies DS, Thorgeirsson S and Dollery CT. Induction of drug metabolising enzymes in man and rat by dichloralphenazone. 4th Int Congr Pharmacol(1969) Basel.

2 Breckenridge A, Orme ML'E, Thorgeirrson S, Davies DS and Brooks RV. Drug interaction with warfarin: studies with dichloralphenazone, chloral hydrate and phenazone (antipyrine). Clin Sci (1971) 40, 351.

3 Breckenridge A and Orme M. Clinical implications of enzyme induction. NY Acad Sci (1971) 179, 421.

Anticoagulants + Diflunisal

Abstract/Summary

There is some limited evidence that diflunisal can increase the anticoagulant effects of nicoumalone (acenocoumarol) and possibly warfarin, but phenprocoumon appears not to be affected. Prothrombin times should be checked if diflunisal is given to patients taking any anticoagulant, and when the diflunisal is withdrawn.

Clinical evidence

Five normal subjects were given subtherapeutic doses of warfarin. When given 500 mg diflunisal daily for two weeks their serum warfarin levels fell by about one third (from 741 to 533 ng/ml) but the anticoagulant response was unaffected. When the diflunisal was withdrawn, the serum warfarin levels rose once more while the anticoagulant response fell.[1]

A brief report states that three out of six subjects on nicoumalone experienced significant increases in prothrombin times when given 750 mg diflunisal daily, but no interaction was seen in two subjects on phenprocoumon.[3]

Mechanism

Uncertain. Diflunisal can displace warfarin from its plasma protein binding sites[1] but this on its own is almost certainly not the full explanation.

Importance and management

This interaction is neither well defined nor well documented. Its importance is uncertain. However the reports cited and the manufacturers literature indicate that an increased anticoagulant effect should be looked for if diflunisal is added to established treatment with any anticoagulant. A decreased effect would be expected if diflunisal is withdrawn. Phenprocoumon is possibly an exception and appears not to interact. The risk of bleeding (because of changes in platelet activity or gastrointestinal irritation) appears to be less than with aspirin.[2]

References

1 Serlin MJ, Mossman S, Sibeon RG, Tempero KF and Breckenridge AM. Interaction between diflunisal and warfarin. Clin PharmacolTher (1980) 28, 493.

2 Tempero KF, Cirillo VJ and Steelman SL. Diflunisal: a review of pharmacokinetic and pharmacodynamic properties, drug interactions, and special tolerability studies in humans. Br J clin Pharmac (1977) 4, 31S.

3 Caruso I et al. Unpublished observations quoted in ref. 2.

Anticoagulants + Dipyridamole

Abstract/Summary

Mild bleeding can sometimes occur when anticoagulants and dipyridamole are used concurrently even though prothrombin times remain stable and well within the therapeutic range.

Clinical evidence

30 patients stabilized on either warfarin (28 patients) or phenindione (two patients) showed no significant changes in prothrombin times when given dipyridamole in doses up to 400 mg daily for a month, but three patients developed mild bleeding (epistaxis, bruising, haematuria) which resolved when either drug was withdrawn or the dosage reduced.[1]

Two other reports state that prothrombin ratios remain unaltered when dipyridamole is given with warfarin, and claim that there is no risk of bleeding.[2,3]

Mechanism

Uncertain. A reduction in platelet adhesiveness or aggregation induced by the dipyridamole may have been responsible.[1]

Importance and management

Information seems to be very limited. However since bleeding can sometimes occur even when prothrombin values are within the therapeutic range, some caution is appropriate. The authors of the study cited[1] suggest that prothrombin activity should be maintained at the upper end of the therapeutic range as a precaution. Only warfarin and phenindione have been implicated, but it would be sensible to apply the same precautions with any anticoagulant.

References

1 Kalowski S and Kincaid-Smith P. Interaction of dipyridamole with anticoagulants in the treatment of glomerulonephritis. Med J Aust (1973) 2, 164.
2 Rajah SM, Sreeharan N, Rao S and Watson D. Warfarin versus warfarin plus dipyridamole on the incidence of arterial thromboembolism in prosthetic heart valve patients. VII Int Cong Thromb Haem London (1979) Abstr 379.
3 Donaldson DR, Sreeharan N, Crow MJ and Rajahs SM. Assessment of the interaction of warfarin with aspirin and dipyridamole. Thromb Haemostas (Stuttgart) (1982) 47, 77.

Anticoagulants + Dipyrone

Abstract/Summary

One report claims that no interaction occurs with phenprocoumon or ethylbiscoumacetate, whereas another describes a rapid but transient increase in the effects of ethylbiscoumacetate.

Clinical evidence, mechanism, importance and management

A study in 11 normal subjects showed that the concurrent use of 1 g dipyrone daily did not alter the anticoagulant effects of either phenprocoumon (five subjects) or ethylbiscoumacetate (six subjects).[1] Another report describes a short-lived but rapid (within 4 h) increase in the effects of ethylbiscoumacetate caused by dipyrone.[2] The reasons are not understood. Monitor the effects if concurrent use is thought appropriate. Dipyrone causes serious blood dyscrasias including agranulocytosis so that its use is very questionable indeed.

References

1 Badian M, Le Normand Y, Rupp W and Zapf R. There is no interaction between dipyrone (metamizol) and the anticoagulants, phenprocoumon and ethylbiscoumacetate, in normal caucasian subjects. Int J Pharmaceut (1984) 18, 9–15.
2 Mehvar SR and Jamali F. Dipyrone-ethylbiscoumacetate interaction in man. Ind J Pharm (1981) 7, 293–9.

Anticoagulants + Disopyramide

Abstract/Summary

The anticoagulant effects of warfarin are reduced to some extent by disopyramide in many patients, but there are two reports of patients who needed less warfarin while taking disopyramide.

Clinical evidence

(a) Reduced warfarin effects

A study in 10 patients with recent atrial fibrillation scheduled for electroconversion, maintained on warfarin and with a British Corrected Ratio of 2–3, showed that disopyramide increased the clearance of warfarin by 21% (from 166.3 to 201.1 ml/h).[5] In another study it was found that two out of three patients needed a warfarin dosage increase of about 10% when concurrently treated with disopyramide (600 mg daily) for atrial fibrillation.[2]

(b) Increased warfarin effects

A report describes a patient who following a myocardial infarction was given 3 mg warfarin daily and 100 mg disopyramide six-hourly with digoxin, frusemide and potassium supplements. When the disopyramide was withdrawn his warfarin requirements doubled over a nine-day period.[1] An increased response to warfarin in the presence of disopyramide has been seen in another patient.[4]

Mechanism

Unknown. One idea is that when the disopyramide controls fibrillation, changes occur in cardiac output and in the flow of blood through the liver. This might have an effect on the synthesis of the blood clotting factors.[2,3] But the discordant response in the two patients remains unexplained.

Importance and management

Very poorly documented and not established. The outcome of concurrent use is uncertain. It would be prudent to monitor the effects of any anticoagulant if disopyramide is given or withdrawn, and appropriate dosage adjustments made if necessary.

References

1 Haworth E and Burroughs AK. Disopyramide and warfarin interaction. Br Med J (1977) 2, 866.
2 Sylven C and Anderson P. Evidence that disopyramide does not interact with warfarin. Br Med J (1983) 286, 1181.
3 Ryll C and Davis LJ. Warfarin-disopyramide interactions. Drug Intell Clin Pharm (1979) 13, 260.
4 Marshall J. Personal communication 1987.
5 Woo KS, Chan K and Pun CO. The mechanisms of warfarin-disopyramide. Circulation (1987) 76, Suppl IV-520.

Anticoagulants + Disulfiram

Abstract/Summary

The anticoagulant effects of warfarin are increased by disulfiram and bleeding can occur if the anticoagulant dosage is not reduced appropriately. Bad breath smelling of bad eggs has also been described during concurrent treatment.

Clinical evidence

Haemorrhage in a patient given warfarin and disulfiram prompted study of this interaction.[1] Eight normal subjects anticoagulated with warfarin were given 500 mg disulfiram daily for 21 days. The plasma warfarin levels of seven of them rose by an average of 20% and their prothrombin activity fell by about 10%.

Other experiments with single doses of warfarin confirm these results,[2-4] and the interaction has been described in other reports.[5,6] Bad breath reminiscent of the smell of bad eggs has also been described in patients taking warfarin and disulfiram.[6]

Mechanism

Not fully understood. The suggestion[2-4] that disulfiram inhibits the liver enzymes concerned with the metabolism of warfarin has not been confirmed by later studies.[7] It is now postulated[7] that disulfiram may chelate with the metal ions necessary for the production of active thrombin from prothrombin, thereby augmenting the actions of warfarin.

Importance and management

An established interaction, although direct information about patients is very limited. What is known suggests that most individuals will demonstrate this interaction. If concurrent use is thought appropriate, the effects of warfarin or any other anticoagulant should be monitored and suitable dosage adjustments made when adding or withdrawing disulfiram.

Patients already on disulfiram should be started on a small dose of anticoagulant.

References

1 Rothstein E. Warfarin effect enhanced by disulfiram. J Amer Med Ass (1968) 206, 1574.
2 O'Reilly RA. Interaction of sodium warfarin and disulfiram. Ann Int Med (1973) 78, 73.
3 O'Reilly RA. Potentiation of anticoagulant effect by disulfiram. Clin Res (1971) 19, 180.
4 O'Reilly RA. Interaction of warfarin and disulfiram in man. Fed Proc (1972) 31, 248.
5 Rothstein E. Warfarin effect enhanced by disulfiram (Antabuse). J Amer Med Ass (1972) 221, 1051.
6 O'Reilly RA and Mothley CH. Breath odor after disulfiram. J Amer Med Ass (1977) 238, 2600.
7 O'Reilly RA. Dynamic interaction between disulfiram and separated enantiomorphs of racemic warfarin. Clin PharmacolTher (1981) 29, 332.

Anticoagulants + Ditazole

Abstract/Summary

Ditazole does not alter the anticoagulant effects of nicoumalone.

Clinical evidence, mechanism, importance and management

50 patients with artificial heart valves taking nicoumalone (acenocoumarol) showed no changes in their prothrombin times while taking 800 mg ditazole daily.[1] There seems to be no information about other anticoagulants.

Reference

1 Jacovella G and Milazzotto F. Ricerca di interazioni fra ditazolo e anticoagulanti in portatori di protesi valvolari intracardache. Clinica Terapeutica (1977) 80, 425.

Anticoagulants + Diuretics

Abstract/Summary

The anticoagulant effects of warfarin are not affected by the concurrent use of bumetanide, frusemide or chlorothiazide. A small reduction in the effects of warfarin, clorindione and phenprocoumon, but not of nicoumalone, occurs with chlorthalidone. Spironolactone reduces the effects of warfarin similarly. On rare occasions a marked increase has been seen with ethacrynic acid. In contrast the anticoagulant effects of ethylbiscoumacetate, nicoumalone and warfarin can be increased by tienilic acid (ticrynafen). Bleeding may occur.

Clinical evidence

(a) Nicoumalone, phenprocoumon or warfarin + chlorthalidone

Six normal subjects given single 1.5 mg/kg doses of warfarin showed reduced hypoprothrombinaemia (from 77 to 58 u) when also given 100 mg chlorthalidone daily, although the plasma warfarin levels remained unaltered.[3] Similarly reduced anticoagulant effects have been described with phenprocoumon, and clorindione but no significant effects were seen on the activity of nicoumalone.[4]

(b) Warfarin + frusemide or bumetanide

A study in 10 normal subjects showed that their response to single 0.8 mg/kg doses of warfarin were unaffected by taking 1 mg bumetanide daily for 14 days.[1] This confirms a previous study in 11 normal subjects given 2 mg daily.[2] A study on six normal subjects showed that warfarin plasma levels, half-lives and prothrombin times in response to a 50 mg oral dose were not significantly altered by the presence of frusemide (80 mg daily).[2]

(c) Warfarin + ethacrynic acid

A case report describes a marked increase in the anti-coagulant effects of warfarin in a woman on two occasions when administered doses of ethacrynic acid ranging from 50 to 300 mg. She had hypoalbuminaemia.[5] A therapeutically significant interaction between warfarin and ethacrynic acid is reported elsewhere, but no details are given.[6]

(d) Warfarin + spironolactone

A study in nine subjects given single 1.5 mg/kg doses of warfarin showed that the concurrent use of 200 mg spironolactone reduced the prothrombin time (expressed as a percentage of the control activity with warfarin alone) from 100 to 76%. Plasma warfarin levels remained unchanged.[8]

(e) Warfarin + thiazides

A study on eight normal subjects given single 40–60 mg oral doses of warfarin and 1 g chlorothiazide daily showed that the mean half-life of the anticoagulant was increased slightly (from 39 to 44 h) but the prothrombin time was barely affected (from 18.9 to 18.6 s).[7]

(f) Ethylbiscoumacetate, nicoumalone and warfarin + tienilic acid

Two patients taking ethylbiscoumacetate began to bleed spontaneously (haematuria, ecchymoses of the legs and gastrointestinal bleeding) when they started to take 250 mg tienilic acid daily. The thrombotest percentage of one of them was found to have fallen below 10%.[10] Increased anti-coagulant effects and/or bleeding, beginning within a few days, have been described in patients or subjects given tienilic acid while taking ethylbiscoumacetate,[10,16] nicoumalone (acenocoumarol)[11,12] or warfarin.[14,16,17]

Mechanism

It has been suggested that the diuresis induced by chlorthalidone and spironolactone reduces plasma water which leads to a concentration of the blood clotting factors.[3,8] Ethacrynic acid can displace warfarin from its plasma protein binding sites,[9] but it is almost certain that this, on its own, does not explain the marked interaction described.[5,6] Tienilic acid reduces the metabolism of S-warfarin (but not R-warfarin) thereby prolonging its stay in the body and increasing its effects.[17] It was originally thought that this was a drug displacement interaction.[10,13,15]

Importance and management

The documentation relating to diuretics other than tienilic acid is very limited indeed and seems to be confined to the reports cited, most of which were single dose studies. This evidence suggests that most of these diuretics either do not interact with the anticoagulants at all, or they do so only to a small extent. This is in general agreement with common experience. Prothrombin times should be monitored if chlorthalidone or spironolactone are started or withdrawn, and anticoagulant dosages adjusted if necessary. Somewhat greater caution should be exercised with ethacrynic acid. Information about other anticoagulants is lacking.

The anticoagulant-tienilic acid interaction is established and of clinical importance. The incidence is uncertain. Concurrent use should be avoided. If that is not possible, prothrombin times should be closely monitored and the anticoagulant dosage reduced as necessary. There seems to be no information about other anticoagulants but it would be prudent to assume that they will interact similarly. Tienilic acid has been withdrawn in many countries because of its hepatotoxicity.

References

1 Nipper H, Kirby S and Iber FL. The effect of bumetanide on the serum disappearance of warfarin sodium. J Clin Pharmacol (1981) 21, 654–6.
2 Nilsson CM, Horton ES and Robinson DS. The effect of furosemide and bumetanide on warfarin metabolism and anticoagulant response. J Clin Pharmacol (1978) 18, 91.
3 O'Reilly RA, Sahud MA and Aggeler PM. Impact of aspirin and chlorthalidone on the pharmacodynamics of oral anticoagulant drugs in man. Ann NY Acad Sci (1971) 179, 173.
4 Vinazzer H. Die Beeinflussungen der Antikoagulantientherapie durch ein Diuretikum. Wien Z Inn Med Ihre Grenzge (1963) 44, 323.
5 Petrick RJ, Kronacher N and Alcena V. Interaction between warfarin and ethacrynic acid. J Amer Med Ass (1975) 231, 843–4.
6 Koch-Weser J. Hemorrhagic reactions and drug interactions in 500 warfarin-treated patients. Clin Pharmacol Ther (1973) 14, 139.
7 Robinson DS and Sylwester D. Interaction of commonly prescribed drugs and warfarin. Ann Int Med (1970) 72, 853.
8 O'Reilly RA. Spironolactone and warfarin interaction. Clin Pharmacol Ther (1980) 27, 198.
9 Sellers EM and Koch-Wester J. Kinetics and clinical importance of displacement of warfarin from albumin by acidic drugs. Ann NY Acad Sci (1971) 179, 213–25.
10 Detilleux M, Caquet R and Laroche C. Potentialisation de l'effet des anticoagulantes comariniques par un nouveaux diuretique, l'acide tienilique. Nouv Presse med (1976) 36, 2395.
11 Portier H, Destaing F and Chavve L. Potentialisation de l'effet des anti-coagulantes coumariniques par l'acide tienilique: un nouvelle observation. Nouv Presse med (1977) 6, 468.

12 Grand A, Drouin B and Arche GJ. Potentialisation de l'action anti-
    coagulante des antivitamines K par l'acide tienilique. Nouv Presse med
    (1977) 6, 2691.
13 Slattery JT and Levy G. Ticrynafen effect on warfarin protein binding
    in human serum. J Pharm Sci (1979) 68, 393.
14 McLain DA, Garriga FJ and Kantor OS. Adverse reactions associated
    with ticrynafen use. J Amer Med Ass (1980) 243, 763.
15 Prandota J, Albengres E and Tillement JP. Effect of tienilic acid
    (Diflurex) on the binding of warfarin ^{14}C to human plasma proteins.
    Int J Clin Pharmacol Ther Toxicol (1980) 18, 158.
16 Prandota J and Pankow-Prandota L. Klinicznie znamienna interakcja
    nowego leku moczopednego kwasu tienylowego z lekami
    przeciwzakrzepowymi pochodnymi kumaryny. Przeglad Lek (1982) 39,
    385–8.
17 O'Reilly RA. Ticrynafen-racemic warfarin interaction: hepatotoxic or
    stereoselective? Clin Pharmacol Ther (1982) 32, 356–61.

Anticoagulants + Erythromycin

Abstract/Summary

*A marked increase in the effects of warfarin with bleeding has
been seen in a small number of patients when concurrently
treated with erythromycin, but most patients are unlikely to
develop a clinically important interaction. This interaction has
also been seen in a patient on nicoumalone (acenocoumarol).*

Clinical evidence

(a) Warfarin

A case report describes an elderly woman on warfarin,
digoxin, hydrochlorothiazide and quinidine who developed
haematuria and bruising within a week of starting to take 2 g
erythromycin stearate daily. Her prothrombin time had risen
to 64 s.[1]

Seven other cases of bleeding and/or hypoprothrombinaemia
have been described[2–8] in patients on warfarin when given
erythromycin (as ethylsuccinate, stearate, estolate, lactobionate or base). A study in 12 normal subjects showed that
the clearance of a single dose of warfarin was reduced by an
average of 14% (range zero to almost one third) after taking
1 g erythromycin daily for eight days.[9] In another study on
eight patients erythromycin caused only a small increase in
the effects of warfarin.[11,12]

(b) Nicoumalone (acenocoumarol)

Haemorrhage occurred in a patient on nicoumalone when
treated with erythromycin.[10]

Mechanism

It is believed that erythromycin can stimulate the liver enzymes to produce metabolites which bind to cytochrome P450
to form inactive complexes, the result being that the metabolism of warfarin is reduced and its effects are thereby increased.[9] But why it only happens in a few individuals is
not clear.

Importance and management

An established interaction, but unpredictable. The incidence
is uncertain but the paucity of reports suggests that it is low.
The effect in a few patients is evidently considerable but in
most it is likely to be small and unimportant. Concurrent use
need not be avoided but it would be prudent to monitor the
effects, especially in those who clear warfarin slowly and who
therefore only need low doses. The elderly in particular
would seem to fall into this higher risk category. Information
about anticoagulants other than warfarin and nicoumalone
seems not to be available but the same precautions would be
advisable.

References

1 Bartle WR. Possible warfarin-erythromycin interaction. Arch Intern
   Med (1980) 140, 985.
2 Schwartz JI and Bachmann K. Erythromycin-warfarin interaction. Arch
   Intern Med (1984) 144, 2094.
3 Husserl FE. Erythromycin-warfarin interaction. Arch Intern Med (1983)
   143, 1831–2.
4 Sato RI, Gray DR and Brown SE. Warfarin interaction with
   erythromycin. Arch Intern Med (1984) 144, 2413–4.
5 Friedman HS and Bonventre MV. Erythromycin-induced digoxin toxicity. Chest (1982) 82, 202.
6 Hansten PD and Horn JR. Erythromycin and warfarin. Drug Interactions Newsletter (1985) 5, 37–40.
7 Hassell D and Utt JK. Suspected interaction: warfarin and
   erythromycin. South Med J (1985) 78, 1015–16.
8 Bussey HI, Knodel LC and Boyle DA. Warfarin-erythromycin interaction. Arch Intern Med (1985) 145, 1736–7.
9 Bachmann K, Schwartz JI, Forney R, Frogameni A and Jauregui LE.
   The effect of erythromycin on the disposition kinetics of warfarin.
   Pharmacology (1984) 28, 171–6.
10 Grau E, Fontenberta J and Felez J. Erythromycin-oral anticoagulants
   interaction. Arch Intern Med (1986) 146, 1639.
11 Weibert RT. Effect of erythromycin in patients receiving long term warfarin therapy. Clin Pharmacol Ther (1987) 41, 224.
12 Weibert RT, Lorentz SM, Townsend RJ, Cook CE, Klauber MR and
   Jagger PI. Effect of erythromycin on patients receiving long-term warfarin. Clin Pharmacy (1989) 8, 210–14.

Anticoagulants + Ethchlorvynol

Abstract/Summary

*The anticoagulant effects of dicoumarol and warfarin (probably
other anticoagulants as well) are reduced by the concurrent use
of ethchlorvynol.*

Clinical evidence

Six patients on dicoumarol showed a rise in their Quick index
from 38 to 55% while taking 1 g ethchlorvynol daily over an
18-day period. Another patient on dicoumarol became over-
anticoagulated and developed haematuria on two occasions
when the ethchlorvynol was withdrawn, once for six days
and the other for four days.[1]

A marked reduction in the anticoagulant effects of warfarin
occurred in another patient when given ethchlorvynol.[2]

Mechanism

Uncertain. The idea that ethchlorvynol increases the metabolism of the anticoagulants by the liver is not confirmed by studies in dogs and rats.[3]

Importance and management

Information is very sparse, but the interaction seems to be established. Anticipate the need to increase the anticoagulant dosage if ethchlorvynol is started. Reduce the anticoagulant dosage if it is stopped. An alternative non-interacting substitute may be found among the benzodiazepines.

References

1 Cullen SI and Catalano PM. Griseofulvin-warfarin antagonism. J Amer Med Ass (1967) 199, 582.
2 Johansson SA. Apparent resistance to oral anticoagulant therapy and influence of hypnotics on some coagulation factors. Acta med Scand (1968) 184, 297.
3 Martin YC. The effect of ethchlorvynol on the drug-metabolising enzymes of rats and dogs. Biochem Pharmacol (1967) 16, 2041.

Anticoagulants + Fenofibrate (Procetofene)

Abstract/Summary

The anticoagulant effects of nicoumalone (acenocoumarol) are increased by fenofibrate and bleeding may occur unless the anticoagulant dosage is reduced by about one-third. Other anticoagulants probably behave similarly.

Clinical evidence and mechanism

Two patients on nicoumalone needed a 30% reduction in their dosage to maintain the same prothrombin time when given 200 mg fenofibrate in the morning and 100 mg in the evening.[1] Six patients taking coumarin anticoagulants (not specifically named) needed an average dosage reduction of 12% (range 0–21%) when treated with fenofibrate.[2] In another study it was found that fenofibrate increased the effects of un-named anticoagulants in four patients by the same amount as that seen with clofibrate (i.e. by about one-third).[4] A patient on an un-named anticoagulant developed haematuria when treated with fenofibrate.[3] The reasons are not understood.

Importance and management

Information seems to be limited to the reports cited but it would appear to be an established and clinically important interaction. Monitor the effects of concurrent use and anticipate the need to reduce the anticoagulant dosage by about a third. Only nicoumalone is specifically named in the reports but expect all the oral anticoagulants to behave similarly.

References

1 Harvengt C, Heller F and Desager JP. Hypolipidemic and hypouricemic action of fenofibrate in various types of hyperlipoproteinemias. Artery (1980) 7, 73–82.
2 Stahelin HB, Seiler W and Pult N. Erfahrungen mit dem Lipidsenker Procetofen (Lipanthyl). Schweiz Rundschau Med (Praxis) (1979) 68, 24–8.
3 Lauwers PL. Effect of procetofene on blood lipids of subjects with essential hyperlipidaemia. Curr Ther Res (1979) 26, 30–8.
4 Raynaud Ph. Un nouvel hypolipidemiant: le procetofene. Revue de Medecine de Tours (1977) 11, 325–30.

Anticoagulants + Feprazone

Abstract/Summary

The anticoagulant effects of warfarin are increased by feprazone which can lead to bleeding.

Clinical evidence

A study on five patients on long-term warfarin treatment showed that after five days treatment with 300 mg feprazone daily, their mean prothrombin time rose from 29 to 38 s, despite a 40% reduction in their warfarin dosage (from 5 to 3 mg daily). Four days after withdrawal of the feprazone, their prothrombin times were almost back to pretreatment levels.[1]

Mechanism

Unknown. Feprazone is highly bound to plasma proteins, so that some of the interaction may be due to displacement from plasma protein binding sites. But this is certainly not the whole story.

Importance and management

Although information is limited to the study quoted, the interaction would appear to be established. Concurrent use should be avoided to prevent bleeding. If that is not possible, the anticoagulant response should be closely monitored and suitable reductions made to the warfarin dosage. Other anticoagulants may be expected to behave similarly.

Reference

1 Chierichetti S, Bianchi G and Cerri B. Comparison of feprazone and phenylbutazone interaction with warfarin in man. Curr Ther Res (1975) 18, 568.

Anticoagulants + Floctafenine or Glafenine

Abstract/Summary

The anticoagulant effects of nicoumalone (acenocoumarol) and phenprocoumon are increased by floctafenine. The anticoagulant effects of phenprocoumon are increased by glafenine but no interaction occurs with nicoumalone (acenocoumarol), ethylbiscoumacetate or 'indanedione'.

Clinical evidence, mechanism, importance and management

(a) Glafenine

A double-blind study on 20 patients stabilized on phenprocoumon showed that a significant increase in thrombotest times occurred within a week of starting to take 600 mg glafenine daily.[2] Another report states that five out of seven patients needed an anticoagulant dosage reduction while taking glafenine.[3] The reason is not understood. Monitor the effects of concurrent use and reduce the anticoagulant dosage appropriately. 10 subjects on nicoumalone (acenocoumarol), ethylbiscoumacetate or 'indanedione' showed no changes in their anticoagulant response when given 800 mg glafenine daily over a four-week period.[4]

(b) Floctafenine

A double-blind study[1] on 10 patients on nicoumalone (acenocoumarol) or phenprocoumon showed that concurrent treatment with 800 mg floctafenine daily prolonged their Thrombotest times by an average of approximately one-third. The anticoagulant dosage of some of the patients was reduced. The reasons are not understood. The effects of concurrent use should be monitored and the anticoagulant dosage reduced as necessary. Information about other anticoagulants is lacking, but the same precautions would seem to be appropriate.

References

1 Boejinga JK, van de Broeke RN, Jochemsen R, Breimer DD, Hoogslag MA and Jeleticka-Bastiaanse A. De invloed van floctafenine (Idalon) op antistollingsbehandeling met coumarinederivaten. Ned T Geneesk (1981) 125, 1931–5.
2 Boejinga JK and van der Vijgh WJF. Double blind study of the effect of glafenine (Glifanan) on oral anticoagulant therapy with phenprocoumon (Marcumar). Europ J clin Pharmacol (1977) 12, 291.
3 Boejinga JK, Gan TB and van der Meer J. De invloed van glafenine (Glifanan) op antistollingsbehandeling met coumarinederivaten. Ned T Geneesk (1974) 118, 1895.
4 Raby C. Recherches sur une eventuelle potentialisation de l'action des anticoagulants de synthese par la glafenine. Therapie (1977) 32, 293.

Anticoagulants + Flutamide

Abstract/Summary

Flutamide can increase the anticoagulant effects of warfarin.

Clinical evidence

Five patients with prostatic cancer and taking warfarin showed increases in their prothrombin times when given flutamide. For example one patient needed reductions in his warfarin dosage from 35 to 22.5 mg weekly over a two month period. Another showed a prothombin time rise from 15 to 37 s within four days of starting 750 mg flutamide daily.[1]

Mechanism

Not understood. Flutamide sometimes causes liver dysfunction.

Importance and management

Information is very limited but the interaction would seem to be established. Monitor prothrombin times if flutamide is given to patients on warfarin, reducing the dosage when necessary. Nothing seems to be known about the effects on other anticoagulants but follow the same precautions.

Reference

1 Chandler R (Schering-Plough). Reports on Company files. Personal communication (1990).

Anticoagulants + Food

Abstract/Summary

The rate of absorption of dicoumarol can be increased by food. Two reports describe antagonism of the effects of warfarin by ice-cream, and another attributes an increase in prothrombin time to the use of aspartame. Soy protein may reduce the effects of warfarin.

Clinical evidence

(a) Dicoumarol

A study with 10 normal subjects showed that the peak serum concentrations of dicoumarol, following a single 250 mg dose, were increased on average by 85% when taken with food. Two subjects showed increases of 242 and 206%.[1]

(b) Warfarin

A woman taking 22.5 mg warfarin in single daily doses failed to show the expected prolongation of her prothrombin times. It was then discovered that she took the warfarin in the evening and she always ate ice-cream before going to bed. When the warfarin was taken in the mornings, the prothrombin times increased.[2] Another patient's warfarin requirements almost doubled when she started to eat very large quantites of ice cream (1 litre each evening) but not while taking normal amounts. She took the warfarin at 6 pm and the ice cream at about 10 pm.[5] Another very brief report states that a patient on warfarin showed a raised prothrombin time, possibly due to the use of aspartame.[3] A study in 10 patients with hypercholesterolaemia found that two weeks' treatment with a soy-protein cholesterol-lowering diet caused a marked reduction (Quick time increase of 114%) in the anticoagulant effects of warfarin.[4]

Mechanism

Uncertain. One suggestion for the dicoumarol/food reaction[1] is that prolonged retention of dicoumarol with food in the upper part of the gut, associated with increased tablet dissolution, may have been responsible for the increased absorption. Soy protein possibly increases the activity of vitamin K at its liver receptors, thereby reducing the effects of warfarin.

Importance and management

None of these interactions is well documented, however they clearly demonstrate that food can sometimes affect the response to the oral anticoagulants, and may account for otherwise unexplained fluctuations or changes in the anticoagulant response which some patients show. Patients on warfarin who are given soy protein should be well monitored.

References

1 Melander A and Wahlin E. Enhancement of dicoumarol bioavailability by concomitant food intake. Europ J Clin Pharmacol (1978) 14, 441.
2 Simon LS and Likes KE. Hypoprothrombinaemic response due to ice-cream. Drug Intell Clin Pharm (1978) 12, 121.
3 Beeley L, Beadle F and Lawrence R (eds). Bulletin of the West Midlands Centre for Adverse Drug Reaction Reporting, Birmingham, England. (1974) 19, 9.
4 Gaddi A, Sangiorigi Z, Ciarrocchi A, Braiato A and Descovich GC. Hypocholesterolemic soy protein diet and resistance to warfarin therapy. Curr Ther Res (1989) 45, 1006–10.
5 Blackshaw C A and Watson V A. Interaction between warfarin and ice cream. Pharm J (1990) 244, 318.

Anticoagulants + Glucagon

Abstract/Summary

The anticoagulant effects of warfarin are rapidly and markedly increased by glucagon in large doses (50 mg or more over two days) and bleeding can occur if the warfarin dosage is not reduced appropriately.

Clinical evidence

Eight out of nine patients on warfarin showed a marked increase in the anticoagulant effects (prothrombin times of 30–50 s or more) when given 50 mg glucagon over two days. Three of them bled. Eleven other patients given a total of 30 mg glucagon over 1–2 days failed to show this interaction.[1]

Mechanism

Unknown. Changes in the production of blood clotting factors and an increase in the affinity of warfarin for its site of action have been proposed.[1] A study in guinea pigs using acenocoumarol suggested that changes in the metabolism of the warfarin or its absorption from the gut are not responsible.[2]

Importance and management

This appears to be an established interaction of clinical importance, although direct information is limited to the report cited.[1] Its authors recommend that if 25 mg glucagon per day or more is given for two or more days, the dosage of warfarin should be reduced in anticipation and prothrombin times closely monitored. Smaller doses (total 30 mg) are reported not to interact.[1]

Information about other anticoagulants is lacking, but it would be prudent to assume that they will interact similarly.

References

1 Koch-Weser J. Potentiation by glucagon of the hypoprothrombinemic action of warfarin. Ann Intern Med (1970) 72, 331.
2 Weiner M and Moses D. The effect of glucagon and insulin on the prothrombin response to coumarin anticoagulants. Proc Soc Biol Med (1968) 127, 761.

Anticoagulants + Glutethimide

Abstract/Summary

The anticoagulant effects of warfarin and dicoumarol are decreased by the concurrent use of glutethimide in many but not all patients.

Clinical evidence

A study on 10 subjects taking warfarin, with prothrombin times of 18–22 s, showed that after taking 500 mg glutethimide daily for four weeks their prothrombin times were reduced by an average of 4 s.[5,6]

Other studies have shown that after taking 1 g glutethimide daily for three weeks the half-life of warfarin is reduced by a third to a half.[1,4] 750 mg glutethimide daily for 10 days can reduce the half-life of dicoumarol by about a third.[2,3]

In contrast, an early study on 25 patients found no evidence of an interaction with dicoumarol.[7] Yet another report describes an *increase* in prothrombin times and haemorrhage in a patient on warfarin after taking 3.5 g glutethimide over a five-day period.[8]

Mechanism

Glutethimide is a liver enzyme inducing agent which increases the metabolism and clearance of the anticoagulants from the body, thereby reducing their effects.[1–6] There is no obvious explanation for the reports of 'no interaction'[7] and of an 'increased effect'[8] cited above.

Importance and management

An established interaction. The incidence is uncertain, but in one study[1] 40% of the subjects failed to show the interaction, and in another[6] one out of 10 did not. The importance of this interaction is uncertain but if concurrent treatment is started, the anticoagulant effects should be monitored and the anticoagulant dosage increased as necessary. The effects of the interaction can appear within a few days and persist for up to three weeks or more after the glutethimide has been withdrawn.[4] Information about anticoagulants other than warfarin and dicoumarol is lacking, but it would be prudent to assume that they will interact similarly. A non-interacting substitute for glutethimide may be found among the benzodiazepines.

References

1 Corn M. Effect of phenobarbital and glutethimide on the biological half-life of warfarin. Thromb Diath Haemorrh (1966) 16, 606.
2 van Dam, FE and Overkamp MJH. The effect of some sedatives (phenobarbital, glutethimide, chlordiazepoxide, chloral hydrate) on the rate of disappearance of ethylbiscoumacetate from the plasma. Folia medica Neerlandica (1967) 10, 141.
3 van Dam FE, Overkamp M and Haanen C. The interaction of drugs. Lancet (1966) ii, 1027.
4 Macdonald MG, Robinson DS, Sylwester D and Jaffe JJ. The effects of phenobarbital, chloral betaine and glutethimide administration on warfarin plasma levels and hypoprothrombinaemic responses in man. Clin Pharmacol Ther (1969) 10, 80.
5 Udall JA. Clinical implications of warfarin interactions with five sedatives. Amer J Cardiol (1975) 35, 67.
6 Udall JA. Warfarin interactions with chloral hydrate and glutethimide. Curr Ther Res (1975) 17, 67.
7 Grilli H. Glutethimide y tiempo de prothrombina. Su aplicion en la terapeutica anticoagulante. Pren med argent (1959) 46, 2867.
8 Taylor PJ. Haemorrhage while on anticoagulant therapy precipitated by drug interaction. Arizona Med (1967) 24, 697.
9 Hunningshake DB and Azarnoff DL. Drug interactions with warfarin. Arch intern Med (1968) 121, 349.

Anticoagulants + Griseofulvin

Abstract/Summary

The anticoagulant effects of warfarin can be reduced by the concurrent use of griseofulvin in some but not all patients.

Clinical evidence

The anticoagulant effects of warfarin were markedly reduced in three out of four individuals (two of them patients) when they were given 1–2 g griseofulvin daily. The fourth subject (a volunteer) showed no interaction, even when the griseofulvin dosage was raised to 4 g daily for two weeks.[1]

In another study[2] only four out of 10 patients on warfarin showed this interaction after taking 1 g griseofulvin daily for two weeks.[2] The average reduction in prothrombin time was 4.2 s. A very brief report describes a coagulation defect in a patient on warfarin and griseofulvin.[3] Yet another describes this interaction in man which took 12 weeks to develop fully.[4] He eventually needed a 41% increase in his daily dose of warfarin.

Mechanism

Not understood. It has been suggested that the griseofulvin acts as a liver enzyme inducer which increases the metabolism of the warfarin, thereby reducing its effects.[1,4]

Importance and management

An established interaction which affects some but not all (three out of four, and four out of ten).[1,2] Because it is not possible to predict who is likely to be affected, the prothrombin times of all patients on warfarin who are given griseofulvin should be monitored, and suitable warfarin dosage increases made as necessary. Information about other anticoagulants is lacking, but it would be prudent to assume that they will interact similarly.

References

1 Cullen SI and Catalano PM. Griseofulvin-warfarin antagonism. J Amer Med Ass (1967) 199, 582.
2 Udall JA. Drug interference with warfarin therapy. Clin Med (1970) 77, 20.
3 McQueen EG. New Zealand Committee on Adverse Drug Reactions: 14th Annual Report. NZ Med J (1980) 91, 226.
4 Okino K and Weibert RT. Warfarin-griseofulvin interaction. Drug Intell Clin Pharm (1986) 20, 291–3.

Anticoagulants + Halofenate

Abstract/Summary

An isolated case report describes a marked increase in the anticoagulant effects of warfarin caused by the concurrent use of halofenate.

Clinical evidence, mechanism, importance and management

A patient, controlled on 10 mg warfarin daily, showed a dramatic increase in his prothrombin time to 103 s when he was given 10 mg/kg halofenate daily. His prothrombin times returned to normal when the warfarin dosage was reduced to 2.5 mg daily.[1] A similar interaction has been seen in dogs and it is suggested that halofenate can affect both the synthesis and destruction of prothrombin, the net effect being a prolongation of the prothrombin time.[2]

Although this interaction appears to be of little or no general importance, it should be borne in mind if these drugs are used together.

References

1 McMahon FG, Jaqin A, Ryan JR and Hague D. Some effects of MK 185 on lipid and uric acid metabolism in man. Univ Mich Med Centre J (1970) 36, 247.
2 Weintraub M and Griner PF. Alterations in the effects of warfarin in dogs by halofenate. An influence upon the kinetics of prothrombin. Thromb Diath Haemorrh (1975) 34, 445.

Anticoagulants + Haloperidol

Abstract/Summary

A single case report describes a marked reduction in the anti-coagulant effects of phenindione caused by the concurrent use of haloperidol.

Clinical evidence, mechanism, importance and management

A man, stabilized on 50 mg phenindione daily, was given haloperidol by injection (5 mg eight-hourly for 24 h) followed by 3 mg twice daily by mouth. Adequate anticoagulation was not achieved even when the phenindione dosage was increased to 150 mg. When the haloperidol dosage was halved, the necessary dose of anticoagulant was 100 mg, and only when the haloperidol was withdrawn was it possible to return to the original anticoagulant dosage.[1] The reasons for this are not understood. Concurrent use need not be avoided, but prescribers should be aware of this case.

Reference

1 Oakley DP and Lautch H. Haloperidol and anticoagulant treatment. Lancet (1963) ii, 1229.

Anticoagulants + Heparinoids

Abstract/Summary

An isolated case report describes bleeding in a patient on nicoumalone after using a heparinoid-impregnated bandage.

Clinical evidence, mechanism, importance and management

A man who was well stabilized on nicoumalone (acenocoumarol) and also taking metoprolol, dipyridamole and isosorbide dinitrate began to bleed within about three days of starting to use a medicated bandage on an inflamed lesion on his hand, probably caused by a mosquito bite. His prothrombin percentage was found to have fallen to less than 10%. The bandage was impregnated with a compound based on xylane acid polysulphate which is a semi-synthetic heparinoid. It would appear that enough of the heparinoid had been absorbed through his skin to increase his anti-coagulation to the point where he began to bleed.

Reference

1 Potel G, Maulaz B, Paboeuf C, Touze MD and Baron D. Potentialisa-tion de l'acenocoumarol apres application cutanee d'un heparinoide semi-synthetique. Therapie (1989) 44, 67–70.

Anticoagulants + Herbal remedies

Abstract/Summary

Some herbal remedies such as tonka beans, melilot and woodruff can contain naturally occurring anticoagulants which may be expected to increase the effects of the anticoagulant drugs.

Clinical evidence, mechanism, importance and management

A woman[1] with unexplained abnormal menstrual bleeding was found to have a prothrombin time of 53 s, and laboratory tests showed that her blood clotting factors were abnormally low. When given parenteral vitamin K her prothrombin time rapidly returned to normal. She strongly denied taking any anticoagulant drugs, but it was eventually discovered that she had been drinking large quantities of a herbal tea containing among other ingredients tonka beans, melilot and sweet woodruff, all of which contain natural coumarins that can be converted into anticoagulants by moulds. The anticoagulant effects of these compounds may have been increased by the paracetamol (acetaminophen) and dextropropoxyphene which she was taking concurrently. The effects of conventional anticoagulants would be expected to be increased by herbal remedies of this kind if taken in sufficient quantities.

Reference

1 Hogan RP. Hemorrhagic diathesis caused by drinking a herbal tea. J Amer Med Ass (1983) 249, 2679–80.

Anticoagulants + Hydrocodone

Abstract/Summary

The anticoagulant effects of warfarin have been shown to be increased by hydrocodone in a patient and in a normal subject.

Clinical evidence, mechanism, importance and management

A patient, well stabilized on warfarin (and also taking digoxin, propranolol, clofibrate and spironolactone) showed a rise in his prothrombin time from about twice to three times his control value when he began to take *Tussionex* (hydro-codone+phenyltoloxamine) for a chronic cough. When the cough syrup was discontinued, his prothrombin time fell. In a subsequent study in a volunteer the equivalent dosage of hydrocodone increased the elimination half-life of warfarin from 30 to 42 h.[1] The reason is not known. Concurrent use need not be avoided but monitor the effects and reduce the warfarin dosage if necessary.

Reference

1 Azarnoff DL. Drug interactions: the potential for adverse effects. Drug Inf J (1972) 6, 19.

Anticoagulants + Indomethacin

Abstract/Summary

The anticoagulant effects of warfarin, phenprocoumon, nicoumalone (acenocoumarol) and clorindione are not normally affected by the concurrent use of indomethacin, but some caution is still necessary because indomethacin can irritate the gut and cause bleeding.

Clinical evidence

A study in 16 normal subjects showed that 100 mg indomethacin daily for five days had no effect on the anticoagulant effects of warfarin. When taken for 11 days by 19 normal subjects neither the anticoagulant effects nor the half-life of warfarin were affected.[1]

Other studies in normal subjects and patients anticoagulated with phenprocoumon,[2-4] clorindione[2] or nicoumalone[5] similarly showed that anticoagulant effects were not changed by indomethacin.

In contrast a handful of somewhat equivocal reports describe possible interactions in patients taking warfarin. One patient was also taking allopurinol which is known to interact with the anticoagulants.[6] Another patient appeared to be inadequately stabilized on the anticoagulant before the indomethacin was given.[7] No details are given in the third case,[8] and only two other isolated cases appear to result from unexplained interactions.[9,10]

Mechanism

None. Indomethacin reduces platelet aggregation and thereby prolongs bleeding when it occurs.

Importance and management

It is well established that normally indomethacin does not alter the anticoagulant effects of warfarin, nicoumalone, phenprocoumon or clorindione. Other anticoagulants would be expected to behave similarly. Concurrent use need not be avoided but some caution is still appropriate because indomethacin can cause gastrointestinal irritation, ulceration and bleeding which may be prolonged. In one case this is reported to have had a fatal outcome.[9]

References

1 Vesell ES, Passananti GT and Johnson AO. Failure of indomethacin and warfarin to interact in normal human volunteers. J Clin Pharmacol (1975) 19, 486.
2 Muller G and Zollinger W. The influence of indomethacin on blood coagulation, particularly with regard to the interference with anticoagulant treatment. Die Entzundung-Grundlagen und Pharmakologische Beeinflussung. International Symposium on Inflammation. Freiburg in Breisgau, May 4–6, 1966. Heister R and Hofmann HF (eds), Urban and Schwarzenburg, Munich (1966).
3 Frost H and Hess H. Concomitant administration of indomethacin and anticoagulants. Ibid.
4 Muller KH and Herrman K. Is simultaneous therapy with anticoagulant and indomethacin feasible? Med Welt (1966) 17, 1553.
5 Gaspardy, Von G, Balint G and Gapsardy G. Wirkung der Kombina-
tion Indomethacin under Syncumar (acenocoumarol) auf der Prothrombinspiegel im Blutplasma. Z Rheumaforsch (1967) 26, 332.
6 Odegaard AE. Undersokelse av interaksjon mellom antikoagulantia og indometacin. Tidsskr Norske Laegeforen (1974) 94, 2313.
7 Koch-Weser J. Haemorrhagic reactions and drug interactions in 500 warfarin-treated patients. Clin Pharmacol Ther (1973) 14, 139.
8 McQueen EG. New Zealand Committee on Adverse Reactions. NZ Med J (1980) 91, 226.
9 Self TH, Soloway MS and Vaughan D. Possible interaction of indomethacin and warfarin. Drug Intell Clin Pharm (1978) 12, 580.
10 Beeley L and Steward P. Bulletin of the West Midlands Centre for Adverse Drug Reaction Reporting (1987) 25, 28.

Anticoagulants + Influenza vaccines

Abstract/Summary

The concurrent use of warfarin and influenza vaccine is usually safe and uneventful, but there are reports of bleeding in three patients (life-threatening in one case) attributed to an interaction. Information about other anticoagulants is lacking.

Clinical evidence

(a) Evidence of no interaction

A study on 21 men on long-term warfarin treatment showed that after vaccination with 1982/3 Trivalent influenza vaccines, Types A and B, their prothrombin times were not significantly altered.[3]

Other studies[4,6] on 13 and 19 elderly men and women, 24,26 and 33 other patients[10-12] found no evidence of an adverse warfarin-influenza vaccine interaction, although a small increase in the prothrombin ratio (from 1.68 to 1.81) was seen in one study[11] and a small prothrombin time decrease in another.[12] No interaction was seen in other studies on four volunteer subjects[7] or on seven and 33 residents in nursing homes.[5,8] One case of gross but transient haematuria occurred, but it was not possible to link this firmly with the vaccination.[5]

(b) Evidence of an interaction

A very brief report describes a patient on long-term warfarin treatment who '...almost bled to death after receiving a 'flu shot...'.[1] No further details are given. An elderly man on long-term warfarin treatment developed bleeding (haematemesis and melaena) shortly after being given an influenza vaccine. His prothrombin time was found to be 36 s. A subsequent study on eight patients showed that vaccination (with Trivalent types A and B) prolonged their prothrombin times by 40%, but no signs of bleeding were seen.[2] A man well-stabilized on warfarin developed a massive gastrointestinal haemorrhage with a prothrombin time of 48 s and diffuse gastric bleeding within 10 days of influenza vaccination.[9]

Mechanism.

Not understood. One suggestion is that when an interaction occurs the synthesis of the blood clotting factors is altered.[2] There is no evidence that the vaccine changes the metabolism of the warfarin[2] although the metabolism of aminopyrine (used as an indicator of changes in metabolism) is reduced.[9]

Importance and management

A well-investigated interaction. The weight of evidence shows that influenza vaccination in those taking warfarin is normally safe and uneventful, nevertheless it would be prudent to be on the alert because very occasionally bleeding may occur. Information about other anticoagulants is lacking but it seems probable that they will behave like warfarin.

References

1 Sumner HW, Holtzman JL and McLain CJ. Drug-induced liver diseases. Geriatrics (1981) 36, no.10, 83.
2 Kramer P, Tsuru M, Cook CE, McLain CJ and Holtzman JL. Effect of influenza vaccine on warfarin anticoagulation. Clin Pharmacol Ther (1984) 35, 416–8.
3 Lipsky BA, Pecoraro RE, Roben NJ, de Baquiere P and Delaney CJ. Influenza vaccination and warfarin anticoagulation. Ann Int Med (1984) 100, 835–7.
4 Gomolin IH, Chapron DJ and Luhan PA. Effects of influenza virus vaccine on theophylline and warfarin clearance in institutionalized elderly. J Amer Ger Soc (1984) 32, April Suppl. S21.
5 Patriara PA, Kendal AP, Stricof RL, Weber JA, Meissner MK and Dateno B. Influenza vaccination and warfarin or theophylline toxicity in nursing home residents. N Eng J Med (1983) 308, 1601–2.
6 Gomolin IH, Chapron DJ and Luhan PA. Lack of effect of influenza vaccine on theophylline levels and warfarin anticoagulation in the elderly. J Am Geriatr Soc (1985) 33, 269.
7 Scott AK, Cannon J and Breckenridge AM. Lack of effect of influenza vaccination on warfarin in healthy volunteers. Br J Clin Pharmacol (1985) 19, 144P.
8 Gomolin IH. Lack of effect of influenza vaccine on warfarin anticoagulation in the elderly. Canada Med Ass J (1986) 135, 39–41.
9 Kramer P and McClain CJ. Depression of aminopyrine metabolism by vaccination. N Engl J Med (1981) 21, 1262–4.
10 Bussey HI and Saklad JJ. Influence of influenza vaccine on warfarin therapy. Drug Intell Clin Pharm (1986) 20, 460.
11 Weibert RT, Lorentz SM, Norcross WA, Klauber MR and Jagger PI. Effect of influenza vaccine in patients receiving long-term warfarin therapy. Clin Pharm (1986) 5, 499–503.
12 Bussey HI and Saklad JJ. Effect of influenza vaccine on chronic warfarin therapy. Drug Intell Clin Pharm (1988) 21, 198–201.

Anticoagulants + Insecticides

Abstract/Summary

A single case has been reported of a patient who totally failed to respond to warfarin after very heavy exposure to an insecticide.

Clinical evidence, mechanism, importance and management

A rancher in the USA on warfarin showed a very marked reduction in his anticoagulant response after dusting his sheep with an insecticide containing 5% camphechlor (toxaphene) and 1% lindane (gamma-benzene hexachloride). Normally 7.5 mg warfarin daily maintained his prothrombin time at 35 s (control 12 s), but after exposure to the insecticide even 15 mg daily failed to have any effect at all.[1] The dusting was done by putting the insecticide in a sack and hitting the sheep with it in an enclosed barn. These compounds are known liver enzyme inducing agents[2] which increase the metabolism and clearance of the warfarin, thereby reducing and even abolishing its effects. Intense exposure of this kind is unusual, but it serves to illustrate the interaction potentialities of the chlorinated hydrocarbon insecticides, particularly for farm workers and others who may be exposed to considerable concentrations over long periods of time.

References

1 Jeffery WH, Ahlin TA, Goreen C and Hardy WR. Loss of warfarin effect after occupational insecticide exposure. J Amer Med Ass (1976) 236, 2881.
2 Conney AH. Environmental factors influencing drug metabolism. In Fundamentals of Drug Metabolism and Disposition. LaDu BN, Mandel HG and Way EL (eds). Williams and Wilkins Co (1971) p 253.

Anticoagulants + Isoxicam and Piroxicam

Abstract/Summary

Isoxicam and piroxicam can increase the effects of warfarin and nicoumalone (acenocoumarol).

Clinical evidence

(a) Isoxicam

Six patients stabilized on warfarin needed a reduction in their warfarin dosage, averaging 20% (range 10–30%) when concurrently treated with 200 mg isoxicam daily over a six week period. The effects of the interaction appeared in the second week and almost reached a maximum after four weeks.[2]

(b) Piroxicam

A man stabilized on warfarin showed a fall in his prothrombin time from 1.7–1.9 times his control value to a value of 1.3 when he stopped taking piroxicam, 20 mg daily. The prothrombin times rose again when he re-started the piroxicam, and fell and rose again when the piroxicam was again stopped and re-started.[1]

20 mg piroxicam daily increased the effects of acenocoumarol (nicoumalone) in four out of 11 subjects, three being considered mild and one being significant.[3] An increased prothrombin ratio has been seen in another patient.[4]

Mechanism

Not understood.

Importance and management

These interactions are established but not well documented. Concurrent use need not be avoided but the effects should be monitored and the anticoagulant dosage reduced if necessary. Remember too that isoxicam and piroxicam can cause gastrointestinal irritation and reduce platelet aggregation. Information about other anticoagulants is lacking but it would be prudent to assume that they will interact similarly.

References

1 Rhodes RS, Rhodes PJ, Klein C and Sintek CD. A warfarin-piroxicam drug interaction. Drug Intell Clin Pharm (1985) 19, 556–8.
2 Farnham DJ. Studies of isoxicam in combination with aspirin, warfarin sodium and cimetidine. Sem Arth Rheum (1983) 12 (Suppl 2) 175–85.
3 Jacotot B. Interaction of piroxicam with oral anticoagulants. IXth Eur Congr Rheumatol, Wiesbaden, September 1979, pp 46–82.
4 Beeley L and Stewart P. Bulletin of the W. Midlands Centre for Adverse Drug Reaction Reporting (1987) 25, 28.

Anticoagulants + Ketoconazole

Abstract/Summary

Three elderly patients have been described who showed an increase in the anticoagulant effects of warfarin when given ketoconazole. There is other evidence which shows that not all individuals will demonstrate this interaction.

Clinical Evidence

An elderly woman, stabilized on warfarin for three years, complained of spontaneous bruising three weeks after starting a course of ketoconazole (200 mg twice daily). Her British comparative ratio (a measure of her anticoagulant response) was found to have risen from 1.9 to 5.4. Her liver function was normal. She was restabilized on her previous warfarin dosage three weeks after the ketoconazole was withdrawn.[1]

The British Committee on the Safety of Medicines has a report of a man of 84 taking warfarin whose British comparative ratio rose to 4.8 when given ketoconazole, and fell to 1.4 when it was withdrawn.[1] Janssen, the manufacturers of ketoconazole, also have a report of an elderly man on warfarin whose prothrombin time climbed from 26–39 s to over 60 s when given 400 mg ketoconazole daily.[3] In contrast, two volunteers showed no changes in their anticoagulant response to warfarin when concurrently treated with ketoconazole (200 mg daily) over a three week period.[2]

Mechanism

Uncertain. It has been suggested[4] that, as in rats,[5] ketoconazole may inhibit human liver enzymes concerned with the metabolism of warfarin so that its effects are increased. It is perhaps noteworthy that all of the cases involved elderly patients whose liver function may already have been poor.

Importance and management

Information about this interaction seems to be limited to the reports cited. Its general importance and incidence is therefore uncertain, but it is probably quite small. However it would now seem prudent to monitor the anticoagulant response of any patient given both drugs, particularly the elderly, to ensure that excessive hypoprothrombinaemia does not occur. Information about other anticoagulants is lacking.

References

1 Smith AG, Potentiation of oral anticoagulants by ketoconazole. Br Med J (1984) 288, 188–9.
2 Stevens DA, Stiller RL, Williams PL and Sugar AM. Experience with ketoconazole in three major manifestations of progressive coccidiomycosis. Am J Med (1983) 74 (1B), 58–63.
3 Simonite J. Janssen Pharmaceuticals. Private communication (1986).
4 Simpson JG, Cunningham C and Whiting P. Potentiation of oral anticoagulants by ketoconazole. Br Med J (1984) 288, 646.
5 Niemegeers CJE, Levron JC, Awouters F and Janssen PAJ. Inhibition and induction of microsomal enzymes in the rat. A comparative study of four antimycotics: miconazole, econazole, clotrimazole and ketoconazole. Arch Int Pharmacodynam (1961) 251, 26–38.

Anticoagulants + Laxatives, Liquid paraffin or Psyllium

Abstract/Summmary

The theoretical possibility that laxatives or liquid paraffin might affect the response to oral anticoagulants appears to be unconfirmed. Psyllium (ispaghula) has been shown not to affect either the absorption or the anticoagulant effects of warfarin.

Clinical evidence, mechanism, importance and management

A study in six normal subjects showed that psyllium, given as a 14 g dose of colloid (*Metamucil*) in a small amount of water with a single 40 mg dose of warfarin, and three further doses of psyllium at 2 h intervals thereafter, did not affect either the absorption or the anticoagulant effects of the warfarin.[1] In theory, laxatives and liquid paraffin (mineral oil) which shorten the transit time along the gut might be expected to decrease the absorption of both vitamin K and the oral anticoagulants, and liquid paraffin might also impair the absorption of the lipid-soluble vitamin. But despite warnings in various books, reviews and lists of drug interactions, there appears to be no direct evidence, as yet, that this is an interaction of any practical importance.

Reference

1 Robinson DS, Benjamin DM and McCormack JJ. Interaction of warfarin and nonsystemic gastrointestinal drugs. Clin Pharmacol Ther (1971) 12, 491.

Anticoagulants + Meclofenamic acid or Mefenamic acid

Abstract/Summary

The anticoagulant effects of warfarin are increased to some extent by meclofenamic acid and a modest reduction in the warfarin dosage may be needed. Mefenamic acid does not interact significantly with warfarin.

Clinical evidence

(a) Meclofenamic acid

A study on seven patients taking warfarin showed that after taking meclofenamic acid (200–300 mg daily) for seven days, the average dose of warfarin required fell from 6.5 to 4.25 mg daily, and by the end of four weeks it was 5.5 mg (a 16% reduction with a 0–25% range).[5] This interaction can be accommodated by making a modest warfarin dosage reduction.

(b) Mefenamic acid

A single cross-over trial on 12 normal subjects on warfarin showed that after taking 2 g mefenamic acid daily for a week their mean prothrombin concentrations (20.03%) fell by 3.49%.[1] Microscopic haematuria were seen in three of them, but no overt haemorrhage. Their prothrombin concentrations were 15–25% of normal, well within the accepted anticoagulant range.

Mechanisms

Mefenamic acid can displace warfarin from its plasma protein binding sites,[2–4] and *in vitro* studies have shown that therapeutic concentrations (equivalent to 4 g daily) can increase the unbound and active warfarin concentrations by 140–340%.[2,3] But this interaction mechanism alone is only likely to have a transient effect.

Importance and management

The warfarin-meclofenamic acid interaction is established but of only moderate clinical importance. A modest reduction in warfarin dosage may be needed. No clinically important warfarin-mefenamic acid interaction has been described, however bear in mind that both of these NSAID's may irritate the gut and cause some bleeding. There seems to be no information about other anticoagulants.

References

1 Holmes EL. Pharmacology of the fenamates: IV. Toleration by normal human subjects. Ann Phys Med (1966) 9 (Suppl) 36.
2 Sellers EM and Koch-Weser J. Displacement by warfarin from human albumin by diazoxide and ethacrynic, mefenamic and nalidixic acids. Clin Pharmacol Ther (1969) 11, 524.
3 Sellers EM and Koch-Weser J. Kinetics and clinical importance of displacement of warfarin from albumin by acidic drugs. Ann NY Acad Sci (1971) 179, 213.
4 McElnay JC and D'Arcy PFD. Displacement of albumin-bound warfarin by anti-inflammatory agent in vitro. J Pharm Pharmacol (1980) 32, 709.
5 Baragar FD and Smith TC. Drug interaction studies with sodium meclofenamate (Meclomen). Curr Ther Res (1978) 23, April Suppl. S51.

Anticoagulants + Meprobamate

Abstract/Summary

The anticoagulant effects of warfarin are not significantly altered by the concurrent use of meprobamate.

Clinical evidence, mechanism, importance and management

Nine men stabilized on warfarin were given 1600 mg meprobamate daily for two weeks. Three of them showed a small increase in prothrombin times, five a small decrease and one remained unaffected.[1] 10 other patients on warfarin showed only a small clinically unimportant reduction in prothrombin times when given 2400 mg meprobamate daily for four weeks.[2] Similar results were found in another study.[3] No particular precautions seem necessary. Other anticoagulants probably behave similarly, but this requires confirmation.

References

1 Udall JA. Warfarin therapy not influenced by meprobamate. A controlled study in nine men. Curr Ther Res (1970) 12, 724.
2 Gould I, Michael A, Fisch S and Gomprecht RF. Prothrombin levels maintained with meprobamate and warfarin. A controlled study. J Amer Med Ass (1972) 220, 1460.
3 DeCarolis PP and Gelfland ML. Effect of tranquillizers on prothrombin times response to coumarin. J Clin Pharmacol (1975) 15, 557.

Anticoagulants + Meptazinol

Abstract/Summary

The anticoagulant effects of warfarin are not altered by meptazinol.

Clinical evidence, mechanism, importance and management

A study[1] on six elderly patients maintained on warfarin (approximately 5 mg daily) showed that the concurrent oral administration of 800 mg meptazinol daily for seven days had no significant effect on their prothrombin times. Information about other anticoagulants is lacking.

Reference

1 Ryd-Kjellen E and Alm A. Effect of meptazinol on chronic anticoagulant therapy. Human Toxicol (1986) 5, 101–2.

Anticoagulants + Methaqualone

Abstract/Summary

Methaqualone can cause a small but clinically unimportant reduction in the anticoagulant effects of warfarin.

Clinical evidence, mechanism, importance and management

10 patients on warfarin given 300 mg methaqualone at bedtime for three weeks showed a small but clinically unimportant fall in their prothrombin times. Their average prothrombin times before, during and after concurrent treatment were 20.9, 20.4 and 19.6 s respectively.[1] Another report describes a patient whose warfarin plasma levels were unaffected by the concurrent use of methaqualone,[2] although there was some evidence that enzyme induction had occurred. It seems probable that the small change in prothrombin times reflects a limited degree of enzyme induction which results in the metabolism and clearance of warfarin being slightly increased. Methaqualone has certainly been shown to have some enzyme-inducing effects in man.[2,3] No special precautions seem to be necessary during the concurrent use of warfarin and methaqualone. Other anticoagulants are expected to behave similarly.

References

1 Udall JA. Clinical implications of warfarin interactions with five sedatives. Amer J Cardiol (1975) 35, 67.
2 Whitfield JB, Moss DW, Neale G, Orme M and Breckenridge A. Changes in plasma gamma-glutamyl transpeptidase activity associated with alterations in drug metabolism in man. Br Med J (1973) i, 316.
3 Nayak RK, Smyth RD and Chamberlain AP. Methaqualone pharmacokinetics after single and multiple dose administration in man. J Pharmacokinet Biopharmaceut (1974) 2, 107.

Anticoagulants + Methylphenidate

Abstract/Summary

Despite some evidence to the contrary, it seems that the anticoagulant effects of ethylbiscoumacetate are not affected by the concurrent use of methylphenidate. There is nothing to suggest that an interaction occurs with any of the other anticoagulants.

Clinical evidence, importance and management

A study[1] in four normal subjects indicated that, after taking 20 mg methylphenidate daily for 3–5 days, the half-life of ethyl biscoumacetate was on average approximately doubled due, it was suggested, to the enzyme inhibitory effects of the methylphenidate. However a subsequent double-blind study on 12 subjects failed to confirm that any interaction occurs.[2]

This interaction has not been confirmed and there seems to be no reason for avoiding concurrent use. Other anticoagulants may be expected to behave similarly.

References

1 Garrettson LK, Perel JM and Dayton PG. Methylphenidate interaction with both anticonvulsants and ethyl biscoumacetate. J Amer Med Ass (1969) 207, 2053.
2 Hague DE, Smith ME, Ryan JR and McMahon FG. The interaction of methylphenidate and prolintane with ethyl biscoumacetate metabolism. Fed Proc (1971) 30, 366 (Abs).

Anticoagulants + Metronidazole

Abstract/Summary

The anticoagulant effects of warfarin are markedly increased by metronidazole, and bleeding can occur if the dosage of warfarin is not reduced appropriately.

Clinical evidence

A study in eight normal subjects showed that 750 mg metronidazole daily for a week increased the half-life of racemic warfarin (i.e. the normal ordinary mixture of R(+) and S(−)) by about one-third (from 35 to 46 h).[1] The anticoagulant effects of S(−) warfarin were virtually doubled and the half-life increased by 60%, but no change in the response to R(+) was seen (except in one subject).

Bleeding has been seen in two patients taking warfarin and metronidazole.[2,3] One of them[2] had severe pain in one leg, ecchymoses and haemorrhage of the legs, and an increase in her prothrombin time from 17/19 s to 147 s within 17 days of starting the metronidazole.

Mechanism

It is suggested[1] that the metronidazole inhibits the activity of the enzymes responsible for the metabolism (ring oxidation) of the S(−) warfarin, but not the R(+) warfarin. As a result the racemate with the more potent activity is retained within the body, and its actions are increased and prolonged.

Importance and management

An established and clinically important interaction, although the documentation is small. If concurrent use cannot be avoided, the warfarin dosage should be reduced appropriately. What is known suggests that a reduction of about one-third to a half may be necessary. Information about other anticoagulants is lacking, but it would be prudent to expect them to behave similarly. Some indirect evidence suggests that metronidazole may possibly not interact with phenprocoumon.[4]

References

1 O'Reilly RA. The stereoselective interaction of warfarin and metronidazole in man. N Engl J Med (1976) 295, 354.
2 Kazmier FJ. A significant interaction between metronidazole and warfarin. Mayo Clin Proc (1976) 51, 782.
3 Dean RP and Talbert RL. Bleeding associated with concurrent warfarin and metronidazole therapy. Drug Intell Clin Pharm (1980) 14, 864.
4 Staiger Von Ch, Wang NS, de Vries J and Weber E. Untersuchungen

zur Wirkung von Metronidazol auf den Phenazon-Metabolismus. Arzneim.-Forsch./Drug Res (1984) 34, 89–91.

Anticoagulants + Miconazole

Abstract/Summary

The anticoagulant effects of nicoumalone (acenocoumarol),
ethylbiscoumacetate, fluindione, phenindione, phenprocoumon,
tioclomarol and warfarin can be markedly increased if micon-
azole is given orally. Bleeding can occur if the anticoagulant
dosage is not reduced appropriately. Some reports indicate that
halving the dose is sufficient. It is doubtful if an interaction
occurs if miconazole pessaries or creams are used but it can
occur with buccal gel formulations.

Clinical evidence

Two patients with prosthetic heart valves,[1] well stabilized
for several months on warfarin, developed haemorrhagic
complications within 10 days of starting to take miconazole
(250 g four times a day). One of the patients developed blood
blisters and bruised easily. Her prothrombin ratio was found
to have risen from 2–3 to 16. The other patient was found
to have a prothrombin ratio of 23.4. He developed two
haematomas soon after both drugs were withdrawn. Both
patients were subsequently restabilized in the absence of
miconazole on their former doses of warfarin. None of the
other drugs being taken are likely to have been responsible
for the increased anticoagulant effects.[1]

The Centres de Pharmacovigilance Hospitaliere in Bordeaux[2]
have on record five cases where miconazole (500 g daily) was
responsible for a marked increase in prothrombin times and/
or bleeding (haematomas, haematuria, gastrointestinal bleeding) in patients taking nicoumalone (two cases),
ethylbiscoumacetate (one case), tioclomarol (one case) and
phenindione (one case). Other cases have been described
elsewhere involving nicoumalone, fluindione, warfarin and
phenprocoumon[3–5,7–9].

Mechanism

Not understood.

Importance and management.

An established interaction of clinical importance. The incidence is not known. In three cases[1,2] bleeding began
within 10–13 days of starting the miconazole whereas
another patient bled within only three days.[4] Oral miconazole should not be given to patients taking any of the anticoagulants cited unless the prothrombin times can be closely
monitored and suitable dosage reductions made. Two reports
indicate that halving the dose may be sufficient,[2,5] but in
some instances the reduction needed may be much greater.
One patient required an increase in her nicoumalone dosage
from 2 mg twice weekly to 3–4 mg daily when miconazole
(dose not stated) was withdrawn.[3] An interaction with
miconazole in the form of a cream or pressary is unlikely

because the concentrations used are low and the systemic absorption is small, however this needs confirmation. Absorption from a buccal gel can apparently be substantial because
three patients taking either warfarin, nicoumalone or fluindione bled or showed prolonged prothrombin times as a
result of an interaction.[7–9] Information about other anticoagulants is lacking, but it would be prudent to assume that
they will interact similarly with miconazole.

References

1 Watson PG, Lochan RG and Redding VJ. Drug interaction with
   coumarin derivative anticoagulants. Br Med J (1982) 285, 1044–5
2 Loupi E, Descotes J, Lery N and Evreux J Cl. Interactions medicamenteuses et miconazole. Therapie (1982) 37, 437–41
3 Anon. New Possibilities in the treatment of systemic mycoses. Reports
   on the experimental and clinical evaluation of miconazole. Round table
   discussion and Chairman's summing up. Proc Roy Soc Med (1977), 70,
   Suppl l, 52.
4 Ponge T, Barrier J, Spreux A, Guillou B, Larousse Cl and Grolleau JY.
   Potentialisation des effets de l'acenocoumarol par le miconazole.
   Therapie (1982) 37, 217–24.
5 Goenen M, Reynaert M, Jaumin P, Chalant Ch.H and Tremoreaux J.
   A case of candida albicans endocarditis three years after an aortic valve
   replacement. J Cardiovasc Surg (1977) 18, 391–6.
6 Deresinski SC, Galgiani JN and Stevens DA. Miconazole treatment of
   human coccidioidomycosis: status report. In Ajello L (ed) Coccidioidomycosis: current clinical and diagnostic status. Proc 3rd Int
   Coccidioidomycosis Symp., Tucson, Arizona, November 1976. Miami
   Symp Specialists. (1977) pp 267–92.
7 Marotel C, Cerisay D, Vasseur P, Rouvier B and Chabanne JP. Potentialisation des effets de l'acenocoumarol par le gel buccal de
   miconazole. La Presse Med (1986) 15, 1684–5.
8 Colquhoun MC, Daly M, Stewart P and Beeley L. Interaction between
   warfarin and miconazole oral gel. Lancet (1987) i, 695.
9 Ponge T, Rapp MJ, Fruneau P, Ponge A, Wassen-Hove L, Larousse Cl
   and Cottin S. Interaction medicamenteuse impliquant le miconazole en
   gel et la fluindione. Therapie (1987) 42, 412–3.

Anticoagulants + Monoamine oxidase inhibitors

Abstract/Summmary

The theoretical possibility that the concurrent use of MAOI
might increase the effects of the oral anticoagulants has not
been confirmed in man.

Clinical evidence, mechanism, importance and management

A number of studies[1–4] have shown that the monoamine
oxidase inhibitors can increase the effects of some oral anticoagulants in animals, but reports of this interaction in man
are lacking and no special precautions seem to be necessary.

References

1 Fumarola D and De Rinaldis P. Ricerche sperimentali sugli inibitori
   della mono-aminossidasi. Influenza della nialmide sulla attivita degli
   anticaogulanti indiretti. Haematolgica (1964) 49, 1263.
2 Reber K and Studer A. Beeinflussung der Wirkung einiger indirekter
   Antikoagulantien durch Monoaminoxydase-Hemmer. Thromb Diath
   Haemorrh (1965) 14, 83.
3 De Nicola P, Fumarola D and De Rinaldis P. Beeinflussung der gerin-

nungshemmenden Wirkung der indirekten Antikoagulantien durch die MAO-Inhibitoren. Thromb Diath Haemorrh (1964) 12 (Suppl), 125.

4 Hrdina P, Rusnakova M and Kovalcik V. Changes of hypoprothrombinaemic activity of indirect anticoagulants after MAO inhibitors and reserpine. Biochem Pharmacol (1953) 12 (Suppl), 241.

Anticoagulants + Nalidixic acid

Abstract/Summary

Three patients, two on warfarin and the other on nicoumalone, developed hypoprothrombinaemia when given nalidixic acid. One of them bled.

Clinical evidence

A woman, well stabilized on warfarin (prothrombin ratio 2.0), developed a purpuric rash and bruising within six days of starting to take 2 g nalidixic acid daily. Her prothrombin time was found to have risen to 45 s.[1]

Another patient on nicoumalone (acenocoumarol) showed hypoprothrombinaemia after receiving 1 g nalidixic acid daily.[2] Another woman, previously well controlled on warfarin, developed a prothrombin time of 60 s 10 days after starting to take 3 g nalidixic acid daily.[5]

Mechanism

Uncertain. *In vitro* experiments[3,4] have shown that nalidixic acid can displace warfarin from its binding sites on human plasma albumin, but this mechanism on its own is almost certainly not the full explanation.

Importance and management

Information seems to be limited to the reports cited. It seems to be an established interaction but uncommon. Concurrent use need not be avoided but it would be prudent to monitor the effects closely, particularly during the first week.

References

1 Hoffbrand BI. Interaction of nalidixic acid and warfarin. Br Med J (1974) 2, 666.
2 Potasman I and Bassan H. Nicoumalone and nalidixic acid interaction. Ann Intern Med (1980) 92, 572.
3 Sellers EM and Koch-Weser J. Kinetics and clinical importance of displacement of warfarin from albumin by acidic drugs. Ann NY Acad Sci (1971) 179, 213.
4 Sellers EM and Koch-Weser J. Displacement of warfarin from human albumin by diazoxide and ethacrynic, mefenamic and nalidixic acids. Clin Pharmacol Ther (1970) 11, 524.
5 Leor J, Levartowsky D and Sharon C. Interaction between nalidixic acid and warfarin. Ann Intern Med (1987) 107, 601.

Anticoagulants + Nizatidine

Abstract/Summary

Nizatidine does not interact with warfarin.

Clinical evidence, mechanism, importance and management

A study in seven normal subjects given enough warfarin (about 5–6 mg daily) to increase their prothrombin times from 11.5 to 17.6 s showed that the concurrent use of 300 mg nizatidine daily for two weeks had no significant effects on their prothrombin times, kaolin-cephalin clotting times, the activity of factors II, VII, XI and X, or on their steady-state serum warfarin levels.[1] This failure of nizatidine to affect warfarin levels is consistent with the fact that it does not inhibit the activity of liver microsomal enzymes, unlike cimetidine. No particular precautions appear to be necessary during concurrent use. There seems to be no direct information about other anticoagulants, but they would also be expected not to be affected by nizatidine.

Reference

1 Cournot A, Berlin I, Sallord JC and Singlas E. Lack of interaction between nizatidine and warfarin during concurrent use. J Clin Pharmacol (1988) 28, 1120–2.

Anticoagulants + Nomifensine

Abstract/Summary

A very brief single case report describes a marked increase in the anticoagulant effects of warfarin attributed to the concurrent use of nomifensine.[1] Nomifensine was withdrawn worldwide in 1986.

Reference

1 Beeley L. Bulletin of the West Midlands Adverse Drug Reaction Study Group. University of Birmingham, England. January (1980) no 10.

Anticoagulants + Non-steroidal antiinflammatory drugs (NSAID's)– Arylalkanoates

Abstract/Summary

The effects of the anticoagulants can be increased by flurbiprofen in a few patients and they may bleed. No interaction normally occurs with ibuprofen in normal doses, and this also would appear to be true for diclofenac, fenbufen, indoprofen, naproxen, oxaprozin, pirprofen and tolmetin, but isolated cases have been described with diclofenac, ketoprofen, tiaprofenoic acid and tolmetin. The manufacturers of fenoprofen say that an interaction is possible, but there seems to be no direct clinical evidence that an interaction actually occurs. All NSAID's cause some gastrointestinal irritation and possible bleeding. Other NSAID's are discussed individually. See Index.

Clinical evidence

(a) Diclofenac

Studies in 32 patients and a further 20 patients on nicoumalone (acenocoumarol) showed that the concurrent use of 100 mg diclofenac daily does not normally alter its anti-coagulant effects,[21,22] however an isolated and unexplained case of pulmonary haemorrhage associated with a very prolonged prothrombin time has also been reported.[20] Other studies confirm that diclofenac does not interact with either nicoumalone, phenprocoumon or warfarin.[23–25,32]

(b) Fenbufen

A study in five subjects on warfarin showed that when given 800 mg fenbufen daily for a week, their prothrombin times within two days were increased by 1.9 s, and the serum warfarin levels fell by 14%.[9] These changes are unlikely to be clinically significant.

(c) Fenoprofen, ketoprofen

In vitro evidence shows that the phenylalkanoic acid derivatives can displace anticoagulants from plasma protein binding sites. There is no direct clinical evidence that this matters with fenoprofen, but there is an isolated case of bleeding in a patient on warfarin (prothrombin time increased from 18 to 41 s) a week after starting to take 75 mg ketoprofen daily.[18]

(d) Flurbiprofen

19 patients on phenprocoumon given 150 mg flurbiprofen daily showed a small but significant fall in prothrombin times. Two patients bled (haematuria, epistaxis, haemorrhoidal bleeding) and three patients showed a fall in prothrombin times below the therapeutic range.[1]

Two patients on nicoumalone showed a rise in thrombotest times and bled (haematuria, melaena, haematomas) within 2–3 days of starting to take 150–300 mg flurbiprofen daily.[2] A necrotising purpuric rash accompanied by an increase in the thrombotest values was seen in two patients on warfarin treated with flurbiprofen.

(e) Ibuprofen

Studies with 19 patients[3,4] and 24 patients[5] on phenprocoumon, and 36 subjects,[6] 50 patients and 30 subjects,[7] and 40 patients[13] on warfarin showed that the effects of these anticoagulants were not altered while concurrently taking 600–2400 mg ibuprofen daily for 7–14 days.

(f) Indoprofen

A study on 18 patients on warfarin given 600 mg indoprofen daily for seven days showed that no changes occurred in any of the blood coagulation measurements made.[8]

(g) Naproxen

A study on 10 subjects showed that 17 days treatment with naproxen (750 mg daily) did not alter the pharmacokinetics of a single dose of warfarin, or its anticoagulant effects.[17] Similar results were found in another study.[14] Yet another study in patients on phenprocoumon showed that 500 mg naproxen daily transiently increased the anticoagulant effects and caused an unimportant change in primary bleeding time.[15]

(h) Oxaprozin

A study in 10 normal subjects stabilized on warfarin for an average of 13 days showed that while taking 1200 mg oxaprozin daily for seven days their prothrombin times were not significantly altered.[31]

(i) Pirprofen

A study in 18 patients on long-term treatment with phenprocoumon showed that there was no change in the anticoagulant effects while taking 600 mg pirprofen daily. Bleeding time was prolonged by about 50%.[12]

(j) Tolmetin

15 subjects on warfarin showed no changes in prothrombin times while taking 1200 mg tolmetin daily over a three-week period.[26] 15 subjects on phenprocoumon similarly showed no changes in prothrombin times when given 800 mg tolmetin daily for 10 days.[27] Bleeding times are also reported not to be significantly altered in subjects or patients on phenprocoumon[27] or nicoumalone[28] when given 800 mg tolmetin daily. However there is a single unexplained case report of a diabetic patient on insulin, digoxin, theophylline, ferrous sulphate, frusemide and sodium polystyrene sulphonate who bled after taking three 400 mg doses of tolmetin. His prothrombin time had risen from 15–22 s to 70 s.[29] The manufacturers of tolmetin and the FDA also have 10 other cases on record.[29,30] However the manufacturers of tolmetin point out that over a 10-year period approximately 10 million patients have received tolmetin so that the risk of an interaction appears to be very small indeed.[30]

(k) Tiaprofenoic acid

A study in six subjects on phenprocoumon showed that while taking 800 mg tiaprofenoic acid daily for two days the anticoagulant effects and the pharmacokinetic profiles of both drugs remained unchanged.[10,11] No significant interaction occurred in nine patients on nicoumalone given 600 mg tiaprofenoic acid daily for two weeks, but a 'rebound' rise in prothrombin percentages occured following its withdrawal.[16] However an elderly man on nicoumalone had severe epistaxis and bruising 4–6 weeks after starting to take 600 mg tiaprofenoic acid daily. His prothrombin time had risen to 129 s.[19]

Mechanism

Drug displacement and enzyme inhibition do not seem to explain the anticoagulant/flubiprofen interactions.[1] Most of the phenylalkanoic acid derivatives can displace the anticoagulants from plasma protein binding sites to some extent, but this mechanism on its own is rarely, if ever, responsible for a clinically important drug interaction.

Importance and management

The absence of an interaction between ibuprofen and either warfarin or phenprocoumon is very well established. Other anticoagulants would be expected to behave similarly. The absence of an interaction also normally appears to be true with diclofenac, indoprofen, fenbufen, naproxen, oxaprozin and pirprofen although the documentation is more limited. In contrast a few patients may bleed when given flurbiprofen or tolmetin. As this is unpredictable and occasionally serious it is important to monitor the effects of concurrent use in all patients. There also seems to be a slight possibility of an interaction with ketoprofen and tiaprofenoic acid, but with fenoprofen it appears at present to be only theoretical. However some caution is appropriate with every non-steroidal anti-inflammatory drug because, to a greater or lesser extent, they irritate the stomach lining and have effects on platelet activity which can result in gastrointestinal bleeding. See the index for interactions with other NSAID's.

References

1 Marbert GA, Duckert F, Walter M, Six P and Airenne H. Interaction study between phenprocoumon and flurbiprofen. Curr Med Res Opin (1977) 5, 26.
2 Stricker BHCh and Delhez JL. Interaction between flurbiprofen and coumarins. Br Med J (1982) 285, 812–13.
3 Thilo D, Nyman F and Duckert F. A study of the effect of the anti-rheumatic drugs ibuprofen (Brufen) on patients being treated with the oral anticoagulant phenprocoumon (Marcoumar). J Int Med Res (1974) 2, 276.
4 Duckert F. The absence of effect of the antirheumatic drug ibuprofen on oral anticoagulation with phenprocoumon. Curr Med Res Opin (1975) 3, 556.
5 Bockhout-Musser MJ and Loeliger EA. Influence of ibuprofen on oral anticoagulation with phenprocoumon. J Int Med Res (1974) 2, 279.
6 Penner JA and Abbreht PH. Lack of interaction between ibuprofen and warfarin. Curr Ther Res (1975) 18, 862.
7 Goncalves L. Influence of ibuprofen on haemostasis in patients on anti-coagulant therapy. J Int Med Res (1973) 1, 180.
8 Jacono A, Passo P, Gualtieri S, Raucci D, Bianchi A, Vigorito C, Bergamini N and Iadevaia V. Clinical study of the possible interactions between indoprofen and oral anticoagulants. Eur J Rheumatol Inflamm (1981) 4, 32–5.
9 Savitsky JP, Terzakis T, Bina P, Chiccarelli F and Hayes J. Fenbufen–warfarin interaction in healthy volunteers. Clin Pharmacol Ther (1980) 27, 284.
10 von Durr J, Pfeiffer MH, Wetzelsberger K and Lucker PW. Unter-suchung zur Frage einter Interaktion von Tiaprofensaure und Phen-procoumon. Arzneim.-Forsch/Drug Res (1981) 31, 2163–7.
11 Luckner PW, Penth B and Wetzelberger K. Pharmacokinetic interaction between tiaprofenoic acid and several other compounds for chronic use. Rheumatology (1982) 7, 99–106.
12 Marbert GA, Duckert F and Schonenberger PM. Eine Untersuchung uber Wechselwirkung zwischen Pirprofen und Phenprocoumon. Fortsch Med (1985) 207–9.
13 Marini U, Cecchi A and Venturino M. Mancanza di interazione tra ibuprofen lisinato e anticoagulanti orali. Clin Ter (1985) 112, 25–9.
14 Jain A, McMahon FG, Slattery JT and Levy G. Effect of naproxen on the steady-state serum concentration and anticoagulant activity of war-farin. Clin Pharmacol Ther (1979) 25, 61.
15 Angelkort B. Zum einfluss von Antikoagulantien-behandlung mit Phenprocoumon. Forschrift Med (1978) 96, 1249.
16 Meurice J. Interaction of tiaprofenoic acid and acenocoumarol. Rheumatol (1982) 7, 111–7.
17 Slattery JT, Levy G, Jain A and McMahon FG. Effect of naproxen on the kinetics of elimination and anticoagulant activity of a single dose of warfarin. Clin Pharmacol Ther (1979) 25, 51.
18 Flessner MF and Knight H. Prolongation of prothrombin time and severe gastrointestinal bleeding associated with combined use of war-farin and ketoprofen. J Amer Med Ass (1988) 259, 353.
19 Whittaker SJ, Jackson CW and Whorwell PJ. A severe, potentially fatal, interaction between tiaprofenoic acid and nicoumalone. Br J Clin Prac (1986) 40, 440.
20 Gomez LMC, Beato EP, Venegas JP and Moro EP. Hemorragia pulmonar debido a la interaccion de acenocoumarina y diclofenac sodico. Rev clin esp (1987) 181, 227–8.
21 Michot F. Bericht uber eine klinische Doppelblindstudie zur Frage der moglichen Interaktion zwischen Voltaren und dem oralen Anti-koagulans Acenocoumarol. J Int Med Res (1975) 3, 153.
22 Michot F, Ajdacic K and Glaus L. A double-blind clinical trial to deter-mine if an interaction exists between diclofenac sodium and the oral anticoagulant acenocoumarol (nicoumalone). J Int Med Res (1975) 3, 153.
23 Wagenhauser F. Research findings with new, non-steroidal anti-rheumatic agents. Scand J Rheum (1975) 4 (Suppl 8) S05–01.
24 Krzywanek HJ and Breddin K. Beeinflusst Diclofenac die orale Anti-koagulantientherapie und die Plattchenaggregation? Med Welt (1977) 28, 1843.
25 Breddin K (1975) Cited as personal communication in 22 above.
26 Whitsett TL, Barry JP, Czerwinski AW, Hall WH and Hampton JW. Tolmetin and warfarin. A clinical investigation to determine if inter-action exists. In 'Tolmetin, A New Non-steroidal Anti-Inflammatory Agent.' Ward JR (ed). Proceedings of a Symposium, Washington DC, April 1975, Excerpta Medica, Amsterdam, New York, p. 160.
27 Rust O, Biland L, Thilo D, Nyman D and Duckert F. Prufung des Anti-rheumatikums Tometin auf Interaktionen mit oralen Antikoagulantien. Schweiz med Wsch (1975) 105, 752.
28 Malbach E. Uber die Beeinflussung der Blutungzeit durch Tolectin. Schweiz Rundschau Med (Praxis) (1978) 67, 161.
29 Koren JF, Cochran DL and Janes RL. Tolmetin-warfarin interaction. Am J Med (1987) 82, 1278–9.
30 Santopolo AC. Tolmetin-warfarin interaction. Am J Med (1987) 82, 1279–80.
31 Davis LJ, Kayser SR, Hubscher J and Williams RL. Effects of oxaprozin on the steady-state anticoagulant activity of warfarin. Clin Pharm (1984) 3, 295–7.
32 Fitzgerald DE and Russell JG. Voltarol and warfarin, an interaction? In Current Themes in Rheumatology, Chiswell RJ and Birdwood GFB (Eds). Cambridge Medical Publications p 26.

Anticoagulants + Omeprazole

Abstract/Summary

Omeprazole causes a small and probably clinically trivial change in the anticoagulant effects of warfarin.

Clinical evidence, mechanism, importance and management

A study in 21 normal healthy subjects anticoagulated with warfarin showed that 20 mg omeprazole daily for two weeks caused a statistically significant though small decrease in the mean thrombotest percentage (from 21.1 to 18.7%). (S)-warfarin serum levels remained unchanged but a slight (12%)

rise in (R)-warfarin levels were seen. The reasons are not understood. No changes in warfarin dosages were needed.[1] These results suggest that no interaction of clinical importance is likely in patients given warfarin, but further confirmation of this is needed.

Reference

1 Sutfin T, Balmer K, Bostrom H, Eriksson S, Hoglund P and Paulsen O. Stereoselective interaction of omeprazole with warfarin in healthy men. Ther Drug Monit (1989) 11, 176–84.

Anticoagulants + Oxametacin

Abstract/Summary

The anticoagulant effects of warfarin and nicoumalone (acenocoumarol) can be increased by the concurrent use of oxametacin. A reduction in the anticoagulant dosage may be necessary.

Clinical evidence, mechanism, importance and management

A study[1] in 12 anticoagulated patients (11 on warfarin and one on nicoumalone) showed that the concurrent use of oxametacin (100 mg three times a day) for 14 days reduced the thrombotest percentage from 11.2 to 7.8%. A third of the patients needed a reduction in the anticoagulant dosage or its withdrawal. Monitor concurrent use closely and reduce the dosage of the anticoagulant if necessary. Information about other anticoagulants is lacking but it would seem prudent to apply the same precautions.

Reference

1 Baele G, Rasquin K and Barbier F. Effects of oxametacin on coumarin anticoagulation and on platelet function in humans. Arzneim.-Forsch/Drug Res (1983) 33, 149–52.

Anticoagulants + Oxpentifylline

Abstract/Summary

The anticoagulant effects of phenprocoumon are not significantly altered by the concurrent use of oxpentifylline (pentoxifylline).

Clinical evidence, mechanism, importance and management

A study[1] in 10 patients showed that the anticoagulant effects of phenprocoumon were slightly but not significantly altered by the concurrent use of 1600 mg oxpentifylline daily for 27 days. No special precautions would seem to be necessary. Information about other anticoagulants seems to be lacking.

Reference

1 Ingerlsev J, Mouritzen C and Stenbjerg S. Pentoxifylline does not interfere with stable coumarin anticoagulant therapy: a clinical study. Pharmatherapeutica (1986) 4, 595–600.

Anticoagulants + Oxyphenbutazone

Abstract/Summary

The anticoagulant effects of warfarin are markedly increased by oxyphenbutazone which can lead to serious bleeding.

Clinical evidence, mechanism, importance and management

A man on warfarin developed gross haematuria within nine days of starting to take 400 mg oxyphenbutazone daily. His prothrombin time had increased to 68 s. A subsequent study on him confirmed that the hypoprothrombinaemia was due to the oxyphenbutazone.[1] Two similar cases have been described elsewhere.[2,3] A clinical study has also shown that oxyphenbutazone slows the clearance of dicoumarol.[4] Oxyphenbutazone is the major metabolite of phenylbutazone within the body and it may be presumed that the explanation for the anticoagulant/phenylbutazone interaction equally applies to oxyphenbutazone (see 'Anticoagulants + Phenylbutazone'). Direct evidence of this interaction seems to be limited to the reports cited, but it is established and of clinical importance. It would be prudent to apply all the precautions suggested for phenylbutazone.

References

1 Hobbs CB, Miller AL and Thornley JH. Potentiation of anticoagulant therapy by oxyphenbutazone. A probable case. Postgrad Med J (1965) 41, 563.
2 Fox SL. Potentiation of anticoagulants caused by pyrazole compounds. J Amer Med Ass (1964) 188, 320.
3 Taylor PJ. Haemorrhage while on anticoagulant therapy precipitated by drug interaction. Arizona Med (1967) 24, 697.
4 Weiner M, Siddiqui AA, Bostanci N and Dayton PG. Drug interactions: the effect of combined administration on the half-life of coumarin and pyrazolone drugs in man. Fed Proc (1965) 24, 153.

Anticoagulants + Paracetamol (Acetaminophen)

Abstract/Summary

The anticoagulant effects of warfarin, dicoumarol, anisindione and phenprocoumon are not affected, or only increased to a small extent, by repeated doses of paracetamol (acetaminophen).

Clinical evidence

A study[1] on 37 patients taking warfarin, dicoumarol, anisindione or phenprocoumon showed that while taking 2.6 g paracetamol daily for two weeks the average increase in their prothrombin times was 3.7 s.

10 patients on warfarin had a 1.2 s increase in their prothrombin times after taking 3.25 g paracetamol daily for two weeks,[3] and a further study on 10 patients given warfarin or phenprocoumon showed that two 650 mg doses of paracetamol had no effect on their prothrombin times.[2] A controlled study[4] on 10 patients on un-named coumarin anticoagulants found that 2 g paracetamol daily for three weeks increased the thrombotest times by approximately 20%. The anticoagulant dosage was reduced in five patients and in one of the 10 control patients.

Mechanism

Not understood

Importance and management

An established interaction but of minimal importance. The weight of clinical evidence and common experience shows that occasional or repeated doses of paracetamol (acetaminophen) either do not change the effects of the oral anticoagulants cited, or only cause a small increase. Any alteration can be accommodated by a modest reduction in the anticoagulant dosage. It seems probable that other anticoagulants will behave similarly. Paracetamol (acetaminophen) is safer than aspirin because it does not affect platelets or cause gastric bleeding.

References

1 Antlitz AM, Mead JA and Tolentino MA. Potentiation of oral anticoagulant therapy by acetaminophen. Curr Ther Res (1968) 10, 501.
2 Antlitz AM and Awalt LF. A double blind study of acetaminophen used in conjunction with oral anticoagulant therapy. Curr Ther Res (1969) 11, 360.
3 Udall JA. Drug interference with warfarin therapy. Clin Med (1978) 77, 20.
4 Boejinga JJ, Boerstra EE, Ris P, Breimer DD and Jeletich-Bastiaanse A. Interaction between paracetamol and coumarin anticoagulants. Lancet (1982) i, 506.

Anticoagulants + Penicillins

Abstract/Summary

The effects of the oral anticoagulants are not normally altered by the penicillins but isolated cases of increased prothrombin times and bleeding have been seen in patients given penicillin G, talampicillin and ampicillin/flucloxacillin. Carbenicillin in the absence of an anticoagulant can prolong prothrombin times and might therefore also do so in the presence of an anticoagulant. In contrast isolated cases of a reduction in the effects of warfarin have been seen with nafcillin and dicloxacillin.

Clinical evidence

(a) Decreased anticoagulant effects

A patient stabilized on warfarin showed a fall in his prothrombin time from a range of 20–25 s down to 14–17 s (despite a doubling of the warfarin dosage) when concurrently treated with 12 g nafcillin daily given intravenously.[1] A few months after the nafcillin was discontinued, the half-life of the warfarin was found to have climbed from 11 to 44 hours. Two other cases of this 'warfarin resistance' have been reported.[15,16] A study in seven patients on warfarin showed that 500 mg dicloxacillin sodium four times daily and at bedtime for seven days reduced their mean prothrombin times by 1.9 s. One patient showed a 5.6 s reduction.[14]

(b) Increased anticoagulant effects

Hypoprothrombinaemia has been described in one patient on warfarin given 24 million units of penicillin G daily intravenously.[2] Penicillin G is also known to be able to increase bleeding times and cause bleeding in the absence of an anticoagulant.[5] An increased prothrombin time has been described in a patient on warfarin when treated with ampicillin and flucloxacillin and both bleeding and an increase in the prothrombin ratio has been described in a patient on warfarin given talampicillin.[3] Increases in bleeding times, bleeding,[4–7,9,12] and extended prothrombin times[9,12] have been described with carbenicillin in the absence of an anticoagulant. Ampicillin, methicillin and ticarcillin are also reported to prolong bleeding times,[8,10,11,13] and in theory they might also increase the effects of both heparin and the oral anticoagulants, but reports of such interactions seem to be lacking.

Mechanisms

The nafcillin–warfarin interaction is possibly due to changes in the metabolism of warfarin by the liver. Changes in bleeding times caused by the other penicillins appear to result from changes in Antithrombin III activity, blood platelet changes and alterations in the fibrinogen-fibrin conversion.

Importance and management

Documented reports of interactions between anticoagulants and penicillins are relatively rare, bearing in mind how frequently these drugs are used. Normally no changes occur, however many individual physicians say that they have seen changes and this is reflected in a statement in the British National Formulary which says that ' . . . common experience in anticoagulant clinics is that prothrombin times can be prolonged by a few seconds following a course of broad-spectrum antibiotic e.g. ampicillin.' Concurrent use should therefore be monitored so that the very occasional and unpredictable cases (increases or decreases in the anticoagulant effects) can be identified and handled accordingly.

References

1 Qureshi GD, Reinders TP, Somori GJ and Evans HJ. Warfarin resistance with nafcillin therapy. Ann Int Med (1984) 100, 527–9.
2 Brown MA, Korschinski ED and Miller DR. Interaction of penicillin-

G and warfarin? Can J Hosp Pharm (1979) 32, 18–19.

3 Beeley L and Daly M. Bull W Mid Centre for Adverse Drug Reaction Reporting (1986) 23, 13.
4 Brown CH, Natelson EA, Bradshaw MW, Williams TW and Alfrey CP. The hemostatic defect produced by carbenicillin, N Engl J Med (1974) 291, 265–70.
5 Roberts PL. High dose penicillin and bleeding. Ann Intern Med (1974) 81, 267–8.
6 McClure PD, Casserly JG, Monsier C and Crozier D. Carbenicillin-induced bleeding disorder. Lancet (1970) ii, 1307–8.
7 Waisbren BA, Evani SV and Ziebert AP. Carbenicillin and bleeding. J Amer Med Ass (1971) 217, 1243.
8 Andrassy K, Ritz E and Weisschedel E. Bleeding after carbenicillin administration. N Engl J Med (1975) 292, 109–10.
9 Yudis M, Mahood WH and Maxwell R. Bleeding problems with carbenicillin. Lancet (1972) ii, 599.
10 Brown CH, Bradshaw MJ, Natelson EA, Alfrey CP and Williams TW. Defective platelet function following the administration of penicillin compounds. Blood (1976) 47, 949.
11 Brown CH, Natelson EA, Bradshaw MW, Alfrey CP and Williams TW. Study of the effects of ticarcillin on blood coagulation and platelet function. Antimicrob Ag Chemother (1975) 7, 652.
12 .Lurie A, Ogilvie M, Townsend R, Gold C, Meyers AM and Goldberg B. Carbenicillin-induced coagulopathy. Lancet (1970) i, 1114–15.
13 .Beeley L and Stewart P. Bull W Mid Centre for Adverse Drug Reaction Reporting (1987) 25, 16.
14 Krstenansky PM, Jones WN and Garewal HS. Effect of dicloxacillin sodium on the hypoprothrombinemic response to warfarin sodium. Clin Pharm (1987) 6, 804–6.
15 Fraser GL, Miller M, Kane K. Warfarin resistance associated with nafcillin therapy. Am J Med (1989) 87, 237–8.
16 Du Pont Pharmaceuticals (1988). Quoted in ref 15 as personal communication.

Anticoagulants + Phenazone (Antipyrine)

Abstract/Summary

The anticoagulant effects of warfarin are reduced by the concurrent use of phenazone.

Clinical evidence

The plasma warfarin concentrations of five patients were halved (from 2.93 to 1.41 µg/ml) and the anticoagulant effects accordingly reduced after taking 600 mg phenazone daily for 50 days.[1] The prothrombin percentage of one patient rose from five to 50%. In an associated study it was found that 600 mg phenazone daily for 30 days caused falls in the warfarin half-lives in two patients from 47 to 27 h and from 69 to 39 h respectively.[1–3]

Mechanism

Phenazone is a potent enzyme inducing agent which increases the metabolism and clearance of warfarin from the body, thereby reducing its effects.[1–3]

Importance and management

An established interaction. The effects of concurrent use should be monitored and the dosage of warfarin increased appropriately. Other anticoagulants may be expected to behave similarly.

References

1 Breckenridge A and Orme M. Clinical implication of enzyme induction. Ann NY Acad Sci (1971) 179, 421.
2 Breckenridge A, Orme ML'E, Thorgeirsson S, Davies DS and Brooks RV. Drug interactions with warfarin: studies with dichloralphenazone, chloral hydrate and phenazone (Antipyrine). Clin Sci (1971) 40, 351.
3 Breckenridge A, Orme ML'E, Thorgeirsson S and Dollery CT. Induction of drug metabolising enzymes in man and rat by dichloralphenazone. 4th Int Cong Pharmacol (Basel) July 14–18 (1969) p 182.

Anticoagulants + Phenothiazines

Abstract/Summary

Chlorpromazine does not interact significantly with nicoumalone.

Clinical evidence, mechanism, importance and management

Although chlorpromazine in doses of 40–100 mg is said to have '...played a slightly sensitizing role...' in two out of eight patients on nicoumalone[1] and is reported to increase its anticoagulant effects in animals,[2] there is nothing to suggest that special precautions should be taken during concurrent use in man. No important interactions appear to occur between the oral anticoagulants and other phenothiazines.

References

1 Johnson R, David A and Chartier Y. Clinical experience with G-23350 (Sintrom). Can Med Ass J (1957) 77, 760.
2 Weiner M. Effect of centrally active drugs on the action of coumarin anticoagulants. Nature (1966) 212, 1599.

Anticoagulants + Phenylbutazone

Abstract/Summary

The anticoagulant effects of warfarin are markedly increased by phenylbutazone. Concurrent use should be avoided because serious bleeding can occur. Bleeding has been seen in patients on phenindione or phenprocoumon when given phenylbutazone, but successful concurrent use has been achieved with both phenprocoumon and nicoumalone (acenocoumarol) apparently achieved by careful reduction of the anticoagulant dosage.

Clinical evidence

(a) Phenylbutazone added to stabilized warfarin treatment

A man, stabilized on warfarin following mitral valve replacement, was later given phenylbutazone for back pain by his general practitioner. On admission to hospital a week later he had epistaxis, and his face, legs and arms had begun to swell. He showed extensive bruising of the jaw, elbow and calves, some evidence of gastrointestinal bleeding, and a prothrombin time of 98 s.[2]

(b) Warfarin added to treatment with phenylbutazone

A man, hospitalized following a myocardial infarction, was given a single 600 mg dose of phenylbutazone. Next day, when coagulation studies were done, his prothrombin time was 12 s and he was given 40 mg warfarin to initiate anti-coagulant therapy. Within 48 h he developed massive gastrointestinal bleeding and was found to have a prothrombin time exceeding 100 s.[3]

There are numerous other reports of this interaction in man involving warfarin,[4–11] phenprocoumon[1,15,20] and nicoumalone.[16] A single unconfirmed report describes this interaction in two patients taking phenindione.[14]

Mechanism

Phenylbutazone inhibits the metabolism of S(−) warfarin (the more potent of the two isomers) so that it is cleared from the body more slowly and its effects are increased and prolonged.[12] Phenylbutazone also very effectively displaces the anticoagulants from their plasma protein binding sites, thereby increasing the concentrations of free and active anticoagulant molecules in plasma water,[4,9,13,17,18] but the importance of this latter mechanism is probably small.

Importance and management

The warfarin-phenylbutazone interaction is very well established and clinically important. Serious bleeding can occur and concurrent use should be avoided. Much less is known about phenindione-phenylbutazone but concurrent use should also be avoided.[14] Direct evidence of a serious phenprocoumon-phenylbutazone interaction seems to be limited to two reports,[1,20] and there is good evidence that successful and apparently uneventful concurrent use is possible, presumably because the response and the anticoagulant dosage were carefully controlled.[19] A study in 357 patients given 600 mg phenylbutazone to which was added nicoumalone (acenocoumarol) from day five onwards found that 25% less nicoumalone was needed than in control group on nicoumalone alone. Clearly concurrent use is possible. Information about other anticoagulants is lacking, but unless there is clear evidence to the contrary expect them to behave like warfarin. Remember too that phenylbutazone affects platelet aggregation and can cause gastrointestinal bleeding whether an anticoagulant is present or not. Alternative non-interacting NSAID's include ibuprofen and naproxen. See Index.

References

1 Sigg A, Pestalozzi H, Clauss A and Koller F. Verstarkung der Anti-koagulantienwirkung durch Butazolidin. Schweiz med Wsch (1956) 86, 1194.

2 Bull J and Mackinnon J. Phenylbutazone and anticoagulant control. Practitioner (1975) 215, 767.

3 Robinson DS. The application of basic principles of drug interaction to clinical practice. J Urology (1975) 113, 100.

4 Aggeler PM, O'Reilly RA, Leong I and Kowitz PE. Potentiation of anticoagulant effect of warfarin by phenylbutazone. N Engl J Med (1967) 276, 196.

5 Udall JA. Drug interference with warfarin therapy. Clin Med (1970) 77, 20.

6 McLaughlin GE, McCarty DJ and Segal BL. Hemarthrosis complicating anticoagulant therapy: report of three cases. J Amer Med Ass (1966) 196, 202.

7 Hoffbrand BI and Kininmonth DA. Potentiation of anticoagulants. Br Med J (1967) 2, 838.

8 Eisen MJ. Combined effect of sodium warfarin and phenylbutazone. J Amer Med Ass (1964) 189, 64.

9 O'Reilly RA. The binding of sodium warfarin to plasma albumin and its displacement by phenylbutazone. Ann NY Acad Sci (1973) 226, 293.

10 Schary WL, Lewis RJ and Rowland M. Warfarin-phenylbutazone interaction in man. A long-term multiple-dose study. Res Comm Chem Pathol Pharmacol (1975) 10, 663.

11 Chierichetti S, Bianchi G and Cerri B. Comparison of feprazone and phenylbutazone intraction with warfarin in man. Curr Ther Res (1975) 18, 568.

12 Lewis RJ, Trager WF, Chan KK, Breckenridge A, Orme M, Rowland M and Schary W. Warfarin. Stereochemical aspects of its metabolism and the interaction with phenylbutazone. J Clin Invest (1974) 53, 1607.

13 Tillement J-P, Zini R, Mattei C and Singlas E. Effect of phenylbutazone on the binding of vitamin K antagonists to albumin. Europ J clin Pharmacol (1973) 6, 15.

14 Kindermann A. Vasculares Allergid nach Butalidon und Gefahren Kombinierter Anwendung mit Athrombon (Phenylindandion) Dermatol Wsch (1961) 143, 172.

15 Seiler K and Duckert F. Properties of 3-(1-phenyl-propyl)-4-oxycoumarin (Marcoumar) in the plasma when tested in normal cases under the influence of drugs. Thromb Diath Haemorrh (1968) 19, 89.

16 Guggisberg W and Montigel C. Erfahrungen mit kombinierter Butazolidin-Sintrom-Prophylaxe und Butazolidin-prophylaxe thromboembolischer Erkrankungen. Ther Umsch (1958) 15, 227.

17 Solomon HM and Schrogie JJ. The effect of various drugs on the binding of warfarin-^{14}C to human albumin. Biochem Pharmacol (1967) 16, 1219.

18 O'Reilly RA. Interaction of several coumarin compounds with human and canine plasma albumin. Mol Pharmacol (1970) 7, 209.

19 Kaufmann P. Vergleich zwischen einer Thromboembolie-prophylaxe mit Antikoagulantien und mit Butazolidin. Schweiz Med Wsch (1957) (Suppl 24) 87, 755.

20 O'Reilly RA. Phenylbutazone and sulfinpyrazone interaction with oral anticoagulant phenproumon. Arch Int Med (1982) 142, 1634.

Anticoagulants + Phenyramidol

Abstract/Summary

The anticoagulant effects of warfarin, dicoumarol and phenindione are increased by phenyramidol. Bleeding can occur if the anticoagulant dosage is not reduced appropriately.

Clinical evidence

Two patients on warfarin showed a marked increase in their prothrombin times when given 1.2–1.6 mg phenyramidol daily. One of them bled. Further study on eight other patients taking warfarin, dicoumarol, or phenindione showed that a marked increase in their prothrombin times occurred within 3–7 days of starting to take 0.8–1.6 g phenyramidol daily.[1] No marked change occurred in a patient on phenprocoumon, but he only took the phenyramidol for three days.

Mechanism

Studies in man, mice and rabbits suggest that phenyramidol inhibits the metabolism of the anticoagulants so that they are cleared from the body more slowly and their effects are thereby increased and prolonged.[2]

Importance and management

An established interaction although the documentation is very limited. Prothrombin times should be closely monitored and suitable anticoagulant dosage reductions should be made if bleeding is to be avoided. Anticoagulants other than those cited may be expected to behave similarly. The failure to demonstrate an interaction with phenprocoumon may have been because the phenyramidol was given for such a short time.

References

1 Carter SA. Potentiation of the effect of orally administered anticoagulants by phenyramidol hydrochloride. N Engl J Med (1965) 273, 423.
2 Solomon HM and Schrogie JJ. The effect of phenyramidol on the metabolism of bishydroxycoumarin. J Pharmacol Exp Ther (1966) 154, 660.

Anticoagulants + Piracetam

Abstract/Summary

A single case report describes a woman on warfarin who began to bleed within a month of starting to take piracetam.

Clinical evidence, mechanism, importance and management

A woman patient on regular treatment with warfarin, insulin, thyroxine and digoxin began to bleed (menorrhagia) within a month of starting to take 600 mg piracetam (*Nootropil*) daily. Her British Corrected Ratio was found to have risen to 4.1 (normal range 2.3 to 2.8). Within 2 days of withdrawing both the warfarin and piracetam her BCR had fallen to 2.07.[1] The reason for this apparent interaction is not known. There is far too little evidence to forbid concurrent use, but prescribers should now be on the alert for this reaction.

Reference

1 Pan HYM and Ng RP. The effect of *Nootropil* in a patient on warfarin. Europ J Clin Pharmacol (1983) 24, 711.

Anticoagulants + Prolintane

Abstract/Summary

The anticoagulant effects of ethyl biscoumacetate are not affected by the concurrent use of prolintane. Information about other anticoagulants is lacking.

Clinical evidence, mechanism, importance and management

The responses to single 20 mg/kg doses of ethylbiscoumacetate were examined in 12 subjects before and after four days' treatment with 20 mg prolintane daily. The mean half-life of the anticoagulant and prothrombin times remained unchanged.[1] Other anticoagulants probably behave similarly, but this requires confirmation.

Reference

1 Hague DE, Smith ME, Ryuan JR and McMahon FG. The interaction of methylphenidate and prolintane with ethylbiscoumacetate metabolism. Fed Proc (1971) 30, 336 (Abs).

Anticoagulants + Propafenone

Abstract/Summary

The anticoagulant effects of warfarin and possibly phenprocoumon are increased by the concurrent use of propafenone. A reduction in the anticoagulant dosage may be necessary.

Clinical evidence

A study in eight normal subjects taking 5 mg warfarin daily showed that while concurrently taking 225 mg propafenone three times daily for a week the mean steady-state serum levels of the warfarin rose by 38% (from 0.98 to 1.36 μg/ml). Five of the eight showed prothrombin time increases of 4–6 s.[1] Another brief report suggests that propafenone increases the anticoagulant effects of phenprocoumon.[2] A possible reason is that the propafenone reduces the metabolism and loss from the body of the anticoagulant, thereby increasing its effects. Information seems to be limited to these reports but they indicate that prothrombin times should be monitored if propafenone is added to patients taking warfarin or phenprocoumon, and the anticoagulant dosage reduced where necessary. It would be prudent to apply the same precautions with any anticoagulant.

References

1 Kates RE, Yee Y-G and Kirsten EB. Interaction between warfarin and propafenone in healthy volunteers. Clin Pharmacol Ther (1987) 42, 305–11.
2 Korst HA, Brandes JW and Littmann KP. Warning: propafenone potentiates the effect of oral anticoagulants. Med Klin (1981) 72, 349–50.

Anticoagulants + Proquazone

Abstract/Summary

The anticoagulant effects of phenprocoumon are not affected by the concurrent use of proquazone. Information about other anticoagulants is lacking.

Clinical evidence, mechanism, importance and management

A double-blind study on 20 patients on phenprocoumon

showed that the concurrent treatment with 300 mg proquazone daily for 14 days had no effect on the plasma levels of factors II, VII, X, prothrombin times or platelet aggregation.[1] Other anticoagulants probably behave similarly but this requires confirmation.

Reference

1 Vinazzer H. On the interaction between the anti-inflammatory substance proquazone (RU 43–715) and phenprocoumon. Int J Pharmacol (1977) 15, 214.

Anticoagulants + Quinidine

Abstract/Summary

The anticoagulant effects of warfarin can be increased (bleeding has been seen), decreased or remain unaltered when quinidine is given concurrently. A decrease in the effects of dicoumarol has also been reported.

Clinical evidence

(a) Anticoagulant effects increased

Three patients stabilized on warfarin with prothrombin levels within the range 18–25% began to bleed within 7–10 days of starting to take 800–1400 mg quinidine daily. Their prothrombin levels were found to have fallen to 6–8%. Bleeding ceased when the warfarin was withdrawn.[3]

There are other reports of haemorrhage associated with the concurrent use of warfarin and quinidine.[2,4,9]

(b) Anticoagulant effects decreased

Four patients on warfarin or dicoumarol needed dosage increases of 7–23% to maintain adequate anticoagulation while receiving 1200 mg quinidine daily.[8]

(c) Anticoagulant effects unaltered

10 patients on long-term treatment with warfarin (2.5–12.5 mg daily) showed no significant alteration in their prothrombin times when given 800 mg quinidine daily for two weeks.[5–7]

Another study on eight patients also failed to find evidence of an interaction.[9]

Mechanism

Quinidine can depress the synthesis of the vitamin-K dependent blood clotting factors and has a direct hypoprothrombinaemic effect of its own.[2] This would account for its additive effects with warfarin,[3] but does not explain why it can apparently also have antagonistic effects,[8] or no effect at all.[5–7]

Importance and management

Since increases[1–4] (with subsequent bleeding) and decreases[8] in the effects of warfarin, as well as the absence of an interaction[5–7,9] have been described, the outcome of concurrent use is clearly very uncertain. It would therefore be prudent to monitor the effects of quinidine closely to ensure that prothrombin times remain within the therapeutic range. The same precautions should apply with all the other anticoagulants, although nothing seems to be documented about any but dicoumarol, cited above.[8]

References

1 Sopher IM and Ming SC. Fatal corpus luteum haemorrhage during anticoagulant therapy. Obst Gynecol (1971) 37, 695.
2 Beaumont JL and Tarrit A. Les accidents haemorrhagiques survenus au cours de 1500 traitments anticoagulants. Sang (1955) 26, 680.
3 Gazzaniga AB and Stewart DR. Possible quinidine-induced haemorrhage in a patient on warfarin sodium. N Engl J Med (1969) 280, 711.
4 Koch-Weser J. Quinidine-induced hypoprothrombinemic haemorrhage in patients on chronic warfarin therapy. Ann Intern Med (1968) 68, 511.
5 Udall J. Quinidine and hypoprothrombinaemia. Ann Intern Med (1968) 69, 403.
6 Udall J. Drug interference with warfarin therapy. Amer J Cardiol (1969) 23, 143.
7 Udall J. Drug interference with warfarin therapy. Clin Med (1970) 77, 20.
8 Sylven C and Anderson P. Evidence that disopyramide does not interact with warfarin. Brit Med J (1983) 286, 1181.
9 Jones FL. More on quinidine induced hypoprothrombinaemia. Ann Intern Med (1986) 69, 1074.

Anticoagulants + Quinine

Abstract/Summary

The effects of the oral anticoagulants are not significantly altered by the concurrent use of quinine.

Clinical evidence, mechanism, importance and management

Two studies,[1,3] using the Page method[4] to measure prothrombin times, showed that marked increases (up to 12 s) could occur when normal doses of quinine (330 mg) were given in the absence of an anticoagulant, but other studies[2,3] using the conventional Quick method showed that the prothrombin times were only prolonged by 0–2.1 s. Common experience would seem to confirm that any quinine-induced increase in the effects of the oral anticoagulants is very small and not clinically important.

References

1 Pirk LA and Engelberg R. Hypoprothrombinemic action of quinine sulphate. J Amer Med Ass (1945) 128, 1093.
2 Quick AJ. Effect of synthetic vitamin K and quinine sulphate on the prothrombin level. J Lab Clin Med (1946) 31, 79.
3 Pirk LA and Engelberg R. Hypoprothrombinemic action of quinine sulphate. Amer J Med Sci (1947) 213, 593.
4 Page RC, de Beer EJ and Orr ML. Prothrombin studies using Russell viper venom: relation of clotting time to prothrombin concentration in human plasma. J Lab Clin Med (1941) 27, 197.

Anticoagulants + Quinolone antibiotics

Abstract/Summary

Enoxacin is reported not to interact with warfarin, nor ciprofloxacin with nicoumalone or ethylbicoumacetate, nor ofloxacin with phenprocoumon. An increase in the anticoagulant effects of warfarin has been seen in a few patients given ciprofloxacin and in one patient given ofloxacin. A single report describes a patient who showed a marked increase in the anticoagulant effects of nicoumalone when treated with pefloxacin and rifampicin, and another single report describes haemorrhage in a very old woman on warfarin when given norfloxacin.

Clinical evidence and mechanism

(a) Anticoagulants + ciprofloxacin

Bayer, the UK manufacturers of ciprofloxacin, have in their records reports of no significant changes in prothrombin times in 40 patients chronically treated with ethylbiscoumacetate or nicoumalone when ciprofloxacin was used concurrently,[2] but elevated warfarin levels in one patient and prolonged prothrombin times in two patients on warfarin have been observed.[2]

(b) Anticoagulants + enoxacin

A study in six normal subjects showed that while taking 400 mg enoxacin twice daily the pharmacokinetics of S-warfarin were unaffected, whereas the clearance of R-warfarin was decreased from 0.22 to 0.15 l/h and its elimination half-life was prolonged from 36.8 to 52.2 h. The overall anticoagulant (hypoprothrombinaemic) response to the warfarin was unaltered.[1] Another report about one patient is in agreement with these findings.[6]

(c) Anticoagulants + norfloxacin

A 91-year-old woman on warfarin and digoxin developed a serious brain haemorrhage within 11 days of starting to take norfloxacin (precise dose not stated but said to be 'full'). Her prothrombin times had risen from 21.6 to 36.5 s. The manufacturers of norfloxacin (MSD) are said to have other reports of a warfarin/norfloxacin interaction but no details are given.[5]

(d) Anticoagulants + ofloxacin

A study in seven normal subjects taking phenprocoumon showed that the concurrent use of 200 mg ofloxacin daily for a week did not significantly affect their prothrombin times.[4] A woman with a mitral valve replacement and under treatment with digoxin, frusemide, spironolactone, verapamil and 5 mg warfarin daily, showed a marked increase in her international normalized ratio (from 2.5 to 4.4) within two days of starting to take 200 mg ofloxacin three times daily. Two days later the ratio had risen to 5.8.[7]

(e) Anticoagulants + pefloxacin

A patient showed a marked increase in the effects of nicoumalone (Quick time reduced from 26 to less than 5%) within five days of starting to take pefloxacin (800 mg daily) and rifampicin (1200 mg daily).[3] Rifampicin is an enzyme inducer which normally causes a reduction in the effects of the anticoagulants, which would suggest that the pefloxacin was responsible for this reaction.

Importance and management

Information about the concurrent use of these quinolone antibiotics and anticoagulants is sparse. If ciprofloxacin, norfloxacin or ofloxacin are given with warfarin, or pefloxacin with nicoumalone the effects should be closely monitored and anticoagulant dosage reductions made if necessary. Until more is known it would also be prudent to monitor the concurrent use of any anticoagulant and every quinolone antibiotic.

References

1 Toon S, Hopokins KJ, Garstang FM, Aarons L, Sedman A and Rowland M. Enoxacin-warfarin interaction: pharmacokinetic and stereochemical aspects. Clin Pharmacol Ther (1987) 42, 33–41.
2 Ansell PJ. Bayer UK Limited. Personal communication (1988).
3 Pertek JP, Helmer J, Vivin P and Kipper R. Potentialisation d'une antivitamine K par l'association pefloxacine-rifampicine. Ann Fr Anesth Reanim (1986) 5, 320–1.
4 Verho M, Malerczyk V, Rosenkrantz B and Grotsch H. Absence of interaction between ofloxacin and phenprocoumon. Curr Med Res Opin (1987) 10, 474–9.
5 Lenville T and Matanin D. Norfloxacin and warfarin. Ann Intern Med (1989) 110, 751.
6 McLeod AD and Burgess C. Drug interaction between warfarin and enoxacin. NZ Med J (1988) 101, 216.
7 Leor J, Matetzki S. Ofloxacin and warfarin. Ann Intern Med (1988) 109, 761.

Anticoagulants + Rifampicin (Rifampin)

Abstract/Summary

The anticoagulant effects of warfarin, nicoumalone (acenocoumarol) and phenprocoumon are markedly reduced by the concurrent use of rifampicin. The anticoagulant dosage will need to be increased (possibly two–threefold) to accommodate this interaction.

Clinical evidence

A study in 18 patients on nicoumalone (acenocoumarol) showed that when concurrently treated with 900 mg rifampicin daily for seven days the anticoagulant dosage needed to be increased to maintain the Quick value within the therapeutic range.[1]

There are numerous other reports and studies of this interaction in man involving a considerable number of patients and subjects on nicoumalone,[6] phenprocoumon[7] or warfarin.[2–5,8–11]

Mechanism

Rifampicin is a liver enzyme inducing agent which accelerates the metabolism and clearance of the anticoagulants from the body, thereby reducing their effects.[12] One study showed that the serum levels of warfarin and the prothrombin response were approximately halved.[3]

Importance and management

A well-documented and clinically important interaction which will occur in most patients. A marked reduction in the anticoagulant effects may be expected within 5–7 days,[1,2] persisting for about the same length of time after the rifampicin has been withdrawn. With warfarin there is evidence that the dosage may need to be doubled[2] or tripled[8] to accommodate this interaction, and reduced by an equivalent amount following withdrawal of the rifampicin.[2,5] It seems probable that other anticoagulants will behave similarly.

References

1 Michot F, Burgi M and Buttner J. Rimactan (Rifampizin) und Anti-koagulantientherapie. Schweiz med Wsch (1970) 100, 583.
2 Romankiewicz JA and Ehrman M. Rifampin and warfarin: a drug interaction. Ann Intern Med (1975) 82, 224.
3 O'Reilly RA. Interaction of sodium warfarin and rifampin. Ann Intern Med (1974) 81, 337.
4 O'Reilly RA. Interaction of rifampicin in man. Clin Res (1973) 21, 207.
5 Self TH and Mann RB. Interaction of rifampicin and warfarin. Chest (1975) 67, 490.
6 Sennwalt G. Etude de l'influence de la rifampicine sur l'effet anticoagulant de l'acenocoumarol. Rev medicale Suisse Romande (1974) 94, 945.
7 Boekhout-Mussert RJ, Bieger R, van Brummelen A and Lemkes HHD. Inhibition by rifampicin of the anticoagulant effect of phenprocoumon. J Amer Med Ass (1974) 229, 1903.
8 Fox P. Warfarin-rifampicin interaction. Med J Aust (1982) 1, 60.
9 O'Reilly RA. Interaction of chronic daily warfarin therapy and rifampin. Ann Intern Med (1975) 83, 506.
10 Felty P. Warfarin–rifampicin interaction. Med J Aust (1952) 62, 60.
11 Beeley L, Daly M and Stewart P. Bull W Med Centre for Adverse Drug Reaction Reporting (1987) 84, 23.
12 Heinmark LD, Gibaldi M, Trager WF, O'Reilly RA and Goulart DA. The mechanism of the warfarin–rifampicin drug interaction in humans. Clin Pharmacol Ther (1987) 42, 388–94.

Anticoagulants + Rioprostil

Abstract/Summary

Rioprostil can reduce the effects of the oral anticoagulants to some extent but the clinical importance of this is uncertain.

Clinical evidence, mechanism, importance and management

The effects of seven days pretreatment with rioprostil (0.3 mg twice daily) on the anticoagulant effects of single doses of nicoumalone (10 mg) or phenprocoumon (0.2 mg/kg) were examined on 13 subjects. The pharmacokinetics of these anticoagulants remained unchanged but their anticoagulant effects were reduced. The thrombotest and factor VII activity percentages rose for reasons which are not understood. For

example those on phenprocoumon showed a rise in the thrombotest percentages on day three from a range of 18–50% (no rioprostil) to 26–100% (on rioprostil). However the authors of this report say that 'the observed interaction can be classed with the pharmacological curiosities because there is poor clinical relevancy.'[1] Until this is confirmed the effects of the concurrent use of rioprostil and any anticoagulant should be monitored for evidence of a reduced anticoagulant effect.

Reference

1 Thijssen HHW, Hamulyak K. The interaction of the prostaglandin E derivative rioprostil with oral anticoagulant agents. Clin Pharmacol Ther (1989) 46, 110–16.

Anticoagulants + Roxithromycin

Abstract/Summary

Roxithromycin does not interact with warfarin.

Clinical evidence, mechanism, importance and management

A double-blind randomized placebo study in 21 normal subjects, given enough warfarin to maintain their thrombotest percentages at 10–20%, found that the concurrent use of 150 mg roxithromycin twice daily for 14 days had no significant effect on the anticoagulant effects of the warfarin. Serum roxithromycin levels also remained unchanged.[1] No special precautions are needed during concurrent use. There is as yet no information about other anticoagulants.

Reference

1 Paulsen O, Nilsson L-G, Saint-Salvi B, Manuel C and Lunell E. No effect of roxithromycin on pharmacokinetic or pharmacodynamic properties of warfarin and its enantiomers. Pharmacol Toxicol (1988) 63, 215–20.

Anticoagulants + Simvastatin

Abstract/Summary

Simvastatin causes a small but probably clinically unimportant increase in the anticoagulant effects of warfarin.

Clinical evidence, mechanism, importance and management

A study in 20 normal subjects taking 5–13 mg warfarin daily and with prothrombin times averaging 19 s showed that the concurrent use of 40 mg simvastatin daily for seven days caused an increase in their prothrombin times of less than 2 s.[1] This is unlikely to be of clinical importance but, until simvastatin has been used much more widely in fully anti-

coagulated patients, it would be prudent to monitor prothrombin times during concurrent use.

References

1 *Zocor* (simvastatin) product monograph, Merck Sharpe and Dhome
   (1988), 25.

Anticoagulants + Sucralfate

Abstract/Summary

*Two case reports describe a marked reduction in the effects of
warfarin in two patients given sucralfate. Other evidence
suggests that this interaction is uncommon.*

Clinical Evidence

An isolated case report describes a man on multiple therapy
(digoxin, frusemide, chlorpropamide, potassium chloride and
warfarin) whose serum warfarin levels were depressed to
about one-third when given sucralfate. When the sucralfate
was withdrawn, his serum warfarin levels rose to their
former levels accompanied by the expected prolongation of
prothrombin times.[2]

Another report describes a patient whose prothrombin times
remained subtherapeutic while taking sucralfate despite warfarin doses of up to 17.5 mg warfarin daily. When the
sucralfate was stopped his prothrombin time rose to 1.5 times
his control, even though the warfarin dose was reduced to
10 mg daily.[4] In contrast an open cross-over study on eight
elderly patients on warfarin showed that while taking
sucralfate (1 g three times a day) over a period of two weeks
their anticoagulant response and serum warfarin levels remained unchanged.[1] No interaction was found in another
study.[3]

Mechanism

Unknown. It is suggested that the sucralfate may possibly
adsorb the warfarin so that its bioavailability is reduced.[4]

Importance and management

The documentation appears to be limited to the reports cited.
This indicates that an adverse interaction can occur but it is
not common. Concurrent use need not be avoided but be
alert for evidence of a reduced anticoagulant response to warfarin. Information about other anticoagulants is lacking, but
it would seem prudent to take the same precautions.
Ranitidine is an alternative non-interacting anti-ulcer agent.

References

1 Neuvonen PJ, Jaakkola A, Totterman J and Penttila O. Clinically significant sucralfate-warfarin interaction is not likely. Br J clin Pharmac
   (1985) 20, 178–9
2 Mungall D, Talbert RL, Phillips C, Jaffe D and Ludden TM. Sulcrate
   and warfarin. Ann Int Med (1983) 98, 557.
3 Talbert RL, Dalmady-Israel C, Bussey HI, Crawford MH and Ludden

TM. Effect of sucralfate on plasma warfarin concentration in patients
requiring chronic warfarin therapy. Drug Intell Clin Pharm (1985) 19,
456.
4 Braverman SE, Marino MT. Sucralfate-warfarin interaction. Drug Intell
   Clin Pharm (1988) 22, 913.

Anticoagulants + Sulindac

Abstract/Summary

*Five patients have shown a marked increase in the anti-
coagulant effects of warfarin when given sulindac (two of them
bled), but it seems probable that only the occasional patient
will develop this interaction.*

Clinical evidence

A patient on warfarin, ferrous sulphate, phenobarbitone and
sulphasalazine showed a marked increase in his prothrombin times (more than three times the control value) after
taking 200 mg sulindac daily for five days.[1,2,4]

There are four similar cases of this interaction on record.[3,4,7]
Two of the patients bled, one of whom did so after taking
only three 100 mg doses of sulindac.[3] In contrast, studies in
patients and normal subjects on warfarin or phenprocoumon
given sulindac failed to demonstrate this interaction.[4–6]

Mechanism

Not understood

Importance and management

An established but unpredictable interaction. The incidence
is not known but it appears only to affect the occasional
patient.[4,5] It should also be borne in mind that sulindac can
irritate the gastric mucosa, affect platelet activity and cause
gastrointestinal bleeding. If concurrent use is thought appropriate it should be monitored for evidence of increased hypoprothrombinaemia and/or bleeding. Other anticoagulants
probably interact similarly but this requires confirmation.
Alternative anti-inflammatory drugs which do not interact include ibuprofen and naproxen (see appropriate synopses).

References

1 Beeley L (ed). Bulletin of the West Midlands Adverse Reaction Group,
   University of Birmingham, England. (1978) No. 6.
2 Beeley L and Baker S. Personal communication (1978).
3 Carter SA. Potential effect of sulindac on response of prothrombin time
   to oral anticoagulants. Lancet (1979) ii, 698.
4 Ross JRY and Beeley L. Sulindac, prothrombin time and anticoagulants. Lancet (1979) ii, 1075.
5 Loftin JP and Vessell ES. Interaction between sulindac and warfarin:
   different results in normal subjects and in an unusual patient with a
   potassium-losing renal tubular defect. J Clin Pharmacol (1979) 11–12,
   733.
6 Schenk H, Klein G, Haralambus J and Goebel R. Coumarintherapie
   unter dem antirheumaticum sulindac. Z Rheumatol (1980) 39, 102.
7 McQueen EG. New Zealand Committee on Adverse Drug Reactions.
   17th Annual Report 1982. NZ Med J (1983) 96, 95–9.

Anticoagulants + Suloctidil or Zomepirac

Abstract/Summary

Suloctidil does not significantly alter the anticoagulant effects of phenprocoumon, nor zomepirac the effects of warfarin.

Clinical evidence, mechanism, importance and management

Eight patients showed no significant changes in the anticoagulant effects of phenprocoumon when treated with 300 mg suloctidil three times a day.[1] The anticoagulant effects of warfarin were similarly unaltered in 16 subjects given 150 mg zomepirac four times a day.[2] No special precautions seem to be necessary. Information about other anticoagulants is lacking.

References

1 Verhaeghe R and Vanhoof A. The concomitant use of suloctidil and a long-acting oral anticoagulant. Acta Clin Belg (1977) 32, 1.
2 Minn FL and Zinny MA. Zomepirac and warfarin: a clinical study to determine if interaction exists. J Clin Pharmacol (1980) 12–13, 418.

Anticoagulants + Sulphinpyrazone

Abstract/Summary

The anticoagulant effects of warfarin and nicoumalone (acenocoumarol) are markedly increased by sulphinpyrazone. Serious bleeding can occur if the anticoagulant dosage is not reduced appropriately. Phenprocoumon does not interact significantly.

Clinical evidence

A study[1] in five patients on warfarin showed that when they were given 800 mg sulphinpyrazone daily their prothrombin ratios rose rapidly over the next 2–3 days and two patients needed vitamin K to combat the excessive hypoprothrombinaemia. The average warfarin requirements fell by 46%. When the sulphinpyrazone was withdrawn, the warfarin requirements rose to their former levels within 1–2 weeks.

This interaction has been described in numerous studies and case reports in those taking warfarin[2,3,6–12,17]and nicoumalone.[13] Severe bleeding occurred in some instances. An increased effect followed by an unexplained reduced effect has been described in one report.[8] In a trial using nicoumalone it was found possible to reduce the anticoagulant dosage by an average of 20% while taking 800 mg sulphinpyrazone daily.[13] Phenprocoumon is reported not to interact.[16,19]

Mechanism

Some early *in vitro* evidence[4,5] suggested that plasma protein binding displacement might explain this interaction, but more recent clinical studies[1,14,15,18] indicate that sulphinpyrazone also inhibits the metabolism of the anticoagulants (the more potent S(−) isomer in the case of warfarin) so that the anticoagulant is cleared from the body more slowly and its effects are increased and prolonged.

Importance and management

A very well established interaction of clinical importance. Prothrombin times should be closely monitored during concurrent use and suitable anticoagulant dosage reductions made. Halving the dosage of warfarin[1,4,17] and reducing the nicoumalone dosage by 20%[13] has proved to be adequate in patients taking 600–800 mg sulphinpyrazone daily. Phenprocoumon is reported not to interact,[16,19] but it would be prudent to expect other anticoagulants to behave like warfarin and nicoumalone. It has been recommended that because of the difficulties of monitoring this interaction and of making the necessary dosage adjustments, concurrent use should not be undertaken unless the patient is hospitalized.[3]

References

1 Miners JO, Foenander T, Wanwimolruk S, Gallus AS and Birkett DJ. Interaction of sulphinpyrazone with warfarin. Europ J Clin Pharmacol (1982) 22, 327–31.
2 Weiss M. Potentiation of coumarin effect by sulphinpyrazone. Lancet (1979) i, 609.
3 Mattingly D, Bradley M and Selley PJ. Hazards of sulphinpyrazone. Br Med J (1978) 2, 1786.
4 Tulloch JA and Marr TCK. Sulphinpyrazone and warfarin after myocardial infarction. Br Med J (1979) ii, 133.
5 Seiler K and Duckert F. Properties of 3-(1-phenyl-propyl)-4-oxycoumarin (Marcoumar) in the plasma when tested in normal cases and under the influence of drugs. Diath Haemorrh (1968) 19, 389.
6 Davis JW and Johns LE. Possible interaction of sulphinpyrazone with coumarins. N Engl J Med (1978) 299, 955.
7 Bailey RR and Reddy J. Potentiation of warfarin action by sulphinpyrazone. Lancet (1980) i, 254.
8 Nenci GG, Agnelli G and Berretini M. Biphasic sulphinpyrazone-warfarin interaction. Br Med J (1981) 282, 1361.
9 Gallus A and Birkett D. Sulphinpyrazone and warfarin: a probable interaction. Lancet (1980) i, 535.
10 Jamil A, Reid JM and Messer M. Interaction between sulphinpyrazone and warfarin. Chest (1981) 79, 375.
11 Girolami A, Schivazappa L, Fabris F and Randi ML. Biphasic sulphinpyrazone interaction. Br Med J (1981) 283, 1338.
12 Thompson PL and Serjeant C. Potentially serious interaction of warfarin with sulphinpyrazone. Med J Aust (1981) 1, 41.
13 Michot F, Holt NF and Fontanilles F. Uber die beeinflussung der gerinnungshemmenden Wirkungen von Acenocoumarol durch Sulphinpyrazon. Schweiz med Wsch (1981) 111, 255.
14 O'Reilly RA and Goulart DA. Comparative interaction of sulphinpyrazone and phenylbutazone with racemic warfarin: alteration *in vivo* of free fraction of plasma albumin. J Pharmacol Exp Ther (1981) 219, 691.
15 O'Reilly RA. Stereoselective interaction of sulfinpyrazone with racemic warfarin and its separated enantiomorphs in man. Circulation (1982) 65, 202–7.
16 O'Reilly RA. Phenylbutazone and sulphinpyrazone interaction with oral anticoagulant phenprocoumon. Arch Intern Med (1982) 142, 1634.
17 Girolami A, Fabris F, Casonata A and Randi ML. Potentiation of anticoagulant response to warfarin by sulphinpyrazone: a double-blind study in patients with prosthetic heart valves. Clin Lab Haemat (1982) 4, 23–6.
18 Toon S, Lawrence KL, Gibaldi M, Trager WF, O'Reilly RA, Motley CH

and Goulart DA. The warfarin-sulfinpyrazone interaction: stereochemical considerations. Clin Pharmacol Ther (1986) 39, 15–24.
19 Heimark LD, Toon S, Gibaldi M, Trager WF, O'Reilly RA and Goulart DA. The effect of sulfinpyrazone on the disposition of pseudoracemic phenprocoumon in humans. Clin Pharmacol Ther (1987) 42, 312–19.

Anticoagulants + Sulphonamides

Abstract/Summary

The anticoagulant effects of warfarin are increased by co-trimoxazole (sulphamethoxazole/trimethoprim). Bleeding may occur if the dosage of the warfarin is not reduced appropriately. Phenindione does not interact with co-trimoxazole. There is also evidence that sulphaphenazole, sulphafurazole (sulfisoxazole) and sulphamethizole may interact like co-trimoxazole.

Clinical evidence

(a) Co-trimoxazole (sulphamethoxazole/trimethoprim)

Six out of 20 patients taking warfarin showed an increase in their prothrombin ratios within 2–6 days of starting to take two tablets of co-trimoxazole daily (each tablet contains 400 mg sulphamethoxazole and 80 mg trimethoprim).[9] One patient bled and needed to be given vitamin K. The warfarin was temporarily withdrawn from four patients and the dosage was reduced in the last patient to control excessive hypoprothrombinaemia.

An increase in the effects of warfarin caused by co-trimoxazole has been described in numerous other reports.[10–12,14–19] In some cases bleeding occurred. Phenindione is reported not to interact.[13]

(b) Sulphafurazole (sulfisoxazole)

A man taking digitalis, diuretics, antacids and warfarin was later started on 500 mg sulphafurazole (sulfisoxazole) six-hourly. After nine days his prothrombin time had risen from 20 to 28 s, and after 14 days he bled (haematuria, haemoptysis, gum bleeding). His prothrombin time was found to be 60 s.[5]

Two other patients bled and demonstrated prolonged prothrombin times when given warfarin and sulphafurazole (sulfisoxazole).[7,8]

(c) Sulphamethizole

A study on two patients showed that the half-life of warfarin was increased over 40% (from 65 to 93 h) after taking 4 g sulphamethizole daily for a week.[6]

(d) Sulphaphenazole

A study in 16 patients given single oral doses of phenindione and 500 mg sulphaphenazole showed that their prothrombin times measured after 24 h were increased by 16.8 s compared with 10.3 s in 12 other patients who had only had phenindione.[2] These patients almost certainly had some hypoalbuminaemia.

Mechanism

Not understood. Plasma protein binding displacement can occur, but on its own it does not provide an adequate explanation.[3,4] Sulphonamides can drastically reduce the intestinal bacterial synthesis of vitamin K, but this is not normally an essential source of the vitamin unless dietary sources are exceptionally low.[1] Evidence suggesting that the metabolism of the anticoagulants is decreased appears not to be fully established.[3,6]

Importance and management

The warfarin/co-trimoxazole interaction is well documented and well established. The incidence appears to be high. If bleeding is to be avoided the warfarin dosage should be reduced and prothrombin times monitored. Information about other anticoagulants is lacking, apart from phenindione which is said not to interact.

The phenidione/sulphaphenazole, warfarin/sulphafurazole (sulfisoxazole) and warfarin/sulphamethizole interactions are poorly documented, but it would seem prudent to follow the precautions suggested for co-trimoxazole if any of these sulphonamides is given. Some caution would be appropriate with any sulphonamide, but direct information is lacking.

References

1 Udall JA. Human sources and absorption of vitamin K in relation to anticoagulation stability. J Amer Med Ass (1965) 194, 107.
2 Varma DR, Gupta RK, Gupta S and Sharma KK. Prothrombin response to phenindione during hypoalbuminaemia. Br J clin Pharmac (1975) 2, 467.
3 Seiler K and Duckert F. Properties of 3-(1-phenyl-propyl)-4-oxycoumarin (Marcoumar) in the plasma when tested in normal cases and under the influence of drugs. Thromb Diath Haemorrh (1968) 19, 89.
4 Solomon HM and Schrogie JJ. The effect of various drugs on the binding of warfarin C14 to human albumin. Biochem Pharmacol (1967) 16, 219.
5 Self TH, Evans W and Ferguson T. Interaction of sulfisoxazole and warfarin. Circulation (1975) 52, 528.
6 Lumholtz B, Siersbaek-Nielsen K, Skovsted L, Kampmann J and Hansen JM. Sulphamethizole-induced inhibition of diphenylhydantoin, tolbutamide and warfarin metabolism. Clin Pharmacol Ther (1976) 17, 731.
7 Sioris LJ, Weibert RT and Pentel PR. Potentiation of warfarin anticoagulation by sulfisoxazole. Arch Int Med (1980) 140, 546–7.
8 Kayser S. Warfarin-sulfonamide interaction. Hospital Pharmacy Bulletin, University of California at San Francisco Hospitals 1978.
9 Hassall C, Feetam CL, Leach RH and Meynell MJ. Potentiation of warfarin by co-trimoxazole. Lancet (1975) ii, 1155.
10 Barnett DB and Hancock BW. Anticoagulant resistance: an unusual case. Br Med J (1975) i, 608.
11 O'Reilly RA and Motley CH. Racemic warfarin and trimethoprim-sulfamethoxazole interaction in humans. Ann Int Med (1979) 91, 34.
12 Hassal C, Feetam CL, Leach RH and Meynell MJ. Potentiation of warfarin by co-trimoxazole. Br Med J (1975) 2, 684.
13 De Swiet J. Potentiation of warfarin by co-trimoxazole. Br Med J (1975) 3, 491.
14 Tilstone WJ, Gray JMB, Nimmo-Smith RH and Lawson DH. Interaction between warfarin and sulphamethoxazole. Postgrad Med J (1977) 53, 388.
15 Kaufman JM and Fauver HE. Potentiation of warfarin by trimethoprim-sulfamethoxazole. Urology (1980) 16, 601.

16 Beeley L, Ballantine N and Beadle F. Bulletin West Midlands Centre for Adverse Drug Reaction Reporting (1983) 16, 7.
17 McQueen EG. New Zealand Committee on Adverse Drug Reactions. 17th Annual Report 1982. NZ Med J (1983) 96, 95–9.
18 Greenlaw CW. Drug interaction between cotrimoxazole and warfarin. Am J Hosp Pharm (1978) 35, 1399.
19 Errick JK and Keyes PW. Co-trimoxazole and warfarin: case report of an interaction. Am J Hosp Pharm (1979) 36, 1155.

References

1 Tenni P, Lalich DL and Byrne MJ. Life threatening interaction between tamoxifen and warfarin. Br Med J (1989) 298, 93.
2 Lodwick R, McConkey B, Brown AM and Beeley L. Life threatening interaction between tamoxifen and warfarin. Br Med J (1987) 295, 1141.
3 Ritchie LD, Grant SM. Tamoxifen-warfarin interaction: the Aberdeen hospitals drug file. Br Med J (1989) 298, 1253.

Anticoagulants + Tamoxifen

Abstract/Summary

The anticoagulant effects of warfarin are markedly increased by tamoxifen. A dosage reduction (about a half, or even more) may be needed to avoid bleeding.

Clinical evidence

A woman on warfarin needed a dosage reduction from five to 1 mg daily to keep her prothrombin time within the range 20–25 s while taking 40 mg tamoxifen daily. A retrospective study of the records of five other patients on tamoxifen revealed that two had shown marked increases in prothrombin times and bleeding shortly after starting warfarin. The other three needed warfarin doses which were about one-third of those taken by other patients not on tamoxifen.[1]

This confirms the first report of this interaction in a woman on warfarin who developed haematemesis, abdominal pain and haematuria six weeks after starting 20 mg tamoxifen daily. Her prothrombin time had risen from 39 to 206 s. She was restabilized on a little over half the warfarin dosage while continuing to take the tamoxifen.[2] The Aberdeen Hospitals Drug File has on record 22 patients given both drugs. 17 of them had no problems but two developed grossly elevated warfarin levels and three haemorrhaged.[3] The manufacturers (ICI) of tamoxifen have another report of this interaction on their files.[2]

Mechanism

Uncertain. It seems possible that these drugs compete for the same metabolizing systems in the liver, the result being that the loss of the warfarin is reduced and its effects increased and prolonged.

Importance and management

An established and clinically important interaction. Monitor the effects closely if tamoxifen is added to treatment with warfarin and reduce the dosage appropriately. The reports cited indicate a reduction of a half to two-thirds. Some may need much larger reductions. The warfarin dosage will need to be increased if the tamoxifen is later withdrawn. The authors of one of the reports[1] postulate that the anti-tumour effects of the tamoxifen may also possibly be reduced. This needs further study. The effect of tamoxifen on other anticoagulants is uncertain but be alert for the same reaction.

Anticoagulants + Terodiline

Abstract/Summary

Terodiline does not alter the anticoagulant effects of warfarin.

Clinical evidence, mechanism, importance and management

A randomized trial in 22 normal subjects taking 2.5–9.4 mg warfarin daily to achieve thrombotest percentages within the 10–20% range showed that the concurrent use of 25 mg terodiline twice daily for two weeks had no effect on the serum levels or the anticoagulant effects of warfarin.[1] No special precautions would seem necessary during concurrent use.

Reference

1 Hoglund P, Paulsen O and Bogentoft S. No effect of terodiline on anti-coagulation effect of warfarin and steady-state plasma levels of warfarin enantiomers in healthy volunteers. Ther Drug Monit (1989) 11, 667–73.

Anticoagulants + Tetracyclic, Tricyclic and other antidepressants

Abstract/Summary

The effects of the oral anticoagulants are not normally altered by the concurrent use of tricyclic antidepressants, nor by maprotiline or mianserin, but the anticoagulant control in the occasional patient may become more difficult. A single case report describes a patient on warfarin whose prothrombin times were increased when given mianserin, and another given lofepramine.

Clinical evidence

A study[1,2] in six volunteers given nortriptyline (0.6 mg/kg daily) for eight days indicated that the mean half-life of dicoumarol was increased from 35 to 106 h, but a later study[3] failed to find a consistent effect of either nortriptyline (40 mg daily) or amitriptyline (75 mg daily), taken over nine days, on the half-lives or elimination of either dicoumarol or warfarin in 12 normal subjects. The half-lives were shortened, prolonged or remained unaffected.

Two reports have briefly noted that the control of anticoagulation may be more difficult in patients taking amitriptyline and other tricyclic antidepressants.[4,5] Another very brief report suggests the possibility of increased warfarin effects in a patient given lofepramine.[11]

The anticoagulant effects of nicoumalone (20 patients) have been shown to be unaffected by the use of maprotiline (150 mg daily),[6] and the effects of phenprocoumon (60 patients) were not affected by mianserin (30–60 mg daily).[7] A single case report describes a man on warfarin whose prothrombin time rose from 20 to 25 s after taking 10 mg mianserin daily for seven days.[8]

Mechanism

Not understood. One suggestion is that the tricyclic antidepressants inhibit the metabolism of the anticoagulant (seen in animals with nortriptyline and amitriptyline on warfarin,[9] but not with desipramine or nicoumalone[10]). Another idea is that the tricyclics slow intestinal motility thereby increasing the time available for the dissolution and absorption of dicoumarol.

Importance and management

There would appear to be no good reason for avoiding the concurrent use of the oral anticoagulants and either the tricyclic antidepressants, maprotiline or mianserin but the effects should be monitored because the occasional patient may show an altered anticoagulant response.

References

1 Vessell ES, Passantanti T and Greene FE. Impairment of drug metabolism in man by allopurinol and nortriptyline. N Engl J Med (1970) 283, 1484.
2 Vessell ES, Passantanti GT and Aurori KC. Anomalous results of studies on drug interaction in man. Pharmacology (1975) 13, 101.
3 Pond SM, Graham GG, Birkett DJ and Wade DN. Effects of tricyclic antidepressants on drug metabolism. Clin Pharmacol Ther (1975) 18, 191.
4 Koch-Weser J. Haemorrhagic reactions and drug interactions in 500 warfarin treated patients. Clin Pharmacol Ther (1973) 14, 139.
5 Williams JRB, Griffin JP and Parkins A. Effect of concomitantly administered drugs on the control of long term anticoagulant therapy. Quart J Med (1976) 45, 63.
6 Michot F, Glaus K, Jack DB and Theobald W. Antikoagulatorische Wirkung von Sintrom und Konzentration von Ludiomil in Blut bei gleichzeitiger Verabreichung beider Praparate. Med Klin (1975) 70, 626.
7 Kopera H, Schenk H and Stulmeijer S. Phenprocoumon requirement, whole blood coagulation time, bleeding time and plasma gamma-GT in patients receiving mianserin. Europ J clin Pharmacol (1978) 13, 351.
8 Warwick HMC and Mindham RHS. Concomitant administration of mianserin and warfarin. Br J Psychiat (1983) 143.
9 Loomis CW and Racz WJ. Drug interactions of amitriptyline and nortriptyline with warfarin in the rat. Res Commun Chem Pathol Pharmacol (1980) 30, 41.
10 Weiner M. Effect of centrally active drugs on the action of coumarin anticoagulants. Nature (1966) 212, 1599.
11 Beeley L, Stewart P and Hickey FM. Bulletin of the W. Midlands Centre for Adverse Drug Reaction Reporting (1988) 26, 21.

Anticoagulants + Tetracyclines

Abstract/Summary

The effects of the anticoagulants are not usually altered by concurrent treatment with the tetracycline antibiotics, but the occasional patient has shown an increase and even bleeding.

Clinical evidence

Six out of nine patients on an un-named anticoagulant showed a fall in their PP% from a range of 10–30% to less than 6% when treated with 250 mg chlortetracycline four times a day for four days.[1] A study[2] on the effects of antibiotics describes one patient out of 20 taking dicoumarol who bled when given tetracycline. An increased anticoagulant effect is briefly mentioned in two other reports,[3,4] and a single report describes a woman on warfarin who bled (menorrhagia) after taking 200 mg doxycycline daily for eight days.[5]

Mechanism

Not understood. Tetracyclines in the absence of anticoagulants can reduce prothrombin activity,[6] and both hypoprothrombinaemia and bleeding have been described.[7,8] The idea that antibiotics can decimate the intestinal flora of the gut thereby depleting the body of an essential source of vitamin K has been shown to be incorrect, apart from exceptional cases where normal dietary sources are extremely low.[9,10]

Importance and management

This interaction (if such it is) is very poorly documented. Concurrent use need not be avoided, but as the occasional patient may show increased anticoagulant effects and even bleeding, the effects should be monitored.

References

1 Magid E. Tolerance to anticoagulants during antibiotic therapy. Scand J clin Lab Invest (1962) 14, 565.
2 Chiavazza F and Merialdi A. Sulle interferenze fra dicumarolo e antibiotici. Minerva Ginecol (1973) 25, 630.
3 Wright IS. Pathogenesis and treatment of thrombosis. Circulation (1952) 5, 178.
4 Scarrone LA, Beck DF and Wright IS. Tromexan and dicumarol in thromboembolism. Circulation (1952) 6, 489.
5 Westfall LK, Mintzer DL and Wiser TH. Potentiation of warfarin by tetracycline. Amer J Hosp Pharm (1980) 37, 1624.
6 Searcy RL, Craig RG, Foreman JA and Bergqvist LM. Blood clotting anomalies associated with intensive tetraycycline therapy. Clin Res (1964) 12, 230.
7 Rios JF. Haemorrhagic diathesis induced by antimicrobials. J Amer Med Ass (1968) 205, 142.
8 Kippel AP and Pitsinger B. Hypoprothrombinaemia secondary to antibiotic therapy and manifested by massive gastrointestinal haemorrhage. Arch Surg (1968) 96, 266.
9 Udall JA. Human sources and absorption of vitamin K in relation to anticoagulation stability. J Amer Med Kss (1965) 194, 107.
10 Pineo GF, Gallus AS and Hirsh J. Unexpected vitamin K deficiency in hospitalized patients. Can Med Ass J (1973) 109, 880–3.

Anticoagulants + Thyroid or Antithyroid compounds

Abstract/Summary

The anticoagulant effects of warfarin, dicoumarol, nicoumalone (acenocoumarol) and phenindione are increased by the concurrent use of thyroid compounds. Bleeding can occur if the anticoagulant is not reduced appropriately. A reduction in the anticoagulant effects may be expected if antithyroid compounds are used.

Clinical evidence

Hypothyroidic patients are relatively resistant to the effects of the oral anticoagulants and need larger doses than hyperthyroidic patients who are relatively sensitive.[6,8,11,14] Drug-induced changes in thyroid status (even in those who are euthyroidic but who are taking thyroxine for hypercholesterolaemia) will alter the response to the oral anticoagulants.

(a) Anticoagulants + thyroid compounds

A patient with myxoedema required a gradual reduction in his dosage of phenindione from 200 to 75 mg daily as his thyroid status was restored by the administration of liothyronine.[3] Seven out of 11 euthyroidic patients on warfarin showed lengthened prothrombin times and needed a small weekly dosage reduction in warfarin (by 2.5 mg to 30 mg) during the first four weeks of treatment with 4–8 mg d-thyroxine daily for hypercholesterolaemia. One patient bled.[1] Hypoprothrombinaemia and bleeding have been described in two patients on warfarin when their thyroid replacement therapy was started or increased.[13] Similar responses have been described in other reports and studies involving warfarin,[4,12,15] dicoumarol[2] and nicoumalone.[3]

(b) Anticoagulants + antithyroid compounds

A hyperthydroidic patient on warfarin showed a marked increase in his prothrombin times on two occasions when his treatment with methimazole was stopped and he became hyperthyroidic again.[6]

Mechanism

In hypothyroidic patients the catabolism (destruction) of the blood clotting factors (II, VII, IX and X) is low and this tends to cancel to some extent the effects of the anticoagulants which reduce blood clotting factor synthesis. Conversely, in hyperthyroidic patients in whom the catabolism is increased, the net result is an increase in the effects of the anticoagulants.[5] It has also been suggested that the thyroid hormones may increase the affinity of the anticoagulants for its receptor sites.[7,4]

Importance and management

A clearly documented and clinically important interaction occurs if oral anticoagulants and thyroid compounds are taken concurrently. Hypothyroidic patients taking an anticoagulant who are subsequently treated with thyroid as replacement therapy will need a changing downward adjustment of the anticoagulant dosage as treatment proceeds if excessive hypoprothrombinaemia and bleeding are to be avoided. Some adjustment may be necessary with euthyroidic (normal) patients given dextrothyroxine for hypercholesterolaemia. All the oral anticoagulants may be expected to behave similarly.

As the thyroid status of hyperthyroidic patients returns to normal by the use of antithyroid drugs (e.g. carbimazole, methimazole, propylthiouracil) an increase in the anticoagulant requirements would be expected. Propylthiouracil in the absence of an anticoagulant has very occasionally been reported to cause hypoprothrombinaemia and bleeding.[9,10]

References

1 Owens JC, Neeley WB and Owen WR. Effect of sodium dextrothyroxine in patients receiving anticoagulants. N Engl J Med (1962) 266, 76.
2 Jones RJ and Cohen L. Sodium dextrothyroxine in coronary disease and hypercholesterolemia. Circulation (1961) 24, 164.
3 Walters MB. The relationship between thyroid function and anticoagulant therapy. Amer J Cardiol (1963) 11, 112.
4 Solomon HM and Schrogie JJ. Change in receptor site affinity: a proposed explanation for the potentiating effect of D-thyroxine on the anticoagulant response to warfarin. Clin Pharmacol Ther (1967) 8, 797.
5 Loeliger EA, van der Esch B, Mattern MJ and Hemker HC. The biological disappearance rate of prothrombin, factors VII, IX and X from plasma in hypothyroidism, hyperthyroidism and during fever. Thromb Diath Haemorrh (1964) 10, 267.
6 Vagenakis AG. Enhancement of warfarin-induced hypoprothrombinemia by thyrotoxicosis. Johns Hopkins Med J (1972) 131, 69.
7 Schrogie JJ and Solomon HM. The anticoagulant reponse to bishydroxycoumarin. II. The effect of D-thyroxine, clofibrate and norethandrolone. Clin Pharmacol Ther (1967) 8, 70.
8 Self TH, Straughan AB and Weisburst MR. Effect of hyperthyroidism on hypoprothrombinemic reponse to warfarin. Amer J Hosp Pharm (1976) 33, 387.
9 D'Angelo G and LeGresley L. Severe hypoprothrombinemia after propylthiouracil therapy. Can Med ASS J (1959) 71, 479.
10 Gotta AW, Sullivan CA, Seaman J and Jaen-Giles B. Prolonged intra-operative bleeding caused by propylthiouracil-induced hypoprothrombinemia. Anesthesiology (1972) 37, 562.
11 McIntosh TJ, Brunk SF and Kolln I. Increased sensitivity to warfarin thyrotoxicosis. J Clin Invest (1970) 49, 63A.
12 Winters WL amd Soloff LA. Observations on sodium d-thyroxine as a hypercholesterolemic agent in persons with hypercholesterolemia with and without ischemic heart disease. Amer J Med Sci (1962) 103, 458.
13 Hansten PD. Oral anticoagulants and drugs which alter thyroid function. Drug Intell Clin Pharm (1980) 14, 331.
14 Rice AJ, McIntosh TJ, Fouts JR, Brunk SF and Wilson WR. Decreased sensitivity to warfarin in patients with myxedema. Amer J Med Sci (1971) 262, 211.
15 Costigan DC, Freedman MH and Ehrlich RM. Potentiation of oral anticoagulant effect of L-thyroxine. Clin Pediatr (1984) 23, 172.

Anticoagulants + Ticlopidine

Abstract/Summary

The concurrent use of warfarin and ticlopidine may possible cause liver damage.

Clinical evidence, mechanism, importance and management

A Japanese study has found evidence that warfarin and ticlopidine together can sometimes cause cholestatic liver injury and severe jaundice. Four out of 132 patients (3%) given both drugs after cardiovascular surgery demonstrated this toxicity. The authors conclude that '...close attention should be paid to the concomitant use of thes drugs.'[1]

Reference

1 Takase K, Fujioka H, Ogasawara M, Aonuma H, Tameda Y, Nakano T and Kosaka Y. Drug-induced hepatitis during combination therapy of warfarin potassium and ticlopidine hydrochloride. Mie Med J (1990) 40, 27–32.

Anticoagulants + Trazodone

Abstract/Summary

An isolated case report describes a woman who needed an increase in her warfarin dosage while taking trazodone, but other studies suggest that concurrent use can be uneventful.

Clinical evidence, mechanism, importance and management

A woman needed a 17% increase (from 6.4 to 7.5 mg) in her daily dosage of warfarin when given 300 mg trazodone daily in order to maintain her prothrombin time at 20 s. Her warfarin requirements fell when the trazodone was later withdrawn.[1] The reasons for this reaction are not understood. In contrast, six anticoagulated patients on heparin or a coumarin anticoagulant showed no significant changes in prothrombin times when given 75 mg trazodone daily.[2] Check the prothrombin times if trazodone is given.

References

1 Hardy J-L and Sirois A. Reduction of prothrombin and partial thromboplastin times with trazodone. Canad Med Ass J (1986) 135, 1372.
2 Cozzolino G, Pazzaglia I, De Gaetano V and Macri M. Clinical investigation on the possible interaction between anticoagulants and a new psychotropic drug (Trazodone). Clin Europa (1972) 593.

Anticoagulants + Vitamin E

Abstract/Summary

There is some very limited evidence that the effects of warfarin may be increased, and of dicoumarol reduced, by the concurrent use of large doses of vitamin E.

Clinical evidence, mechanism, importance and management

A patient on warfarin (and also taking digoxin, frusemide, clofibrate, potassium chloride and phenytoin, later substituted by quinidine) began to bleed as a result of secretly taking 1200 IU vitamin E daily over a period of two months. His prothrombin time was found to be 36 s. A later study showed that 800 IU vitamin E daily reduced his blood clotting factor levels and caused bleeding.[1] Another study on three normal subjects showed that 42 IU vitamin E daily for a month reduced the response to a single dose of dicoumarol after 36 h from 52 to 33%.[2] The reasons are not fully understood. One suggestion is that vitamin E interferes with the activity of vitamin K in producing the blood clotting factors[1] Another idea is that it increases the dietary requirements of vitamin K.[3,4] This interaction is poorly documented and its importance uncertain. There seems to be no clear reason for avoiding vitamin E in normal doses, but large doses may cause problems.[1] The effects should be monitored.

References

1 Corrigan JJ and Marcus FI. Coagulopathy associated with vitamin E ingestion. J Amer Med Ass (1974) 230, 1300.
2 Schrogie JJ. Coagulopathy and fat-soluble vitamins. J Amer Med Ass (1975) 232, 341.
3 Anon. Vitamin K, vitamin E and the coumarin drugs. Nutr Rev (1982) 40, 180.
4 Anon. Megavitamin E supplementation and vitamin K-dependent carboxylation. Nutr Rev (1983) 41, 268–70.

Anticoagulants + Vitamin K

Abstract/Summary

The effects of the anticoagulants can be reduced or abolished by the concurrent use of vitamin K. This can be used as an effective antidote for overdosage, but unintentional and unwanted antagonism has occurred in patients after taking some proprietary chilblain preparations, health foods, food supplements, enteral feeds or exceptionally large amounts of some green vegetables (such as spinach, brussel sprouts or broccoli) which contain significant amounts of vitamin K.

Clinical evidence

A woman on nicoumalone showed a fall in her British corrected anticoagulant ratio to 1.2 (normal range 1.8–3.0) within two days of starting to take an over-the-counter chilblain preparation (*Gon*) containing 10 mg acetomenaphthone per tablet. She took a total of 50 mg vitamin K over 48 h.[1]

Similar antagonism has been described in patients on warfarin taking liquid dietary supplements such as *Ensure*,[2,7,14,16] *Ensure-Plus*,[6,9] *Isocal*[12] and *Osmolite*.[8,13,15] A reduction in the effects of dicoumarol, nicoumalone and warfarin (described as 'warfarin resistance') has been seen in those whose diets contained exceptionally large amounts of green vegetables (up to 0.75–1.1 lbs daily)[3,4,10] such as spinach,[5,17] brussel sprouts[18,20] or broccoli[17] or liver[19] which are rich in vitamin K.

Mechanism

The oral anticoagulants compete with the normal supply of vitamin K from the gut to reduce the synthesis by the liver of blood clotting factors. If this supply is boosted by an unusually large intake of vitamin K, the competition swings in favour of the vitamin and the synthesis of the blood clotting factors begins to return to normal. As a result the prothrombin time also begins to fall to its normal value. Brussel sprouts increase the metabolism of warfarin to a small extent which would also decrease its effects.[20]

Importance and management

A very well established, well documented and clinically important interaction. It would be expected to occur with every oral anticoagulant because they have a common mode of action. The drug intake and diet of any patient who shows 'warfarin resistance' should be investigated for the possibility of this interaction. It can be accommodated either by increasing the anticoagulant dosage, or by reducing the increased intake of vitamin K. It is estimated that a normal Western diet contains 300–500 μg vitamin K daily, and that the minimum daily requirement is 0.30–1.50 μg/kg body weight (about 100 μg in a 10 stone/140 lb/63 kg individual). Table 6.2 gives the vitamin K content of some vegetables. Other tables listing the vitamin K content of the enteral feeds have been published,[12–14,18] but the situation is continually changing as manufacturers reformulate their products,(in some instances to accommodate the problem of this interaction).

Table 6.2 Vitamin K content of some vegetables

Vegetable	Vitamin K content
Turnip greens	650 μg/100 g
Broccoli	200 μg/100 g
Lettuce	129 μg/100 g
Cabbage	125 μg/100 g
Spinach	89 μg/100 g
Green beans	14 μg/100 g
Potatoes	3 μg/100 g

Data from Olson[11] and others.

References

1 Heald GE and Poller L. Anticoagulants and treatment for chilblains. Br Med J (1974) 2, 455.
2 O'Reilly RA and Ryland DA. 'Resistance' to warfarin due to unrecognized vitamin K supplementation. N Engl J Med (1980) 303, 160.
3 Quick AJ. Leafy vegetables in diet alter prothrombin time in patients taking anticoagulant drugs. J Amer Med Ass (1964) 187 (11) 27.
4 Qureshi GD, Reinders P, Swint JJ and Slate MB. Acquired warfarin resistance and weight-reducing diet. Arch Intern Med (1981) 141, 507.
5 Udall JA and Krock LB. A modified method of anticoagulant therapy. Curr Ther Res (1968) 10, 207.
6 Zallman JA, Lee DP and Jeffrey PL. Liquid nutrition as a cause of warfarin resistance. Amer J Hosp Pharm (1981) 38, 1174.
7 Westfall LK. An unrecognized cause of warfarin resistance. Drug Intell Clin Pharm (1981) 15, 131.
8 Lader EW, Yang L and Clarke A. Warfarin dosage and vitamin K in Osmolite. Ann Intern Med (1980) 93, 373.
9 Michaelson R, Kempson SJ, Naria B and Gold JWM. Inhibition of the hypoprothrombinemic effect of warfarin (Coumadin) by Ensure-Plus, a dietary supplement. Clin Bull (1980) 10, 171–2.
10 Kempin SJ. Warfarin resistance caused by broccoli. N Engl J Med (1983) 308, 1229–30.
11 Olson RE. Vitamin K. In: Modern nutrition in health and disease. Goodhart RS and Shils ME (eds.) Lea and Febiger, Philadelphia (1980) p 170–180.
12 Watson AJM, Pegg M and Green JRB. Enteral feeds may antagonize warfarin. Br Med J (1984) 288, 557.
13 Parr MD, Record KE, Griffith GL, Zeok JV and Todd EP. Effect of enteral nutrition on warfarin therapy. Clin Pharm (1982) 1, 274–6.
14 Howards PA and Hannaman KN. Warfarin resistance linked to enteral nutrition products. J Amer Diet Ass (1985) 85, 713–15.
15 Lee M, Schwart RN and Sharifi R. Warfarin resistance and vitamin K. Ann Intern Med (1981) 94, 140.
16 McIntire B and Wright RA. Enteral alimentation: an update on new products. Nutr Supp Serv (1981) 1, 7.
17 Karlson B, Leijd B and Hellstrom A. On the influence of vitamin K-rich vegetables and wine on the effectiveness of warfarin treatment. Acta Med Scand (1986) 220, 347–50.
18 Kutsop JJ. Update on vitamin K content of enteral products. Am J Hosp Pharm (1984) 41, 1762.
19 Kalra PA, Cooklin M, Wood G, O'Shea GM and Holmes AM. Dietary modification as a cause of anticoagulation instability. Lancet (1988) ii, 803.
20 Ovesen L, Lyduch S, Idorn ML. The effect of diet rich in brussel sprouts on warfarin pharmacokinetics. Eur J Clin Pharmacol (1988) 34, 521–4.

Heparin + Aspirin

Abstract/Summary

Although concurrent use is effective in the prevention of postoperative thromboembolism, the risk of bleeding in patients receiving heparin is increased almost two and a half times by the use of aspirin.

Clinical evidence

Eight out of 12 patients developed serious bleeding when treated with heparin (5000 u subcutaneously every 12 h) and aspirin (600 mg twice daily) as prophylaxis for deep vein thrombosis following operations for fracture of the hip. Haematomas of the hip and thigh occurred in three patients, bleeding through the wound in four, and uterine bleeding in the other patient.[1]

An epidemiological study of 2656 patients given heparin and aspirin (doses not stated) revealed that the incidence of bleeding was almost 2.5 times that which was seen in patients not given aspirin.[2] A striking prolongation of bleeding times is described elsewhere[3] in patients on heparin after treatment with aspirin.

Mechanism

Heparin suppresses the normal blood clotting mechanisms and prolongs bleeding times.[3] Aspirin decreases platelet aggregation so that any heparin-induced bleeding is exaggerated and prolonged.[3]

Importance and management

An established and important interaction. Although concurrent use is effective in the prevention of post-operative thromboembolism,[4] the risks of this interaction need to be very carefully considered, and the advantages and disadvantages carefully weighed. The assertion[5] made in 1969 that aspirin '...should be scrupulously avoided in patients on heparin...' is an overstatement, but it emphasises the need for care. Concurrent use should certainly be carefully monitored. If an analgesic is required, paracetamol (acetaminophen) is a safer substitute.

References

1 Yett HS, Skillman JJ and Salzman EW. The hazards of aspirin plus heparin. N Engl J Med (1978) 298, 1092.
2 Walker AM and Jick H. Predictors of bleeding during heparin therapy. J Amer Med Ass (1980) 244, 1209.
3 Heiden D, Rodrien R and Mieckle CH. Heparin bleeding, platelet dysfunction and aspirin. J Amer Med Ass (1981) 246, 330.
4 Vinazzer H, Loew D, Simma W and Brucke P. Prophylaxis of postoperative thromboembolism by low dose heparin and by acetylsalicylic acid given simultaneously: a double blind study. Thromb Res (1980) 17, 177.
5 Deykin D. The use of heparin. N Engl J Med (1976) 294, 1122.

Importance and management

Direct documentation is limited, but the interaction seems to be established. Uneventful concurrent use[5,6] has been described with dextran 40 which suggests that the interaction may possibly be confined to the use of dextran 70, but this requires confirmation. If concurrent use is undertaken the effects should be very closely monitored and the dosage of heparin reduced as necessary (a third to a half has been recommended[1]).

References

1 Atik M. Potentiation of heparin by dextran and its clinical implication. Thromb Haemorrh (1977) 38, 275.
2 Atik M. Personal communication (1980).
3 Bloom WL and Brewer SS. The independent yet synergistic effects of heparin and dextran. Acta Chir Scand (1968) 387 (Suppl) 53.
4 Morrison N D, Stephenson CBS, Maclean D and Stanhope JM. Deep vein thrombosis after femoropopliteal bypass grafting with observations on the incidence of complications following the use of dextran 70. NZ Med J (1976) 84, 233.
5 Schondorf TH and Weber V. Prevention of deep venous thrombosis in orthopedic surgery with the combination of low dose heparin plus either dihydroergotamine or dextran. Scand J Haematol (1980) 36 (Suppl) 126.
6 Serjeant JCB. Mesenteric embolus treated with low-molecular weight dextran. Lancet (1965) i, 139.

Heparin + Dextran

Abstract/Summary

Although concurrent use can be successful and uneventful, there is evidence that the anticoagulant effects of heparin can be increased by some dextrans. It has been suggested that the heparin dosage may need to be reduced to a third or a half during concurrent use to prevent bleeding.

Clinical evidence

A study on nine patients with peripheral vascular disease showed that the mean clotting time 1 h after the infusion of 10,000 u heparin was increased from 36 to 69 s when given at the same time as 500 ml dextran. Dextran alone had no effect, but the mean clotting time after 5,000 u heparin with dextran was almost the same as after 10,000 u heparin alone.[1,2]

The abstract quoted[1] contains some confusing typographical errors but the correct text has been confirmed.[2] This study would seem to explain two other reports of an increase in the incidence of bleeding in those given both heparin and dextran.[3,4]

Mechanism

Both heparin and dextran prolong coagulation time, but by a number of different and independent mechanisms. When given together their effects would seem to be additive.[3]

Heparin + Glyceryl trinitrate (Nitroglycerin)

Abstract/Summary

There is good evidence that the effects of heparin are reduced by the concurrent infusion of glyceryl trinitrate but one study failed to confirm this interaction.

Clinical evidence

(a) Heparin effects reduced

A study in seven patients with coronary artery disease showed that while receiving intravenous glyceryl trinitrate they needed an increased dose of intravenous heparin to achieve satisfactory anticoagulation (activated partial thromboplastin times (APTT) of 1.5–2.5 × control values). When the glyceryl trinitrate was stopped six out of the eight showed an marked increase in APTT values to 3.5. One patient had transient haematuria.

This study confirms a previous report, the authors of which attributed this response to an interaction with the propylene glycol diluent of the glyceryl trinitrate infusion.[2] However this interaction has been shown to occur when glyceryl trinitrate is given without propylene glycol.[1] Another study in 27 patients given heparin found that the partial thromboplastin time (PTT) was approximately halved (from 130 to about 60 s) when additionally given 2–5 mg/h glyceryl trinitrate intravenously. The heparin levels measured in nine patients were unchanged. The PTT rose again when the glyceryl trinitrate was stopped.[4,5]

212

(b) Heparin effects unchanged

A study in 10 patients following angioplasty found no significant APTT changes over a 30 min period following the addition of intravenous glyceryl trinitrate (41–240 μg/ml) to infusions of heparin.[3]

Mechanism

Not understood.

Importance and management

The discord between these reports is not understood. Until the situation is fully resolved it would seem prudent to monitor the effects of concurrent use closely, being alert for the need to use higher doses of heparin. If this occurs, remember to reduce the heparin dosage when the glyceryl trinitrate infusion is stopped. More study is needed.

References

1 Habbab MA and Haft JI. Heparin resistance induced by intravenous nitroglycerin. A word of caution when both drugs are used concomitantly. Arch Intern Med (1987) 147, 857–60.
2 Col J, Col-Debeys C and Lavenne-Pardonge E. Propylene glycol-induced heparin resistance. Am Heart J (1985) 110, 171–3.
3 Lepor NE, Amin DK, Berberian L and Shah PK. Does nitroglycerin induce heparin resistance? Clin Cardiol (1989) 12, 432–4.
4 Pizzulli L, Nitsch J and Luederitz B. Nitroglycerin inhibition of the heparin effect. Eur Heart J (1989) 10 (Abstr Suppl) 116.
5 Pizzulli L, Nitsch J and Luederitz B. Hemmung der Heparinwirkung durch Glyceroltrinitrat. Dtsch Med Wochensch (1988) 113, 1837–40.

Heparin + Probenecid

Abstract/Summary

Some very limited evidence suggests that the effects of heparin may be possibly increased by probenecid and bleeding may occur.

Clinical evidence, mechanism, importance and management

In 1950 (but not reported[1] until 1975) a woman with subacute bacterial endocarditis was treated with probenecid orally and penicillin by intravenous drip, kept open with minimal doses of heparin. After a total of 215 mg (about 20,000 u) heparin had been given over a 3-week period, increasing epistaxes developed and the clotting time was found to be 24 min (normal 5–6). This was controlled with protamine. It had previously been observed[2] that carinamide, the predecessor of probenecid, prolonged clotting times in the presence of heparin. The general importance of this possible interaction is uncertain, but it would seem prudent to monitor the effects of concurrent use.

References

1 Sanchez G. Enhancement of heparin effects by probenecid. N Engl J Med (1975) 292, 48.
2 Sirka HD, McCleery RS and Artz CP. The effect of carinamide with heparin on the coagulation of human blood: a preliminary report. Surgery (1948) 24, 811.

7

ANTICONVULSANT
DRUG INTERACTIONS

The anticonvulsant drugs listed in Table 7.1 find their major application in the treatment of various kinds of epilepsy, although some of them are also used for other conditions. The list is not exclusive by any means, but it contains the anticonvulsant drugs which are discussed either in this chapter or elsewhere in this book. In addition, some of the barbiturates which are not used as anticonvulsants are also included in this chapter. The Index should be consulted for a full list of interactions involving all of these drugs.

Table 7.1 Anticonvulsant drugs

Generic or non-proprietary names	Proprietary names
Acetazolamide	*Acetamide, Atenezol, Diamox, Defiltran, Didoc, Diuramid, Diurawas, Edemox, Glaucomide, Glauconox, Glaupax, Inidrase, Oratrol*
Carbamazepine	*Convuline, Hermolepsin, Karbamazepin, Nordotold, Tegretal, Tegretol, Timonil*
Clonazepam	*Clonopin, Iktorivil, Rivotril*
Dipropylacetamide (valpromide)	*Depamide, Vistora*
Ethosuximide	*Emeside, Ethymal, Petinimid, Petnidan, Pyknolepsinum, Simatin, Suxinutin, Thetamid, Zarodan, Zarontin*
Methylphenobarbitone (mephobarbital)	
Pheneturide	*Benuride*
Phenobarbitone (phenobarbital)	
Phenytoin (diphenylhydantoin)	*Antisacer, Apamin, Dantoin, Difhydan, Di-Hydan, Dilantin, Dintoina, Diphantoine, Diphenylan, Ditan, Epanutin, Epilantin, Epinat, Fenantoin, Fenytoin, Hydantol, Labopal, Lehydan, Neosidantoina, Phenhydan, Phentoin, Pyoredol, Solantyl, Tacosal, Toin Unicelles, Zentropil*
Progabide	
Primidone	*Dilon, Liskantin, Majdolsin, Midone, Mylepsin, Mylepsinum, Mysoline, Prosoline, Resimatil, Sertan*
Stiripentol	
Sulthiame	*Ospolot*
Valproic acid (sodium valproate, dipropylacetate)	*Convulex, Convulexette, Depakene, Depakin, Depakine, Deprakine, Epilim, Logical (magnesium valproate), Orfiril, Propymal*
Valpromide (dipropylacetamide)	*Depamide, Vistora*

Anticonvulsants + Acetazolamide

Abstract/Summary

Severe osteomalacia and rickets have been seen in patients on phenytoin, phenobarbitone and primidone when concurrently treated with acetazolamide. A marked reduction in serum primidone levels with a loss in seizure control, and rises in serum carbamazepine levels with toxicity have also been described.

Clinical evidence

(a) Osteomalacia

Two young women on phenytoin, primidone or phenobarbitone developed severe osteomalacia while taking 750 mg acetazolamide daily, despite a normal intake of calcium. When the acetazolamide was withdrawn, the hyperchloraemic acidosis shown by both patients abated and the high urinary excretion of calcium fell by 50%.[1]

This interaction has been described in two adults[3] and in three children[2] who developed rickets.

(b) Reduced serum primidone levels

A patient on primidone showed an increase in fit-frequency and a virtual absence of primidone (or phenobarbitone) in the serum when treated with acetazolamide. Primidone absorption recommenced when the acetazolamide was withdrawn. A subsequent study in two other patients showed that acetazolamide reduced the absorption of primidone in one but not in the other.[5]

(c) Increased serum carbamazepine levels

A girl of 9 and two boys of 14 and 19, all of them on the highest dosages of carbamazepine tolerable without side-effects, developed signs of toxicity after taking acetazolamide (250–750 mg daily) and were found to have serum carbamazepine levels which were elevated 30–50%. In one instance toxicity appeared within 48 h.[6]

Mechanisms

Uncertain. (a) Mild osteomalacia induced by anticonvulsants is a recognized phenomenon.[4] This, it seems, is exaggerated by acetazolamide which increases urinary calcium excretion, possibly by causing systemic acidosis which results from the reduced absorption of bicarbonate by the kidney. (b and c) The acetazolamide-induced changes in primidone absorption and the rises in serum carbamazepine levels are not understood.

Importance and management

The documentation of all of these interactions is very limited, and their incidence uncertain. The effects of concurrent use should be closely monitored for the possible development of these adverse interactions and steps taken to accommodate them. Withdraw the acetazolamide if necessary, or in the case of the anticonvulsants, adjust the dosage appropriately. In the case of the children cited[2] the acetazolamide was withdrawn and 10,000 U of vitamin D were given. It seems possible that other carbonic anhydrase inhibitors may behave like acetazolamide.

References

1 Mallette LE. Anticonvulsants, acetazolamide and osteomalacia. N Engl J Med (1975) 292, 668.
2 Matsuda I, Takekoshi Y, Shida N, Fujieda K, Nagai B, Arashima S, Anakura M and Oka Y. Renal tubular acidosis and skeletal demineralization in patients on long-term anticonvulsant therapy. J Pediatr (1975) 87, 202.
3 Mallette LE. Acetazolamide-accelerated anticonvulsant osteomalacia. Arch InternMed (1977) 137, 1013.
4 Anast CS. Anticonvulsant drugs and calcium metabolism. N Engl J Med (1975) 292, 567.
5 Syversen GB, Morgan JP, Weintraub M and Myers GJ. Acetazolamide-induced interference with primidone absorption. Arch Neurol (1977) 34, 80.
6 McBride MC. Serum carbamazepine levels are increased by acetazolamide. Ann Neurol (1984) 16, 393.

Anticonvulsants + Aspartame

Abstract/Summary

Aspartame can cause convulsions in some susceptible individuals.

Clinical evidence, mechanism, importance and management

Grand mal seizures have been reported in 80 people associated with the consumption of aspartame (*Nutrasweet*) as a sweetening agent. Three of them were taking phenytoin. Petit mal and psychomotor attacks were also seen in another 18 subjects taking aspartame.[1] Another 149 cases of aspartame-associated convulsions have been reported to the FDA.[1] The reasons for this adverse reaction are not understood. It may be prudent for patients taking anticonvulsants to avoid aspartame.

Reference

1 Roberts HJ. Aspartame (*Nutrasweet*)-associated epilepsy. Clin Res (1988) 36, 349A.

Anticonvulsants + Calcium channel blockers

Abstract/Summary

Verapamil can cause a marked rise in serum carbamazepine levels resulting in intoxication. The same effect has been seen in two patients given diltiazem. Nifedipine appears not to interact with carbamazepine but it caused phenytoin intoxication in one patient. The serum levels of felodipine are very markedly reduced by carbamazepine, phenobarbitone and phenytoin, and verapamil levels are also very much reduced by phenobarbitone.

Clinical evidence

Anticonvulsant and toxic effects increased

(a) Carbamazepine + diltiazem or nifedipine

An epileptic patient on 1 g carbamazepine daily developed signs of toxicity (dizziness, nausea, ataxia and diplopia) within two days of starting to take 60 mg diltiazem three times a day. His serum carbamazepine levels had risen about 50% (from 13 to 21 mg/l) but fell once again when the diltiazem was stopped. No interaction occurred when the diltiazem was replaced by nifedipine, 20 mg three times a day.[1]

Another report describes carbamazepine toxicity in a patient given diltiazem associated with a 50% rise in serum levels.[3]

(b) Carbamazepine + verapamil

Sixileptic patients developed mild carbamazepine intoxication within 36–96 h of starting 120 mg verapamil three times a day. The symptoms disappeared when the verapamil was withdrawn. Total carbamazepine serum levels had risen by 46% (33% in free plasma carbamazepine concentrations). Rechallenge of two of the patients with less verapamil (120 mg twice a day) caused a similar rise in serum verapamil levels. This report also describes another patient with elevated serum carbamazepine levels while taking verapamil.[2]

Two reports describe carbamazepine toxicity in three patients caused by verapamil. The verapamil was successfully replaced by nifedipine in one patient.[4,8]

(c) Phenytoin + nifedipine

An isolated report describes intoxication in a man on phenytoin three weeks after starting to take 30 mg nifedipine daily. His serum phenytoin levels had risen to 30.4 μg/ml. Two weeks after stopping the nifedipine his serum phenytoin levels had fallen to 10.5 μg/ml and all the symptoms had gone two weeks later.[5]

Calcium channel blocker effects reduced

(a) Felodipine + carbamazepine, phenobarbitone and phenytoin

After taking 10 mg felodipine daily for four days, 10 epileptics on carbamazepine or phenytoin or phenobarbitone or carbamazepine with phenytoin had markedly reduced serum felodipine levels (peak levels of 1.6 nmol/l compared with 8.9 nmol/l in 12 control subjects). The AUC (area under the time-concentration curve) was reduced to about 7%.[7]

(b) Nifedipine + phenobarbitone

A study in 15 normal subjects showed that after taking 100 mg phenobarbitone daily for two weeks the clearance of a single 20 mg dose of nifedipine in a 'cocktail' also contain-

ing sparteine, mephenytoin and antipyrine was increased almost threefold (from 1088 to 2981 ml/min) and the nifedipine AUC (area under the concentration-time curve was reduced about 60% (from 343 to 135 ng.h/ml).[9]

(c) Verapamil + phenobarbitone

A study in seven normal subjects showed that after taking 100 mg phenobarbitone daily for three weeks the clearance of verapamil (80 mg orally six-hourly) was increased fourfold (from 22 to 91 ml/min/kg) and the bioavailability was reduced fivefold (from 0.59 to 0.12).[6]

Mechanism

It would appear that the calcium channel blockers inhibit the metabolism of carbamazepine and phenytoin by the liver, thereby reducing their loss from the body and increasing serum levels. In contrast, the anticonvulsants are well recognized as enzyme inducers which can increase the metabolism of the calcium channel blockers by the liver, resulting in a very rapid loss from the body.

Importance and management

(I) Information about the effects of calcium channel blockers on carbamazepine is limited, but what is known indicates that if verapamil and possibly diltiazem are given the carbamazepine dosage will need to be reduced to avoid intoxication. Nifedipine appears to be a non-interacting alternative, but may not be safe with phenytoin. There appears to be no information about the effects of calcium channel blockers on other anticonvulsants.

(II) Carbamazepine, phenobarbitone and phenytoin markedly reduce felodipine levels, phenobarbitone has the same effect on verapamil and possibly on nifedipine also. A considerable increase in the dosage of these calcium channel blockers will be needed in epileptic patients taking these drugs. There is no direct information of interactions with other calcium channel blockers, but be alert for evidence of reduced effects with others metabolized in a similar way (nifedipine, nicardipine, nitrendipine).

References

1 Brodie MJ and Macphee GJA. Carbamazepine neurotoxicity precipitated by diltiazem. Brit Med J (1986) 292, 1170–1.
2 Macphee GJA, McInnes GT, Thompson GG and Brodie MJ. Verapamil potentiates carbamazepine neurotoxicity: a clinically important inhibitory interaction. Lancet (1986) i, 700–3.
3 Eimer M and Carter BL. Elevated serum carbamazepine concentrations following diltiazem initiation. Drug Intell Clin Pharm (1987) 21, 340–2.
4 Beattie B, Biller J, Mehlaus B and Murray M. Verapamil-induced carbamazepine neurotoxicity. Eur Neurol (1988) 28, 104–5.
5 Ahmad S. Nifedipine-phenytoin interaction. J Am Coll Cardiol (1984) 3, 1582.
6 Rutledge DR, Pieper JA, Sirmans SM and Mirvis DM. Verapamil disposition after phenobarbital treatment. Clin Pharmacol Ther (1987) 41, 245.
7 Capewell S, Freestone S, Critchley JAJH, Pottage A and Prescott LF. Reduced felodipine bioavailability in patients taking anticonvulsants. Lancet (1988) ii, 480–2.
8 Price WA and Di Marzio LR. Verapamil-carbamazepine neurotoxicity. J Clin Psychiatry (1988) 49, 80.

9 Schellens JHM, van der Wart JHF, Brugman M and Breimer DD. Influence of enzyme induction and inhibition on the oxidation of nifedipine, sparteine, mephenytoin and antipyrine in humans assessed by a 'cocktail' study design. J Pharmacol Exp Ther (1989) 249, 638–45.

Anticonvulsants + Cinromide

Abstract/Summary

Cinromide can depress the serum levels of phenytoin, carbamazepine and sodium valproate.

Clinical evidence, mechanism, importance and management

A very brief report states that during concurrent use cinromide was seen to reduce serum concentrations of phenytoin by 18%, of carbamazepine by 31% and (in one patient) of sodium valproate by 41%.[1] The clinical importance of these interactions is uncertain.

Reference

1 Cramer JA and Mattson RH. Cinromide pharmacokinetics and interactions. Epilepsia (1981) 22, 235.

Anticonvulsants + Cytotoxic drugs

Abstract/Summary

Phenytoin serum levels have been seen to be markedly reduced during concurrent treatment with some cytotoxic drug regimens (cisplatinum, bleomycin, vinblastine; methotrexate, vinblastine, carmustine) and seizures can occur if the phenytoin dosage is not raised appropriately. A similar interaction has also been seen in a patient on phenytoin, carbamazepine and sodium valproate when treated with cisplatin and doxorubicin (adriamycin).

Clinical evidence

Two reports[1,2] describe two patients who showed a marked fall in serum phenytoin levels (from an estimated 15 to 2 μg/ml in one case accompanied by seizures) when concurrently treated with cisplatinum, bleomycin and vinblastine. A subsequent study[1] showed that the phenytoin absorption from the gut was reduced to 22–32%. Another report described a similar interaction in a patient on vinblastine, methotrexate and carmustine.[3,4] On two occasions an epileptic woman treated with phenytoin, carbamazepine and sodium valproate had seizures within 2–3 days of starting a *Chap-V* course (intravenous doxorubicin, 35 mg/m^2 on day one and cisplatin 20 mg/m^2 for days 1–5). The serum levels of all three anticonvulsants were found to be depressed and below therapeutic levels.[5] On a third occasion the trough serum levels of carbamazepine and sodium valproate from days 5/7 to 13 were seen to decrease from 3.6 to 1.2 and from

40.9 to 10 mg/l respectively when given these cytotoxic drugs.[5]

Mechanism

Not fully established but a suggested reason is that these cytotoxic drugs damage the intestinal wall which reduces the absorption of the anticonvulsants, but other mechanisms may also have some part to play.

Importance and management

Although the evidence for these interactions is very limited, it would be prudent to monitor serum anticonvulsant levels closely both during treatment with these cytotoxics.

References

1 Sylvester RK, Lewis FB, Caldwell KC, Lobell M, Perri R and Sawchuk RA. Impaired phenytoin bioavailability secondary to cisplatinum, vinblastine and bleomycin. Ther Drug Monit (1984) 6, 302–5.
2 Fincham RW and Schottelius DD. Case report. Decreased phenytoin levels in antineoplastic therapy. Ther Drug Monit (1979) 1, 277.
3 Riva R, Albani F and Baruzzi A. On the interaction between phenytoin and antineoplastic agents. Ther Drug Monit (1985) 7, 123–6.
4 Bollini P, Riva R, Albani F, Ida N, Cacciari L, Bollini C and Baruzzi A. Decreased phenytoin level during antineoplastic therapy: a case report. Epilepsia (1983) 24, 75–8.
5 Neef C and de Voogd-van der Straaten I. An interaction between cytostatic and anticonvulsant drugs. Clin Pharmacol Ther (1988) 43, 372–5.

Anticonvulsants + Denzimol

Abstract/Summary

Very marked and rapid rises in the serum levels of carbamazepine and phenytoin occur, accompanied by acute toxicity, if denzimol is given concurrently. No interaction seems to occur with either sodium valproate or primidone.

Clinical evidence, mechanism, importance and management

All six patients on carbamazepine showed very marked rises in serum concentrations within 5–30 days and acute toxicity when concurrently treated with denzimol (150–450 mg daily). Despite a reduction in the carbamazepine dosage in four of the six, serum levels rose by 114% (range 50–142%). Two patients on phenytoin showed rises of 97 and 174% respectively over a five-week period. Seven other patients taking sodium valproate or primidone showed no significant changes in their serum levels.[1] It is suggested that the serum anticonvulsant level rises occur because denzimol inhibits the metabolism of carbamazepine and phenytoin by the liver. More study is needed to assess whether it can safely be given routinely with carbamazepine or phenytoin.

Reference

1 Patsalos PN, Shorvon SD, Elyas AA and Smith G. The interaction of denzimol (a new anticonvulsant) with carbamazepine and phenytoin. J Neurol Neurosurg Psychiatry (1985) 48, 374–7.

Anticonvulsants + Dextropropoxyphene

Abstract/Summary

Carbamazepine serum levels can be raised by the concurrent use of dextropropoxyphene. Toxicity may develop unless suitable dosage reductions are made. A trivial or only modest rise in serum phenytoin or phenobarbitone levels may occur but the development of toxicity is unlikely in most patients.

Clinical evidence

(a) Carbamazepine + dextropropoxyphene

The observation of toxicity (headache, dizziness, ataxia, nausea, tiredness) during the concurrent use of carbamazepine and dextropropoxyphene prompted further study. Five subjects given 65 mg dextropropoxyphene three times a day showed a mean rise in serum carbamazepine levels of 65%. Three of them showed evidence of carbamazepine toxicity.[1-2]

In another study the same workers found a 66% rise in other subjects after six days treatment with dextropropoxyphene.[3] Intoxication due to this interaction is reported elsewhere.[4,5,7]

(b) Phenobarbitone + dextropropoxyphene

A study in four epileptic patients on phenobarbitone showed that they averaged a 20% rise in serum levels after taking dextropropoxyphene 65 mg three times a day for a week.[3]

(c) Phenytoin + dextropropoxyphene

A study in six patients on phenytoin showed that only a very small rise in serum levels occurred when concurrently treated with dextropropoxyphene (65 mg three times a day) for 6–13 days.[3]

In contrast one patient is reported to have experienced a marked elevation in serum phenytoin levels while taking dextropropoxyphene.[6]

Mechanisms

Uncertain. It is suggested that the dextropropoxyphene inhibits the metabolism of the carbamazepine by the liver enzymes, leading to its accumulation in the body,[1-2] and this may also be true for the phenobarbitone.

Importance and management

The carbamazepine–dextropropoxyphene interaction is established and clinically important. Concurrent use should be avoided. If dextropropoxyphene is absolutely necessary, the serum carbamazepine levels should be closely monitored and suitable dosage reductions made to prevent the development of intoxication. In most cases it would seem simpler to use an alternative non-interacting analgesic although the occasional single dose may not matter.

The concurrent use of dextropropoxyphene and either phenytoin or phenobarbitone need not be avoided, but because rises in the serum levels of both anticonvulsants can occur it would be prudent to monitor the outcome.

References

1 Dam M and Christiansen J. Interaction of propoxyphene with carbamazepine. Lancet (1977) ii, 509.
2 Dam M, Kristensen B, Hansen BS and Christiansen J. Interaction between carbamazepine and propoxyphene in man. Acta Neurol Scand (1977) 56, 603.
3 Hansen BS, Dam M, Brandt J, Hvidberg EF, Angelo H, Christensen JM and Lous P. Influence of dextropropoxyphene on steady state serum levels and protein binding of three anti-epileptic drugs in man. Acta Neurol Scand (1980) 61, 357.
4 Yu YL, Huang CY, Chin E, Woo E and Chang CM. Interaction between carbamazepine and dextropropoxyphene. Postgrad Med J (1986) 62, 231–3.
5 Kubacka RT and Ferrante JA. Carbamazepine-propoxyphene interaction. Clin Pharm (1983) 2, 104.
6 Kutt H. Biochemical and genetic factors regulating Dilantin metabolism in man. Ann NY Acad Sci (1971) 179, 704.
7 Risinger MW. Carbamazepine toxicity with concurrent use of propoxyphene: a report of five cases. Neurology (1987) 37 (Suppl 1) 87.

Anticonvulsants + Disulfiram

Abstract/Summary

Phenytoin serum levels are markedly and rapidly increased by the concurrent use of disulfiram. Phenytoin intoxication can develop. There is evidence that phenobarbitone and carbamazepine are not affected by disulfiram, and that calcium carbimide does not interact with phenytoin.

Clinical evidence

The serum phenytoin levels of four patients on long-term treatment showed rises of 100–500% over a nine day period when concurrently treated with 400 mg disulfiram daily, with no signs of levelling off until the disulfiram was withdrawn. Two of them developed signs of mild intoxication.[1] In a follow-up study on two patients, one of them showed ataxia and a serum phenytoin rise of 55% (from 18 to 28 μg/ml) within five days.[1,2]

A study in 10 normal subjects showed that disulfiram increased the half-life of phenytoin from 11 to 19 h.[3] There are case reports describing this interaction.[4-7]

Mechanism

The disulfiram inhibits the liver enzymes concerned with the metabolism of the phenytoin thereby prolonging its stay in the body and resulting in a rise in its serum levels (to toxic concentrations in some instances). One study concluded that the inhibition was non-competitive.[7]

Importance and management

An established, moderately well documented, clinically important and potentially serious interaction. The evidence available indicates that it occurs in most patients and develops rapidly. Recovery may take 2–3 weeks when the disulfiram is withdrawn. Olesen[1,2] offers the opinion that the dosage of phenytoin '. . .could of course be reduced [to accommodate the interaction] but it would be difficult to maintain the precise balance required. . .'.

Alternative anticonvulsants include phenobarbitone which in one study[2,3] (paralleling those cited above) showed only minor (10%) serum level fluctuations with disulfiram. Three of the patients were taking primidone and one phenobarbitone. Carbamazepine also appears not to interact. Signs of toxicity disappeared in a patient when phenytoin was replaced by carbamazepine,[6] and this observation was confirmed in a study on five non-alcoholic patients.[8]

A different solution is to replace the disulfiram with calcium carbimide. A study in four patients showed that 50 mg daily for a week followed by 100 mg for two weeks had no effect on serum phenytoin levels.[2]

References

1 Olesen OV. Disulfiramum (Antabuse) as inhibitor of phenytoin metabolism. Acta pharmacolet toxicol (1966) 24, 317.
2 Olesen OV. The influence of disulfiram and calcium carbimide on the serum diphenylhydantoin excretion of HPPH in the urine. Arch Neurol (1967) 16, 642.
3 Svendsen TL, Kristensen MB, Hansen JM and Skovsted L. The influence of disulfiram on the half-life and metabolic clearance rate of diphenylhydantoin and tolbutamide in man. Europ J clin Pharmacol (1976) 9, 439.
4 Kiorboe E. Phenytoin intoxication during treatment with Antabuse. Epilepsia (1966) 7, 246.
5 Kiorboe E. Antabus som arsag til forgiftning med fenytoin. Ugeskr laeg (1966) 128, 1531.
6 Dry J and Pradalier A. Intoxication par la phenytoin au cours d'une association therapeutique avec le disulfirame. Therapie (1973) 28, 799.
7 Taylor JW, Alexander B and Lyon LW. Mathematical analysis of a phenytoin-disulfiram interaction. Amer J Hosp Pharm (1981) 38, 93.
8 Krag B, Dam M, Helle A and Christensen JM. Influence of disulfiram on the serum concentrations of carbamazepine in patients with epilepsy. Acta neurol Scand (1981) 63, 395.

Anticonvulsants + Felbamate

Abstract/Summary

Preliminary evidence indicates that felbamate can raise serum phenytoin levels but reduce serum carbamazepine levels.

Clinical evidence, mechanism, importance and management

A very brief report of a study in four patients, associated later with a further study in five normal subjects, showed that felbamate increases serum phenytoin levels. Despite a 20% reduction in the phenytoin dosage before the felbamate (30–54.9 mg/kg/day) was given, one subject needed a slight increase in dosage whereas two others needed a further reduction in phenytoin dosage. The reason is thought to be that the felbamate inhibits the metabolism of the phenytoin, thereby reducing its loss from the body and increasing its serum levels. Be alert for the need to reduce the phenytoin dosage if felbamate is added to avoid possible phenytoin toxicity. Related studies suggested that felbamate increases the loss of carbamazepine from the body so that an increase in the dosage may possibly be needed. Trough serum carbamazepine levels after seven days of felbamate were reduced from 6.2 to 4.6 μg/ml.[1,2]

References

1 Fuerst RH, Graves NM, Leppik IE, Remmel RP, Rosenfeld WE and Sierzant TL. A preliminary report on alteration of carbamazepine and phenytoin metabolism by felbamate. Drug Intell Clin Pharm (1986) 20, 465–6.
2 Fuerst RH, Graves NM, Leppik IE, Brundage RC, Holmes GB and Remmel RP. Felbamate increases phenytoin but decreases carbamazepine concentrations. Epilepsia (1988) 29, 488–91.

Anticonvulsants + Folic acid

Abstract/Summary

If folic acid supplements are given to treat the folate deficiency which can be caused by the use of anticonvulsants (phenytoin, phenobarbitone, primidone and possibly pheneturide), the serum anticonvulsant levels may fall, leading to decreased seizure control in some patients.

Clinical evidence

A study on 50 folate-deficient epileptics (taking phenytoin with phenobarbitone and primidone) showed that after one month's treatment with 5 mg folic acid daily, the serum phenytoin levels of one group (10 patients) had fallen from 20 to 10 μg/ml, and of another group taking 15 mg daily from 14 to 10 μg/ml. Only one patient showed a marked increase in fit frequency and severity.[1]

Another long-term study on 26 patients with folic acid deficiency (less than 5 ng/ml) due to anticonvulsant treatment with two or more drugs (phenytoin, phenobarbitone, primidone) showed that when they were given 15 mg folic acid daily the mental state of 22 of them improved to a variable degree, but the frequency and severity of fits in 13 (50%) increased to such an extent that the vitamin had to be withdrawn.[2]

Similar results have been described in other studies and reports.[2,3,8]

Mechanism

Patients on anticonvulsants not infrequently have subnormal serum folic acid levels (frequencies of 27–58% have been reported[4]) due, so it is believed, to the enzyme-inducing characteristics of the anticonvulsants which make excessive demands on folate for the synthesis of the cytochromic enzymes concerned with drug metabolism. Ultimately drug metabolism becomes limited by the lack of folate, and patients may also experience a depression in their general mental health[2] and even frank megaloblastic anaemia.[7] If however folic acid is given to treat this deficiency, the metabolism of the anticonvulsant increases once again,[9] resulting in a reduction in serum anticonvulsant levels which, in some instances, may become so low that seizure control is partially or totally lost.

Importance and management

A very well documented and clinically important interaction (only a few references are listed here). Reductions in serum phenytoin levels of 16-50% after taking 5-15 mg folic acid daily for 2-4 weeks have been described.[2-5] The incidence is uncertain (reports range from 0-50%[1,2,6]). Folic acid supplements should only be given to folate-deficient epileptics taking phenytoin, phenobarbitone, primidone and possibly pheneturide if their serum anticonvulsant levels can be well monitored so that suitable dosage increases can be made.

References

1 Baylis EM, Crowley JM, Preece JM, Sylvester PE and Marks V. Influence of folic acid on blood-phenytoin levels. Lancet (1971) i, 62.
2 Reynolds EH. Effects of folic acid on the mental state and fit-frequency of drug-treated epileptics. Lancet (1967) i, 1086.
3 Strauss RG and Bernstein R. Folic acid and Dilantin antagonism in pregnancy. Obstet Gynecol (1974) 44, 345.
4 Davis RE and Woodliff HJ. Folic acid deficiency in patients receiving anticonvulsant drugs. Med J Aust (1971) 2, 1070.
5 Furlanut M, Benetello P, Avogaro A and Dainese R. Effects of folic acid on phenytoin kinetics in healthy subjects. Clin Pharmacol Ther (1978) 24, 294.
6 Grant RHE and Stores OPR. Folic acid in folate-deficient patients with epilepsy. Brit Med J (1970) 4, 644.
7 Ryan GMS and Forshaw JWB. Megaloblastic anaemia due to phenytoin sodium. Brit Med J (1955) 11, 242.
8 Latham AN, Millbank L, Richens A and Rowe DJF. Liver enzyme induction by anticonvulsant drugs, and its relationship to disturbed calcium and folic acid metabolism. J Clin Pharmacol (1973) 13, 337.
9 Berg MJ, Fischer LJ, Rivey MP, Vern BA, Lantz RK and Schottelius DD. Phenytoin and folic acid interaction: a preliminary report. Ther Drug Monit (1983) 5, 389-94.

Anticonvulsants + Influenza vaccines

Abstract/Summary

Influenza vaccine can cause a rise in serum phenobarbitone levels, but carbamazepine is unaffected. See also 'Phenytoin + Influenza vaccines'.

Clinical evidence, mechanism, importance and management

Serum phenobarbitone levels rose by 30% in 11 out of 27 children (very prolonged in some individuals) when given 0.5 ml of an influenza vaccine, USP, types A and B, whole virus (Squibb), but no significant changes occurred in the serum carbamazepine levels of another 20 children.[1] The suggested reason is the vaccine inhibits the liver enzymes concerned with the metabolism of phenobarbitone, thereby reducing its loss from the body. The effects of giving influenza vaccines to patients treated with phenobarbitone should be monitored. See also 'Phenytoin + Influenza vaccines'.

Reference

1 Jann MW and Fidone GS. Effect of influenza vaccine on serum anticonvulsant concentrations. Clin Pharm (1986) 5, 817-20.

Anticonvulsants + Nafimidone

Abstract/Summary

Nafimidone causes a marked rise in the serum levels of carbamazepine and phenytoin. Dosage reductions are necessary to prevent toxicity.

Clinical evidence

Two epileptics with intractable partial seizures, stabilized on carbamazepine and phenytoin, showed a rise in the serum levels of both drugs within a day of additionally starting to take nafimidone (3 mg/kg daily in three divided doses). By the second day carbamazepine toxicity had developed. In four other patients, similarly treated, the dosages of carbamazepine and phenytoin were reduced to prevent excessively high serum levels. Carbamazepine elimination was reduced 76-87% and phenytoin elimination by 38-77% while taking nafimidone. Serum levels fell to normal within a day of stopping the nafimidone.[1]

Mechanism

Not understood. It seems possible that nafimidone inhibits the metabolism of carbamazepine and phenytoin by the liver, thereby reducing their loss from the body.

Importance and management

Information is limited but the interaction would appear to be established. The dosages of carbamazepine and phenytoin will need to be markedly reduced if nafimidone is added, and increased when it is withdrawn.

Reference

1 Treiman DM and Ben-Menachem E. Inhibition of carbamazepine and phenytoin metabolism by nafimidone, a new antiepileptic drug. Epilepsia (1987) 28, 699-705.

Anticonvulsants + Progabide

Abstract/Summary

Serum phenytoin levels can rise if progabide is used concurrently. A reduction in the dosage of phenytoin may be required. A rise in serum phenobarbitone levels has been seen. Changes in the serum levels of other anticonvulsants (carbamazepine, sodium valproate, clonazepam) caused by progabide and their effects on serum progabide levels appear to be small.

Clinical evidence, mechanism, importance and management

Marked increases in serum phenytoin levels have been seen in a few patients given progabide concurrently.[1,2] In one study[3,6] in epileptic patients, 17 out of 26 needed a reduction in the dosage of phenytoin to keep the levels within +25% of the serum levels before progabide was given, and this occurred within 4–10 weeks of starting concurrent treatment. Most of the patients needing a dosage reduction showed a maximum increase of 40% or more. In contrast only small changes were seen in another study.[7] Yet another described a small increase in the clearance of progabide in the presence of phenytoin.[8]

Information about other anticonvulsants is limited, but progabide is reported not to change carbamazepine[3,4,7,8] or sodium valproate[4,7,8] serum levels, nor to affect clonazepam levels significantly,[5] while a small increase in serum phenobarbitone levels has been seen.[4,7,9] An increase in carbamazepine-epoxide levels has been reported.[9] Some reduction in serum progabide levels is reported with sodium valproate.[8]

The possibility that the dosage of phenytoin and phenobarbitone may need to be reduced should be borne in mind if progabide is used concurrently. The significance of the increased levels of carbamazepine-epoxide is uncertain.

References

1 Dam M, Gram L, Philbert A, Hansen BS, Blatt Lyon B, Christensen JM and Angelo HR. Progabide: a controlled trial in partial epilepsy. Epilepsia (1983) 24, 127–34.
2 Van der Linden GJ, Meinardi H, Meijer JWA, Bossi L and Gomeni C. A double-blind cross-over trial with progabide (SL 76002) against placebo in patients with secondary generalized epilepsy. In: Advances in Epileptology: XIIth Epilepsy Int Symp. Dam M, Gram L and Penry JK (eds). Raven Press, New York. (1981) pp 141–4.
3 Cloyd JC, Brundage RC, Leppik IE, Graves NM and Welty TE. Effect of progabide on serum phenytoin and carbamazepine concentrations: a preliminary report. In: LERS Monograph series, volume 3. Edited by Bartholini G. Epilepsy and GABA receptor agonists: basic and therapeutic research. Meeting, Paris, March 1984. Raven Press, New York. (1985) pp 271–8.
4 Thenot JP, Bianchetti G, Abriol C, Feuerstein J, Lambert D, Thebault JJ, Warrington SJ and Rowland M. Interactions between progabide and antiepileptic drugs. Ibid (1985) pp 259–69.
5 Warrington SJ, O'Brien C, Thiercelin JF, Orofiamma B and Morselli PL. Evaluation of pharmacodynamic interaction between progabide and clonazepam in healthy men. Ibid (1985) pp 279–86.
6 Cloyd JC, Brundage RC, Leppik IE, Graves NM and Welty TE. Effect of progabide on phenytoin pharmacokinetics. Epilepsia (1984) 5, 656–7.
7 Bianchetti G, Thiercelin JF, Thenot JP, Feuerstein D, Lambert D, Rulliere JJ, Thebault JJ and Morselli PL. Effect of progabide on the phamacokinetics of various antiepileptic drugs. Neurology (1984) 34 (Suppl 1) 213.
8 Thiercelin JF, Padovani P, Thenot JP, Rowland M, Warrington S and Morselli PL. Effect of various antiepileptic drugs on the pharmacokinetics of progabide and its acid metabolite. Neurology (1984) 34 (Suppl 1) 266.
9 Bianchetti G, Padovani P, Thenot JP, Thiercelin JF and Morselli PL. Pharmacokinetic interactions of progabide with other antiepileptic drugs. Epilepsia (1987) 28, 68–73.

Anticonvulsants + Pyridoxine

Abstract/Summary

Large doses of pyridoxine (200 mg daily) can cause marked reductions (40–50%) in the serum phenytoin and phenobarbitone levels of some patients.

Clinical evidence, mechanism, importance and management

A study in epileptic patients on phenytoin or phenobarbitone showed that 200 mg pyridoxine daily for four weeks reduced the phenobarbitone serum levels of five patients by about 50%. Reductions in serum phenytoin levels of almost 40% (range 8–66%) were also seen when given pyridoxine (80–200 mg daily) for 2–4 weeks. A number of other patients were not affected.[1] It is suggested that the pyridoxine increases the activity of the liver enzymes concerned with the metabolism of the these anticonvulsants. The documentation of this interaction is very limited, but what is known suggests that concurrent use should be monitored if large doses of pyridoxine like this are used. It seems unlikely that small doses (as in multivitamin preparations) will interact to any great extent.

Reference

1 Hansson O and Sillanpaa M. Pyridoxine and serum concentrations of phenytoin and phenobarbitone. Lancet (1976) i, 256.

Anticonvulsants + Quinolone antibiotics

Abstract/Summary

Ciprofloxacin and enoxacin very occasionally cause convulsions and the makers advise caution or avoidance in epileptic subjects.

Clinical evidence, mechanism, importance and management

The makers of ciprofloxacin and enoxacin suggest that these antibiotics should be used with caution or avoided in epileptics because a very small number of patients have developed convulsions. Ciprofloxacin has been associated with convulsions in both epileptic[1-3] and non-epileptic[1] patients. Blood levels of phenytoin and valproic acid appear to be unaffected.[1] Enoxacin may also possibly lower the convulsive threshold in patients predisposed to seizures.[4] Particular care should therefore be exercised if these antibiotics are given to epileptic patients. This is strictly speaking a disease–drug interaction rather than a drug–drug interaction.

References

1 Slavich IL, Gleffe R and Haas EJ. Grand mal seizures during ciprofloxacin therapy. J Amer Med Ass (1989) 261, 558–9.
2 Beeley L, Magee P and Hickey F. Newsletter of the W.Midlands Centre for Adverse Drug Reaction Reporting, January (1989).
3 Schacht P, Arcieri G, Branolte J, Bruck H, Chysky V, Griffith E, Gruenwald G, Hullmann R, Konopka CA, O'Brien B, Rahm V, Ryoki T, Westwood A and Weuta H. Worldwide clinical data on efficacy and safety of ciprofloxacin. Eur J Clin Study Treat Infect (1988) Suppl 1, 29–43.
4 Comprecin (enoxacin) Clinical Information Manual. Parke Davis (1989).

Anticonvulsants + Stiripentol

Abstract/Summary

Stiripentol causes marked rises in the serum levels of carbamazepine, phenobarbitone and phenytoin. Reduce their dosages to avoid the development of toxicity.

Clinical evidence

A study was undertaken on six epileptic patients taking two or three anticonvulsants (phenytoin, phenobarbitone, carbamazepine, primidone, nitrazepam) who were additionally given stiripentol (600–2400 mg daily). All five on phenytoin showed a reduction in the phenytoin clearance from 29.5 to 18.5 litre daily while taking 1200 mg stiripentiol daily, and to 6.48 litre daily while on 2400 mg stiripentol. These changes in clearance were reflected in marked rises in the steady-state serum levels of the anticonvulsants: for example the serum phenytoin levels of one patient rose from 14.4 mg/l to 27.4 mg/l over 30 days while taking stiripentol, despite a halving of his phenytoin dosage. Phenytoin toxicity was seen in two subjects.[1]

The clearance of carbamazepine in one subject fell from 209 to 128 litre daily while on 1200 mg stiripentol daily and to 61 litre daily while on 2400 mg stiripentol daily. Phenobarbitone clearance in two subjects fell from 3.8 and 5 litre daily to 2.3 and 3.4 litre daily while taking 2400 mg stiripentol daily.[1] Another study in adults and children confirmed that stiripentol halved the clearance of carbamazepine.[2]

Mechanism

Uncertain. It seems probable that stiripentol inhibits the activity of the liver enzymes concerned with the metabolism of these anticonvulsants so that their loss from the body is reduced and their serum levels rise accordingly.

Importance and management

These interactions would seem to be established and of clinical importance. The dosages of phenytoin, phenobarbitone and carbamazepine should be reduced to avoid the development of elevated serum levels and possible toxicity during concurrent use. In the case of phenytoin halving the dose may not be enough. One study suggests that the carbamazepine dosage should be decreased incrementally over 7–10 days as soon as the stiripentol is started and, regardless of age, the maintenance dose of carbamazepine should be 4.4 to 8.7 mg/kg/day to give serum levels of 5–10 μg/ml.

References

1 Levy RH, Loiseau P, Guyot M, Blehaut HM, Tor J and Morland TA. Stiripentol kinetics in epilepsy: non-linearity and interactions. Clin Pharmacol Ther (1984) 36, 661–9.
2 Levy RH, Kerr BM, Farwell J, Anderson GD, Martinez-Lage M and Tor J. Carbamazepine/stiripentol interaction in adult and paediatric patients. Epilepsia (1989) 30, 701.

Anticonvulsants + Tobacco smoking

Abstract/Summary

Smoking appears to have no important effect on the serum levels of phenytoin, phenobarbitone or carbamazepine.

Clinical evidence, mechanism, importance and management

A comparative study in 88 epileptic patients taking anticonvulsants (phenobarbitone, phenytoin and carbamazepine alone and in combination) showed that although smoking had a tendency to lower the steady-state serum concentrations of these drugs, a statistically significant effect was only shown on the concentration-dose ratios of the phenobarbitone-treated patients.[1] In practical terms smoking appears to have only a negligible effect on the serum levels of these anticonvulsants and epileptics are unlikely to need higher doses than non-smokers.

Reference

1 Benetello P, Furlanut M, Pasqui L, Carmillo L, Perlotto N and Testa G. Absence of effect of cigarette smoking on serum concentrations of some anticonvulsants in epileptic patients. Clin Pharmacokinetics (1987) 12, 302–4.

Anticonvulsants + Vigabatrin

Abstract/Summary

Vigabatrin lowers serum phenytoin levels but not those of phenobarbitone or carbamazepine.

Clinical evidence, mechanism, importance and management

A study in epileptic patients showed that 2–3 g vigabatrin daily did not change the serum levels of phenobarbitone (26 patients), carbamazepine (12 patients) or valproic acid (two patients). The mean serum phenytoin levels (19 patients) were about 20% lower during concurrent use (for reasons which are not understood) and in two patients they fell below the therapeutic range. Seizure frequency remained unaltered.[1] This confirms the findings of two other studies.[2,3] There seems to be no reason for avoiding concurrent use.

References

1 Tassinari CA, Michelucci R, Ambrosetto G and Salvi F. Double-blind study of vigabatrin in the treatment of drug-resistant epilepsy. Arch Neurol (1987) 44, 907–10.
2 Rimmer EM and Richens A. Double-blind study of gamma-vinyl GABA in patients with refractory epilepsy. Lancet (1984) i, 189–90.
3 Browne TR, Mattson RH, Penry JK, Smith DB, Treimann DM, Wilder BJ, Ben-Menachem E, Napolieloo MJ, Sherry KM and Szabo GK. Vigabatrin for refractory complex partial seizures; multicenter single-blind study with long-term follow up. Neurology (1987) 37, 184–9.

Anticonvulsants + Viloxazine

Abstract/Summary

Carbamazepine serum levels can rise by 50% if viloxazine is given concurrently. Intoxication may occur if the carbamazepine dosage is not reduced appropriately. Viloxazine can also raise serum phenytoin to toxic levels.

Clinical evidence

(a) Carbamazepine + viloxazine

Seven patients on carbamazepine showed a 50% rise (from 8.1 to 12.1 μg/ml) in their serum carbamazepine levels after taking 300 mg viloxazine daily for three weeks.[1] Five of them showed signs of mild intoxication (dizziness, ataxia, fatigue, drowsiness). These symptoms disappeared and the serum carbamazepine levels fell when the viloxazine was withdrawn.[1]

Another study confirmed this interaction. Intoxication was seen.[4] The pharmacokinetics of viloxazine are unaffected by carbamazepine.[3]

(b) Phenytoin + viloxazine

The manufacturers of viloxazine warn that phenytoin serum levels may be raised during concurrent use and that phenytoin intoxication may occur. No further details are given.[2] The pharmacokinetics of viloxazine are unaffected by phenytoin.[3]

Mechanism

Uncertain. What is known suggests that the viloxazine inhibits the metabolism of the anticonvulsants, thereby reducing their clearance from the body.

Importance and management

Information seems to be limited to the reports cited. What is known indicates that if concurrent use is undertaken, both serum carbamazepine and phenytoin levels should be monitored closely and suitable dosage reductions made as necessary to avoid the possible development of intoxication.

References

1 Pisani F, Narbone MC, Fazio A, Cristafulli P, Primerano G, D'Angostino AA, Oteri G and Perri R. Effect of viloxazine on serum carbamazepine levels in epileptic patients. Epilepsia (1984) 25, 482–5.
2 Bell J (ICI Pharmaceuticals). Personal communication (1984).
3 Pisani F, Fazio A, Spina E, Artesi C, Pisani B, Russo M, Trio R and Perucca E. Pharmacokinetics of the antidepressant drug viloxazine in normal subjects and in epileptic patients receiving chronic anticonvulsant treatment. Psychopharmacology (1986) 90, 295–8.
4 Pisani F, Fazio A, Oteri G, Perucca E, Russo M, Trio R, Pisani B and Di Perri R. Carbamazepine-viloxazine interaction in patients with epilepsy. J Neurol Neurosurg Psychiatry (1986) 49, 1142–5.

Barbiturates + Caffeine

Abstract/Summary

The hypnotic effects of pentobarbitone (-al) are reduced or abolished by the concurrent use of caffeine. Caffeine-containing drinks should be avoided at bedtime if satisfactory hypnosis is to be achieved.

Clinical evidence

A controlled study on 42 patients given either a placebo, or 250 mg caffeine, or 100 mg pentobarbitone, or both caffeine and pentobarbitone, showed that the caffeine totally abolished the hypnotic effects of the barbiturate. The effects of the pentobarbitone–caffeine combination were indistinguishable from the placebo.[1]

Mechanism

Caffeine stimulates the cerebral cortex and impairs sleep, whereas pentobarbitone depresses the cortex and promotes sleep. These mutually opposing actions would seem to explain this interaction.

Importance and management

There seems to be only one direct study of this interaction, but it is well supported by common experience and the numerous studies of the properties of each of these compounds. Patients given barbiturate hypnotics should avoid caffeine-containing drinks (tea, coffee, Coca-Cola, etc.) at or near bedtime if the hypnotic is to be effective. The same is probably true for other non-barbiturate hypnotics, but this needs confirmation.

Reference

1 Forrest WH, Bellville JW and Brown BW. The interaction of caffeine with pentobarbital as a night-time hypnotic. Anesthesiology (1972) 36, 37.

Barbiturates + Cimetidine

Abstract/Summary

Phenobarbitone reduces the absorption of cimetidine, and cimetidine increases the metabolism of pentobarbitone, but both interactions seem to be of very limited clinical importance.

Clinical evidence, mechanism, importance and management

In vitro studies with human liver microsomes showed that cimetidine in above clinical concentrations reduced the metabolism of pentobarbitone, whereas ranitidine does not interact.[2] A study on eight normal subjects showed that 100 mg phenobarbitone daily for three weeks reduced the AUC (area under the curve) of a single 400 mg oral dose of cimetidine by 15%, and the time during which the plasma concentrations of the cimetidine exceeded 0.5 μg/ml (regarded as therapeutically desirable) was reduced by 11%.[1] The mechanisms underlying these interactions are that cimetidine is an enzyme inhibitor which reduces the rate of metabolism of pentobarbitone, whereas phenobarbitone apparently stimulates the enzymes in the gut wall so that the metabolism of the cimetidine is increased. Thus the amount absorbed and released into the circulation is reduced.

Direct information is limited. Mutual interactions take place between these drugs but the effects are small and unlikely to be of clinical importance. No special precautions seem to be necessary. Direct information about other barbiturates is lacking but it seems probable that they will behave similarly.

References

1 Somogyi A, Thielscher S and Gugler R. Influence of phenobarbital treatment on cimetidine kinetics. Eur J clin Pharmacol (1981) 19, 343.
2 Knodell RG, Holtzmann JL, Crankshaw DL, Steele NM and Stanley LN. Drug metabolism by rat and human hepatic microsomes in response to interaction with H_2-receptor antagonists. Gastroenterol (1982) 82, 84–88.

Barbiturates + Miconazole

Abstract/Summary

Miconazole increases serum pentobarbitone levels.

Clinical evidence, mechanism, importance and management

Five patients in intensive care given pentobarbital to decrease intracranial pressure showed marked rises in serum pentobarbital levels, and falls in total plasma clearance of 50–90% when concurrently treated with miconazole. The reason is thought to be that the miconazole inhibits the liver enzymes concerned with the metabolism of the barbiturate, thereby reducing its clearance from the body.[1] It would be prudent to monitor the effects of concurrent use to ensure that serum barbiturate levels do not rise too high. There seems to be no information about other barbiturates.

Reference

1 Heinemeyer G, Roots I, Schultz H and Dennhardt R. Hemmung der Pentobarbital-Elimination durch Miconazol bei Intesivtherapie des erhohten intracraniellen Druckes. Intensivmed (1988) 22, 164–7.

Barbiturates + Rifampicin (Rifampin)

Abstract/Summary

Rifampicin markedly increases the clearance of hexobarbitone(-al) from the body, and phenobarbitone possibly increases the clearance of rifampicin. The effects of each drug may be expected to be reduced.

Clinical evidence

(a) Effect of rifampicin on hexobarbitone

A study in six healthy subjects showed that after taking 1200 mg rifampicin daily for eight days the average elimination half-life of hexobarbitone had decreased from 407 to 171 min, and the metabolic clearance had increased about threefold.[1]

Similar results have been found in other studies with normal subjects[2] and those with cirrhosis or cholestasis.[3]

(b) Effect of phenobarbitone on rifampicin

Conflicting evidence: one study showed no effect[4] whereas another indicated that the serum levels of rifampicin were reduced.[5]

Mechanism

Rifampicin is a potent liver enzyme inducing agent which accelerates the metabolism of the hexobarbitone. Whether phenobarbitone (also a potent enzyme-inducing agent) can affect the metabolism of rifampicin in a similar way is not clear.

Importance and management

The documentation for both of these interactions is very limited, but the effects seen are consistent with what is known about these drugs. Concurrent use need not be avoided, but it would be prudent to be on the alert for a reduced response to both drugs. Increase the dosages as necessary. Whether rifampicin interacts with other barbiturates is uncertain.

References

1 Breimer DD, Zilly W and Richter E. Influence of rifampicin on drug metabolism: differences between hexobarbital and antipyrine. Clin Pharmacol Ther (1977) 21, 470.

2 Breimer DD, Zilly W and Richter E. Induction of drug metabolism in man after rifampicin treatment measured by increased hexobarbital and tolbutamide clearance. Eur J Clin Pharmacol (1975) 9, 219.

3 Breimer DD, Zilly W and Richter E. Stimulation of drug metabolism by rifampicin in patients with cirrhosis or cholestasis measured by increased hexobarbital and tolbutamide clearance. Eur J Clin Pharmacol (1977) 11, 287.

4 Acocella G, Bonollo L, Mainardi M, Margaroli P and Nicolis FB. Kinetic studies on rifampicin. III. Effect of phenobarbital on the half-life of the antibiotic. Tijdschrift Gastro-Enterologie (1974) 17, 151.

5 De la Roy Y de R, Beauchant G, Breuil K and y Patte F. Diminution de taux serique de rifampicine par le phenobarbital. Presse Med (1971) 79, 350.

Barbiturates + Sodium valproate

Abstract/Summary

Serum phenobarbitone levels can be increased by the concurrent use of sodium valproate which may result in excessive sedation and lethargy. A reduction in the dosage of the phenobarbitone by a third to a half can be safely carried out without loss of seizure control.

Clinical evidence

A 9-month study in 11 epileptics on phenobarbitone (90–400 mg daily) showed that when they were additionally given sodium valproate (11–42 mg/kg/day) they complained of sedation and, on average, the dosage of phenobarbitone could be reduced to 54% with continued good seizure control. Two other patients on a constant dose of phenobarbitone showed significantly increased phenobarbitone levels (12 and 48% respectively).[1]

Another study showed that 1200 mg sodium valproate raised serum phenobarbitone levels by an average of 27%.[2] This interaction has been described in numerous other reports.[3–17,19] Sodium valproate levels are also reported to be reduced about 25%.[18]

Mechanism

The evidence indicates that sodium valproate inhibits the metabolism of the phenobarbitone by the liver, leading to its accumulation in the body.

Importance and management

An extremely well documented and well established interaction of clinical importance. The incidence seems to be high.

The effects of concurrent use should be well monitored and suitable phenobarbitone dosage reductions made when necessary to avoid toxicity (sedation and lethargy). It would seem that the dosage can be safely reduced by a third to a half with full seizure control.[1]

References

1 Wilder BJ, Willmore LJ, Bruni J and Villarreal HJ. Valproic acid: interaction with other anticonvulsant drugs. Neurology (1978) 28, 892.

2 Richens A and Ahmad S. Controlled trial of sodium valproate in severe epilepsy. Brit Med J (1975) 3, 255.

3 Meinardi H and Bongers E. Analytical data in connection with the clinical use of di-n-propylacetate. In Clinical Pharmacology of Antiepileptic Drugs, edited by Schneider H et al. Springer-Verlag, NY and Berlin (1975) p. 235.

4 Schobben F, Van der Kleijn E and Gabreels FJM. Pharmacokinetics of di-n-propylacetate in epileptic patients. Eur J clin Pharmacol (1975) 8, 97.

5 Gram L, Wulff K and Rasmussen KE. Valproate sodium: a controlled clinical trial including monitoring of drug levels. Epilepsia (1977) 18, 141.

6 Jeavons PM and Clark JE. Sodium valproate in treatment of epilepsy. Brit Med J (1974) 2, 584.

7 Volzke E and Doose H. Dipropylacetate (Depakine, Ergenyl) in the treatment of epilepsy. Epilepsia (1973) 14, 185.

8 Millet Y, Sainty JM, Galland MC, Sidoine R and Jonglard J. Problemes poses par l'association therapeutique phenobarbital de sodium a propos d'un cas. Eur J Toxicol (1976) 9, 381.

9 Jeavons PM, Clark JE and Maheshwari MC. Treatment of generalized epilepsies of childhood and adolescence with sodium valproate ('Epilim'). Dev Med Child Neurol (1977) 19, 9.

10 Vakil SD, Critchley EMR, Phillips JC, Haydock C, Cocks A and Dyer T. The effect of sodium valproate (Epilim) on phenytoin and phenobarbitone blood levels. In Clinical and Pharmacological Aspects of Sodium Valproate (Epilim) in the Treatment of Epilepsy. Proceedings of a Symposium held at the University of Nottingham, September 1975, p75.

11 Scott DF, Boxer CM, and Herzberg JL. A study of the hypnotic effects of Epilim and its possible interaction with phenobarbitone. Ibid p 155.

12 Richens A, Scoular IT, Ahamad S and Jordan BJ. Pharmacokinetics and efficacy of Epilim in patients receiving long-term therapy with other antiepileptic drugs. Ibid p 78.

13 Loiseau P, Orgogozo JM, Brachet-Liermain A and Morselli PL. Pharmacokinetic studies on the interaction between phenobarbital and valproic acid. In Adv Epileptol Proc Cong Int League Epilepsy 13th. Edited by Meinardi H and Rowan A. (1977/8) p 261.

14 Fowler GW. Effect of dipropylacetate on serum levels of anticonvulsants in children. Proc West Pharmacol (1978) 21, 37.

15 Patel IH, Levy RH and Cutler RE. Phenobarbital-valproic acid interaction. Clin Pharmacol Ther (1980) 27, 515.

16 Coulter DL, Wu H and Allen RJ. Valproic acid therapy in childhood epilepsy. J Amer Med Ass (1980) 244, 785.

17 Kapetanovic IM, Kupferberg HJ, Porter RJ, Theodore W, Schulman E and Penry JK. Mechanism of valproate-phenobarbital interaction. Clin Pharmacol Ther (1981) 29, 480.

18 May T and Rambeck B. Serum concentrations of valproic acid: influence of dose and comedication. Ther Drug Monit (1985) 7, 387–90.

19 de Gatta MRF, Gonzalez ACA, Sanchez MJC, Hurle AD-G, Borbujo JS and Corral LM. Effect of sodium valproate on phenobarbital serum levels in children and adults. Ther Drug Monitor (1986) 8, 416–20.

Barbiturates + Triacetyloleandomycin

Abstract/Summary

A patient showed a fall in his serum phenobarbitone levels when concurrently treated with triacetyloleandomycin.

Clinical evidence, mechanism, importance and management

A patient on phenobarbitone and carbamazepine showed a fall in serum phenobarbitone levels (from about 40 to 31 μg/ml) over a three-day period when treated with triacetyloleandomycin.[1] The general importance of this single report is uncertain, but it would now seem prudent to be alert for changes in seizure control if this antibiotic is used.

Reference

1 Dravet C, Mesdjian E, Cenraud B and Roger J. Interaction between carbamazepine and triacetyloleandomycin. Lancet (1977) i, 810.

Carbamazepine or Phenobarbitone + Benzodiazepines

Abstract/Summary

Serum barbiturate and carbamazepine levels are not affected by clonazepam, but carbamazepine can lower serum clonazepam levels. This is possibly of limited clinical importance. Barbiturate intoxication has been attributed in a single case report to the concurrent use of chlordiazepoxide.

Clinical evidence, mechanism, importance and management

Clonazepam in slowly increasing doses up to a maximum of 4–6 mg/day given over a six-week period to patients on phenobarbitone or carbamazepine, alone or in combination, had no effect on either phenobarbitone or carbamazepine serum levels.[2] On the other hand a study in seven subjects given 1 mg clonazepam daily showed that carbamazepine (200 mg daily) over a three-week period reduced clobazam serum levels and its half-life.[3] A similar reduction in steady-state clonazepam levels but a rise in norclobazam levels in normal subjects is described in another study.[4] Since norclobazam retains some anticonvulsant activity the effect of carbamazepine may possibly have no clinical significance, but this needs further study.

A single case report describes a man given phenobarbitone and chlordiazepoxide who demonstrated drowsiness, unsteadiness, slurred speech, nystagmus, poor memory and hallucinations, all of which disappeared once the phenobarbitone was withdrawn. Substantial doses of chlordiazepoxide were well tolerated.[1]

References

1 Kane FJ and McCurdy RL. An unusual reaction to combined Librium-barbiturate therapy. Am J Psychiatry (1964) 120, 816.
2 Johannessen SI, Strandjord RE and Muthe-Kaas AW. Lack of effect of clonazepam on serum levels of diphenylhydantoin, phenobarbital and carbamazepine. Acta Neurol Scand (1977) 55, 506.
3 Lai AA, Levy RH and Cutler RE. Time course of interaction between carbamazepine and clonazepam. Clin Pharmacol Ther (1978) 24, 316.
4 Levy RH, Lane EA, Guyot M, Brachet-Lierman A, Cenraud G and Loiseau P. Analysis of parent drug-metabolite relationship in the

presence of an inducer. Application to the carbamazepine-clobazam interaction in normal man. Drug Metab Dispos (1983) 11, 286–92.

Carbamazepine + Cimetidine or Ranitidine

Abstract/Summary

Epileptic patients and subjects chronically treated with carbamazepine show a transient increase in serum levels, possibly accompanied by an increase in side-effects, for the first few days after starting to take cimetidine, but these side-effects rapidly disappear. Ranitidine appears not to interact.

Clinical evidence

In a study in eight normal subjects who had been taking 900 mg carbamazepine daily for six weeks it was observed that the steady-state carbamazepine levels increased by 17% after taking 1200 mg cimetidine daily for two days. Six of the eight experienced side-effects, but after seven days treatment the carbamazepine levels had fallen again and the side-effects disappeared.[8]

A study in seven epileptic patients on long-term treatment with carbamazepine showed that after taking 1 g of cimetidine daily (200 mg three times a day and 400 mg at night) for a week, their steady-state carbamazepine serum levels remained unaltered.[6] No interaction was seen in another study in 11 epileptic patients.[7] A very elderly woman, aged 89, developed signs of carbamazepine toxicity within two days of starting to take 400 mg cimetidine daily, and showed a rise in serum carbamazepine levels which fell once again when the cimetidine was withdrawn.[5]

The results of these studies in patients and subjects taking carbamazepine chronically differ from the single dose studies and short-term studies in normal subjects. For example, a 33% rise in serum levels,[1] a 20% fall in clearance[2] and a 26% increase in the AUC[3] have been reported.

Mechanism

Not fully understood. It is thought that cimetidine can inhibit the activity of the liver enzymes concerned with the metabolism of carbamazepine, resulting in its reduced clearance from the body, but the effect is short-lived because it is opposed by the auto-inducing effects of the carbamazepine. This would explain why the single-dose and short-term studies in normal subjects suggest that a clinically important interaction could occur, but in practice in patients on long-term treatment it causes few problems.

Importance and management

An established interaction but of minimal importance. Patients on chronic treatment with carbamazepine should be warned that for the first few days after starting to take cimetidine they may experience some increase in the carbamazepine side-effects (nausea, headache, dizziness, fatigue, drowsiness, ataxia, an inability to concentrate, a bitter taste) because the serum levels are transiently increased, but these side-effects will subside and disappear by the end of a week. Ranitidine appears to be a non-interacting alternative to cimetidine.[4]

References

1 Macphee GJA, Thompson GG, Scobie G, Agnew E, Parke BK, Murray T, McColl KEL and Brodie MJ. Effects of cimetidine on carbamazepine auto- and hetero-induction in man. Br J clin Pharmac (1984) 18, 411–19.
2 Webster LK, Mihaly GW, Jones DB, Smallwood RA, Phillips JA and Vajda FJ. Effect of cimetidine and rantidine on carbamazepine and sodium valproate pharmacokinetics. Eur J Clin Pharmacol (1984) 27, 341–3.
3 Dalton MJ, Powell JR and Messenheimer JA. The influence of cimetidine on single dose carbamazepine pharmacokinetics. Epilepsia (1985) 26, 127–30.
4 Dalton MJ, Powell JR and Messenheimer JA. Ranitidine does not alter single-dose carbamazepine pharmacokinetics in healthy adults. Drug Intell Clin Pharm (1985) 19, 941–4.
5 Telerman-Topet N, Duret ME and Coers C. Cimetidine interaction with carbamazepine. Ann InternMed (1981) 94, 544.
6 Sonne J, Luhdorf K, Larsen NE and Andreasen PB. Lack of interaction between cimetidine and carbmazepine. Acta Neurol Scand (1983) 68, 253–6.
7 Levine M, Jones MW and Sheppard I. Differential effect of cimetidine on serum concentrations of carbamazepine and phenytoin. Neurology (1985) 35, 562-5
8 Dalton MJ, Powell JR, Messenheimer JA and Clark J. Cimetidine and carbamazepine: a complex drug interaction. Epilepsia (1986) 27, 553–8.

Carbamazepine + Danazol

Abstract/Summary

Serum carbamazepine levels can be doubled by the concurrent use of danazol. Carbamazepine toxicity may occur unless the dosage is reduced appropriately.

Clinical evidence

A patient taking 800 mg carbamazepine daily showed a rise in serum levels from 10 to 21 μg/ml within two weeks of starting to take danazol. This interaction was seen in five other patients. The anticonvulsant effects of carbamazepine were improved without (perhaps somewhat surprisingly) disturbing side effects.[1] The serum carbamazepine levels of six other epileptic patients were observed to be approximately doubled within 7–30 days of being treated with danazol (500 mg). Acute carbamazepine toxicity (dizziness, drowsiness, blurred vision, ataxia, nausea) was experienced by five out of the six.[2] Steady-state carbamazepine serum levels were found to be increased 50–100% by danazol in five other patients.[4] Other single cases of this interaction are described elsewhere.[3,4] A study showed that during danazol treatment the clearance of carbamazepine was reduced by 60% and the half-life doubled.[4]

Mechanism

Danazol inhibits the metabolism of the carbamazepine by the liver, thereby reducing its loss from the body.[1,4,5]

Importance and management

This interaction is established and of clinical importance. Concurrent use should be avoided unless the carbamazepine serum levels can be monitored and the dosage reduced as necessary.

References

1 Kramer G, Besser R, Theisohn M and Eichelbaum M. Carbamazepine-danazol drug interaction: mechanism and usefulness. Acta Neurol Scand (1984) 70, 249.
2 Zielinski JJ, Lichten EM and Haidukewych D. Clinically significant danazol-carbamazepine interaction. Ther Drug Monit (1987) 9, 24–7.
3 Ramsy RE, McJilton JS, Vasquez D and Marcos J. Increase in the protein binding of carbamazepine from danazol co-administration. Abstracts of the 16th Epilepsy International Congress, Hamburg, Sept 6–9, 1986.
4 Kramer G, Theisohn M, von Unruh GE and Eichelbaum M. Carbamazepine-danazol interaction: its mechanism examined by a stable isotope technique. Ther Drug Monitor (1986) 8, 387–92.
5 Kramer G and Theisohn M. Therapeutische nutzbare Arzneimittelinterinteraktionen mit Carbamazepin? Psycho (1983) 9, 366–8.

Carbamazepine and Diuretics

Abstract/Summary

Two patients on carbamazepine developed hyponatraemia when given hydrochlorothiazide or frusemide.

Clinical evidence, mechanism, importance and management

Two epileptic patients developed symptomatic hyponatraemia while on carbamazepine, one while taking hydrochlorothiazide and the other while taking frusemide.[1] The reasons are uncertain but all three drugs can cause sodium to be lost from the body. This seems to be an uncommon interaction but be aware that it can occur.

Reference

1 Ramzy Y, Nastase C, Camille Y, Henderson M, Belzile L and Beland F. Carbamazepine, diuretics and hyponatremia: a possible interaction. J Clin Psychiatry (1987) 48, 281–3.

Carbamazepine + Erythromycin

Abstract/Summary

Carbamazepine serum levels can very rapidly rise to toxic concentrations if erythromycin is given concurrently. Intoxication has been described in many reports. Erythromycin appears not to interact with phenytoin.

227

Clinical evidence

A girl of eight taking 50 mg phenobarbitone and 800 mg carbamazepine daily was additionally given 500 mg and later 1000 mg erythromycin daily. Within two days she began to experience balancing difficulties and ataxia which were eventually attributed to carbamazepine intoxication. Her serum carbamazepine levels were found to have risen from a little below 10 μg/ml to over 25 μg/ml (therapeutic range 2–10 μg/ml).[1]

Marked rises in serum carbamazepine levels[11] and/or intoxication following the addition of erythromycin have been described. At least 24 cases of carbamazepine intoxication have been reported.[3–10,13–16] A study in eight normal subjects showed that 1 g erythromycin daily for five days reduced the clearance of carbamazepine by an average of 20% (range 5–41%).[2] Another study confirmed this interaction.[17]

Mechanism

It is suggested that erythromycin has a high affinity for the active site on the liver enzymes concerned with the metabolism of the carbamazepine so that the metabolism of the latter is rapidly and markedly inhibited, resulting in its rapid accumulation which leads to toxicity.[11]

Importance and management

A well-documented and established interaction. Its incidence is uncertain. Concurrent use should be avoided unless the effects can be very closely monitored (measurement of serum carbamazepine levels) and suitable dosage reductions made. Toxic symptoms (ataxia, vertigo, drowsiness, lethargy, confusion, diplopia) can develop very rapidly (within 24 h), and serum carbamazepine levels can return to normal within 8–12 h of withdrawing the antibiotic.[10] It has been suggested that '...the interaction may be more intense at higher erythromycin dosing rates (for instance 500 mg every six hours).'[2] Erythromycin appears not to interact with phenytoin.[12]

References

1 Amedee-Manesme O, Rey E, Brussieux J, Goutieres F and Aicardi J. Antibiotiques a ne jamais associer a la carbamazepine. Arch Fr Pediatr (1982) 39, 126.
2 Wong YY, Ludden TM and Bell RD. Effect of erythromycin on carbamazepine kinetics. Drug Intell Clin Pharm (1983) 16, 484.
3 Straughan J. Erythromycin-carbamazepine interaction? S Afr Med J (1982) 61, 420–1.
4 Mesdjian E, Dravet C, Cenraud B and Roger J. Carbamazepine intoxication due to triacetyloleandomycin administration in epileptic patients. Epilepsia (1980) 21, 489–96.
5 Vajda FJE and Bladin PF. Carbamazepine-erythromycin base interaction. Med J Aust (1984) 2, 81.
6 Hedrick R, Williams F, Morin R, Lamb WA and Cate JC. Carbamazepine-erythromycin interaction leading to carbamazepine toxicity in four epileptic children. Ther Drug Monit (1983) 5, 405–7.
7 Miller SL. The association of carbamazepine intoxication and erythromycin use. Ann Neurol (1985) 18, 413.
8 Berrettini WH. A case of erythromycin-induced carbamazepine toxicity. J Clin Psychiatry (1986) 47, 147.
9 Carranco E, Kareus J and Co S, Peak V and Al-Rajeh S. Carbamazepine toxicity induced by concurrent erythromycin therapy. Arch Neurol (1985) 42, 187–8.
10 Goulden KJ, Camfield P, Dooley JM, Fraser A, Meek DC, Renton KW and Tibbles JAR. Severe carbamazepine intoxication after coadministration of erythromycin. J Pediatr (1986) 109, 135–8.
11 Wroblewski BA, Singer WD and Whyte J. Carbamazepine-erythromycin interaction. Case studies and clinical significance. J Amer Med Ass (1986) 255, 1165–7.
12 Bachmann K, Schwartz JI, Forney RB and Jauregui L. Single dose phenytoin clearance during erythromycin treatment. Res Comm Chem Path Pharmacol (1984) 46, 207–17.
13 Kessler JM. Erythromycin-carbamazepine interaction. S Afr Med J (1985) 67, 1038.
14 Jaster PJ and Abbas D. Erythromycin-carbamazepine interaction. Neurology (1986) 36, 594–5.
15 Loiseau P, Guyot M, Pautrizel B, Vincon G and Albin H. Intoxication par la carbamazepine due a l'interaction carbamazepine-erythromycine. La Presse Med (1985) 14, 162.
16 Zitelli BJ, Howrie DL, Altman H and Marcon TJ. Erythromycin-induced drug interactions. Clin Ped (1987) 26, 117–19.
17 Miles MV and Tennison MB. Erythromycin effects on multiple-dose carbamazepine kinetics. Ther Drug Monit (1989) 11, 47–52.

Carbamazepine + Isoniazid

Abstract/Summary

Carbamazepine serum levels are markedly and very rapidly increased by the concurrent use of isoniazid. Intoxication can occur if the carbamazepine dosage is not reduced appropriately.

Clinical evidence

A study describes 10 out of 13 patients, stabilized on carbamazepine, who developed disorientation, listlessness, aggression, lethargy and, in one case, extreme drowsiness when concurrently treated with 200 mg isoniazid daily. Serum carbamazepine levels were measured in three of the patients and they were found to have risen above the normal therapeutic range.[3]

Carbamazepine toxicity, associated with marked rises in serum carbamazepine levels, has been described in other reports.[1,2,4,5] Some of the patients were also taking sodium valproate. There is also some evidence that carbamazepine increases the hepatotoxicity of isoniazid.[6]

Mechanism

It seems probable that the isoniazid inhibits the activity of the liver enzymes concerned with the metabolism and clearance of carbamazepine, so that it accumulates in the body.

Importance and management

The documentation is limited, but a clinically important and potentially serious interaction is established. Toxicity can develop quickly (the reports indicate within 1–5 days) and also disappear quickly if the isoniazid is withdrawn. Concurrent use should not be undertaken unless the effects can be closely monitored and suitable downward dosage adjustments made (a reduction to a half or a third can be effective[3]). It seems probable that those who are 'slow' metabolizers of isoniazid may show this interaction more quickly and to a greater extent than fast metabolizers.[1]

References

1 Wright JM, Stokes EF and Sweeney VP. Isoniazid-induced carbamazepine toxicity and vice versa: a double drug interaction. N Engl J Med (1982) 307, 1325–7.
2 Block SH. Carbamazepine-isoniazid interaction. Pediatr (1982) 69, 494–5.
3 Valsalan VC and Cooper GL. Carbamazepine intoxication caused by interaction with isoniazid. Br Med J (1982) 285, 261–2.
4 Arguelles PP, Riera JMS, Tahull JMG and Bori AV. Interaccion carbamacepina-tuberculostaticos. Med Clin (1984) 83, 867–8.
5 Beeley L and Ballantine N. Bulletin of the West Midlands Adverse Drug Reaction Group. (1981) 13, 8.
6 Barbare JC, Lallement PY, Vorhauer W and Veyssier P. Hepatotoxicite de l'isoniazide: influence de la carbamazepine? Gastroenterol Clin Biol (1986) 10, 523–4.

Carbamazepine + Macrolide antibiotics

Abstract/Summary

Carbamazepine serum levels are markedly and very rapidly increased by the concurrent use of triacetyloleandomycin. Intoxication can often develop within 1–3 days. Flurithromycin and josamycin appears to interact to a lesser extent and roxithromycin not at all. See also 'Carbamazepine + Erythromycin'.

Clinical evidence

Eight epileptics on carbamazepine developed signs of intoxication (dizziness, nausea, vomiting, excessive drowsiness) within 24 h of starting to take triacetyloleandomycin. The only two patients available for examination showed a sharp rise in serum carbamazepine levels (from 5 to 28 $\mu g/ml$) over three days, and a rapid fall following withdrawal.[1,5]

Another report[2] by the same authors describes a total of 17 similar cases of intoxication caused by triacetyloleandomycin. Some of the patients demonstrated three or fourfold increases in serum carbamazepine levels. Other cases have been described elswhere.[3,4] In most instances the serum carbamazepine levels returned to normal within about 3–5 days of withdrawing the antibiotic.[2]

Mechanism

It seems probable that the triacetyloleandomycin slows the rate of metabolism of the carbamazepine by the liver enzymes so that the anticonvulsant accumulates within the body.

Importance and management

The carbamazepine–triacetyloleandomycin interaction is established, clinically important and potentially serious. The incidence is high. The rapidity of its development (24 h in some cases) and the extent of the rise in serum carbamazepine levels suggest that it would be difficult to control carbamazepine levels by reducing its dosage. Concurrent use should be avoided if possible. Josamycin (2 g daily for a week) and flurithromycin (500 mg daily for a week) have

been found to reduce the clearance of carbamazepine by about 20%[6,7,9] so that they both appear to be safer alternatives to either triacetyloleandomycin or erythromycin, nevertheless a reduction in the dosage of the carbamazepine may be needed. Monitor the effects of concurrent use closely. Roxithromycin has been shown not to interact.[8]

References

1 Dravet C, Mesdjian E, Cenraud B and Roger J. Interaction between carbamazepine and triacetyloleandomycin. Lancet (1977) i, 810.
2 Mesdjian E, Dravet C, Cenraud B and Roger J. Carbamazepine intoxication due to triacetyloleandomycin administration in epileptic patients. Epilepsia (1980) 21, 489–496.
3 Amedee-Manesme O, Rey E, Brussieux J, Gontiers F and Aicardi J. Antibiotiques a ne jamais associer a la carbamazepine. Arch Fr Pediatr (1982) 39, 126.
4 Bavoux F, Dreyfus-Brisac C, Lanfranchi C and Ponsot G. Interaction carbamazepine-troleandomycine et interaction carbamazepine-erythromycine. BIR Creteil (1980) 4, 1.
5 Dravet C, Mesdjian E, Cenraud B and Roger J. Interaction carbamazepine triacetyloleandomycine: une nouvelle interaction medicamenteuse? Nouv Presse Med (1977) 6, 467.
6 Albin H, Vincon G, Pehourcq F and Dangoumau J. Influence de la josamycine sur la pharmacocinetique de la carbamazepine. Therapie (1982) 37, 151–6.
7 Vincon G, Albin H, Demotes-Mainard F, Guyot M, Brachet-Liermain A and Loiseau P. Pharmacokinetic interaction between carbamazepine and josamycin. Proc Eur Congr Biopharmaceutics Pharmacokinetics vol III: Clinical Pharmacokinetics. Edited by Aiache JM and Hirtz J. Published by Imprimerie de l'Universite de Clermont-Ferrand. (1984) pp 270–6.
8 Saint-Salive B, Tremblay D, Surjus A and Lefebvre MA. A study of the interaction of roxithromycin with theophylline and carbamazepine. J Antimicrob Chemother (1987) 20, Suppl B, 121–9.
9 Barzaghi N, Gatti G, Crema F, Faja A, Monteleone E, Amione C, Leone L and Perucca E. Effect of flurithromycin, a new macrolide antibiotic, on carbamazepine disposition in normal subjects. Int J Clin Pharm Res (1988) VIII, 101–5.

Carbamazepine + Miconazole

Abstract/Summary

An isolated report describes an adverse response in a patient on carbamazepine when given miconazole.

Clinical evidence, mechanism, importance and management

A patient on long-term treatment with carbamazepine (400 mg daily) developed malaise, myoclonia and tremor within three days of being given 1.125 g miconazole, and on each subsequent occasion when given miconazole. These toxic effects disappeared when the miconazole was withdrawn.[1] The general importance of this reaction is unknown.

Reference

1 Loupi E, Descotes J, Lery N and Evreux JCl. Interactions medicamenteuses et miconazole. A propos de 10 observations. Therapie (1982) 37, 437–41.

Carbamazepine + Monoamine oxidase inhibitors (MAOI)

Abstract/Summary

Tranylcypromine appears not to interact adversely with carbamazepine

Clinical evidence, mechanism, importance and management

No adverse interaction has been reported but the manufacturers of carbamazepine say that concurrent use should be avoided because of the close structural similarity between carbamazepine and the tricyclic antidepressants. However a report describes a woman taking 600 mg carbamazepine daily (blood level 9.7 mg/l) who was additionally given up to 40 mg tranylcypromine daily. After two weeks her carbamazepine levels were 6.3 mg/l and her depressive symptoms improved substantially.[1] Two other patients similarly treated also experienced no adverse effects and no substantial changes in the serum levels of carbamazepine were seen.[1,2] Bearing in mind that the MAOI and the tricyclics can be administered together, under certain well controlled conditions, without problems (see 'Monoamine oxidase inhibitors + Tricyclic antidepressants'), the warning may prove to be overcautious. As yet there seems to be no direct information about other MAOI.

References

1 Lydiard RB, White D, Harvey B and Taylor A. Lack of pharmacokinetic interaction between tranylcypromine and carbamazepine. J Clin Psychopharmacol (1987) 7, 360.
2 Joffe RT, Post RM and Uhde TW. Lack of pharmacokinetic interaction of carbamazepine and tranylcypromine. Arch Gen Psychiatry (1985) 42, 738.

Carbamazepine + Phenobarbitone

Abstract/Summary

Carbamazepine serum levels are reduced to some extent by the concurrent use of phenobarbitone, but seizure control remains unaffected.

Clinical evidence

A comparative study in epileptic patients showed that on average those taking both carbamazepine and phenobarbitone (44 patients) had carbamazepine serum levels which were 18% lower than those taking only carbamazepine (43 patients).[1]

Similar results were found in other studies in both adult and child patients treated with both drugs.[2,3] The seizure control remained unaffected.

Mechanism

It seem probable that phenobarbitone stimulates the liver enzymes concerned with the metabolism of the carbamazepine, resulting in its more rapid clearance from the body.

Importance and managment

An established interaction, but of no practical importance since the seizure control is not diminished, despite the small fall in serum carbamazepine levels.

References

1 Christiansen J and Dam M. Influence of phenobarbital and diphenylhydantoin on plasma carbamazepine levels in patients with epilepsy. Acta Neurol Scandinav (1973) 49, 543–6.
2 Cereghino JJ, Brock JT, Van Meter JC, Penry JK, Smith LD and White BG. The efficacy of carbamazepine combinations in epilepsy. Clin Pharmacol Ther (1975) 18, 733.
3 Rane A, Hojer B and Wilson JT. Kinetics of carbamazepine and its 10,11-epoxide metabolite in children. Clin Pharmacol Ther (1976) 19, 276.

Carbamazepine + Primidone

Abstract/Summary

A single case report describes markedly reduced serum carbamazepine levels, accompanied by poor seizure control, in a patient concurrently treated with primidone.

Clinical evidence

The complex partial seizures of a 15-year-old boy failed to be controlled despite treatment with primidone (12 mg/kg daily in three doses) and carbamazepine (10 mg/kg daily in three doses). Even when the carbamazepine dosage was increased from 10 to 20 and then to 30 mg daily his serum carbamazepine levels only rose from 3.5 to 4.0 and then to 4.8 μg/ml, and his seizures continued. When the primidone was gradually withdrawn his serum carbamazepine levels climbed to 12 μg/ml and his seizures completely disappeared.[1]

Mechanism

When the primidone was stopped, the clearance of the carbamazepine decreased by about 60%. This is consistent with the known enzyme-inducing effects of primidone (converted in the body to phenobarbitone) which can increase the metabolism of other drugs by the liver.

Importance and management

Direct information seems to be limited to this report so that its general importance is uncertain, but be alert for evidence of reduced carbamazepine levels in any patient given primidone. More study is needed.

Reference

1 Benetello P and Furlanut M. Primidone-carbamazepine interaction: clinical consequences. Int J Clin Pharm Res (1987) VII, 165–8.

Carbamazepine + Sodium valproate

Abstract/Summary

The serum levels of both drugs may possibly fall by 20–25% during concurrent use, but the rise in the levels of carbamazepine-epoxide which also has anticonvulsant activity may possibly offset the effects of this interaction.

Clinical evidence

(a) Serum carbamazepine levels reduced

A study on seven adult epileptics who had been taking carbamazepine (8.3–13.3 mg/kg) for more than two months showed that their steady-state serum carbamazepine levels fell by an average of 24% (range 3–59%) over a six-day period when concurrently treated with sodium valproate (2 g daily). The levels fell in six of the patients and remained unchanged in one.[1,2]

Other reports state that falls,[4,5,7] no changes[5,6,9] and even a slight rise[7] have been seen in some patients. One report described a 100% rise in the serum levels of carbamazepine-10,11-epoxide.[9] Acute psychosis occurred in one patient when carbamazepine was added to sodium valproate treatment.[10]

(b) Serum sodium valproate levels reduced

A study on the kinetics of sodium valproate in six normal subjects showed that the concurrent use of carbmazepine, 200 mg daily, over a three week period reduced the minimum steady-state sodium valproate levels by about 20% and increased the clearance by 30%.[3]

Another report states that lower sodium valproate levels were seen in patients on carbamazepine than those who were not.[8]

Mechanism

The evidence suggests that each drug increases the metabolism of the other so that both are cleared from the body more quickly. The levels of the metabolite of carbamazepine, carbamazepine-epoxide, increase during concurrent use.

Importance and management

Documentation is not great, but both interactions seem to be established. Be alert for falls in the serum levels of both drugs. However the clinical importance of this is uncertain because the metabolite of carbamazepine (carbamazepine-epoxide) also has anticonvulsant activity so that it may possibly not be necessary to increase the dosages of the drugs to maintain adequate seizure control.

References

1 Levy RH, Morselli PL, Bianchetti G, Guyot M, Brachet-Liermain A and Loiseau P. Interaction between valproic acid and carbamazepine in epileptic patients. In 'Metabolism of Antiepileptic Drugs' edited by RH Levy et al. Raven Press, New York (1984) pp 45–51.
2 Levy RH, Moreland TA, Morselli PL, Guyot M, Brachet-Liermain and Looseau P. Carbamazepine/valproic acid interaction in man and rhesus monkey. Epilepsia (1984) 25, 338–45.
3 Bowdle TA, Levy RH and Cutler RE. Effects of carbamazepine on valproic acid kinetics in normal subjects. Clin Pharmacol Ther (1979) 26, 629.
4 Jeavons PM and Clark JE. Sodium valproate in the treatment of epilepsy. Brit Med J (1974) 2, 584.
5 Wilder BJ, Willmore LJ, Bruni J and Villarreal HJ. Valproic acid: interaction with other anticonvulsant drugs. Neurology (1978) 28, 892.
6 Fowler GW. Effects of dipropylacetate on serum levels of anticonvulsants in children. Proc West PharmacolSoc (1978) 21, 37.
7 Varma R, Michos GA, Varma RS and Hoshino AY. Clinical trials of Depakene (valproic acid) coadministered with anticonvulsants in epileptic patients. Res Comm Pscyhol Psychiat Behav (1980) 5, 265.
8 Reunanen MI, Luoma P, Myllyla VV and Hokkanen M. Low serum valproic acid concentrations in epileptic patients on combination therapy. Curr Ther Res (1980) 28, 455–62.
9 Pisani F, Fazio A, Oteri G, Ruello C, Gitto C, Russo R and Perucca E. Sodium valproate and valpromide: differential interactions with carbamazepine in epileptic patients. Epilepsia (1986) 27, 548–52.
10 McKee RJW, Larkin JG, Brodie MJ. Acute psychosis with carbamazepine and sodium valproate. Lancet (1989) i, 167.

Carbamazepine + Valpromide

Abstract/Summary

Carbamazepine intoxication can occur if valpromide is substituted for sodium valproate in patients taking carbamazepine. The serum levels of carbamazepine may not rise but the levels of its active metabolite, carbamazepine-epoxide, can be markedly increased. It has been suggested that this may possibly increase the teratogenic, mutagenic and carcinogenic risks.

Clinical evidence

Five out of seven epileptic patients taking carbamazepine exhibited symptoms of carbamazepine intoxication when concurrent treatment with sodium valproate was replaced by valpromide (*Depamide*), despite the fact that their serum carbamazepine levels did not increase.[1] The intoxication appeared to be connected with a fourfold increase in the serum levels of the metabolite of carbamazepine (carbamazepine-10,11-epoxide) which rose to 8.5 µg/ml.

In another study on six epileptic patients the serum levels of this metabolite rose threefold (range 2–9-fold) within a week of concurrent use and two of the patients developed confusion, dizziness and vomiting. The symptoms disappeared and serum carbamazepine-epoxide levels fell when the valpromide dosage was reduced to two-thirds.[2]

Mechanism

Valpromide reduces the metabolism by the liver of carbamazepine and its metabolite, carbamazepine-epoxide, because it inhibits epoxide hydrolase.[4] This metabolite has anti-convulsant activity but it may also be toxic if its serum levels become excessive.[2,3]

Importance and management

An established interaction. It is suggested that both carba-mazepine and carbamazepine-epoxide serum levels should be monitored during concurrent use.[3] The dosages should be reduced appropriately if necessary. There is also some debate about whether this combination should be avoided, not only because of the risk of intoxication but also because inhibition of epoxide hydrolase may be undesirable.[1] This enzyme is thought to be important for the detoxification of a number of teratogenic, mutagenic and carcinogenic epoxides.[1,3]

References

1 Meijer JWA, Binnie CD, Debets RMChr, Van Parys JAP and de Beer-Pawlikowski NKB. Possible hazard of valpromide-carbamazepine combination therapy in epilepsy. Lancet (1984) i, 802.
2 Pisani F, Fazio A, Oteri G, Ruello C, Gitto C, Russo R and Perucca E. Sodium valproate and valpromide: differential interactions with carba-mazepine in epileptic patients. Epilepsia (1986) 27, 548–52.
3 Levy RH, Kerr BM, Loiseau P, Guyot M and Wilensky AJ. Inhibition of carbamazepine epoxide elimination by valpromide and valproic acid. Epilepsia (1986) 27, 592.
4 Pisani F, Fazio A, Oteri G, Spina E, Perucca E and Bertilsson L. Effect of valpromide on the pharmacokinetics of carbamazepine-10,11-epoxide. Br J clin Pharmac (1988) 25, 611–13.

Ethosuximide + Barbiturates, Phenytoin or Primidone

Abstract/Summary

Falls in serum ethosuximide levels can occur if primidone or phenytoin are used concurrently, whereas methylphenobarbitone can cause a rise. Ethosuximide is also reported to have caused phenytoin intoxication.

Clinical evidence, mechanism, importance and management

A study[1] on 198 epileptic patients showed that the concurrent use of phenytoin or primidone depressed serum ethosuximide levels, whereas a report describes a rise when methylphenobarbitone was used.[2] Three cases have occurred in which ethosuximide appeared to have been responsible for the development of phenytoin intoxication,[3–5] but primidone serum levels are reported not to be affected.[6] The concurrent use of anticonvulsant agents is common and often advantageous, but these reports emphasize the need to monitor the effects to ensure that seizure control remains good and that toxicity does not develop.

References

1 Battino D, Cusi C, Franceschetti S, Moise A, Spina S and Avanzini G. Ethosuximide plasma concentrations: influence of age and concomitant therapy. Clin Pharmacokinet (1982) 7, 176–80.

2 Smith GA, McKauge L, Dubetz D, Tyrer JH and Eadie MJ. Factors influencing plasma concentrations of ethosuximide. Clin Pharmacokinet (1979) 4, 38.
3 Lander CM, Eadie MJ and Tyrer JH. Interactions between anticonvulsants. Proc Aust Assoc Neurol (1975) 12, 111.
4 Dawson GW, Brown HW and Clark BG. Serum phenytoin after ethosuximide. Ann Neurol (1978) 4, 583.
5 Franzten E, Hansen JM and Hansen OE. Phenytoin (Dilantin) intoxication. Acta Neurol Scand (1967) 43, 440.
6 Schmidt D. The effect of phenytoin and ethosuximide on primidone metabolism in patients with epilepsy. J Neurol (1975) 209, 115.

Ethosuximide + Carbamazepine

Abstract/Summary

Serum ethosuximide levels are reduced by carbamazepine, but whether this adversely affects seizure control is uncertain.

Clinical evidence

A study in normal subjects taking 500 mg ethosuximide daily showed that the mean serum levels were reduced by 17% (from 32 to 27 µg/ml) after taking 200 mg carbamazepine daily for 18 days. One patient showed a 35% reduction.[1] A reduction in serum levels has also been described in patients.[3] In contrast, no interaction was seen in another study on epileptic patients taking several anticonvulsants.[2] The most probable explanation for this interaction is that the carbamazepine—a recognized enzyme inducing agent—increases the metabolism and clearance of the ethosuximide. The evidence for this interaction is very limited and its clinical importance is uncertain, but until it is more clearly defined it would prudent to be alert for any signs of reduced seizure control.

References

1 Warren JW, Benmaman JD, Wannamaker BBB and Levy RH. Kinetics of a carbamazepine-ethosuximide interaction. Clin Pharmacol Ther (1980) 28, 646.
2 Smith GA, McKauge L, Dubetz D, Tyrer JH and Eadie MJ. Factors influencing plasma concentrations of ethosuximide. Clin Pharmacokinet (1979) 4, 38.
3 Battino D, Cusi C, Franceschetti S, Moise A, Spina S and Avanzini G. Ethosuximide plasma concentrations: influence of age and associated concomitant therapy. Clin Pharmacokinet (1982) 7, 176–80.

Ethosuximide + Isoniazid

Abstract/Summary

A single report describes a patient who developed psychotic behaviour and signs of ethosuximide intoxication when concurrently treated with isoniazid.

Clinical evidence, mechanism, importance and management

An epileptic patient, well controlled on ethosuximide and sodium valproate for two years, developed persistent hiccoughing, nausea, vomiting, anorexia and insomnia within a week of starting to take 300 mg isoniazid daily. Psychotic behaviour gradually developed over the next five weeks. The appearance and subsequent disappearance of these symptoms appeared to be related to the sharp rise (up to 198 μg/ml) and later the fall in serum ethosuximide levels. It is suggested that the isoniazid may have inhibited the metabolism of the ethosuximide, leading to accumulation and intoxication. The general importance of this reaction is uncertain, but it would now seem prudent to monitor concurrent use.

Reference

1 Van Wieringen A and Vrijlandt CM. Ethosuximide intoxication caused by interaction with isoniazid. Neurology (1983) 33, 1227–8.

Ethosuximide + Sodium valproate

Abstract/Summary

Some studies have shown that ethosuximide serum levels can rise significantly if sodium valproate is given concurrently. Other studies have failed to demonstrate this interaction.

Clinical evidence

Four out of five patients taking ethosuximide (averaging 27 mg/kg) showed an approximately 50% increase in serum levels (from an average of 73 to 112 μg/ml) within three weeks of starting to take sodium valproate (averaging 42 mg/kg). Other anticonvulsants being taken included phenytoin, phenobarbitone, primidone and clonazepam.[1] Nine days treatment with sodium valproate is reported in a single dose study in six normal subjects to have raised serum ethosuximide levels, the clearance being reduced by 15%,[2] but other studies have described no changes[3,4] or even reduced serum levels.[5] The reason for these discordant results is not understood. The concurrent use of anticonvulsant agents is common and often advantageous, but these reports emphasize the need to monitor the effects to ensure that toxicity does not develop and that good seizure control is maintained.

References

1 Mattson RH and Cramer JA. Valproic acid and ethosuximide interaction. Ann Neurol (1980) 7, 583.
2 Pisani F, Narbone MC, Trunfio C, Fazio A, La Rosa G, Oteri G and Di Perri R. Valproic acid-ethosuximide interaction: a pharmacokinetic study. Epilepsia (1984) 23, 229–33.
3 Fowler GW. Effect of dipropylacetate on serum levels of anticonvulsants in children. Proc West Pharmacol Soc (1978) 21, 37.
4 Bauer LA, Harris C, Wilensky AJ, Raisys VA and Levy RH. Ethosuximide kinetics: possible interaction with valproic acid. Clin Pharmacol Ther (1982) 31, 741–5.
5 Battino D, Cusi C, Franceschetti S, Moise A, Spina S and Avanzini G. Ethosuximide plasma concentrations: influence of age and associated concomitant therapy. Clin Pharmacokinet (1982) 7, 167–80.

Phenytoin + Alcohol

Abstract/Summary

Chronic heavy drinking reduces serum phenytoin concentrations and above-average doses of phenytoin may be needed to maintain adequate levels. Excessive drinking also seems to increase the frequency of seizures in epileptics. Moderate and occasional drinking has little effect.

Clinical evidence

A comparative study showed that blood phenytoin levels measured 24 h after the last dose of phenytoin of a group of 15 drinkers (consuming a minimum of 200 g ethanol daily for at least three weeks) was approximately half that of 76 nondrinkers. The phenytoin half-life was reduced 30% (from 23.5 to 16.3 h).[1]

Another study confirmed that alcoholics have lower than usual plasma levels of phenytoin after taking standard doses while drinking,[2] and a report describes a chronic alcoholic who was resistant to large doses of phenytoin.[3] The metabolism of phenytoin is not affected by acute ingestion of alcohol.[4]

Mechanism

Supported by animal data,[5] the evidence suggests that alcohol induces liver microsomal enzymes so that the rate of metabolism and clearance of phenytoin from the body is increased.

Importance and management

An established interaction although the documentation is limited. Those who drink heavily may need above average doses of phenytoin to maintain adequate serum levels. Epileptics should be encouraged to limit their drinking because heavy drinking appears to increase the frequency of seizures.[6] Occasional moderate drinking appears to be safe.

References

1 Kater RMH, Roggin G, Tobon F, Zieve P and Iber FL. Increased rate of clearance of drugs from the circulation of alcoholics. Amer J Med Sci (1969) 258, 35.
2 Sandor P, Sellers EM, Dumbrell M and Khouw V. Effect of short- and long-term alcohol use on phenytoin kinetics in chronic alcoholics. Clin Pharmacol Ther (1981) 30, 390–7.
3 Birkett DJ, Graham GG, Chinwah PM, Wade DN and Hickie JB. Multiple drug interactions with phenytoin. Med J Aust (1977) 2, 467–8.
4 Schmidt D. Effect of ethanol intake on phenytoin metabolism on volunteers. Experentia (1975) 31, 1313.
5 Rubin E and Lieber CS. Hepatic microsomal enzymes in man and rat: induction and inhibition by ethanol. Science (1968) 162, 690.
6 Lambie DG, Stanaway L and Johnson RH. Factors which influence the effectiveness of treatment of epilepsy. Aust NZ Med J (1986) 16, 779–84.

Phenytoin + Allopurinol

Abstract/Summary

A single case report describes phenytoin intoxication in a boy when given allopurinol.

Clinical evidence, mechanism, importance and management

A 13-year-old boy with Lesch-Nyhan syndrome who was taking phenobarbitone, clonazepam, sodium valproate and phenytoin (200 mg daily) became somnolent within seven days of starting to take allopurinol (150 mg daily). His serum phenytoin levels were found to have almost tripled (from 7.5 to 20 μg/ml).[1]

The reason for this reaction is not known (possibly inhibition of liver enzymes?) and its general importance is uncertain—probably very small—but it might be prudent to monitor the effects of concurrent use to confirm that no toxic effects develop.

Reference

1 Yokochi K, Yokochi A, Chiba K and Ishizaki T. Phenytoin-allopurinol interaction: Michaelis-Menten kinetic parameters of phenytoin with and without allopurinol in a child with Lesch-Nyhan syndrome. Ther Drug Monit (1982) 4, 353–7.

Phenytoin + Amiodarone

Abstract/Summary

Serum phenytoin levels can be raised, markedly so in some individuals, by the concurrent use of amiodarone. Phenytoin intoxication may occur if the dosage of phenytoin is not reduced appropriately. Amiodarone serum levels are reduced.

Clinical evidence

(a) Phenytoin serum levels increased

Three patients showed a marked rise in serum phenytoin levels when concurrently treated with amiodarone (400–1200 mg daily). One of them developed phenytoin intoxication (ataxia, lethargy, vertigo) within four weeks of starting to take amiodarone and had a serum phenytoin level of 40 μg/ml, representing a 3–4-fold rise. Levels restabilized when the phenytoin dosage was reduced from 400 to 200 mg daily. The serum phenytoin levels of the other two were approximately doubled by the amiodarone.[1]

A threefold rise in serum phenytoin levels with toxicity caused by amiodarone (400 mg daily) was described in another report,[2] and a study in normal subjects showed that after taking 200 mg amiodarone daily for three weeks the AUC (area under the concentration-time curve) of phenytoin was increased by 31%.[3] An elderly man showed evidence of

intoxication within two weeks of starting to take amiodarone.[4]

(b) Amiodarone serum levels reduced

A study in five subjects given 200 mg amiodarone daily showed that over a 5-week period the serum amiodarone levels gradually increased. When phenytoin (3–4 mg/kg daily) was added for a period of two weeks, the serum amiodarone levels fell to concentrations which were 32.5%–48.7% below those predicted.[5]

Mechanisms

Uncertain. (a) It seems possible that amiodarone inhibits the liver enzymes concerned with the metabolism of phenytoin, resulting in a rise in its serum levels. Amiodarone also binds extensively to serum and tissue proteins and a displacement interaction may have had some part to play. (b) Phenytoin is an enzyme-inducing agent which possibly increases the metabolism of the amiodarone by the liver.

Importance and management

Information seems to be limited to the reports cited but both interactions appear to be clinically important. Concurrent use should not be undertaken unless the effects can be well monitored. (a) Phenytoin dosage reductions should be made as necessary. The phenytoin levels in some individuals can be doubled after only 10 days concurrent use.[1] One patient described above was restabilized on half the dosage of phenytoin.[1] Amiodarone is cleared from the body very slowly so that this interaction will persist for weeks after its withdrawal so that continued monitoring is important. Be aware that ataxia due to phenytoin intoxication may be confused with amiodarone-induced ataxia.[1,4] (b) Increase the amiodarone dosage as necessary.

References

1 McGovern B, Geer VR, LaRaia PJ, Garan H and Ruskin JN. Possible interaction between amiodarone and phenytoin. Ann InternMed (1984) 101, 650–1.
2 Gore JM, Haffajee CI and Alpert JS. Interaction of amiodarone and diphenylhydantoin. Amer J Cardiol (1984) 54, 1145.
3 Nolan PE, Marus FI, Hoyer G, Bliss M, Mayersohn MP and Gear K. Pharmacokinetic interaction between amiodarone and phenytoin. J Amer Coll Cardiol (1987) 9, (2 Suppl A) 47A.
4 Shackleford EJ and Watson FT. Amiodarone-phenytoin interaction. Drug Intell Clin Pharm (1987) 21, 921.
5 Nolan PE, Marcus FI, Karol MD, Hoyer GL and Gear K. Evidence for an effect of phenytoin on the pharmacokinetics of amiodarone. Pharmacotherapy (1988) 8, 121.

Phenytoin + Antacids

Abstract/Summary

Some, but not all, studies have shown that antacids can reduce phenytoin serum levels and this may have been responsible for some loss of seizure control in a few patients, but usually no clinically important interaction occurs.

Clinical evidence

(a) Evidence of an interaction

Three patients taking phenytoin were found to have low serum phenytoin levels (2–4 µg/ml) when given phenytoin and un-named antacids at the same time, but when the antacid administration was delayed 2–3 h the serum phenytoin levels rose 2–3-fold.[1]

A controlled study in six epileptics showed that *Gelusil* (magnesium trisilicate and aluminium hydroxide) could cause a 12% reduction in serum phenytoin levels.[2] Two epileptics are reported elsewhere to have shown inadequate seizure control which coincided with their ingestion of antacids for dyspepsia.[3] Reduced levels of phenytoin (AUC's reduced about one-third) occurred in eight subjects given either aluminium hydroxide, magnesium hydroxide or calcium carbonate,[5] and a reduction (greater than 30%) occurred in three subjects given *Asilone* (dimethicone, aluminum hydroxide, magnesium oxide).[6]

(b) Evidence of no interaction

A study in six normal subjects given aluminium hydroxide or magnesium hydroxide failed to show any change in the rate or extent of absorption of a single dose of phenytoin.[3] Another study on two subjects[4] found no alteration in the absorption of phenytoin due to magnesium hydroxide, aluminium hydroxide–magnesium trisilicate mixture or calcium carbonate. No statistically significant decrease in absorption was seen in six subjects given *Asilone*.[6]

Mechanism

Not understood. One suggestion is that diarrhoea and a general increase in peristalsis caused by some antacids may cause a reduction in phenytoin absorption. Another is that antacids may cause changes in gastric acid secretion which could affect phenytoin solubility.

Importance and management

This possible interaction is fairly well documented, but the results are conflicting. In practice it appears not to be important in most patients, although some loss of seizure control has been seen to occur in a few. Whether an interaction occurs is not predictable because it seems to depend on the individual patient and the antacid being taken. Concurrent use need not be avoided but if there is any hint that an epileptic patient is being affected, separation of the dosages by 2–3 h may minimize the effects.

References

1 Pippinger L. Quoted by Kutt H in 'Interactions of antiepileptic drugs.' Epilepsia (1975) 16, 393.
2 Kulshreshtha VK, Thomas M, Wadsworth J and Richens A. Interaction between phenytoin and antacids. Br J clin Pharmac (1978) 6, 177.
3 O'Brien LS, Orme ML'E and Breckenridge AM. Failure of antacids to alter the pharmacokinetics of phenytoin. Br J clin Pharmac (1978) 6, 176.
4 Chapron DJ, Kramer PA, Mariano SL and Hohnadel DC. Effect of calcium and antacids on phenytoin bioavailability. Arch Neurol (1979) 36, 436.
5 Carter BL, Garnett WR, Pellock JM, Stratton MA and Howell JR. Effect of antacids on phenytoin bioavailability. Ther Drug Monit (1981) 3, 333–40.
6 McElnay JC, Uprichard G and Collier PS. The effect of activated dimethicone and a proprietary antacid preparation containing this agent on the absorption of phenytoin. Br J clin Pharmac (1982) 13, 501.

Phenytoin + Anticoagulants

Abstract/Summary

The serum levels of phenytoin can be increased by dicoumarol (intoxication seen) and phenprocoumon, but they are usually unchanged by warfarin and phenindione. However a single case of phenytoin intoxication has been seen with warfarin. Phenytoin can reduce the anticoagulant effects of dicoumarol and increase the effects of warfarin, whereas the effects of phenprocoumon normally appear to be unaltered.

Clinical Evidence

Effects of Oral Anticoagulants on Phenytoin

(i) Phenytoin + dicoumarol

A study on six subjects taking 300 mg phenytoin daily showed that when additionally given dicoumarol (doses adjusted to give prothrombin values of about 30%) their serum phenytoin levels rose on average over seven days by almost 10 µg/ml (+ 126%).[4] Similar results are described in another study.[7]

A patient on dicoumarol developed phenytoin intoxication within only six days of starting to take 300 mg phenytoin daily.[6]

(ii) Phenytoin + phenprocoumon or pheninidione

A study in four patients on 300 mg phenytoin daily showed that when additionally given phenprocoumon (doses adjusted to give PP values within the therapeutic range) their serum phenytoin levels rose from 10 to 14 µg/ml over seven days.[7] The phenytoin half-life increased from 9.9 to 14 h. No changes were seen in an associated study when pheninidione was used instead of phenprocoumon.[7]

(iii) Phenytoin + warfarin

A study in two patients on 300 mg phenytoin daily found that serum phenytoin levels were unaffected by the concurrent use of warfarin over seven days, and the half-life of phenytoin in four other patients was unaffected.[7] However a patient on 300 mg phenytoin daily has been described who developed signs of intoxication within a short time of starting to take warfarin.[5]

Effects of Phenytoin on Oral Anticoagulants

(i) Dicoumarol + phenytoin

Six subjects on constant daily doses of dicoumarol (40–160 mg) were given 300 mg phenytoin daily for a week. Serum dicoumarol levels started to fall within five days and continued to do so for five days after the phenytoin was stopped. They fell from 29 to 21 µg/ml. No significant changes in the PP% occurred until three days after stopping the phenytoin when it climbed from 20 to 50%. Four other subjects on 60 mg dicoumarol daily showed a fall in serum levels from 20 to 5 µg/ml over a six week period while taking 300 mg phenytoin daily for the first week and then 100 mg daily for five weeks. The PP% after two weeks had risen from 20 to 70% and only fell to previous levels five and a half weeks after stopping the phenytoin.[1]

(ii) Phenprocoumon + phenytoin

An investigation in patients on long-term phenprocoumon treatment showed that in the majority of cases phenytoin had no significant effect on either serum phenprocoumon levels or the anticoagulant control, although a few patients showed a fall and others a rise in serum anticoagulant levels.[2]

(iii) Warfarin + phenytoin

The prothrombin time of a patient on warfarin increased from 21 to 32 sec over a month when given 300 mg phenytoin daily, despite a 22% reduction in the warfarin dosage. He was restabilized on the original warfarin dosage when the phenytoin was withdrawn. Another patient is said to have shown this interaction but no details are given.[8] Three other reports describe this interaction.[9–11] The last one[11] describes a patient who had an increased anticoagulant response for six days, after which it was reduced.

Table 6.2 Summary of interactions between phenytoin and anticoagulants

Concurrent treatment with phenytoin and anticoagulant	Effect on serum anticoagulant levels	Effect on serum phenytoin levels
Dicoumarol	Reduced[1]	Markedly increased[4,6,7]
Phenprocoumon	Usually unchanged[2]	Increased[7]
Warfarin	Increased[8–11]	Usually unchanged[7]
	Single case of increase followed by decrease[11]	Single case of increase[5]
Phenindione	Not documented	Usually unchanged[4,7]
Other anticoagulants	Not documented	Not documented

Mechanisms

Multiple and complex. Dicoumarol and phenprocoumon (but not normally warfarin) appear to inhibit the metabolism of phenytoin by the liver so that its loss from the body is reduced. Phenytoin appears to increase the metabolism of dicoumarol, reduce the metabolism of warfarin, but has no effect on the metabolism of phenprocoumon. Phenytoin possibly also has a diverse depressant effect on the liver which lowers blood clotting factor production.[3]

Importance and management

None of these interactions has been extensively studied, but what is known suggests that the use of dicoumarol with phenytoin should be avoided. Serum phenytoin levels should be well monitored if phenprocoumon is used, and both the phenytoin levels and anticoagulant control should be well monitored if warfarin is given. Dosage adjustments may be needed to accommodate these interactions. Information about other anticoagulants (apart from phenindione) appears to be lacking, but it would clearly be prudent to monitor the effects of concurrent use.

References

1 Hansen JM, Siersbaek-Nielsen K, Kristensen M, Skovsted L and Christensen LK. Effect of diphenylhydantoin on the metabolism of dicoumarol in man. Acta Med Scand (1971) 189, 15.
2 Chrishe HW, Tauchert M and Hilger HH. Effect of phenytoin on the metabolism of phenprocoumon. Eur J Clin Invest (1974) 4, 331.
3 Solomon GE, Hilgartner MW and Kutt H. Coagulation defects caused by diphenylhydantoin. Neurology (1972) 22, 1165.
4 Jansen JM, Kristensen M, Skovsted L and Christensen LK. Dicoumarol induced diphenylhydantoin intoxication. Lancet (1966) ii, 265.
5 Rothermich NO. Diphenylhydantoin intoxication. Lancet (1966) ii, 640.
6 Franzten E, Hansen JM, Hansen OE and Kristensen M. Phenytoin (Dilantin) intoxication. Acta Neurol Scand (1967) 43, 440.
7 Skovsted L, Kristensen M, Hansen JM and Siersbaek-Nielsen K. The effect of different oral anticoagulants on diphenylhydantoin (DPH) and tolbutamide metabolism. Acta Med Scand (1976) 199, 513.
8 Nappi JM. Warfarin and phenytoin interaction. Ann InternMed (1979) 90, 852.
9 Koch-Weser J. Haemorrhagic reactions and drug interactions in 500 warfarin treated patients. Clin Pharmacol Ther (1973) 14, 139.
10 Taylor JW and Lyon LW. Oral anticoagulant-phenytoin interactions. Drug Intell Clin Pharm (1980) 14, 669–73.
11 Levine M and Sheppard I. Biphasic interaction of phenytoin and warfarin. Clin Pharm (1984) 3, 200–3.

Phenytoin + Aspirin

Abstract/Summary

Phenytoin toxicity has been seen in one patient on phenytoin while concurrently taking aspirin, but it seems very unlikely that this adverse interaction normally occurs in most patients.

Clinical evidence

It has been claimed that if a '...patient has been taking large quantities of aspirin for headache...the dilantin (phenytoin) is potentiated',[1] but this remains unconfirmed apart from an isolated report of phenytoin toxicity in a patient associated with taking 975 mg of an enteric-coated aspirin.[5] While it is known that the salicylates are able to displace phenytoin from its plasma protein binding sites,[2-7] it is very doubtful if this normally causes a clinically important interaction. Bearing in mind the extremely common use of aspirin, the almost total silence in the literature about an adverse phenytoin–aspirin interaction implies that no special precautions are normally needed.

References

1 Toakley JG. Dilantin overdosage. Med J Aust (1968) 2, 639.
2 Ehrnebo M and Odar-Cederlof I. Distribution of phenobarbital and diphenylhydantoin between plasma and cells in blood: effect of salicylic acid, temperature and total drug concentration. Eur J clin Pharmacol (1977) 11, 37.
3 Fraser DG, Ludden TM, Evans RP and Sutherland EW. Displacement of phenytoin from plasma binding sites by salicylate. Clin Pharmacol Ther (1980) 27, 165.
4 Paxton JW. Effects of aspirin on salivary and serum phenytoin kinetics in healthy subjects. Clin Pharmacol Ther (1980) 27, 170.
5 Leonard RF, Knott PJ, Rankin GO and Melnick DE. Phenytoin-salicylate interaction. Clin Pharmacol Ther (1981) 29, 260.
6 Olanow CW, Finn A and Prussak C. The effect of salicylate on phenytoin pharmacokinetics. Trans Am Neurol Ass (1979) 104, 109.
7 Inoue F and Walsh RJ. Folate supplements and phenytoin-salicylate interaction. Neurology (1983) 33, 115–16.

Phenytoin + Azapropazone

Abstract/Summary

Serum phenytoin levels can be markedly increased by the concurrent use of azapropazone. Phenytoin intoxication can develop rapidly. It is inadvisable for patients to take these drugs concurrently.

Clinical evidence

The observation of phenytoin intoxication in a patient within a fortnight of starting to take azapropazone (1200 mg daily) prompted further study in five normal subjects given 125–250 mg phenytoin daily. When additionally given 1200 mg azapropazone daily their mean serum phenytoin levels fell briefly from 5 to 3.7 μg/ml before rising steadily over the next seven days to 10.6 μg/ml. At this point the phenytoin was withdrawn because two subjects complained of severe drowsiness.[1]

An extension of this study is described elsewhere.[3] Another report describes phentyoin intoxication in a woman when fenclofenac was replaced by 1200 mg azapropazone daily.[2]

Mechanism

The most likely explanation is that azapropazone inhibits the liver enzymes concerned with the metabolism of phenytoin, resulting in its accumulation in the body. It also seems possible that azapropazone displaces phenytoin from its plasma protein binding sites so that levels of unbound (and active) phenytoin is increased. This means that intoxication may

therefore occur at serum levels which would be well tolerated in the absence of azapropazone.

Importance and management

Information seems to be limited to the reports cited, but it appears to be a clinically important interaction. The incidence is uncertain, but it was demonstrated by all the five subjects examined in the study cited.[1,3] As intoxication may possibly occur at serum levels which would be well tolerated in the absence of azapropazone, concurrent use is potentially hazardous and the manufacturers (Robins) state that azapropazone should not be given to patients taking phenytoin.

References

1 Geaney DP, Carver JG, Aronson JK and Warlow CP. Interaction of azapropazone with phenytoin. Brit Med J (1982) 284, 1373.
2 Roberts CJC, Daneshmend TK, Macfarlane D and Dieppe PA. Anticonvulsant intoxication precipitated by azapropazone. Postgrad Med J (1981) 57, 191.
3 Geaney DP, Carver JG, Davies CL and Aronson JK. Pharmacokinetic investigation of the interaction of azapropazone with phenytoin. Br J clin Pharmac (1983) 15, 727–34.

Phenytoin + Barbiturates

Abstract/Summary

Concurrent use is common, advantageous and normally uneventful. Changes in serum phenytoin levels (often decreases but sometimes increases) can occur if phenobarbitone is added but seizure control is not usually affected. Phenytoin intoxication following barbiturate withdrawal has been seen. Increased phenobarbitone levels and possibly toxicity may result from the addition of phenytoin to phenobarbitone treatment.

Clinical evidence

(a) Phenytoin treatment to which phenobarbitone is added

A study in 12 epileptics treated with phenytoin (3.7 to 6.8 mg/kg daily) showed that while taking phenobarbitone (1.4–2.5 mg/kg daily) their serum phenytoin levels were depressed. Five patients showed a mean reduction of two thirds (from 15.7 to 5.7 μg/ml). In most cases phenytoin levels rose again when the phenobarbitone was withdrawn. In one patient this was so rapid and steep that he developed ataxia and a cerebellar syndrome with phenytoin levels up to 60 μg/ml, despite a reduction in phenytoin dosage.[1]

This interaction has been described in other reports.[2-6] However a rise[4-7] or no alteration[3-6] in serum phenytoin levels have also been described.

(b) Phenobarbitone treatment to which phenytoin is added

Elevated serum phenobarbitone levels occurred in 40 epileptic children when additionally given phenytoin. In five patients illustrated the phenobarbitone levels approximately doubled.

In some cases mild ataxia was seen but the relatively high barbiturate levels were well tolerated.[2]

Mechanism

Phenobarbitone can have a dual effect on phenytoin metabolism: it may cause enzyme induction which results in a more rapid clearance of the phenytoin from the body, or with large doses it may inhibit metabolism by competing for enzyme systems. The total effect will depend on the balance between the two. The reason for the elevation of serum phenobarbitone levels is not fully understood.

Importance and management

These interactions are well documented and well established. Concurrent use is common and can be therapeutically valuable. Some manufacturers market fixed-dose combinations of both drugs (e.g. *Epanutin* with *Phenobarbitone, Garoin*). Changes in dosage or the addition or withdrawal of either drug need to be well monitored to ensure that drug intoxication does not occur, or that seizure control is worsened. Other barbiturates are also enzyme-inducing agents and may be expected to interact similarly.

References

1 Morselli PL, Rizzo M and Garattini S. Interaction between phenobarbital and diphenylhydantoin in animals and in epileptic patients. Ann NY Acad Sci (1971) 179, 88.
2 Cucinell SA, Conney AH, Sansur M and Burns JJ. Drug interactions in man. I. Lowering effect of phenobarbital on plasma levels of bishydroxycoumarin (Dicumarol) and diphenylhydantoin (Dilantin). Clin Pharmacol Ther (1965) 6, 420.
3 Buchanan RA, Heffelfinger JC and Weiss CF. The effect of phenobarbital on diphenylhydantoin metabolism in children. Paediatrics (1969) 43, 114.
4 Kutt H, Hayes J, Verebeley K and McDowell F. The effect of phenobarbital on plasma diphenylhydantoin level and metabolism in man and rat liver microsomes. Neurology (1969) 19, 611.
5 Diamond WD and Buchanan RA. A clinical study of the effect of phenobarbital on diphenylhydantoin plasma levels. J Clin Pharmacol (1970) 10, 306.
6 Garrettson LK and Dayton PG. Disappearance of phenobarbital and diphenylhydantoin from serum of children. Clin Pharmacol Ther (1970) 11, 674.
7 Booker HE, Tormay A and Toussaint J. Concurrent administration of phenobarbital and diphenylhydantoin: lack of interference effect. Neurology (1971) 21, 383.

Phenytoin + Benzodiazepines

Abstract/Summary

Reports are inconsistent: benzodiazepines can cause serum phenytoin levels to rise (intoxication has been seen), fall, or remain unaltered. In addition phenytoin may cause clonazepam, oxazepam and diazepam serum levels to fall.

Clinical evidence

(a) Serum phenytoin levels increased

The observation of intoxication in patients on phenytoin when given chlordiazepoxide or diazepam prompted more detailed study. 25 patients on 300–400 mg phenytoin daily and one of these benzodiazepines demonstrated serum phenytoin levels which were 80–90% higher than those not taking a benzodiazepine. Some individuals demonstrated even greater increases.[1]

Increased phenytoin serum levels and intoxication have also been attributed in other reports to the concurrent use of diazepam,[4,5,11,12] clonazepam,[2,7,15,16] chlordiazepoxide[3] and possibly, but not certainly, to nitrazepam.[6]

(b) Serum phenytoin levels decreased

24 patients given phenytoin and 4–6 mg clonazepam daily over a two month period showed a mean 18% fall in their serum phenytoin levels.[9]

Other studies describe similar findings with clonazepam[13,20] and diazepam.[8,10]

(c) Serum phenytoin levels unaltered, serum benzodiazepine levels reduced

Clonazepam is reported not to alter serum phenytoin levels.[13,14] In addition, a study in patients given 250–400 mg phenytoin daily showed that serum clonazepam levels were reduced by more than 50% (from 183 to 81 ng/ml).[17] Diazepam and oxazepam may be similarly affected in epileptic patients given phenytoin or phenobarbitone.[18,19]

Mechanisms

The inconsistency of these reports is not understood. Benzodiazepine-induced changes in the metabolism of the phenytoin, both enzyme induction and inhibition,[9,10,13] as well as alterations in the apparent volume of distribution have been discussed. Enzyme induction may possibly account for the fall in serum benzodiazepine levels.

Importance and management

A confusing picture. Concurrent use certainly need not be avoided (it has proved to be valuable in many cases) but the serum phenytoin levels should be monitored so that undesirable changes can be detected. Only diazepam, chlordiazepoxide, nitrazepam and clonazepam have been implicated, but it seems possible that other benzodiazepines will interact similarly.

References

1 Vajda FJ E, Prineas RJ and Lovell RRH. Interaction between phenytoin and the benzodiazepines. Lancet (1971) i, 346.
2 Eeg-Oloffson O. Experiences with Rivotril in treatment with epilepsy—particular minor motor epilepsy—in mentally retarded children. Acta Neurol Scand (1973) 49 (Suppl 53) 29.
3 Kutt H and McDowell FJ. Management of epilepsy with diphenylhydantoin sodium. J Amer Med Ass (1968) 203, 969.

4 Rogers HJ, Halsam RA, Longstreth J and Lietman PS. Diphenylhydantoin-diazepam interaction: a pharmacokinetic analysis. Pediatr Res (1975) 9, 286.

5 Ibid. Phenytoin intoxication during concurrent diazepam therapy. J Neurol Neurosurg Psychiat (1977) 40, 890.

6 Treasure T and Toseland PA. Hyperglycaemia due to phenytoin toxicity. Arch Dis Child (1971) 46, 563.

7 Windorfer C. Drug interactions during anticonvulsive therapy. Int J Clin Pharmacol (1976) 14, 231.

8 Siris JH, Pippenger CE, Werner WL and Masland RL. Anticonvulsive drug serum levels in psychiatric patients with seizure disorders. NY State J Med (1974) 74, 1554.

9 Edwards VE and Eadie MJ. Clonazepam—a clinical study of its effectiveness as an anticonvulsant. Proc Aus Assoc Neurol (1973) 10, 61.

10 Houghton GW and Richens A. The effects of benzodiazepines and pheneturide on phenytoin metabolism in man. Br J Clin Pharmacol (1974) 1, P344.

11 Kaviks J, Berry SW and Wood D. Serum folic acid and phenytoin levels in permanently hospitalized patients receiving anticonvulsant therapy. Med J Aust (1971) 2, 369.

12 Shuttleworth E, Wise G and Paulson G. Choreoathetosis and diphenylhydantoin intoxication. J Amer Med Ass (1974) 230, 1170.

13 Huang CY, McLeod JG, Sampson D and Hensley WJ. Clonazepam in the treatment of epilepsy. Med J Aust (1974) 2, 5.

14 Johannessen SI, Strandjord EE and Munthe-Kaas AW. Lack of effect of clonazepam on serum levels of diphenylhydantoin, phenobarbital and carbamazepine. Acta Neurol Scand (1977) 55, 506.

15 Janz D and Schneider H. Bericht uber Wodadiboff II. In 'Antiepileptische Langzeitmedikation'. Biblthea Psychiatr (1975) 151, 55. Karger Verlag, Basel.

16 Windorfer A and Sauer W. Drug interactions during anticonvulsant therapy in childhood: diphenylhydantoin, primidone, phenobarbitone, clonazepam, nitrazepam, carbamazepine and dipropylacetate. Neuropaediatr (1977) 8, 29.

17 Sjo O, Hvidberg EF, Naestroft J and Lund M. Pharmacokinetics and side-effects of clonazepam and its 7-amino metabolite in man. Europ J Clin Pharmacol (1975) 8, 249.

18 Hepner GW, Vesell ES, Lipton A, Harvey HA, Wilkinson GR and Schenker S. Disposition of aminopyrine, antipyrine, diazepam and indocyanin green in patients with liver disease or on anticonvulsant therapy: diazepam breath test and correlations in drug elimination. J Lab Clin Med (1977) 90, 440–56.

19 Scott AK, Khir ASM, Steele WH, Hawksworth GM and Petrie JC. Oxazepam pharmacokinetics in patients with epilepsy treated long-term with phenytoin alone or in combination with phenobarbitone. Br J clin Pharmacol (1983) 16, 441–4.

20 Saavedra IN, Aguilera LI, Faure E and Galdames DG. Case report. Phenytoin/clonazepam interaction. Ther Drug Monit (1985) 7, 481.

Phenytoin + Carbamazepine

Abstract/Summary

The reports are inconsistent. Some describe rises in serum phenytoin levels (with toxicity) whereas others describe falls in both phenytoin and carbamazepine serum levels. Concurrent use should be monitored.

Clinical evidence

(a) Reduced serum phenytoin levels

600 mg carbamazepine daily for 4–14 days reduced the serum phenytoin levels of three out of seven patients from 15 to 7 μg/ml, 18 to 12 μg/ml and 16 to 10 μg/ml respectively. Phenytoin serum levels rose again 10 days after withdrawal of the carbamazepine.[1]

Reduced serum phenytoin levels have been described in other reports.[2,3,6]

(b) Raised serum phenytoin levels

A study in six epileptics treated with phenytoin (350–600 mg daily) showed that the addition of carbamazepine (600–800 mg daily) increased the phenytoin serum levels by 35%, increased its half-life by 41% and reduced its clearance by 36.5% over a 12-week period. Five of the six showed developed additional signs of toxicity (sedation, ataxia, nystagmus, etc). Neurotoxicity increased by 204%. The phenytoin dosage remained unchanged throughout the period of the study.[15]

Increases in serum phenytoin levels have been described in other reports.[4,9–14] Rises of 81% and up to 100% have been reported.[12,9]

(c) Reduced serum carbamazepine levels

A series of multiple regression analyses on data from a large number of patients (precise number is not clear from the report), showed that phenytoin reduces serum carbamazepine on average by 0.9 μg/ml for each 2 mg/kg phenytoin taken each day.[4]

Reduced serum carbamazepine levels have been described in other studies.[7,8,13]

Mechanisms

Not understood. A reduction in phenytoin metabolism and an increase in carbamazepine metabolism have been suggested.[14]

Importance and management

These contradictory reports makes assessment of this interaction difficult. What is known indicates that it would be wise to monitor anticonvulsant levels during concurrent use so that steps can be taken to avoid the development of toxicity. Not all patients appear to demonstrate an adverse interaction, but it is not possible to identify those potentially at risk. The risk of carbamazepine-induced water intoxication is reported to be reduced in patients concurrently taking phenytoin.[8]

References

1 Hansen JM, Siersboek-Nielsen K and Skovsted L. Carbamazepine-induced acceleration of diphenylhydantoin and warfarin administration in man. Clin Pharmacol Ther (1971) 12, 539.

2 Cereghino JJ, van Meter JC, Brock JT, Penry JK, Smith LD and White BG. Preliminary observations of serum carbamazepine concentration in epileptic patients. Neurology (1973) 23, 357.

3 Hooper WD, Dubetz DK, Eadie MJ and Tyrer JH. Preliminary observations on the clinical pharmacology of carbamazepine ('Tegretol'). Proc Aust Ass Neurol (1974) 11, 189.

4 Lander CM, Eadie MJ and Tyrer JH. Interactions between anticonvulsants. Proc Aust Ass Neurol (1975) 12, 111.

5 Christiansen J and Dam M. Influence of phenobarbital and diphenylhydantoin on plasma carbamazepine levels in patients with epilepsy. Acta Neurol Scandinav (1973) 49, 543.

6 Windorfer A and Sauer W. Drug interactions during anticonvulsant therapy in childhood: diphenylhydantoin, primidone, phenobarbitone,

clonazepam, nitrazepam, carbamazepine and dipropylacetate. Neuropadiatrie (1977) 8, 29.

7 Cereghino JJ, Block JT, van Meter JC, Penry JK, Smith LD and White
BG. The efficacy of carbamazepine combinations in epilepsy. Clin Pharmacol Ther (1975) 18, 733.

8 Perucca E and Richens A. Reversal by phenytoin of carbamazepine-induced water intoxication: a pharmacokinetic interaction.
J Neurol Neurosurg Psychiat (1980) 43, 540.

9 Gratz ES, Theodore WH, Newmark ME, Kuppferberg HJ, Porter RJ
and Qu Z. Effect of carbamazepine on phenytoin clearance in patients
with complex partial seizures. Neurology (1982) 32, A223.

10 Browne TR, Evans JE, Szabo GK, Evans BA and Greenblatt DJ. Effect
of carbamazepine on phenytoin pharmacokinetics determined by stable
isotope technique. J Clin Pharmacol (1984) 24, 396.

11 Leppik IE, Pepin SM, Jacobi J and Miller KW. Effect of carbamazepine
on the Michaelis-Menten parameters of phenytoin. In Metabolism of
Antiepileptic Drugs (ed Levy RH et al) Raven Press, New York. (1984)
pp 217–22.

12 Zielinski JJ, Haidukewych D and Leheta BJ. Carbamazepine-phenytoin
interaction: elevation of plasma phenytoin concentrations due to carbamazepine comedication. Ther Drug Monit (1985) 7, 51–3.

13 Hidano F, Obata N, Yahaba Y, Unno K and Fukui R. Drug interactions
with phenytoin and carbamazepine. Fol Psych Neurol Japon (1983) 37,
342–4.

14 Zielinski JJ and Haidukewych D. Dual effects of carbamazepine-phenytoin interaction. Ther Drug Monitor (1987) 9, 21–3.

15 Browne TR, Szabo GK, Evans JE, Evans BA, Greenblatt DJ and Mikati
MA. Carbamazepine increases phenytoin serum concentration and
reduces phenytoin clearance. Neurology (1988) 38, 1146–50.

Phenytoin + Chloramphenicol

Abstract/Summary

*Serum phenytoin levels can be raised by the concurrent use of
chloramphenicol. Phenytoin toxicity may occur unless the
phenytoin dosage is reduced appropriately. Other evidence
indicates that phenytoin may reduce or raise serum
chloramphenicol levels in children.*

Clinical evidence

(a) Serum phenytoin levels increased

A man on phenytoin (400 mg daily) developed signs of
toxicity within a week of additionally taking chloramphenicol
(four six-hourly doses of 1 g intravenously followed by 2 g
six-hourly). His serum phenytoin levels had risen approximately threefold (from about 7 to 24 μg/ml).[2]

This interaction has been described in a number of other
reports.[1,3,4,6–10,13] One study showed that chloramphenicol
more than doubled the half-life of phenytoin.[1]

(b) Serum chloramphenicol levels reduced or increased

A child on a six-week course of chloramphenicol (100 mg/
kg/day intravenously in four divided doses) showed a reduction in peak and trough serum levels of 46 and 74% respectively within two days of beginning additional treatment with
phenytoin (4 mg/kg/day). Levels were further reduced by 63
and 87% respectively when additionally treated with phenobarbitone (4 mg/kg/day).[11]

In contrast, six children (aged 1 month to 12 years) developed
raised chloramphenicol levels into the toxic range while concurrently receiving phenytoin.[12]

Mechanisms

It seems probable that chloramphenicol, a known enzyme inhibitor, depresses the liver enzymes concerned with the
metabolism of phenytoin, thereby reducing its rate of
clearance from the body.[5] The changes in the pharmacokinetics of chloramphenicol in children is not understood.

Importance and management

The rise in serum phenytoin levels (a) in adults is well-
documented and clinically important. A two- to fourfold rise
can occur within a few days of beginning concurrent treatment. Concurrent use should be avoided unless the effects
can be closely monitored and appropriate phenytoin dosages
reduction made as necessary. The general clinical importance
of the changes in serum chloramphenicol levels in children
(b) is uncertain, but the effects of concurrent use should certainly be monitored. More study is needed. It seems doubtful
if enough chloramphenicol would be absorbed from eye-drop
solutions for an interaction to occur, but this needs confirmation.

References

1 Christensen LK and Skovsted L. Inhibition of drug metabolism by
chloramphenicol. Lancet (1969) ii, 1397.

2 Ballek RE, Reidenberg MM amd Orr L. Inhibition of DPH metabolism
by chloramphenicol. Lancet (1973) i, 150.

3 Houghton GW and Richens A. Inhibition of phenytoin metabolism by
other drugs used in epilepsy. Int J Clin Pharmacol (1975) 12, 210.

4 Rose JQ, Choi HK, Schentag JJ, Kinkel WR and Jusko WJ. Intoxication
caused by interaction of chloramphenicol and phenytoin. J Amer Med
Ass (1977) 237, 2630.

5 Dixon RL and Fouts JR. Inhibition of microsomal drug metabolism
pathway by chloramphenicol. Biochem Pharmacol (1962) 11, 715.

6 Koup JR, Gibaldi M, McNamara P, Hilligoss DM, Colburn WA and
Bruck E. Interaction of chloramphenicol with phenytoin and phenobarbital. Clin Pharmacol Ther (1978) 24, 571.

7 Vincent FM, Mills L and Sullivan JK. Chloramphenicol-induced phenytoin intoxication. Ann Neurol (1978) 3, 469.

8 Harper JM, Yost RL, Stewart RB and Ciezkowski J. Phenytoin-
chloramphenicol interaction. Drug Intell Clin Pharm (1979) 13, 425.

9 Greenlaw CW. Chloramphenicol-phenytoin drug interaction. Drug
Intell Clin Pharm (1979) 13, 609.

10 Saltiel MS and Stephens NM. Phenytoin-chloramphenicol interaction.
Drug Intell Clin Pharm (1980) 14, 221.

11 Powell DA, Nahata M, Durrell DC, Glazer JP and Hilty MD. Interactions among chloramphenicol, phenytoin and phenobarbitone in a
pediatric patient. J Pediat (1981) 98, 1001.

12 Karasinski K, Kusmiesz H and Nelson JD. Pharmacological interactions
among chloramphenicol, phenytoin and phenobarbital. Pediatr Infect
Dis (1982) 1, 232–5.

13 Cosh DG, Rowett DS, Lee PC and McCarthy PJ. Case report—
phenytoin therapy complicated by concurrent chloramphenicol and
enteral nutrition. Aust J Hosp Pharm (1987) 17, 51–3.

Phenytoin + Chlorpheniramine

Abstract/Summary

Phenytoin intoxication in two patients has been attributed to the concurrent use of chlorpheniramine.

Clinical evidence, mechanism, importance and management

A week or so after starting to take chlorpheniramine (12 g daily), a woman on phenytoin and phenobarbitone developed phenytoin intoxication and was found to have serum phenytoin levels of about 65 μg/ml. The toxic symptoms disappeared and phenytoin levels fell when the chlorpheniramine was withdrawn.[1] Another woman on anticonvulsants, including phenytoin, developed slight grimacing of the face and involuntary jaw movements (but no speech slurring, ataxia or nystagmus) within 12 days of starting to take 12–16 mg chlorpheniramine daily. Her serum phenytoin levels were found to be 30 μg/ml which fell when the chlorpheniramine was withdrawn.[2] The reason for these reactions is not clear but it has been suggested that chlorpheniramine may have inhibited the metabolism of phenytoin by the liver. These are isolated cases so there would seem to be no good reason for avoiding concurrent use in all patients, but it would be reasonable to monitor the effects. There seem to be no reports of interactions between phenytoin and other antihistamines.

References

1 Pugh RNH, Geddes AM and Yeoman WB. Interaction of phenytoin with chlorpheniramine. Br J clin Pharmac (1975) 2, 173.
2 Ahmad S, Laidlaw J, Houghton GW and Richens A. Involuntary movements caused by phenytoin intoxication in epileptic patients. J Neurol Neurosurg Psychiat (1975) 38, 225.

Phenytoin + Cholestyramine or Colestipol

Abstract/Summary

Neither cholestyramine nor colestipol affect the absorption of phenytoin from the gut.

Clinical evidence, mechanism, importance and management

A study in six normal subjects showed that neither cholestyramine (5 g) nor colestipol (10 g) had a significant effect on the absorption of a single 500 mg dose of phenytoin.[1] Another study in six normal subjects found that 4 g cholestyramine four times daily had no significant effect on the extent of the absorption of 400 mg phenytoin, although it was absorbed a little more rapidly.[2] No special precautions would seem to be necessary if either of these drugs and phenytoin is taken concurrently.

References

1 Callaghan JT, Tsuru M, Holtzman JL and Hunningshake DB. Effect of cholestyramine and colestipol on the absorption of phenytoin. Eur J Clin Pharmacol (1983) 24, 675–8.
2 Barzaghi N, Monteleone M, Amione C, Lecchini S, Perucca E and Frigo GM. Lack of effect of cholestyramine on phenytoin bioavailability. J Clin Pharmacol (1988) 28, 1112–4.

Phenytoin + Cimetidine, Famotidine and Ranitidine

Abstract/Summary

Phenytoin serum levels are raised by the use of cimetidine and toxicity may occur unless the phenytoin dosage is reduced appropriately. Ranitidine does not interact with phenytoin and this also appears to be true for famotidine

Clinical evidence

(a) Phenytoin + cimetidine

Nine patients showed a 60% rise (from 5.7 to 9.1 μg/ml) in serum phenytoin levels after taking cimetidine (1 g daily) concurrently for three weeks. The serum phenytoin fell to its former levels within two weeks of withdrawing the cimetidine.[1,2,5,6]

This interaction has been described in many reports and studies involving numerous patients and subjects.[3,4,8,9,11–15] Phenytoin toxicity developed in some individuals. The extent of the rise is very variable (13–33% over six days in one report[3] and 22–280% over two weeks in another[10]). A case of severe and life-threatening neutropenia and another of agranulocytosis attributed to the concurrent use of high doses of both drugs have also been reported.[7]

(b) Phenytoin + famotidine or ranitidine

Studies in four patients given ranitidine for two weeks[17] showed that no interaction occurred, and a study in 10 subjects given famotidine demonstrated that the phenytoin pharmacokinetics remained unaltered.[16,18]

Mechanism

Cimetidine is a potent enzyme inhibitor which depresses the activity of the liver enzymes concerned with the metabolism of phenytoin, thus allowing it to accumulate in the body and, in some instances, to reach toxic concentrations. Neither famotidine nor ranitidine affect these enzymes.

Importance and management

The phenytoin–cimetidine interaction is well documented and clinically important. It is not possible to identify those who will show the greatest response, but those with serum levels at the top end of the therapeutic range are most at risk. Cimetidine should not be given to patients taking phenytoin unless the serum levels can be monitored and suitable dosage reductions made if necessary. Ranitidine is clearly an alternative non-interacting H_2-blocker, and what is known so far about famotidine indicates that it also does not interact.

References

1 Neuvonen PJ, Ritta A, Tokola R and Kaste M. Cimetidine-phenytoin interaction: effect of serum phenytoin concentration and antipyrine test in man. Nauyn-Schmied Arch Pharmacol (1980) 313 (Suppl) R60.
2 Sazie E and Jaffe JP. Severe granulocytopenia with cimetidine and phenytoin. An InternMed (1980) 93, 151.
3 Hetzel DJ, Bochner F, Hallpike JF, Shearman DJC and Hann CS. Nimetidine interaction with phenytoin. Brit Med J (1981) 282, 1512.
4 Algozzine GJ, Steward RB and Springer PK. Decreased clearance of phenytoin with cimetidine. Ann InternMed (1981) 95, 244.
5 Neuvonen PJ, Tokola R and Kaste M. Cimetidine interaction with phenytoin. Brit Med J (1981) 283, 501.
6 Ibid. Cimetidine-phenytoin interaction: effect on serum phenytoin concentration and antipyrine test. Eur J Clin Pharmacol (1981) 21, 215–20.
7 Al-Kawas FH, Lenes BA and Sacher RA. Cimetidine and agranulocytosis. Ann InternMed (1979) 90, 992–3.
8 Bartle WK, Walker SE and Shapero I. Effect of cimetidine on phenytoin metabolism. Clin Pharm Ther (1982) 31, 202.
9 Bartle WK, Walker SE and Shapero I. Dose-dependent effect of cimetidine on phenytoin kinetics. Clin Pharmacol Ther (1983) 33, 649–55.
10 Watts RW, Hetzel DJ, and Bochner F. Lack of interaction between ranitidine and phenytoin. Brit J clin Pharmac (1983) 15, 499–500.
11 Phillips P and Hansky J. Phenytoin toxicity secondary to cimetidine administration. Med J Aust (1984) 141, 602.
12 Griffin JW, May JR and DiPiro JT. Drug interactions: theory versus practice. Amer J Med (1984) 77 (Suppl 5B) 85–9.
13 Frigo GM, Lecchini S, Caravaggi M, Gatti G, Tonini M, D'Angelo L, Perucca E and Crema A. Reduction of phenytoin clearance caused by cimetidine. Europ J Clin Pharmacol (1983) 25, 135–7.
14 Salem RB, Breland BD, Mishra SK and Jordan JE. Effect of cimetidine on phenytoin serum levels. Epilepsia (1983) 24, 284–8.
15 Iteogu MO, Murphy JE, Shleifer N and Davis R. Effect of cimetidine on single-dose phenytoin kinetics. Clin Pharm (1983) 2, 302–3.
16 Sambol NC, Upton RA, Chremos AN, Lin ET and Williams RL. A comparison of the influence of famotidine and cimetidine on phenytoin elimination and hepatic blood flow. Br J clin Pharmac (1989) 27, 83–7.
17 Hetzel DJ, Watts RW, Bochner F and Shearman. Ranitidine, unlike cimetidine, does not interact with phenytoin. Aust NZ J Med (1983) 13, 324.
18 Sambol NC, Upton RA, Chremos AN, Lin E, Gee W and Williams RL. Influence of famotidine and cimetidine on the disposition of phenytoin and indocyanine green. Clin Pharmacol Ther (1986) 39, 225.

Phenytoin + Cloxacillin

Abstract/Summary

A marked reduction in serum phenytoin levels in a patient has been attributed to the concurrent use of cloxacillin.

Clinical evidence, mechanism, importance and management

An epileptic woman taking 400 mg phenytoin daily, hospitalized for second degree burns sustained during a generalized seizure, showed an '...astonishing drop...' in serum phenytoin levels (from 21.8 to 3.5 μg/ml) which was attributed to the concurrent use of cloxacillin, 0.5 g six-hourly. Serum phenytoin values within the original range

and using the original dosage were only satisfactorily restored when the cloxacillin was withdrawn. The authors of the report advise a 'watchful awareness' if both drugs are used. This seems to be the only report of an adverse interaction between phenytoin and a penicillin. Its incidence and general importance would seem to be very small if viewed against the very wide-spread use of the pencillins.

Reference

1 Fincham RW, Wiley DE and Schottelius DD. Use of phenytoin levels in a case of status epilepticus. Neurology (1976) 26, 879.

Phenytoin + Diazoxide

Abstract/Summary

Four children showed very marked reductions in serum phenytoin levels when diazoxide was given and seizure control was lost in one case. There is some evidence that the effects of diazoxide may also be reduced.

Clinical evidence

Two children receiving 17 and 30 mg/kg/day phenytoin respectively failed to achieve therapeutic phenytoin serum levels when given diazoxide. When the diazoxide was withdrawn, satisfactory serum phenytoin levels were achieved with dosages of only 6.6 and 10 mg/kg/day. When diazoxide was restarted experimentally in one child, the serum phenytoin fell to undetectable levels over three days and seizures occurred.[1,2]

Two other reports describe this interaction.[3,5] In addition it appears that the effects of the diazoxide can also be reduced.[3,4]

Mechanism

What is known[1–3] suggests that diazoxide increases the metabolism and the clearance of phenytoin from the body. The half-life of diazoxide is reduced by phenytoin.[4]

Importance and management

Information is limited to these reports concerning children, but the interaction would appear to be established. Increased dosages of phenytoin would appear to be necessary if seizure control is to be maintained, and reduced dosages following its withdrawal. Concurrent use should be well monitored. The clinical importance of the reduced diazoxide effects is uncertain.

References

1 Roe TF, Podosin RL and Blaskovics ME. Drug interaction. Diazoxide and diphenylhydantoin. Pediatr Res (1975) 9, 285.
2 Roe TF, Podison RL and Blascovics ME. Drug Interaction. Diazoxide and diphenylhydantoin. J Pediatr (1975) 87, 480.
3 Petro DJ, Vannucci RC and Kulin HE. Diazoxide-diphenylhydantoin interaction. J Pediatr (1976) 89, 331.

4   Pruitt AW, Dayton PG and Patterson JH. Disposition of diazoxide in children. Clin Pharmacol Ther (1973) 14, 73.
5   Turck D, Largilliere C, Depuis B and Farriaux JP. Interaction entre le diazoxide et la phenytoine. Presse Med (1986) 15, 31.

Phenytoin + Dichloralphenazone

Abstract/Summary

Serum phenytoin levels may be reduced by the concurrent use of dichloralphenazone. Some loss in seizure control is possible.

Clinical evidence, mechanism, importance and management

A study in five normal subjects showed that after taking 1 g dichloralphenazone each night for 13 nights their total body clearance of phenytoin (single dose given intravenously) was doubled. The phenazone component of dichloralphenazone is a known enzyme-inducer and the increased clearance of phenytoin may be due to an enhancement of its metabolism. There seem to be no reports of adverse effects in patients given both drugs so that the clinical importance of this interaction is uncertain, however it would seem prudent to watch for falling serum phenytoin levels if dichloralphenazone is added to established treatment with phenytoin.

Reference

1   Riddell JG, Salem SAM and McDevitt DG. Interaction between phenytoin and dichloralphenazone. Br J clin Pharmacol (1980) 9, 118P.

Phenytoin + Fluconazole

Abstract/Summary

Phenytoin serum levels can rise rapidly if fluconazole is given. Toxicity will develop unless the phenytoin dosage is reduced appropriately.

Clinical evidence

A patient on 300 mg phenytoin daily developed signs of toxicity (dizziness, nystagmus, ataxia) within two days of starting to take 400 mg fluconazole daily. His serum phenytoin levels had risen from a range of 30–40 μmol/l to 140 μmol/l. Serum levels fell and the toxicity rapidly disappeared when the phenytoin dosage was reduced.[2]

10 subjects on 200 mg phenytoin daily for three days and 200 mg fluconazole for 14 days were compared with 10 other subjects not given fluconazole. Fluconazole was found to increase the phenytoin AUC_{0-24} (area under the concentration-time curve over 24 h) by 75%, and the trough phenytoin serum levels were raised by 128%. Phenytoin appeared not to affect fluconazole trough serum levels.[1] At least three other cases of phenytoin toxicity caused by fluconazole have been documented.[3,4]

Mechanism

Not established. A reduction in the metabolism and clearance of the phenytoin by the fluconazole is a probable explanation.[1,2] It is suggested that fluconazole causes a dose related inhibition of the human cytochrome P450 system.[2]

Importance and management

Information is limited but the interaction would appear to be established. The phenytoin dosage should be reduced to prevent toxicity if fluconazole is added. In the case report cited above[2] a reduction from 300 to 200 mg phenytoin daily controlled this interaction.

References

1   Blum RA, Wilton JH, Hilligoss DM, Gardner MJ, Chin EB and Schentag JJ. Effect of fluconazole on the disposition of phenytoin. Clin Pharmacol Ther (1990) 47, 182.
2   Mitchell AS and Holland JT. Fluconazole and phenytoin: a predictable interaction. Br Med J (1989) 298, 1315.
3   Howittt KM and Oziemski MA. Phenytoin toxicity induced by fluconazole. Med J Aust (1989) 151, 603–4.
4   Wooller HO (Pfizer). Personal communication quoted in reference 3.

Phenytoin + Food

Abstract/Summary

The absorption of phenytoin can be affected some foods. A very marked reduction in phenytoin absorption has been described when given with enteral feeds (e.g. Fortison, Isocal, Osmolite) administered by nasogastric tube.

Clinical evidence

(a) Phenytoin + food eaten normally

A study showed that serum drug levels were low when the phenytoin was disguised in vanilla pudding and given to mentally retarded children, but were doubled when mixed with apple sauce. Three out of 10 patients developed serum phenytoin levels within the toxic range.[5] An epileptic patient showed a marked fall in his serum phenytoin levels accompanied by an increased seizure frequency when the phenytoin was given at bedtime with a food supplement (*Ensure*).[10] Absorption of phenytoin as the acid in a micronized form (*Fentoin*, ACO, Sweden) may be increased by 27% and peak serum levels can average 40% higher when given with food.[2] One single dose study found that when taken with a meal the total absorption of phenytoin was was not affected, although it was slightly delayed.[1]

(b) Phenytoin + food by nasogastric tube

A patient on 300 mg phenytoin daily who was being fed with *Fortison* through a nasogastric tube achieved a phenytoin serum level of only 1.0 mg/l until the phenytoin was given diluted in water and separated from the food by 2 h. Using this method and with an increase in the dose to 420 mg daily a serum level of 6 mg/l was achieved.[6] This report describes a similar reaction in another patient.[6]

A study in 20 patients and five normal subjects showed that a 73–75% reduction in phenytoin absorption occurred when given by nasogastric tube with an enteral food product (*Isocal*).[3] Other reports describe the same interaction in patients given *Osmolite*, *Fortison* or other enteral foods.[4,7,8,12–14]

Mechanism

Uncertain. It seems that the phenytoin can bind to some food substances.[9] This has been demonstrated with *Osmolite*.[11]

Importance and management

(a) Phenytoin is often taken with water or food to reduce gastric irritation. This normally appears not to have a marked effect on absorption but the studies cited above show that some formulations and some foods can interact. If there are problems with the control of convulsions or evidence of toxicity, review how and when the patient is taking the phenytoin.

(b) The interaction between phenytoin and enteral foods given by nasogastric tube is well established and clinically important. The markedly reduced bioavailability has been successfully managed by giving the phenytoin diluted in water 2 h after stopping the feed, flushing with 60 ml of water, and waiting another 2 h before restarting the feed.[3,6,12] Some increase in the phenytoin dosage may also be needed. Monitor concurrent use closely.

References

1 Kennedy MC and Wade DN. The effect of food on the absorption of phenytoin. Aust NZ J Med (1982) 12, 258–61.
2 Melander A, Brante G, Johansson O and Wahlin-Boll E. Influence of food on the absorption of phenytoin in man. Eur J Clin Pharmacol (1979) 15, 269.
3 Bauer LA. Interference of oral phenytoin absorption by continuous nasogastric feedings. Neurology (1982) 32, 570–2.
4 Hatton RC. Dietary interaction with phenytoin. Clin Pharm (1984) 3, 110–1.
5 Jann MW, Bean J and Fidone G. Interaction of dietary pudding with phenytoin. Pediatrics (1986) 78, 952–3.
6 Summers VM and Grant R. Nasogastric feeding and phenytoin interaction. Pharm J (1989) 243, 181.
7 Weinryb J and Cogen R. Interaction of nasogastric phenytoin and enteral feeding solution. J Amer Geriatr Soc (1989) 37, 195–6.
8 Pearce GA. Apparent inhibition of phenytoin absorption by an enteral nutrient formula. Aust J Hosp Pharm (1988) 18, 289–92.
9 Millar SW and Strom JG. Stability of phenytoin in three enteral nutrient formulas. Am J Hosp Pharm (1988) 45, 2529–32.
10 Longe RL and Smith OB. Phenytoin interaction with an oral feeding results in loss of seizure control. J Amer Geriatr Soc (1988) 36, 542–4.
11 Hooks MA, Longe RL and Taylor AT. Recovery of phenytoin from an enteral nutrient formula. Am J Hosp Pharm (1986) 43, 685.
12 Summers VM and Grant R. Nasogastric feeding and phenytoin interaction. Pharm J (1989) 243, 181.
13 Worden JP, Wood CA and Workman CH. Nasogastric feeding and phenytoin interaction. Neurology (1984) 34, 132.
14 Fitzsimmons WE, Garnett WR and Kreuger KA. Phenytoin and enteral feeding. Drug Intell Clin Pharm (1988) 22, 920.

Phenytoin + Gabapentin

Abstract/Summary

The pharmacokinetics of both phenytoin and gabapentin remain unchanged during concurrent use.

Clinical evidence, mechanism, importance and management

The pharmacokinetics of both phenytoin and gabapentin remained unchanged in eight epileptics when given 400 mg gabapentin three times daily for eight days. The patients had been taking phenytoin for at least two months.[1]

Reference

1 Anhut H, Leppik I, Schmidt B and Thomann P. Drug interaction study of a new anticonvulsant gabapentin with phenytoin in epileptic patients. Naunyn-Schmied Arch Pharmacol (1988) 337, Suppl R127.

Phenytoin + Hypoglycaemic agents

Abstract/Summary

Large and toxic doses of phenytoin have been observed to cause hyperglycaemia, but normal therapeutic doses do not usually affect the control of diabetes. Two isolated cases of phenytoin intoxication have been attributed to the use of tolazamide and tolbutamide.

Clinical evidence

(a) The effect of phenytoin on the response to hypoglycaemic agents

Phenytoin has been shown in a number of reports[1–4,7,8] to raise the blood sugar levels of both diabetics and non-diabetics, but in virtually all the cases on record the phenytoin dosage was large or even in the toxic range, and there is no evidence that a hyperglycaemic response to usual doses of phenytoin is normally large enough to interfere with the control of diabetes either with diet alone or with conventional hypoglycaemic agents. In a single case[2] involving hyperglycaemia in which both insulin and phenytoin were used, the situation was complicated by the use of other drugs and by kidney impairment.

(b) The effect of hypoglycaemic agents on the response to phenytoin

17 patients on phenytoin (100–400 mg daily) who were given tolbutamide (500 mg three times a day) showed a transient rise in the amount of non-protein-bound phenytoin, but no signs of intoxication appeared.[11] A man concurrently treated with phenytoin and tolazamide developed phenytoin toxicity which disappeared when the tolazamide was replaced by insulin.[10] A woman previously successfully treated with phenytoin and tolbutamide developed intoxication on a later occasion when again given tolbutamide.[13]

Mechanisms

Studies in animals and man[5,6,9] suggest that phenytoin-induced hyperglycaemia occurs because the release of insulin from the pancreas is impaired. This implies that no interaction is possible without functional pancreatic tissue. Just why the phenytoin–tolazamide and –tolbutamide interactions occurred is not understood.[12]

Importance and management

The weight of evidence shows that no interaction of clinical importance normally occurs between phenytoin and the hypoglycaemic agents. No special precautions seem normally to be necessary. There appear to be only two unexplained cases on record of a sulphonylurea–phenytoin interaction.

References

1 Klein JP. Diphenylhydantoin intoxication associated with hyperglycaemia. J Paediatr (1966) 69, 463.
2 Goldberg EM and Sanbar SS. Hyperglycaemic, non-ketotic coma following administration of Dilantin (diphenylhydantoin). Diabetes (1969) 18, 101.
3 Peters BH and Samaan NA. Hyperglycaemia with relative hypo-insulinaemia in diphenylhydantoin intoxication. N Engl J Med (1969) 281, 91.
4 Millichap JG. Hyperglycaemic effect of diphenylhydantoin. N Engl J Med (1969) 281, 447.
5 Kizer JS, Cordon-Vargas M, Brendel K and Bressler R. The in vitro inhibition of insulin secretion by diphenylhydantoin. J Clin Invest (1970) 49, 1942.
6 Levin SR, Booker J, Smith DF and Grodsky M. Inhibition of insulin secretion by diphenylhydantoin in the isolated perfused pancreas. J Clin Endocrinol Metab(1970) 30, 400.
7 Farfiss BL and Lutcher CL. Diphenylhydantoin-induced hyperglycaemia and impaired insulin release. Diabetes (1971) 46, 563.
8 Treasure T and Toseland PA. Hyperglycaemia due to phenytoin toxicity. Arch Dis Child (1971) 46, 563.
9 Malherbe C, Burrill KC, Levin SR, Karam JH and Forsham PH. Effect of diphenylhydantoin on insulin secretion in man. N Engl J Med (1972) 286, 339.
10 Pannekoek JH (1969) cited in 11.
11 Wesseling II and Mols-Thurkow I. Diphenylhydantoin (DPH) and tolbutamide in man. Eur J clin Pharmacol (1975) 8, 75.
12 Wesseling H, Mols-Thurkow I and Mulder GJ. Effect of sulphonylureas (tolazamide, tolbutamide and chlorpropamide) on the metabolism of diphenylhydantoin in the rat. Biochem Pharmacol (1973) 22, 3033.
13 Beech E, Mathur SV and Harrold BP. Phenytoin toxicity produced by tolbutamide. Br Med J (1988) 297, 1613–4.

Phenytoin + Ibuprofen

Abstract/Summary

The weight of evidence suggests that ibuprofen does not normally interact adversely with phenytoin, although there is a single case report of phenytoin intoxication during concurrent use.

Clinical evidence, mechanism, importance and management

Studies[1,2] in normal subjects have shown that the pharmacokinetics of single doses of phenytoin (300–900 mg) are not altered by 1200–2400 mg ibuprofen daily, however a single report describes a woman stabilized on 300 mg phenytoin daily who developed phenytoin intoxication within a week of starting to take 1600 mg ibuprofen daily.[3] Her serum phenytoin levels had risen from a range of 40–70 to 101 mmol/l. The reasons are not understood. Her phenytoin serum levels fell when the ibuprofen was withdrawn. Both phenytoin and ibuprofen have been available for a number of years and this case seems to be the first and only report of an adverse interaction. It seems most unlikely therefore that this is an interaction of general importance, nevertheless prescribers should bear it in mind if both drugs are given.

References

1 Bachmann KA, Schwartz JI, Forney RB, Jauregui L and Sullivan TJ. Inability of ibuprofen to alter single dose phenytoin disposition. Br J clin Pharmac (1986) 21, 165–9.
2 Townsend R, Fraser DG, Scavone JM and Cox SR. The effects of ibuprofen on phenytoin pharmacokinetics. 6th Annual Meeting of the American College of Clinical Pharmacy (Abstract) 1985.
3 Sandyk R. Phenytoin toxicity induced by interaction with ibuprofen. S Afr Med J (1982) 62, 592.

Phenytoin + Influenza vaccines

Abstract/Summary

Influenza vaccine is reported to increase, decrease or to have no effect on the serum levels of phenytoin. The efficacy of the vaccine remains unchanged.

Clinical evidence

(a) Phenytoin serum levels increased

Eight epileptic children on phenytoin showed an approximately 50% increase in their serum phenytoin levels (from 9.5 to 15.16 μg/ml) seven days after being given 0.5 ml influenza virus vaccine, USP, types A and B, whole virus (Squibb). Four patients in a group cited below[2] whose phenytoin levels were unchanged after immunization, showed serum phenytoin increases ranging from 46 to 170% over weeks 4–17 after being immunized with 0.5 ml inactivated whole-virion trivalent vaccine.[2]

(b) Phenytoin serum levels decreased

A study on seven patients showed that within four days of receiving 0.5 ml subviron, trivalent influenza vaccine their serum phenytoin levels were reduced 11–14%.[1]

(c) Phenytoin serum levels unchanged

A study on 16 patients given 0.5 ml inactivated whole-virion trivalent influenza vaccine showed that 7 and 14 days later their mean serum phenytoin levels were not significantly altered.[2] The efficacy of influenza vaccine is reported to be unchanged by phenytoin.[3]

Mechanism

Where an interaction occurs it is suggested that it may be due to the inhibitory effect of the vaccine on the liver enzymes concerned with the metabolism of the phenytoin, resulting in a reduced clearance from the body.[4]

Importance and management

The outcome of immunization with influenza vaccine is uncertain. Concurrent use need not be avoided but it would be prudent to monitor the effects closely.

References

1 Sawchuk RJ, Rector TS, Fordice JJ and Leppik IE. Case report. Effect of influenza vaccination on plasma phenytoin concentrations. Ther Drug Monit (1979) 1, 285–8.
2 Levine M, Jones MW and Gribble M. Increased serum phenytoin concentration following influenza vaccination. Clin Pharm (1984) 3, 505–9.
3 Levine M, Beattie BL, McLean DM and Corman D. Phenytoin therapy and immune response to influenza vaccine. Clin Pharm (1985) 4, 191–4.
4 Jann MW and Fidone GS. Effect of influenza vaccine on serum anticonvulsant concentrations. Clin Pharm (1986) 5, 817–20.

Phenytoin + Isoniazid

Abstract/Summary

Phenytoin serum levels can be raised by the concurrent use of isoniazid. Those who are 'slow metabolizers' of isoniazid (10–25%) may develop phenytoin intoxication if the dosage of phenytoin is not reduced appropriately.

Clinical evidence

A study in 32 patients on phenytoin (300 mg daily) showed that, within a week of starting to take isoniazid (300 mg daily) and para-aminosalicylic acid (15 g daily), six of them had phenytoin levels almost 5 μg/ml higher than the rest of the group, and on the following days when levels climbed above 20 μg/ml the typical signs of phenytoin toxicity were seen. All six had unusually high serum isoniazid serum levels.[1,2]

Rises in serum phenytoin levels and toxicity induced by the concurrent use of isoniazid has been described in numerous other reports involving large numbers of patients, one of which describes a fatality.[3–13] It occurs in those who are 'slow metabolizers (acetylators)' of isoniazid (see 'Mechanism' below) and the incidence is between 10 and 25%.

Mechanism

Isoniazid inhibits the liver microsomal enzymes which metabolize phenytoin. As a result the phenytoin accumulates and its serum levels rise.[1,2] Only those who are 'slow metabolizers (acetylators)' of isoniazid (this is genetically determined) attain blood levels of isoniazid which are sufficiently

high to cause extensive inhibition of the phenytoin metabolism, whereas the 'fast metabolizers' remove the isoniazid too quickly for this to occur. Thus some individuals will show a rapid rise in phenytoin levels which eventually reaches toxic concentrations, whereas others will show only a relatively slow and unimportant rise to a plateau within, or only slightly above the therapeutic range.

Importance and management

A well-documented, well-established, clinically important and potentially serious interaction. About 50% of the population are slow or relatively slow metabolizers of isoniazid, but not all of them develop serum phenytoin levels in the toxic range (20 μg/ml plus). The reports indicate that somewhere between 10 and 25% are at risk.[1–4,10] This adverse interaction may take only a few days to develop fully in some patients, but several weeks in others so that concurrent use should be very closely monitored. Serum phenytoin levels should be monitored and suitable dosage reductions made as necessary. One patient is reported to have had better seizure control with fewer side-effects while taking both drugs than with phenytoin alone.[14] See also 'Phenytoin + Rifampicin, Isoniazid and Ethambutol'.

References

1 Kutt H, Brennan R, Dehejia H and Verebeley K. Diphenylhydantoin intoxication. A complication of isoniazid therapy. Amer Rev Resp Dis (1970) 101, 377.
2 Brennan RW, Dehejia H, Kutt H, Verebelely K and McDowell F. Diphenylhydantoin intoxication attendant to slow inactivation of isoniazid. Neurology (1970) 20, 687.
3 Murray FJ, Outbreak of unexpected reactions among epileptics taking isoniazid. Amer Rev Resp Dis (1962) 86, 729.
4 Kutt H, Winters W, McDowell FH. Depression of parahydroxylation of diphenylhydantoin by antituberculosis chemotherapy. Neurol (1966) 16, 594.
5 Manigand G, Thieblot Ph and Deparis M. Accidents de la diphenylhydantoine induits par les traitements antituberculeux. Presse Med (1971) 79, 815.
6 Beauvais P, Mercier D, Hanoteau J and Brissand H-E. Intoxication a la diphenylhydantoine induite par l'isoniazide. Arch Franc Ped (1973) 30, 541.
7 Johnson J. Epanutin and isoniazid interaction. Br Med J (1975) 1, 152.
8 Johnson J and Freeman HL. Death due to isoniazid (INH) and phenytoin. Br J Psychiatr (1975) 129, 511.
9 Geering JM, Ruch W and Dettli L. Diphenylhydantoin-Intoxikation durch Diphenylhydantoin-Isoniazid Interaktion. Schweiz med Wsch (1974) 104, 1224.
10 Miller RR, Porter J and Greenblatt DJ. Clinical importance of the interaction of phenytoin and isoniazid. A report from the Boston Collaborative Drug Surveillance Program. Chest (1979) 75, 356.
11 Witmer DR and Ritschel WA. Phenytoin-isoniazid interaction: a kinetic approach to management. Drug Intell Clin Pharm (1984) 18, 483–6.
12 Perucca E and Richens A. Anticonvulsant drug interactions. In: Tyrer J (ed) The treatment of epilepsy. MTP Lancaster. (1980) pp 95–128.
13 Sandyk R. Phenytoin toxicity induced by antituberculous drugs. S Afr Med J (1982) 332.
14 Thulasimnay M and Kela AK. Improvement of psychomotor epilepsy due to interaction of phenytoin-isoniazid. Tubercle (1984) 65, 229–30.

Phenytoin + Loxapine

Abstract/Summary

A single case report describes depressed serum phenytoin levels during concurrent treatment with loxapine.

Clinical evidence

The serum phenytoin levels of an epileptic patient were depressed by the concurrent use of loxapine, and showed a marked rise when it was withdrawn.[1] The general importance of this is uncertain, but it would now seem prudent to monitor the effects in any patient, particularly as loxapine can lower the convulsive threshold. More study is needed.

Reference

1 Ryan GM and Matthews PA. Phenytoin metabolism stimulated by loxapine. Drug Intell Clin Pharm (1977) 11, 428.

Phenytoin + Methylphenidate

Abstract/Summary

Raised serum phenytoin levels and phenytoin toxicity have been seen in three patients when given methylphenidate, but it is an uncommon reaction. One of the patients also showed raised serum primidone and phenobarbitone levels.

Clinical evidence

A hyperkinetic epileptic boy of five taking 8.9 mg/kg phenytoin and 17.7 mg/kg primidone daily, developed ataxia without nystagmus when additionally treated with 20–40 mg methylphenidate daily. Serum levels of the anticonvulsants were found to be at toxic concentrations and only began to fall when the methylphenidate dosage was reduced.[1]

A further case of phenytoin intoxication occurred in another child when given methylphenidate,[5] but only one other case was seen in other clinical studies and observations on three subjects,[2] 11 patients,[3] and over 100 other patients.[4] A patient who demonstrated phenytoin intoxication on one occasion when given methylphenidate later failed to do so.[2]

Mechanism

Not fully understood. The suggestion is that methylphenidate acts as an enzyme inhibitor, slowing the metabolism of the phenytoin by the liver and leading to its accumulation in those few individuals whose drug metabolizing system is virtually saturated by large doses of phenytoin.

Importance and management

An established but uncommon interaction. Concurrent use need not be avoided but be alert for any evidence of phenytoin intoxication, particularly if the dosage is high.

References

1 Garrettson KJ, Perel JM and Dayton PG. Methylphenidate interaction with both anticonvulsants and ethyl biscoumacetate. A new action of methylphenidate. J Amer Med Ass (1969) 207, 2053.

2 Mirkin BL and Wright F. Drug interactions: effect of methylphenidate on the disposition of diphenylhydantoin in man. Neurology (1971) 21, 1123.

3 Kupferberg HJ, Jeffery W and Hunningshake DB. Effect of methylphenidate on plasma anticonvulsant levels. Clin Pharmacol Ther (1972) 13, 201.

4 Oettinger L. Interaction of methylphenidate and diphenylhydantoin. Drug Ther (1976) 5, 107.

5 Ghofrani M. Possible phenytoin-methylphenidate interaction. Dev Med Child Neurol (1988) 30, 267–8.

Phenytoin + Metronidazole

Abstract/Summary

A small and usually clinically unimportant rise in serum phenytoin levels may occur if metronidazole is used concurrently although a few patients have developed toxic levels.

Clinical evidence, mechanism, importance and management

A pharmacokinetic study[1] in normal subjects found that metronidazole (750 mg daily) increased the half-life of a single 300 mg intravenous dose of phenytoin by 44% (from 16 to 23 h) and reduced the clearance by 14.75%. In another study in normal subjects the pharmacokinetics of a single 300 mg oral dose of phenytoin were unaffected by 800 mg metronidazole daily for five days.[2] An anecdotal report describes '...several patients...' who developed toxic phenytoin serum levels when given metronidazole.[3] The reason for these discordant reports is not clear, but if and when metronidazole affects serum phenytoin levels, the rise seems to be relatively small, usually of minimal clinical importance except possibly in those whose levels are already high and close to the toxic threshold. Monitor the outcome. More study is needed.

References

1 Blyden GT, Scavone JM and Greenblatt DJ. Metronidazole impairs clearance of phenytoin but not of alprazolam or lorazepam. Clin Pharmacol Ther (1988) 28, 240–5.

2 Jensen JC and Gugler R. Interaction between metronidazole and drugs eliminated by oxidative metabolism. Clin PharmacolTher (1985) 37, 407–10.

3 Picard EH. Side effects of metronidazole. Mayo Clin Proc (1983) 58, 401.

Phenytoin + Miconazole

Abstract/Summary

Two reports describe phenytoin intoxication in two patients when concurrently treated with miconazole

Clinical evidence, mechanism, importance and management

An epileptic man,[1] well controlled on phenytoin, developed signs of intoxication within a day of starting treatment with intravenous miconazole (500 mg eight-hourly) and flucytosine. After a week of concurrent treatment his serum phenytoin levels had climbed by 50% (from 29 to 43 μg/ml). He had some signs of very mild phenytoin intoxication even before the antifungal treatment was started. Another patient[2] became intoxicated (nystagmus, ataxia) within five days of starting to take 500 mg miconazole daily. His serum phenytoin climbed to 41 μg/ml. A probable explanation is that the miconazole can depress the metabolism and clearance of the phenytoin by the liver, resulting in its accumulation in the body. Evidence for this interaction seems to be limited to these reports, even so it would be prudent to avoid concurrent use unless serum phenytoin levels can be closely monitored and appropriate reductions made in the phenytoin dosage. The interaction apparently develops very rapidly.

References

1 Rolan PE, Somogyi AA, Drew MJR, Cobain WG, South D and Bochner F. Phentyoin intoxication during parenteral treatment with miconazole. Brit Med J (1983) 287, 1760.
2 Loupi E, Descotes J, Lery N and Evereux J Cl. Interactions medicamenteuses et miconazole. A propos de 10 observations. Therapie (1982) 37, 437–41.

Phenytoin + Omeprazole

Abstract/Summary

The loss of phenytoin from the body is reduced by omeprazole and serum phenytoin levels are expected to rise to some extent.

Clinical evidence

A double-blind cross-over study in 10 normal subjects showed that after taking 40 mg omeprazole daily for nine days the AUC (area under the time-concentration curve) of a single 300 mg dose of phenytoin was increased by 25% (from 122 to 151 μg/ml/hr) and the half-life was increased by 45% (from 17.9 to 25.9 h).[1]

In another study the clearance of an intravenous dose of phenytoin was reduced by 15% by omeprazole.[2]

Mechanism

Not understood. A possible explanation is that the omeprazole reduces the metabolism of the phenytoin by the liver, thereby reducing its loss from the body.

Importance and management

Information is very limited. The clinical importance of this interaction is uncertain but anticipate the need to reduce the phenytoin dosage.

References

1 Prichard PJ, Walt RP, Kitchingman GK, Somerville KW, Langman MJS, Williams J and Richens A. Oral phenytoin pharmacokinetics during omeprazole therapy. Br J clin Pharmac (1987) 24, 534–5.
2 Gugler R and Jensen JC. Omeprazole inhibits oxidative drug metabolism. Gastroenterology (1985) 89, 1235–41.

Phenytoin + Pheneturide

Abstract/Summary

Phenytoin serum levels can be increased by about 50% if pheneturide is used concurrently.

Clinical evidence, mechanism, importance and management

A study in nine patients showed that the half-life of phenytoin was prolonged from 32 to 47 h by pheneturide. Mean serum levels were raised about 50% (from 35 to 53 μM) but fell rapidly when the pheneturide was withdrawn.[1] This study confirms a previous report of this interaction.[2] The reason for this reaction is uncertain, but since the two drugs have a similar structure it is possible that they compete for the same metabolizing enzymes in the liver, thereby resulting, at least initially, in a reduction in the metabolism of the phenytoin. If concurrent use is undertaken the outcome should be well monitored. Reduce the phenytoin dosage as necessary.

References

1 Houghton GW and Richens A. Inhibition of phenytoin metabolism by other drugs used in epilepsy. Int J Clin Pharmacol (1975) 12, 210.
2 Hulsman JW, van Heycop Ten Ham MW and van Zijl CHW. Influence of ethylphenacemide on serum levels of other anticonvulsant drugs. Epilepsia (1970) 11, 207.

Phenytoin + Phenothiazines

Abstract/Summary

The serum levels of phenytoin can be raised or lowered by the use of chlorpromazine, thioridazine or prochlorperazine.

Clinical evidence, mechanism, importance and management

The reports are inconsistent. A patient on phenytoin, primidone and sulthiame showed a doubling in his serum phenytoin levels (from 7 to 15 μg/ml) after taking 50 mg chlorpromazine daily for a month. Four other patients on 50–100 mg chlorpromazine showed no interaction.[1] In another report[2] one out of three patients showed a fall in serum phenytoin levels when given chlorpromazine, and a fall is described in a further report.[5] Yet another report[3] states (without giving details) that in rare instances chlorpromazine and prochlorperazine have been noted to impair phenytoin metabolism. One out of six patients on phenytoin, phenobarbitone and thioridazine showed a marked rise in serum phenytoin levels, whereas four others showed a fall.[2] Phenytoin intoxication has also been described in two patients on thioridazine.[4] A retrospective study on 27 patients on phenytoin showed that four had an increase, two had a decrease and the rest demonstrated no changes in phenytoin serum levels when given thioridazine.[6]

The mechanism of these interactions is uncertain, but it may be related to changes in the metabolism of the phenytoin caused by the phenothiazines. The concurrent use of phenytoin and the phenothiazines cited need not be avoided, but it would be prudent to watch for any signs of changes in serum phenytoin levels which would affect anticonvulsant control. Whether other phenothiazines interact similarly is uncertain.

References

1 Houghton GW and Richens A. Inhibition of phenytoin metabolism by other drugs used in epilepsy. Int J clin Pharmacol (1975) 12, 221.
2 Siris JH, Pippenger CE, Werner WL and Masland RL. Anticonvulsant drug-serum levels in psychiatric patients with seizure disorders. Effects of certain psychotropic drugs. NY State M Med (1974) 74, 1554.
3 Kutt H and McDowell F. Management of epilepsy with diphenylhydantoin sodium. Dosage regulation for problem patients. J Amer Med Ass (1968) 203, 969.
4 Vincent FM. Phenothiazine-induced phenytoin intoxication. Ann Int Med (1980) 93, 56.
5 Haidukewych D and Rodin EA. Effect of phenothiazines on serum antiepileptic drug concentrations in psychiatric patients with seizure disorder. Ther Drug Monit (1985) 7, 401.
6 Sands CD, Robinson JD, Salem RB, Stewart RB and Muniz C. Effect of thioridazine on phenytoin serum concentration: a retrospective study. Drug Intell Clin Pharm (1987) 21, 267–72.

Phenytoin + Phenylbutazone

Abstract/Summary

Phenytoin serum levels can be increased by phenylbutazone. Intoxication may occur if the phenytoin dosage is not reduced appropriately. It seems likely that oxyphenybutazone will interact similarly.

Clinical evidence

Six epileptic patients on phenytoin (200–250 mg daily) given 300 mg phenylbutazone daily showed a mean fall in their phenytoin serum levels from 15 to 13 μg/ml over the first three days, after which the levels climbed steadily to 19 μg/ml over the next 11 days.[1] One patient developed signs of toxicity.

Mechanism

The predominant effect of phenylbutazone seems to be the inhibition of the enzymes concerned with the metabolism of phenytoin (half-life increased from 13.7 to 22 h.[3]), leading to its accumulation in the body and a rise in its serum levels. The initial transient fall may possibly be related in some way to the displacement by the phenylbutazone of the phenytoin from its plasma protein binding sites.[2]

Importance and management

An established interaction, although the documentation is very small. Patients on both drugs should be monitored and suitable phenytoin dosage reductions made where necessary to ensure that intoxication does not occur. There is no direct evidence that oxyphenbutazone interacts like phenylbutazone, but since it is the main metabolic product of phenylbutazone in the body and has been shown to prolong the half-life of phenytoin[4] it would be expected to interact similarly.

References

1 Neuvonen PJ, Lehtovaara R, Bardy A and Elomaa E. Antipyretic analgesics in patients on anti-epileptic drug therapy. Eur J Clin Pharmacol (1979) 15, 263.
2 Lunde PKM. Plasma protein binding of diphenylhydantoin in man: interaction with other drugs and the effect of temperature and plasma dilution. Clin Pharmacol Ther (1970) 11, 846.
3 Andreasen PB, Froland A, Skovsted L, Andersen SA and Haugue M. Diphenylhydantoin half-life in man and its inhibition by phenylbutazone: the role of genetic factors. Acta Med Scand (1973) 193, 561.
4 Soda DM and Levy G. Inhibition of drug metabolism by hydroxylated metabolites: cross-inhibition and specificity. J Pharm Sci (1975) 64, 1928.

Phenytoin + Phenyramidol

Abstract/Summary

Serum phenytoin levels can be markedly increased (as much as threefold) by the concurrent use of phenyramidol. Phenytoin toxicity may occur unless the phenytoin dosage is reduced appropriately.

Clinical evidence, mechanism, importance and management

The observation that poorly controlled epileptics taking phenytoin improved when given phenyramidol prompted more detailed study. Five subjects given phenytoin (100 mg three times daily) doubled their serum phenytoin levels (from

6.6 to 12.0 μg/ml) after taking 1200 mg phenyramidol daily for six days.[1] The evidence suggests that phenyramidol inhibits the liver microsomal enzymes concerned with the metabolism of the phenytoin, thereby prolonging its stay in the body (phenytoin half-life increased from 26 to 55 h).[1]

Information seems to be limited to this study, but interaction would seem to be established. The incidence is uncertain, but all five subjects demonstrated rises in serum levels ranging from about 40 to 200%.[1] Phenytoin serum levels should be closely monitored if phenyramidol is given concurrently, and the phenytoin dosage reduced appropriately to ensure that intoxication does not occur.

Reference

1   Solomon HM and Schrogie JJ. The effect of phenyramidol on the metabolism of diphenylhydantoin. Clin Pharmacol Ther (1967) 8, 554–6.

Phenytoin + Rifampicin (Rifampin)

Abstract/Summary

The clearance of phenytoin is doubled by the concurrent use of rifampicin or rifampicin with isoniazid and ethambutol. Serum phenytoin levels will fall accordingly.

Clinical evidence

Studies in six patients showed that the clearance of phenytoin (100 mg given intravenously) doubled (from 46.7 to 97.8 ml/min) after taking 450 mg rifampicin daily for two weeks, and also doubled (from 47.1 to 81.3 ml/min) in 14 other patients given 450 mg rifampicin, 300 mg isoniazid and 1200 mg ethambutol daily for two weeks. No further changes occurred in the kinetics of phenytoin after three months antitubercular treatment.[1]

A man on phenytoin needed a dosage reduction to keep his serum phenytoin levels within the therapeutic range when his treatment with rifampicin came to an end.[2]

Mechanism

The evidence is consistent with the belief that the rifampicin (a known potent liver enzyme-inducing agent) increases the metabolism and clearance of the phenytoin from the body. These enzyme-inducing effects are apparently only slightly counteracted by the enzyme-inhibiting effects of isoniazid (which would be expected to reduce the clearance of phenytoin).

Importance and management

Direct information seems to be limited to these reports, but the interaction appears to be established and of clinical importance. Monitor the serum phenytoin levels and increase the dosage appropriately if rifampicin is started. Reduce the dosage if the rifampicin is stopped. See also 'Phenytoin + Isoniazid'.

References

1   Kay L, Kampmann, Svendsen TL, Vergman B, Hansen JEM, Skovsted L and Kristensen M. Influence of rifampicin and isoniazid on the kinetics of phenytoin. Br J clin Pharmac (1985) 20, 323–6.
2   Abajo FJ. Phenytoin interaction with rifampicin. Br Med J (1988) 297, 1048.

Phenytoin + Sodium valproate

Abstract/Summary

Concurrent use is common and usually uneventful. Initially total serum phenytoin levels may fall but this is offset by a rise in the levels of free (and active) phenytoin which may very occasionally cause some toxicity. After continued use the serum phenytoin levels rise again.

Clinical evidence

A study extending over a year on eight patients taking phenytoin and sodium valproate showed that by the end of 10 weeks the serum phenytoin levels of six of them had fallen by as much as 50%, but had returned to their original levels by the end of the year.[1]

Similar results were found in another study.[13] In another it was noted that within 4–7 days the total serum phenytoin levels had fallen from 19.4 to 14.6 μg/ml.[7] A number of reports clearly show that total serum phenytoin levels fall during early concurrent use while the concentrations of free phenytoin rise.[7–12] The occasional patient may show signs of phenytoin toxicity during this period and the dosage may need to be reduced.[2] Delerium was seen in one patient on sodium valproate when given phenytoin.[10] Sodium valproate levels are reduced by the presence of phenytoin.[3,4] Very occasionally (and inexplicably) the fit-frequency has increased in patients on phenytoin given sodium valproate.

Mechanism

The initial fall in serum phenytoin levels appears to result from the displacement of phenytoin by the sodium valproate from its protein binding sites (the extent being subject to diurnal variation[5]).[7–12] This allows more of the unbound drug to be exposed to metabolism by the liver and the total phenytoin levels fall. After several weeks the metabolism of the phenytoin is inhibited by the valproate and its levels rise.[8,11] Phenytoin reduces sodium valproate levels, probably because it increases its metabolism by the liver.[3]

Importance and management

An extremely well-documented interaction (only a selection of the references being listed here). Concurrent use is common and usually advantageous, the adverse effects of the interactions between the drugs usually being of only minor practical importance, however the effects should be monitored. A few patients may experience mild and transient toxicity if sodium valproate is started, but most patients on phenytoin do not need a dosage change. During the first few weeks total serum phenytoin levels may fall by 20–50%, but usually no increase in the dosage is needed because it is balanced by an increase in the levels of free (active) phenytoin levels. In the period which follows, the phenytoin levels may rise again 40–50%. Saliva sampling which measures free phenytoin is more reliable in this situation than total serum levels.[6] When monitoring concurrent use it is important to understand fully the implications of changes in 'total' and 'free' or 'unbound' serum phenytoin concentrations.

References

1 Vakil SD, Critchley EMR, Philips JC, Haydock D, Cocks A and Dyer T. The effect of sodium valproate (Epilim) on phenytoin and phenobarbitone blood levels. In 'Clinical and Pharmacological Aspects of Sodium Valproate (Epilim) in the Treatment of Epilepsy'. Proceedings of a symposium held at Nottingham University, September 1975, MCS Consultants, England, p 75.
2 Haigh D and Forsythe WI. The treatment of childhood epilepsy with sodium valproate. Dev Med Child Neurol (1975) 17, 743–8.
3 Rambeck B and May T. Serum concentrations of valproic acid: influence of dose and co-medication. Ther Drug Monit (1985) 7, 387–90.
4 Sackellares JC, Sato S, Dreifuss FE and Penry JK. Reduction of steady-state valproate levels by other antiepileptic drugs. Epilepsia (1981) 22, 437–41.
5 Riva R, Albani F, Contin M, Perucca E, Ambrosetto G, Gobbi G, Santucci M, Procaccianti G and Baruzzi A. Time-dependent interaction between phenytoin and valproic acid. Neurology (1985) 35, 510–15.
6 Knott C, Hamshaw-Thomas A and Reynolds F. Phenytoin-valproate interaction: importance of saliva monitoring in epilepsy. Br Med J (1982) 284, 13–16.
7 Mattson RH, Cramer JA, Williamson PD and Novelly RA. Valproic acid in epilepsy: clinical and pharmacological effects. Ann Neurol (1978) 3, 20–5.
8 Perucca E, Hebdige S, Frigo GM, Gatti G, Lecchini S and Crema A. Interaction between phenytoin and valproic acid: plasma protein binding and metabolic effects. Clin Pharmacol Ther (1980) 28, 779–89.
9 Tsanaclis LM, Allen J, Perucca E, Routledge PA and Richens A. Effect of valproate on free plasma phenytoin concentrations. Br J clin Pharmac (1984) 18, 17–20.
10 Tollefson GD. Delerium induced by the competitive interaction between phenytoin and dipropylacetate. J Clin Psychopharmacol (1981) 1, 154–8.
11 Bruni J, Gallo JM, Lee CS, Pershalski RJ and Wilder BJ. Interactions of valproic acid with phenytoin. Neurology (1980) 30, 1233–6.
12 Friel PN, Leal KW and Wilensky AJ. Valproic acid-phenytoin interaction. Ther Drug Monit (1979) 1, 243–8.
13 Bruni J, Wilder BJ, Willmore LJ and Barbour B. Valproic acid and plasma levels of phenytoin. Neurology (1979) 29, 904–5.

Phenytoin + Sucralfate

Abstract/Summary

The absorption of phenytoin can be reduced about 7–20% by the concurrent use of sucralfate. There is indirect evidence that the interaction can be avoided by giving the phenytoin 2 h after the sucralfate.

Clinical Evidence

In a double-blind cross-over study with eight normal subjects, the concurrent administration of l g sucralfate was found to reduce the absorption of a single 300 mg dose of phenytoin by 20%, measured over a 48 h period.[1] Peak serum phenytoin levels were also reduced, but this was said not to be statistically significant.

Another study demonstrated an absorption reduction of 7.7–9.5%.[2] A similar interaction has been demonstrated in dogs.[3]

Mechanism

Uncertain.

Importance and management

Information is limited, but this interaction would appear to be established. The reduction in absorption is small, but it might be enough to reduce the steady-state serum concentrations of phenytoin in some patients to levels where seizure control is lost. Concurrent use should be monitored. A study in dogs[2] showed that no change in absorption occurred if the phenytoin was given 2 h after the sucralfate, so it seems possible that the same precaution could prevent this interaction in man.

References

1 Smart HL, Somerville KW, Williams J, Richens A and Langman MJS. The effects of sucralfate upon phenytoin absorption in man. Br J clin Pharmac (1985) 20, 238–40.
2 Hall TG, Cuddy PG, Glass CJ and Melethil S. Effect of sucralfate on phenytoin bioavailability. Drug Intell Clin Pharm (1986) 20, 607–11.
3 Lacz JP, Groschang AG, Giesing DH and Browne RK. The effect of sucralfate on drug absorption in dogs. Gastroenterology (1982) 82, 1108.

Phenytoin + Sulphinpyrazone

Abstract/Summary

Some limited evidence indicates that phenytoin serum levels may be markedly increased by the concurrent use of sulphinpyrazone. Toxicity may possibly occur unless the phenytoin dosage is reduced appropriately.

Clinical evidence

The serum phenytoin levels of two out of five patients on phenytoin (250–350 mg daily) were doubled (from approximately 10 to 20 μg/ml) within 11 days of starting to take 800 mg sulphinpyrazone daily. One of the remaining patients showed a small increase and the other two no changes at all. When the sulphinpyrazone was withdrawn, the serum phenytoin concentrations fell to their former levels.[1]

A clinical study in patients showed that 800 mg sulphinpyrazone daily for a week increased the phenytoin half-life from 10 to 16.5 h and reduced the metabolic clearance from 59 to 32 ml/min.[2]

Mechanism

Uncertain. It seems probable that sulphinpyrazone inhibits the metabolism of the phenytoin by the liver, thereby allowing it to accumulate in the body and leading to a rise in its serum levels. Displacement of phenytoin from its plasma protein binding sites may also have some part to play.

Importance and management

Information seems to be limited to just two reports (one is an abstract and the other an indirect reference) which await further confirmation. A similar interaction is reported with phenylbutazone with which sulphinpyrazone has a very close chemical relationship. Thus what is known suggests that concurrent use should be monitored and suitable phenytoin dosage reductions made where necessary. The incidence is uncertain, but two out of the five patients studied[1] are reported to have demonstrated this interaction. More study is needed.

References

1 Hansen JM, Busk G, Niemi G, Haase NJ, Lumholtz B, Skovsted L and Kampmann JP. Inhibition of phenytoin metabolism by sulphinpyrazone. In: Turner P and Padgham C (eds). Abstracts of the world conference on clinical pharmacology and therapeutics. London. (Macmillan, London) (1980) Abstract 584.
2 Simonsen K, Busk G, Niemi G, Haase HNJ, Lumholtz B, Skovsted L, Kampmann JP and Hansen JM. Influence of sulphinpyrazone on the metabolism of antipyrine, phenytoin and tolbutamide. Clin Pharmacol Ther (1982) in press. Quoted thus by Pedersen AK, Kacobsen P, Kampmann JP and Hansen JM. Clinical pharmacokinetics and potentially important drug interactions of sulphinpyrazone. Clin Pharmacokinet (1982) 7, 42–56.

Phenytoin + Sulphonamides

Abstract/Summary

Phenytoin serum levels can be raised by the concurrent use of co-trimoxazole, sulphamethizole, sulphamethoxazole, sulphaphenazole and trimethoprim. Phenytoin intoxication may develop. Sulphadimethoxine, sulphamethoxypyridazine, sulphamethoxydiazine and sulphafurazole (sulfisoxazole) are reported not to interact.

Clinical evidence

(a) Phenytoin + co-trimoxazole (sulphamethoxazole + trimethoprim)

A patient on 400 mg phenytoin daily developed intoxication (ataxia, nystagmus, loss of balance) within two weeks of starting to take 960 mg co-trimoxazole twice daily. His serum levels were found to have climbed to 152 μmol/1 (normal range 40–80 μmol/l).[6]

A child developed phenytoin intoxication within 48 h of starting co-trimoxazole. She was also taking sulthiame.[7] A clinical study showed that co-trimoxazole and trimethoprim

can increase the phenytoin half-life by 30 and 51% respectively, and decrease the mean metabolic clearance by 27–30%.[5] Sulphamethoxazole alone had only a small effect.

(b) Phenytoin + sulphamethizole

The development of phenytoin intoxication in a patient given sulphamethizole prompted a study of this interaction in eight patients. After seven days' treatment with sulphamethizole (1 g four times daily) the phenytoin half-life had lengthened from 11.3 to 20.5 h. Three out of four patients showed rises in serum phenytoin levels from 22 to 33, from 19 to 23 and from 4 to 7 μg/ml respectively. The fourth patient was not affected.[1,2]

Another single-dose study showed that the half-life of phenytoin was similarly increased and the mean metabolic clearance reduced by 36%.[5]

(c) Phenytoin + sulphaphenazole or sulphadiazine

After taking 2 g sulphaphenazole (13 patients) or 4 g sulphadiazine (eight patients) daily for a week, the half-life of single IV doses of phenytoin were found to have increased by 237 and 80% respectively. The mean metabolic clearance decreased by 67 and 45% respectively.[5]

(d) Phenytoin + other sulphonamides

Sulphadimethoxine, sulphamethoxypyridazine, sulphamethoxydiazine and sulphafurazole (sulfisoxazole) have been found not to interact with phenytoin significantly.[2,4,7]

Mechanism

The sulphonamides which interact appear to do so by inhibiting the metabolism of the phenytoin by the liver, resulting in its accumulation in the body. This would also seem to be true for trimethoprim.[3]

Importance and management

The documentation seems to be limited to the reports cited, but the interaction is established. Co-trimoxazole, sulphamethizole, sulphadiazine, sulphaphenazole and trimethoprim can increase serum phenytoin levels. It probably occurs in most patients but the small number of adverse reaction reports suggest that the risk of intoxication is small. It is clearly most likely in those with serum phenytoin levels at the top end of the range. If concurrent use is thought appropriate, the serum phenytoin levels should be closely monitored and the phenytoin dosage reduced if necessary. Alternatively use a non-interacting sulphonamide (see (d) above). There seems to be no information about other sulphonamides but it would be prudent to be alert for this interaction if any are given with phenytoin.

References

1 Lumholtz B, Siersbaek-Nielsen K, Skovsted L, Kampmann J and Hansen JM. Sulfamethizole-induced inhibition of diphenylhydantoin, tolbutamide and warfarin metabolism. Clin Pharmacol Ther (1975) 17, 731.

2 Siersbaek-Nielsen K, Hansen M, Skovsted L, Lumholtz B and Kampmann J. Sulphamethizole-induced inhibition of diphenylhydantoin and tolbutamide metabolism in man. Clin Pharmacol Ther (1973) 14, 148.

3 Hansen JM, Siersbaek-Nielsen K, Skovsted L, Kampmann JP and Lumholtz B. Potentiation of warfarin by co-trimoxazole. Br Med J (1975) 1, 684.

4 Hansen JM, Kristensen M, Skovsted L and Christensen LK. Dicoumarol-induced diphenylhydantoin intoxication. Lancet (1966) ii, 265.

5 Hansen JM, Kampmann JP, Siersbaek-Nielsen K, Lumholtz B, Arroe M, Abildgaard U and Skovsted L. The effect of different sulphonamides on phenytoin metabolism in man. Acta Med Scand (1979) Suppl, 264, 106.

6 Wilcox JB. Phenytoin intoxication and co-trimoxazole. NZ Med J (1981) 96, 235–6.

7 Gillman MA and Sandyk R. Phenytoin intoxication and co-trimoxazole. Ann InternMed (1985) 102, 559.

Phenytoin + Sulthiame

Abstract/Summary

Serum phenytoin levels can be approximately doubled by the concurrent use of sulthiame. Phenytoin intoxication may occur unless suitable phenytoin dosage reductions are made.

Clinical evidence

The serum phenytoin levels of six out of seven epileptic patients approximately doubled within 5–25 days of starting to take 400 mg sulthiame daily. All of them experienced an increase in side effects and definite phenytoin intoxication occurred in two of them. Phenytoin serum levels fell once again when the sulthiame was withdrawn.[1]

A number of other reports confirm this interaction,[2–8] some of which describe the development of phenytoin intoxication.

Mechanism

The evidence suggests that sulthiame interferes with the metabolism of the phenytoin by the liver, leading to its accumulation in the body. In one study the phenytoin half-life almost doubled (from 28 to 52 h) during treatment with sulthiame.

Importance and management

A reasonably well-documented, established and clinically important interaction. The incidence seems to be high. If sulthiame is added to established treatment with phenytoin, increases in serum phenytoin levels of up to 75% may be expected.[3,7] Phenytoin serum levels should be closely monitored and appropriate dosage reductions made to prevent the development of intoxication.

References

1 Olesen OV and Jensen ON, Drug-interaction between sulthiame (Ospolot) and phenytoin in the treatment of epilepsy. Dan Med Bull (1969) 16, 154.

2 Houghton GW and Richens A. Inhibition of phenytoin metabolism by sulthiame. Br J Pharmac (1973) 49, 157P.

3 Houghton GW and Richens A. Inhibition of phenytoin metabolism by sulthiame in epileptic patients. Br J clin Pharmac (1974) 1, 59.

4 Richens A and Houghton GW. Phenytoin intoxication caused by sulthiame. Lancet (1973) ii, 1442.

5 Houghton GW and Richens A. Inhibition of phenytoin metabolism by other drugs during epilepsy. Int J Clin Pharmacol (1975) 12, 210.

6 Frantzen E, Hansen JM, Hansen OE and Kristensen M. Phenytoin (Dilantin) intoxication. Acta Neurol Scandinav (1967) 43, 440.

7 Houghton GW and Richens A. Phenytoin intoxication induced by sulthiame in epileptic patients. J Neurol Neurosurg Psychiat (1974) 37, 275.

8 Hansen JM, Kristensen L and Skovsted L. Sulthiame (Ospolot) as inhibitor of diphenylhydantoin metabolism. Epilepsia (1968) 9, 17.

Phenytoin + Terfenadine

Abstract/Summary

Terfenadine does not interact adversely with phenytoin.

Clinical evidence, mechanism, importance and management

A study in 12 epileptic patients on phenytoin showed that single and chronic daily doses of 60 mg terfenadine had no effect on the pharmacokinetics of the phenytoin.[1] No special precautions are needed.

Reference

1 Coniglio AA, Garnett WR, Pellock JH, Tsidonis O, Hepler CD, Serafin R, Small RE, Driscoll SM and Karnes HT. Effect of acute and chronic terfenadine on free and total serum phenytoin concentrations in epileptic patients. Epilepsia (1989) 30, 611–16.

Phenytoin + Theophylline

Abstract/Summary

The serum levels of each drug and their therapeutic effects can be markedly reduced by the presence of the other. Dosage increases may be needed to maintain adequate concentrations. Separating the oral dosage by 1–2 h can minimize the effects of theophylline on phenytoin.

Clinical evidence

(a) Reduced phenytoin serum levels

The seizure frequency of an epileptic woman on phenytoin (400 mg daily) increased when she was given intravenous and later oral theophylline. Her serum phenytoin levels had more than halved (from 15.7 to 5–8 μg/ml). An increase in the phenytoin dosage to 600 mg daily raised her serum phenytoin levels to only 7–11 μg/ml until the drugs were given 1–2 h apart. The patient then developed phenytoin intoxication with a serum level of 33 μg/ml. A subsequent study in four normal subjects confirmed that separating the dosages raised the serum levels of both drugs.[1]

A study on 14 subjects showed that, after two weeks of concurrent use, withdrawal of the theophylline resulted in a 40% rise in the mean serum phenytoin levels of five of the subjects and a mean rise of 30% in the total group.[2]

(b) Reduced theophylline serum levels

The observation that a patient on phenytoin needed an increase in the dosage of theophylline prompted a study in 10 normal subjects. After taking phenytoin for 10 days (serum levels 10–20 μg/ml) the clearance of theophylline was increased by 73%, and both the area under the time-concentration curve and the half-life were reduced about 50%.[3] A study in six normal subjects showed that after taking 300 mg phenytoin daily for three weeks the mean clearance of theophylline was increased by 45% (range 31–65%).[4] Other reports on individual asthmatic patients and normal subjects have shown that phenytoin can cause a two to threefold increase in the clearance of theophylline.[5,6,9,10] Another study found that the effects of phenytoin on theophylline were additive with the effects of smoking.[8]

Mechanisms

(a) Uncertain. The evidence suggests that theophylline inhibits the absorption of phenytoin from the gut. (b) It seems probable that the phenytoin, a known enzyme-inducing agent, increases the metabolism of the theophylline by the liver, thereby hastening its clearance from the body.

Importance and management

These mutual interactions are established and of clinical importance. Patients given both drugs should be monitored to confirm that therapy remains effective. Ideally the serum levels should be measured to confirm that they remain within the therapeutic range. Dosage increases of up to 50% or more may be required.[7] Separating the oral dosages by 1–2 h apparently minimizes the effects of theophylline on phenytoin.

References

1   Fincham RW, Schottelius DD, Wyatt R, Hendeles L and Weinberger M. Phenytoin-theophylline interaction: a case report. In Advances in Epileptology. Xth Epilepsy Int Symp. Wada JA and Perry JK (eds) Raven Press, NY (1980) p 505.
2   Taylor JW, Hendeles L, Weinberger M, Lyon LW, Wyatt R and Riegelman S. The interaction of phenytoin and theophylline. Drug Intell Clin Pharm (1980) 14, 638.
3   Marquis J-F, Carruthers SG, Spense JD, Brownstone YS and Toogood JH. Phenytoin-theophylline interaction. N Engl J Med (1982) 307, 1189–90.
4   Miller M, Cosgriff J, Kwong T and Morken DA. Influence of phenytoin on theophylline clearance. Clin Pharmacol Ther (1984) 35, 656–9.
5   Sklar SJ and Wagner JC. Enhanced theophylline clearance secondary to phenytoin therapy. Drug Intell Clin Pharm (1985) 19, 34–6.
6   Reed RC and Schwartz HJ. Phenytoin-theophylline-quinidine interaction. N Engl J Med (1983) 308, 724–5.
7   Slugg PH and Pippenger CE. Theophylline and its interactions. Cleve Clin Q (1985) 52, 417–24.
8   Crowley JJ, Cusack BJ, Jue SG, Koup JR and Vestal RE. Cigarette smoking and theophylline metabolism: effects of phenytoin. Clin Pharmacol Ther (1987) 42, 334–40.
9   Landsberg K and Shalansky S. Interaction between phenytoin and theophylline. Can J Hosp Pharm (1988) 41, 31–2.
10 Adebayo GI. Interaction between phenytoin and theophylline in healthy volunteers. Clin Exp Pharmacol Physiol (1988) 15, 883–7.

Phenytoin + Tienilic acid (Ticrynafen)

Abstract/Summary

Phenytoin intoxication occurred in two patients when they were additionally treated with tienilic acid.

Clinical evidence, mechanism

An epileptic patient, well controlled on phenobarbitone and phenytoin for six years, developed various adverse effects within three weeks of starting to take tienilic acid (250 mg daily) and, despite a reduction in the phenytoin dosage from 300 mg to 100 mg daily, developed clear signs of phenytoin intoxication a week later. His serum phenytoin levels had increased threefold (to 30.2 μg/ml). Three weeks after stopping the tienilic acid, his serum phenytoin levels had fallen again, and all adverse symptoms had disappeared at the end of a further three weeks.[1] Phenytoin intoxication is described elsewhere in another patient treated with tienilic acid.[2] The mechanism is not understood. Tienilic acid is highly protein bound and may displace phenytoin from its binding sites, but it seems more likely that the interaction results from it inhibition of the metabolism of the phenytoin which allows it to accumulate in the body.

Importance and management

Although information seems to be limited to only two patients, concurrent use should be avoided unless the serum phenytoin levels can be monitored and suitable downward adjustments made if necessary. More study is needed. Tienilic acid has been withdrawn in some countries because it can cause serious liver damage.

References

1   Ahmad S. Ticrynafen-induced phenytoin toxicity: an interaction. J Roy Soc Med (1981) 74, 162.
2   Weber KT and Fisherman AP. In 'A new class of diuretics with uricosuric activity'. Postgrad Med Comm (1979) pp 57–63.

Phenytoin + Trazodone

Abstract/Summary

A single case report describes phenytoin intoxication in a patient when concurrently treated with trazodone.

Clinical evidence, mechanism, importance and management

A patient taking 300 mg phenytoin daily developed signs of phenytoin intoxication after taking 500 mg trazodone daily for six weeks. His serum phenytoin levels had risen from 17.5 to 46 μg/ml.[1] Therapeutic phenytoin serum levels were restored by reducing the phenytoin dosage to 200 mg daily and the trazodone to 400 mg daily. The reasons for this apparent interaction are not understood. Concurrent use need not be avoided but patients should be monitored if given both drugs.

Reference

1 Dorn JM. A case of phenytoin toxicity possibly precipitated by trazodone. J Clin Psychiatry (1986) 47, 89–90.

Phenytoin + Tricyclic antidepressants

Abstract/Summary

Some very limited evidence suggests that imipramine can raise serum phenytoin levels but nortriptyline and amitriptyline appear not to interact. Phenytoin possibly reduces serum desipramine levels. The reduction in the seizure threshold caused by the tricyclic antidepressants should also be borne in mind if concurrent treatment is considered.

Clinical evidence

(a) Serum phenytoin levels increased or unchanged

The serum phenytoin levels of two patients rose over a three-month period when concurrently treated with imipramine, 75 mg daily. One of them showed an increase from 30 to 60 μmol/l and developed mild intoxication. These signs disappeared and the phenytoin serum levels of both patients fell when the imipramine was withdrawn. One of them was also taking nitrazepam and clonazepam, and the other sodium valproate and carbamazepine.[1]

Other studies have shown that nortriptyline, 75 mg daily, had a small but non-significant effect on the serum phenytoin levels of five patients,[2] and that amitriptyline had no effect on the elimination of phenytoin in three subjects.[3]

(b) Serum tricyclic antidepressant levels reduced

A report describes two patients who had low serum desipramine levels, despite taking standard dosages, while concurrently taking phenytoin.[5]

Mechanisms

One suggestion is that imipramine inhibits the metabolism of the phenytoin by the liver which results in its accumulation in the body. The reduced desipramine levels may be a result of enzyme induction by the phenytoin.

Importance and management

The documentation is very limited indeed and none of these interactions is adequately established. The tricyclic antidepressants as a group lower the seizure threshold[4] which raises the question of the advisability of giving them to epileptic patients. If concurrent use is undertaken the effects should be very well monitored.

References

1 Perucca E and Richens A. Interaction between phenytoin and imipramine. Br J clin Pharmac (1977) 4, 485.
2 Houghton GW and Richens A. Inhibition of phenytoin metabolism by other drugs used in epilepsy. Int J clin Pharmacol (1975) 12, 210.
3 Pond SM, Graham GG, Birkett DJ and Wade DN. Effects of tricyclic antidepressants on drug metabolism. Clin Pharmacol Ther (1975) 18, 191.
4 Dallos V and Heathfield K. Iatrogenic epilpesy due to antidepressant drugs. Brit Med J (1969) 4, 80.
5 Fogel BS and Haltzman S. Desipramine and phenytoin: a potential drug interaction of relevance. J Clin Psychiatry (1987) 48, 387–8.

Primidone + Barbiturates

Abstract/Summary

Elevated serum phenobarbitone levels may develop if primidone and phenobarbitone are given concurrently.

Clinical evidence, mechanism, importance and management

Primidone is substantially converted into phenobarbitone within the body. For example, a group of patients taking primidone without phenobarbitone developed serum primidone levels of 9 μg/ml and serum phenobarbitone levels of 31 μg/ml.[1] If phenobarbitone is given at the same time the serum levels may become excessive. This effect may be possibly exacerbated if phenytoin is also being given. If concurrent use is undertaken be particularly alert for any evidence of phenobarbitone intoxication.

Reference

1 Booker HE, Hosokowa K and Burdette RD. A clinical study of serum primidone levels. Epilepsia (1970) 11, 395.

Primidone + Carbamazepine, Clonazepam or Clorazepate

Abstract/Summary

Carbamazepine is reported to reduce, whereas clonazepam is reported to raise serum primidone levels. Clorazepate with primidone may possibly cause personality changes.

Clinical evidence, mechanism, importance and management

An extremely brief report on 155 epileptic children indicated that the serum levels of primidone may be reduced by carbamazepine but no details were given.[1] The same report stated that in children aged 3–15 the concurrent use of clonazepam increased the concentrations of primidone to toxic levels.[1] Another report suggested that the concurrent use of primidone and clorazepate may have been responsible for the development of irritability, aggression and depression in a group of patients.[2] None of these effects appears to be well documented or confirmed but some caution would seem appropriate during concurrent use.

References

1 Windorfer A and Sauer W. Drug interactions during anticonvulsant therapy in childhood: diphenylhydantoin, primidone, phenobarbitone, clonazepam, nitrazepam, carbamazepine and dipropylacetate. Neuropadiatrie (1977) 8, 29.
2 Feldman RG. Clorazepate in temporal lobe epilepsy. J Am Med Ass (1976) 236, 2603.

Primidone + Isoniazid

Abstract/Summary

A single case report describes elevated serum primidone levels and reduced phenobarbitone levels during concurrent treatment with primidone and isoniazid.

Clinical evidence, mechanism, importance and management

A patient on primidone showed raised serum primidone levels and reduced serum phenobarbitone levels due, it was demonstrated, to the concurrent use of isoniazid which inhibited the metabolism of the primidone by the liver. The half-life of primidone rose from 8.7 to 14 h while taking isoniazid and steady-state primidone levels rose by 83%. The importance of this interaction is uncertain but prescribers should be aware that it can occur if concurrent treatment is undertaken.[1]

Reference

1 Sutton G and Kupferberg HJ. Isoniazid as an inhibitor of primidone metabolism. Neurology (1975) 25, 1179.

Primidone + Phenytoin

Abstract/Summary

Serum phenobarbitone levels are increased in patients on primidone when concurrently treated with phenytoin. This is normally an advantageous interaction, but phenobarbitone intoxication occurs occasionally.

Clinical evidence

A study in 44 epileptic patients taking primidone and phenytoin showed that their serum phenobarbitone:primidone ratio was high (4.35) compared with 15 other patients (1.05) who were only taking primidone.[1]

Similar results are described in other studies.[2-4,7,8] A few patients may develop intoxication.[6,7]

Mechanism

Phenytoin increases the metabolic conversion of primidone to phenobarbitone while possibly depressing the subsequent metabolic destruction of the phenobarbitone. The net effect is a rise in phenobarbitone levels.[5]

Importance and management

Well documented. Concurrent use is common. This is normally an advantageous interaction since a metabolic product of primidone is phenobarbitone which is itself an active anticonvulsant. However it should be borne in mind that phenobarbitone serum levels can sometimes reach toxic concentrations,[6] particularly if a quite small dose of phenobarbitone is added.[1]

References

1 Fincham RW, Schottelius DD and Sahs AL. The influence of diphenylhydantoin on primidone metabolism. Arch Neurol (1974) 30, 259.
2 Fincham RW, Schottelius DD and Sahs AL. The influence of diphenylhydantoin on primidone metabolism. Trans Am Neurol Ass (1973) 98, 197.
3 Schmidt D. The effect of phenytoin and ethosuximide on primidone metabolism in patients with epilepsy. J Neurol (1975) 209, 115.
4 Reynolds EH, Fenton G, Fenwick P, Johnson AL and Laundy M. Interaction of phenytoin and primidone. Br Med J (1975) 2, 594.
5 Porro MG, Kupferberg HJ, Porter RJ, Theodore WH and Newmark ME. Phenytoin: an inhibitor and inducer of primidone metabolism in an epileptic patient. Br J clin Pharmac (1982) 14, 294–7.
6 Galdames P, Ortizo M, Saavedra S and Aguilera O. Interaccion fenitoina-primidona: intoxicacion por fenobarbital, en un adulto tratado con ambas drogas. Rev Med Chile (1980) 108, 716.
7 Gallagher BB, Baumel IP, Mattson RH and Woodbury SG. Primidone, diphenylhydantoin and phenobarbital. Aspects of acute and chronic toxicity. Neurology (1973) 23, 145–9.
8 Callaghan N, Feeley M, Duggan F, O'Callaghan M and Seldrup J. The effect of anticonvulsant drugs which induce liver microsomal enzymes on derived and ingested phenobarbitone levels. Acta Neurol Scan (1977) 56, 1–6.

Primidone + Sodium valproate

Abstract/Summary

Serum levels of primidone may be increased or decreased by the concurrent use of sodium valproate. After continued use the interaction may cease to have any effect.

Clinical evidence

(a) Increased serum primidone levels

The serum primidone levels of seven children taking 10–18 mg/kg daily were seen to have risen by a factor of 2–3 when sodium valproate (dosage not stated) was given concurrently. After 1–3 months the effect of the sodium valproate had almost disappeared in three of the patients but persisted in one. The effects on the other three are not recorded.[1]

This interaction is described in other reports: ataxia, drowsiness and marked sedation were seen.[2–5]

(b) Reduced serum primidone levels or no changes

Five patients failed to show any significant changes in serum primidone or phenobarbitone levels when concurrently treated with sodium valproate,[6] whereas another study in two patients found a reduction in serum primidone levels of 24 and 42% respectively when treated with sodium valproate.[7]

Mechanism

Not understood. One suggestion is that the sodium valproate initially slows or blocks the metabolism of the primidone, but later this effect is lost.[1]

Importance and management

There seems to be no consistency about the response of patients to concurrent use. More study is needed. If concurrent use is undertaken, the outcome should be well monitored. Be alert for any signs of primidone intoxication.

References

1 Windorfer A, Sauer W and Gadeke R. Elevation of diphenylhydantoin and primidone serum concentrations by addition of dipropylacetate, a new anticonvulsant drug. Acta Paediatr Scand (1975) 64, 771.
2 Wilder BJ, Willmore LJ, Bruni J and Villarreal HJ. Valproic acid: interaction with other anticonvulsant drugs. Neurology (1978) 28, 892.
3 Haigh D and Fosytahe WI. The treatment of childhood epilepsy with sodium valproate. Dev Med Child Neurol (1975) 17, 743.
4 Richens A and Ahmad S. Controlled trial of sodium valproate in severe epilepsy. Br Med J (1975) 3, 255.
5 Volzke E and Doose H. Dipropylacetate (Depakine, Ergenyl) in the treatment of epilepsy. Epilepsia (1973) 14, 185.
6 Bruni J. Valproic acid and plasma levels of primidone and derived phenobarbital. Can J Neurol Sci (1981) 8, 91.
7 Varma R, Michos GA, Varma RS and Hoshino AY. Clinical trials of Depakene (valproic acid) coadministered with other anticonvulsants in epileptic patients. Res Comm PsycholPsychiat Behav (1980) 5, 265.

Sodium valproate + Antacids

Abstract/Summary

The absorption of sodium valproate is slightly increased by **Maalox** *(aluminium-magnesium hydroxide) but not by magnesium trisilicate or calcium carbonate suspension.*

Clinical evidence, mechanism, importance and management

The area under the time-absorption curve of a single dose of sodium valproate (given 1 h after breakfast) was increased by 12% (range 3–28%) in normal subjects given 62 ml *Maalox* 1 and 3 h after breakfast and at bedtime. Neither magnesium trisilicate suspension (*Trisogel*) nor calcium carbonate suspension (*Titralac*) had a significant effect on absorption.[1] No special precautions would seem necessary during concurrent use.

Reference

1 May CA, Garnett WR, Small RE and Pellock JM. Effects of three antacids on the bioavailability of valproic acid. Clin Pharm (1982) 1, 244–7.

Sodium valproate + Aspirin

Abstract/Summary

Sodium valproate toxicity developed in three patients when given large and repeated doses of aspirin.

Clinical evidence

A girl of 17 taking 21 mg/kg sodium valproate daily was prescribed 18 mg/kg of aspirin daily for lupus arthritis. Within a few days she developed a disabling tremor which disappeared when the aspirin was stopped. Total serum valproate levels were not significantly changed, but the free fraction fell from 24 to 14% when the aspirin was withdrawn. Similar toxic reactions (tremor, nystagmus, drowsiness, ataxia) were seen in two children of six and four given 12–20 mg/kg aspirin four-hourly while taking sodium valproate (25–48 mg/kg daily).[1]

Mechanism

Aspirin displaces sodium valproate from its protein binding sites[2] and also decreases its metabolism by the liver[3] so that the levels of free (and pharmacologically active) sodium valproate rise. This would be expected to increase both the therapeutic and toxic effects of the sodium valproate.

Importance and management

Direct information seems to be limited to the studies cited. It would be prudent to avoid giving repeated doses of aspirin to patients taking sodium valproate, unless the response can be monitored and the dosage adjusted appropriately, but the occasional single dose probably does not matter. More study is needed.

References

1 Goulden KJ, Dooley JM, Camfield PR and Fraser AD. Clinical valproate toxicity induced by acetylsalicylic acid. Neurology (1987) 37, 1392–4.
2 Orr JM, Abbott FS, Farrell K, Ferguson S, Sheppard I and Godolphin W. Interaction between valproic acid in epileptic children: serum protein binding and metabolic effects. Clin Pharmacol Ther (1982) 31, 642–9.
3 Abbott FS, Kassam J, Orr JM and Farrell K. The effect of aspirin on valproic acid metabolism. Clin Pharmacol Ther (1986) 40, 94–100.

Sodium valproate + Benzodiazepines

Abstract/Summary

The concurrent use of sodium valproate and clonazepam may cause an increase in side effects but some patients are benefitted. Diazepam serum levels may be raised by sodium valproate.

Clinical evidence, mechanism, importance and management

A study in epileptic children and adolescents showed that the addition of clonazepam increased the unwanted effects (drowsiness, absence status) in nine out of the 12 patients. The authors suggested that this combination should be avoided.[1] However it has been pointed out in a very brief letter that neither affects the the serum concentrations of the other drug and that '...it would be improper to conclude that clonazepam and valproic acid should never be given together in patients with absence seizures since some patients with refractory absence seizures have an excellent response to this combination of drugs.'[3] Enhanced sedation has been briefly described during the concurrent use of sodium valproate and other unnamed benzodiazepines.[2] Sodium valproate can also increase the serum levels of diazepam but the importance of this is uncertain.[4]

References

1 Jeavons PM, Clark JE and Mahashwari MC. Treatment of generalized epilepsies of childhood and adolescence with sodium valproate ('Epilim'). Dev Med Child Neurol (1977) 19, 9.
2 Volzke E and Doose H. Dipropylacetate (Depakine, Ergenyl) in the treatment of epilepsy. Epilepsia (1973) 14, 185.
3 Browne TR. Interaction between clonazepam and sodium valproate. N Engl J Med (1979) 300, 678.
4 Dhillon SA and Richens A. Valproic acid and diazepam interaction *in vivo*. Br J Clin Pharmacol (1982) 13, 553.

Sodium valproate + Chlorpromazine or Haloperidol

Abstract/Summary

Serum levels of sodium valproate are slightly raised in patients given chlorpromazine, but this appears to be of minimal clinical importance. No interaction occurs between sodium valproate and haloperidol.

Clinical evidence, mechanism, importance and management

A study in six patients on 400 mg sodium valproate showed that while taking 100–300 mg chlorpromazine daily their steady-state trough serum valproate levels were raised by 22%, the half-life increased by 14% and the clearance reduced by 13% (possibly due to some reduction in the metabolism by the liver)[1]. This interaction would seem to be of minimal importance. A parallel study in six other patients given 6–10 mg haloperidol daily showed no significant interaction with sodium valproate[1].

Reference

1 Ishizaki T, Chiba K, Saito M, Kobayashi K and Iizuka R. The effects of neuroleptics (haloperidol and chlorpromazine) on the pharmacokinetics of valproic acid in schizophrenic patients. J Clin Psychopharmacol (1984) 4, 254–61.

Sodium valproate + Cimetidine or Ranitidine

Abstract/Summary

Ranitidine does not interact with sodium valproate, and cimetidine interacts only minimally.

Clinical evidence, mechanism, importance and management

A study in six patients showed that the clearance of sodium valproate was reduced to a small extent (2–17%) in the presence of cimetidine, but not by ranitidine.[1] It seems doubtful if the sodium valproate–cimetidine interaction is of clinical importance.

Reference

1 Webster LK, Mihaly GW, Jones DB, Smallwood RA, Phillips JA and Vajda FJ. Effect of cimetidine and ranitidine on carbamazepine and sodium valproate pharmacokinetics. Eur J Clin Pharmacol (1984) 27, 341–3.

8

ANTIHYPERTENSIVE
DRUG INTERACTIONS

Hypertension (elevated blood pressure) can be controlled by the use of a very wide spectrum of drugs acting either centrally within the brain or peripherally. The drugs dealt with in this chapter include the centrally acting drugs (clonidine, methyldopa), adrenergic neurone blockers (guanethidine), vasodilators (alpha-1 blockers such as prazosin, indoramin and others whose mode of action is uncertain—e.g. hydralazine, diazoxide),

angiotensin-converting enzyme (ACE) inhibitors and diuretics. The beta-blockers, calcium channel blockers, and pargyline (MAOI) are dealt with in separate chapters. Table 8.1 lists the drugs dealt with in this chapter and some of their proprietary names. Where these drugs are the affecting agent rather than the drug affected, the interactions are described elsewhere. The index must be consulted for a full listing of all the interactions.

Table 8.1 Antihypertensive drugs

Non-proprietary names	Proprietary names
ACE inhibitors	
Captopril	*Acepril, Alopresin, Capoten, Captolane, Cesplon, Cor Tensobon, Dilabar, Garranil, Loprin, Lopril, Tensoprel*
Enalapril	*Converten, Enapren, Innovace, Naprilene, Pres, Reniten, Vasotec, Xanef*
Lisinopril	*Carace, Zestril*
Quinapril	
Pentopril	
Ramipril	
Adrenergic neurone blockers	
Bethanidine	*Bendogen, Esbatal, Batel, Benzoxine, Betaling, Eusmanid, Hypersin, Regulin*
Guanadrel	*Hylorel*
Guanethidine	*Ganda, Ismelin(e), Antipres, Dopom, Ipotidina, Normoten, Solo-ethidine, Visutensil*
Guanfacine	*Entulic, Estulic, Tenex*
Guanoclor	*Vatensol*
Guanoxan	*Envacar*
Alpha-blocking agents	
Indoramin	*Baratol, Indorene, Wydora*
Phenoxybenzamine	*Dibenyline, Dibenzyline, Dibenzyran*
Phentolamine	*Rogitine, Regitine,*
Prazosin	*Hypovase, Duramipress, Eurex, Hexapress, Perpress, Pratsiol*
Centrally-acting agents	
Clonidine	*Catapres(s)(an), Clonilou, Clonistada, Drylon, Ipotensium, Tensinova, Tenso-Timelets*
Debrisoquine	*Declinax, Equitonil*
Methyldopa	*Aldomet, Dopamet, Hydromet, Alphamex, Dimal, Elanpres, Equibar, Grospisk, Hyperpax, Hypodopa, Medomet, Medopren, Methoplain, Novomedopa, Sembrina, Sinepress*

259

Table 8.1 *continued*

Non-proprietary names	Proprietary names
Directly-acting vasodilators	
Diazoxide	*Eudemine, Hyperstat, Hypertonalum, Proglicem, Proglycem*
Hydralazine	*Apresolin(e), Alphapress, Aprelazine, Dralzine, Hydrapres, Hyperazin, Hyperex, Hyperphen, Ipolina, Rolazine, Supres, Vasodur*
Minoxidil	*Loniten, Regaine, Alopexil, Alostil, Minodyl, Rogaine*
Diuretics	
Potassium depleters	
Bumetanide	
Ethacrynic acid	
Frusemide (furosemide)	
Thiazides	
Potassium-sparers	
Amiloride	
Spironolactone	
Triamterene	
Rauwolfia alkaloids	
Reserpine	
Serotonin Blockers	
Ketanserin	*Sufrexal*

ACE inhibitors + Allopurinol

Abstract/Summary

Three cases of serious Stevens-Johnson syndrome (one fatal) and another case of hypersensitivity have been attributed to the concurrent use of captopril and allopurinol.

Clinical evidence, mechanism, importance and management

An elderly man with hypertension, chronic renal failure and mild polyarthritis on multiple drug treatment which included captopril (50 mg daily) and diuretics developed fatal Stevens-Johnson syndrome within five weeks of starting to take 200 mg allopurinol daily.[1] Two other patients similarly treated developed the syndrome 3–5 weeks after allopurinol was added to their treatment with captopril.[1] A later report describes fever, arthralgia and myalgia in a man similarly treated. He improved when the captopril was withdrawn.[2] It is not known whether this is an interaction or not because allopurinol alone can cause severe hypersensivity reactions particularly in the presence of renal failure and the use of diuretics. Captopril is also capable of inducing a hypersensitivity reaction. All that can be constructively said at the moment is that patients on both drugs should be very closely monitored for any signs of hypersensitivity and, if necessary, the drugs should be withdrawn at once.

References

1 Pennell DJ, Nunan TO, O'Doherty MJ and Croft DN. Fatal Stevens-Johnson syndrome in a patient on captopril and allopurinol. Lancet (1984) i, 463.
2 Samanta A and Burden AC. Fever, myalgia and arthralgia in a patient on captopril and allopurinol. Lancet (1984) i, 679.

ACE inhibitors + Antacids

Abstract/Summary

An antacid has been found to reduce the absorption of captopril by one-third.

Clinical evidence, mechanism, importance and management

A study in 10 normal subjects showed that when 50 mg captopril was taken with an antacid containing aluminium hydroxide, magnesium carbonate and magnesium hydroxide the bioavailability was reduced by about one-third.[1] The clinical significance of this is uncertain. More study is needed.

Reference

1 Mantyla R, Mannisto PT, Vuorela A, Sundberg S and Ottoila P. Impairment of captopril bioavailability by concomitant food and antacid intake. Int J Clin Pharmacol Ther Toxicol (1984) 22, 626–9.

ACE inhibitors + Azathioprine

Abstract/Summary

The concurrent use of captopril and azathioprine occasionally results in leucopenia.

Clinical evidence, mechanism, importance and management

Both captopril and azathioprine given alone can cause bone marrow depression which results in a fall in the white cell count, and sometimes these effects appear to be additive. A patient whose white cell count fell sharply when treated with captopril and azathioprine together, showed no leucopenia when given each drug separately.[1] Another patient previously treated with azathioprine developed leucopenia when later given captopril.[2] Other patients have similarly shown leucopenia when given both drugs, in one case leucopenia did not develop when he was rechallenged with captopril alone.[3,4] As the development of this interaction is not predictable, it would be prudent to monitor the white cell count during concurrent use.

References

1 Kirchetz EF, Grone HJ, Rieger J, Holscher M and Scheler F. Successful low dose captopril rechallenge following drug induced leucopenia. Lancet (1981) i, 1363.
2 Case DB, Whitman HH, Laragh JH and Spiera H. Successful low dose captopril rechallenge following drug induced leucopenia. Lancet (1981) i, 1362–3.
3 Elijovisch F and Krakoff OR. Captopril associated with granulocytopenia in hypertension after renal transplant. Lancet (1980), i, 927–8.
4 Edwards CRW, Drury P, Penketh A and Damnlinji SA. Successful reintroduction of captopril after neutropenia. Lancet (1981) i, 723.

ACE inhibitors + Diuretics

Abstract/Summary

Captopril combined with diuretics can be safe and effective but (a) a few patients may feel dizzy or lightheaded within an hour of taking the first dose, and acute hypotension can occur. (b) Hyperkalaemia is possible if potassium-sparing diuretics (e.g. amiloride, spironolactone, triamterene) and/or potassium supplements are used. (c) Hypokalaemia may occur if potassium-depleting diuretics (frusemide, ethacrynic acid, etc.) are used. (d) Severe renal deterioration and failure has been seen in patients with renal arterial stenosis.

Clinical evidence, mechanism, importance and management

(a) High doses, hypovolaemia, sodium depletion

Normally concurrent use is safe and effective but hypotensive symptoms such as dizziness and lightheadedness occasionally occur, particularly in those on high diuretic doses, within an hour or so of taking the first dose of captopril. Those most at risk appear to be those patients with hypovolaemia and sodium depletion caused by the use of a diuretic. The effects should be closely monitored. A case of renal failure has been described in a patient with congestive heart failure when treated with captopril and metolazone.[7]

(b) Potassium-sparing diuretics and/or potassium supplements

Five patients on potassium-sparing diuretics (not named) and/or potassium supplements showed a serum potassium level increase from 3.88 to 4.84 mEq/l when concurrently treated with captopril. Serum potassium levels climbed out of the normal clinical range in three of the patients, but no signs or symptoms of hyperkalaemia occurred.[6] Increased serum potassium levels have been seen with captopril alone so it would seem that the effects are additive. Potassium-sparing diuretics such as amiloride, spironolactone or triamterene and/or potassium supplements should not be given with captopril unless the serum potassium levels can be closely monitored. It may be necessary to reduce the dosages or withdraw one of the drugs. However a comparative study has shown that enalapril added to frusemide and amiloride did not affect serum potassium levels, and no differences were seen when compared with patients taking frusemide and amiloride alone.[10]

(c) Potassium-depleting diuretics

Although ACE inhibitors can maintain body potassium, the concurrent use of potassium-depleting diuretics can result in hypokalaemia. A patient with ischaemic heart disease developed hypokalaemia over a two-month period (a fall from 4.9 to 3.4 mmol/l) accompanied by acute pulmonary oedema, ventricular tachycardia and multifocal premature beats when given on captopril, frusemide, amiodarone and isosorbide dinitrate.[9] Another patient on captopril, frusemide, flecainide, digoxin and allopurinol also developed hypokalaemia (a fall from 4.2 to 3.1 mmol/l) and cardiac arrhythmias despite a potassium supplement.[9] The authors of this report advise regular monitoring of the serum potassium levels if congestive heart failure is treated with ACE inhibitors and diuretics of this kind (i.e. frusemide, bumetanide, ethacrynic acid, etc.).

(d) Renal arterial stenosis

Six studies describe renal deterioration or failure (rises in blood urea and serum creatinine levels) in patients with renal arterial stenosis given captopril or enalapril with frusemide, bendrofluazide, hydrochlorothiazide-amiloride, chlorthalidone or spironolactone.[1-5,8] In one study there was evidence that captopril caused no renal deterioration except when combined with the diuretic. Stopping or starting the diuretic initiated or reversed the deterioration. The reasons are not understood.[5] The outcome of using this drug combination should be very closely monitored in patients with renal arterial stenosis. Withdrawal of the diuretic and a reduction in the dosage of the captopril may be needed.

References

1 Curtis JJ, Luke RG, Whelchel JD, Dietheim AG, Jones P and Dunstan HP. Inhibition of angiotensin-converting enzyme in renal transplant recipients with hypertension. N Engl J Med (1983) 308, 377–81.

2 Silas JH, Klenza Z, Solomon SA and Bone MJ. Captopril induced reversible renal failure: a marker of renal stenosis affecting a solitary kidney. Br Med J (1983) 286, 1702–3.

3 Hricik DE, Browning PJ, Kopelman R, Goorno WE, Madia NE and Dzau VJ. Captopril-induced functional renal insufficiency in patients with bilateral renal artery stenosis. N Engl J Med (1983) 308, 373–6.

4 Watson ML, Bell GM, Muir AL, Buist TAS, Kellett RJ and Padfield PL. Captopril/diuretic combinations in severe renovascular disease: a cautionary note. Lancet (1983) ii, 404–5.

5 Hoefnagels WHL, Strijk SP and Thien T. Reversible renal failure following treatment with captopril and diuretics in patients with renovascular hypertension. Neth J Med (1984) 27, 269–74.

6 Burnakis TG and Mioduch HJ. Combined therapy with captopril and potassium supplementation. A potential for hyperkalaemia. Arch Intern Med (1984) 144, 2371–2.

7 Hogg KJ and Hillis WS. Captopril/metolazone induced renal failure. Lancet (1986) i, 501–2.

8 O'Donnell D. Renal failure due to enalapril and captopril in bilateral artery stenosis: greater awareness needed. Med J Aust (1988) 148, 525–7.

9 Begg EJ. Dosing regimens of captopril and enalapril in elderly patients and those with renal insufficiency. NZ Med J (1987) 100, 695.

10 Radley AS and Fitzpatrick RW. An evaluation of the potential interaction between enalapril and amiloride. J Clin Pharmacy Ther (1987) 12, 319–23.

ACE inhibitors + Miscellaneous drugs

Abstract/Summary

No clinically important interactions have been seen between captopril, quinapril or pentopril and cimetidine; between quinapril and propranolol; between captopril and probenecid or procainamide, or between lisinopril and nifedipine.

Clinical evidence, mechanism, importance and management

Cimetidine in normal subjects does not seem to alter the pharmacokinetics or pharmacological effects of captopril,[1] nor the pharmacokinetics of quinapril.[4] Cimetidine can reduce the clearance of pentopril by 11–14% and pentopril can reduce the clearance of cimetidine by 21%,[5] but it seems doubtful if either of these two effects is clinically important. The pharmacokinetics of captopril and procainamide are unaffected by concurrent use.[2] Steady-state levels of captopril are only slightly increased by the use of probenecid and no interaction of clinical importance seems to occur.[3] No evidence of either a pharmacokinetic or pharmacodynamic interaction was seen in 12 normal subjects given single doses of nifedipine (20 mg) and lisinopril (20 mg).[6] 80 mg propranolol three times daily was found not to affect the pharmacokinetics of a single 20 mg dose of quinapril in 10 normal subjects.[7]

References

1 Richer C, Bah M, Cadilhalez C and Giudicelli JF. Cimetidine does not alter free unchanged captopril pharmacokinetics and biological effects in healthy volunteers. J Pharmacol (Paris) (1986) 17, 338–42.

2 Sugerman AA and McKown J. Lack of kinetic interaction of captopril (CP) and procainamide (PA) in healthy subjects. J Clin Pharmacol (1985) 25, 455–74.

3 Singhvi SM, Duchin KL, Willard DA, McKinstry DN and Migdalof BH. Renal handling of captopril: effect of probenecid. Clin Pharmacol Ther (1982) 32, 182–9.

4 Ferry JJ, Cetnarowski AB, Sedman AJ, Thomas RW and Horvath AM. Multiple-dose cimetidine administration does not influence the single-dose pharmacokinetics of quinapril and its active metabolite (CI-928). J Clin Pharmacol (1988) 28, 48–51.

5 Kochak GM, Rakhit A, Thompson TN and Hurley ME. Pentopril-cimetidine interaction caused by a reduction in hepatic blood flow. J Clin Pharmacol (1988) 28, 222–7.

6 Lees KR and Reid JL. Lisinopril and nifedipine: no acute interaction in normotensives. Br J clin Pharmac (1988) 25, 307–13.

7 Horvath AM, Blake DS, Ferry JJ and Colburn WA. Proprandol does not influence quinapril pharmacokinetics in healthy volunteers. J Clin Pharmacol (1987) 27, 719.

ACE inhibitors + Non-steroidal anti-inflammatory drugs

Abstract/Summary

The antihypertensive effects of captopril can be reduced or abolished by indomethacin, ibuprofen and aspirin, whereas sulindac only has a very small effect. Indomethacin only interacts minimally with the blood pressure lowering effects of enalapril and lisinopril.

Clinical evidence

(a) Captopril + aspirin

Eight patients with essential hypertension showed a 20 mm Hg fall in diastolic blood pressure when given a single 25–100 mg dose of captopril. When additionally given aspirin (600 mg every 6 h for 24 h) the diastolic blood pressures of four of the patients rose by an average of 7 mm Hg.[1]

The same interaction has been mentioned in another report.[4]

(b) Captopril + indomethacin or ibuprofen

Five patients with essential hypertension demonstrated a fall in blood pressure from 178/116 to 132/92 mm Hg when treated with 100–200 mg captopril twice daily. The addition of 50 mg indomethacin twice daily caused a blood pressure rise to 144/103 mm Hg.[2] This same interaction has been described in patients with hypertension and in normal subjects given indomethacin in doses ranging from 50 to 250 mg.[3-8] One of these studies found that 50 mg captopril lowered the mean blood pressure of eight normal subjects when lying from 85 to 74 mm Hg. The addition of either 50 mg indomethacin or 800 mg ibuprofen caused the blood pressure to rise to 84 mm Hg.[7]

(c) Captopril + sulindac

In the study detailed above[2] it was also found that 200 mg sulindac twice daily given to patients taking captopril caused only a small rise in blood pressure: from 132/92 to 137/95 mm Hg.[2]

(d) Enalapril, lisinopril, pentopril + indomethacin or sulindac

In a study in 29 patients with essential hypertension given enalapril (40 mg daily) it was found that indomethacin (100 mg daily) caused a small rise in blood pressure (from 134/89 to 143/93 mm Hg) whereas sulindac (400 mg daily) had little or no effect.[9] Another study by the same workers found that indomethacin did not interact significantly with enalapril.[10] In another study it was found to have little effect on the hypotensive effects of lisinopril[11] whereas another study found a small increase in blood pressure.[13] No change in the disposition of pentopril occurs if indomethacin is used, but the effects on blood pressure do not seem to have been assessed.[12]

Mechanism

The antihypertensive effects of some ACE inhibitors can be interfered with by drugs which block prostaglandin synthesis, but where and how is as yet not fully understood.

Importance and management

The captopril–indomethacin interaction is well established. The incidence is reported to be high (nine out of ten in one study[1]). Not enough is known about the captopril–ibuprofen interaction for its incidence to be known, whereas half of the patients showed an effect with aspirin.[1] Occasional doses of aspirin or ibuprofen probably do not matter, but if aspirin, ibuprofen or indomethacin are used regularly the blood pressure should be monitored. Sulindac appears not to interact significantly. It seems possible that this interaction may occur with other NSAID's but information so far is lacking. Information about enalapril is very limited but any interaction with indomethacin seems to be small. Lisinopril is not affected by indomethacin. Information about pentopril is very limited.

References

1 Moore TJ, Crantz FR, Hollenberg NK, Koletsky RJ, Leboff MS, Swartz SL, Levine L, Podolsky S, Dluhy RG and Williams GH. Contribution of prostaglandins to the antihypertensive action of captopril in essential hypertension. Hypertension (1981) 3, 168–73.

2 Salvetti A, Pedrinelli R, Magagna A and Ugenti P. Differential effects of selective and non-selective prostaglandin-synthesis inhibition on the pharmacological responses to captopril in patients with essential hypertension. Clin Sci (1982) 63, 261S–263S.

3 Silberbauer K, Stanek B and Templ H. Acute hypotensive effect of captopril in man modified by prostaglandin synthesis inhibition. Br J Clin Pharmacol (1982) 14, 87–93S.

4 Swartz SL and Williams GH. Angiotensin-converting enzyme inhibition and prostaglandins. Am J Cardiol (1982) 49, 1405–9.

5 Witzgall H, Hirsch F, Schere B and Weber PC. Acute haemodynamic and hormonal effects of captopril are diminished by indomethacin. Clin Sci (1982) 62, 611–5.

6 Dzau VJ, Packer M, Lilly LS, Swartz SL, Hollenberg NK and Williams GH. Prostaglandins in severe congestive heart failure. Relation to activation of the renin-angiotensin system and hyponatremia. N Engl J Med (1984) 310, 347–52.

7 Goldstone R, Martin K, Zipser R and Horton R. Evidence for a dual action of converting enzyme inhibitor on blood pressure in normal man. Prostaglandins (1981) 22, 587–98.
8 Ogihara T, Maruyama A, Hata T, Mikami H, Nakamaru M, Naka T, Ohde H and Kumahara Y. Hormonal responses to long term converting enzyme inhibition in hypertensive patients. Clin Pharmacol Ther (1981) 30, 328–5.
9 Oparil S, Horton R, Wilkins LH, Irvin J, Hammett DK and Dustan HP. Antihypertensive effect of enalapril (MK-421) in low renin essential hypertension: role of vasodilatory prostaglandins. Clin Res (1983) 31, 538A.
10 Oparil S, Horton R, Wilkins LH, Irvin J and Hammett DK. Antihypertensive effect of enalapril in essential hypertension: role of prostacyclin. Am J Med Sci (1987) 294, 395–402.
11 Shae W, Shapiro D, Antonello J, Cressman M, Vlasses P and Oparil S. Indomethacin does not blunt the antihypertensive effect of lisinopril. Clin Pharmacol Ther (1987) 41, 219.
12 Lin S, Rahkit A, Redalieu E, Hurley M, Garg D and Weidler D. Effect of indomethacin on the disposition of pentopril in man. J Clin Pharmacol (1986) 26, 546.
13 Salvetti A, Abdel-Haq B, Magagna A and Pedrinelli R. Indomethacin reduces the antihypertensive action of enalapril. Clin and Exp Theory and Practice (1987) A9 (2 and 3) 559–67.

ACE inhibitors + Other anti-hypertensives

Abstract/Summary, clinical evidence, mechanism, importance and management

There is some evidence that the effects of captopril may be delayed when patients are switched from clonidine.[1] The hypotensive effects of captopril and either minoxidil or sodium nitroprusside appear to be additive and it may be necessary to reduce the dosages to avoid excessive hypotension.[2,3]

References

1 Grone H-J, Kirchertz EJ and Rieger J. Mogliche Komplikationenen und Probleme der Captopriltherapie bei Hypertonikern mit ausgepraten Gefassschaden. Therpiewoche (1981) 31, 5280–7.
2 Jennings GL, Gelman JS, Stockigt JR and Korner PI. Accentuated hypotensive effect of sodium nitroprusside in man after captopril. Clin Sci (1981) 61, 521–6.
3 Traub YM and Levey BA. Combined treatment with minoxidil and captopril in refractory hypertension. Arch Intern Med (1983) 143, 1142–4.

Acetazolamide + Beta-blockers

Abstract/Summary

The concurrent use of acetazolamide and timolol eye-drops resulted in severe mixed acidosis in a patient with chronic obstructive lung disease.

Clinical evidence, mechanism, importance and management

An elderly man with severe chronic obstructive lung disease was given 750 mg acetazolamide daily orally and 0.5% timolol maleate eye-drops, one drop in each eye twice daily, as operative premedication to reduce ocular hypertension before surgery for glaucoma. Five days later a progressive worsening of dyspnoea was seen and he was found to have a severe mixed acidosis.[1] The reason seems to have been the additive effects of acetazolamide which blocked the excretion of hydrogen ions in the kidney, and the bronchoconstrictor effects of the timolol which was sufficiently absorbed systemically to exacerbate the airway obstruction in this patient and thereby reduced the respiration. This isolated case emphasizes the potential risks of using beta-blockers in patients with obstructive lung disease and of concurrent use with acetazolamide even if kidney function is normal.

Reference

1 Boada JE, Estopa R, Izquierdo J, Dorca J and Manresa F. Severe mixed acidosis by combined therapy with acetazolamide and timolol eye drops. Eur J Resp Dis (1986) 68, 226–8.

Amiloride + Cimetidine

Abstract/Summary

Cimetidine does not alter serum amiloride levels or its diuretic effects but amiloride can cause some reduction in the cimetidine levels.

Clinical evidence, mechanism, importance and management

A study in eight normal subjects given 5 mg amiloride daily found that the concurrent use of 400 mg cimetidine twice daily for 12 days reduced the renal clearance of amiloride by 17% (from 358 to 299 ml/min) and the urinary excretion of amiloride from 65 to 53% of the administered dose. The amiloride also reduced the excretion of the cimetidine from 43 to 32% of the dose and the AUC was reduced by 14%.[1] No changes in the diuretic effects (urinary volume, Na+ or K+ excretion) occurred. It seems that each drug reduces the gastrointestinal absorption of the other drug by as yet unidentified mechanisms. The overall serum levels of the amiloride remain unchanged because the reduced absorption is offset by a reduction in its renal excretion.

These mutual interactions seem to be clinically unimportant but confirmation from studies in patients is needed.

Reference

1 Somogyi AA, Hovens CM, Muirhead MR and Bochner F. Renal tubular secretion of amiloride and its inhibition by cimetidine in humans and in an animal model. Drug Metab Disp (1989) 17, 190–6.

Antihypertensives + Alcohol

Abstract/Summary

Chronic moderate to heavy drinking raises the blood pressure and reduces to some extent the effectiveness of antihypertensive drugs. A few patients may experience postural hypotension, dizziness and fainting shortly after having a drink.

Clinical evidence, mechanisms, importance and management

(a) Hypertensive reaction

A study in 44 men with essential hypertension, treated with diuretics, beta-blockers, verapamil, prazosin, captopril or methyldopa and who were moderate to heavy drinkers, showed that when they reduced their drinking over a six-week period from an average of 450 ml ethanol weekly (about six drinks daily) to 64 ml ethanol weekly, their average blood pressure fell by 5.0/3.0 mm Hg.[1] The reasons are uncertain. These findings are consistent with those of other studies.[2,3] It seems likely that this effect will occur with any antihypertensive. Patients with hypertension should be encouraged to reduce their intake of alcohol. It may then become possible to reduce the dosage of the antihypertensive.

(b) Hypotensive reaction

A few patients taking some antihypertensives feel dizzy, begin to 'black out' or faint if they stand up quickly or after exercise. This orthostatic and exertional hypotension may be exaggerated in some patients shortly after drinking alcohol because it causes vasodilatation and can lower the output of the heart (noted in patients with various types of heart disease[4,5,6]). Patients just beginning hypertensive treatment should be warned.

References

1 Puddey IB, Beilin LJ and Vandongen R. Regular alcohol use raises blood pressure in treated hypertensive subjects. A randomized controlled trial. Lancet (1987) i, 647–51.
2 Potter JF and Beevers DG. Pressor effect of alcohol in hypertension. Lancet (1984) i, 119–22.
3 Puddey IB, Beilin LJ, Vandongen R, Rouse IL and Rogers P. Evidence for a direct effect of alcohol on blood pressure in normotensive men—a randomized controlled trial. Hypertension (1985) 7, 707–13.
4 Gould L, Zahir M, DeMartino A and Gomerbrecht RF. Cardiac effects of a cocktail. J Amer Med Ass (1971) 218, 1799.
5 Conway N. Haemodynamic effects of ethyl alcohol in patients with coronary heart disease. Brit Heart J (1968) 30, 638.
6 Noble EP, Parker E, Alkana R, Cohen H and Birch H. Propranolol-ethanol interaction in man. Fed Proc (1973) 32, 724.

Antihypertensives + Bupropion, Mianserin or Maprotiline

Abstract/Summary, Clinical evidence, mechanism, importance and management

Mianserin does not affect the control of blood pressure with propranolol, hydralazine, clonidine, guanethidine, bethanidine[1,2,3,6] or methyldopa.[4,6] Bupropion and maprotiline do not reduce the antihypertensive effects of clonidine.[5,7]

References

1 Burgess CD, Turner P and Wadsworth J. Cardiovascular responses to mianserin hydrochloride: a comparison with tricyclic antidepressant drugs. Br J clin Pharmac (1978) 5, 215.
2 Coppen A, Ghose K, Swade C and Wood K. Effect of mianserin hydrochloride on peripheral uptake mechanisms for noradrenaline and 5-hydroxytryptamine in man. Br J clin Pharmac (1978) 5, 135.
3 Elliott HL, Mc Lean K, Reid JL and Sumner DJ. Pharmacodynamic studies on mianserin and its interaction with clonidine. Br J clin Pharmac (1981) 11, 122P.
4 Elliott HL, Whiting B and Reid JL. Assessment of the interaction between mianserin and centrally-acting antihypertensive drugs. Br J clin Pharmac (1983) 15, 323–8S.
5 Gundert-Remy U, Amann E, Hildbrandt R and Weber E. Lack of interaction between the tetracyclic antidepressant maprotiline and the centrally acting antihypertensive drug clonidine. Eur J Clin Pharmacol (1983) 25, 595–9.
6 Elliot HL, McLean K, Sumner DJ and Reid JL. Absence of effect of mianserin on the actions of clonidine or methyldopa in hypertensive patients. Eur J Clin Pharmacol (1983) 24, 15–19.
7 Cubeddu LX, Cloutier G, Gross K, Grippo PA-CR, Tanner L, Lerea L, Shakarjian M, Knowlton G, Harden TK, Arendshorst W and Rogers JF. Bupropion does not antagonize cardiovascular actions of clonidine in normal subjects and spontaneously hypertensive rats. Clin Pharmacol Ther (1984) 35, 576–84.

Antihypertensives + Fenfluramine

Abstract/Summary

Fenfluramine can cause a small but clinically unimportant increase in the blood pressure lowering effects of antihypertensive agents.

Clinical evidence, mechanism, importance and management

Fenfluramine has some hypotensive activity, but in a number of trials with considerable numbers of obese hypertensive patients given 60 mg fenfluramine daily, the changes in blood pressure in those taking beta-blockers, bethanidine, debrisoquine, guanethidine, methyldopa, reserpine or diuretics were small and, in the context of adverse interactions, of little or no clinical importance.[1–3]

References

1 Waal-Manning J and Simpson FO. Fenfluramine in obese patients on various antihypertensive drugs. Double-blind controlled trial. Lancet (1969) ii, 1392.
2 Simpson FO and Waal-Manning J. Use of fenfluramine in obese

patients on antihypertensive therapy. S Afr Med J (1971) 45 (Suppl), 47.

3 General Practitioner Clinical Trials. Hypotensive effect of fenfluramine in the treatment of obesity. Practitioner (1971) 207, 101.

8 Burch GE, Phillips JH and Wood W. The high-pork diet of the Negro of the Southern United States (Editorial). Arch Intern Med (1957) 100, 859.

9 Burch GE. Pork and hypertension. Am Heart J (1973) 86, 713.

Antihypertensives + Food

Abstract/Summary

The ingestion of food has little or no effect on the absorption of spironolactone, captopril, enalapril or pentopril. Hypertension has been seen in negroes after eating large amounts of pork.

Clinical evidence, mechanism, importance and management

Some early studies suggested that food reduced the bioavailability of captopril and delayed its antihypertensive effects,[1,2] but long-term work has shown that the absorption and bioavailability are not significantly changed.[5,6] Other studies show that food has little or no effect on either enalapril[3] or pentopril.[4] A study in subjects given 100 mg spironolactone showed that food did not affect steady-state levels, blood pressure or heart rate. This supports the recommendation that it should be taken with breakfast to avoid gastric irritation.[7] Studies in negroes in southern USA have shown that those who eat extremely large amounts of pork can experience unpleasant symptoms including dizziness, nausea, vomiting, headache, diarrhoea, blurred vision, fainting, scotoma, lacrimation and general malaise.[8] Two members of one family experienced very marked hypertension and one of them died after eating a considerable amount of pork.[9] Salt pork possibly represents an additional problem. This is not, strictly speaking, an interaction, but rather an undesirable reaction in those under treatment for hypertension or cardiac failure. Whether it is confined to negroes is uncertain. More study is needed.

References

1 Mantyla R, Mannisto PT, Vuorela A, Sundberg S and Ottoila P. Impairment of captopril bioavailability by concomitant food and antacid intake. Int J Clin Pharmacol Ther Toxicol (1984) 22, 626–9.

2 Singhvi SM, McKinstry DN, Shaw JM, Willard DA and Migdalof BH. Effect of food on the bioavailability of captopril in healthy subjects. J Clin Pharmacol (1982) 22, 135–40.

3 Swanson BN, Vlasses PH, Ferguson RK, Bergquist PA, Till AE, Irvin JD and Harris K. Influence of food on the bioavailability of enalapril. J Pharm Sci (1984) 73, 1655–7.

4 Rahkhit A, Hurley ME, Redalieu E, Kochak G, Tipnis V, Coleman J and Rommel A. Effect of food on the bioavailability of pentopril, an angiotensin-converting-enzyme inhibitor, in healthy subjects. J Clin Pharmacol (1985) 25, 424–8.

5 Ohman KP, Kagedal B, Larsson R and Karlberg BE. Pharmacokinetics of captopril and its effect on blood pressure during acute and chronic administration and in relation to food intake. J Cardiovasc Pharmacol (1985) 7, S20–4.

6 Salvetti A, Pedrinelli R, Magagna A, Abdel-Haq B and Graziadei L. Influence of food on acute and chronic effects of captopril in essential hypertensive patients. J Cardiovasc Pharmacol (1985) 7, S25–9.

7 Thulin T, Wahlin-Boll E, Liedholm H, Lindholm L and Melander A. Influence of food intake on antihypertensive drugs: spironolactone. Drug-Nutrient Interactions (1983) 2, 169–73.

Antihypertensives + Phenothiazines

Abstract/Summary

The hypotensive side-effects of the phenothiazines may increase the effects of some antihypertensive agents and patients may feel faint if they stand up quickly. Guanethidine-like drugs are the exception because their effects are opposed by the phenothiazines. An isolated report describes hypertension in a patient given methyldopa and trifluoperazine.

Clinical evidence, mechanism, importance and management

Many of the phenothiazines such as chlorpromazine cause postural hypotension so that patients feel faint and dizzy if they stand up quickly. It is particularly marked with methotrimeprazine. This reaction may be exaggerated in the presence of an antihypertensive agent and may prove to be problematical. For example, one report describes dizziness and hypotension (systolic pressure of 70 mm Hg) in a man a little over an hour after being given 100 mg chlorpromazine, 0.1 mg clonidine and 40 mg frusemide.[2] For this reason the reaction of patients to the use of both types of drug should be monitored, particularly during the first period of treatment. Dosage adjustment may be necessary. There is also an isolated and unexplained case on record of a psychotic patient on fluphenazine decanoate who began to demonstrate delerium, agitation, disorientation, short-term memory loss, confusion and clouded consciousness within 10 days of starting to take 0.2 mg clonidine daily. These symptoms disappeared when the clonidine was stopped and returned when the clonidine was re-started.[3] Guanethidine-like drugs behave differently because their antihypertensive actions can be opposed by the phenothiazines (see 'Guanethidine and related drugs+Phenothiazines'). An isolated report describes a paradoxical rise in blood pressure in a patient with systemic lupus erythematosus and renal disease when treated with methyldopa and trifluoperazine. The suggested explanation is that the phenothiazine blocked the uptake of the 'false transmitter' (alpha-methyl noradrenaline) produced during therapy with methyldopa.[1]

References

1 Westhervelt FB and Atuk NO. Methyldopa-induced hypertension. J Amer Med Ass (1974) 227, 557.

2 Fruncillo RJ, Gibbons WJ, Vlasses PH and Ferguson RK. Severe hypotension associated with concurrent clonidine and antipsychotic medication. Am J Psychiatry (1985) 142, 274.

3 Allen RM and Flemenbaum A. Delirium associated with combined sulphenazine-clonidine therapy. J Clin Psychiatry (1979) 236, 55.

Antihypertensives + Pyrazolone compounds

Abstract/Summary

Phenylbutazone and kebuzone reduce the antihypertensive effects of guanethidine and chlorothiazide. This would be expected to occur with other antihypertensive agents.

Clinical evidence, mechanism, importance and management

15 patients on 75 mg guanethidine daily showed a mean blood pressure rise of 13 mm Hg (from 123 to 136 mm Hg, i.e. diastolic+one-third pulse pressure) when concurrently treated with 750 mg phenylbutazone or kebuzone daily.[1] A similar rise in pressure was seen in 20 other patients taking 50 mg hydrochlorothiazide daily when given phenylbutazone.[1] These rises represent an approximately two-thirds reduction in the antihypertensive effects of guanethidine and hydrochlorothiazide. The mechanism of this interaction is uncertain but it is probably due to salt and water retention by these pyrazolone compounds. Direct evidence of this interaction seems to be limited to this report but it is in line with what is known about these anti-inflammatory compounds. Patients taking any anti-hypertensive agent should be monitored if phenylbutazone, kebuzone or oxyphenbutazone are given concurrently. A number of other NSAID's do not interact like this.

Reference

1 Polak F. Die hemmende Wirkung von Phenylbutazon auf die durch einige Antihypertonika hervorgerufene Blutdrucksenkung bei Hypertonikern. Zsch inn Med (1976) 22, 375.

Antihypertensives + Salbutamol

Abstract/Summary

Severe hypotension attributed to the use of a salbutamol infusion in the presence of methyldopa has been reported.

Clinical evidence, mechanism, importance and management

The manufacturers of salbutamol issued a general warning in 1979 about the concurrent use of salbutamol infusion with either methyldopa or any other drug with an acute hypotensive effect.[1] Three reports had been received of acute hypotension following the use of salbutamol infusion to postpone delivery in premature labour in women already taking 2–2.5 g methyldopa daily for the hypertension of pregnancy.[1] The suggested reason is that it results from peripheral vasodilation due to stimulation of the beta-receptors by the salbutamol. There is as yet nothing to suggest that salbutamol given orally will interact similarly.

Reference

1 Allen and Hanbury Ltd. Letter, 16th February 1979.

Clonidine + Beta-blockers

Abstract/Summary

The combined use of clonidine and the beta-blockers can be therapeutically valuable, but (a) a sharp and serious rise in blood pressure ('rebound hypertension') can follow sudden withdrawal of the clonidine which may be worsened by the presence of a beta-blocker. (b) There are also two reports describing abolition by the beta-blockers of the hypotensive effects of clonidine and even hypertension.

Clinical evidence

(a) Exacerbation of the clonidine-withdrawal hypertensive rebound

A woman with a blood pressure of 180/140 mm Hg was treated with clonidine and timolol. When the clonidine was stopped in error, she developed a violent throbbing headache and became progressively confused, ataxic and semicomatose during which she also had a grand mal convulsion. Her blood pressure was found to have risen to 300 + /185 mm Hg.[3]

Other reports describe similar cases of hypertensive rebound (a sudden and serious rise in blood pressure) within 24 and 72 h of stopping the clonidine, apparently worsened by the presence of propranolol[5–8,10] or timolol.[3] The symptoms resemble those of phaeochromocytoma, and include tremor, apprehension, flushing, nausea, vomiting, severe headache and a serious rise in blood pressure. One patient died from a cerebellar haemorrhage.[8]

(b) Antagonism of the hypotensive effects

When sotalol in daily doses of 160 mg was given to 10 hypertensive patients taking 0.45 mg clonidine daily, the fall in blood pressure caused by the clonidine was abolished in six of the patients. Two of the other patients had blood pressures which were lower than with either drug alone, and the remaining two patients were unresponsive to treatment.[1]

Two cases of hypertension involving clonidine with propranolol have also been described.[2]

Mechanism

The normal additive hypotensive effects of these drugs result from the two acting in concert at different but complementary sites in the cardiovascular system. Just why antagonism sometimes occurs is unexplained. The reliability of one of the reports[1] has been questioned. The marked hypertension (hypertensive rebound) which can occur when clonidine is withdrawn is thought to be due to an increase in the levels of circulating catecholamines. With the beta (vasodilator) effects blocked by a beta-blocker, the alpha (vasoconstrictor) effects of the catecholamines are unopposed and the hypertension is further exaggerated.

Importance and management

Since the 'rebound hypertension' which can follow sudden withdrawal of clonidine can be seriously worsened by a beta-blocker, the beta-blocker should be stopped several days before the clonidine is gradually withdrawn.[4] A successful alternative is to replace the clonidine and the beta-blocker with labetalol[9] which is both an alpha- and a beta-blocker. If this is done, the blood catecholamine levels still rise markedly (20×) and the patient may experience tremor, nausea, apprehension and palpitations, but no serious blood pressure rise or headaches occur.[9] The dosage of labetalol (800–1200 mg) will need to be titrated for the patient, with regular checks on the blood pressure over 2–3 days. In those situations where clonidine is stopped and a hypertensive episode develops, the blood pressure can be controlled with an alpha-blocking agent such as phentolamine (5 mg IV).[5] Diazoxide has also been used.[3,8] Re-introduction of the clonidine, given orally or intravenously, should also stabilize the situation. It is clearly important to emphasize to patients taking clonidine and beta-blockers that they must keep taking their drugs.

What are the advantages and disadvantages of combined treatment? Studies in patients, treated with clonidine and either propranolol[11] or atenolol[12] (non-selective blockers), showed that the hypotensive effects were additive, and smaller doses of clonidine could be used which decreased its troublesome side-effects (sedation and dry mouth). In contrast, with nadolol[12] (cardio-selective) the blood pressure reductions were the same as with either drug alone. The weight of evidence is that adverse reactions (abolition of the blood pressure lowering effects or even hypertension) are rare.[1,2] The authors of one of these reports suggest that clonidine and propranolol should not be used together in cases of refractory hypertension.[2]

References

1 Saarimaa H. Combination of clonidine and sotalol in hypertension. Br Med J (1976) 1, 810.
2 Warren SE, Ebert E, Swerdlin A-H, Steinerger SM and Stone R. Clonidine and propranolol paradoxical hypertension. Arch Intern Med (1979) 139, 252–3.
3 Bailey RR and Neale TJ. Rapid clonidine withdrawal with blood pressure overshoot exaggerated by beta-blockade. Br Med J (1976) 1, 942.
4 Harris AL. Clonidine withdrawal and beta-blockade. Lancet (1976) i, 596.
5 Bruce DL, Croley TF and Less JS. Preoperative clonidine withdrawal syndrome. Anesthesiology (1979) 51, 90–2.
6 Cairns SA and Marshall AJ. Clonidine withdrawal. Lancet (1976) i, 368.
7 Strauss FG, Franklin SS, Lewin AJ and Maxwell MH. Withdrawal of hypertensive therapy (1977) 238, 1734–6.
8 Vernon C and Sakula A. Fatal rebound hypertension after abrupt withdrawal of clonidine and propranolol. Br J Clin Pract (1979) 33, 112.
9 Rosenthal T, Rabinowitz B, Boichis H, Elazar E, Brauner A and Neufeld A. Use of labetalol in hypertensive patients during discontinuation of clonidine therapy. Eur J Clin Pharmacol (1981) 20, 237–40.
10 Reid JL, Wing LMH, Dargie HJ, Hamilton CA, Davies DS and Dollery CT. Clonidine withdrawal in hypertension. Changes in blood pressure and plasma and urinary noradrenaline. Lancet (1977) i, 1171–4.
11 Lilja M, Jounela AJ, Juustila H and Mattila MJ. Interaction of clonidine and beta-blockers. Acta Med Scand (1980) 207, 173–6.
12 Fogari R and Corradi L. Interaction of clonidine and beta blocking agents in the treatment of essential hypertension. In 'Low dose oral and transdermal therapy of hypertension' (Proceedings of Conference 1984), edited by Weber MA, Drayer JIM and Kolloch R. Springer-Verlag, 1985, pp. 118–21.

Clonidine or Apomorphine + Oral contraceptives

Abstract/Summary

The sedative effects of clonidine are increased by the concurrent use of the pill, but those of apomorphine are decreased.

Clinical evidence, mechanism, importance and management

An experimental study[1] on alpha-2-receptors in a group of women showed that the sedative effects of clonidine and of apomorphine were increased and decreased respectively while taking an oral contraceptive (ethinyloestradiol 30 μg, levonorgestrel 150 or 250 μg). The clinical importance of this is uncertain.

Reference

1 Chalmers JS, Fulli-Lemaire I and Cowen PJ. Effects of the contraceptive pill on sedative responses to clonidine and apomorphine in normal women. Psych Med (1985) 15, 363–7.

Clonidine + Prazosin

Abstract/Summary

There is some evidence that prazosin may possibly reduce the antihypertensive effects of clonidine whereas other evidence suggests that this does not occur.

Clinical evidence

A study in 18 patients with essential hypertension showed that the hypotensive effects of an intravenous dose of clonidine were reduced by the presence of prazosin.[1] Other studies failed to find this effect.[2–4] In the presence of prazosin the rebound hypertension following clonidine withdrawal is only moderate (a rise from 145/85 to 169/104 mm Hg).[4] More work is needed to establish what happens with certainty but it seems possible that concurrent use may not always be favourable. Monitor the effects.

References

1 Kapocsi J, Farsang C and Vizi ES. Prazosin partly blocks clonidine-induced hypotension in patients with essential hypertension. Eur J Clin Pharmacol (1987) 32, 331–4.
2 Kuokkanen K and Mattila MJ. Antihypertensive effects of prazosin in combination with methyldopa, clonidine or propranolol. Ann Clin Res (1979) 11, 18–24.

3 Stokes GS, Gain JM, Mahoney JE, Raaftos J and Steward JH. Long term use of prazosin in combination or alone for treating hypertension. Med J Aust (1977) 2 (Suppl) 13–16.
4 Andrejak M, Fievet P, Makdassi R, Conroy E, de Fremont JF, Coevoet B and Fournier A. Lack of antagonism in the antihypertensive effects of clonidine and prazosin in man. Clin Sci (1981) 61, 453–5S.

Clonidine + Rifampicin (Rifampin)

Abstract/Summary

Rifampicin does not interact with clonidine

Clinical evidence, mechanism, importance and management

600 mg rifampicin twice daily for seven days had no effect on the elimination kinetics of clonidine nor on the pulse rates or blood pressures of six normal subjects taking 0.4 mg clonidine daily.[1] No special precautions would seem necessary.

Reference

1 Affrime MB, Lowenthal DT and Rufo M. Failure of rifampicin to induce the metabolism of clonidine in normal volunteers. Drug Intell Clin Pharm (1981) 15, 964–6.

Clonidine + Tricyclic antidepressants

Abstract/Summary

Clomipramine, desipramine and imipramine reduce or abolish the antihypertensive effects of clonidine. Other tricyclics are expected to behave similarly. A hypertensive crisis developed in a woman on clonidine when given imipramine, and severe pain in a man on amitriptyline and diamorphine when given clonidine intrathecally.

Clinical evidence

Four out of five hypertensive patients on 600–1800 ug clonidine daily (with chlorthalidone or hydrochlorothiazide) showed blood pressures rises averaging 22/15 mm Hg when lying and 12/10 mm Hg when standing after taking 75 mg desipramine daily for two weeks.[2]

This interaction has been seen in other patients taking clomipramine, desipramine and imipramine.[1,2,3,10–12] The antihypertensive effects of clonidine were reduced about 50% in six patients given desipramine.[10] A man on 800 μg clonidine daily showed a blood pressure rise from 150/90 to 220/130 mm Hg within four days of starting 75 mg clomipramine daily.[11] An elderly woman on 200 μg clonidine daily developed severe frontal headache, dizziness, chest and neck pain and tachycardia (120 bpm) with hypertension (230/140–130 mm Hg) on the second day of taking 50 mg

imipramine for incontinence.[4] The effects of the withdrawal of clonidine from another elderly patient may also have been made worse by the presence of amitriptyline.[5] In a study in eight normal subjects it was seen that the concurrent use of 75 mg imipramine daily reduced the antihypertensive effects of single 300 μg doses of clonidine by 40–50%.[9] A man with severe pain, well controlled with amitriptyline, sodium valproate and intrathecal boluses of diamorphine, experienced severe pain within 5 min of an intrathecal test dose of 75 μg clonidine.[13]

Mechanism

Not understood. One idea is that the tricyclics block the uptake of clonidine into neurones within the brain.[6] Another is that the tricyclics desensitize alpha-2-receptors.

Importance and management

The clonidine-tricyclics interaction is established and clinically important. The incidence is uncertain but it is not seen in all patients.[2] Avoid concurrent use unless the effects can be monitored. Increasing the dosage of clonidine may possibly be effective. 'Titration' of the clonidine dosage was apparently done successfully in 10 out of 11 hypertensive patients already on amitriptyline or imipramine.[7] Only clomipramine, desipramine and imipramine have been implicated so far, but other tricyclics would be expected to behave similarly (seen in animals with amitriptyline, nortriptyline and protriptyline[8]). Alternative antidepressants which do not interact with clonidine are maprotiline, mianserin and bupropion (see appropriate synopsis).

References

1 Conolly ME, Paterson JW and Dollery CT. In 'Catapres in Hypertension', Conolly ME (ed), Butterworths, London (1969) p 167.
2 Briant RH, Reid JL and Dollery CT. Interaction between clonidine and desipramine in man. Br Med J (1973) 1, 522.
3 Coffler DE. Antipsychotic drug interaction. Drug Intell Clin Pharm (1976) 10, 114.
4 Hui KK. Hypertensive crisis induced by interaction of clonidine with imipramine. J Amer Ger Soc (1983) 31, 164–5.
5 Stiff JL and Harris DB. Clonidine withdrawal complicated by amitriptyline therapy. Anesthesiology (1983) 59, 73–4.
6 van Spanning HW and van Zwieten PA. The interference of tricyclic antidepressants with the central hypotensive effect of clonidine. Eur J Pharmacol (1973) 24, 402.
7 Raftos J, Bauer GE, Lewis RG, Stokes GS, Mitchell AS, Young AA and Maclachalan I. Clonidine in the treatment of severe hypertension. Med J Aust (1973) 1, 786–93.
8 van Zwieten PA. Interaction between centrally active hypotensive drugs and tricyclic antidepressants. Arch Int Pharmacodyn Ther (1975) 214, 12.
9 Cubeddu LX, Cloutier G, Gross K, Grippo PA-CR, Tanner L, Lerea L, Shakarjian M, Knowlton G, Harden TK, Arendshorst W and Rogers JF. Bupropion does not antagonize cardiovascular actions of clonidine in normal subjects and spontaneously hypertensive rats. Clin Pharmacol Ther (1984) 35, 576–84.
10 Checkley SA, Slade AP, Shur E and Dawling S. A pilot study on the mechanism of action of desipramine. Br J Psychol (1981) 138, 248–51.
11 Andrjak M, Fournier A, Hardin JM, Coevoet B, Lambrey G, De Fremont JF and Quichaud J. Suppression de l'effet antihypertenseur de la clonidine par la prise simultanee d'un antidepresseur tricyclique. Nouv Presse med (1977) 6, 2603.
12 Lacomblez L, Warot D, Bouche P, Derousesne C. Suppression de l'effet antihypertenseur de la clonidine par la clomipramine. Rev Med Interne (1988) 9, 291–3.

13 Hardy PA, Wells JC. Pain after spinal intrathecal clonidine. An adverse interaction with tricyclic antidepressants? Anaesthesia (1988) 43, 1026–7.

Diazoxide + Hypoglycaemic agents and Hypotensive agents

Abstract/Summary

(a) Severe hypotension, in some cases fatal, has followed the administration of diazoxide before or after hydralazine. (b) Excessive hyperglycaemia is possible if diazoxide is given with other drugs with hyperglycaemic activity (e.g. the thiazides, chlorpromazine).

Diazoxide has two main effects and two main therapeutic uses: it lowers blood pressure and is used to control severe hypertension, and it raises blood sugar levels and is used for intractable hypoglycaemia. If other drugs are used which either increase or oppose either of these two effects (antihypertensives, diuretics, hypo- or hyperglycaemics) the sum of the responses should be monitored and controlled to ensure that an overall balance is maintained, bearing in mind that some of these other drugs may also have dual activity. The hypotensive and hyperglycaemic effects of diazoxide may represent an unwanted side-effect when the other therapeutic use is being exploited.

(a) Diazoxide + Hydralazine

Clinical evidence

A previously normotensive 25-year old woman had a blood pressure of 250/150 mm Hg during the 34th week of pregnancy which failed to respond to magnesium sulphate given intravenously. It fell transiently to 170/120 mm Hg when given 15 mg hydralazine. One hour later intravenous diazoxide, 5 mg/kg resulted in a blood pressure fall to 60/0 mm Hg. Despite large doses of noradrenaline, the hypotension persisted and the woman died.[1]

Other cases of severe hypotension are described in other studies and reports.[1-8] In some instances the patients had also had other antihypertensive agents such as methyldopa[3,4] or reserpine.[8] At least three of the cases had a fatal outcome.[8]

Mechanism

Not fully understood. The hypotensive effects (vasodilatory) of the two drugs are additive, and it would seem that in some instances the limit of the normal compensatory responses of the cardiovascular system to maintain an adequate blood pressure is reached.

Importance and management

An established, adequately documented and clinically important interaction. Concurrent use should be extremely cautious and thoroughly monitored. The authors of one of the reports cited[1] warn that '…diazoxide should be administered with caution to patients being concurrently treated with other potential vasodilatory or catechol-amine depleting agents.' The concurrent use of diazoxide and beta-blockers seems to be safe and effective (see 'Beta-blockers + Hydralazine').

(b) Diazoxide + Chlorpromazine and Bendrofluazide

Clinical evidence, mechanism, importance and management

An isolated report[8] describes a child on long-term treatment of hypoglycaemia with diazoxide, 8 mg/kg, and bendrofluazide, 1.25 mg daily, who developed a diabetic precoma and severe hyperglycaemia after a single 30 mg dose of chlorpromazine. The reason is not understood but one idea is that all three drugs had additive hyperglycaemic effects. Enhanced hyperglycaemia has been seen in other patients given diazoxide and thiazide diuretics.[9] Caution is clearly needed to ensure that the hyperglycaemic effects do not become excessive.

References

1 Henrich WL, Cronin R, Miller PD and Anderson RJ. Hypotensive sequelae of diazoxide and hydralazine therapy. J Am Med Ass (1977) 237, 264–5.
2 Miller WE, Gifford RW, Humphrey DC and Vidt DG. Management of severe hypertension with intravenous injections of diazoxide. Am J Cardiol (1969) 24, 870–5.
3 Kumar GK, Pastoor FC, Robayo JR and Razzaque MA. Side effects of diazoxide. J Am Med Ass (1973) 225, 275–6.
4 Tansey WA, Williams EG, Landerman RH and Schwartz MJ. Diazoxide. J Am Med Ass (1973) 225, 749.
5 Saker BM, Mathew TH, Eremin J and Kincaid-Smith P. Diazoxide in the treatment of the acute hypertensive emergency. Med J Aust (1968) 1, 592–3.
6 Finnerty FA. Hypertensive encephalopathy. Am J Med (1972) 52, 672–8.
7 Davey M, Moodley J and Soutter P. Adverse effects of a combination of diazoxide and hydralazine therapy. SA Med J (1981) 59, 496.
8 Aynsely-Green A and Illig R. Enhancement by chlorpromazine of hyperglycaemic action of diazoxide. Lancet (1975) ii, 658.
9 Seltzer HS and Allen EW. Hyperglycaemia and inhibition of insulin secretion during administration of diazoxide and trichlormethiazide in man. Diabetes (1969) 18, 19.

Diuretics (Potassium-sparing) + Potassium supplements and Salt substitutes

Abstract/Summary

The concurrent use of potassium-sparing diuretics (spironolactone, triamterene, amiloride) and potassium supplements can result in severe and even life-threatening hyperkalaemia unless the potassium levels are well-monitored and controlled. Potassium-containg salt substitutes can be equally hazardous.

Clinical evidence

One study showed that hyperkalaemia occurred in 5.7% patients on spironolactone alone and 15.4% of those also taking a potassium supplement. The incidence rose to 42% in those on spironolactone with a potassium supplement and who also had azotemia.[1] A retrospective survey of another group of patients given spironolactone and potassium chloride supplements showed that about half of them developed hyperkalaemia.[2] The pacemaker of a patient failed because of hyperkalaemia caused by the concurrent use of *Dyazide* (triamterene + hydrochlorothiazide) and 'Slow-K'.[3] Another patient on spironolactone became hyperkalaemic because he took a potassium-containing salt-substitute ('No Salt')[4] and two other patients on spironolactone became hyperkalaemic and developed heart arrhythmias because they also used a salt substitute.[5]

Mechanism

The effects of these potassium conserving diuretics and the potassium supplements are additive, resulting in hyperkalaemia.

Importance and management

A well-established and well-documented interaction (particularly in the case of spironolactone) of clinical importance. Triamterene and amiloride would be expected to behave similarly. Potassium supplements should not be given to patients on potassium-conserving diuretics except in cases of marked potassium depletion and where the effects can be closely monitored. Patients should also be warned about the risks of using potassium-containing salt substitutes which may increase the potassium intake by 50–60 mEq daily.[5] The signs and symptoms of hyperkalaemia include muscular weakness, fatigue, parasthesia, flaccid paralysis of the extremities, bradycardia, shock and ECG abnormalities which may develop slowly and insidiously.

References

1 Greenblatt DJ and Koch-Weser J. Adverse reactions to spironolactone. A report from the Boston Collaborative Drug Surveillance Program. Clin Pharmacol Ther (1973) 14, 136–7.
2 Simborg DN. Medication prescribing on a university medical service—the incidence of drug combinations with potential adverse interactions. Johns Hopkins Med J (1976) 139, 23.
3 O'Reilly MV, Murnaghan DP and Williams MB. Transvenous pacemaker failure induced by hyperkalemia. J Amer Med Ass (1974) 228, 336–7.
4 McCaughan D. Hazards of non-prescription potassium supplements. Lancet (1984) i, 513–14.
5 Yap V, Patel A and Thomsen J. Hyperkalemia with cardiac arrhythmia. Induction by salt substitutes, spironolactone and azotemia. J Am Med Ass (1976) 236, 2775.

Diuretics + Trimethoprim

Abstract/Summary

Excessively low serum sodium levels have been seen a few patients taking thiazide diuretics when given trimethoprim or co-trimoxazole.

Clinical evidence

A 75-year-old woman with multiple medical conditions and taking methyldopa, thyroxine and *Moduretic* (hydrochlorothiazide + amiloride) experienced nausea and anorexia and was found to have hyponatremia (107 mmol/l) within four days of starting to take trimethoprim. The problem resolved when the *Moduretic* and trimethoprim were stopped and she was later discharged on methyldopa, thyroxine and *Moduretic*. When rechallenged four months later with trimethoprim in the absence of *Moduretic* no hyponatraemia occurred, but it developed rapidly when the *Moduretic* was added.[1] The authors of this report say that they have seen several other patients who developed hyponatraemia within 4–12 days of taking trimethoprim or co-trimoxazole (sulphamethoxazole + trimethoprim), all of whom were elderly and all but one was taking a diuretic.

Two other patients are described in another report who developed hyponatraemia when co-trimoxazole was added to treatment with *Moduret* (hydrochlorothiazide + amiloride) or hydrochlorothiazide/triamterene.[2]

Mechanism

Both the thiazides and trimethoprim can cause sodium loss and in these cases their additive effects were sufficient to cause extreme hyponatraemia.

Importance and management

Information is limited but it would seem prudent to be on the alert for any signs of hyponatremia (nausea, anorexia, etc.) in any patient in this category while taking these drugs.

References

1 Eastall R and Edmonds CJ. Hyponatraemia associated with trimethoprim and a diuretic. Br Med J (1984) 289, 1658–9.
2 Hart TL, Johnston LJ, Edmonds MW and Brownscombe L. Hyponatremia secondary to thiazide–trimethoprim interaction. Can J Hosp Pharm (1989) 42, 243–6.

Frusemide (Furosemide) + Chloral hydrate

Abstract/Summary

The intravenous injection of frusemide after treatment with chloral may cause sweating, hot flushes, a variable blood pressure, tachycardia and uneasiness.

Clinical evidence

Six patients in a coronary care unit given an intravenous bolus of 40–120 mg frusemide and who had had chloral hydrate during the previous 24 h developed sweating, hot flushes, variable blood pressure, tachycardia and uneasiness. The reaction was immediate and lasted about 15 min.[1]

A retrospective study of hospital records revealed that out of 43 patients who had had both drugs, one patient developed this reaction and two others may have done so.[2]

Mechanism

Not understood. One suggestion is that frusemide displaces trichloroacetic acid (the metabolite of chloral) from its protein binding sites, which in its turn displaces thyroxine or alters the serum pH so that the levels of free thyroxine rise. There is as yet no experimental confirmation of this idea.

Importance and management

An established interaction, but information is limited to two reports. The incidence is uncertain but probably low. Concurrent use need not be avoided, but it would be prudent to given intravenous frusemide cautiously if chloral has been given recently. It seems probable that variants of chloral hydrate (dichloralphenazone, petrichloral, chloral betaine) will interact similarly. There is no evidence that frusemide given orally or chloral given to patients already on frusemide initiates this reaction.[2]

References

1 Malach M and Berman N. Furosemide and chloral hydrate. Adverse drug interaction. J Amer Med Ass (1975) 232, 638.
2 Pevonka MP, Yost RL, Marks RG, Howell WS and Steward RB. Interaction of chloral hydrate and furosemide. A controlled retrospective study. Drug Intell Clin Pharm (1977) 11, 332.

Frusemide (Furosemide) + Clofibrate

Abstract/Summary

Additional treatment with clofibrate in patients with nephrotic syndrome already receiving frusemide has led to marked diuresis and muscular symptoms.

Clinical evidence, mechanism, importance and management

Six patients with hypoalbuminaemia and hyperlipoproteinaemia secondary to nephrotic syndrome, receiving 80–500 mg frusemide daily, developed muscle pain, low lumbar backache, stiffness and general malaise with pronounced diuresis within three days of receiving additional treatment with 1–2 g clofibrate daily.[1]

Mechanism

Not understood. The marked diuresis may have been due to competition and displacement of the frusemide by the clofibrate from its plasma protein binding sites. Clofibrate occasionally causes a muscular syndrome which could have been exacerbated by (a) the urinary loss of Na+ and K+ and (b) the increase in the half-life of clofibrate (from 12 to 36 h).

Importance and management

The clinical documentation seems to be limited to this report. The authors of this report suggest that serum proteins and renal function should be checked before giving clofibrate. If serum albumins are low, the total daily dosage of clofibrate should not exceed 0.5 g for each 1 g per 100 ml of the albumin concentration. More study is needed.

Reference

1 Bridgeman JF, Rosen SM and Thorp JM. Complications during clofibrate treatment of nephrotic syndrome hyperlipoproteinaemia. Lancet (1972) ii, 506.

Frusemide (Furosemide) + Food

Abstract/Summary

Food reduces the bioavailability of frusemide and its diuretic effects.

Clinical evidence

10 normal subjects were given 40 mg frusemide at 8.00 am with and without breakfast (milk, roll, cheese, butter, egg). The food reduced the peak serum levels by 55% (from 933 to 423 ng/ml) and the bioavailability was reduced approximately 30%.[1] The results were almost identical in five other subjects given a heavy meal (avacado with cream, fish, potatoes, fruit salad).[1] The diuresis over 10 h was reduced by 21% (from 2072 to 1640 ml) and over 24 h by 15% (from 2668 to 2270 ml).[1] When these figures were compared with urinary output of other subjects who were not given frusemide, the increased amount of urine when the frusemide was given without breakfast was about 600 ml whereas the increase was only 200 ml when given with breakfast, representing an approximately two-thirds reduction.

Another study also found a reduction in the urinary recovery of frusemide.[2]

Mechanism

Not understood.

Importance and management

Information is limited. The authors of the first study cited say that frusemide should not be given with food. A two-thirds reduction is very considerable.

References

1 Beerman B and Midskov C. Reduced bioavailability and effect of furosemide given with food. Eur J Clin Pharmacol (1986) 29, 725–7.
2 Manarlund MM, Paalzow LK and Odlind B. Pharmacokinetics of furosemide in man after intravenous and oral administration. Application of moment analysis. Eur J Clin Pharmacol (1984) 26, 197–207.

Frusemide (Furosemide) or Bumetanide + Indomethacin and other NSAID's

Abstract/Summary

The antihypertensive and diuretic effects of frusemide can be reduced or even abolished by the concurrent use of indomethacin. Diclofenac, diflunisal, flurbiprofen, naproxen, piroxicam and tolfenamic acid also appear to interact similarly although much less information is available. Azapropazone, ibuprofen, pirprofen, mofebutazone, sulindac and tenoxicam may possibly not interact or may do so to a lesser extent. Bumetanide appears to behave like frusemide.

Clinical evidence

(a) Frusemide + azapropazone

10 normal subjects showed no change in their urinary excretion caused by frusemide (40 mg daily) when they were concurrently given azapropazone (1200 mg daily). The frusemide did not antagonize the uricosuric effects of the azapropazone.[21]

(b) Frusemide + diclofenac

A study in patients with heart failure and cirrhosis showed that 150 mg diclofenac daily reduced the frusemide-induced excretion of sodium by 38%, but the excretion of potassium was unaltered.[19]

(c) Frusemide + diflunisal

A study in 12 normal subjects showed that 500 mg diflunisal twice daily interacted with frusemide like indomethacin: sodium excretion was reduced 59% but potassium excretion remained unchanged.[17]

In patients with heart failure and cirrhosis treated with frusemide, 500–700 mg diflunisal daily decreased the sodium excretion by 36% and the potassium excretion by 47%.[19] However another study failed to find an interaction.[22]

(d) Frusemide + flurbiprofen

A study in seven normal subjects showed that the increase in renal osmolal clearance of a standard water load, in response to 40 mg frusemide given orally or intravenously, fell from 105 to 19% and from 140 to 70% respectively following concurrent treatment with 100 mg flurbiprofen.[6]

A single dose study in normal subjects showed that 100 mg flubiprofen reduced by 10% the urinary volume and sodium and potassium excretion following 80 mg frusemide orally.[7]

(e) Frusemide + ibuprofen

An elderly man with cardiac failure treated with digoxin, isosorbide and 80 mg frusemide daily, developed congestive heart failure with ascites when given 1200 mg ibuprofen daily. His serum urea and creatinine levels climbed and no diuresis occurred even when the frusemide dosage was doubled. Two days after withdrawing the ibuprofen, brisk diuresis took place, renal function returned to normal and his condition improved steadily.[5] Another elderly patient similarly showed a poor response to frusemide (and later to metolazone as well) until ibuprofen (600 mg four times daily) and at least two aspirin daily were stopped.[24] This was due to hyponatraemic hypovolaemia.

(f) Frusemide or bumetanide + indomethacin

A study in four normal subjects and six patients with essential hypertension showed that frusemide alone (240 mg daily) reduced the mean blood pressure by 13 mm Hg, but when given with indomethacin (200 mg daily) the blood pressures returned to virtually pretreatment levels. Moreover the normal urinary sodium loss induced by the frusemide was significantly reduced.[1]

A study in normal subjects and patients with congestive heart failure given frusemide showed that 100 mg indomethacin reduced the urinary output by 53% and also reduced the excretion of Na^+, K^+ and Cl^- by 64%, 48% and 62% respectively.[8] Another study found a 20–30% reduction in urinary output.[3] 100 mg indomethacin was also found to reduce the bumetanide-induced output of urine, Na^+ and Cl^- (but not K^+) by about 25%.[10,13] There are other reports confirming the interaction between frusemide or bumetanide and indomethacin, some of which are detailed clinical studies whereas others describe individual patients who have developed cardiac failure as a result of this interaction.[2,11,12,15,16]

(g) Frusemide + mofebutazone

A study in 10 normal subjects showed that 600 mg mofebutazone had no effect on the diuretic effects of 40 mg furosemide. The urinary volume and excretion of sodium, potassium and chloride were unchanged.[18]

(h) Frusemide + naproxen

Two elderly women with congestive heart failure failed to respond to treatment with frusemide and digoxin until the naproxen they were taking was withdrawn.[5]

A single dose study in patients with cardiac failure showed that the volume of urine excreted in response to frusemide was reduced about 50% by naproxen.[3]

(i) Frusemide + piroxicam

A 96-year old woman with congestive heart failure failed to respond adequately to frusemide until the dosage of piroxicam she was taking was reduced from 20 to 10 mg daily.[23]

(j) Frusemide + pirprofen

A study in eight patients showed that 800 mg pirprofen did not significantly affect the diuresis induced by frusemide or the urinary excretion of sodium.[20]

(k) Frusemide or bumetanide + sulindac or tolfenamic acid

A study in eight normal subjects showed that tolfenamic acid (300 mg) reduced the diuretic response (volume, sodium, potassium and chloride) to a single 1 mg dose of bumetanide by 34% at 2 h, whereas the effects of 300 mg sulindac were smaller and not statistically significant.[14]

Another study showed that in patients with cirrhosis and ascites that 150 mg sulindac reduced the diuretic effects (volume, sodium, potassium) of 80 mg frusemide given intravenously by 75%, 84% and 42% respectively.[9]

(l) Frusemide + tenoxicam

A study in 12 patients showed that 20–40 mg tenoxicam daily had no significant effect on the urinary excretion of sodium or chloride due to 40 mg frusemide, and blood pressure, heart rate and body weight also were not affected.[25]

Mechanism

Uncertain and complex. It seems almost certain that a number of different mechanisms come into play. One possible mechanism is concerned with the synthesis of renal prostaglandins which occurs when the loop diuretics cause sodium excretion. If this synthesis is blocked by drugs such as the NSAID's, then both natriuresis and renal blood flow will be altered. Indomethacin is a non-specific inhibitor of cyclo-oxygenase, whereas sulindac selectively inhibits cyclo--oxygenase outside the kidney which might explain why it interacts to a lesser extent.

Importance and management

The frusemide-indomethacin interaction is very well documented and of clinical importance, whereas far less is known about the interactions with other NSAID's. Concurrent use often need not be avoided but the effects should be checked. Patients at greatest risk are likely to be the elderly with cardiac failure and/or renal insufficiency. Some of the data comes from studies in normal subjects rather than patients so that the total picture is still far from clear. Diclofenac, diflunisal, flurbiprofen, naproxen, piroxicam and tolfenamic acid are known to interact in some individuals, but not necessarily to the same extent as indomethacin. If raising the diuretic dosage is ineffective, another NSAID such as azapropazone, ibuprofen, pirprofen, sulindac or tenoxicam may prove not to interact significantly (this is not necessarily true for patients with cirrhosis and ascites[9]). Not every NSAID seems to have been investigated but be alert for this interaction with any of them. Phenylbutazone and oxyphenbutazone would be expected to interact because they cause sodium retention and oedema.

References

1 Patal RV, Moorkerjee BK, Bentzel CJ, Hysert PE, Babej M and Lee JB. Antagonism of the effects of frusemide by indomethacin in normal and hypertensive man. Prostaglandins (1975) 10, 649.
2 Allan SG, Knox J and Kerr F. Interaction between diuretics and indomethacin. Br Med J (1981) 283, 1611.
3 Faunch R. Non-steroidal anti-inflammatory drugs and frusemide-induced diuresis. Br Med J (1981) 283, 988.
4 Aggernaes KH. Indometacinehaemning of bumetaniddiurese. Ugeskr Laeg (1980) 142, 691.
5 Laiwah ACY and Mactier RA. Antagonistic effect of non-steroidal anti-inflammatory drugs on frusemide-induced diuresis in cardiac failure. Br Med J (1981) 283, 714.
6 Rawles JM. Antagonism between non-steroidal anti-inflammatory drugs and diuretics. Scott Med J (1982) 27, 37–40.
7 Symmons D and Kendall MJ. Non-steroidal anti-inflammatory drugs and frusemide-induced diuresis. Br Med J (1981) 283, 989.
8 Sorgel F, Koob R, Gluth WP, Kruger B and Lang E. The interaction of indomethacin and furosemide in patients with congestive heart failure. Clin Pharmacol Ther (1985) 37, 231.
9 Kronborg I, Daskalopuolos D, Katkov W and Zipser RD. The influence of sulindac and indomethacin on renal function and furosemide-induced diuresis in patients with cirrhosis and ascites. Clin Res (1984) 32, 14A.
10 Brater C and Chennavasin P. Indomethacin and the response to bumetanide. Clin Pharmacol Ther (1980) 27, 421–5.
11 Ahmad S. Indomethacin-bumetanide interaction: an alert. Am J Cardiol (1984) 54, 246–7.
12 Poe TE, Scott RB and Keith JF. Interaction of indomethacin with furosemide. J Fam Pract (1983) 16, 610–16.
13 Brater DC, Fox WR and Chennavasin P. Interaction studies with bumetanide and furosemide. Effects of probenecid and of indomethacin on response to bumetanide in man. J Clin Pharmacol (1981) 21, 647–53.
14 Pentikainen PJ, Tokola O and Vapaatalo H. Non-steroidal anti-inflammatory drugs and bumetanide response in man. Comparison of tolfenamic acid and sulindac. Clin Pharmacol Ther (1986) 39, 219.
15 Ritland S. Alvorlig interaksjon mellom indometacin og furosemid. Tidsskr Nor Laegeforen (1983) 103, 2003.
16 Nordrehaug JE. Alvorlig interaksjon mellom indometacin og furosemid. Tisskr Nor Laegeforen (1983) 103, 1680–1.
17 Favre L, Glasson PH, Riondel A and Vallotton MB. Interaction of diuretics and non-steroidal anti-inflammatory drugs in man. Clin Sci (1983) 64, 407–15.
18 Matthei U, Grabensee B and Loew D. The interaction of mofebutazone and furosemide. Curr Med Res Op (1987) 10, 638–44.
19 Jean G, Meregalli G, Vasiloco M, Silvani A, Scapiaticci R, Della Ventura GF, Baiocchi C and Thiella G. Interazioni tra terapia diuretica e farmaci antiinfiammatori nonsteroidei. Clin Ter (1983) 105, 471–5.
20 Sorgel F, Hemmerlein M and Lang E. Wirkung von Pirprofen und Indometacin auf die Effekte von Oxprenolon und Furosemid. Arzneim-Forsch/Drug Res (1984) 34, 1330–2.
21 Williamson PJ, Enen MD and Roberts CJC. A study of the potential interactions between azapropazone and frusemide in man. Br J clin Pharmac (1984) 18, 619–23.
22 Tobert JA, Ostazewski T, Reger B, Mesinger MAP and Cook TJ. Diflunisal-furosemide interaction. Clin Pharmacol Ther (1980) 27, 290.
23 Baker DE. Piroxicam-furosemide interaction. Drug Intell Clin Pharm (1988) 22, 505–6.
24 Goodenough GK and Lutz LJ. Hyponatremic hypervolemia caused by a drug-drug interaction mistaken for syndrome of inappropriate ADH. J Amer Geriatr Soc (1988) 36, 285–6.
25 Hartmann D, Kleinbloesem CH, Lucker PW and Vetter G. Study on the possible interaction between tenoxicam and furosemide. Arzneim-Forsch/Drug Res (1987) 37, 1072–6.

Frusemide (Furosemide) + Phenytoin

Abstract/Summary

The diuretic effects of frusemide can be reduced by as much as 50% if phenytoin is used concurrently.

Clinical evidence

The observation that dependent oedema in a group of epileptics was higher than expected, and the response to diuretic treatment seemed to be reduced, prompted further study. 30 patients taking 200–400 mg phenytoin daily with 60–180 mg phenobarbitone produced a maximal diuresis in reponse to 20 or 40 mg frusemide after 3–4 h instead of the usual 2 h, and the total diuresis was reduced 68 and 51% respectively. When given 20 mg frusemide intravenously the total diuresis was reduced 50%. Some of the patients were also taking carbamazepine, pheneturide, ethosuximide, diazepam or chlordiazepoxide.[1]

Another study in five normal subjects given 300 mg phenytoin daily for 10 days showed that the maximal serum frusemide levels when given 20 mg frusemide, orally or intravenously, were reduced by 50%.[2]

Mechanism

Not fully understood. One suggestion is that the phenytoin causes changes in the jejunal Na^+ pump activity which reduces the absorption of the frusemide, but this is not the whole story because an interaction also occurs when frusemide is given intravenously.[3] Another suggestion is that the phenytoin generates a 'liquid membrane' which blocks the transport of the frusemide to its active site.[4]

Importance and management

Information is limited but the interaction is established. A reduced diuretic response should be expected in the presence of phenytoin and a dosage increase may be needed.

References

1 Ahmad S. Renal insensitivity to frusemide caused by chronic anticonvulsant therapy. Br Med J (1974) 3, 657.
2 Fine A, Henderson JS, Morgan DR and Tilstone WJ. Malabsorption of frusemide caused by phenytoin. Br Med J (1977) 2, 1061.
3 Noach EL, Rees H and de Wolff PA. Effects of diphenylhydantoin (DPH) on absorptive processes in the rat jejunum. Arch Int Pharmacodyn Ther (1973) 206, 392.
4 Srivastava RC, Bhise SB, Sood R and Rao MNA. On the reduced furosemide response in the presence of diphenylhydantoin. Colloids and Surfaces (1986) 19, 83–8.

Frusemide (Furosemide) or Bumetanide + Probenecid

Abstract/Summary

Probenecid can reduce the urinary loss of sodium caused by frusemide but it appears not to affect bumetanide.

Clinical evidence, mechanism, importance and management

(a) Frusemide

Concurrent use has been closely studied to sort out renal pharmacological mechanisms. One study in patients given 40 mg frusemide daily found that the addition of 0.5 g probenecid twice daily for three days reduced their urinary excretion of sodium by almost 40% (from 56.7 to 35.9 mmol daily).[5] Other studies have also found some changes in diuresis (a fall in some studies, a rise in others).[1–4] The clinical importance of these interactions is uncertain.

(b) Bumetanide

A study in eight normal subjects showed that 1 g probenecid did not affect their response to 0.5–1.0 mg bumetanide.[6] Another study reported a fall in natriuresis and in the clearance of bumetanide, but of minimal clinical importance.[7]

References

1 Brater DC. Effects of probenecid on furosemide response. Clin Pharmacol Ther (1978) 24, 548.
2 Homeida M, Roberts C and Branch RA. Influence of probenecid and spironolactone on furosemide kinetics and dynamics in man. Clin Pharmacol Ther (1977) 22, 402.
3 Honari J, Blair AD and Cutler RE. Effects of probenecid on furosemide kinetics and natriuresis in man. Clin Pharmacol Ther (1977) 22, 395.
4 Smith DE, Gee WL, Brater DC, Lin ET and Behet LZ. Preliminary evaluation of furosemide-probenecid interaction in humans. J Pharm Sci (1980) 571–5.
5 Hsieh Y-Y, Hsieh B-S, Lien W-P and Wu T-L. Probenecid interferes with the natriuretic action of furosemide. J Cardiovasc Pharmacol (1987) 10, 530–4.
6 Brater DC and Chennavasin P. Effect of probenecid on response to bumetanide in man. J Clin Pharmacol (1981) 21, 311–15.
7 Lant AF. Effects of bumetanide on cation and anion transport. Postgrad Med J (1975) 51 (Suppl 6) 35.

Guanethidine and related drugs + Haloperidol or Thiothixene

Abstract/Summary

The antihypertensive effects of guanethidine can be reduced by the concurrent use of haloperidol or thiothixene.

Clinical evidence

Three hypertensive patients, controlled on guanethidine (60–150 mg daily) showed a rise in their blood pressures when additionally treated with haloperidol (6–9 mg daily). It rose from 132/95 to 149/99 mm Hg in the first patient; from 125/84 to 148/100 mm Hg in the second; and from 138/91 to 154/100 mm Hg in the third. One of the patients was subsequently tested with 60 mg thiothixene daily and his blood pressure rose from 126/87 to 156/110 mm Hg.[1] These results have been described elsewhere.[2,3]

Mechanism

Haloperidol and thiothixene prevent the entry of guanethidine into the adrenergic neurones of the sympathetic nervous system so that its blood pressure lowering effects are lost. This is essentially the same mechanism of interaction as that seen with the tricyclic antidepressants and chlorpromazine.

Importance and management

Information seems to be limited to this report, but it is supported by the well-documented pharmacology of these drugs. It appears to be clinically important. If haloperidol or thiothixene are given to patients on guanethidine, their blood pressures should be monitored. It has been suggested that the guanethidine dosage may need to be increased.[3] There is no direct evidence of an interaction between guanethidine or related drugs and other butyrophenones or thioxanthenes but it would be prudent to adopt the same precautions. More study is needed.

References

1 Janowsky DS, El-Yousef MK, Davis JM, Fann WE and Oates JA. Guanethidine antagonism by antipsychotic drugs. J Tenn State Med Ass (1972) 65, 620.
2 Davis JM. Psychopharmacology in the aged. Use of psychotropic drugs in geriatric patients. J Geriatric Psychiatry (1974) 7, 145.
3 Janowsky DS, El-Yousef MK, Davis JM and Fann WE. Antagonism of guanethidine by chlorpromazine. Am J Psychiatry (1973) 130, 808.

Guanethidine and related drugs + Indirectly-acting sympathomimetic amines and related drugs

Abstract/Summary

The antihypertensive effects of guanethidine-like drugs (bethanidine, debrisoquine, guanoclor, etc.) can be reduced or abolished by the concurrent use of indirectly-acting sympathomimetics and related drugs which are contained in cough, cold and influenza remedies or are used as appetite suppressants (amphetamines, ephedrine, pseudoephedrine, phenylpropranolamine, mazindol, methylphenidate, etc.). The blood pressure may even rise higher than before treatment with the antihypertensive.

Clinical evidence

When 16 hypertensive patients on 25–35 mg guanethidine daily were additionally given dextroamphetamine (10 mg orally), ephedrine (90 mg orally), methamphetamine (30 mg IM) or methylphenidate (20 mg orally), the effects of the guanethidine were completely abolished and in some instances the blood pressures rose higher than before treatment with the guanethidine.[1]

Other reports describe the same interaction between guanethidine and dextroamphetamine[6] or methamphetamine;[6] bethanidine and phenylpropanolamine[2] or mazindol;[13] bretylium and amphetamine;[3] debrisoquine and mazindol;[14] and an unnamed adrenergic blocker and ephedrine.[4]

Mechanism

Indirectly-acting sympathomimetic amines not only prevent guanethidine-like drugs from entering the adrenergic neurones of the sympathetic nervous system, but they can also displace the antihypertensive drug already there.[10] As a result the blood pressure lowering effects are lost. In addition these amines release noradrenaline from the neurones which raises the blood pressure. Thus the antihypertensive effects are not only opposed, but the pressure may even be raised higher than before treatment.[7–12] Mazindol is related to the tricyclic antidepressants and probably interacts solely by blocking the entry of the guanethidine-like drugs into adrenergic neurones.

Importance and management

Well-documented, well-established and clinically important interactions. Patients taking guanethidine and related drugs (bretylium, bethanidine, debrisoquine, guanoclor, guanacline, guanadrel, etc.) should avoid indirectly-acting sympathomimetics and they should be warned not to use any of the proprietary over-the-counter remedies for coughs, colds and influenza if they contain any of these amines. They may be tempted to do so because nasal stuffiness is a common side-effect of guanethidine and related drugs. The same precautions apply to the drugs with sympathomimetic activity and others which are used as appetite suppressants. However diethylpropion appears not to interact with guanethidine or bethanidine.[15] Not every guanethidine-like antihypertensive-sympathomimetic combination has been investigated in man, but from their well-understood pharmacology they are expected to behave similarly.

References

1 Gulati OD, Dave BT, Gokhale SD and Shah KM. Antagonism of adrenergic neurone blockade in hypertensive subjects. Clin Pharmacol Ther (1966) 7, 510.
2 Misage JR and McDonald RH. Antagonism of hypotensive action of bethanidine by 'common cold' remedy. Br Med J (1970) 2, 347.
3 Wilson R and Long C. Action of bretylium antagonized by amphetamine. Lancet (1960) ii, 262.
4 Starr KJ and Petrie JC. Drug interactions in patients on long-term oral anticoagulant and antihypertensive adrenergic neurone-blocking drugs. Br Med J (1972) 2, 133.
5 Laurence DR and Rosenheim ML. Ciba Foundation Symposium on adrenergic mechanisms. London (1960) p 201.
6 Ober KF and Wang RIH. Drug interactions with guanethidine. Clin Pharmacol Ther (1973) 14, 190.
7 Day MD and Rand MJ. Antagonism of guanethidine and bretylium by various agents. Lancet (1962) i, 1282.
8 Day MD and Rand MJ. Evidence for a competitive antagonism of guanethidine by dexamphetamine. Br J Pharmacol (1963) 20, 17.
9 Day MD. Effect of sympathomimetic amines on the blocking action of guanethidine, bretylium and xylocholine. Br J Pharmacol (1962) 18, 421.
10 Feagin OT, Morgan DH, Oates JA and Shand DG. The mechanism of the reversal of the effect of guanethidine by amphetamines in cat and man. Br J Pharmacol (1970) 39, 253.
11 Starke K. Interactions of guanethidine and indirectly-acting sympathomimetic amines. Arch Int Pharmacodyn Ther (1972) 195, 309.
12 Boura ALA and Green AF. Comparison of bretylium and

guanethidine: tolerance and effects on adrenergic nerve function and responses to sympathomimetic amines. Br J Pharmacol (1962) 19, 31.

13 Boakes AJ. Antagonism of bethanidine by mazindol. Br J clin Pharmacol (1977) 4, 486.

14 Parker J. Wander Pharmaceuticals, England. Personal communication (1976).

15 Seedat YK and Roddy J. Diethylpropion hydrochloride (Tenuate, Dospin) in the treatment of obese hypertensive patients. S Afr med J (1974) 48, 569.

dent to monitor the effects if an MAOI is given to patients on any guanethidine-like drug.

Reference

1 Gulati OD, Dave BT, Gokhale SD and Shah KM. Antagonism of adrenergic neuron blockade in hypertensive subjects. Clin Pharmacol Ther (1966) 7, 510.

Guanethidine and related drugs + Levodopa

Abstract/Summary

When additionally given levodopa it was possible to reduce the dosage of guanethidine in one patient, and another patient was able to stop using a diuretic.

Clinical evidence, mechanism, importance and management

A brief report describes a patient on guanethidine and a diuretic who, when given levodopa (dose not stated but said to be within the ordinary therapeutic range) required a reduction in his daily dose of guanethidine from 60 to 20 mg. Another patient similarly treated was able to discontinue the diuretic.[1] The suggested reason is that the hypotensive side-effects of the levodopa are additive with the effects of the guanethidine. Direct information seems to be limited to this report but it would be a wise precaution to confirm that excessive hypotension does not develop if levodopa is added to treatment with guanethidine or guanethidine-like drugs.

Reference

1 Hunter KR, Stern GM and Laurence DR. Use of levodopa with other drugs. Lancet (1970) ii, 1283.

Guanethidine and related drugs + Monoamine oxidase inhibitors

Abstract/Summary

The antihypertensive effects of guanethidine can be reduced by nialamide

Clinical evidence, mechanism, importance and management

Four out of five hypertensive patients on guanethidine (25–35 mg daily) showed a blood pressure rise from 140/85 to 165/100 mm Hg 6 h after being given a single 50 mg dose of nialamide.[1] The reason is not understood but one idea is that MAOI's possibly oppose the guanethidine-induced loss of noradrenaline from sympathetic neurones. Direct information seems to be limited to this single dose study so that the outcome of long-term use is uncertain, but it would be pru-

Guanethidine and related drugs + Phenothiazines

Abstract/Summary

Large doses of chlorpromazine can reduce or even abolish the antihypertensive effects of guanethidine.

Clinical evidence

Two severely hypertensive patients, well controlled on 80 mg guanethidine daily, were additionally given 200–300 mg chlorpromazine. The diastolic blood pressure of one rose over 10 days from 94 to 112 mm Hg and continued to climb to 116 mm Hg even when the chlorpromazine was withdrawn. The diastolic pressure of the other patient rose from 105 to 127 mm Hg, and then on to 150 mm Hg even after the chlorpromazine had been withdrawn.[1]

Other reports similarly describe a marked rise in blood pressure in patients on guanethidine when given chlorpromazine (100–400 mg daily).[2–4]

Mechanism

Chlorpromazine prevents the entry of guanethidine into the adrenergic neurones of the sympathetic nervous system so that its blood pressure lowering effects are lost. This is essentially the same mechanism of interaction as that seen with the tricyclic antidepressants.

Importance and management

Direct information is very limited but the interaction is established and can be clinically important. It may take several days to develop. Not all patients may react to the same extent.[2,6] Concurrent use should be monitored and the dosage of guanethidine increased if necessary. It is uncertain how much chlorpromazine is needed before a significant effect occurs but the smallest dose of chlorpromazine used in the documented studies was 100 mg with 90 mg guanethidine which raised the blood pressure from 113/82 to 153/105 mm Hg. The inherent hypotensive effects of the chlorpromazine may possibly mask this interaction. Other guanethidine-like antihypertensives (bethanidine, debrisoquine, guanoclor, etc.) would be expected to interact similarly but nobody seems to have checked on the effects of phenothiazines other than chlorpromazine. The effects should be monitored. Molindone is reported not to interact.[5]

References

1 Fann WE, Janowsky DS, Davis JM and Oates JA. Chlorpromazine reversal of the antihypertensive action of guanethidine. Lancet (1971) ii, 436.
2 Janowsky DS, El-Yousef MK, Davis JM, Fann WE and Oates JA. Guanethidine antagonism by antipsychotic drugs. J Tenn State Med Ass (1972) 65, 620.
3 Janowsky DS, El-Yousef MK, Davis JM and Fann WE. Antagonism of guanethidine by chlorpromazine. Am J Psychiatry (1973) 130, 808.
4 Davis JM. Psychopharmacology in the aged. Use of psychotropic drugs in geriatric patients. J Geriatric Psychiatry (1974) 7, 145.
5 Simpson LL. Combined use of molindone and guanethidine in patients with schizophrenia and hypertension. Am J Psychiatry (1979) 136, 1410.
6 Tuck D, Hamberger B and Sjoqvist F. Drug interactions: effect of chlorpromazine on the uptake of monoamines into adrenergic neurones in man. Lancet (1972) ii, 492.

Guanethidine and related drugs + Pizotifen

Abstract/Summary

An isolated report describes the abolition of the antihypertensive effects of debrisoquine by pizotifen.

Clinical evidence, mechanism, importance and management

A man with severe focal glomerulonephritis and hypertension, well controlled on debrisoquine, 30 mg daily, timilol 10 mg and frusemide 40 mg eight-hourly, was additionally given pizotifen (*Sandomigran*) as a prophylactic for migraine. Over the next few weeks his blood pressure climbed from 130/90 to 195/145 mm Hg. It was found impossible to lower the pressure with either diazoxide or prazosin, but within 48 h of withdrawing the pizotifen the pressure had fallen to 105/82 mm Hg and later stabilized at 140/90 mm Hg.[1] The reason is not known but Sandoz, the manufacturers of pizotifen, suggest that as it is structurally similar to the tricyclic antidepressants, it may possibly oppose the actions of debrisoquine in a similar way by blocking the entry of the antihypertensive into the adrenergic neurones of the sympathetic nervous system.[1] Information is limited to this report but it would be wise to check for this interaction in any patient on debrisoquine or any other guanethidine-like hypertensive if pizotifen is given.

Reference

1 Bailey RR. Antagonism of debrisoquine sulphate by pizotifen (*Sandomigran*). NZ Med J (1976) 1, 449.

Guanethidine and related drugs + Tricyclic antidepressants

Abstract/Summary

The antihypertensive effects of guanethidine, bethanidine, bretylium and debrisoquine are reduced or abolished by the concurrent use of tricyclic antidepressants such as amitriptyline, desipramine, imipramine, nortriptyline, protriptyline and others. Doxepin in doses of more than 200–250 mg daily interacts similarly, but in smaller doses appears not to do so.

Clinical evidence

Five hypertensive patients, controlled on 50–150 mg guanethidine daily, showed a blood pressure rise of 27 mm Hg (diastolic pressure + one-third pulse pressure) when given 50–75 mg desipramine or 20 mg proptriptyline daily for 1–9 days. The full antihypertensive effects of the guanethidine were not re-established until five days after the antidepressants were withdrawn.[1]

The same interaction has been described in other reports between guanethidine and desipramine,[2,3] imipramine,[4,5] amitriptyline,[6–8] protriptyline[3] and nortriptyline;[17] between bethanidine and desipramine,[1–3,9] imipramine,[8,10] amitriptyline,[10,20] and nortriptyline;[10,20] and between debrisoquine and desipramine[3] and amitriptyline.[8,10] In some cases it develops rapidly and fully within a few hours and lasts for many days (e.g. two 25 mg doses of imipramine—less than a day's dosage—completely abolished the effects of bethanidine for an entire week[2]), whereas the interaction with guanethidine may take several days to develop fully. Tricyclic antidepressants have also been deliberately used to return the blood pressure to normal in patients taking bretylium, without reducing its antiarrhythmic efficacy.[21]

Mechanism

Before the guanethidine-like drugs can exert their hypotensive actions they must first enter the adrenergic nerve endings associated with blood vessels using the noradrenaline (norepinephrine) uptake mechanism. The tricyclics successfully compete for the same mechanism so that the antihypertensives fail to reach their site of action, and as a result the blood pressure rises once again.[19] The differences in the rate of development, duration and extent of the interactions reflect the differences between the various guanethidine-like drugs and the various tricyclics, as well as individual differences between patients.

Importance and management

A very well-documented and well-established interaction of clinical importance. Not every combination of guanethidine-like drug and tricyclic antidepressant has been studied but all are expected to interact similarly. Concurrent use should be avoided unless the effects are very closely monitored and the interaction balanced by raising the dosage of the antihypertensive. Alternative and probably better solutions are as follows:

(a) Choose a different antidepressant

Maprotiline only appears to interact in a few patients[8,11] but there seems to be no way of predicting the outcome. Doxepin does not interact until doses of about 200–250 mg daily are used, but with 300 mg or more daily it interacts to the same extent as other tricylics.[9,12–16] Mianserin is reported not to interact (see 'Antihypertensives + Bupropion, Mianserin or Maprotiline') and theoretically iprindole should not, but this needs confirmation.

(b) Choose a different antihypertensive

Clonidine should be avoided because it interacts similarly (see 'Clonidine + Tricyclic antidepressants'). Depression is also associated with methyldopa and the rauwolfia alkaloids which makes them unsuitable, but beta-blockers appear not to be affected.[18]

References

1 Mitchell JR, Arias L and Oates JA. Antagonism of the antihypertensive actions of guanethidine sulfate by desipramine hydrochloride. J Am Med Ass (1967) 202, 973.

2 Oates JA, Mitchell JR, Feagin OT, Kaufmann JS and Shand DG. Distribution of guanidium antihypertensives—mechanism of their selective action. Ann NY Acad Sci (1971) 197, 302.

3 Mitchell JR, Cavanaugh JH, Arias L and Oates JA. Guanethidine and related agents. III. Antagonism by drugs which inhibit the norepinephrine pump in man. J Clin Ivest (1970) 49, 1596.

4 Leishmann AWD, Matthews HL and Smith AJ. Antagonism of guanethidine by imipramine. Lancet (1963) i, 112.

5 Boston Collaborative Drug Surveillance Program. Adverse reactions to the tricyclic antidepressant drugs. Lancet (1972) i, 529.

6 Meyer JF, McAllister CK and Godlberg LI. Insidious and prolonged antagonism of guanethidine by amitriptyline. J Am Med Ass (1970) 213, 1487.

7 Ober KF and Wang RIH. Drug interactions with guanethidine. Clin Pharmacol Ther (1973) 14, 190.

8 Smith AZJ and Bant WP. Interactions between post-ganglionic sympathetic blocking drugs and antidepressants. J Int Med Res (1975) 3, (Suppl 2) 55.

9 Oates JA, Fann WE and Cavanaugh JH. Effect of doxepin on the norepinephrine pump. A preliminary report. Psychosomatics (1969) 10 (Suppl), 12.

10 Skinner C, Coull DC and Johnston AW. Antagonism of the hypotensive action of bethanidine and debrisoquine by tricyclic antidepressants. Lancet (1969) ii, 564.

11 Briant RH and George CF. The assessment of potential drug interaction with a new tricyclic antidepressant drug. Br J clin Pharmac (1974) 1, 113.

12 Fann WE, Cavanaugh JH, Kaufmann JS, Griffith JD, Davis JM, Janowsky DS and Oates JA. Doxepin: effects on transport of biogenic amines in man. Psychopharmacologica (1971) 22, 111.

13 Gerson IM, Friedman R and Unterberg H. Non-antagonism of antiadrenergic agents by dibenzoxepine (preliminary report). Dis Nerv Syst (1970) 31, 780.

14 Ayd FI. Long-term administration of doxepin (Sinequan). Dis Nerv Syst (1971) 32, 617.

15 Ayd FJ. Doxepin with other drugs. South med J (1973) 66, 465.

16 Ayd FJ. Maintenance doxepin (Sinequan) therapy for depressive illness. Dis Nerv Syst (1975) 36, 109.

17 Mc Queen EG. New Zealand Committee on Adverse Reactions: Ninth Annual Report 1974. NZ Med J (1974) 2, 305.

18 Cocco G and Ague C. Interactions between cardioactive drugs and antidepressants. Eur J Clin Pharmacol (1977) 11, 389.

19 Cairncross KD. On the peripheral pharmacology of amitriptyline. Arch Int Pharmacodyn (1965) 154, 438.

20 La Corte WStJ, Ryan JR, McMahon FG, Jain AK, Ginzler F, Duncan W and Morley E. Titrating nortriptyline with bethanidine to eliminate the hypotensive effects in normal males. Clin Pharmacol Ther (1982) 31, 241.

21 Woosley RL, Stots B, Keele MD, Roden DM, Nies AM and Oates JA. Pharmacological reversal of hypotensive effect complicating anti-arrhythmic therapy with bretylium. Clin Pharmacol Ther (1982) 32, 313–21.

Guanethidine and related drugs + Tyramine-rich foods

Abstract/Summary

One study found no interaction between debrisoquine and tyramine, but a single case report describes a serious hypertensive reaction in a patient who ate 50 g Gruyére cheese.

Clinical evidence

(a) No interaction

A study in four hypertensive patients taking 40–60 mg debrisoquine daily showed that when they were given oral doses of tyramine in water only a moderate and unimportant increase in their sensitivity occurred. Intestinal MAO-activity remained unchanged.[1]

Hypertensive reaction

A hypertensive woman, treated for a week with doses of debrisoquine progressively increased to 70 mg daily, was given 50 g Gruyere cheese to eat. Within 5 min her blood pressure had risen from 135/85 mm Hg to 170/90 mm Hg, and by the end of an hour it had climbed to 195/165 mn Hg. It fell to 160/95 mm Hg when 2 mg phentolamine was given, but rose again to 200/110 mm Hg during the next hour.[2]

Mechanism

Not understood. Debrisoquine has some MAO-inhibitory activity but (unlike the antidepressant MAO-inhibitors) it appears not to affect the MAO in the gut wall so that tyramine is metabolized normally.[1,3] For a detailed account of the MAO-tyramine interaction see 'Tyramine-rich foods+MAO-Inhibitors'. In the isolated case cited it may have been that the cheese contained particularly large amounts of tyramine which were absorbed through the mucosal lining of the mouth while being chewed. If this is what happened, the tyramine by-passed the gut and liver and was able to release the noradrenaline from the adrenergic sympathetic neurones resulting in a rise in blood pressure.

Importance and management

Information seems to be limited to the reports cited. The absence of other reports of a hypertensive reaction would seem to be a measure of its rarity. Prescribers may feel it prudent to warn their patients about tyramine-rich foods. A list of these is to be found in the synopsis 'Tyramine-rich foods+MAO-Inhibitors'. No interaction would be expected with the other guanethidine-like drugs.

References

1 Pettinger WA, Korn A, Spiegel H, Solomon HM, Pocelinko R and Abrams WB. Debrisoquin, a selective inhibitor of intraneuronal monoamine oxidase in man. Clin Pharmacol Ther (1969) 10, 667.
2 Amery A and Deloof W. Cheese reaction during debrisoquine treatment. Lancet (1970) ii, 613.
3 Pettinger WA and Horst WD. Quantifying metabolic effects of antihypertensive and other drugs at the sympathetic neuron level: clinical and basic correlations. Ann NY Acad Sci (1971) 179, 310.

Hydralazine + Indomethacin or Diclofenac

Abstract/Summary

It is uncertain whether indomethacin does or does not reduce or abolish the hypotensive effects of hydralazine, whereas diclofenac appears to oppose dihydralazine.

Clinical evidence, mechanism, importance and management

One study in normal subjects reported that, after taking 200 mg indomethacin, the hypotensive response to 0.15 mg/kg hydralazine given intravenously was abolished, and the subjects only responded when given another dose 30 min later.[1] In contrast another study, also in normal subjects, reported that 100 mg indomethacin did not affect the hypotensive response to 0.2 mg/kg hydralazine given intravenously.[2] So it is not clear if indomethacin interacts with hydralazine given intravenously, and equally uncertain if an interaction occurs when hydralazine is given orally. On the other hand a study in four hypertensive subjects showed that the actions of dihydralazine (hypotensive, urinary excretion, heart rate, sodium clearance) are reduced by diclofenac.[3] Concurrent use should be monitored.

References

1 Cinquegrani MP and Liang C-s. Indomethacin attenuates the hypotensive action of hydralazine. Clin Pharmacol Ther (1986) 39, 564–70.
2 Jackson SH D and Pickles H. Indomethacin does not attenuate the effects of hydralazine in normal subjects. Eur J Clin Pharmacol (1983) 25, 303–5.
3 Reimann IW, Ratge D, Wisser H and Frohlich JC. Are prostaglandins involved in the antihypertensive effect of dihydralazine? Clin Sci (1981) 61, 319–21S.

Indoramin + Alcohol

Abstract/Summary

The serum levels of both indoramin and alcohol may be raised by concurrent use. The increased drowsiness may possibly increase the risk of driving.

Clinical evidence

A double-blind study in 10 normal subjects given 50 mg indoramin and 0.5 g/kg alcohol in 600 ml alcohol-free lager showed that the AUC (area under the concentration/time curve) of the indoramin was increased by 25% and the peak levels raised by 58%. When given alcohol intravenously (0.175 mg/kg) the indoramin caused a 26% rise in blood alcohol levels during the first hour-and-a-quarter after dosing. Both alcohol and indoramin caused sedation[1,2].

Mechanism

Uncertain. Increased absorption of the indoramin from the gut or reduced liver metabolism may be responsible for the raised indoramin serum levels.

Importance and management

Information is limited but the interactions appear to be established. The clinical importance of the raised serum indoramin and alcohol levels is uncertain, however since indoramin sometimes causes drowsiness when it is first given, there is the possibility that alertness will be reduced which could increase the risks of driving or handling other machinery. Patients should be warned if they drink. More study is needed.

References

1 Abrams SML, Pierce DM, Franklin RA, Johnston A, Marrott PK, Cory EP and Turner P. Effect of ethanol on indoramin pharmacokinetics. Br J clin Pharmac (1984) 18, 294P.
2 Abrams SM, Pierce DM, Johnston A, Hedges A, Franklin RA and Turner P. Pharmacokinetic interaction between indoramin and ethanol. Hum Toxicol (1989) 8, 237–41.

Ketanserin + Beta-blockers

Abstract/Summary

The pharmacokinetics of neither drug appears to be affected by the presence of the other but additive hypotensive effects may occur. Very marked and acute hypotension has been seen in two patients on atenolol when first given ketanserin.

Clinical evidence, mechanism, importance and management

A study in six patients and two normal subjects given ketanserin (40 mg thrice daily for three weeks) showed that the concurrent use of propranolol (80 mg twice daily for six days) did not significantly alter the steady-state serum levels of ketanserin.[1] Another study on normal subjects, using single doses of both drugs, showed that the pharmacokinetics of neither drug was affected by the presence of the other.[3] The hypotensive effects of the ketanserin were slightly increased by the propranolol in the study already cited[1] and additive hypotensive effects were seen in a study in patients with essential hypertension.[2] Acute hypotension is reported to have occurred in two patients taking atenolol within an hour of additionally being given a 40 mg oral dose of ketanserin. One of them briefly lost consciousness.[4] Concurrent use can be valuable and uneventful but a few patients may experience marked hypotensive effects when first given ketanserin. Patients should be warned. Information about other beta-blockers seems not to be available.

References

1 Trenk D, Luh A, Radkow N and Jahnchen E. Lack of effect of propranolol on the steady-state plasma levels of ketanserin. Arzneim-Forsch/Drug Res (1985) 35, 1286–8.
2 Hedner T and Persson B. Antihypertensive properties of ketanserin in combination with beta-adrenergic blocking agents. J Cardiovasc Pharmac (1985) 7 (Suppl 7) S161–3.
3 Williams FM, Leeser JE and Rawlins MD. Pharmacodynamics and pharmacokinetics of single doses of ketanserin and propranolol alone and in combination in healthy volunteers. Br J clin Pharmac (1986) 22, 301–8.
4 Waller PC, Cameron HA and Ramsey LE. Profound hypotension after the first dose of ketanserin. Postgrad Med J (1987) 63, 305–7.

Ketanserin + Diuretics

Abstract/Summary

Sudden deaths, probably from heart rhythm abnormalities, are very markedly increased in patients taking potassium-losing diuretics if they are concurrently treated with ketanserin. Potassium-sparing diuretics do not appear to interact in this way.

Clinical evidence, mechanism, importance and management

A large multi-national study involving 3899 patients showed that a harmful and potentially fatal interaction could occur in those given ketanserin (40 mg three times daily) and potassium-losing diuretics. 35 of 249 patients on both drugs died (16 suddenly) compared with only 15 of 260 (five suddenly) taking a placebo and potassium-losing diuretics. No significant increase in the number of deaths occurred in those on ketanserin and potassium-sparing diuretics. The reason for the deaths seems to be that the ketanserin accentuates and exaggerates the harmful effects of the potassium-losing diuretics on the heart which can worsen arrhythmias. It was found that the corrected QT interval of the heart was prolonged as follows: ketanserin alone (18 ms), ketanserin + potassium-sparing diuretics (24 ms), ketanserin+potassium-losing diuretics (30 ms). In some individuals this can apparently have a fatal outcome.

Potassium-losing diuretics (thiazides, frusemide, etc.) with ketanserin should be avoided but potassium-sparing diuretics (amiloride, triamterene, etc.) seem to be safe.

Reference

1 Prevention of Atherosclerotic Complications with Ketanserin Trial Group. Prevention of atherosclerotic complications: controlled trial of ketanserin. Br Med J (1989) 298, 424–30.

Methyldopa + Barbiturates

Abstract/Summary

The effects of methyldopa are not altered by the use of phenobarbitone.

Clinical evidence, mechanism, importance and management

Indirect evidence from one study in man suggested that phenobarbitone could reduce methyldopa levels,[1] but later work which directly measured the blood levels of methyldopa failed to find any evidence of an interaction.[2]

References

1 Kaldor A, Juvancz P, Demeczky M, Sebestynen and Palotas J. Enhancement of methyldopa metabolism with barbiturate. Br Med J (1971) 3, 518.
2 Kristensen M, Jorgensen M and Hansen T. Plasma concentration of alphamethyldopa and its main metabolite, methyldopa-O-sulphate, during long term treatment with alphamethyldopa with special reference to possible interaction with other drugs given simultaneously. Clin Pharmacol Ther (1973) 14, 139.

Methyldopa + Cephalosporins

Abstract/Summary

Two reports describe the development of pustular eruptions in two women taking methyldopa when they were given cephradine or cefazolin.

Clinical evidence, mechanism, importance and management

A black woman aged 74 on methyldopa and insulin developed pruritis on her arms and legs within 2 h of starting to take cephradine. Over the next two days fever and a widespread pustular eruption developed.[1] Another black woman of 65 on methyldopa and frusemide experienced severe pruritis within 8 h of starting to take 1 g cefazolin sodium every 12 h. Over the next two days superficial and coalescing pustules appeared on her trunk, arms and legs.[2] The reasons are not understood. There seem to be no other reports of this reaction. The concurrent use of methyldopa may possibly have been purely coincidental.

References

1 Kalb RE and Grossman ME. Pustular eruption following administration of cephradine. Cutis (1986) 38, 58–60.
2 Stough D, Guin JD, Baker GF and Haynie L. Pustular eruptions following administration of cefazolin: a possible interaction with methyldopa. J Amer Acad Dermatol (1987) 16, 1051–2.

Methyldopa + Disulfiram

Abstract/Summary

An isolated report describes a patient whose hypertension failed to respond to methyldopa in the presence of disulfiram.

Clinical evidence, mechanism, importance and management

The hypertension of an alcoholic patient on disulfiram failed to respond to moderate to high doses of intravenous methyldopa, but did so when given oral low dose clonidine. The postulated reason is that disulfiram blocks the activity of dopamine beta-hydroxylase, the enzyme responsible for the conversion of the methyldopa to its active form.[1] The general importance of this alleged interaction is uncertain.

Reference

1 McCord RW and LaCorte WS. Hypertension refactory to methyldopa in a disulfiram-treated patient. Clin Res (1984) 32, 923A.

Methyldopa + Haloperidol

Abstract/Summary

Three cases of dementia have been attributed to the use of methyldopa and haloperidol, but concurrent use without serious problems has also been described.

Clinical evidence.

Two patients on long term treatment with methyldopa (1–1.5 g daily) without problems developed a dementia syndrome (mental retardation, loss of memory, disorientation, etc.) within three days of starting to take 6–8 mg haloperidol daily. The symptoms cleared within 72 h of withdrawing the haloperidol.[1]

Another patient treated with these drugs showed severe irritability and aggressive behaviour.[3]

Mechanism

Not understood. Among the side-effects of methyldopa relevant to this interaction are sedation, depression and dementia; and of haloperidol, drowsiness, dizziness and depression.

Importance and management

These three cases must be viewed alongside another report of a four-week trial in 10 schizophrenics given 500 mg methyldopa and 10 mg haloperidol daily. Among the important side-effects were somnolence (eight patients) and dizziness (six patients) but no serious interaction of the kind described above.[2] Concurrent use need not be avoided but it would be prudent to be on the alert for the development of adverse effects.

References

1 Thornton WE. Dementia induced by methyldopa with haloperidol. N Engl J Med (1976) 243, 1222.
2 Chouinard G, Pinard G, Serrano M and Tetreault L. Potentiation of haloperidol by alpha-methyldopa in the treatment of schizophrenic patients. Curr Ther Res (1973) 15, 473.
3 Nadel I and Wallach M. Drug interaction between haloperidol and methyldopa. Br J Psychiatry (1979) 135, 484.

Methyldopa + Iron salts

Abstract/Summary

The antihypertensive effects of methyldopa can be reduced by the concurrent use of ferrous sulphate. Ferrous gluconate appears to interact similarly.

Clinical evidence

Arising out of a metabolic study of the interaction between methyldopa and ferrous sulphate, five hypertensive patients who had been taking 500–1500 mg methyldopa daily for more than a year were additionally given 325 mg ferrous sulphate three times daily. After two weeks the blood pressures of all of them had risen. The systolic pressures of three of them had risen by more than 15 mm Hg. Four had diastolic pressure rises, two of them exceeding 10 mm Hg.[1]

Mechanism

Uncertain. One suggestion is that the iron chelates with the methyldopa in the gut, thereby reducing its absorption (reduced 50%).[1] The increase in the metabolic sulphonation of the methyldopa also seems to have had a part to play.

Importance and management

Information seems to be limited to this report so that this interaction is as yet unconfirmed and its clinical importance is uncertain. Monitor the effects of concurrent use and increase the methyldopa dosage if necessary. Ferrous gluconate appears to interact like ferrous sulphate.

Reference

1 Campbell N, Paddock V and Sundaram R. Alteration of methyldopa absorption, metabolism, and blood pressure control caused by ferrous sulphate and ferrous gluconate. Clin Pharmacol Ther (1988) 43, 381–6.

Methyldopa + Phenoxybenzamine

Abstract/Summary

An isolated case report describes total urinary incontinence in a patient treated with methyldopa and phenoxybenzamine after bilateral lumbar sympathectomy.

Clinical evidence, mechanism, importance and management

A woman who had previously had bilateral lumbar sympathectomy for Reynauds disease developed total urinary incontinence when given 500–1500 mg methyldopa and 12.5 mg phenoxybenzamine daily, but not with either drug alone. This would seem to be the outcome of the additive effects of the sympathectomy and the two drugs on the sympathetic control of the bladder sphincters.[1] Stress incontinence has previously been described with these drugs. The general importance of this interaction is probably small.

Reference

1 Fernandez PG, Shani S, Galway BA, Granter S and McDonald J. Urinary incontinence due to interaction of phenoxybenzamine and alpha-methyldopa. Can Med Ass J (1981) 124, 174.

Methyldopa + Tricyclic antidepressants

Abstract/Summary

The antihypertensive effects of methyldopa are not normally adversely affected by the concurrent use of desipramine but an isolated report describes hypertension, tachycardia, tremor and agitation in man on methyldopa when additionally treated with amitriptyline.

Clinical evidence

A hypertensive man, controlled on 700 mg methyldopa daily with a diuretic, experienced tremor, agitation, tachycardia (148 beats/min) and hypertension (a rise from 120–150/80–90 mm Hg to 170/110 mm Hg) within 10 days of starting to take 75 mg amitriptyline daily. A week after stopping the amitriptyline his pulse rate was 100 and his blood pressure 160/90 mm Hg.[1] In contrast, a double-blind cross-over study in five volunteers (one with mild hypertension) showed that 75 mg desipramine daily for three days had no significant effect on the hypotensive effects of single 750 mg doses of methyldopa.[5] Another study in three hypertensive patients on methyldopa (2.5–3.0 g daily) showed that when given 75 mg desipramine daily for 5–6 days, the blood pressure (diastolic + one-third pulse pressure) fell by five mm Hg.[2]

Mechanism

Not understood. Antagonism of the antihypertensive actions of methyldopa by tricyclic antidepressants is seen in animals and it seems to occur within the brain, possibly within the rhombencephalon.[3,4]

Importance and management

Normally no adverse interaction occurs, nevertheless it would seem prudent to monitor the effects of concurrent use if amitriptyline or any other tricyclic antidepressant is given to patients taking methyldopa. Methyldopa sometimes induces depression so that it may not be the best choice of antihypertensive in depressed patients.

References

1 White AG. Methyldopa and amitriptyline. Lancet (1965) ii, 441.
2 Mitchell JR, Cavanaugh JH, Arias L and Oates JA. Guanethidine and related agents. III. Antagonism by drugs which inhibit the norepinephrine pump in man. J Clin Invest (1970) 49, 1596.
3 Van Spanning HW and van Zwieten PA. The interaction between alpha-methyldopa and tricyclic antidepressants. Int J Clin Pharmacol (1975) 11, 65.
4 Van Zwieten PA. Interaction between centrally acting hypotensive drugs and tricyclic antidepressants. Arch Int Pharmacodyn Ther (1975) 214, 12.
5 Reid JL, Porsius AJ, Zambulis C, Polak G, Hamilton CA and Dean CR. The effects of desmethylimipramine on the pharmacological actions of alpha-methyldopa in man. Eur J Clin Pharmacol (1979) 16, 75.

Prazosin + Beta-blockers

Abstract/Summary

Prazosin causes some patients to faint when they first start treatment, and it is more likely to occur if the patient is already taking a beta-blocker.

Clinical evidence. mechanism, importance and management

Some patients experience acute postural hypotension, tachycardia and palpitations when they begin to take prazosin, and a few even collapse in a sudden faint. It usually happens within 30–90 min of the first dose. This can be exacerbated if they are already taking beta-blockers. Three out of six hypertensive patients taking 0.8 mg alprenolol daily experienced this 'first dose' hypotensive reaction when given 0.5 mg prazosin. Other patients already taking prazosin showed no unusual fall in blood pressure when given the first of several doses of alprenolol.[1] The severity and the duration of this first dose response was also found to be increased in normal subjects taking propranolol or primidolol when they were given prazosin.[2] The pharmacokinetics of prazosin are not affected by either atenolol[1] or propranolol.[3]

Just why this adverse reaction occurs is not clear, but it seems to be related to an impaired venous return associated with the dilatation of the arterioles and venules, and some factor which causes heart slowing. The normal cardiovascular responses which follow a sudden fall in blood pressure are apparently compromised by the presence of a beta-blocker. The problem is usually only short-lasting because within hours or days some physiological compensation occurs which allows the blood pressure to be lowered without falling precipitously.

Concurrent use need not be avoided, but it has been recommended that patients already taking beta-blockers should start on a dose of prazosin which is less than 0.5 mg.[1] They should also be told what may happen and what to do. Giving the first dose at bedtime seems sensible. No particular precautions seem necessary in patients already taking prazosin who are additionally given beta-blockers.

References.

1 Seideman P, Grahnen A, Haglund K, Lindstrom B and von Bah C. Prazosin first dose phenomenon during combined treatment with a beta-adrenoceptor in hypertensive patients. Br J clin Pharmacol (1982) 13, 865–70.
2 Elliott HL, McLean K, Sumner DJ, Meredith PA and Reid JL. Immediate cardiovascular reponses to oral prazosin—effects of beta-blockers. Clin Pharmacol Ther (1981) 29, 303–9.
3 Rubin P, Jackson G and Blaschke T. Studies on the clinical pharmacology of prazosin. II: The influence of indomethacin and of propranolol on the action and the disposition of prazosin. Br J clin Pharmacol (1980) 10, 33–9.

Prazosin + Calcium channel blockers

Abstract/Summary

The blood pressure may fall sharply if calcium channel blockers are given to patients already taking prazosin. Only administer together if the response can be closely monitored.

Clinical evidence

(a) Prazosin + nifedipine

Two patients with severe hypertension given prazosin (2–5 mg) experienced a sharp fall in blood pressure shortly after being given nifedipine sublingually. One of them had a fall in standing blood pressure from 200/120 to 88/48 mm Hg about 20 min after being given a total of 15 mg nifedipine. He complained of dizziness. Eight other patients with hypertension given prazosin showed falls in blood pressure 20 min after nifedipine from 198/108 to 173/96 mm Hg when lying and from 192/114 to 168/97 mm Hg when standing.[1]

(b) Prazosin + verapamil

A study in eight normal subjects given single 1 mg doses of prazosin showed that the average serum prazosin levels were raised 86% (from 5.2 to 9.6 ng/ml) when given with 160 mg verapamil, and the prazosin AUC (area under the curve) increased by 62%. The standing blood pressure fell from 114/82 to 99/81 mm Hg after the prazosin and after both drugs to 89/60 mm Hg at 4 h.[2]

Mechanism

Uncertain. One of the likely reasons would seem to be that the vasodilatory effects of prazosin and the calcium channel blockers are additive. The increase in serum prazosin levels resulting from the interaction with verapamil is possibly because the metabolism of the prazosin by the liver is reduced.[3]

Importance and management

The interaction of prazosin with both of these calcium channel blockers would appear to be established and of clinical importance although the documentation is limited. Marked additive hypotensive effects can occur. It has been suggested that concurrent use should only be undertaken if the effects can be closely monitored.[1] When nifedipine is added to prazosin treatment, a 5 mg test dose of nifedipine should be given with the patient lying down. If the patient is already taking nifedipine, a test dose of 0.5 mg prazosin should be given.[1] The same precautions would also seem applicable with verapamil and any other calcium channel blocker.

References

1 Jee LD and Opie LH. Acute hypotensive response to nifedipine added to prazosin in treatment of hypertension. Br Med J (1983) 287, 1514.
2 Pasanisi F, Meredith PA, Elliott HL and Reid JL. Verapamil and prazosin: pharmacodynamic and pharmacokinetic interactions in normal man. Br J clin Pharmac (1984) 18, 290P.
3 Meredith PA, Elliott HL, Pasanisi F and Reid JL. Prazosin and verapamil: a pharmacokinetic and pharmacodynamic interaction. Br J clin Pharmac (1986) 21, 85P.

Rauwolfia alkaloids + Tricyclic antidepressants

Abstract/Summary

The rauwolfia alkaloids cause depression and are not usually used in patients needing treatment for depression, but there are a few reports of their successful use in some resistant forms of depression when combined with the tricyclic antidepressants.

Clinical evidence, mechanism, importance and management

Depression and sedation are among the very well-recognized side effects of rauwolfia treatment. For example, out of a total of 270 patients given treatment for hypertension with rauwolfia, 23% developed depressive episodes within seven months of starting treatment.[1] Animals treated with reserpine have been widely used by pharmacologists as experimental models of depression when testing the effectiveness of new compounds with potential antidepressant activity. The rauwolfia alkaloids cause adrenergic (noradrenaline-releasing) and serotoninergic (5-HT-releasing) neurones to become depleted of their normal stores of neurotransmitter, the result being that very reduced amounts are available for release by nerve impulses. Because of this action at adrenergic sympathetic nerve endings the blood pressure falls. The brain possesses both types of neurone and failure in transmission is believed to be responsible for the sedation and depression which can occur. However one study describes 14 out of 15 patients with endogenous depression resistant to imipramine who responded well when given up to 300 mg imipramine and 7.5–10.0 mg reserpine daily after an initial manic response.[2] Other reports describe the use of reserpine with desipramine[3,5] and imipramine[4] although the authors of the latter question the advantages claimed by other workers. However, in general, concurrent use should be avoided. Only in well-controlled situations and with patients unresponsive to other forms of treatment should this combination be used.

References

1 Bolte E, Marc-Aurele J, Brouillet J, Beauregard P, Verdy M and Genest J. Mental depressive episodes during rauwolfia therapy for arterial hypertension with special reference to dosage. Can Med Ass J (1959) 80, 291.

2 Haskovec L and Rysanek K. The action of reserpine in imipramine-resistant depressive patients. A clinical and biochemical study. Psychopharmacologica (1967) 11, 18.

3 Poldinger W. Combined administration of desipramine and reserpine or tetrabenazine in depressed patients. Psychopharmacologia (1963) 4, 308.

4 Carney MWP, Thakurdas H and Sebastian J. Effects of imipramine and reserpine in depression. Psychopharmacologia (1969) 14, 349.

5 Amsterdam JD and Berwish N. Treatment of refractory depression with combination reserpine and tricyclic antidepressant therapy. J Clin Psychopharmacol (1987) 7, 238–42.

Spironolactone + Aspirin and Salicylates

Abstract/Summary

The antihypertensive effects of spironolactone are unaffected by the concurrent use of aspirin in patients with hypertension, although there is evidence that the spironolactone-induced loss of sodium in the urine is reduced in normal subjects.

Clinical evidence

(a) Effects in hypertensive patients

Five patients with low-renin essential hypertension, well-controlled for four months or more with 100–300 mg spironolactone daily, were examined in a double blind crossover trial. Daily doses of aspirin of 2.4 to 4.8 g given over six-week periods had no effect on blood pressure, serum electrolytes, body weight, urea nitrogen or plasma renin activity.[4]

(b) Effects in normal subjects

A six-week crossover study in 10 normal subjects given single 25, 50 and 100 mg doses of spironolactone showed that 600 mg of aspirin reduced the urinary excretion of electrolyte. The effectiveness of the spironolactone was reduced 70%, and the overnight sodium excretion reduced by a third in seven of 10 subjects given 25 mg spironolactone daily and a single 600 mg dose of aspirin.[1]

Reductions in sodium excretion are described in other studies.[2,3] In one of these the sodium excretion was completely abolished when aspirin was given one-and-a-half hours after the spironolactone, but only partially reduced when administered in the reverse order.[3]

Mechanism

Uncertain. There is evidence that the active secretion of canrenone (the active metabolite of spironolactone) is blocked by aspirin, but the significance of this is not entirely clear.[2]

Importance and management

An adequately but not extensively documented interaction. Despite the results of the studies in normal subjects, the study in hypertensive patients shows that the blood pressure lowering effects of spironolactone are not affected by aspirin. Concurrent use need not be avoided, but it would be prudent nonetheless to monitor the response to confirm that no adverse interaction is taking place.

References

1 Tweedale MG and Ogilvie RI. Antagonism of spironolactone-induced natriuresis by aspirin in man. N Engl J Med (1973) 289, 198.

2 Ramsay LE, Harrison IR, Shelton JR and Vose CW. Influence of acetylsalicylic acid on the renal handling of a spironolactone metabolite in healthy subjects. Eur J clin Pharmacol (1976) 10, 43.

3 Elliott HC. Reduced adrenocortical steroid excretion rates in man following aspirin administration. Metabolism (1962) 11, 1015.

4 Hollifield JW. Failure of aspirin to antagonize the antihypertensive effect of spironolactone in low-renin hypertension. South Med J (1976) 69, 1034.

Spironolactone + Dextropropoxyphene

Abstract/Summary

A single case report describes the development of gynecomastia and a rash in a man on spironolactone when he was given dextropropoxyphene.

Clinical evidence, mechanism, importance and management

A patient who had been taking spironolactone uneventfully for four years developed swollen and tender breasts and a rash on his chest and neck a fortnight after starting to take *Darvon*, a compound preparation containing dextropropoxyphene, aspirin, phenacetin and caffeine. The problem disappeared when both drugs were withdrawn but the rash reappeared when the *Darvon* alone was given. It disappeared again when it was withdrawn. No problems occurred when the spironolactone was given alone, but both the rash and the gynecomastia recurred when the *Darvon* was added. The reasons for this reaction are not understood. Gynecomastia is a known side-effect of spironolactone (incidence 1.2%). The authors of this report surmise that the dextroproxyphene component of *Darvon* was responsible in some way. Concurrent use need not be avoided but prescribers should be aware of this case.

Reference

1 Licata AA and Bartter FC. Spironolactone-induced gynecomastia related to allergic reaction to 'darvon compound'. Lancet (1976) ii, 905.

Thiazides + Calcium carbonate

Abstract/Summary

Hypercalcaemia and metabolic alkalosis (milk–alkali syndrome) can develop if very large amounts of calcium carbonate are taken while receiving thiazide diuretics.

Clinical evidence

A 47-year-old man was admitted to hospital complaining chiefly of dizziness and general weakness which had begun two months previously. He was taking 500 mg chlorothiazide daily for hypertension, 120 mg thyroid daily for hypothyroidism and 7.5–10.0 g calcium carbonate daily for 'heartburn'. On examination he was found to have metabolic alkalosis with respiratory compensation, a total serum calcium concentration of 6.8 meq/l (normal 4.3–5.2 meq/l) and an abnormal ECG. He was diagnosed as having the milk–alkali syndrome. He rapidly recovered when the thiazide and calcium carbonate were withdrawn and he was given sodium chloride by infusion, frusemide and oral phosphates.[1]

Another patient developed similar symptoms while taking large amounts of calcium carbonate and hydrochlorothiazide.[2]

Mechanism

The hypercalcaemia developed because of the ingestion of the large amounts of calcium carbonate, associated with the reduced calcium excretion caused by the thiazide diuretic. The alkalosis came about because of the high intake of calcium carbonate and the use of the thiazide which limited the bicarbonate excretion. This milk–alkali syndrome (hypercalcaemia, alkalosis, renal insufficiency) was originally associated with the ingestion of large amounts of alkali and milk for the treatment of peptic ulcer before other and better treatments became available.

Importance and management

An established and well understood interaction, but uncommon. Patients should be warned about the ingestion of very large amounts of calcium carbonate (readily available over the counter) if they are taking thiazide diuretics. It is unlikely to occur unless the calcium carbonate intake is particularly excessive.

References

1 Gora ML, Seth SK, Bay WH and Visconti JA. Milk-alkali syndrome associated with use of chlorothiazide and calcium carbonate. Clin Pharm (1989) 8, 227–9.
2 Hakim R, Tolis G, Goltzman A, Meltzer S and Friedman R. Severe hypercalcaemia associated with hydrochlorothiazide and calcium carbonate therapy. Can Med Ass J (1979) 8, 591–4.

Thiazides + Cholestyramine or Colestipol

Abstract/Summary

The absorption of hydrochlorothiazide from the gut can be reduced by a third if colestipol is given concurrently, and two-thirds by cholestyramine. The diuretic effects are reduced accordingly. Separating the dosages of the thiazide and the cholestyramine by 4 h can reduce but not overcome the effects of this interaction.

Clinical evidence

The blood levels of the hydrochlorothiazide were reduced to about one-third in six subjects taking 8 g cholestyramine 2 min before and 6 and 12 h after a single 75 mg oral dose. Total urinary excretion fell to 15%. In a parallel study with 10 mg colestipol, the blood levels of the thiazide fell to about two-thirds and the total urinary excretion fell to 57%.[1]

A further study showed that giving the cholestyramine 4 h after the hydrochlorothiazide reduced the effects of the interaction but the absorption was still reduced by a third.[3] Another study demonstrated a 42% reduction when using chlorothiazide and colestipol.[2]

Mechanism

Hydrochlorothiazide becomes bound to these non-absorbable anionic exchange resins within the gut, and less is available for absorption.

Importance and management

An established interaction of clinical importance. The best dosing schedule would appear to be to give the hydrochorothiazide 4 h before the cholestyramine to minimize mixing in the gut. Even so a one-third reduction in thiazide absorption occurs.[3] The optimum time-interval with colestipol has not been investigated but it would be reasonable to take similar precautions. Information about other thiazides is lacking although it is probable that they will interact similarly.

References

1 Hunninghake DB, King S and La Croix K. The effect of cholestyramine and colestipol on the absorption of hydrochlorothiazide. Int J Clin Pharmacol Ther Toxicol (1982) 20, 151–4.
2 Kauffmann RE and Azarnoff DL. Effect of colestipol on gastrointestinal absorption of chlorothiazide in man. Clin Pharmacol Ther (1973) 14, 886.
3 Hunninghake DB and Hibbard DM. Influence of time intervals for cholestyramine dosing on the absorption of hydrochlorothiazide. Clin Pharmacol Ther (1986) 39, 329–4.

Thiazides + Indomethacin and other NSAID's

Abstract/Summary

The antihypertensive effects of the thiazides can be reduced to some extent by indomethacin, but it appears to be of only moderate clinical importance and may possibly only be a transient interaction. Ibuprofen appears to interact to a lesser extent or not at all, but no adverse interaction occurs with diclofenac, diflunisal, naproxen or sulindac.

Clinical evidence

(a) Thiazides + indomethacin

A double-blind controlled trial in seven patients with hypertension, treated with thiazide diuretics (5–10 mg bendrofluazide or amiloride 5 mg + hydrochlorothiazide 50 mg) showed that when they were additionally treated with 100 mg indomethacin daily for three weeks, their systolic/diastolic blood pressures rose by 13/9 mm Hg when lying and by 16/9 mm Hg when standing. Body weight increased by 1.1 kg.[1]

A later study found a 6/3 mm Hg blood pressure rise in patients given indomethacin for two weeks which had gone after four weeks.[7] Only a 5/1 mm Hg blood pressure rise was seen in another study in hypertensive patients on hydrochlorothiazide given 100 mg indomethacin daily,[4] whereas no significant changes in blood pressure were seen in healthy subjects.[3] 100 mg indomethacin was found to reduce the urinary excretion of sodium and chloride caused by bemetizide by 47 and 44% respectively in normal subjects,[5] but it had no effect on the sodium excretion caused by hydrochlorothiazide.[2] Indomethacin does not affect the pharmacokinetics of hydrochlorothiazide.[2,3]

(b) Thiazides + other NSAID's

375 mg diflunisal twice daily caused the plasma levels of hydrochlorothiazide to rise by 25–30%, but this appears to be clinically unimportant.[8,9] Diflunisal also has uricosuric activity which counteracts the uric acid retention which occurs with hydrochlorothiazide. Diclofenac, sulindac and naproxen do not reduce either the hypotensive or diuretic effects of hydrochlorothiazide, and may even slightly enhance the antihypertensive effects.[4,6,7,10] Ibuprofen (1200 mg daily) caused a small rise in systolic but not in diastolic pressures in one study,[10] but not in another involving bendrofluazide.[11] 3200 mg ibuprofen daily for a week had little effect on blood pressures controlled with hydrochlorothiazide in yet another study.[13] Both ibuprofen and diclofenac can cause a weight rise.[10]

Mechanism

Not understood. Since the prostaglandins have a role to play in kidney function, drugs such as the NSAID's which inhibit their synthesis might be expected to have some effect on the actions of diuretics whose effects may depend on the activity of the prostaglandins. A study in rats suggested that indomethacin may oppose the thiazides by reducing chloride delivery to the site of thiazide action in the distal tubule.[12]

Importance and management

The thiazide–indomethacin interaction is well documented although the findings are not entirely consistent. It seems to be of only moderate clinical importance but the effects of concurrent use should be monitored and the thiazide dosage modified if necessary. Ibuprofen interacts to a lesser extent or not at all, and no adverse interaction appears to occur with naproxen, sulindac or diflunisal. The uricosuric effects of diflunisal may be usefully exploited to counteract the uric acid retention which occurs with hydrochlorothiazide. The effects of other NSAID's do not seem to have been studied.

References

1 Watkins J, Abbott EC, Hensby CN, Webster J and Dollery CT. Attenuation of hypotensive effect of propranolol and thiazide diuretics by indomethacin. Br Med J (1980) 281, 702–5.
2 Williams RL, Davies RO, Berman RS, Holmes GI, Huber P, Gee WL, Lin ET and Benet LZ. Hydrochlorothiazide pharmacokinetics and pharmacologic effect: the influence of indomethacin. J Clin Pharmacol (1982) 22, 32–41.
3 Koopmans PP, Wim GPM, Tan Y, van Ginneken CAM and Gribnau FWJ. Effects of indomethacin and sulindac on hydrochlorothiazide kinetics. Clin Pharmacol Ther (1985) 37, 625–8.
4 Koopmans PP, Thien Th, Thomas CMG, van den Berg RJ and Gribnau FWJ. The effects of sulindac and indomethacin on the antihypertensive and diuretic action of hydrochlorothiazide in patients with mild to moderate essential hypertension. Br J clin Pharmac (1986) 21, 417–23.
5 Dusing R, Nicolas V, Glatte B, Glanzer K, Kipnowski J and Kramer HJ. Interaction of bemetizide and indomethacin in the kidney. Br J clin Pharmac (1983) 377–84.
6 Steiness E and Waldorff S. Different interactions of indomethacin and sulindac with thiazides in hypertension. Br Med J (1982) 285, 1702–3.
7 Koopmans PP, Thien Th and Gribnau FWJ. Influence of non-steroidal anti-inflammatory drugs on diuretic treatment of mild to moderate essential hypertension. Br Med J (1984) 289, 1492–4.
8 Tempero KF, Cirillo VJ and Steelman SL. Diflunisal: a review of the pharmacokinetic and pharmacodynamic properties, drug interactions and special tolerability studies in humans. Br J clin Pharmac (1977) 31S.
9 Tempero KF, Cirillo VJ, Steelman SL, Besselaar GH, Smit Sibinga CTh, De Schepper P, Tjandramaga TB, Dresse A and Gribnau FW J. Special studies on diflunisal, a novel salicylate. Clin Res (1975) 23, 224A.
10 Koopmans PP, Thien Th and Gribnau FWJ. The influence of ibuprofen, dicolfenac and sulindac on the blood pressure lowering effect of hydrochlorothiazide. Eur J Clin Pharmacol (1987) 31, 553–7.
11 Davies JG, Rawlins DC and Busson M. Effect of ibuprofen on blood pressure control by propranolol and bendrofluazide. J Int Med Res (1988) 16, 173–81.
12 Kirchner KA, Brandon S, Mueller RA, Smith MJ and Bower JD. Mechanism of attenutated hydrochlorothiazide response during indomethacin administration. Kidney Int (1987) 31, 1097–1103.
13 Wright JT, McKenney JM, Lehany AM, Bryan DL, Cooper LW and Lambert CM. The effect of high-dose short-term ibuprofen on antihypertensive control with hydrochlorothiazide. Clin Pharmacol Ther (1989) 46, 440–4.

Thiazides + Propantheline

Abstract/Summary

Propantheline can substantially increase the absorption of hydrochlorothiazide from the gut.

Clinical evidence, mechanism, importance and management

The absorption of hydrochlorothiazide in six normal subjects was delayed but substantially increased (+40%) by the concurrent use of 60 mg propantheline, due, it is suggested, to a slower delivery of the drug to its areas of absorption.[1] The clinical importance of this is uncertain, but some increase in the diuretic effects would be expected.

Reference

1 Beerman B and Groschinsky-Grind M. Enhancement of the gastrointestinal absorption of hydrochlorothiazide by propantheline. Eur J Clin Pharmacol (1978) 13, 385.

Triamterene + Cimetidine or Ranitidine

Abstract/Summary

Ranitidine reduces the absorption and the diuretic effects of triamterene but the clinical importance of this is uncertain. Cimetidine appears not to interact with triamterene significantly.

Clinical evidence

(a) Cimetidine

A study in six normal subjects given 100 mg triamterene daily for four days showed that although 800 mg cimetidine daily increased the triamterene AUC by 22%, reduced its metabolism (hydroxylation) by 32% and its renal clearance by 28% as well as its absorption, the loss of sodium in the urine was not significantly changed nor were its potassium-sparing effects altered.[2]

(b) Ranitidine

A study in eight normal subjects showed that taking 300 mg ranitidine daily for four days approximately halved the absorption of triamterene, 100 mg daily (as measured by its renal clearance). Its metabolism was also reduced, the total effect being a 24% reduction in the AUC (area under the time-concentration curve). As a result of the reduced serum triamterene levels the urinary sodium loss was reduced to some extent but potassium excretion remained unchanged.[1]

Mechanism

These changes are due to reduced triamterene absorption from the gut and reduced liver metabolism and renal excretion caused by the these H_2-blockers.

Importance and management

Information about the triamterene–ranitidine interaction is limited and the clinical importance remains uncertain. Nobody seems to have measured whether this interaction significantly reduces the diuretic effects of triamterene in patients. The outcome of concurrent use should therefore be monitored. Cimetidine also interacts with triamterene but this appears to be clinically unimportant because its diuretic effects are minimally changed.[2] No dosage changes are likely to be necessary.

References

1 Muirhead M, Bochner F and Somogyi A. Pharmacokinetic drug interactions between triamterene and ranitidine in humans: alterations in renal and hepatic clearances and gastrointestinal absorption. J Pharmacol exp Ther (1988) 244, 734–9.
2 Muirhead MR, Somoygi AA, Rolan PE and Bochner F. Effect of cimetidine on renal and hepatic drugs elimination: studies with triamterene. Clin Pharmacol Ther (1986) 40, 400–7.

Triamterene + Indomethacin

Abstract/Summary

Concurrent use can rapidly lead to acute renal failure.

Clinical evidence

A study in four normal subjects showed that the concurrent use of indomethacin (150 mg daily) and triameterene (200 mg daily) over a three-day period reduced the creatinine clearance of two of them by 62 and 72% respectively. Kidney function returned to normal after a month. Indomethacin alone caused an average 10% fall in creatinine clearance, but triamterene alone caused no consistent change in kidney function. No adverse reactions were seen in 18 other subjects treated in the same way with indomethacin and three other diuretics (frusemide, chlorothiazide, spironolactone).[1,2]

Five patients have been described who rapidly developed acute renal failure after receiving indomethacin and triamterene either concurrently or sequentially.[3–6]

Mechanism

Uncertain. One suggestion is that triamterene causes renal ischaemia for which the kidney compensates by increasing prostaglandin (PGE_2) production, thereby preserving renal blood flow. Indomethacin opposes this by inhibiting prostaglandin synthesis, so that the damaging effects of triamterene on the kidney continue unchecked.

Importance and management

Information is limited to these reports, but the interaction is established. The incidence is uncertain but it occurred in two of the four subjects in the study cited.[1,2] Since acute renal failure can apparently develop very rapidly it would be prudent to avoid concurrent use.

References

1 Favre L, Glasson P and Vallotton MB. Reversible acute renal failure from combined triamterene and indomethacin. A study in healthy subjects. Ann Intern Med (1982) 96, 317–20.

2 Favre L, Glasson PH, Riondel A and Vallotton MB. Interaction of diuretics and non-steroidal anti-inflammatory drugs in man. Clin Sci (1983) 64, 407–15.

3 McCarthy JT, Torres VE, Romero JC, Wochos DN and Velosa JA. Acute intrinsic renal failure induced by indomethacin: role of prostaglandin synthetase inhibition. Mayo Clin Proc (1982) 57, 289–96.

4 McCarthy JT. Drug induced renal failure. Mayo Clin Proc (1982) 57, 463.

5 Weinberg MS, Quigg RJ, Salant DJ and Bernard DB. Anuric renal failure precipitated by indomethacin and triamterene. Nephron (1985) 40, 216–18.

6 Mathews A amd Baillie GR. Acute renal failure and hyperkalaemia associated with triamterene and indomethacin. Vet Hum Toxicol (1986) 28, 224–5.

9
ANTIPARKINSONIAN DRUG INTERACTIONS

The drugs in this chapter are classified together because their major therapeutic application is in the treatment of Parkinson's disease. This disease is named after Dr James Parkinson who a century-and-a-half ago described the four mains signs of the disease—muscle rigidity, tremor, muscular weakness and hypokinesia. Similar symptoms may also be displayed as the unwanted side-effects of therapy with certain drugs.

The basic cause of the disease lies in the basal ganglia of the brain, particularly the corpus striatum and the substantia nigra, where the normal balance between dopaminergic nerve fibres (those which use dopamine as the chemical transmitter) and the cholinergic (acetylcholine-using) nerve fibres is lost because the dopaminergic fibres degenerate. As a result the cholinergic fibres come to be in dominant control. Much of the treatment of Parkinson's disease is based on an attempt to redress the balance, either by limiting the activity of the cholinergic fibres with anticholinergic (atropine-like) drugs, and/or by 'topping up' the dopaminergic system with dopamine in the form of levodopa, or with other agents such as amantadine or bromocriptine which increase dopaminergic activity in the brain. Dopamine cannot penetrate the blood-brain barrier so that its precursor, dopa, is given instead. These days it is common to include with dopa an enzyme-inhibitor such as carbidopa (in *Sinemet*) or benserazide (in *Madopar*) which prevents the 'wasteful' enzymic metabolism of the levodopa outside the brain and thereby allows the use of lower oral doses which have fewer side-effects.

In addition to the interactions discussed in this chapter, some of the drugs are involved in interactions described elsewhere. Consult the index for a full listing.

Table 9.1 *Antiparkinsonian drugs*

Non-proprietary names	Proprietary names
Anticholinergics	
Benazpryzine	*Brizin*
Benzhexol (trihexiphenidyl)	*Antispas, Aparkane, Apo-Trihex, Artane, Artilan, Bentex, Novoheidyl, Paralest, Pargitan, Parkinane Retard, Peragit, Tremin, Trixyl*
Benztropine	*Bensylate, Cogentin(e)(ol)*
Biperiden	*Akineton, Akinophyl, Tasmolin*
Bornaprine	*Sormodren*
Caramiphen	*Rescaps-d, Tuss-ade, Tuss-ornade*
Chlorphenoxamine	*Clorevan, Phenoxene, Systral(leten)*
Cycrimine	*Pagitan(e)*
Dexetimide	*Tremblex*
Diethazine	
Ethopropazine (profenamine)	*Lysivane, Parkin, Parsidol, Parsitan, Parsotil*

Table **9.1** *continued.*

Non-proprietary names	Proprietary names
Ethylbenztropine	*Ponalid*
Ethylbenzhydramine	*PKM*
Mazaticol	*Pentona*
Methixene	*Methyloxan, Tremaril, Tremarit, Tremonil, Tremoquil, Trest*
Orphenadrine (mephenamine)	*Biophen, Brocadispal, Distalene, Euflex, Lysantin, Mefeamina, Myotrol, Norflex, Orpadrex, Orphenate, Tega-flex, X-otag*
Piroheptine	*Trimol*
Procyclidine	*Arpicolin, Kemadrin(e), Kemadren, Osnervan Procyclid*
Tigloidine	*Mepidium*
Tropatepine	*Lepticur*
Amantadine	*Amantan, Amazolon, Antadine, Aontenton, Mantadan(e), Mantadix, PK-Merz, Solu-Contenon, Symmetrel, Trivaline, Virofal, Virosol*
Bromocriptine	*Bagren, Lactismine, Parlodel, Pravidel*
Levodopa (L-Dopa)	*Bendopa, Berkdopa, Brocadopa, Cidandopa, Dopaidan, Dopaken, Dopalfher, Dopar, Doparkine, Doparl, Dopasol, Dopaston, Dopastral, Eldopal, Eldopa, Eldopatec, Larodopa, Levopa, Syndopa, Veldopa*
Levodopa + benserazide	*Madopar*
Levodopa + carbidopa	*Sinemet*
Pergolide	
Piribedil	*Circularina, Trivastal, Trivastan*

Amantadine + Miscellaneous drugs

Abstract/Summary

The use of amantadine in patients taking amphetamines, other CNS stimulants, or having treatment with other drugs for epilepsy, gastrointestinal ulceration, Parkinson's disease or congestive heart failure may cause problems.

Clinical evidence, mechanism, importance and management

Geigy, the manufacturers of amantadine, say[1] that although adverse interactions have not been reported, they recommend that amantadine should be given with caution if amphetamines or other CNS stimulants are being used. They advise that amantadine is not given to those who are subject to convulsions or with a history of gastric ulceration. They also warn that amantadine can aggravate the CNS, gastro-intestinal and other side-effects of drugs used in the treatment of Parkinson's disease (anticholinergics, levodopa). Amantadine sometimes causes peripheral oedema which may possibly have an adverse effect on the control of congestive heart failure.

Reference

1 ABPI Data Sheet Compendium 1985–6. Datapharm Publications, London 1985, p 505.

Amantadine + Thiazides

Abstract/Summary

Concurrent use can be successful and uneventful but two patients have been described who developed amantadine toxicity when given hydrochlorothiazide-triamterene or cyclopenthiazide-K.

Clinical evidence

A patient developed signs of amantadine toxicity (ataxia, agitation, hallucinations) within a week of additionally starting treatment with two tablets of *Dyazide* (hydrochlorothiazide-triamterene) daily. The symptoms rapidly disappeared when all the drugs were withdrawn. In a later study this patient showed a 50% rise in amantadine serum levels (from 156 to 243 ng/ml) after taking the diuretic for seven days.[1]

Another very brief report describes confusion and hallucinations in a patient given amantadine and cyclopenthiazide K.[2] In contrast, the successful and apparently uneventful concurrent use of amantadine and diuretics (named as a thiazide in one of them)[3] has also been described.[3,4]

Mechanism

Uncertain. Amantadine is largely excreted unchanged in the urine and it seems probable that these diuretics reduce the renal clearance.

Importance and management

Information about an adverse interaction appears to be limited to these two reports. Its incidence is uncertain. There seems to be no reason for avoiding concurrent use, but the effects should be well monitored.

References

1 Wilson TW and Rajput AH. Amantadine–Dyazide interaction. Can Med Ass J (1983) 129, 974–5.
2 New Zealand Committee on Adverse Drug Reactions. 11th year. April 1975–March 1976. Serial no 5476.
3 Birdwood GFB, Gilder SSB and Wink CAS (eds). Parkinson's Disease. A new approach to treatment. Int Clin Symp Report on Symmetrel in Parkinsonism. London June 1971. Academic Press (1971) p 66.
4 Parkes JD, Marsden CD and Price P. Amantadine-induced heart failure. Lancet (1977) i, 904.

Anticholinergics + Betel nuts

Abstract/Summary

The control of the extrapyramidal (parkinsonian) side-effects of fluphenazine and flupenthixol by procyclidine was lost in two patients when they began to chew betel nuts.

Clinical evidence

An Indian patient on depot fluphenazine (50 mg every three weeks) for schizophrenia, and mild parkinsonian tremor controlled with procyclidine (5 mg twice daily), developed marked rigidity, bradykinesia and jaw tremor when he began to chew betel nuts. The symptoms were so severe he could barely speak. When he stopped chewing the nuts his stiffness and abnormal movements disappeared. Another patient on flupenthixol developed marked stiffness, tremor and akathisia, despite taking up to 20 mg procyclidine daily, when he began to chew betel nuts. The symptoms vanished within four days of stopping the nuts.[1]

Mechanism

Betel nuts contain arecoline which mimics the actions of acetylcholine. It seems that the arecoline opposed the actions of the anticholinergic procyclidine which was being used to control the extrapyramidal side-effects of the two neuroleptics, thereby allowing these side-effects to emerge.

Importance and management

Direct information seems to be limited to this report but the interaction would seem to be established and clinically important. Patients taking anticholinergic drugs for the control of drug-induced extrapyramidal (Parkinson-like) symptoms or Parkinson's disease should avoid betel nuts. The authors of this report suggest that a dental inspection for the characteristic red stains of the betel may possibly provide a simple explanation for the sudden and otherwise mysterious deterioration in the symptoms of patients from Asia and the East Indies.

Reference

1 Deahl M. Betel nut-induced extrapyramidal syndrome: an unusual drug interaction. Movement Disorders (1989) 4, 330–3.

Bromocriptine + Alcohol

Abstract/Summary

There is some very limited evidence that the adverse effects of bromocriptine may possibly be increased by alcohol.

Clinical evidence, mechanism, importance and management

Intolerance to alcohol has been briefly mentioned in a report about patients taking bromocriptine for acromegaly.[1] In another report two patients with high prolactin levels are said to have developed the side-effects of bromocriptine even in low doses while continuing to drink.[2] When they abstained, the frequency and the severity of the side-effects fell, even with higher doses of bromocriptine. This, it is suggested, may be due to some alcohol-induced increase in the sensitivity of dopamine receptors.[1] No other reports of this interaction have been traced.[3] There would seem to be little reason, on the basis of this extremely sparse evidence, to tell all patients on bromocriptine not to drink, but it would be reasonable to warn them to avoid alcohol if side-effects develop.

References

1 Wass JAH, Thorner MO, Morris DV, Rees LH, Mason AE and Besser EM. Long-term treatment of acromegaly with bromocriptine. Br Med J (1977) 1, 875.
2 Ayres J and Maisey MN. Alcohol increases bromocriptine side-effects. N Engl J Med (1980) 302, 806.
3 Hunt M (Sandoz). Personal communication (1990).

Bromocriptine + Griseofulvin

Abstract/Summary

Evidence from a single case where bromocriptine was being used for acromegaly suggests that its effects can be opposed by griseofulvin.

Clinical evidence, mechanism, importance and management

The effects of bromocriptine, used for the treatment of acromegaly, were blocked when a patient was given griseofulvin for the treatment of a mycotic infection.[1] The mechanism of this interaction and its general importance are unknown, but prescribers should be aware of it when treating patients with bromocriptine.

Reference

1 Schwinn G, Dirks H, McIntosh C and Kobberling J. Metabolic and clinical studies in patients with acromegaly treated with bromocriptine over 22 months. Eur J Clin Invest (1977) 7, 101.

Bromocriptine + Macrolide antibiotics

Abstract/Summary

Bromocriptine toxicity occurred in an elderly man when given josamycin. A study found that erythromycin causes a very marked increase in serum bromocriptine levels.

Clinical evidence

(a) Erythromycin

A study in five normal subjects found that 250 mg erythromycin estolate four times daily for four days caused a marked change in the pharmacokinetics of a single 5 mg oral dose of bromocriptine. The clearance of the bromocriptine was decreased by 70.6% while the peak serum levels were raised by 460%.[2]

(b) Josamycin

An elderly man with Parkinson's disease, well-controlled for 10 months on daily treatment with levodopa (and benserazide) 200 mg, bromocriptine 70 mg and domperidone 60 mg, was additionally given 2 g josamycin daily for a respiratory infection. Shortly after the first dose he became drowsy with visual hallucinations, and began to show involuntary movements of his limbs similar to the dystonic and dyskinetic movements seen in choreo-athetosis. These adverse effects (interpreted as bromocriptine toxicity) disappeared within a few days of withdrawing the antibiotic.[1]

Mechanism

Not understood. One suggestion is that the macrolide antibiotic inhibits the metabolism of the bromocriptine by the liver, thereby reducing its loss from the body and raising its serum levels.[1]

Importance and management

Information seems to be limited to these reports, nevertheless there is enough evidence to warrant close monitoring if either of these macrolide antibiotics is added to bromocriptine treatment. There seems to be no direct evidence about any other macrolides, but some of them certainly inhibit liver metabolism and can raise the serum levels of other drugs.

References

1 Montastruc JL and Rascol A. Traitement de la maladie de Parkinson par doses elevees de bromocriptine. Interaction possible avec josamycine. La Presse Med (1984) 13, 2267–8.

2   Nelson MV, Berchon RC, Kareti D and Lewitt PA. Pharmacokinetic evaluation of erythromycin and caffeine administered with bromocriptine in normal subjects. Clin Pharmacol Ther (1990), 47, 66.

Levodopa + Antacids

Abstract/Summary

Antacids appear not to interact significantly with levodopa, except possibly with one slow-release preparation the bioavailability of which is reduced.

Clinical evidence, mechanism, importance and management

Levodopa can be metabolized in the stomach so that, in theory at least, antacids which increase gastric emptying might decrease this 'wasteful' metabolism and increase the amounts available for absorption. This would seem to be confirmed by one study which found that an aluminium-magnesium hydroxide antacid raised peak serum levodopa levels and they occurred sooner.[2,3] However no interaction was seen when magaldrate was used,[4] nor in a study in 15 parkinsonian patients taking bromocriptine, levodopa and carbidopa who were given six 30 ml doses of aluminium hydroxide (*Mylanta*) daily. No effect was seen on the fluctuations in response to levodopa which normally occur.[1] However in another study using *Madopar HBS*, a sustained release preparation of levodopa and benserazide, the concurrent use of an un-named antacid reduced the bioavailability by about one third.[5] The overall picture is that concurrent use need not be avoided, but the outcome should be monitored.

References

1   Lau E, Waterman K, Glover R, Schulzer M and Calne DB. Effect of antacid on levodopa therapy. Clin Neuropharmacol (1986) 9, 477–9.
2   Rivera-Calimlim L, Dujovne CA, Morgan JO, Lasagna L and Bianchine JR. Absorption and metabolism of L-dopa by the human stomach. Eur J Clin Invest (1971) 1, 313.
3   Pocelinko GBT and Solomon HM. The effect of an antacid on the absorption and metabolism of levodopa. Clin Pharmacol Ther (1972) 13, 149.
4   Leon AS and Spiegel HE. The effect of antacid administration on the absorption and metabolism of levodopa. J Clin Pharmacol (1972) 12, 263.
5   Malcolm SL, Allen JG, Bird H, Quinn NP, Marion MH and Marsden CD. Single dose pharmacokinetics of *Madopar* HBS in patients and effect of food and antacid on the absorption of Madopa HBS in volunteers. Eur Neurol (1987) 27, 28–35.

Levodopa + Anticholinergics

Abstract/Summary

Although anticholinergic drugs are very widely used in conjunction with levodopa, they may reduce the absorption of levodopa and reduce its therapeutic effects to some extent.

Clinical evidence

A study in six normal subjects and six patients with Parkinson's disease showed that the administration of benzhexol (trihexyphenidyl) lowered the peak serum levels and reduced the absorption of levodopa in about half of the subjects by an average of 16–20%.[1]

A patient who needed 7 g levodopa daily while taking homatropine developed levodopa toxicity when the homatropine was withdrawn, and he was subsequently restabilized on 4 g levodopa daily.[2] This interaction is described in another report.[3]

Mechanism

Anticholinergics delay gastric emptying which gives the gastric mucosa more time to metabolize the levodopa 'wastefully' so that less is available for absorption in the small intestine.[4]

Importance and management

Anticholinergics are almost certainly the most commonly co-administered drugs with levodopa (one study suggests that the incidence may be as much as 50%[1]). Prescribers should be alert for evidence of a reduced levodopa response if anticholinergics are added, or for levodopa toxicity if they are withdrawn.

References

1   Algeri S, Cerletti C, Curcio M, Morselli PL, Bonollo L, Buniva M, Minazzi M and Minoli G. Effect of anticholinergic drugs on gastrointestinal absorption of L-dopa in rats and man. Eur J Pharmacol (1976) 35, 293.
2   Fermaglich J and O'Doherty DS. Effect of gastric motility on levodopa. Dis Nerv Syst (1972) 33, 624.
3   Birket-Smith E. Abnormal involuntary movements in relation to anticholinergics and levodopa therapy. Acta Neurol Scand (1975) 52, 158.
4   Rivera-Calimlim L, Morgan JP, Dujovne CA, Bianchine JR and Lasagna L. L-dopa absorption and metabolism by the human stomach. J Clin Invest (1970) 49, 79.

Levodopa + Benzodiazepines

Abstract/Summary

The therapeutic effects of levodopa can be reduced or abolished in some patients by the concurrent use of chlordiazepoxide, diazepam or nitrazepam.

Clinical evidence

Eight patients on levodopa were concurrently treated with various benzodiazepines, mostly in unstated doses but said to be within the normal therapeutic range. No adverse interaction occurred in three given chlordiazepoxide or one given oxazepam, but a dramatic deterioration in the control of parkinsonism was seen in a man given 5 mg diazepam twice daily, from which he spontaneously recovered. Two out of three given nitrazepam also showed marked deterioration but failed to react in the same way when rechallenged with nitrazepam in three further tests.[1]

There are other reports of a loss in the control of the parkinsonism in nine patients given chlordiazepoxide[2-6] and three patients given diazepam.[5] However another report says that diazepam and especially flurazepam are valuable for sleep induction and maintenance in patients on levodopa.[7]

Mechanism

Not understood.

Importance and management

Established and clinically important interactions but the incidence is uncertain. Apparently it only affects some patients. Concurrent use need not be avoided but monitor the outcome closely for any sign of deterioration in the control of the parkinsonism. Information about other benzodiazepines is lacking but it would seem reasonable to apply the same precautions. 75 mg hydroxyzine daily was found to be a non-interacting substitute for chlordiazepoxide in one patient.[6]

References

1 Hunter KR, Stern GM and Laurence DR. Use of levodopa with other drugs. Lancet (1970) ii, 1283.
2 Mackie L. Drug antagonism. Br Med J (1971) 2, 651.
3 Schwartz GA and Fahn S. Newer medical treatments in parkinsonism. Med Clin N Amer (1970) 54, 773.
4 Brogden RN, Speight TM and Avery GS. Levodopa: a review of its pharmacological properties and therapeutic use with particular reference to Parkinsonism. Drugs (1971) 2, 262.
5 Wodak J, Gilligan BS, Veale JL and Dowty BJ. Review of 12 months' treatment with L-dopa in Parkinson's disease with remarks on usual side-effects. Med J Aust (1972) 2, 1277.
6 Yosselson-Superstine S and Lipman AG. Chlordiazepoxide interaction with levodopa. Ann Intern Med (1982) 96, 259.
7 Kales A, Ansel RD, Markham CH, Scharf MB and Tan T-L. Sleep in patients with Parkinson's disease and normal subjects prior to and following levodopa administration. Clin Pharmacol Ther (1971) 12, 397–406.

Levodopa + Beta-blockers

Abstract/Summary

Concurrent use normally appears to be favourable, but the long-term effects of the elevated growth hormone levels are uncertain.

Clinical evidence, mechanism, importance and management

Most of the effects of combined use seem to be favourable. Dopamine derived from levodopa stimulates beta-receptors in the heart which can cause heart arrhythmias. These receptors are blocked by propranolol.[1] An enhancement of the effects of levodopa and a reduction in tremor in some[2] but not all patients[3,5] have been described. However there is evidence that growth hormone levels are substantially raised,[4] but to what extent this might prove to be an adverse response during long-term treatment appears not to have been assessed.

References

1 Goldberg LI and Whitsett TL. Cardiovascular effects of levodopa. Clin Pharmacol Ther (1971) 12, 376.
2 Kissel P, Tridon P and Andre JM. Levodopa-propranolol therapy in parkinsonian tremor. Lancet (1974) ii, 403.
3 Sandler M, Fellows LE, Calne DB and Findley LJ. Oxprenolol and levodopa in parkinsonian patients. Lancet (1975) i, 168.
4 Camanni F and Massara F. Enhancement of levodopa-induced growth hormone stimulation by propranolol. Lancet (1974) i, 942.
5 Marsden CD, Parkes JD and Rees JE. Propranolol in Parkinson's disease. Lancet (1974) ii, 410.

Levodopa or Piribedil + Clonidine

Abstract/Summary

Clonidine is reported to oppose the effects of levodopa or piribedil used to control Parkinson's disease.

Clinical evidence

A study in seven patients (five taking piribedil and two taking levodopa with benserazide) showed that concurrent treatment with 1.5 mg clonidine daily for 10–24 days caused a worsening of the symptoms of Parkinson's disease (an exacerbation of rigidity and akinesia). The concurrent use of anticholinergic drugs reduced the effects of this interaction.[1]

Another report on 10 hypertensive and three normotensive patients with Parkinson's disease, some of them taking levodopa and some of them not, claimed that concurrent treatment with clonidine did not affect the control of the parkinsonism, although two patients stopped taking the clonidine because of an increase in tremor and gait disturbance.[2]

Mechanism

Not understood. A suggestion is that the clonidine opposes the antiparkinson effects by stimulating alpha-receptors in the brain. Another idea is that the clonidine directly stimulates post-synaptic dopaminergic receptors.

Importance and management

Information seems to be limited to these reports. Be alert for a reduction in the control of the Parkinson's disease during concurrent use. The effects of this interaction appear to be reduced if anticholinergic drugs are also being used.

References

1 Shoulson I and Chase TN. Clonidine and the antiparkinsonian response to L-dopa or piribedil. Neuropharmacology (1976) 15, 25–7.
2 Tarsy D, Parkes JD and Marsden CD. Clonidine in Parkinson's disease. Arch Neurol (1975) 32, 134–6.

Levodopa + Ferrous sulphate

Abstract/Summary

Ferrous sulphate markedly reduces the bioavailability of levodopa.

Clinical evidence

Eight normal subjects, three men and five women, were given a single 250 mg dose of levodopa, with and without a single 325 mg dose of ferrous sulphate, and the serum levodopa levels were measured for the following 6 h. Peak serum levodopa levels were reduced by 55% (from 3.6 to 1.6 nmol/l) and the AUC was reduced by 51% (from 257 to 125 nmol.min/ml). Those subjects who had the highest peak levels and greatest absorption showed the greatest reductions when given ferrous sulphate.[1]

Mechanism

Ferrous iron rapidly oxidizes to ferric iron at the pH values found in the intestine which then binds strongly to the levodopa to form chelation complexes which are poorly absorbed.[1]

Importance and management

Information appears to be limited to this report. The clinical importance of this interaction in patients awaits study but the extent of the reduction in absorption (50%) suggests that the control of parkinsonism may be worsened. Be alert for any evidence of this. Increasing the levodopa dosage or separating the dosages as much as possible may prove to be effective. More study is needed.

Reference

1 Campbell NRC and Hasinoff B. Ferrous sulfate reduces levodopa bioavailability: chelation as a possible mechanism. Clin Pharmacol Ther (1989) 45, 220–5.

Levodopa + Food

Abstract/Summary

The fluctuations in response to levodopa experienced by some patients may be due to timing of meals and the kind of diet, particularly the protein content, both of which can reduce the effects of levodopa.

Clinical evidence

(a) Changes in absorption

A study in patients with Parkinson's disease treated with levodopa showed that if taken with a meal, the mean absorption of the levodopa from the gut and the peak plasma levels were reduced by 27 and 29% respectively, and the peak serum level was delayed by 34 min.[1] Another study showed that peak serum levodopa levels were reduced if taken with food rather than when fasting.[2]

(b) Changes in response

A study showed that glycine and lysine given to four patients receiving levodopa as a constant IV infusion had no effect, but phenylalanine, leucine and isoleucine reduced the clinical response although the serum levodopa levels remained unchanged.[1]

Other studies have shown that a high daily intake of protein reduces the effects of levodopa, compared with the situation when the intake of protein is low.[3,4]

Mechanism

(a) Meals which delay gastric emptying allow the levodopa to be exposed to 'wasteful' metabolism in the gut which reduces the amount available for absorption. In addition (b) some large neutral amino acids arising from the digestion of proteins can compete with levodopa for transport into the brain so that the therapeutic response may be reduced, whereas other amino acids do not have this effect.[1,4]

Importance and management

An established interaction, but unpredictable. Since the fluctuations in the response of patients to levodopa may be influenced by what is eaten, and when, a change in the pattern of drug and food administration on a trial-and-error basis may be helpful. Multiple small doses of levodopa and distributing the intake of proteins may also iron out the effects of these interactions. Diets which conform to the recommended daily allowance of protein (0.8 g/kg body weight) are reported to eliminate this adverse drug-food interaction.[4]

References

1 Anon. Timing of meals may affect clinical response to levodopa. Am Pharm (1985) 25, 34–5.
2 Morgan JP, Bianchine JR, Spiegel HE, Nutley NJ, Rivera-Calimlim L and Hersey RM. Metabolism of levodopa in patients with Parkinson's disease. Arch Neurol (1971) 25, 39–44.
3 Gillespie NG, Mena I and Cotzias GC. Diets affecting treatment of parkinsonism with levodopa. J Am Diet Ass (1973) 62, 525–8.
4 Juncos JL, Fabbrini G, Mouradian MM, Serrati C and Chase TN. Dietary influences on the antiparkinsonian response to levodopa. Arch Neurol (1987) 44, 1003–5.

Levodopa + Methionine

Abstract/Summary

The effects of levodopa can be reduced by methionine.

Clinical evidence

14 patients with Parkinson's disease and treated with levodopa were given a low-methionine diet for a period of eight days. Five out of seven then given 4.5 g methionine daily showed a definite worsening of the symptoms (gait, tremor, rigidity, etc) which ceased when the methionine was withdrawn. Three out of seven given a placebo showed some subjective improvement.[1]

This report confirms the results of a previous study.[2]

Mechanism

Uncertain. One idea is that the methionine competes with the levodopa for active transport into the brain so that its effects are reduced.

Importance and management

Information is very limited but it indicates that large doses of methionine should be avoided in patients being treated with levodopa.

References

1 Pearce LA and Waterbury LD. L-methionine: a possible levodopa antagonist. Neurology (Minneap) (1974) 24, 640.
2 Pearce LA and Waterbury LD. L-methionine: a possible levodopa antagonist. Neurology (Minneap) (1971) 21, 410.

Levodopa + Methyldopa

Abstract/Summary

Methyldopa can increase the effects of levodopa and permit a reduction in the dosage in some patients, but it can also worsen dyskinesias in others. A small increase in the hypotensive actions of methyldopa may also occur.

Clinical evidence

(a) Effects on the response to levodopa

A double-blind cross-over trial in 10 patients with Parkinson's disease who had been taking levodopa for 12–40 months, showed that the optimum daily dose of levodopa, 5.5 g, fell by 78% when using the highest doses of methyldopa studied (1920 mg daily) and by 50% with 800 mg methyldopa daily.[1]

A one-third[2] and a two-thirds[3] reduction in the levodopa dosage during concurrent treatment with methyldopa have been described in other reports. Another report states that the control of Parkinson's disease in some patients improved during concurrent use, but worsened the dyskinesias in others.[9] Methyldopa on its own can cause a reversible parkinsonian-like syndrome.[6–8]

(b) Effects on the response to methyldopa

A study in 18 patients with Parkinson's disease showed that levodopa and methyldopa taken together lowered the blood pressure in doses which, when given singly, did not alter the pressure. Daily doses of 1–2.5 g levodopa with 500 mg methyldopa caused a 12/6 mm Hg fall in blood pressure. No change in the control of the Parkinson's disease was seen, but the study lasted only a few days.[4]

Mechanism

Not understood.[5] (a) One idea is that the methyldopa inhibits the enzymic destruction of levodopa outside the brain so that more is available to exert its therapeutic effects. Another is that a false neurotransmitter produced from methyldopa opposes the effects of levodopa. (b) The increased hypotension may simply be due to the additive effects of the two drugs.

Importance and management

Well documented, but the picture presented is a little confusing. Concurrent use need not be avoided but the outcome should be well monitored. The use of methyldopa may allow a reduction in the dosage of the levodopa (the reports cited[1–3] quote figures of between 30 and 78%) and enhance the control of Parkinson's disease, but it should also be borne in mind that in some patients the control may be worsened. The increased hypotensive effects seem to be small but they too should be checked.

References

1 Fermaglich J and Chase TN. Methyldopa or methyldopa hydrazine as levodopa synergists. Lancet (1973) i, 1261.
2 Mones KJ. Evaluation of alpha-methyldopa and alpha-methyldopa hydrazine with L-dopa therapy. NY State J Med (1974) 74, 47.
3 Fermaglich J and O'Doherty DS. Second generation of l-dopa therapy. Neurology (1971) 21, 408.
4 Gibberd FB and Small E. Interaction between levodopa and methyldopa. Br Med J (1973) 2, 90.
5 Smith SE. The pharmacological actions of 3.4-dihydroxy-phenyl-alpha-methylalanine (alpha-methyldopa), an inhibitor of 5-hydroxytryptophan decarboxylase. Br J Pharmacol (1960) 15, 319.
6 Groden BM. Parkinsonism occurring with methyldopa treatment. Br Med J (1963) 2, 1001.
7 Peaston MJT. Parkinsonism associated with alpha-methyldopa therapy. Br Med J (1964) 2, 168.
8 Strang RR. Parkinsonism occurring during methyldopa therapy. Can Med Ass J (1966) 95, 928.
9 Sweet RD, Lee JE and McDowell FH. Methyldopa as an adjunct to levodopa treatment of Parkinson's disease. Clin Pharmacol Ther (1972) 13, 23–7.

Levodopa + Metoclopramide

Abstract/Summary

Some of the effects of levodopa are increased by metoclo-pramide and other effects are opposed. The outcome of concurrent use is uncertain.

Clinical evidence, mechanism, importance and management

Metoclopramide is a dopamine antagonist and occasionally it causes extrapyramidal disturbances (parkinson-like symptoms) especially in children.[1] On the other hand metoclopramide opposes the effects of levodopa on stomach emptying which can result in an increase in the bioavailability of levodopa.[2,3] The outcome of these two opposite effects (reduced effects and increased bioavailability) is uncertain, but it would be prudent to monitor concurrent use. There seem to be no clinical reports describing an adverse interaction.

References

1 Castells-Van Daele M, Jaeken J and Van der Schueren P. Dystonic reactions in children caused by metoclopramide. Arch Dis Child (1970) 45, 130–3.
2 Berkowitz DM and McCallum RW. Interaction of levodopa and metoclopramide on gastric emptying. Clin Pharmacol Ther (1980) 27, 415–20.
3 Mearrick PT et al. Metoclopramide, gastric emptying and L-dopa absorption. Aust NZ J Med (1974) 4, 144.

Levodopa or Whole broad beans + Monoamine oxidase inhibitors (MAOI)

Abstract/Summary

A rapid, serious and potentially life-threatening hypertensive reaction can occur in patients being treated with MAOI for hypertension or depression if they are concurrently given levodopa, or if they eat whole broad beans which contain dopa. An interaction with compound levodopa preparations containing carbidopa or benserazide (Sinemet, Madopar) is unlikely. Selegiline (Deprenyl) does not interact adversely with levodopa.

Clinical evidence

(a) Levodopa + monoamine oxidase inhibitor

A patient who had been taking phenelzine daily for 10 days was given 50 mg levodopa by mouth. Within an hour his blood pressure had risen from 135/90 to about 190/130 mm Hg, and despite the IV injection of 5 mg phentolamine it continued to rise over the next 10 min to 200/135 mm Hg, before falling in reponse to a further 4 mg injection of phentolamine. Next day the experiment was repeated with 25 mg levopa but no blood pressure changes were seen, and three weeks after withdrawal of the phenelzine even 500 mg levodopa had no effect on the blood pressure.[1]

Similar cases of severe hypertension, accompanied in most instances by flushing, throbbing and pounding in the head, neck and chest, and lightheadedness have been described in other case reports and studies involving the concurrent use of levodopa with pargyline,[2] nialamide,[3,4] tranylcypromine,[4,5,7] phenelzine[6,14] and isocarboxazid.[12]

(b) Whole broad beans + monoamine oxidase inhibitor

A similar hypertensive reaction can occur in patients taking MAOI who have eaten WHOLE cooked broad beans (*Vicia faba L*), that is to say the beans with pods, the latter normally containing dopa.[10] The reports involve pargyline[8] and phenelzine.[9]

Mechanism

Not fully understood. Levodopa is enzymically converted in the body, firstly to dopamine and then to noradrenaline (norepinephrine), both of which are normally under enzymic attack by monoamine oxidase. But in the presence of a monoamine oxidase inhibitor this attack is suppressed which means that the total levels of dopamine and noradrenaline are increased. Precisely how this then leads to a sharp rise in blood pressure is not clear, but either dopamine or noradrenaline, or both, directly or indirectly stimulate the alpha-receptors of the cardiovascular system.

Importance and management

A well-documented, serious and potentially life-threatening interaction. Patients should not be given levodopa during treatment with any of the older MAOI cited here, whether used for depression or hypertension, and for a period of 2–3 weeks after their withdrawal. The same precautions apply to the eating of WHOLE cooked broad beans, the dopa being in the pods but not in the beans. If accidental ingestion occurs the hypertensive reaction can be controlled by the IV injection of an alpha-blocker such as phentolamine. This interaction has been shown to be inhibited in man by the presence of dopa decarboxylase inhibitors[5] such as carbidopa (in *Sinemet*) and benserazide (in *Madopar*) so that a serious interaction is unlikely to occur with these preparations. Even so the manufacturers of both list the MAOI among their contraindications. Selegiline (*Deprenyl*) which is an inhibitor of MAO-B does not interact adversely with levodopa.[11,13]

References

1 Hunter KR, Boakes AJ, Laurence DR and Stern GM. Monoamine oxidase inhibitors and L-dopa. Br Med J (1970) 3, 388.
2 Hodge JV. Use of monoamine oxidase inhibitors. Lancet (1965) i, 764.
3 Friend DG, Bell WR and Kline NS. The action of L-dihydroxyphenyl-alanine in patients receiving nialamide. Clin Pharmacol Ther (1965) 362.
4 Horowitz D, Goldberg LI and Sjoerdsma A. Increased blood pressure responses to dopamine and norepinephrine produced by monoamine oxidase inhibitors in man. J Lab Clin Med (1960) 56, 747.
5 Teychenne PF, Calne DB, Lewis PJ and Findley LJ. Interactions of levodopa with inhibitors of monoamine oxidase and L-aromatic amino acid decarboxylase. Clin Pharmacol Ther (1975) 18, 273.

6 Schildkraut JJ, Klerman G, Friend I and Greenblatt M. Biochemical and pressor effects of oral D,L-dihydroxyphenylalanine in patients pretreated with antidepressant drugs. Ann NY Acad Sci (1963) 107, 1005.

7 Sharpe J, Marquez-Julio A and Ashby P. Idiopathic orthostatic hypotension treated with levodopa and MAO inhibitor: a preliminary report. Can Med Ass J (1972) 107, 296.

8 Hodge JV, Nye ER and Emerson GW. Monoamine oxidase inhibitors, broad beans and hypertension. Lancet (1964) i, 1108.

9 Bromley DJ. Monoamine oxidase inhibitors. Lancet (1964) i, 1181.

10 McQueen EG. Interactions with monoamine oxidase inhibitors. Br Med J (1975) 3, 101.

11 Birkmayer W, Riederer P, Ambrozi I and Youdim MBH. Implications of combined treatment with 'Madopar' and L-deprenil in Parkinson's disease. Lancet (1977) i, 439.

12 Birkmayer W, Hornykiewicz O. Archiv fur Psychiatrie und der Nervenkrankheiten vereinigt mit Zeitschrift fur die gasamte Neurologie und Psychiatrie (1962) 203, 560. Quoted in ref 1.

13 Elsworth JD, Glover V, Reynolds GP, Sandler M, Lees AJ, Phuapradit P, Shaw KM, Stern GM and Kumar P. Deprenyl administration in man: a selective monoamine oxidase B inhibitor without a 'cheese effect'. Psychopharmacology (1978) 57, 33.

14 Kassirer JP, Kopleman RI. A modern medical Descartes. Hosp Prac (1987) September 15th, 17–25.

Levodopa + Papaverine

Abstract/Summary

There are case reports of a deterioration in the control of parkinsonism in patients treated with levodopa when given papaverine, but a controlled trial failed to confirm this interaction.

Clinical evidence

(a) Reduced levodopa effects

A woman with long-standing parkinsonism, well controlled on levodopa and later levodopa with benserazide, began to show a steady worsening of her parkinsonism within a week of additionally starting to take 100 mg papaverine daily. The deterioration continued until the papaverine was withdrawn. The normal response to levodopa returned within a week. Four other patients showed a similar response.[1]

Two other similar cases have been described in another report.[2]

(b) No change in levodopa effects

A double-blind cross-over trial was carried out on nine patients with parkinsonism being treated with levodopa (range 100–750 mg daily) plus a decarboxylase inhibitor. Two of them were also taking bromocriptine (40 mg daily) and two benzhexol (15 mg daily). No changes in the control of their disease were seen when they were concurrently treated with 150 mg papaverine hydrochloride daily for three weeks.[5]

Mechanism

Not understood. One suggestion is that papaverine blocks the dopamine receptors in the striatum of the brain, thereby inhibiting the effects of the levodopa.[1,3] Another is that papaverine may have a reserpine-like action on the vesicles of adrenergic neurones.[1,4]

Importance and management

Direct information seems to be limited to the reports cited. The situation is controversial but concurrent use can apparently be uneventful. However in the light of the reports of adverse interactions it would be prudent to monitor the outcome closely. Carefully controlled trials can provide a good picture of the general situation, but may not necessarily pick out the occasional patient who may be affected by an interaction.

References

1 Duvoisin RC. Antagonism of levodopa by papaverine. J Amer Med Ass (1975) 231, 845.

2 Posner DM. Antagonism of levodopa by papaverine. J Amer Med Ass (1975) 233, 768.

3 Gonzalez-Vegas JA. Antagonism of dopamine-mediated inhibition in the nigro-striatal pathway: a mode of action of some catatonia-inducing drugs. Brain Res (1974) 80, 219.

4 Cebeddu LX and Weiner JA. Relationship between a granular effect and exocytic release of norepinephrine by nerve stimulation. Pharmacologist (1974) 16, 190.

5 Montastruc JL, Rascol O, Belin J, Ane M and Rascol A. Does papaverine interact with levodopa in Parkinson's disease? Ann Neurol (1987) 22, 558–9.

Levodopa + Phenothiazines or Butyrophenones

Abstract/Summary

Phenothiazines and butyrophenones can oppose the effects of levodopa. The antipsychotic effects and extrapyramidal side-effects of the phenothiazines can be opposed by levodopa.

Interaction, mechanism, importance and management

Phenothiazines (such as chlorpromazine) and butyrophenones (haloperidol, droperidol) block the dopamine receptors in the brain and can therefore upset the balance between cholinergic and dopaminergic components within the corpus striatum and substantia nigra. As a consequence they may not only induce the development of extrapyramidal (parkinson-like) symptoms, but they can aggravate parkinsonism and antagonize the effects of levodopa used in its treatment.[1–3] Antiemetics such as prochlorperazine[1,2] and trifluoperazine[2] can behave in this way. For this reason drugs of this kind are generally regarded as contraindicated in patients under treatment for Parkinson's disease or they are only to be used with great caution in carefully controlled conditions. Non-phenothiazine antiemetics which do not antagonize the effects of levodopa include cyclizine (*Marzine*) and diphenidol (*Vontrol*).

The extrapyramidal symptoms which frequently occur with the phenothiazines have been treated with varying degrees of success with levodopa, but the levodopa may also antagonize the antipsychotic effects of the phenothiazines.[5]

References

1 Duvoisin R.C. Diphenidol for levodopa-induced nausea and vomiting. J Amer Med Ass (1972) 221, 1408.
2 Campbell JB. Long-term treatment of Parkinson's disease with levodopa. Neurology (1970) 20 (December Suppl), 18.
3 Klawans HL and Weiner WJ. Attempted use of haloperidol in the treatment of L-dopa induced dyskinesias. J Neurol Neurosurg Psychiatry (1974) 37, 427–30.
4 Yaryura-Tobias JA. Action of L-dopa in drug-induced extrapyramidalism. Dis Nerv Syst (1970) 1, 60.
5 Hunter KR, Stern GM, Laurence DR. Use of levodopa and other drugs. Lancet (1970) ii, 1283.

Levodopa + Phenylbutazone

Abstract/Summary

A single case report describes antagonism of the effects of levodopa by phenylbutazone.

Interaction, mechanism, importance and management

A patient who was very sensitive to levodopa found that only by taking frequent small doses (0.125 g) was he able to prevent the involuntary movements of his tongue, jaw, neck and limbs. If these developed he was able to suppress them with phenylbutazone, but this also lessened the beneficial effect.[1] The reason is not understood. This interaction has not been confirmed by anyone else and its general importance is not known, but prescribers should be aware of this isolated case.

Reference

1 Wodak J, Gilligan BS, Veale JL and Dowty BJ. Review of 12 months treatment with L-dopa in Parkinson's disease, with remarks on unusual side effects. Med J Aust (1972) 2, 1277–82.

Levodopa + Phenytoin

Abstract/Summary

The therapeutic effects of levodopa can be reduced or abolished by the concurrent use of phenytoin.

Clinical evidence, mechanism, importance and management

In a study on five patients treated with levodopa (630–4600 mg plus 150–225 mg carbidopa daily) for Parkinson's disease, it was found that when they were additionally given phenytoin (100–500 mg daily) for 5–19 days the levodopa dyskinesias were relieved but the beneficial effects of the levodopa were also reduced or abolished. The patients became slow, rigidity re-emerged and some of them became unable to get out of a chair. Within two weeks of stopping the phenytoin, their parkinsonism was again well controlled by the levodopa.[1] The mechanism of this interaction is not understood. Information seems to be limited to this study, nevertheless it would seem prudent to avoid giving phenytoin to patients already taking levodopa. If both drugs are used it may be necessary to increase the dosage of the levodopa.

Reference

1 Mendez JS, Cotzias GC, Mena I and Papavasiliou PS. Diphenylhydantoin blocking of levodopa effects. Arch Neurol (1975) 32, 44.

Levodopa + Piperidine

Abstract/Summary

Piperidine hydrochloride opposes both the dyskinesia associated with the use of levodopa and the beneficial effects of levodopa.

Clinical evidence, mechanism, importance and management

A study on 11 patients with Parkinson's diseases and levodopa-induced dyskinesia showed that piperidine hydrochloride, in daily doses of 700–6300 mg over periods of 10–33 days, diminished the dyskinesia, but it also opposed the effects of the levodopa so that the parkinsonian symptoms re-emerged.[1] This is probably because piperidine has cholinergic effects which upset the cholinergic/dopaminergic balance for which the levodopa had originally been given. This was essentially an experimental study undertaken in the hope that piperidine might prove to be beneficial. It would seem that there is no therapeutic value in the concurrent use of these drugs.

Reference

1 Tolosa ES, Cotzias GC, Papavasilou PS and Lazarus CB. Antagonism by piperidine of levodopa effects in Parkinson's disease. Neurology (1977) 27, 875.

Levodopa + Pyridoxine (Vitamin B6)

Abstract/Summary

The effects of levodopa are reduced or abolished by the concurrent use of pyridoxine, but no interaction occurs with levodopa-carbidopa or levodopa-benserazide preparations (e.g. Sinemet, Madopar).

Clinical evidence

(a) Levodopa + pyridoxine

A study in 25 patients being treated with levodopa showed that if they were given high doses of pyridoxine (750–1000 mg daily) the effects of the levodopa were completely abolished within 3–4 days, and some reduction in the effects were evident within 24 h. Daily doses of 50–100 mg also reduced or abolished the effects of levodopa, and an increase in the signs and symptoms of parkinsonism occurred in eight out of 10 patients taking only 5–10 mg pyridoxine daily.[1]

The antagonism of the effects of levodopa by pyidoxine has been described in numerous other reports.[2–11]

(b) Levodopa-carbidopa + pyridoxine

A study on six chronic levodopa-treated patients with Parkinson's disease showed that when given 250 mg levodopa with 50 mg pyridoxine their mean levodopa plasma levels fell by 70% (from 356 to 109 ng/ml). With levodopa-carbidopa their mean plasma levels rose almost three-fold (to 845 ng/ml) and with 50 mg pyridoxine as well a further slight increase occurred (to 891 ng/ml), although the plasma-integrated area fell 22% from that obtained with levodopa-carbidopa.[11]

The absence of an interaction is confirmed in another report.[12]

Mechanism

The conversion of levodopa to dopamine within the body requires the presence of pyridoxal-5-phosphate (derived from pyridoxine) as a co-factor. When dietary amounts of pyridoxine are high, the 'wasteful' metabolism of levodopa outside the brain is increased so that less is available for entry into the CNS and its effects are reduced accordingly. Pyridoxine may also alter levodopa metabolism by Schiff-base formation. However in the presence of dopa-decarboxylase inhibitors such as carbidopa or benserazide, this 'wasteful' metabolism of levodopa is reduced and much larger amounts are available for entry into the CNS, even if quite small doses are given. So even in the presence of large amounts of pyridoxine, the peripheral metabolism remains unaffected and the serum levels of levodopa are virtually unaltered.

Importance and management

The levodopa-pyridoxine interaction is clinically important, well-documented and well-established. Doses of pyridoxine as low as 5 mg daily can reduce the effects of levodopa, and should be avoided. Patients should be warned about the self-administration of proprietary pyridoxine-containing preparations. Martindale's Extra Pharmacopoeia lists numerous over-the-counter preparations containing varying amounts of pyridoxine (ranging from 0.1 to 25 mg in each tablet or capsule) many of which could undoubtedly interact to a significant extent. Some breakfast cereals are fortified with pyridoxine and other vitamins, but the amounts are usually too small to matter. For example, a normal serving of Kellogg's Corn Flakes or Rice Krispies (UK preparations) contains only about 0.6 mg pyridoxine, and a whole 500 g packet contains only 9 mg. There is no good clinical evidence to suggest that a low-pyridoxine diet is desirable, and indeed it may be harmful since the normal dietary requirements are about 2 mg daily. The problem of this interaction can be totally solved by using levodopa-carbidopa or levodopa-benserazide preparations (e.g. *Sinemet* or *Madopar*) which are unaffected by pyridoxine.

References

1 Duvoisin RC, Yahr MD and Cote LD. Pyridoxine reversal of L-dopa effects in parkinsonism. Trans Amer Neurol Ass (1969) 94, 81.
2 O'Reilly S. Pyridoxine reversal of L-dopa effects in parkinsonism. Trans Amer Neurol Ass (1969) 94, 81.
3 Markham CH. Pyridoxine reversal of L-dopa effects in parkinsonism. Trans Amer Neurol Ass (1969) 94, 81.
4 Schwab RS. Pyridoxine reversal of L-dopa effects in parkinsonism. Trans Amer Neurol Ass (1969) 94, 81.
5 Celesia GG and Barr AN. Psychosis and other psychiatriac manifestations of levodopa therapy. Arch Neurol (1970) 23, 193.
6 Carter AB. Pyridoxine and parkinsonism. Br Med J (1973) 4, 236.
7 Cotzias GC and Papavasiliou PS. Blocking the negative effects of pyridoxine on patients receiving levodopa. J Amer Med Ass (1971) 215, 1504.
8 Leon AS, Spiegel HE, Thomas G and Abrams WB. Pyridoxine antagonism of levodopa in parkinsonism. J Amer Med Ass (1971) 218, 1924.
9 Hildick-Smith M. Pyridoxine in parkinsonism. Lancet (1973) ii, 1029.
10 Yahr MD and Duvoisin RC. Pyridoxine and levodopa in the treament of parkinsonism. J Amer Med Ass (1972) 220, 861.
11 Mars H. Levodopa, carbidopa and pyridoxine in Parkinson's disease: metabolic interactions. Arch Neurol (1974) 30, 444.
12 Papavasiliou PS, Cotzias GC, Duby SE, Steck AJ, Fehling C and Bell MA. Levodopa in parkinsonism: potentiation of central effects with a peripheral inhibitor. N Engl J Med (1972) 286, 8–14.

Levodopa + Rauwolfia alkaloids

Abstract/Summary

The effects of levodopa are opposed by the concurrent use of rauwolfia alkaloids such as reserpine.

Clinical evidence, mechanism, importance and management

Reserpine and other rauwolfia alkaloids deplete the brain of monoamines, including dopamine, thereby reducing and preventing the effects of dopamine.[1] This opposes the effects of administered levodopa. There are sound pharmacological reasons for believing that this is an interaction of clinical importance and a reduction in the antiparkinsonian activity of levodopa by reserpine has been observed.[2] The rauwolfia alkaloids should be avoided in patients with Parkinson's disease, whether or not they are taking levodopa.

References

1 Bianchine JR and Sunyapridakul L. Interactions between levodopa and other drugs: significance in the treatment of Parkinson's disease. Drugs (1973) 6, 364.
2 Yahr MD. Personal communication (1977).

301

Levodopa + Tricyclic antidepressants

Abstract/Summary

Concurrent use is usually uneventful although a small reduction in the effects of levodopa may occur. Two unexplained hypertensive crises have also occurred when both drugs were used.

Clinical evidence

(a) Reduced levodopa effects

A study in man showed that the concurrent use of imipramine, 100 mg daily for three days, reduced the absorption of a single 500 mg dose of levodopa. Peak serum concentrations of levodopa were reduced about 50% although the 24-h cumulative excretion was not significantly different from the control.[1]

(b) Hypertensive crises

A hypertensive crisis (blood pressure 210/110 mm Hg) associated with agitation, tremor and generalized rigidity developed in a woman taking six tablets of *Sinemet* (levodopa 100 mg + 10 mg carbidopa) when she started to take 25 mg imipramine three times a day. It occurred again when she was later accidentally given the same dosage of amitriptyline.[5]

A similar hypertensive reaction (a rise from 190/110 to 270/140 mm Hg) occurred over 36 h in another woman taking amitriptyline when given half a tablet of *Sinemet* and 10 mg metoclopramine three times a day.[2]

Mechanisms

(a) The tricyclics have anticholinergic activity which slows gastric emptying, and this allows more time for the gastric mucosa to metabolize the levodopa 'wastefully', thereby reducing the amount available for entry into the brain.

(b) The hypertensive reactions are not understood.

Importance and management

Information seems to be limited to these reports. Concurrent use is normally successful and uneventful[3,4,6] but it would be prudent to check that the effects of the levodopa are not undesirably reduced. Also be alert for the possibility of a hypertensive reaction which resolves if the tricyclic antidepressant is withdrawn.

References

1 Morgan JP, Rivera-Calimlim L, Messiha F, Sandaresan PR and Trabert N. Imipramine-mediated interference with levodopa absorption from the gastrointestinal tract in man. Neurology (1975) 25, 1029.
2 Rampton DS. Hypertensive crisis in a patient given Sinemet, metoclopramine and amitriptyline. Br Med J (1977) 3, 607.
3 Yahr MD. The treatment of Parkinsonism—Current concepts. Med Clin N Amer (1972) 56, 1377.
4 Calne DB and Reid JL. Antiparkinsonian drugs: pharmacological and therapeutic aspects. Drugs (1972) 4, 49.
5 Edwards M. Adverse interaction of levodopa with tricyclic antidepressants. The Practitioner (1982) 226, 1448.
6 van Wiegeren A and Wright J. Observations on patients with Parkinson's disease treated with L-dopa. Trial and evaluation of L-dopa therapy. SA Med J (1972) 46, 1262.

10
BETA-BLOCKER
DRUG INTERACTIONS

The adreno-receptors of the sympathetic nervous system are of two main types, namely alpha (α) and beta (β). The beta-adreno-receptor blocking drugs—better known as the beta-blockers—are sufficiently selective to block only the beta-receptors and this property is therapeutically exploited to reduce, for example, the normal sympathetic stimulation of the heart. The activity of the heart in response to stress and exercise is reduced, its consumption of oxygen is diminished, and in this way the angina of effort can be treated. The beta-blockers can also be used in the treatment of cardiac arrhythmias, hypertension, and in the form of eye-drops for glaucoma and ocular hypertension.

Some of the beta-blockers are sufficiently selective to show that all beta-receptors are not identical but can be further subdivided into two groups, beta-1 and beta-2. The former are found in the heart and the latter in the bronchi. Since one of the unwanted side-effects of generalized beta-blockade can be the loss of the normal noradrenaline-stimulated bronchodilation (leading to bronchospasm), there was clear therapeutic advantage in the development of the cardioselective beta-1 blocking drugs (e.g. practolol, metoprolol) which leave the beta-2 receptors virtually unaffected. These cardioselective beta-blockers are therefore particularly valuable in patients such as asthmatics where bronchospasm is clearly unacceptable, although it should be pointed out that the selectivity is not absolute because a few asthmatics even develop bronchospasm with these drugs. Tables 10.1 and 10.2 list most of the beta-blockers currently available.

In addition to the interactions with the beta-blockers detailed in this chapter, there are others discussed elsewhere. See the Index for a full listing.

Table 10.1 Cardioselective beta-blockers (beta-1 receptors only)

Non-proprietary names	Proprietary names
Acebutolol	*Acecor, Alol, Diasectral, Molson, Neptal, Prent, Rhodiasectral, Secadrex, Sectral, Westfalin*
Atenolol	*Atenol, Beta-Adalat, Blokium, Ibinolo, Kalten, Myocord, Neatenol, Prenormine, Seles beta, Telvodin, Tenif, Tenoret(ic), Tenormin(e), Vericordin*
Betaxolol	*Betoptic, Betoptima, Kerlone*
Bevantolol	
Bisoprolol	*Concor, Detensiel, Emcor, Monocor*
Celiprolol	*Selectol*
Esmolol	*Brevibloc*
Metoprolol	*Beloc, Beprolo, Betaloc, Co-betaloc, Lopres(s)or, Metoros, Novometoros, Prelis, Selokeen, Selo-Zok*
Pindolol	*Barbloc, Betadren, Carvisken, Decreten, Durapindol, Hexapindol, Pectobloc, Pinbetol, Viskaldix, Viskeen, Visken(e)*
Practolol	*Dalzic, Eraldin(a)*

Table 10.2 *see overleaf*

Table 10.3 Drugs with both alpha and beta-blocking activity

Non-proprietary names	Proprietary names
Labetolol	*Abetol, Alfabetal, Amipress, Ipolab, Labrocol, Lolum, Mitalolo, Normodyne, Presdate, Pressalolo, Trandate*
Medraxolol	

303

Table 10.2 Non-selective beta-blockers (block beta-1 and beta-2 receptors)

Non-proprietary names	Proprietary names
Alprenolol	*Apllobal, Aptin(e), Aptol, Gubernal, Regletin, Sinalol, Vasoton*
Befunolol	*Bentos, Glauconex*
Bopindolol	*Sandonorm*
Bucindolol	
Bufetolol	*Adobiol*
Bufuralol	
Bunitrolol	*Stresson*
Bupranolol	*Betadran, Betadrenol, Looser, Monobeltin, Ophtorenin, Panimit*
Butofilolol	*Cafide*
Carazolol	*Conducton*
Carteolol	*Arteolol, Arteoptic, Carteol, Endak, Mikelan, Teoptic*
Indenolol	*Pulsan, Securpres*
Levobunolol	*Betagan, Vistagan*
Moprolol	*Levotensin, Omeral*
Mepindolol	*Betagon, Corindolan, Mepicor*
Metipranolol	*Betamann, Betanol, Beta-ophthiole, Disorat, Glauline, Turoptin*
Nadolol	*Corgard, Corgaretic, Solgol*
Nifenalol	*Impeasel, Inpea*
Oxprenolol	*Apsolox, Captol, Laracor, Lo-Tone, Oxanol, Slow-Pren, Trasicor, Trasidex*
Penbutolol	*Betapressin(e), Blocotin, Ipobar, Lasipressin*
Propranolol	*Angilol, Apsolol, Avlocardyl, Bedranol, Beprane, Berkolol, Beta-neg, Betaryl, Beta-Tablinen, Beta-Timelets, Blocardyl, Cartdinol, Cardispare, Caridolol, Deralin, Detensol, Dociton, Efekotolol, Elbrol, Euprovasin, Frekven, Herzul, Inderal(ici), Indobloc, Kemi, Noloten, Novopranol, Pranolol, Prano-puren, Prolol, Pronovan, Propabbloc, Propalong, Propayerst, Propranur, Pur-bloka, Pylapron, Rexigen, Sagittol, Sumial, Tensiflex, Tesnol*
Sotalol	*Beta-cardone, Betades, Sotacor, Sotalex, Sotapor*
Tertatolol	*Artex*
Timolol	*Betim, Blocadren, Blocanol, Cusimolol, Oftan-timolol, Proflax, Temserin, Tenopt, Timacor, Timoptic, Timoptol*

Beta-blockers + Alcohol

Abstract/Summary

The effects metoprolol and atenolol are not changed by the concurrent use of alcohol, nor does propranolol change the effects of alcohol.

Clinical evidence, mechanism, importance and management

A study in eight normal subjects showed that when they were given single 100 mg doses of atenolol or metoprolol 6 h after drinking the equivalent of 200 ml absolute alcohol, no statistically significant changes took place in the pharmacokinetics of either of these beta-blockers, or in blood pressures or pulse rates.[1] A study in 12 normal subjects showed that 160 mg propranolol did not significantly change the performance of a number of psychomotor tests when given with 50 ml/70 kg body weight of alcohol.[2] Another study with propranolol and alcohol suggested that concurrent use may have some effect on divided attention.[3] There do not seem to be any strong reasons for avoiding concurrent use, however your attention is drawn to the synopsis, 'Antihypertensives+Alcohol'.

References

1 Kirch W, Spahn H, Hutt HJ, Ohnhaus EE and Mutschler E. Interaction between alcohol and metoprolol or atenolol in social drinking. Drugs (1983) 25 (Suppl 2) 152.
2 Lindenschmidt R, Brown D, Cerimele B, Walle T and Forney RB. Combined effects of propranolol and ethanol on human psychomotor performance. Toxicol Appl Pharmacol (1983) 67, 117–21.
3 Noble EP, Parker E, Alkana R, Cohen H and Birch H. Propranolol-ethanol interaction in man. Fed Proc (1973) 32, 724.

Beta-blockers + Allopurinol

Abstract/Summary, clinical evidence, mechanism, importance and management.

Allopurinol does not affect the pharmacokinetics of atenolol.[1]

References

1 Schafer-Korting M, Kirch W, Axthelm T, Kohler H and Mutschler E. Atenolol interaction with aspirin, allopurinol, and ampicillin. Clin Pharmacol Ther (1983) 33, 283–8.

Beta-blockers + Antacids

Abstract/Summary

Although some antacids and antidiarrhoeals may cause a modest reduction in the absorption of propranolol, atenolol and other beta-blockers, and possibly an increase in the absorption

of metoprolol, the clinical importance of these interactions is uncertain. It is probably minimal.

Clinical evidence

(a) Propranolol + aluminium hydroxide

A study in six normal subjects given 40 mg propranolol showed that 30 ml aluminium hydroxide gel affected neither the plasma concentrations nor the increases in heart rates caused by exercise.[1]

In contrast, a study in five subjects showed that 30 ml aluminium hydroxide gel given with single 80 mg doses of propranolol caused a reduction in the plasma concentrations of the propranolol and the AUC (area under the plasma-concentration time curve) of almost 60%.[2] Some studies in *animals* have shown that bismuth subsalicylate, kaolin-pectin and magnesium trisilicate can also reduce the absorption of propranolol.[5,6]

(b) Atenolol or metoprolol + aluminium hydroxide or calcium gluconate/carbonate

A study in six normal subjects showed that 5.6 g aluminium hydroxide caused an insignificant fall (20%) in plasma atenolol levels, following a single 100 mg dose. Six hypertensive subjects, given 500 mg calcium as the lactate, gluconate or carbonate, showed a reduction in the absorption of atenolol following a single 100 mg dose, but the half-life was prolonged and the beta-blocking effects were not significantly changed.[3]

Another study showed that an aluminium and magnesium-containing antacid reduced the bioavailability of atenolol 37% but increased that of metoprolol by 25%.[4]

(c) Indenolol + aluminium/magnesium hydroxide/simethicone or kaolin/pectin

A study in *rats* showed that when given indenolol with either *Simeco* or *Kaopectate*, the 6 h AUC (area under the concentration/time curve) were reduced 15 and 30% respectively.[7]

Mechanism

Uncertain. The reduction in absorption could possibly be related to a delay in gastric emptying caused by the antacid, or to some complexation between the two drugs in the gut which reduces absorption.

Importance and management

The documentation of these interactions is limited and in some instances somewhat contradictory. It is also largely confined to single dose or animal studies which may have limited clinical relevance. Although some changes in absorption may occur, nobody seems to have shown that it has a significant effect on the therapeutic use of the beta-blockers. Nevertheless it might be prudent to be on the alert for any changes in the response to beta-blockers during concurrent use. Separating the dosages would seem a simple way of avoiding any problems. There seems to be no information about other beta-blockers or antacids.

References

1 Hong CY, Hu SC, Lin SJ and Chiang BN. Lack of influence of aluminium hydroxide on the bioavailability and beta-adrenoceptor blocking activity of propranolol. Int J Clin Pharmacol Ther Toxicol (1985) 23, 244–46.

2 Dobbs JH, Skoutakis VA, Acchardio SR and Dobbs BR. Effects of aluminium hydroxide on the absorption of propranolol. Curr Ther Res (1977) 21, 887.

3 Kirch W, Schafer-Korting M, Axthelm T, Kohler H and Mutschle E. Interaction of furosemide and calcium and aluminium salts. Clin Pharmacol Ther (1981) 30, 429–35.

4 Regardh CG, Lundborg P and Persson BA. The effect of antacid, metoclopramide and propantheline on the bioavailability of metoprolol and atenolol. Biopharm Drug Dispos (1981) 2, 79–87.

5 Moustafa MA, Gouda MW and Tariq M. Decreased bioavailability of propranolol due to interactions with adsorbent antacids and anti-diarrhoeal mixtures. Int J Pharmaceutics (1986) 30, 225–8.

6 McElnay JC, D'Arcy PF and Leonard JK. The effect of activated dimethicone, other antacid constituents, and kaolin on the absorption of propranolol. Experentia (1982) 38, 605–7.

7 Tariq M and Babhair SA. Effect of antacid and antidiarrhoeal drugs on the bioavailability of indenolol. IRCS Med Sci (1984) 12, 87–8.

Beta-blockers + Anticholinesterases

Abstract/Summary

A small number of reports describe marked bradycardia and hypotension during the recovery period from anaesthesia and neuromuscular blockade in patients on beta-blockers when given anticholinesterase drugs.

Clinical evidence

A patient taking nadolol and recovering from surgery during which succinylcholine had been used for tracheal intubation and pancuronium for general muscular relaxation, developed prolonged bradycardia (32–36 bpm) and hypotension (systolic pressure 60–70 torr) when neostigmine and atropine were given to reverse the neuromuscular blockade.[1] Another patient on propranolol and anaesthetized with N_2O/O_2 and alcuronium also developed severe bradycardia (a fall from 65 to 40 bpm) and hypotension (systolic pressure 70 mmHg) when given physostigmine.[2] Prolonged bradycardia and hypotension were seen in an elderly woman on atenolol when given neostigmine and atropine for the reversal of muscle relaxation at the end of general anaesthesia.[6] Other reports similarly describe this effect when neostigmine was used.[3–5] The reason appears to be due to the additive heart-slowing effects of the beta-blockers and the acetylcholine-like effects of these anticholinesterase drugs which, in the instances cited, were not adequately controlled by the use of atropine. There seem to be few reports describing these adverse effects.

References

1 Seidl DC and Martin DE. Prolonged bradycardia after neostigmine administration in a patient taking nadolol. Anesth Analg (1984) 63, 365–7.

2 Baraka A and Dajani A. Severe bradycardia following physostigmine in the presence of beta-adrenergic blockade. Middle Eastern J Anaesthesiology (1984) 7, 291–3.

3 Sprague DH. Severe bradycardia after neostigmine in a patient taking propranolol to control paroxsymal atrial tachycardia. Anesthesiology (1975) 42, 208–10.

4 Wagner DL, Moorthy SS and Stoertling RK. Administration of anti-cholinesterase drugs in the presence of beta-blockade. Anesth Analg (1982) 61, 153–4.

5 Prys-Roberts C. Cardiovascular responses to anaesthesia and surgery in patients receiving beta-receptor antagonists. In 'Beta-blockade and Anaesthesia', Poppers PJ, van Dijk B and van Elzakker AH M. (eds). Rijswijk, Netherlands: Astra Pharmaceutica (1980) 164–70.

6 Eldor J, Hoffmann B and Davidson JT. Prolonged bradycardia and hypotension after neostigmine administration in a patient receiving atenolol. Anaesthesia (1987) 42, 1294–7.

Beta-blockers + Barbiturates

Abstract/Summary

The serum levels and the therapeutic effects of those beta-blockers which are mainly removed from the body by liver metabolism (e.g. propranolol, alprenolol, metoprolol, etc.) are reduced by the concurrent use of barbiturates. Alprenolol concentrations are halved, but the others are possibly not affected as much. Beta-blockers which are mainly lost unchanged in the urine (e.g. atenolol, sotalol, nadolol, etc.) are not affected by the barbiturates.

Clinical evidence

A study in six patients with essential hypertension, treated with 400 mg alprenolol twice daily, showed that while taking 100 mg pentobarbitone at bedtime for 10 days their alprenolol serum levels were reduced by 59%. Mean pulse rates at rest rose by 6% (from 67 to 75 bpm) and blood pressures rose 8–9% (from 138/93 to 143/97 mm Hg). In a further study on the same patients, resting pulse rates rose from 70 to 74 bpm, and their blood pressures rose from 134/89 to 145/97 mm Hg within 4–5 days of starting the barbiturate, and fell once again within 8–9 days of stopping.[6]

These results confirm previous studies by the same authors and others: Pentobarbitone was found to cause a 40% reduction in serum alprenolol levels after a single 200 mg dose of alprenolol. There was also a 20% reduction in the effects of the beta-blocker on the heart rate during exercise.[2] The AUC (area under the time/concentration curve) of alprenolol was reduced by about 80% after 100 mg pentobarbitone daily for 10–14 days.[1] Other studies have shown that 100 mg pentobarbitone for 10 days reduced the AUC of metoprolol by 32% (eight normal subjects),[3] and 100 mg phenobarbitone daily for seven days reduced the AUC of timolol by 24% (12 normal subjects).[4] Phenobarbitone also seems to increase the clearance of propranolol, but not sotalol.[5]

Mechanism

Barbiturates are potent liver enzyme inducing agents which can increase the metabolism and clearance of other drugs from the body. Those beta-blockers which are removed from the body principally by liver metabolism (e.g. alprenolol, propranolol, metoprolol, timolol, etc.) can therefore be cleared more quickly in the presence of a barbiturate, whereas other beta-blockers which are lost mainly unchanged in the urine (e.g. sotalol) are not affected.

Importance and management

The alprenolol–pentobarbitone interaction is well documented and of clear clinical importance when the beta-blocker is being used to treat hypertension, and possibly angina. Since blood levels are roughly halved, it seems reasonable to expect that the dosage will need to be doubled to accommodate this interaction. This needs confirmation. All of the barbiturates would be expected to do the same. A reduced response is likely with any of the beta-blockers which are extensively metabolized (e.g. propranolol, metoprolol, alprenolol, timolol, etc.), but the effects on the AUC's of metoprolol and timolol are less than with alprenolol (32%, 24% and 80% respectively) so that the dosage increases needed may also be less. Detailed information about propranolol and other beta-blockers is lacking. The interaction can almost certainly be avoided by using one of the beta-blockers which are primarily lost unchanged in the urine (e.g. atenolol, sotalol, nadolol, etc.).

References

1 Alvan G, Piafsky K, Lind M and von Bah C. Effect of pentobarbital on the disposition of alprenolol. Clin Pharmacol Ther (1977) 22, 316.
2 Collste P, Seideman P, Borg K-O, Haglund K and von Bah C. Influence of pentobarbital on effects and plasma levels of alprenolol and 4-hydroxy-alprenolol. Clin Pharmacol Ther (1979) 25, 423–7.
3 Haglund K, Seiderman P, Collste P, Borg K-O and von Bah C. Influence of pentobarbital on metoprolol plasma levels. Clin Pharmacol Ther (1979) 26, 326.
4 Mantyla R, Mannisto P, Nykanen S, Kopenen A and Lamminsivu U. Pharmacokinetic interactions of timolol with vasodilating drugs, food and phenobarbitone in healthy volunteers. Eur J Clin Pharmacol (1983) 24, 227–30.
5 Sotaniemi EA, Anttila M, Pelkonen RO, Jarvensivu P and Sundquist H. Plasma clearance of propranolol and sotalol and hepatic drug-metabolizing activity. Clin Pharmacol Ther (1979) 26, 153–161.
6 Seideman P, Borg K-O, Haglund K and von Bah C. Decreased plasma concentrations and clinical effects of alprenolol during combined treatment with pentobarbitone in hypertension. Br J clin Pharmac (1987) 23, 267–71.

Beta-blockers + Calcium channel blockers

Abstract/Summary

Concurrent use appears to be common and useful. Felodipine raises serum metoprolol levels and nisoldipine raises serum propranolol levels but this does not appear to be clinically undesirable. (See also other synopses about beta-blockers + diltiazem, nifedipine, verapamil.)

Clinical evidence

(a) Felodipine

A double-blind crossover study in eight normal subjects showed that, over a five-day period, metoprolol (100 mg twice daily) did not affect the pharmacokinetics of felodipine (10 mg twice daily). On the other hand the bioavailability of metoprolol was increased by 30% and its peak serum levels by 38%.[1] Another study in 10 normal subjects given 10 mg felodipine with either 100 mg metoprolol, 5 mg pindolol, 80 mg propranolol or 10 mg timolol found no changes in heart rate, PR interval or blood pressure which was considered to be harmful to patients with hypertension or angina,[2] however seven of the ten reported some increase in adverse reactions.

(b) Nisoldipine

12 normal subjects were given single oral doses of 20 mg nisoldipine and 40 mg propranolol. The propranolol AUC was increased by 43% and the peak serum concentration by 68%. The degree of beta-blockade was increased. The nisoldipine AUC was increased by 30% and the peak serum concentration by 57%.[3]

Mechanism

Not understood. A possible reason is that the metabolism of the beta-blockers is changed by changes in blood flow through the liver.

Importance and management

The concurrent use of beta-blockers and calcium channel blockers is common and normally valuable but not always entirely free of problems. Serious cardiodepression has been seen in a few patients on beta-blockers given nifedipine, diltiazem and particularly verapamil (see 'Beta-blockers + Diltiazem', 'Beta-blockers + Nifedipine', 'Beta-blockers + Verapamil'). Information about other calcium channel blockers and beta-blockers is much more limited but against this background it would seem prudent to monitor concurrent use for any evidence of undesirable cardiodepression.

References

1 Smith SR, Wilkins MR, Jack DB, Kendall MJ and Laugher S. Pharmacokinetic interactions between felodipine and metoprolol. Eur J Clin Pharmacol (1987) 31, 575–8.
2 Carruthers SG and Bailey DG. Tolerance and cardiovascular effects of single dose felodipine/beta-blocker combinations in healthy subjects. J Cardiovasc Pharmacol (1987) 10 (Suppl 1) S169–77.
3 Levine MAH, Ogilvie RI and Leenen FHH. Pharmacokinetic and pharmacodynamic interactions between nisoldipine and propranolol. Clin Pharmacol Ther (1988) 43, 39–48.

Beta-blockers + Cholestyramine or Colestipol

Abstract/Summary

Although both cholestyramine and colestipol can reduce the absorption of propranolol to some extent, this does not seem to reduce its effects.

Clinical evidence

(a) Cholestyramine

A study on six normal subjects showed that when single 120 mg doses of propranolol and 8 g doses of cholestyramine were taken together, peak propranolol serum levels were reduced by almost 25% and the area under the curve (AUC) was reduced 13%. When given an additional dose of cholestyramine 12 h before the propanolol, the AUC was reduced by 43%. No changes in blood pressures or pulse rates were observed.[2] A study on five patients with type II hyperlipidaemia on 160 mg propranolol daily demonstrated no significant changes in blood levels of propranolol after being given a single (unstated) dose of cholestyramine.[1]

(b) Colestipol

A study in six normal subjects showed that when single 120 mg doses of propranolol and 10 mg doses of colestipol were taken together, the peak serum propranolol levels were raised. But they were decreased if an additional 10 mg dose of colestipol was taken 12 h before the propranolol, and the AUC was reduced by about 30%. No changes in blood pressure or pulse rates were seen.[2]

Mechanism

Uncertain. It seems probable that both the cholestyramine and colestipol can bind to the propranolol in the gut, thereby reducing its absorption.

Importance and management

Information is limited. Even though both cholestyramine and colestipol can apparently reduce the absorption of propranolol, no changes in its pharmacological effects were reported[2] which suggests that the interaction is clinically unimportant. There is no obvious reason for avoiding concurrent use. There seems to be no information about other beta-blockers.

References

1 Schwartz DE, Schaeffer E, Brewer HB and Franciosa JA. Bioavailability of propranolol following administration of cholestyramine. Clin Pharmacol Ther (1982) 31, 268.
2 Hibbard DM, Peters JR and Hunninghake DB. Effects of cholestyramine and colestipol on the plasma concentrations of propranolol. Br J clin Pharmac (1984) 18, 337–42.

Beta-blockers + Cimetidine

Abstract/Summary

The blood levels of beta-blockers which are extensively metabolized by the liver (e.g. metoprolol, propranolol) can be doubled by the concurrent use of cimetidine, but normally this appears to be clinically unimportant. No important interaction normally seems to occur with other beta-blockers. An isolated report describes profound bradycardia (heart rate 36 beats/min) in a patient given atenolol and cimetidine, and marked postural hypotension occurred in another patient on labetalol and cimetidine.

Clinical evidence

(a) Propranolol + cimetidine

12 normal subjects were given 1.2 g cimetidine daily for a week. From day 3 onwards they were also given two 80 mg daily doses of propranolol, morning and evening, until the end of the week. The mean steady-state blood levels of propranolol were raised 57%, the AUC (area under the concentration-time curve) increased 47% and the half-life was prolonged by 17%, but heart rates remained unchanged.[1]

A number of other single-dose and steady-state studies confirm that cimetidine can cause marked rises (up to 100%) in blood levels of propranolol[2–7] but no changes occur in either resting or exercised heart rates,[3,5–7] nor in blood pressures.[5,7] In contrast, one study showed a reduction in pulse rates.[16] One patient given 1 g cimetidine daily for six weeks showed an approximately threefold increase in serum propranolol level (AUC + 340%) when given a single 80 mg dose of propranolol.[11]

(b) Atenolol, betaxolol, nadolol, penbutolol or pindolol + cimetidine

A report describes a patient taking atenolol for angina who developed profound sinus bradycardia (36 beats/min) and hypotension when additionally treated with cimetidine.[11,12] The original report does not specifically name atenolol, but it is identified elsewhere in a letter.[12] In contrast, well-controlled studies in other subjects have shown that cimetidine does not normally significantly alter blood levels of atenolol[6,8–10], nor does it affect heart rates whether resting or exercised.[9,10] Blood levels of betaxolol[21] and nadolol[5] are similarly unaffected. Pindolol and penbutolol plasma levels are slightly raised or unaffected, but exercise-induced heart rates are not changed.[17,19]

(c) Metoprolol + cimetidine

A study in six normal subjects given 100 mg metoprolol daily for a week showed that the concurrent use of 1 g cimetidine daily[6] increased the peak plasma levels by 70% and the AUC rose by 61%, but there were no changes in resting or exercised heart rates, nor in blood pressures.[6] Some other studies confirm that cimetidine increases metoprolol serum levels[8,13,14,20] whereas another did not.[9] No changes in exercised heart rates were seen.[14,20]

(d) Labetalol (an alpha- and beta-blocker) + cimetidine

A study in three normal subjects showed that the bioavailability of labetalol was increased about 80% after four days treatment with cimetidine (1 g daily).[15] One subject in a related study developed postural hypotension (70/40 mm Hg), felt lightheaded and almost fainted on standing.[18]

Mechanism

The blood levels of beta-blockers extensively metabolized by liver (propranolol, metoprolol and penbutolol) are increased because cimetidine reduces their metabolism, both by inhibiting the activity of the liver enzymes and by reducing the flow of blood to the liver.[6,17] Those beta-blockers which are not metabolized to a significant extent (atenolol, nadolol) are not affected because they are largely excreted unchanged in the urine.[5,10] Pindolol[17] falls between these two groups of drugs.

Importance and management

The concurrent use of beta-blockers and cimetidine has been well studied yet, despite the very considerable rises in blood levels which can occur with some beta-blockers, the effects of these interactions normally appear—perhaps surprisingly—to be clinically unimportant. Concurrent use is common but only one case of profound bradycardia involving atenolol (see case cited above) appears to have been reported. Marked hypotension also seems to be rare. Combined use need not be avoided, however it has been suggested that patients with impaired liver function who are given beta-blockers which are extensively metabolized (metoprolol, propranolol, etc.) might possibly develop grossly elevated blood levels which could cause adverse effects. This needs confirmation.

References

1 Donn KH, Powell JR, Rogers JF and Eshelman FN. The influence of H$_2$-receptor antagonists on steady-state concentrations of propranolol and 4-hydroxypropranolol. J Clin Pharmacol (1984) 24, 500–8.

2 Kirsch W, Kohler H, Spahn H and Mutschler I. Interaction of cimetidine with metoprolol, propranolol or atenolol. Lancet (1981) ii, 531

3 Reimann IW, Klotz U and Frohlich JC. Effects of cimetidine and ranitidine on steady-state propranolol kinetics and dynamics. Clin Pharmacol Ther (1982) 32, 749–57.

4 Reimann IW, Klotz U, Siems B and Frohlich JC. Cimetidine increases steady-state plasma levels of propranolol. Br J clin Pharmac (1981) 12, 785–90.

5 Duchin KL, Stern MA, Willard DA and McKinstry DN. Comparison of kinetic interactions of nadolol and propranolol with cimetidine. Am Heart J (1984) 108, 1084–6.

6 Kirch W, Spahn H, Kohler H and Mutschler E. Accumulation and adverse effects of metoprolol and propranolol after concurrent administration of cimetidine. Arch Toxicol (1983) Suppl 6, 379–83.

7 Markiewicz A, Hartleb M, Lelek A, Boldys H and Nowak A. The effect of treatment with cimetidine and ranitidine on bioavailability of, and circulatory response to, propranolol. Zbl Pharm (1984) 123, 516–8.

8 Kirch W, Spahn H, Kohler H and Mutschler E. Interaction of metoprolol, propranolol and atenolol with cimetidine. Clin Sci (1982) 63, 451s-53s.

9 Houtzagers JJR, Streurman O, and Regardh CG. The effect of pretreatment with cimetidine on the bioavailability and disposition of atenolol and metoprolol. Br J clin Pharmac (1982) 14, 67–72.

10 Ellis ME, Hussain M, Webb AK, Barker NP and Fitzsimons TJ. The effect of cimetidine on the relative cardioselectivity of atenolol and metoprolol in asthmatic patients. Br J clin Pharmac (1984) 17, 59S-64S.

11 Donovan MA, Heagerty AM, Patel L, Castleden M and Pohl JEF. Lancet (1981) i, 164.

12 Rowley-Jones D and Flind AC. Drug interactions with cimetidine. Pharm J (1981) 283, 659.

13 Kendall MJ, Laugher SJ and Wilkins MR. Ranitidine, cimetidine and metoprolol. Gastroenterol (1986) 90, 1490.

14 Kirch W, Ramsch K, Janisch HD and Ohnhaus EE. The influence of two histamine H$_2$-receptor anagonists, cimetidine and ranitidine, on

15 Daneshmend TK and Roberts CJC. Cimetidine and bioavailability of labetolol. Lancet (1981), i, 505.

16 Feeley J, Wilkinson GR and Wood AJJ. Reduction in liver blood flow and propranolol metabolism by cimetidine. N Engl J Med (1981) 304, 692–5.

17 Spahn H, Kirch W and Mutschler E. The interaction of cimetidine with metoprolol, atenolol, propranolol, pindolol and penbutolol. Br J clin Pharmac (1983) 15, 500–1.

18 Daneshmend TK and Roberts CJC. The effects of enzyme induction and enzyme inhibition on labetalol pharmacokinetics. Br J clin Pharmac (1984) 18, 393–400.

19 Spahn H, Kirsch W, Hajdu P, Mutschler E and Ohnhaus EL. Penbutolol pharmacokinetics: the influence of concomitant administration of cimetidine. Eur J Clin Pharmacol (1986) 29, 555–60.

20 Toon S, Davidson EM, Garstang FM, Batra H, Bowers RJ and Rowland M. The racemic metoprolol H2-antagonist interaction. Clin Pharmacol Ther (1988) 43, 283–9.

21 Rey E, Jammet P, d'Athis P, de Lauture D, Christoforov B, Weber S, Olive G. Effect of cimetidine on the pharmacokinetics of the new beta-blocker betaxolol. Arzneim-Forsch./Drug Res (1987) 37, 953–6.

plasma levels and clinical effect of nifedipine and metoprolol. Arch toxicol (1984) Suppl 7, 256–9.

Beta-blockers + Cimetidine + Phenylephrine

Abstract/Summary

A patient undergoing surgery had a low blood pressure probably resulting from an exaggeration of the effects of labetalol due to an interaction with cimetidine. Bronchospasm occurred later, probably as a result of the combined actions of labetalol and phenylephrine.

Clinical evidence, mechanism, importance and management

An elderly asthmatic patient, treated with nitrates and labetalol (650 mg) for unstable angina and hypertension before surgery for double aortocoronary vein grafting, was given cimetidine (400 mg) as part of his premedication. During the surgery, hypotension (40–45 mm Hg) occurred despite phenylephrine 14 mg. This was followed during rewarming by a rise in pressure to 150 mm Hg, and on cessation of bypass, protracted bronchospasm was seen.[1] The possible reasons are that the cimetidine reduced the metabolism and clearance of the labetalol (see 'Beta-blockers + Cimetidine'). The increase in its alpha-blocking (vasodilating) effects opposed the alpha-stimulating (vasoconstrictor) effects of the phenylephrine so that the blood pressure was low. Later the beta-blocking effects of the labetalol and the alpha-stimulating effects of the phenylephrine combined to cause bronchospasm. The authors of the report point out that higher doses of phenylephrine may be needed in the presence of labetalol, but that this may carry an increased risk of bronchospasm in asthmatic patients.

Reference

1 Durant PAC and Joucken K. Bronchospasm and hypotension during cardiopulmonary bypass after preoperative cimetidine and labetalol therapy. Br J Anaesth (1984) 56, 917–20.

Beta-blockers + Contraceptives (oral)

Abstract/Summary

The blood levels of metoprolol are increased in women taking oral contraceptives, but the clinical importance is uncertain.

Clinical evidence

A study[1] in 12 women on a low-dose combined oral contraceptive showed that the peak serum level and the area under the concentration-time curve of metoprolol, following a single 100 mg oral dose, were increased by 36 and 70% respectively when compared with a similar group not taking the pill. It seems likely that this is because the pill inhibits the metabolism of the metoprolol.

The clinical effects of interaction seem not to have been studied, but changes of this size caused by interactions of other drugs with beta-blockers do not usually have clinically important effects. Beta-blockers such as propranolol which are metabolized similarly are possibly affected in the same way, but not those which are largely excreted unchanged in the urine (e.g. atenolol).

Reference

1 Kendall MJ, Quarterman CP, Jack DB and Beeley L. Metoprolol pharmacokinetics and the oral contraceptive pill. Br J clin Pharmacol (1982) 14, 120–2.

Beta-blockers + Dextromoramide

Abstract/Summary

Two patients developed marked bradycardia and severe hypotension when given propranolol and dextromoramide following the induction of anaesthesia.

Clinical evidence, mechanism, importance and management

Two women about to undergo partial thyroidectomy were given 30 mg propranolol and dextromoramide (1.25 and 4 mg respectively) by injection during the pre-operative period following the induction of anaesthesia with a barbiturate. Each developed marked bradycardia and severe hypotension which responded rapidly to the intravenous injection of atropine.[1] The reasons for this response are not understood.

Reference

1 Cabanne F, Wilkening M, Caillard B, Foissac JC and Aupecle P. Interferences medicamenteuses induites par l'association propranolol-dextromoramide. Anesth Anal Rean (1973) 30, 369–75.

Beta-blockers + Dextropropoxyphene

Abstract/Summary

A single dose study has shown that the bioavailability of metoprolol is markedly increased—and of propranolol to a lesser extent—by the concurrent use of dextropropoxyphene. There seem to be no reports of adverse reactions when both drugs are used.

Clinical evidence, mechanism, importance and management

A single dose study in normal subjects showed that after taking dextropropoxyphene for a day (dose not stated) the bioavailability of metoprolol (100 mg orally) was increased almost fourfold and the total body clearance was reduced 18%. The bioavailability of propranolol (40 mg orally) was increased by about 70%.[1] The probable reason is that the dextropropoxyphene inhibits the metabolism of these beta-blockers by the liver so that they are cleared from the body more slowly. From this it would be expected that the effects of these beta-blockers would be markedly increased, but there seems to be no other evidence that concurrent use presents any problems. Nevertheless it would seem prudent to monitor the effects of giving both drugs. No interaction would be expected with those beta-blockers which, unlike metoprolol and propranolol, are largely excreted unchanged in the urine (e.g. nadolol, sotalol, atenolol, etc.)

Reference

1 Lundborg P and Regard CG. The effect of propoxyphene pretreatment on the disposition of metoprolol and propranolol. Clin Pharmacol Ther (1981) 29, 263–4.

Beta-blockers + Diltiazem

Abstract/Summary

Concurrent use is normally safe and uneventful but a patient on pindolol and another on sotalol have been described who developed profound bradycardia when given diltiazem.

Clinical evidence

The concurrent use of beta-blockers and diltiazem is common, appears to be valuable and is normally without major problems,[1–4] but adverse effects have also been described.

Profound bradycardia and unconsciousness occurred in a 68-year-old woman, treated with 320 mg sotalol daily for supraventricular tachycardia and ventricular premature beats, two days after starting to take 60 mg diltiazem three times a day. Her pulse rate fell to 15 bpm and her blood pressure was unrecordable. Another woman of 77 on 30 mg pindolol three times daily became cold and dizzy 2 h after taking a first 60 mg dose of diltiazem. Her pulse rate fell to 25 bpm and systolic blood pressure to 70 mm Hg.[5]

These responses seem to be extreme examples of the brady-arrhythmias seen in some patients when given propranolol and diltiazem.[6]

Mechanism

Other calcium channel blockers such as verapamil, and to a lesser extent nifedipine, when combined with beta-blockers also occasionally cause marked bradycardia, hypotension and even asystole (see appropriate synopses). The probable reason is that the heart slowing effects of the beta-blocker are additive with the effects of the delay in conduction through the atrioventricular node caused by the calcium channel blockers.

Importance and management

Information about serious adverse effects when beta-blockers and diltiazem are given together seems to be confined to the reports cited here. There seems to be no compelling reason for avoiding the concurrent use of beta-blockers and diltiazem but the outcome should be well monitored.

References

1 Tilmant PY, Lablanche JM, Thieuleux FA, Dupuis BA and Bertrand ME. Detrimental effect of propranolol in patients with coronary arterial spasm countered by combination with diltiazem. Am J Cardiol (1983) 52, 230–33.
2 Rocha P, Baron B, Delestrain A, Pathe M, Cazor J-L and Kahn J-C. Hemodynamic effects of intravenous diltiazem in patients treated chronically with propranolol. Am Heart J (1986) 111, 62.
3 Humen DP, O'Brien P, Puves P, Johnson D and Kostuk WJ. Effort angina with adequate beta-receptor blockade: comparison with diltiazem alone and in combination. J Am Coll Cardiol (1986) 7, 329–35.
4 Kostuk WJ and Plugfelder P. Comparative effects of calcium entry blocking drugs, beta-blocking drugs and their combination in patients with chronic stable angina. Circulation (1987) 75, (Suppl V), 114–21.
5 Hassell AB and Creamer JE. Profound bradycardia after the addition of diltiazen to a beta-blocker. Br Med J (1989) 298, 675.
6 O'Hara MJ, Khurmi NS, Bowles MJ and Raftery BB. Diltiazem and propranolol combination for the treatment of chronic stable angina pectoris. Clin Cardiol (1987) 10, 115–23.

Beta-blockers + Enprostil

Abstract/Summary

Enprostil is reported not to interact with propranolol.

Clinical evidence, mechanism, importance and management

A double-blind crossover study in nine healthy subjects showed that after taking 70 μg enprostil twice daily for six days the elimination of propranolol given orally or intravenously was not affected (whereas it was affected by cimetidine).[1] No special precautions seem necessary during concurrent use. Direct information about other beta-blockers is lacking, but it seems likely that they will behave similarly.

Reference

1 Reilly CS, Biollaz J, Koshakji RP and Wood AJJ. Enprostil, in contrast to cimetidine, does not inhibit propranolol metabolism. Clin Pharmacol Ther (1986) 40, 37–41.

Beta-blockers + Ergotamine or Methysergide

Abstract/Summary

The concurrent use of beta-blockers and ergotamine for the treatment of migraine is usually safe and effective, but three cases of severe peripheral vasoconstriction have been described. There is also an isolated case of an exacerbation of migraine.

Clinical evidence

A man with recurrent migraine headaches, reasonably well-controlled over a six-year period with two daily suppositories of *Cafergot* (ergotamine tartrate 2 g, caffeine 100 mg, butalbital 100 mg, belladonna leaf alkaloids 250 μg) developed progressively painful and purple feet a short while after additionally starting to take 30 mg propranolol daily. When he eventually resumed taking the *Cafergot* alone there was no further evidence of peripheral vasoconstriction.[1]

A similar situation occurred in a woman taking oxprenolol and ergotamine tartrate (dosages unknown) for some considerable time, as well as a number of other drugs.[4] Another report describes a similar reaction in a man after taking 3 mg methysergide and 120 mg propranolol daily for two weeks.[4] It was necessary to amputate both his legs below the knee because of gangrene.

These reports contrast with another stating that concurrent use in 50 patients was both effective and uneventful.[3] The exacerbation of migraine has also been described in a single patient.[2]

Mechanism

Uncertain. One suggestion to explain the vasoconstriction is that the effects of the two drugs are additive.[1,4] Ergot causes vasoconstriction. The beta-blockers do the same by blocking the normal (beta-2-stimulated) sympathetic vasodilatation. The beta-blockers also reduce blood flow by reducing cardiac output.

Importance and management

Concurrent use is usually safe and effective, and there are only three reports of adverse interactions. However it would clearly be prudent to be on the alert for any signs of an adverse response.

References

1 Baumarucker JF. Drug interaction—propranolol and cafergot. N Engl J Med (1973) 288, 916.

2 Blank NK and Rieder MJ. Paradoxical response to propranolol in migraine. Lancet (1973) ii, 1336.
3 Diamond S. Propranolol and ergotamine tartrate (cont.) N Engl J Med (1973) 289, 159.
4 Venter CP, Joubert PH and Buys AC. Severe peripheral ischaemia during concomitant use of beta-blockers and ergot alkaloids. Brit Med J (1984) 2, 289.

Beta-blockers + Erythromycin or Neomycin

Abstract/Summary

Erythromycin and neomycin can increase the serum concentrations of nadolol, but the clinical importance of this is not known.

Clinical evidence, mechanism, importance and management

In eight normal subjects given either 0.5 g neomycin or 0.5 g erythromycin, four times a day for two days, the peak serum nadolol concentration after a single 80 mg oral dose more than doubled (from 146 to 397 ng/ml). The AUC (area under the concentration/time curve) stayed the same but its half-life fell from 17.3 to 11.6 h.[1] The reasons are not understood. More study is needed to find out whether this interaction is of clinical importance. The effects of concurrent use should be monitored. No information seems to be available about other beta-blockers.

Reference

1 du Souich P, Caille G and Larochelle P. Enhancement of nadolol elimination by activated charcoal and antibiotics. Clin Pharmacol Ther (1983) 33, 585–90.

Beta-blockers + Etintidine

Abstract/Summary

The serum levels of propranolol can be markedly increased by etintidine.

Clinical evidence

A study in 12 normal subjects given single 40 mg oral doses of propranolol showed that after taking 400 mg etintidine twice daily for four days the AUC (area under the propranolol concentration time curve) increased by almost 300% (from 146 to 573 ng.h/ml). The elimination half-life and peak serum concentrations doubled and the clearance fell from 102 to 441 l/h.[1]

Mechanism

The probable explanation is that etintidine which is a chemical analogue of cimetidine can (like cimetidine) inhibit the metabolism of the propranolol by the liver, thereby reducing its loss from the body.

Importance and management

Direct information seems to be limited to this single dose study. Its clinical importance is uncertain but the changes seen are so large that increased propranolol effects would be expected. Monitor the effects if etintidine is added or withdrawn. Ranitidine is a non-interacting alternative (see 'Beta-blockers+Ranitidine') and neither nizatidine nor famotidine would be expected to interact. The beta-blockers which interact with cimetidine (see 'Beta-blockers+Cimetidine') would also be expected to interact with etintidine. Thus metoprolol, penbutolol and labetolol are metabolized like propranolol and would be expected to interact similarly, but not nadolol or atenolol.

Reference

1 Huang S-M, Weintraub HS, Marriott TB, Marinan B and Abels R. Etintidine-propranolol interaction study in humans. J Pharmacokinet Biopharm (1987) 15, 557–67.

Beta-blockers + Flecainide

Abstract/Summary

Propranolol and flecainide do not appear to interact together adversely.

Clinical evidence, mechanism, importance and management

A study in 10 normal subjects on cardiac function and drug clearance found that the AUC's (areas under the concentration-time curves) of propranolol and flecainide were increased 20–30% when given together, and they had some additive negative inotropic effects on the heart. The only caution suggested by the authors of the report is if treatment with these drugs is initiated in patients with impaired left ventricular function.[1]

Reference

1 Holtzman JL, Kvam DC, Berry DA, Mottonen L, Borrell G, Harrison LI and Conard GJ. The pharmacodynamic and pharmacokinetic interaction of flecainide acetate with propranolol: effects on cardiac function and drug clearance. Eur J Clin Pharmacol (1987) 33, 97–9.

Beta-blockers + Food

Abstract/Summary

Food can increase, decrease or not affect the bioavailability of beta-blockers, but none of the changes has been shown to be of importance.

Clinical evidence, mechanism, importance and management

Food increases the bioavailability of propranolol and metoprolol by 30–80%,[1–3] and of labetalol by about 40%[4] by changing the extent of their metabolism during their first pass through the liver. Food has very little effect on the absorption of oxprenolol[5,6] or pindolol,[8] whereas the bioavailability of atenolol is reduced about 20%.[7] None of these changes has been shown to be of clinical importance, and it is not clear whether it matters if patients take these drugs in a regular pattern in relation to meals.

References

1 Melander A, Danielson K, Schersten B and Wahlin E. Enhancement of the bioavailability of propranolol and metoprolol by food. Clin Pharmacol Ther (1977) 22, 108–12.
2 Liedholm H and Melander A. Concomitant food intake can increase the bioavailability of propranolol by transient inhibition of its presystemic primary conjugation. Clin Pharmacol Ther (1986) 40, 29–36.
3 McLean AJ, Isbister C, Bobik A and Dudley F. Reduction of first-pass hepatic clearance of propranolol by food. Clin Pharmacol Ther (1981) 30, 31–4.
4 Daneshmend TK and Roberts CJC. The influence of food on the oral and intravenous pharmacokinetics of a high clearance drug: a study with labetalol. Br J Clin Pharmacol (1982) 14, 73–8.
5 Dawes CP, Kendall MJ and Welling PG. Bioavailability of conventional and slow-release oxprenolol in fasted and non-fasted individuals. Br J clin Pharmac (1979) 7, 299–302.
6 John VA and Smith SE. Influence of food intake on plasma oxprenolol concentrations following oral administration of conventional and Oros preparations. Br J clin Pharmac (1985) 19, 191–5S.
7 Melander A, Stenberg P, Liedholm H, Schersten B and Wahlin-Boll E. Food-induced reduction in bioavailability of atenolol. Eur J Clin Pharmacol (1979) 16, 327–30.
8 Kiger JL, Lavene D, Guillaume MF, Guerret M and Longchampt J. The effect of food and clopamide on the absorption of pindolol in man. Int J Clin Pharmacol (1976) 13, 228–32.

Beta-blockers + Halofenate

Abstract/Summary

The serum levels and the therapeutic effects of propranolol can be reduced by the concurrent use of halofenate.

Clinical evidence

In a cross-over study four healthy subjects were given 1 g halofenate or a placebo daily for 21 days. During the last two days they were given either 80 or 160 mg of propranolol. Their steady-state plasma levels of propranolol were reduced by 74 and 81% respectively. The reduction in the beta-blocking effects were checked using isoprenaline and the cardiac response correlated with the reduction in beta-blockade in three of the four subjects.[1]

Mechanism

Unknown. One idea is that the halofenate increases the metabolism and clearance of the propranolol from the body.[1]

Importance and management

Information seems to be confined to this study, but this interaction would seem to be established.[1] Such a large reduction in serum propranolol levels would be expected to cause a reduction in the control of hypertension and angina. If both drugs are given, the response should be monitored, anticipating the need to increase the propranolol dosage. If the mechanism of interaction suggested above is true, then an interaction with other beta-blockers which are extensively metabolized (e.g. alprenolol, metoprolol, timolol) also seems a possibility.

References

1 Huffman DH, Azarnoff DL, Shoeman DW and Dujorne CA. The interaction between halofenate and propranolol. Clin Pharmacol Ther (1976) 19, 807.

Beta-blockers + Haloperidol

Abstract/Summary

An isolated case report describes severe hypotension and cardiopulmonary arrest in a woman on three occasions shortly after being given haloperidol and propranolol.

Clinical evidence, importance and management

A middle-aged woman with schizophrenia and hypertension experienced three episodes of severe hypotension within 30–120 min of being given propranolol (40–80 mg) and haloperidol (10 mg)[1]. On two of the occasions cardiopulmonary arrest took place. She fainted each time, became cyanotic, had no palpable pulses and showed severe hypotension, but rapidly responded to cardiopulmonary resuscitation. She suffered no adverse consequences. The reasons for this reaction are not understood, but one suggestion[1] is that this patient was unduly sensitive to the additive relaxant effect of both drugs on peripheral blood vessels.

This seems to be the only case of this interaction on record. Bearing in mind the very wide-spread use of propranolol, other beta-blockers and haloperidol this interaction is obviously rare. There would seem to be little reason for avoiding concurrent use.

Reference

1 Alexander HE, McCarty K and Giffen MB. Hypotension and cardiopulmonary arrest associated with concurrent haloperidol and propranolol therapy. J Amer Med Ass (1984) 252, 87–8.

Beta-blockers + Hydralazine

Abstract/Summary

Concurrent use is not uncommon in the treatment of hypertension. Serum levels of propranolol and other extensively metabolized beta-blockers (metoprolol, oxprenolol) are increased but no adverse effects seem to have been reported.

Clinical evidence

(a) Effect of hydralazine on beta-blockers

A study in five normal subjects given single 40 mg oral doses of propranolol showed that the concurrent use of 25 and 50 mg doses of hydralazine increased the AUC (area under the concentration/time curve) by 60% and 110%, and raised the peak serum levels by 144 and 240% respectively.

Other studies confirm that hydralazine increases the bioavailability of propranolol by 31–57%,[3] of oxprenolol by 41%,[4] of metoprolol by 30%[2], but not acebutolol or nadolol.[2] The increased levels of oxprenolol[4] did not significantly reduce either diastolic or systolic blood pressures.

(b) Effect of beta-blockers on hydralazine

Oxprenolol was found not to have a significant effect on the pharmacokinetics of hydralazine.[4]

Mechanism

Originally it was believed[3] that hydralazine inhibited the liver enzymes concerned with the metabolism of propranolol (and other extensively metabolized beta-blockers such as metoprolol), thereby increasing their bioavailability, but more recent evidence suggests that the hydralazine reduces metabolism by reducing the blood flow into the liver.[1] Beta-blockers which are not extensively metabolized (nadolol, acebutolol, etc.) would not be expected to be affected because they are largely excreted unchanged in the urine.

Importance and management

Moderately well-documented and established interactions. The rise in the serum levels of some beta-blockers caused by hydralazine appears to be of minimal clinical importance. Concurrent use is common and usually valuable in the treatment of hypertension. No particular precautions seem to be necessary.

References

1 Schnek DW and Vary JE. Mechanism by which hydralazine increases propranolol bioavailability. Clin Pharmacol Ther (1984) 35, 447–53.
2 Jack DB, Kendall MJ, Dean S, Laugher SJ, Zaman R and Tenneson ME. The effect of hydralazine on the pharmacokinetics of three different beta-adrenoceptor antagonists: metoprolol, nadolol and acebutolol. Biopharm Drug Dispos (1982) 3, 47–54.
3 McLean AJ, Skews H, Bobik A and Dudley FJ. Interaction between oral propranolol and hydralazine. Clin Pharmacol Ther (1980) 27, 726–32.
4 Hawksworth GM, Dart AM, Chiang K, Parry K and Petrie JC. Effect of oxprenolol on the pharmacokinetics and pharmacodynamics of hydralazine. Drugs (1983) 25 (Suppl 2) 136–40.

Beta-blockers + Indomethacin and other NSAID's

Abstract/Summary

Indomethacin reduces the antihypertensive effects of the beta-blockers. This interaction can be accommodated either by raising the dosage of the beta-blocker or by using a non-interacting NSAID. Piroxicam interacts similarly while normally imidazole salicylate, isoxicam, naproxen, pirprofen and sulindac do not interact. Isolated cases have been reported with naproxen and ibuprofen. The situation with aspirin is uncertain. Indomethacin has also been reported to cause a marked hypertensive response in women with eclampsia.

Clinical evidence

(a) Beta-blockers + aspirin and other salicylates

A study in 11 patients taking a number of antihypertensives which included propranolol and pindolol showed that 1950 mg aspirin daily did not affect the control of their blood pressure.[12] In contrast another study found that aspirin reduced the hypotensive effects of pindolol and propranolol.[19] Sodium salicylate was found to affect neither the pharmacokinetics of alprenolol nor its effects on heart rate and blood pressure during exercise.[18] Another study in six normal subjects showed that aspirin did not affect the kinetics of atenolol.[17] Imidazole salicylate does not affect the blood pressure control of patients treated with atenolol.[21]

(b) Beta-blockers + ibuprofen

The antihypertensive effects of pindolol and possibly metoprolol were antagonized by the concurrent use of ibuprofen in two patients,[14] but no changes in the control of blood pressure with propranolol were seen in another study.[16]

(c) Beta-blockers + indomethacin

The diastolic blood pressures of seven hypertensive patients treated with pindolol (15 mg daily) or propranolol (80–160 mg daily) rose from 82 to 96 mm Hg when they were also given indomethacin, 100 mg daily, over a 10 day period. Changes in systolic pressures were not statistically significant.[1]

In other studies 100 mg indomethacin raised systolic/diastolic blood pressures of patients on propranolol by 14/5 mm Hg when lying and 16/9 mm Hg when standing.[2] This interaction has also been seen in other patients on propranolol,[4] oxprenolol[3,5] and atenolol.[9,10] Two women with eclampsia treated with pindolol and propranolol became markedly hypertensive (rises from 135/85 to 240/140 mm Hg, and from 130/70 to 230/130 mm Hg) within 4–5 days of being given indomethacin because of premature contractions.[22]

(d) Beta-blockers + isoxicam

A study in 10 normal subjects showed that 200 mg isoxicam daily did not alter the effects of propranolol on either blood pressure or heart rate.[15]

(e) Beta-blockers + naproxen or pirprofen

A study in hypertensive patients treated with timolol, hydrochlorothiazide and amiloride showed that 500 mg naproxen daily caused an insignificant rise in blood pressures,[7] but three cases of poor blood pressure control attributed to the use of naproxen have been described. Another study found that naproxen caused no changes in hypertension controlled with propranolol.[20] Pirprofen in daily doses of 800 mg was found not to affect the antihypertensive effects of oxprenolol.[5]

(f) Beta-blockers + piroxicam

An extensive study[11] found that about a quarter of the patients given 20 mg piroxicam daily and propranolol developed diastolic pressure rises of 10 mm Hg or more when lying or standing.[11] Increases in both systolic and diastolic pressures (+ 8.1/5.2 mm Hg lying and + 8.5/8.9 mm Hg standing) were seen in another study.[13] In contrast, patients taking propranolol and piroxicam for four weeks (doses not stated) showed systolic/diastolic blood pressure rises of 5.8/2.4 mm Hg when lying and 0.5/3.5 mm Hg when standing,[8] but these were said not to be statistically significant. No significant rises were seen in another study in patients given timolol and 20 mg piroxicam daily.[7]

(g) Beta-blockers + sulindac

Sulindac, 400 mg daily, had little effect on the control of hypertension in patients taking timolol, hydrochlorothiazide and amiloride.[7] No statistically significant rises in blood pressure occurred in other patients on propranolol given 400 mg sulindac daily.[11] No change in the hypertensive response to propranolol was seen in other studies.[13,20] In contrast, another study claimed that patients given propranolol and sulindac for four weeks (doses not stated) showed systolic/diastolic blood pressure rises of 4.8/10.3 mm Hg and 2.4/7.1 mm Hg when standing or lying,[8] but these were said not to be statistically significant.[4]

Mechanism

Indomethacin alone can raise blood pressure (13 hypertensive patients given three days treatment with 150 mg indomethacin daily showed a mean systolic blood pressure rise from 118 mm Hg to 131 mm Hg).[6] The probable reason is that it inhibits the synthesis and release into the circulation of two prostaglandins (pgA and pgE) from the kidney medulla which have a potent dilating effect on peripheral arterioles throughout the body. In their absence the blood pressure rises. Thus the hypotensive actions of the beta-blockers are opposed by the hypertensive actions of indomethacin. Other physiological and pharmacological mechanisms may also have a part to play. It seems probable that those NSAID's which behave like indomethacin interact by similar mechanisms.

Importance and management

Some of the beta-blocker/NSAID interactions have been well studied and are of clinical importance but others are not. The concurrent use of beta-blockers and indomethacin need not be avoided (except in patients with eclampsia) but anticipate the need to increase the dosage of the beta-blocker. Alternatively exchange the indomethacin for a non-interacting NSAID. Piroxicam interacts similarly while normally imidazole salicylate, isoxicam, naproxen, pirprofen and sulindac only interact minimally or not at all. The situation with aspirin is unresolved. Because the occasional patient may show a marked interaction even with NSAID's which normally do not interact (e.g. naproxen, ibuprofen), it would be prudent to monitor the effects when any NSAID is given. Direct information about other NSAID's seems not to be available. Many of the antihypertensive agents appear to be affected by this interaction so that exchanging one for another may not avoid the problem.

References

1 Durao V, Prata MM and Goncalves LMP. Modification of antihypertensive effects of beta-adrenoceptor blocking agents by inhibition of endogenous prostaglandin synthesis. Lancet (1977) ii, 1005–7.
2 Watkins J, Abbott EC, Hensby CN, Webster J and Dollery CT. Attenuation of hypotensive effects of propranolol and thiazide diuretics by indomethacin. Br Med J (1980) 281, 702–5.
3 Salvetti A, Arzillis F, Pedrinelli R, Beggi P and Motolese M. Interaction between oxprenolol and indomethacin on blood pressure in essential hypertensive patients. Eur J Clin Pharmacol (1982) 22, 197–201.
4 Lopez-Overjero JA, Weber MA, Drayer JIM, Sealey JE and Laragh JH. Effects of indomethacin alone and during diuretic or beta-adrenoceptor blockade therapy on blood pressure and the renin system in essential hypertension. Clin Sci Mol Med (1978) 55, 203–5s.
5 Sorgel F, Hemmerlein M and Lang E. Wirkung von Pirprofen und Indometacin auf die Effekte von Oxprenolol und Furosemid. Arneim-Forsch./Drug Res (1984) 34, 1330–2.
6 Barrientos A, Alcazar V, Ruilope L, Jarillo D and Rodicio JL. Indomethacin and beta-blockers in hypertension. Lancet (1978) i, 277.
7 Wong DG, Spence JD, Lamki L, Freeman D and McDonald JWD. Effect of non-steroidal anti-inflammatory drugs on control of hypertension by beta-blockers and diuretics. Lancet (1986) i, 997–1001.
8 Alvarez CR, Baez MA and Weidler DJ. Effect of sulindac and piroxicam adminstration on the antihypertensive effect of propranolol. J Clin Pharmacol (1986) 26, 544.
9 Ylitalo P, Pitkajavvi T, Pyykonen M-L, Nurmi A-K, Seppala E and Vapaatal H. Inhibition of prostaglandin synthesis by indomethacin interacts with the antihypertensive effect of atenolol. Clin Pharmacol Ther (1985) 38, 443–9.
10 Salvetti A, Pedrinelli R, Alberci A, Magagna A and Abdel-Haq B. The influence of indomethacin and sulindac on some pharmacological actions of atenolol in hypertensive patients. Br J clin Pharmacol (1984) 17, 108–llS.
11 Ebel DL, Rhymer AR and Stahl E. Effect of sulindac, piroxicam and placebo on the hypotensive effect of propranolol in patients with mild to moderate essential hypertension. Adv Ther (1985) 2, 131–42.
12 Mills EH, Whitworth JA, Andrews J and Kincaid-Smith P. Non-steroidal anti-inflammatory drugs and blood pressure. Aust NZ J Med (1982) 12, 478–82.
13 Pugliese F, Simonetti BM, Cinotte GA, Ciabattoni G, Catella F, Vastano S, Ghidini Ottonelli A and Pierucci A. Differential interaction of piroxicam and sulindac with the anti-hypertensive effect of propranolol. Eur J Clin Invest (1984) 14, 54.
14 Reid ALA. Antihypertensive effect of thiazides. Med J Aust (1981) 2, 109–10.
15 Staiger J, Gharieb AK and Keul J. Zur interaktion von Betablockern (Propranolol) und Antirheumatika (Isoxicam). Herz/Krauslauf (1983) 15, 141–3.
16 Davies JG, Rawlins DC and Busson M. Effect of ibuprofen on blood pressure control by propranolol and bendrofluazide. J Int Med Res (1988) 16, 173–81.
17 Schafer-Korting M, Kirch W, Axthelm T, Kohler H and Mutschler E. Atenolol interaction with aspirin, allopurinol, and ampicillin. Clin Pharmacol Ther (1983) 33, 283–8.
18 Johnsson G, Regardh CG and Solvell L. Lack of biological interaction

of alprenolol and salicylate in man. Eur J clin Pharmacol (1973) 6, 9–14.

19 Sziegoleit W, Rausch J, Polak Gy, Gyorgy M, Dekov E, Bekes M. Influence of acetylsalicylic acid on acute circulatory effects of the beta-blocking agents pindolol and propranolol in humans. Int J Clin Pharmac Ther Tox (1982) 20, 423–30.

20 Schuna AA, Vejraska BD, Hiatt JG, Kochar M, Day R, Goodfriend TL. Lack of interaction between sulindac or naproxen and propranolol in hypertensive patients. J Clin Pharmacol (1989) 29, 524–8.

21 Abdel-Haq B, Magagna A, Avilla S and Salvetti A. The interference of indomethacin and of imidazole salicylate on blood pressure control of essential hypertensive patients treated with atenolol. Int J Clin Pharmacol Ther Toxicol (1987) 25, 598–600.

22 Schoenfeld A, Freedman S, Hod M, Ovadia Y. Antagonism of antihypertensive drug therapy in pregnancy by indomethacin? Am J Obst Gynecol (1989) 161, 1204–5.

Beta-blockers + Morphine

Abstract/Summary

Morphine can raise the serum levels of esmolol. The fatal dose of morphine is markedly reduced in animals by propranolol, but whether this also occurs in man is uncertain.

Clinical evidence, mechanism, importance and management

A study in 10 normal men showed that after being given an injection of 3 mg morphine the steady-state levels of esmolol (an infusion of 300 μg/kg/min over 4 h) were generally higher, but were only statistically significantly higher (by 46%) in two of the subjects. The pharmacokinetics of morphine were unchanged.[1] This interaction should be borne in mind if both drugs are given. There seems to be no information about other interactions with other beta-blockers. Studies in animals have shown that the fatal dose of morphine is reduced 2–7-fold in mice[2] and 15–16-fold in rats[3] by propranolol. The same interaction has also been seen in dogs.[3] So far there seems to be no confirmation that this occurs in man with propranolol or any other beta-blocker but it would seem prudent to use this drug combination cautiously until more is known.

References

1 Lowenthal DT, Porter RS, Saris SD, Bies CM, Slegowski MB and Staudacher A. Clinical pharmacology, pharmacodynamics and interactions of esmolol. Am J Cardiol (1985) 56, 14–14·18F.

2 Murmann W, Almirante L and Saccani-Guelfi M. Effects of hexobarbital, ether, morphine and urethane upon the acute toxicity of propranolol and D-(-)-INPEA. J Pharm Pharmacol (1966) 18, 692–4.

3 Davis WM and Hatoum NS. Possible toxic interaction of propranolol and narcotic analgesics. Drug Intell Clin Pharm (1981) 15, 290.

Beta-blockers + Nicardipine

Abstract/Summary

No pharmacokinetic interaction occurs between propranolol and nicardipine in healthy subjects but the response in patients should be checked.

Clinical evidence, mechanism, importance and management

A study in 12 normal subjects given 80 mg propranolol and 30 mg nicardipine daily for six days showed that no changes in the pharmacokinetics of either drug occurred.[1] However some patients have shown adverse effects (hypotension, heart failure) when beta-blockers and other calcium channel blockers were used together (see 'Beta-blockers + Nifedipine', 'Beta-blockers + Verapamil') so that the outcome of using beta-blockers and nicardipine should be well monitored.

Reference

1 Macdonald FC, Dow RJ, Wilson RAG, Yee KF and Finlayson J. A study to determine potential interactions between nicardipine and propranolol in healthy volunteers. Br J clin Pharmac (1987), 626–7P.

Beta-blockers + Nifedipine

Abstract/Summary

Concurrent use is common in the treatment of hypertension and angina, and usually both beneficial and uneventful, but a few cases of excessive hypotension and heart failure have been reported.

Clinical evidence

Some reports indicate that nifedipine interacts with beta-blockers such as propranolol, atenolol, betaxolol or metoprolol to affect their pharmacokinetics or pharmacodynamics, whereas others found little or no interaction, but there is usually no evidence of haemodynamic deterioration.[5–7,9–12] However there are a few reports of adverse effects.

Two patients with angina under treatment with beta-blockers (alprenolol, propranolol) developed heart failure when additionally given 10 mg nifedipine three times a day. The signs of heart failure disappeared when the nifedipine was withdrawn.[1] One out of 15 patients with hypertension and exertional angina developed hypotension when given 10 mg nifedipine twice daily in addition to treatment with atenolol (50–100 mg), prazosin (9 mg) and diuretics. The situation was controlled by withdrawing the nifedipine.[2] Severe and prolonged hypotension developed in a patient treated with propranolol and nifedipine which may have been a factor which led to fatal myocardial infarction.[3] Cardiac failure is also described in another patient on atenolol when additionally given nifedipine.[4]

Mechanism

Nifedipine depresses the contractility of the heart muscle. This is counteracted by a sympathetic reflex increase in heart rate due to a nifedipine-induced peripheral vasodilation so that the ventricular output stays the same or is even improved. The presence of a beta-blocker may oppose this to some extent by slowing the heart rate which allows the negative inotropic effects of nifedipine to go unchecked.

Importance and management

The concurrent use of beta-blockers and nifedipine in the treatment of hypertension and angina pectoria is normally beneficial, safe and uneventful. A number of clinical studies confirm the value of this combination, however the existence of a handful of reports of adverse reactions emphasizes the need for some care during combined use. Patients should be monitored for any signs of excessive hypotension or cardiac depression. Those likely to be particularly at risk are patients with impairment of left ventricular function[8] and/or those taking beta-blockers in high dosage.

References

1 Anastassiades CJ. Nifedipine and beta-blocker drugs. Br Med J (1980) 281, 1251.
2 Opie LH and White DA. Adverse interaction between nifedipine and beta-blockade. Br Med J (1980) 281, 1462.
3 Staffurth JS and Emery P. Adverse interaction between nifedipine and beta-blockade. Br Med J (1981) 282, 225.
4 Robson RH and Vishwanath MC. Nifedipine and beta-blockade as a cause of cardiac failure. Br Med J (1982) 284, 104.
5 Gangji D, Juvent M, Niset G, Wathieu M, Degreve M, Bellens R, Poortmans J, Degre S, Fitzsimons TJ and Herchuelz A. Study of the influence of nifedipine on the pharmacokinetics and pharmacodynamics of propranolol, metoprolol and atenolol. Br J clin Pharmac (1984) 17, 29–35S.
6 Kendall MJ, Jack DB, Laugher SJ, Lobo J and Smith R. Lack of a pharmacokinetic interaction between nifedipine and the beta-adrenceptor blockers metoprolol and atenolol. Br J clin Pharmac (1984) 18, 331–5.
7 Rowland E, Razis P, Sugrue D and Krikler DM. Acute and chronic haemodynamic and electrophysiological effects of nifedipine in patients receiving atenolol. Br Heart J (1983) 50, 383–9.
8 Brooks N, Cattell M, Pigeon J, Balcon R. Unpredictable response to nifedipine in severe cardiac failure. Br Med J (1980) 281, 1324.
9 Elkayam U, Roth A, Weber L, Kulick D, Kawanishi D, McKay C and Rahimtoola SH. Effects of nifedipine on hemodynamic and cardiac function in patients with left ventricular ejection fraction already treated with propranolol. Am J Cardiol (1986) 58, 536–40.
10 Vineneux Ph, Canal M, Domart Y, Roux A, Cascio B, Orofiamma B, Larribaud J, Flouvat B and Carbon C. Pharmacokinetic and pharmacodynamic interactions between nifedipine and propranolol or betaxolol. Int J Clin Pharmacol Ther Toxicol (1986) 24, 153–8.
11 Rosenkranz B, Ledermann H and Frolich JC. Interaction between nifedipine and atenolol: pharmacokinetics and pharmacodynamics in normotensive volunteers. J Cardiovasc Pharmacol (1986) 8, 943–9.
12 Vetrovec GW and Parker VE. Nifedipine, beta-blocker interaction: effect on left ventricular function. Clin Res (1984) 32, 833A.

Beta-blockers + Omeprazole

Abstract/Summary

Omeprazole does not interact with propranolol.

Clinical evidence, mechanism, importance and management

A randomized double-blind trial with eight normal subjects showed that 20 mg omeprazole daily for eight days had no effect on the steady-state serum levels of propranolol (160 mg daily) nor on its clinical effects (resting and exercised heart rates, blood pressure).[1]

Reference

1 Henry D, Brent P, Whyte I, Mihaly G and Devenish-Meares S. Propranolol steady-state pharmacokinetics are unaltered by omeprazole. Eur J Clin Pharmacol (1987) 33, 369–73.

Beta-blockers + Penicillins

Abstract/Summary

Serum atenolol levels are halved by the concurrent use of 1 g doses of ampicillin. The clinical importance of this is uncertain, but possibly not large. No important interaction occurs if the ampicillin is given in divided doses.

Clinical evidence

A study in six normal subjects showed that when 100 mg atenolol was given with 1 g ampicillin daily for six days, the mean steady-state serum atenolol levels were reduced by 52% (from 199 to 95 ng/ml).[1] The AUC (area under the concentration/time curve) was also reduced by 52%. The blood pressure lowering effects of atenolol at rest were not affected by the presence of ampicillin, but after exercise a small rise in systolic pressures occurred. The effects of atenolol on heart rate during exercise were diminished (from 24% to 11% at 12 h).[1]

Another study showed that when 50 mg atenolol and 1 g ampicillin were given concurrently by mouth, the AUC was reduced by 51.5%, whereas when the ampicillin was given as four 250 mg doses over 24 h, the AUC was only reduced by 18.2%.[1]

Mechanism

Uncertain. Ampicillin apparently affects the absorption of the atenolol.

Importance and management

An established interaction although information is limited. If the minimal effects on blood pressure and heart rate can be taken as a measure, it would appear to be of only moderate or minor clinical importance. It is not clear therefore why the authors of the paper cited[1] say that the atenolol dosage may need to be doubled to achieve the desired antihypertensive effect, and are adamant that doubling the dosage is necessary in the treatment of angina. The second study[2] showed that if the ampicillin is given divided into four 250 mg doses instead of as a single 1 g dose, the effects of the interaction are almost certainly trivial. If a large dose of ampicillin is needed, it has been suggested that the atenolol is given first.[2] Information about other beta-blockers is lacking, although it seems possible that other penicillins will interact like ampicillin.

References

1 Schafer-Korting M, Kirch W, Axthelm T, Kohler H and Mutschler E. Atenolol interaction with aspirin, allopurinol, and ampicillin. Clin Pharmacol Ther (1983) 33, 283–8.
2 McLean AJ, Tonkin A, McCarthy P and Harrison P. Dose-dependence of atenolol-ampicillin interaction. Br J clin Pharmac (1984) 18, 969–71.

Beta-blockers + Phenothiazines

Abstract/Summary

The concurrent use of chlorpromazine and propranolol can result in a marked rise in the serum levels of both drugs. Excessive hypotension has been seen. Two patients showed 3–5-fold increases in serum thioridazine levels when given propranolol.

Clinical evidence

(a) Serum propranolol or pindolol levels raised

The mean steady-state propranolol levels (dosage 80 mg eight-hourly) of four normal subjects and one patient were raised 70% (from 41.5 to 70.2 ng/ml) when additionally given 50 mg chlorpromazine eight-hourly.[1] The increase was considerable in some subjects but barely detectable in others. Another subject on propranolol climbed out of bed after the first dose of chlorpromazine and promptly fainted. He was found to have a pulse rate of 35–40 per min and a blood pressure of 70/0 mm Hg. He rapidly recovered with a pulse rate of 85 and blood pressure of 120/70 when given 3 mg atropine.[1]

Another case of hypotension during the concurrent use of chlorpromazine and sotalol has been reported.[2] Thioridazine also increases serum pindolol levels.[9]

(b) Serum chlorpromazine levels raised

A long-term cross-over study on seven schizophrenic patients given an average of 6.7 mg/kg chlorpromazine, administered three times a day, showed that the concurrent use of propranolol (mean dose 8.1 mg/kg) increased the serum chlorpromazine levels by 100–500% and raised the plasma levels of the active metabolites of chlorpromazine by 50–100%.[4]

The same or similar work by the same authors is described elsewhere.[5] One of the patients was withdrawn from the study because he suffered a cardiovascular collapse while taking both drugs.[5] It has been suggested that the value of propranolol in the treatment of schizophrenia probably results from the rise in serum chlorpromazine levels.[5,6] A schizophrenic patient taking chlorpromazine and thiothixene experienced delerium, grand mal seizures and skin photosensitivity, attributed to the a rise in serum levels of the neuroleptic drugs, after additionally being given propranolol.[7]

(c) Serum thioridazine levels raised

Two patients stabilized on 600 or 800 mg daily showed rises in serum thioridazine levels from 0.3 to 1.6, and from 0.4 to 1.5 μg/ml respectively when concurrently treated over 26–40 days with propranolol given in increasing doses up to a total of 800 mg daily. No thioridazine toxicity was seen although serum levels had risen into the toxic range.[8] Another study confirmed that thioridazine levels rise markedly.[10] Pindolol also increases serum thioridazine levels by up to 50%.[9]

Mechanism

Pharmacokinetic evidence[1] and animal studies[3] suggest that propranolol and chlorpromazine mutually inhibit the liver metabolism of the other drug so that both accumulate within the body. The hypotensive episodes reported[1,2,5] are presumably due to the additive hypotensive effects of both drugs. The mechanism of the propranolol-thioridazine interaction is not understood.

Importance and management

The propranolol-chlorpromazine interactions appear to be established, although information is limited. Concurrent use should be well monitored. The drug dosages should be reduced if necessary. The same precautions apply with propranolol and thioridazine.[8] There seems to be no information about any other beta-blocker/phenothiazine interactions, but if the mechanism of interaction suggested above is true, it seems possible that other beta-blockers which are mainly cleared from the body by liver metabolism (e.g. alprenolol, metoprolol) might interact similarly with chlorpromazine, whereas those mainly cleared unchanged in the urine (e.g. atenolol, nadolol) are less likely to do so.

References

1 Vestal RE, Kornhauser DM, Hollifield JW and Shand DG. Inhibition of propranolol metabolism by chlorpromazine. Clin Pharmacol Ther (1979) 25, 19.
2 Baker L, Barcai A, Kaye R and Haque N. Beta-adrenergic blockade and juvenile diabetes: acute studies and long-term therapeutic trial. J Pediat (1969) 75, 19.
3 Shand DG and Oates JA. The metabolism of propranolol by rat liver microsomes and its inhibition by phenothiazine and tricyclic antidepressants. Biochem Pharmacol (1971) 20, 1720.
4 Peet M, Middlemiss DN and Yates RA. Pharmacokinetic interaction between propranolol and chlorpromazine in schizophrenic patients. Lancet (1980) ii, 978.
5 Peet M, Middlemiss DN and Yates RA. Propranolol in schizophrenia, II. Clinical and biochemical aspects of combining propranolol with chlorpromazine. Br J Psychiat (1981) 138, 112.
6 Lindstrom IH and Persson E. Propranolol in chronic schizophrenia: a controlled study in neuroleptic treated patients. Br J Psychiat (1980) 137, 126.
7 Miller FA and Rampling D. Adverse effects of combined propranolol and chlorpromazine therapy. Am J Psychiat (1982) 139, 1198–9.
8 Silver JM, Yudofsky SC, Kogan M and Katz BL. Elevation of thioridazine plasma levels by propranolol. Am J Psychiatry (1986) 143, 1290–2.
9 Greendyke RM and Gulya A. Effect of pindolol administration on serum levels of thioridazine, haloperidol and phenobarbital. J Clin Psychiatry (1988) 49, 105–7.

10 Greendyke RM and Kanter DR. Plasma propranolol levels and their effect on plasma thioridazine and haloperidol concentrations. J Clin Psychopharmacol (1987) 7, 178–82.

Beta-blockers + Propafenone

Abstract/Summary

Serum metoprolol and propranolol levels can be markedly raised (2–5-fold) by the concurrent use of propafenone.

Clinical evidence

A study in four patients under treatment for ventricular arrhythmias and taking 150–200 mg metoprolol daily found that, when given 150 mg propafenone three times a day, their steady-state serum metoprolol levels rose 2–5-fold. One of the patients suffered distressing nightmares and the other had acute left ventricular failure with pulmonary oedema and haemoptysis which disappeared when the metoprolol dosage was reduced or stopped. Single dose studies in normal subjects demonstrated a twofold decrease in the clearance of metoprolol and a 20% reduction in the heart rate increase due to exercise at one-and-a-half hours. Serum propafenone levels in four other patients were found to be unaffected by metoprolol.[1]

Another study in 12 normal subjects given 50 mg propranolol eight-hourly showed that 225 mg propafenone daily more than doubled their steady-state propranolol levels. The beta-blocking effects were only modestly increased. The propafenone pharmacokinetics remained unchanged.[2]

Mechanism

Uncertain, but it is suggested that the propafenone reduces the metabolism of the metoprolol and propranolol by the liver, thereby reducing clearance and raising serum levels.[1,2]

Importance and management

Information is limited but the interaction would seem to be established. Concurrent use need not be avoided but the dosage of metoprolol and propranolol may need to be reduced. Monitor closely because some patients may experience adverse effects. If the suggested mechanism of interaction is correct it is possible that other beta-blockers which undergo liver metabolism will interact similarly but not those largely excreted unchanged in the urine (e.g. atenolol, nadolol). This needs confirmation.

References

1 Wagner F, Kalusche D, Trenk D, Jahnchen E and Roskamm H. Drug interaction between propafenone and metoprolol. Br J clin Pharmac (1987) 24, 213–20.
2 Kowey PR, Kirsen EB, Fu C-HJ, Mason WD. Interaction between propranolol and propafenone in healthy volunteers. J Clin Pharmacol (1989) 29, 512–17.

Beta-blockers + Ranitidine

Abstract/Summary

Ranitidine does not alter the steady-state plasma levels of atenolol, metoprolol or propranolol, and their therapeutic effects remain unchanged.

Clinical evidence

A study in five normal subjects showed that after taking 300 mg ranitidine daily for six days, the steady-state plasma levels of propranolol (160 mg daily) were unaffected. Exercise-induced heart rate increases and blood pressures also remained unchanged.[1] Similarly no changes in plasma propranolol levels, pulse rates or blood pressures were seen in other studies.[2–6]

A randomized cross-over study on 12 normal subjects showed that the serum levels of metoprolol, 100 mg daily, were unaffected by the concurrent use of 300 mg ranitidine daily over a seven-day period.[7] Some studies confirm these findings,[8,9,13] but other single doses studies report increases in serum metoprolol levels and AUC's (+ 50%) by ranitidine.[10–12] No changes in exercise-induced heart rates were found.[8,13] No changes in the pharmacokinetics of atenolol by ranitidine were reported in a study.[10]

Mechanism

The rises in metoprolol serum levels caused by ranitidine in the single dose studies are not understood.

Importance and management

The possible effects of ranitidine on the serum levels and effects of propranolol and metoprolol have been well studied, but less is known about atenolol. No clinically important interaction has been seen. There is nothing to suggest that the concurrent use of ranitidine and any beta-blocker should be avoided, or that there is any need to take particular precautions.

References

1 Reimann IW, Klotz U and Frohlich JC. Effects of cimetidine and ranitidine on steady-state propranolol kinetics and dynamics. Clin Pharmacol Ther (1982) 32, 749–57.
2 Donn KH, Powell JR, Rogers JF and Eshelman FN. The influence of H₂-receptor antagonists on steady-state concentrations of propranolol and 4-hydroxypropranolol. J Clin Pharmacol (1984) 24, 500–8.
3 Markiewicz A, Hartler M, Lelek H, Boldys H and Nowak A. The effect of treatment with cimetidine and ranitidine on bioavailability of, and circulatory response to, propranolol. Zbl Pharm (1984) 123, 516–18.
4 Heagerty AM, Castleden CM and Patel L. Failure of ranitidine to interact with propranolol. Br Med J (1982) 284, 1304.
5 Heagerty AM, Donovan MA, Castleden CM, Pohl JEF and Patel L. The influence of histamine (H₂) antagonists on propranolol pharmacokinetics. Int J clin Pharmac Res (1986) 2, 203–5.
6 Patel L and Weerasuriya K. The effect of cimetidine and ranitidine on propranolol clearance. Br J clin Pharmac (1983) 15, 152P.
7 Toon S, Batra HK, Garstang FM and Rowland M. Comparative effects of ranitidine and cimetidine on metoprolol in man. Br J Pharmacol (1987). Abstract presented to the British Pharmacological Society meeting, September 1986.

8 Kelly JG, Salem SAM, Kinney CD, Shanks RG and McDevitt DG. Effects of ranitidine on the disposition of metoprolol. Br J clin Pharmac (1985) 19, 219–24.
9 Kendall MJ, Laugher SJ and Wilkins MR. Ranitidine, cimetidine and metoprolol—a pharmacokinetic interaction study. Gastroenterol (1986) 90, 1490.
10 Spahn H, Mutschler E, Kirch W, Ohnhaus EE and Janisch HD. Influence of ranitidine on plasma metoprolol and atenolol concentrations. Br Med J (1983) 286, 1546–7.
11 Kelly JG, Shanks RG and McDevitt DG. Influence of ranitidine on plasma metoprolol concentrations. Br Med J (1983) 287, 1218–19.
12 Kirch W, Ramsch K, Janisch HD and Ohnhaus EE. The influence of two histamine H_2 antagonists, cimetidine and ranitidine, on the plasma levels and clinical effect of nifedipine and metoprolol. Arch Toxicol (1984) 7, 256–9.
13 Tom S, Davidson EM, Garstang FM, Batra H, Bowers RJ and Rowland M. The racemic metoprolol H_2-antagonist interaction. Clin Pharmacol Ther (1988) 43, 283–9.

Beta-blockers + Rifampicin (Rifampin)

Abstract/Summary

Rifampicin increases the loss of propranolol, metoprolol and bisoprolol from the body and reduces their serum levels. The extent to which this affects the therapeutic response to these beta-blockers is uncertain.

Clinical evidence

A study in six normal subjects showed that while taking 600 mg rifampicin daily for three weeks the oral clearance of propranolol was increased from 35.7 to 96.1 ml min[-1] kg[-1]. Increasing the dose of rifampicin to 900 or 1200 mg daily did not increase the clearance. Four weeks after withdrawing the rifampicin the blood levels of propranolol had returned to normal.[1]

A similar interaction occurs with metoprolol. 600 mg rifampicin daily for 15 days given to 10 normal subjects was found to reduce peak serum metoprolol levels (after single 100 mg doses) by 33% and the AUC by 40%.[2] Another study showed that the AUC of bisoprolol was reduced by 34% in subjects given 600 mg rifampicin daily.[3]

Mechanism

Rifampicin is a potent liver enzyme inducing agent which increases the metabolism and loss of the these beta-blockers from the body.

Importance and management

The interactions of rifampicin with propranolol, metoprolol and bisoprolol are established, but their clinical importance is uncertain. Concurrent use should be monitored. Increase the dosage of the beta-blocker if there is any evidence that the therapeutic response is inadequate. Only those beta-blockers which undergo extensive liver metabolism would be expected to be affected by rifampicin (e.g. propranolol, metoprolol, alprenolol, etc.), unlike those mainly lost unchanged in the urine (atenolol, nadolol, etc.).

References

1 Herman RJ, Nakamura K, Wilkinson GR and Wood AJJ. Induction of propranolol metabolism by rifampicin. Br J clin Pharmac (1983) 16, 565–9.
2 Bennett PN, John VA and Whitmarsh VB. Effects of rifampicin on metoprolol and antipyrine kinetics. Br J clin Pharmac (1982) 13, 387.
3 Kirsch W, Rose I, Klingmann I, Pabst J and Ohnhaus EE. Interaction of bisoprolol with cimetidine and rifampicin. Eur J Clin Pharmacol (1986) 31, 59–62.

Beta-blockers + Sulphinpyrazone

Abstract/Summary

The antihypertensive effects of oxprenolol can be reduced or abolished by the concurrent use of sulphinpyrazone.

Clinical evidence

10 hypertensive patients were given 80 mg oxprenolol twice daily, as a result of which their mean supine blood pressures were reduced from 161/101 to 149/96 mm Hg, and their heart rates fell from 72 to 66 beats per minute. When additionally given 400 mg sulphinpyrazone twice daily, their blood pressures climbed again to approximately their former levels. Heart rates remained unaffected.[1] Cardiac workload (Systolic blood pressure × heart rate) was only slightly increased (+8%).

Mechanism

Not understood. One idea is that the sulphinpyrazone inhibits the production of prostaglandins by the kidney which have vasodilatory (antihypertensive) activity. This would oppose the actions of the oxprenolol. Another idea is that the sulphinpyrazone increases the metabolism of the oxprenolol, thereby increasing its loss from the body and reducing its effects.

Importance and management

Information seems to be limited to this study. If sulphinpyrazone is given to patients taking oxprenolol for hypertension, the effects should be monitored. It seems likely that this interaction could be accommodated by raising the dosage of the oxprenolol. The effects of this interaction on cardiac workload appear to be minimal but it would still be prudent to monitor concurrent use if oxprenolol is used for angina. It is not known whether other beta-blockers interact similarly but it would seem wise at the moment to assume that they do.

Reference

1 Ferrara LA, Mancini M, Marotta T, Pasanisi F and Fasano ML. Interference by sulphinpyrazone with the antihypertensive effects of oxprenolol. Eur J Clin Pharmacol (1986) 29, 717–19.

Beta-blockers + Thallium scans

Abstract/Summary

Beta-blockers may falsify the results of stress thallium scans used for the diagnosis of coronary heart disease.

Clinical evidence, mechanism, importance and management

A comparative study in patients, given 201-thallous chloride during exercise for the diagnosis of coronary heart disease, showed that there was a marked reduction in the sensitivity to stress thallium scans in those on beta-blockers when compared with other patients not taking beta-blockers. The suggestion was made that consideration should be given to discontinuing beta-blockers before evaluating these patients.[1] Strictly speaking this is not an interaction in the usual sense of the word.

Reference

1 Henkin RE, Chang W and Provus R. The effect of beta-blockers on thallium scans. J Nucl Med (1982) 23, P35.

Beta-blockers + Tobacco smoking and/or Coffee and tea drinking

Abstract/Summary

The beta-blockers reduce the heart rate and the blood pressure. These therapeutically useful effects are exploited in the treatment of angina and hypertension and they are reduced to some extent if patients smoke. Drinking tea or coffee may have the same but smaller effect. Some increase in the dosage of the beta-blocker may be necessary.

Clinical evidence

(a) Beta-blockers + tobacco smoking

A double blind study in 10 smokers with angina pectoris, taking daily doses of either 240 mg propranolol, 100 mg atenolol or a placebo, showed that when they smoked their plasma propranolol levels were reduced 25%. Plasma atenolol levels were not significantly altered. Both of the beta-blockers reduced heart rates at rest and when exercised, but the reductions were less when they smoked (rises of 8–14%).[1]

Other studies confirm that smoking reduces serum propranolol levels.[2,3] Serum propranolol levels were 200% higher in those who did not smoke.[2] In addition to these pharmacokinetic effects, smoking can abolish the beneficial effects of propanolol on ST segment depression in patients with angina.[6]

(b) Beta-blockers + caffeine

A study in 12 subjects with normal blood pressures showed that while taking 240 mg propranolol, 300 mg metoprolol or a placebo, both their systolic and diastolic blood pressures rose after drinking two 150 ml cups of coffee (made from 24 g coffee). Systolic/diastolic blood pressure rises were +7%/+22% (propranolol), +7%/+19% (metoprolol) and +4%/+16% mm Hg (placebo). The beta-blockers and placebo were given in divided doses over 15 h before the test.[4]

(c) Beta-blockers + tobacco smoking + caffeine

A study of these interactions was made in eight patients with mild hypertension who, while taking daily doses of either propranolol (160 mg), oxprenolol (160 mg) or atenolol (100 mg) over a six week period, were additionally tested with two tipped cigarettes and coffee (200 mg caffeine) over 15 min. Their mean systolic/diastolic blood pressure rises over the following 2 h were 8.5/8/0 mm Hg (propranolol), 12.1/9.1 mm Hg (oxprenolol) and 5.2/4.4 mm Hg (atenolol).[5]

Mechanism

Smoking on its own increases the heart rate, the blood pressure and the severity of myocardial ischaemia (oxygen starvation of the heart muscle).[6] These actions oppose and may even totally abolish the beneficial actions of the beta-blockers. In addition, smoking stimulates the liver enzymes concerned with the metabolism of some beta-blockers (e.g. propranolol, metoprolol) so that their serum levels and their effects are reduced. Smoking also reduces the oxygen-carrying capacity of the blood which may also be significant in those with angina. Caffeine on its own causes the release into the blood of catecholamines, such as adrenaline, which could account for the increases in heart rate and blood pressure which are seen.[5] The blood pressure rise may be exaggerated in the presence of beta-blockers which block vasodilatation, leaving the alpha (vasoconstrictor) effects of adrenaline unopposed. This too opposes the actions of the beta-blockers.

Importance and management

These interactions are established. Smoking tobacco and (to a very much lesser extent) drinking tea or coffee oppose the effects of the beta-blockers in the treatment of angina or hypertension. Patients should be encouraged to stop smoking because, quite apart from its other toxic effects, it aggravates myocardial ischaemia, increases heart rates and can change satifactorily controlled blood pressures into those which are not. If this encouragement is unsuccessful it may be necessary to raise the dosages of the beta-blockers. The effects of atenolol (a selective beta-1 blocker) are opposed less than those of propranolol,[5] and it seems possible that this will also be true for other beta-blockers which are largely cleared unchanged in the urine (e.g. nadolol, pindolol, etc.). The effects of the caffeine in tea, coffee, Coca-Cola, etc. are quite small and there seems to be no strong reason to forbid them, but the excessive consumption of large amounts may not be a good idea, particularly in those who also smoke.

References

1 Fox K, Deansfield J, Krikler S, Ribeiro P and Wright C. The interaction of cigarette smoking and beta-adrenoceptor blockade. Br J clin Pharmac (1984) 17, 92–93S.
2 Vestal RE, Wood AJJ, Branch RA, Shand DG and Wilkinson GR. Effects of age and cigarette smoking on propranolol disposition. Clin Pharmacol Ther (1979) 26, 8–15.
3 Gardner MJ, Cady WJ, Ong YS. Effect of smoking on the elimination of propranolol hydrochloride. Int J Clin Pharmacol Ther Toxicol (1980) 18, 421–4.
4 Smits P, Hoffmann H, Thien T, Houben H and van't Laar, A. Hemodynamic and humoral effects of coffee after beta $_1$-selective and nonselective beta-blockade. Clin Pharmacol Ther (1983) 34, 153–8.
5 Freestone S and Ramsay LE. Effect of beta-blockade on the pressor response to coffee plus smoking in patients with mild hypertension. Drugs (1983) 25 (Suppl 2) 141–5.
6 Fox KM, Jonathan A, Williams H and Selwyn A. Interaction between cigarettes and propranolol in the treatment of angina pectoris. Br Med J (1980) 3, 191–3.

Beta-blockers + Verapamil

Abstract/Summary

Although beta-blockers and verapamil have been used together very successfully and uneventfully, serious cardiodepression (bradycardia, asystole, sinus arrest) sometimes occurs and it has been suggested that the combination should only be given to those who can initially be closely supervised. An adverse interaction can occur even with beta-blockers given as eye drops (timolol).

Clinical evidence

(a) Adverse interactions

A study of 50 patients, given 100 mg atenolol and 360 mg verapamil daily over a mean period of 10 months, showed that 40 of the patients experienced fewer anginal episodes while taking both drugs. 16 patients needed a reduced dosage or withdrawal. Three had bradyarrhythmias (drugs withdrawn) and seven experienced dyspnoea (four withdrawals and three dosage reductions) presumed to be secondary to left ventricular failure. Other complications were tiredness (two patients), postural hypotension (one patient) and dizziness (one patient), all of which were dealt with by reducing the dosage.[15]

In another study[16] on 15 patients given atenolol and verapamil, four experienced profound lethargy, one had left ventricular failure and four had bradyarrhythmias. Other reports describe cardiac failure, sinus arrest,[6,20] ventricular asystole,[1,16] heart block,[12] hypotension,[13,19] and bradycardia[11,13,16,19] in patients on atenolol,[6,20] practolol,[1,2] metoprolol,[8,11,13] propranolol[3,5,7,9,10,19] or pindolol[8] and verapamil. In two cases the patients were using timolol in the form of eye drops.[16–18]

(b) Pharmacokinetic interactions

A study in 10 patients showed that when verapamil was added to metoprolol, the metoprolol AUC (area under the concentration/time curve) was increased by 33% and the peak serum levels were raised 41%.[13] Pulse rates and blood pressures were also less than with metoprolol alone. The pharmacokinetics of atenolol were not altered by verapamil in a study on a single patient.[14]

Mechanism

Both drugs have negative inotropic (i.e. cardiac depressant) effects on the heart which can be additive (see the mechanism of interaction suggested for Beta-blockers + Nifedipine). The beta-blockers reduce the sympathetic drive to the heart. Given together they can cause marked bradycardia, and they may even depress the contraction of the ventricle completely. Verapamil can also raise the serum levels of the beta-blockers which are extensively metabolized in the liver by inhibiting their metabolism (e.g. metoprolol, propranolol).

Importance and management

Well-documented and well-established interactions. Although both drugs have been used together uneventfully and successfully, the reports cited here amply demonstrate that concurrent use may not always be safe, the difficulty being to identify the patients most at risk. The manufacturers list the following among their contraindications and warnings with verapamil alone: hypotension associated with cardiogenic shock, marked bradycardia, uncompensated heart failure, second or third degree atrioventricular block and sick sinus syndrome.[4] These and high doses of either drug are likely predisposing factors. Some practitioners think that the initiation of treatment should be restricted to hospital practice where the dose of each drug can be carefully titrated[15,16] and the patient closely supervised, particularly during the first few days when adverse effects are most likely to develop. If adverse haemodynamic effects occur, the drug dosage should be reduced or withdrawn.[11] One method is to give 50 mg atenolol and 240 mg verapamil daily. If after two weeks no adverse effects develop and the symptoms persist, the verapamil dosage is raised to 360 mg.[15] Beta-blockers which are extensively metabolized (e.g. metoprolol, propranolol) may possibly carry some additional risk because the verapamil raises the serum levels.[14]

References

1 Boothby CB, Garrard CS and Pickering D. Verapamil in cardiac arrhythmias. Br Med J (1972) 2, 349.
2 Seabia-Gomes R, Richards A and Sutton R. Hemodynamic effects of verapamil and practolol. Eur J Cardiol (1976) 4, 79.
3 Livesley B, Catley PF, Campbell RC and Oram S. Double-blind evaluation of verapamil, propranolol, and isosorbide dinitrate against a placebo in the treatment of angina pectoris. Br Med J (1973) 1, 375.
4 ABPI Data Sheet Compendium. Datapharm Publications Ltd (1985) p 1.
5 Ljungstrom A and Aberg H. Interaktion mellan betareceptorblockerare och verapamil. Lakartidningen (1973) 70, 3548.
6 McQueen EG. New Zealand Committee on Adverse Reactions: 14th Annual Report 1979. NZ Med J (1980) 91, 226.
7 McAllister RG, Todd GD, Slack JD, Shearer ME and Hobbs PJ.

Hemodynamic and pharmacokinetic aspects of the interaction between propranolol and verapamil. Clin Res (1981) 29, 755A.

8 Wayne VS, Harper RW, Laufer E, Federman J, Anderson ST and Pitt A. Adverse interaction between beta-adrenergic blocking drugs and verapamil—report of three cases. Aust NZ J Med (1982) 12, 285–9.

9 Balasubramian V, Bowles M, Davies AB and Raferty EB. Combined treatment with verapamil and propranolol in chronic stable angina. Br Heart J (1981) 45, 349–50.

10 Leon MB, Rosing DR, Bonow RO and Epstein HSE. Clinical efficacy of verapamil alone and combined with propranolol in treating patients with chronic stable angina pectoris. Circulation (1980) 62, (Suppl III) 87.

11 Eisenberg JNH and Oakley GDG. Probable adverse interaction between oral metoprolol and verapamil. Postgrad Med J (1984) 60, 705–6.

12 Hutchison SJ, Lorimer AR, Lakhdar A and McAlpine SG. Beta-blockers and verapamil: a cautionary tale. Br Med J (1984) 289, 659–60.

13 Keech AC, Harper RW, Harrison PM, Pitt A and McLean AJ. Pharmacokinetic interaction between oral metoprolol and verapamil for angina pectoris. Am J Cardiol (1986) 58, 551–2.

14 McLean AJ, Knight R, Harrison PM and Harper RW. Clearance-based oral drug interaction between verapamil and metoprolol and comparison with atenolol.

15 Ugourty JC and Silas JH. Beta-blockers and verapamil: a cautionary tale. Br Med J (1984) 289, 1624.

16 Findlay I, McInnes GT and Dargie HJ. Beta-blockers and verapamil: a cautionary tale. Br Med J (1984) 289, 1074.

17 Sinclair NI and Benzie JL. Timolol eye drops and verapamil—a dangerous combination. Med J Aust (1983) 1, 548.

18 Pringle SD and MacEwen CJ. Severe bradycardia due to interaction of timolol eye drops and verapamil. Br Med J (1987) 294, 155–6.

19 Zatuchini J. Bradycardia and hypotension after propranolol HCl and verapamil. Heart and Lung (1985) 14, 94–5.

20 Misra M, Thakur R and Bhandari K. Sinus arrest caused by atenolol-verapamil combination. Clin Cardiol (1987) 10, 365–7.

Beta-blockers + X-ray contrast media

Abstract/Summary

Severe hypotension has been seen in two patients taking beta-blockers when given sodium meglumine diatrizoate as a contrast agent.

Clinical evidence, mechanism, importance and management

Two patients, one taking nadolol and the other propranolol, developed severe hypotensive reactions when given sodium meglumine diatrizoate as a contrast agent for X-ray urography. Both patients developed slowly progressive erythema on the face and arms followed by tachycardia and a weak pulse. Each was treated with subcutaneous adrenaline and hydrocortisone, and placed in the Trendelenburg position. It is suggested that the reaction was due to the release of histamine by the contrast medium, the ability of the body to cope with the hypotension being compromised by the beta-blockade.[1]

Reference

1 Hamilton G. Severe adverse reactions to urography in patients taking beta-adrenergic blocking agents. Can Med Ass J (1985) 133, 122.

11
CALCIUM CHANNEL
BLOCKER INTERACTIONS

This chapter is concerned with those interactions where the activity of the calcium channel blockers (sometimes called calcium antagonists) is changed by the presence of another drug. The table below lists all the calcium channel blockers whose interactions are described in this book, but not all are necessarily dealt with in this chapter because, where the calcium channel blocker is the affecting agent, the relevant synopsis is categorized under the heading of the drug affected. The index should be consulted for a full listing.

The calcium channel blockers have an increasingly wide application and are used for paroxysmal supraventricular tachycardia and angina, arrhythmias, hypertension, congestive heart failure, pulmonary disorders, gastrointestinal disorders and migraine headaches.

Table 11.1

Non-proprietary names	Proprietary names	Non-proprietary names	Proprietary names
Amlodipine		Nisoldipine	
Bepridil	Bepadil, Cordium, Cruor, Vascor	Nitrendipine	Bayotensin, Baypress
Diltiazem	Cardizem	Prenylamine	Angormin, Angoran, Bismetin,
Felodipine			Carditin-same, Crespasin, Daxauten,
Gallopamil	Procorum		Epocol, Eucardion, Herzcon,
Isradipine			Hostagina, Incoran, Lactamine,
Nicardipine	Angioflebil, Cardene, Dagan,		Nyuple, Onlemin, Piboril, Reocorin,
	Flusemide, Lecibral, Lincil, Loxen,		Sedolatan, Segontin(e), Synadrin,
	Nerdipina, Nicardal, Nicodel,		Wasangor
	Perdipina, Perdipine, Ranvil, Vasodin,	Tiapamil	
	Vasonase, Vastrasin	Verapamil	Azupamil, Berkatens, Calan,
Nifedipine	Adalat(e), Anifed, Aprical, Citilat,		Cardiagutt, Cardibeletin, Cardimil,
	Coral, Cordicant, Cordilan, Corotrend,		Cavartil, Coridilox, Durasoptin,
	Dilcor, Duranifin, Fedipina, Hinoxon,		Geangin, Hexasoptin, Isoptin(e/o),
	Nifecor, Nifedicor, Nifedin, Nifedipat,		Manidon, Praecicor, Securon, Univer,
	Nifelat, Nifeniastron, Nife-Puren,		Vasolan, Verakard, Veraloc, Veramex,
	Nifical, Pidilat, Procardia, Tibricol		Veramil, Veroptinstada.

Calcium channel blockers + Aspirin

Abstract/Summary

The antiplatelet effects of the calcium channel blockers may be increased by the concurrent use of aspirin. Abnormal bruising has been seen.

Clinical evidence, mechanism, importance and management

It is recognized that calcium channel blockers such as verapamil, nifedipine and diltiazem can inhibit platelet aggregation because they interfere with the movement of calcium ions through cell membranes. These effects may be additive with those of other antiplatelet drugs. One report describes abnormal bruising and prolonged bleeding times in a patient taking 240 mg verapamil daily while taking two 325 mg aspirin tablets several times a week for headaches. The bruising ceased when the aspirin was stopped.[1] A healthy volunteer taking the same dose of verapamil observed the new appearance of petechiae when also taking aspirin.[1] Concurrent use need not be avoided unless the outcome is clearly adverse.

Reference

1 Ring ME, Martin G V and Fenster PE. Clinically significant antiplatelet effects of calcium-channel blockers. J Clin Pharmacol (1986) 26, 719–20.

Calcium channel blockers + Calcium channel blockers

Abstract/Summary

Blood levels of nifedipine are increased by diltiazem.

Clinical evidence

Pretreatment of six normal subjects with 30 mg or 90 mg of diltiazem three times daily for three days was found to increase the AUC (area under the concentration-time curve) of single 20 mg doses of nifedipine two- and threefold respectively. With the placebo the AUC was 637 ng.h.ml^{-1}; with 30 mg diltiazem 1365 ng.h.ml^{-1} and with 90 mg diltiazem 2005 ng.h.ml^{-1}.

Mechanism

A reduction in the metabolism of the nifedipine by the diltiazem is suggested.[1]

Importance and management

Information is very limited and the clinical importance is uncertain, however be alert for evidence of increased nifedipine effects if diltiazem is given concurrently.

Reference

1 Tateish T, Ohashi K, Toyosaki N, Hosada S, Sugimoto K, Kumagai Y, Kotegawa T, Ebihara A and Tono-oka T. The effect of diltiazem on plasma nifedipine concentration in human volunteers. Jap Circ J (1987) 51, 921.

Calcium channel blockers + Calcium salts

Abstract/Summary

The therapeutic effects of verapamil can be antagonized by calcium.

Clinical evidence, mechanism, importance and management

An elderly woman, successfully treated for over a year with verapamil, re-developed atrial fibrillation within a week of starting to take 1.2 g calcium adipate and 3000 IU calciferol daily for diffuse osteoporosis. Her serum calcium levels had risen from 2.45 to 2.7 mmol/l. Normal sinus rhythm was restored by giving 500 ml saline and repeated doses of 20 mg frusemide and 5 mg verapamil by injection.[1] Verapamil acts by inhibiting the passage of calcium ions into cardiac muscle cells which is antagonized by an increased concentration of calcium ions outside the cells (intravenous calcium has been successfully used to treat verapamil poisoning[2]). Although there is only this single case of an adverse interaction on record, the known pharmacology of verapamil would suggest that this interaction may be of general importance. Calcium should be used with caution in patients taking verapamil.

References

1 Bar-Or D and Yoel G. Calcium and calciferol antagonize effect of verapamil in atrial fibrillation. Brit Med J (1981) 282, 1585.
2 Perkins CN. Serious verapamil poisoning: treatment with intravenous calcium gluconate. Brit Med J (1978) 2, 1127.

Calcium channel blockers + Cimetidine or Ranitidine

Abstract/Summary

The serum levels of diltiazem and nifedipine are increased by cimetidine and it may be necessary to reduce the dosages. Serum nisoldipine and nitrendipine levels are also increased but this seems to be clinically unimportant. It is uncertain whether cimetidine interacts significantly with verapamil. Ranitidine appears to interact minimally with calcium channel blockers but famotidine may possibly reduce heart activity undesirably.

Clinical evidence

(a) Diltiazem

A study in six normal subjects showed that 1200 mg cimetidine daily for a week increased the AUC (area under the curve) of a single 60 mg oral dose of diltiazem by 50% (from 14637 to 22435 ng min/ml) and peak serum levels by 57% (from 46.4 to 73.1 ng/ml). 300 mg ranitidine daily for a week increased the AUC by 15% (statistically insignificant).[11]

Serum diltiazem increases of 40% and AUC increases of 25–50% were seen in another study using cimetidine.[12]

(b) Nifedipine

A study in six normal subjects given 40 mg nifedipine daily showed that the concurrent use of 1 g cimetidine daily for a week increased the maximum serum nifedipine levels by about 80% (from 46.1 to 87.7 ng/ml) and the AUC (area under the curve) by about 60%. 300 mg ranitidine daily for a week caused a non-significant rise of about 25% in maximum nifedipine serum levels and AUC. Seven hypertensive patients showed a fall in mean blood pressure from 127 to 109 mm Hg after taking 40 mg nifedipine daily for four weeks, and a further fall to 95 mm Hg after additionally taking 1 g cimetidine daily for two weeks. When they took 300 mg ranitidine instead, there was a non-significant fall to 103 mm Hg.[1,2,17]

Other studies clearly confirm that cimetidine causes a very significant rise in serum nifedipine levels and an increase in its effects, whereas ranitidine interacts only minimally.[3–6,19,20] A study found no pharmacokinetic interaction between nifedipine and famotidine, but the famotidine reversed the effects of nifedipine on systolic time intervals and significantly reduced the stroke volume and cardiac output.[18]

(c) Nisoldipine and nitrendipine

A study in eight normal subjects showed that after taking 1200 mg cimetidine for a day the bioavailability of a single 10 mg dose of nisoldipine was increased by about 50%, but the haemodynamic effects of the nisoldipine were unaltered.[13]

Another study showed that ranitidine increased the AUC of a single oral dose of nitrendipine by about 50% and decreased its clearance, but no changes in the haemodynamic measurements taken were seen (systolic time intervals, impedance cardiography).[14]

(d) Verapamil

A study in eight normal subjects showed that after taking 300 mg cimetidine six-hourly for eight days no changes occurred in the pharmacokinetics of a single 10 mg intravenous dose of verapamil, but the bioavailability of a 120 mg oral dose increased from 26 to 49%. A small insignificant change in clearance occurred but no change in AUC. The changes in the PR interval caused by the verapamil were unaltered in the presence of cimetidine.[10]

Another study found that 1200 mg cimetidine daily for five days reduced the clearance of verapamil by 21% and increased it elimination half-life by 50%.[7] 800 mg cimetidine daily for a week increased its bioavailability from 35 to 42% and its clearance fell from 45.9 to 33.2 ml/min/kg in another study.[21] Yet another found a small increase in the bioavailability of both enantiomers of verapamil.[8] In contrast, other studies found that the pharmacokinetics of verapamil were unaffected by cimetidine.[6,7,9]

Mechanism

It is believed that cimetidine increases nifedipine levels by inhibiting its oxidative metabolism by the liver. Like ranitidine it may also increase the bioavailability of nifedipine by lowering gastric acidity.[4] The mechanisms of the other interactions are probably similar.

Importance and management

(a) The diltiazem-cimetidine interaction is established. Concurrent use need not be avoided but it has been suggested that the diltiazem dosage may need to be reduced by 30–35%.[15] More study is needed to confirm this. (b) The nifedipine-cimetidine interaction is established. Concurrent use need not be avoided but the increase in the nifedipine effects should be taken into account. A reduction in the nifedipine dosage of 40% has been suggested.[15,16] (c) The limited evidence available suggests that although cimetidine increases the serum levels of nisoldipine and nitrendipine, the haemodynamic changes are unimportant. This needs confirmation. (d) The verapamil–cimetidine interaction is not well established, but until more is known it would seem prudent to monitor the effects of concurrent use. Ranitidine does not to interact significantly with diltiazem or nifedipine and is possibly a non-interacting alternative for cimetidine with other calcium channel blockers. However it is suggested that although famotidine does not have a pharmacokinetic interaction with nifedipine, its negative inotropic effects may possibly be undesirable in the elderly or those with heart failure.[18]

References

1 Kirch W, Janisch HD, Heidemann H, Ramsch K and Ohnhaus EE. Einfluss von Cimetidin und Rantidin auf Pharmakokinetik und antihypertensiven Effekt von Nifedipin. Dtsch Med Wsch(1983) 108, 1757–61.
2 Kirch W, Ramsch K, Janisch HD and Ohnhaus EE. The influence of two histamine H₂-receptor antagonists, cimetidine and ranitidine, on the plasma levels and clinical effect of nifedipine and metoprolol. Arch Toxicol (1984) Suppl 7, 256–9.
3 Smith SR, Kendall MJ, Lobo J, Beerahee A, Jack DB and Wilkins MR. Ranitidine and cimetidine: drug interactions with single dose and steady-state nifedipine administration. Br J clin Pharmac (1987) 23, 311–5.
4 Adams LJ, Antonow DR, McClain CJ and McAllister R. Effect of ranitidine on bioavailability of nifedipine. Gastroenterology (1986) 90, 1320.
5 Kirch W, Ohnhaus EE, Hoensch H and Janisch HD. Ranitidine increases bioavailability of nifedipine. Clin Pharmacol Ther (1985) 37, 204.
6 Abernethy DR, Schwartz JB and Todd EL. Lack of interaction between verapamil and cimetidine. Clin Pharmacol Ther (1985) 38, 342–9.
7 Loi C-M, Rollins DE, Dukes GE and Peat MA. Effect of cimetidine on verapamil disposition. Clin Pharmacol Ther (1985) 37, 654–7.
8 Mikus G, Kroemer HK, Klotz U and Eichelbaum M. Stereochemical

considerations of the cimetidine-verapamil interaction. Clin Pharmacol Ther (1988) 43, 134.

9 Wing LMH, Miners JO and Lillywhite KJ. Verapamil disposition—effects of sulphinpyrazone and cimetidine. Br J clin Pharmac (1985) 19, 385–91.

10 Smith MS, Benyunes MC, Bjornsson TD, Shand DG and Pritchett MD. Influence of cimetidine on verapamil kinetics and dynamics. Clin Pharmacol Ther (1984) 36, 551–4.

11 Winship LC, McKenney JM, Wright JT, Wood JH and Goodman RP. The effect of ranitidine and cimetidine on single-dose diltiazem pharmacokinetics. Pharmacotherapy (1985) 5, 16–9.

12 Mazhar M, Popat KD and Sanders C. Effect of cimetidine on diltiazem blood levels. Clin Res (1984) 32, 741A.

13 Van Harten J, van Brummelen P, Lodewijks M Th M, Danhof M and Breimer DD. Pharmacokinetics and hemodynamic effects of nisoldipine and its interaction with cimetidine. Clin Pharmacol Ther (1988) 43, 332–41.

14 Kirch W, Nahoui R and Ohnhaus EE. Ranitidine/nitrendipine interaction. Clin Pharmacol Ther (1988) 43, 149.

15 Piepho RW, Culbertson VL and Rhodes RS. Drug interactions with the calcium entry blockers. Circulation (1987) 75 (Suppl V) V-181–94.

16 Piepho RW. Individualization of calcium-entry blocker dosage for systemic hypertension. Am J Cardiol (1985) 56, 105H.

17 Kirch W, Hoensch H and Ohnhaus EE. Ranitidin-Nifedipin-Interaktion. Dtsch med Wsch(1984) 109, 1223.

18 Halabi A, Ohnhaus EE and Kirch W. Influence of famotidine on non-invasive haemodynamic parameters and nifedipine plasma levels. Eur J Clin Invest (1988) 18, A23.

19 Schwartz JB, Upton RA, Lin ET, Williams RL and Benet LZ. Effect of cimetidine or ranitidine administration on nifedipine pharmacokinetics and pharmacodynamics. Clin Pharmacol Ther (1988) 43, 673–80.

20 Renwick AG, Le Vie J, Challenor VF, Waller DG, Gruchy B and George CF. Factors affecting the pharmacokinetics of nifedipine. Eur J Clin Pharmacol (1987) 32, 351–55.

21 Mikus G and Stuber H. Influence of cimetidine treatment on the physiological disposition of verapamil. Naunyn-Schmied Arch Pharmacol (1987) 335, Suppl R106.

Calcium channel blockers + Dantrolene

Abstract/Summary

Acute hyperkalaemia and cardiovascular collapse can occur if dantrolene is given in the presence of verapamil or diltiazem, but possibly not with nifedipine.

Clinical evidence, mechanism, importance and management

A 90-year-old man with coronary artery disease taking 80 mg verapamil three times daily, with a history of malignant hyperthermia and undergoing surgery, showed myocardial depression and hyperkalaemia (7.1 mmol/l) within 2 h of being given dantrolene intravenously.[1] Six months later similar preoperative and intraoperative procedures were undertaken uneventfully when the verapamil was replaced by nifedipine. Hyperkalaemia and cardiovascular collapse have been seen in pigs and dogs given dantrolene and verapamil or diltiazem, but not with nifedipine.[2–5]

References

1 Rubin AS and Zablocki AD. Hyperkalaemia, verapamil and dantrolene. Anesthesiology (1987) 66, 246–9.

2 Lynch C, Durbin CG, Fisher NA, Veselis RA and Althaus JS. Effects of dantrolene and verapamil on atrioventricular conduction and cardiovascular performance in dogs. Anesth Analg (1986) 65, 252–8.

3 San Juan AC, Port JD and Wong KC. Hyperkalaemia after dantrolene administration in dogs. Anesth Analg (1986) 65, S131.

4 Saltzman LS, Kates RA, Corke BC, Norfleet EA and Heath KR. Hyperkalaemia and cardiovascular collapse after verapamil and dantrolene administration in swine. Anesth Analg (1984) 63, 473–8.

5 Saltzman LS, Kates RA, Norfleet EA, Corke BC and Heath KR. Hemodynamic interactions of diltiazem-dantrolene and nifedipine and nifedipine-dantrolene. Anaesthesiology (1984) 61, A11.

Calcium channel blockers + Food

Abstract/Summary

Food appears not to have an important effect on the absorption of bepridil or nifedipine.

Clinical evidence, mechanism, importance and management

A study in 15 normal subjects showed that the absorption of two 200 mg capsules of bepridil was delayed by food (peak serum times prolonged from 2.6 to 3.8 h) but the amount absorbed was unchanged.[1] It seems likely that steady-state levels will be unaffected by food. Some single dose studies have suggested that food may delay the absorption of nifedipine and reduce its peak levels,[2–4] but a multiple dose study indicates that food does not have an important effect on the steady-state levels.[5]

References

1 Easterling DE, Stellar SM, Nayak RK and Desiraju RK. The effect of food on the bioavailability of bepridil. J Clin Pharmacol (1984) 24, 416.

2 Ochs HR, Ramsch KD, Verburg-Ochs B, Greenblatt DJ and Gerloff J. Nifedipine: kinetics and dynamics after a single oral dose. Klin Wsch(1984) 62, 427–9.

3 Reitberg DP, Love SJ, Quercia GT and Zinny MA. Effect of food on nifedipine pharmacokinetics. Clin Pharmacol Ther (1987) 42, 72–5.

4 Challenor VF, Waller DG, Gruchy BS, Renwick AG and George CF. Food and nifedipine pharmacokinetics. Br J clin Pharmac (1987) 23, 248–9.

5 Rimoy GH, Idle JR, Bhaskar NK and Rubin PC. The influence of food on the pharmacokinetics of 'biphasic' nifedipine at steady state in normal subjects. Br J clin Pharmac (1989) 28, 612–5.

Calcium channel blockers + Indomethacin or Clonidine

Abstract/Summary

Indomethacin appears not to reduce the hypotensive effects of nifedipine or felodipine, whereas clonidine has a small additive hypotensive effect.

Clinical evidence, mechanism, importance and management

A study in a total of 21 patients with mild to moderate essential hypertension, given 20 mg nifedipine twice daily, showed that 100 mg indomethacin daily for a week did not significantly change the hypotensive effects of the nifedipine, whereas 250 μg clonidine daily for a week increased the hypotensive effects by about 5 mm Hg (mean blood pressure).[1] Another study in normal subjects found that indomethacin did not interact with felodipine.[2]

References

1 Slavetti A, Pedrinelli R, Magagna A, Stornello M and Scapellato L. Calcium antagonists: interactions in hypertension. Am J Nephrol (1986) 6 (Suppl 1) 95–99.
2 Hardy BG, Bartle WR, Myers M, Bailey DG and Edgar B. Effect of indomethacin on the pharmacokinetics and pharmacodynamics of felodipine. Br J clin Pharmac (1988) 26, 557–62.

Calcium channel blockers + Local anaesthetics

Abstract/Summary

Severe hypotension and bradycardia have been seen in patients taking verapamil after epidural anaesthesia with bupivacaine, but not with lignocaine (lidocaine).

Clinical evidence

Four patients on long-term verapamil treatment developed severe hypotension (systolic pressures as low as 60 mm Hg) and bradycardia (48 bpm) after epidural block with bupivacaine (0.5% with adrenaline). This was totally resistant to atropine and ephedrine, and responded only to calcium gluconate or chloride. No such interaction was seen in a similar group of patients when epidural lignocaine was used.[1]

Animal experiments have shown that the presence of verapamil increases the toxicity of lignocaine, and increases toxicity of bupivacaine even more.[2]

Mechanism

Not understood.

Importance and management

Information seems to be limited to these studies involving verapamil. In the absence of more information it would be prudent to assume that other calcium channel blockers may possibly behave similarly. Lignocaine would appear to be preferable to bupivacaine for epidural blockade. Intravenous calcium effectively controls the hypotension and bradycardia produced by verapamil.[3]

References

1 Collier C. Verapamil and epidural bupivacaine. Anaesth Intens Care (1985) 13, 101.
2 Tallman RD, Rosenblatt RM, Weaver JM and Wang Y. Verapamil increases the toxicity of local anaesthetics. J Clin Pharmacol (1988) 28, 317–21.
3 Coaldrake LA. Verapamil overdose. Anaesth Intens Care (1984) 12, 174–5.

Calcium channel blockers + Magnesium salts

Abstract/Summary

A pregnant woman with premature uterine contractions developed muscle weakness and paralysis when given nifedipine and magnesium sulphate concurrently.

Clinical evidence, mechanism, importance and management

A pregnant woman at 32 weeks' gestation was effectively treated for premature uterine contractions with nifedipine, 60 mg orally over 3 h, and later 20 mg over 8 h. 12 h later when contractions began again she was given 500 mg magnesium sulphate intravenously. She developed jerky movements of the extremities, complained of difficulty in swallowing, paradoxical respirations and an inability to lift her head from the pillow. The magnesium was stopped and the muscle weakness disappeared over the next 25 min.[1] The reasons for this reaction are not fully understood. Magnesium ions have neuromuscular blocking activity on skeletal muscle, and both agents can affect the intracellular flow of calcium ions in both skeletal and smooth muscle. Information seems to be limited to this report. The authors recommend that both drugs should not be used for tocolysis in the same patient.

Reference

1 Snyder SW, Cardwell MS. Neuromuscular blockade with magnesium sulphate and nifedipine. Am J Obst Gynecol (1989) 161, 35–6.

Calcium channel blockers + Miscellaneous drugs

Abstract/Summary

The concurrent use of prenylamine and other drugs with negative inotropic effects such as beta-blockers and quinidine, procainamide, amiodarone or lignocaine should be avoided because of the risk of the development of torsades de pointes.

Clinical evidence, mechanism, importance and management

The manufacturers of prenylamine say that prenylamine

should not be given with negative inotropic drugs such as beta-blockers, quinidine, procainamide, amiodarone or lignocaine because there is the risk of the development of torsades de pointes associated with a prolongation of the Q-T interval. Other risk factors are hypokalaemia[5] and conduction disorders.[5] The recommendation is based on reports of atypical ventricular tachycardia (AVT or torsades de pointes) occurring in patients taking prenylamine and propranolol,[1,2] sotalol[3] and other beta-blockers or quinidine-like compounds such as lignocaine (lidocaine).[6,7] The extent of the risk seems not to have been measured but there is evidence that some of these drugs (propranolol, acebutalol, atenolol, oxprenolol, sotalol) have been used concurrently without problems although the Q-T interval was observed to be prolonged.[4]

References

1 Evans TR for Krikler DM. Drug-aggravated sinoatrial block. Proc Roy Soc Med (1975) 68, 808–9.
2 Puritz R, Henderson MA, Baker SN and Chamberlain DA. Ventricular arrhythmias caused by prenylamine. Br Med J (1977) 2, 608–9.
3 Kontopoulos A, Filindris A, Manoudis F and Metaxas P. Sotalol-induced torsades de pointes. Postgrad Med J (1981) 57, 321–3.
4 Oakley D, Jennings K, Puritz R, Krikler D and Chamberlain D. The effect of prenylamine on the QT interval of the resting electrocardiogram in patients with angina pectoris. Postgrad Med J (1980) 56, 753–6.
5 Warembourg H, Pauchant M, Ducloux G, Delbecque M, Vermeersch M and Tonnel-Levy M. Les torsades de pointe. A propos de 30 observations. Lille med (1974) 19, 1–11.
6 Grenadier E, Alpan G, Keidar S and Palant A. Atrio-ventricular block after administation of lignocaine in patients treated with prenylamine. Postgrad Med J (1982) 58, 175–7.
7 Cantle J (Hoechst UK Ltd). Personal communication (1981).

Calcium channel blockers + Rifampicin (Rifampin)

Abstract/Summary

Verapamil serum levels are markedly reduced by the concurrent use of rifampicin and may become therapeutically ineffective unless the dosage is raised appropriately. An isolated report also describes reduced serum nifedipine levels and reduced antianginal effects in a patient when given rifampicin.

Clinical evidence

The observation of a patient whose hypertension was not reduced by verapamil while on antitubercular drugs, prompted a study in four other patients.[1] No verapamil could be detected in the plasma of three of them similarly treated for tuberculosis (rifampicin 450–600 mg daily; isoniazid 5 mg/kg daily; ethambutol 15 mg/kg daily) after receiving a single 40 mg dose of verapamil. A maximum of 20 ng/ml was found in the fourth patient. Six other subjects not taking antitubercular drugs had a maximum verapamil serum concentration of 35 ng/ml after being given a single 40 mg dose.

Essentially the same results are reported in an extended study by the same workers.[3] Supraventricular tachycardia was inadequately controlled in a patient taking 600 mg rifam-

picin and 300 mg isoniazid, despite the administration of 480 mg verapamil every 6 h.[2] Substitution of the rifampicin by ethambutol resulted in a four-fold rise in serum verapamil levels. A later study in six normal subjects showed that after taking rifampicin for two weeks the oral bioavailability of verapamil given orally was reduced from 26 to 2%, and the effects of verapamil on the ECG were abolished.[4] An isolated report describes reduced nifedipine levels (peak levels and AUCs roughly halved) and an increase in anginal attacks in a patient when given rifampicin.[5]

Mechanism

The most likely explanation is that the rifampicin (known to be a potent liver enzyme inducing agent) increases the metabolism of the verapamil and nifedipine by the liver, thereby increasing their clearance from the body.

Importance and management

An established interaction but the documentation is limited. Monitor the effects closely if verapamil or nifedipine and rifampicin are given concurrently, anticipating the need to make a very marked verapamil dosage increase. Ethambutol is a non-interacting alternative antitubercular. There seems to be no information about other calcium channel blockers.

References

1 Rahn KH, Mooy K, Bohm R and van den Vet, A. Reduction of bioavailability of verapamil by rifampin. N Eng J Med (1985) 312, 920–21.
2 Barbarash RA. Verapamil-rifampin interaction. Drug Intell Clin Pharm (1985) 19, 559–60.
3 Mooy J, Bohm R, van Baak M, Kemenade J, v d Vet A and Rahn RH. The influence of antituberculosis drugs on the plasma level of verapamil. Eur J Clin Pharmacol (1987) 32, 107–9.
4 Barbarash RA, Bauman JL, Fischer JH, Kondos G and Batenhorst RL. Near total reduction in verapamil bioavailability by rifampin: electrocardiographic correlates. J Amer Coll Cardiol (1988) 11, 205A.
5 Tsuchihashi K, Fukami K, Kishimoto H, Sumiyoshi T, Haze K, Saito M and Hiramori K. A case of variant angina exacerbated by administration of rifampicin. Heart Vessels (1987) 3, 214–7.

Calcium channel blockers + Sulphinpyrazone

Abstract/Summary

The clearance of verapamil is markedly increased by sulphinpyrazone.

Clinical evidence, mechanism, importance and management

A study in eight normal subjects showed that after taking 800 mg sulphinpyrazone daily for a week, the clearance of a single oral dose of verapamil was increased about threefold (from 4.27 to 13.77 l/h/kg), possibly due to an increase in its liver metabolism.[1] The clinical importance of this is uncertain, but be alert for reduced verapamil effects. It seems probable that the dosage may need to be increased.

Reference

1 Wing LMH, Miners JO and Lillywhite KJ. Verapamil disposition—effects of sulphinpyrazone and cimetidine. Br J clin Pharmac (1985) 19, 385–91.

Calcium channel blockers + Vancomycin

Abstract/Summary

An isolated case report suggests that the hypotensive effects of the rapid infusion of vancomycin may occur more readily in those who are already vasodilated with nifedipine.

Clinical evidence, mechanism, importance and management

A man with severe systemic sclerosis was hospitalized for Raynaud's phenomenon and dental extraction. After being started on 40 mg nifedipine daily, he was given intravenous vancomycin (1 g in 200 ml 5% dextrose) over 30 min. After 20 min he experienced a severe headache and was found to have a marked macular erythema on the upper trunk, head, neck and arms. His blood pressure fell to 100/60 mm Hg and his pulse rate was 90. He recovered spontaneously.[1] The suggested reason is that the vasodilatory effects of the nifedipine were additive with those of the vancomycin (known to cause hypotension and erythema if infused quickly). The authors of this report suggest that vasodilators should be discontinued several days before giving vancomycin, and the blood pressure should be well monitored during infusion.

Reference

1 Daly BM and Sharkey I. Nifedipine and vancomycin-associated red man syndrome. Drug Intell Clin Pharm (1986) 20, 986.

Calcium channel blockers + X-ray contrast media

Abstract/Summary

The hypotensive effects of an intravenous bolus of ionic X-ray contrast medium are increased by the presence of calcium channel blockers (diltiazem, nifedipine, verapamil, etc.). No interaction or only a small interaction appears to occur with non-ionic contrast media. A case report describes serious ventricular tachycardia in a patient on prenylamine when given sodium iothalamate.

Clinical evidence, mechanism, importance and management

(a) Hypotensive effects increased

It is well recognized that ionic X-ray contrast media used for ventriculography reduce the systemic blood pressure due to peripheral vasodilation. They also have a direct depressant effect on the heart muscle. A comparative study of the haemodynamic response of 65 patients showed that the hypotensive effect of a bolus dose of an ionic agent (0.5 ml/kg diatrizoate meglumine and diatrizoate sodium with edetate sodium or disodium) was increased by the concurrent use of nifedipine or diltiazem: it occurred earlier (3.1 s instead of 12.9 s), was more profound (a fall in systolic pressure of 48.4 instead of 36.9 mm Hg) and more prolonged (62 s instead of 36 s).[1] A similar interaction was seen in dogs given verapamil.[2] No interaction or only a minimal interaction was seen in the patients and dogs when non-ionic contrast media (iopamidol or iohexol) were used instead.[1,2] Concurrent use should be undertaken with care.

(b) Ventricular arrhythmia precipitated

An elderly man who had been taking 60 mg prenylamine and 10 mg nifedipine three times a day for two years experienced cardiorespiratory arrest a few seconds after a bolus intravenous injection of 80 ml sodium iothalamate 70% (*Contray 420*), and a further arrest 90 seconds later. On the second occasion the rhythm was identified as ventricular tachycardia, converted to sinus rhythm by a 100 Joule DC shock.[3] The reason is thought to be the additive effects of the prenylamine and sodium iothalamate both of which can prolong the QT_c (corrected QT interval of the heart) which predisposes the development of serious ventricular arrhythmias. Concurrent use should be avoided or undertaken with great care.

References

1 Morris DL, Wisneski JA, Gertz EW, Wexman M, Axelrod R and Langberg JJ. Potentiation by nifedipine and diltiazem of the hypotensive response after contrast angiography. J Am Coll Cardiol (1985) 6, 785–91.
2 Higgins CB, Kuber M and Slutsky RA. Interaction between verapamil and contrast media in coronary arteriograpy: comparison of standard ionic and new non-ionic media. Circulation (1983) 68, 628-35
3 Duncan JS and Ramsay LE. Ventricular tachycardia precipitated by sodium iothalamate (*Contray 420*) injection during prenylamine treatment: a predictable adverse drug interaction. Postgrad Med J (1985) 61, 415–7.

12
ORAL CONTRACEPTIVE AND RELATED SEX HORMONE DRUG INTERACTIONS

The oral contraceptives are of two main types: (i) the combined oestrogen-progestogen preparations, and the combined sequential preparations with the doses of each steroid varied throughout the cycle; (ii) the progestogen-only preparations. The oestrogens used are either ethinyloestradiol in doses of 20–50 μg, or mestranol in doses of 50–100 μg. The progestogens are either those derived from 19-norethisterone (e.g. norethynodrel, ethynodiol acetate, norgestrel, norethisterone, lynoestrenol) or more rarely from 17 alpha-hydroxyprogesterone (e.g. megestrol) in doses ranging from about 0.25–5.0 mg. There are now very many different oral contraceptive preparations available throughout the world but most seem to be variants on these two broad themes.

The combined and sequential preparations are taken for 20–21 days, followed by a period of seven days during which withdrawal bleeding occurs. Some of them include six or seven tablets of lactose to be taken during this period so that the daily habit of taking a tablet is not broken. These contraceptives act in several ways: the oestrogenic component suppresses ovulation and the progestogen acts to change the endometrial structure so that even if conception were to occur, implantation would be unlikely. In addition the cervical mucus become unusually viscous which inhibits the free movement of the sperm.

The progestogen-only or 'mini-pills' are taken continuously. They do not inhibit ovulation but probably act by increasing the viscosity of the cervical mucus so that movement of the sperm is retarded. They may also causes changes in the endometrium which inhibit successful implantation.

Almost all of the interactions described here in this chapter and elsewhere in this book involve the combined oral contraceptives. Very little seems to be known about the interactions with the progestogen-only contraceptives. One should not therefore uncritically assume that interactions known to occur with the former type of contraceptive also occur with the latter, but there may possibly be some overlap. Much more study is needed to define the situation more clearly.

Oral contraceptives + Alcohol

Abstract/Summary

The detrimental effects of alcohol may be reduced to some extent in women on oral contraceptives, but blood alcohol levels are possibly unaltered.

Clinical evidence

A controlled study in 54 women[1] showed that those on oral contraceptives (30, 35 or 50 μg oestrogen) tolerated the effects of alcohol better than those not taking oral contraceptives (as measured by a reaction-time test and a bead-threading test) but their blood-alcohol levels and its rate of clearance were unchanged. Two other studies suggest that blood alcohol levels may be reduced in those taking oral contraceptives.[2,3] The authors of the report cited[1] say that they do not recommend women on oral contraceptives to drink more than usual, and they point out that the risks of prosecution for driving while over the legal blood-alcohol limits remain the same.

References

1 Hobbes J, Boutagy J and Shenfield GM. Interactions between ethanol and oral contraceptive steroids. Clin Pharmacol Ther (1985) 38, 371–80.
2 Jones MK and Jones BM. Ethanol metabolism in women taking oral contraceptives. Alcoholism (1984) 8, 24–8.
3 Zeiner AR and Kegg PS. Effects of sex steroids on ethanol pharmacokinetics and autonomic reactivity. Prog Biochem Pharmacol (1981) 18, 130–42.

Oral contraceptives + Antacids

Abstract/Summary

Despite some in vitro evidence that magnesium trisilicate might possibly reduce the effects and the reliability of the oral contraceptives, other evidence from human studies suggests that concurrent use is safe.

Clinical evidence, mechanism, importance and management

Although *in vitro* studies[1] have clearly shown that 0.5 and 1.0% suspensions of magnesium trisilicate in water adsorb very considerable amounts (50–90%) of ethisterone, mestranol and norethisterone, a single-dose study[2] in 12 women given a single pill (30 μg ethinyloestradiol and either norethisterone acetate 1 mg or levenorgestrel 150 μg) with a single tablet containing magnesium trisilicate (0.5 g) and aluminium hydroxide (0.25 g) showed that the bioavailability of the contraceptive remained unchanged. This is in line with common experience. Nor does there appear to be an important interaction with any other antacid or adsorbent.

References

1 Khalil SAH. The *in vitro* uptake of some oral contraceptive steroids by magnesium trisilicate. J Pharm Pharmac (1976) 28, (Suppl). 47P.
2 Joshi JV, Sankolli GM, Shah RS and Joshi UM. Antacid does not reduce the bioavailability of oral contraceptive steroids in women. Int J Clin Pharmac Ther Toxicol (1986) 24, 192–5.

Oral contraceptives + Anti-asthmatic preparations

Abstract/Summary

There are no recorded interactions, but asthma is included by some manufacturers of oral contraceptives among their 'special precautions' because the asthmatic condition may be worsened. Sometimes it may be improved.

Clinical evidence, mechanism, importance and management

There have been instances in which women have developed allergic conditions such as rhinitis, atopic eczema, urticaria or asthma while taking oral contraceptives.[1–3] In contrast there are other instances where pre-existing asthma and other allergic conditions have improved.[2] For this reason it has been claimed that '. . . it is always worth while giving an oral contraceptive a trial for patients with any of these complaints [eczema, asthma, vasomotor rhinitis, migraine] as there is an even chance that she will be improved; if the condition is aggravated, it will return to its previous state as soon as the medication is stopped.'[1]

References

1 Mears E. Oral contraceptives. Lancet (1964) i, 980.
2 Falliers CJ. Oral contraceptives and allergy. Lancet (1974) ii, 515.
3 Horan JD and Lederman JJ. Possible asthmogenic effect of oral contraceptives. Can Med Ass J (1968) 99, 130.

Oral contraceptives + Antibiotics and Anti-infective agents

Abstract/Summary

Failure of oral contraceptives to prevent pregnancy has been attributed to the concurrent use of a tetracycline in 18 cases. One or two cases of failure have been reported with each of the following: chloramphenicol, cephalexin with clindamycin, dapsone, erythromycin, isoniazid, nitrofurantoin with sulphamethoxypyridazine, sulphonamides and metronidazole.

Clinical evidence

(a) Tetracyclines

A woman on *Microgynon 30* (ethinyloestradiol + D-norgestrel) became pregnant. The evidence indicated that she must have conceived while taking a course of tetracycline (500 mg tetracycline six-hourly for three days and then 250 mg six-hourly for two days) or in the week following. There was no evidence of either nausea or vomiting which might have been alternative explanations for the contraceptive failure.[1] A case of break-through bleeding and another pregnancy attributed to the concurrent use of tetracycline are also described in this report.[1,2] The British Committee on the Safety of Medicines (CSM) has reports of 12 cases of contraceptive failure with tetracyclines (tetracycline, oxytetracycline).[3,9] Another survey describes six failures due to doxycycline, lymecycline or minocycline.[8] Yet another describes two failures with tetracycline.[10]

(b) Chloramphenicol, cephalexin with clindamycin, dapsone, erythromycin, isoniazid, nitrofurantoin, sulphamethoxypyridazine and trimethoprim

Two women on oral contraceptives are briefly reported to have shown break-through bleeding and to have become pregnant. One was taking chloramphenicol and the other sulphamethoxypyridazine.[4,5] One or two cases of failure have been attributed to concurrent treatment with each of the following: chloramphenicol, cephalexin with clindamycin, dapsone, erythromycin, isoniazid, nitrofurantoin, sulphonamides and trimethoprim.[3,9,10] The CSM also has on record five cases implicating co-trimoxazole in contraceptive failure—see 'Contraceptives, oral + Co-trimoxazole'.

(c) Metronidazole

Three out of 25 women on oral contraceptives are stated to have ovulated while taking metronidazole, but no cases of pregnancy were reported.[6] A pregnancy occurred in one woman taking metronidazole, but she was also taking doxycycline.[8] Another study found no evidence that metronidazole affected the reliability of the combined oral contraceptives,[7] but the CSM has three cases of pregnancy on their records attributed to an interaction with metronidazole,[9] and another occurs in another report.[10]

Mechanism

Not understood. Suppression of intestinal bacteria is a possible explanation (see 'Mechanism' in the synopsis dealing with 'Oral contraceptives + Penicillins').

Importance and management

The cases cited appear to be the sum of the reports involving these drugs. The incidence would seem to be very low indeed. It is likely that the majority of women are not at risk, but there is no way as yet of predicting who is likely to be affected. The precautions suggested for 'Oral contraceptives + Penicillins' should be followed.

References

1 Bacon JF and Shenfield GM. Pregnancy attributable to interaction between tetracycline and oral contraceptives. Br Med J (1980) 1, 293.
2 Lesqueux A. Grossesse sous contraceptif oral apres prise de tetracycline. Louvain Med (1980) 99, 413.
3 Back DJ, Breckenridge AM, Crawford FE, MacIver M, Orme L'E and Rowe PH. Interindividual variation and drug interactions with hormonal steroids. Drugs (1981) 21, 46.
4 Hempel E, Bohm W, Carol W and Klinger G. Medikamentose Enzyminduktion und hormonal Kontrazeption. Zbl Gynak (1973) 95, 1451.
5 Hempel E. Personal communication (1975).
6 Joshi JV, Gupta KC, Joshi UM, Krishna U and Saxena BN. Interactions of oral contraceptives with other drugs and nutrition. Contracept Delivery Syst (1982) 3, 60.
7 Viswanathan MK and Govindarajulu P. Metronidazole therapy on the efficacy of oral contraceptive steroid pills. J Reprod Biol Comp Endocrinol (1985) 5, 69–72.
8 Sparrow MJ. Pill method failures. NZ J Med (1987) 100, 102–5.
9 Back DJ, Grimmer FM, Orme L'E, Proudlove C, Mann RD and Breckenridge AM. Evaluation of Committee on Safety of Medicines yellow card reports on oral contraceptive-drug interactions with anticonvulsants and antibiotics. Br J clin Pharmac (1988) 25, 527–32.
10 Kovacs GT, Riddoch G, Duncombe P, Welberry L, Chick P, Weisberg E, Leavesley GM and Baker G. Inadvertent pregnancies in oral contraceptive users. Med J Aust (1989) 150, 549–51.

Oral contraceptives + Anticonvulsants

Abstract/Summary

Oral contraceptives are unreliable during concurrent treatment with phenytoin, primidone, barbiturates and carbamazepine. Failure of contraceptive implants has also been reported. Intermediate break-through bleeding and spotting can take place and pregnancies have occurred. Seizure control may sometimes be disturbed. Sodium valproate appears not to interact.

Clinical evidence

(a) Contraceptive failure

An epileptic woman taking 200 mg phenytoin and 50 mg sulthiame daily (with ferrous gluconate and folic) became pregnant despite the regular use of an oral contraceptive containing 0.05 mg ethinyloestradiol and 3 mg norethisterone acetate.[1]

Since this first report[1] in 1972, at least 27 pregnancies have been reported in epileptic women taking a range of oral contraceptives and anticonvulsants which have included either phenytoin, a barbiturate or primidone.[2–6,10,11,15,25,28] Carbamazepine has also been clearly implicated[13,25–29] and possibly ethosuximide.[26] The Committee on the Safety of Medicines in the UK has received another 43 reports[12,26] making a total of at least 70 cases in the 1968–89 period.[12] It is also reported that subdermal contraceptive implants containing levonorgestrel (*Norplant*) failed to prevent pregnancy in three women taking phenytoin.[21,22] In addition to these interactions, a report describes a menopausal woman on replacement treatment with conjugated oestrogens (*Premarin*), 1.25 mg daily, which became inadequate when she began to take 300 mg phenytoin daily.[16]

(b) Disturbance of seizure control

Epilepsy is included by most oral contraceptive manufacturers among the 'special precautions' to be observed because seizure control may sometimes be made worse, but it also may remain unaltered or even improve:

An epileptic woman under treatment with phenytoin and phenobarbitone became much worse while taking *Lyndiol* but improved when *Gynovlar* and later *Ovulen* were substituted.[7]

Another report describes 20 epileptics taking a variety of anticonvulsants whose condition was unaltered by *Norinyl-1*.[8] A woman on phenytoin and phenobarbitone was completely fit free until she discontinued the oral contraceptive (unnamed) she had been taking.[9]

Mechanism

The most probable explanation is that these anticonvulsants act as potent liver enzyme inducing agents which increase the metabolism and clearance of the contraceptives from the body, thereby reducing their effects and in some instances allowing ovulation to occur. Changes in seizure control have been attributed to changes in fluid retention which can influence seizure frequency.[7,8]

Importance and management

Contraceptive failure in the presence of phenobarbitone, phenytoin, primidone and carbamazepine is established, but uncertain with ethosuximide. The incidence is not known. It may be quite small (a failure-rate of 3.1 per 100 woman years is reported[24]). On the other hand the incidence of spotting and break-through bleeding is known to be high.[17-19] One study found the following: seven out of eleven patients on phenobarbitone, one out of two on phenytoin, and four out of six on carbamazepine.[17] Another study reported a 60% incidence in adolescent women taking un-named anticonvulsants.[18] The unsolved problem is the identification of those women whose menstrual cycles are sufficiently disturbed to allow pregnancy to take place.

Several practical solutions have been suggested. One is to use contraceptives containing 50 μg ethinyloestradiol.[12,13,17] If break-through bleeding still occurs, to give in addition a preparation containing 30 or even 50 μg ethinyloestradiol.[12,14] Another worker reports that two daily doses of an oral contraceptive containing less than 50 μg ethinyloestradiol can be effective,[17] however the advisability of giving such large doses has been questioned.[23] An alternative is to use a mechanical form of contraception or a non-interacting anticonvulsant. There is good evidence that sodium valproate does not normally interact with the oral contraceptives.[17,20] It is also important to be on the alert for changes in seizure control if the interacting anticonvulsants are used.

References

1 Kenyon IE. Unplanned pregnancy in an epileptic. Br Med J (1972) 1, 686.
2 Hempel von E, Bohm W, Carol W and Klinger G. Medikamentose Enzyminduktion und hormonale Kontrazeption. Zbl Gynak (1973) 95, 1451–7.
3 Janz D and Schmidt D. Anti-epileptic drugs and failure of oral contraceptives. Lancet (1974) i, 1113.
4 Janz D and Schmidt D. Anti-epileptic drugs and the safety of oral contraceptives. Paper delivered to the German Section of the International League against Epilepsy. Berlin, 1st September 1974.
5 Belaisch J, Driguez P and Janaud A. Influence de certains medicaments due l'action des pilules contraceptives. Nouv Presse Med (1976) 5, 1645.
6 Gagnaire JC, Tchertchian J, Revol A and Rochet Y. Grossesses sous contraceptifs oraux chez les patientes recevant des barbituriques. Nouv Presse Med (1975) 4, 3008.
7 McArthur J. Notes and comments. Oral contraceptives and epilepsy. Br Med J (1967) 3, 162.
8 Espir M, Wallace ME and Lawson JP. Epilepsy and oral contraception. Br Med J (1969) 1, 294.
9 Copeman H. Oral contraceptives. Med J Aust (1963) 2, 969.
10 Back DJ and Orme ML'E. Drug interactions with oral contraceptive steroids. Prescribers Journal (1977) 17, 137.
11 Coulam CB and Annegers JF. Do anticonvulsants reduce the efficacy of oral contraceptives? Epilepsia (1979) 20, 519.
12 Editorial. Drug interaction with oral contraceptive steroids. Br Med J (1980) 3, 93.
13 Hempel E and Klinger W. Drug stimulated biotransformation of hormonal contraceptive steroids. Clinical implications. Drugs (1976) 12, 442.
14 Back DJ, Bates M, Bowden A, Breckenridge AM, Hall MJ, Jones H, MacIver M, Orme M, Perucca E, Richens A, Rowe PH and Smith E. The interaction of phenobarbital and other anticonvulsants with oral contraceptive steroid therapy. Contraception (1980) 22, 495.
15 Fanoe E. P-pillesvigt-antagelig pa grund af interaktion me fenemal. Ugeskr Laege (1977) 139, 1485.
16 Notelovitz M, Tjapkes A and Ware M. Interaction between estrogen and Dilantin in a menopausal woman. N Engl J Med (1981) 304, 788.
17 Sonnen AEH. Sodium valproate and the pill. In 'Advances in Epileptology', XIIIth Epilepsy Int Symp. Akimoto H, Kazamatsuri H, Seino M and Ward A (Eds). Raven Press, NY (1982) 4229–32.
18 Diamond MP and Thompson JM. Oral contraceptive use in epileptic adolescents. J Adolesc Health Care (1981) 2, 82.
19 Diamond MP, Greene JW, Thompson JM, VanHooydonk JE and Wentz AC. Interaction of anticonvulsants and oral contraceptives in epileptic adolescents. Contraception (1985) 31, 623–32.
20 Crawford P, Chadwick D, Cleland P, Tjia J, Cowie A, Back DJ and Orme ML'E. Sodium valproate and oral contraceptive steroids. Brit J Clin Pharmacol (1985) 20, 288P.
21 Odlind V and Olsson S-E. Enhanced metabolism of levonorgestrel during phenytoin treatment in a woman with Norplant implants. Contraception (1986) 33, 257–61.
22 Haukkamaa M. Contraception by Norplant subdermal capsules is not reliable in epileptic patients on anticonvulsant treatment. Contraception (1986) 33, 559–65.
23 Elkington KW. Use of oral contraceptives by women with epilepsy. J Amer Med Ass (1986) 256, 2961.
24 Kay CR. Progestogen and arterial disease. Evidence from the Royal college of General Practitioners study. Am J Obst Gynecol (1982) 142, 762–6.
25 Sparrow MJ. Pill method failures. NZ J Med (1987) 100, 102–5.
26 Back DJ, Grimmer FM, Orme L'E, Proudlove C, Mann RD and Breckenridge AM. Evaluation of Committee on Safety of Medicines yellow card reports on oral contraceptive-drug interactions with anticonvulsants and antibiotics. Br J clin Pharmac (1988) 25, 527–32.
27 Beeley L, Magee P and Hickey FM. Bulletin of the West Midlands Centre for Adverse Drug Reaction Reporting (1989) 28, 21.
28 Kovacs GT, Riddoch G, Duncombe P, Welberry L, Chick P, Weisberg E, Leavesley GM, Baker G. Inadvertent pregnancies in oral contraceptive users. Med J Aust (1989) 150, 549–51.
29 Rapport DJ and Calabrese JR. Interactions between carbamazepine and birth control pills. Psychosomatics (1989) 30, 462–3.

Oral contraceptives + Antihypertensive agents

Abstract/Summary

The hypertension caused by the oral contraceptives is frequently resistant to antihypertensive therapy with guanethidine or methyldopa.

Clinical evidence, mechanism, importance and management

Virtually all women who take oestrogen-containing oral contraceptives show some rise in blood pressure. One study[1] on 83 women showed that the average rises in systolic/diastolic pressures were 9.2/5.0 mm Hg, and it is about twice as likely to occur as in those not taking an oral contraceptive. There are many reports confirming this response but, despite extensive work, the reason for it is not understood although much of the work has centred around the increases seen in the activity of the renin-antgiotensin system. Once the contraceptive is withdrawn, the blood pressure usually returns to its former levels.[2]

Attempts to control gross rises in pressure using guanethidine or methyldopa have been unsatisfactory[3–5] and one report[3] states that '. . .concurrent medication with guanethidine and oral contraceptives made satisfactory control of hypertension difficult or impossible.' It seems therefore that hypertension associated with, or exacerbated by, the use of oral contraceptives may not respond to drugs whose major actions are at adrenergic neurones.

References

1 Weir RJ, Briggs E, Mack A, Naismith L, Taylor L and Wilson E. Blood pressure in women taking oral contraceptives. Br Med J (1974) 1, 533.
2 Editorial (Anon.) Hypertension and oral contraceptives. Br Med J (1978) 1, 1570.
3 Clezy TM. Oral contraceptives and hypertension: the effect of guanethidine. Med J Aust (1970) 1, 638.
4 Wallace MR. Oral contraceptives and severe hypertension. Aust NZ J Med (1971) 1, 49.
5 Woods JW. Oral contraceptives and hypertension. Lancet (1967) iii, 653.

Oral contraceptives + Antimalarial drugs

Abstract/Summary

Chloroquine and primaquine do not reduce the serum levels of the combined oral contraceptives and there is no evidence that they affect their contraceptive reliability. Chloroquine serum levels remain unchanged during concurrent use and its efficacy appears to be unaltered. Oral contraceptives appear not to affect the treatment of falciparum malaria with mefloquine.

Clinical evidence, mechanism, importance and management

(a) Effect of chloroquine and primaquine on oral contraceptives

A detailed pharmacokinetic study[1] in two groups of women (12 and 7) taking low-dose oral contraceptives (ethinyl-oestradiol + norethisterone) showed that the prophylactic use of chloroquine phosphate, 500 mg once a week for four weeks, caused a small increase in blood levels of the oestrogen (AUC + 15%), but there was nothing to suggest that the normal effects of the contraceptives were changed in any way. Chloroquine blood levels remained unaltered. Another study[2] in six women given a single dose of *Microgynon* (ethinyloestradiol + levonorgestrel) confirmed that neither chloroquine (300 mg) nor primaquine (45 mg) had a significant effect on the pharmacokinetics of either the oestrogen or the progestogen. Further confirmation of the absence of an interaction comes from studies in rhesus monkeys infected with malaria in which it was shown that the efficacy of chlorquine was not altered by the use of either *Norinyl* or *Ovral-28*.[3]

(b) Effect of oral contraceptives on mefloquine

A study in 12 Thai women with falciparum malaria found that their response (parasite and fever clearance) to treatment with mefloquine was not affected by the concurrent use of oral contraceptives. However the half-life and residence time of mefloquine were found to be shorter than in six normal healthy Thai women taking oral contraceptives.[4]

References

1 Gupta KC, Joshi JV, Desai NK, Sankolli GM, Chowdhary VN, Joshi UM, Chitalange S and Satoskar RS. Kinetics of chloroquine and contraceptive steroids in oral contraceptive users during concurrent chloroquine prophylaxis. Indian J Med Res (1984) 80, 658–662.
2 Back DJ, Breckenridge AM, Grimmer SFM, Orme ML'E and Purba HS. Pharmacokinetics of oral contraceptive steroids following the administration of the antimalarial drugs primaquine and chloroquine. Contraception (1984) 30, 289–295.
3 Dutta GP, Puri SK, Kamboj KK, Srivastava SK and Kamboj VP. Interactions between oral contraceptives and malaria infections in rhesus monkeys. Bull WHO (1984) 62, 931–9.
4 Karbwang J, Looareesuwan S, Back DJ, Migasana S, Bunnag D and Breckenridge AM. Effect of oral contraceptive steroids on the clinical cause of malaria infection and on the pharmacokinetics of mefloquine in Thai women. Bull WHO (1988) 66, 763–7.

Oral contraceptives + Antischistosomal drugs

Abstract/Summary

Early schistosomiasis and the use of praziquantel or metriphonate do not appear to have any effect on the oral contraceptives.

Clinical evidence, mechanism, importance and management

Women with advanced schistosomal infections which affect the liver are not given oral contraceptives because their impaired liver function can affect the metabolism of drugs, but there seems to be no reason for withholding these contraceptives from those with only urinary or intestinal infections.[1,2] A study in 25 women with early active schistosomiasis (*S. haematobium* or *S. mansoni*) showed that neither the disease itself nor the concurrent use of antischistosomal drugs (a single 40 mg/kg dose of praziquantel, or metriphonate in three doses of 10 mg/kg at fortnightly intervals) had any effect on their serum oral contraceptive steroid levels when given *Ovral* (50 μg ethinyloestradiol + 500 μg levonorgestrel).[3]

References

1 Shaaban MM, Hammad WA, Fathalla MF, Ghaneimah SA, El-Sharkawy MM, Salim TH, Liaso WC and Smith SC. Effects of oral contraception on liver function tests and serum protein in women with active schistosomiasis. Contraception (1982) 26, 65–74.
2 El-Raghy I, Back DJ, Osman F, Nafeh MA and Orme ML'E. The pharmacokinetics of antipyrine in patients with graded severity of schistosomiasis. Br J clin Pharmac (1985) 20, 313–6.
3 El-Raghy I, Back DJ, Osman F, Orme ML'E and Fathalla M. Contraceptive steroid concentrations in woman with early active schistosomias: lack of effect of antischistosomal drugs. Contraception (1986) 33, 373–7.

Oral contraceptives + Cimetidine or Ranitidine

Abstract/Summary

Cimetidine, but not ranitidine, raises endogenous serum oestradiol levels but whether it raises serum contraceptive steroid levels is uncertain.

Clinical evidence, mechanism, importance and management

800 mg cimetidine twice daily for two weeks was found to increase the serum oestradiol (endogenous) levels of nine men by about 20%, due apparently to the well-recognised inhibitory effects of cimetidine on the metabolism of oestradiol (2-hydroxylation) by the liver. 400 mg twice daily for a week had the same effect in another six men.[1] These raised levels are a possible explanation of the signs and symptoms of oestrogen excess (gynecomastia, sexual dysfunction) which sometimes occurs in men after taking cimetidine for some time. Ranitidine, 150 mg twice daily, was found not to raise serum oestradiol levels.

Whether cimetidine has the same effect on administered oestradiol or other oestrogens (in oral contraceptives for instance) is uncertain but the possibility of increased effects should be borne in mind during concurrent use.

Reference

1 Galbraith RA, Michnovicz JJ. Effects of cimetidine on the oxidative metabolism of estradiol. N Eng J Med (1989) 321, 269–74.

Oral contraceptives + Co-trimoxazole

Abstract/Summary

A human study has shown that co-trimoxazole would be expected to increase the effectiveness of the oral contraceptives, yet there are 12 cases on record of contraceptive failure attributed to the concurrent use of co-trimoxazole.

Clinical evidence

A study in nine women taking a triphasic contraceptive (*Trinordiol*) containing ethinyloestradiol and levonorgestrel showed that while taking two tablets of co-trimoxazole daily (320 mg trimethoprim + 1600 mg sulphamethoxazole in each tablet) their blood levels of ethinyloestradiol rose 30–50% (from 29.3 to 38.2 ng/ml at 12 h and from 18.9 to 27.8 ng/ml at 24 h). Levonorgestrel levels remained unaltered.[1]

In contrast the Committee on the Safety of Medicines in the UK has on its records five cases of oral contraceptive failure attributed to the use of co-trimoxazole,[2,4] and another is reported elsewhere.[5] Two other surveys describe six cases of contraceptive failure while taking co-trimoxazole and trimethoprim.[3,6]

Mechanism

The rise in ethinyloestradiol levels[1] is probably due to inhibition by the sulphamethoxazole of the liver enzymes concerned with the metabolism and clearance of the oestrogen from the body. It is not clear why co-trimoxazole should sometimes paradoxically seem to be the cause of contraceptive failure.

Importance and management

The picture is confusing and contradictory. The authors of the study cited[1] say that '... the effects of contraceptive steroid preparations are enhanced rather than reduced by co-trimoxazole; and it is unlikely that clinical problems will arise in women taking long-term oral contraceptive steroids who are given short courses of co-trimoxazole.' This study appears to have been carefully carried out and controlled whereas the CSM and other reports are simply uncontrolled individual case reports. However some risk, however small, seems to exist and the precautions suggested for 'Oral contraceptives + Penicillins' would seem to be appropriate.

References

1 Grimmer SFM, Allen WL, Back DJ, Breckenridge AM, Orme M, and Tjia T. The effect of co-trimoxazole on oral contraceptive steroids in women. Contraception (1983) 28, 53–9.
2 Back DJ, Breckenridge AM, Crawford FE, MacIver M, Orme ML'E,

Rowe PH. Interindividual variation and drug interactions with hormonal steroid contraceptives. Drugs (1981) 21, 46–61.

3 Sparrow MJ. Pill method failures. NZ Med J (1987) 100, 102–5.

4 Back DJ, Grimmer FM, Orme L'E, Proudlove C, Mann RD and Breckenridge AM. Evaluation of Committee on Safety of Medicines yellow card reports on oral contraceptive-drug interactions with anticonvulsants and antibiotics. Br J clin Pharmac (1988) 25, 527–32.

5 Beeley L, Magee P and Hickey FM. Bull W Midl Centre for Adverse Drug Reaction Reporting (1989) 28, 32.

6 Kovacs GT, Riddoch G, Duncombe P, Welberry L, Chick P, Weisberg E, Leavesley GM and Baker G. Inadvertent pregnancies in oral contraceptive users. Med J Aust (1989) 150, 549–51

Oral contraceptives + Enprostil

Abstract/Summary

Enprostil appears not to interact with the oral contraceptives.

Clinical evidence, mechanism, importance and management

A double-blind cross-over study on 22 normal women taking *Norinyl 1+35* (norethindrone 1 mg + ethinyloestradiol 0.035 mg) showed that the concurrent use of 35 μg enprostil for seven days had no significant effect on the pharmacokinetics of either of the contraceptive steroids. The bioavailability of the oral contraceptives remained unaltered.[1]

Reference

1 Winters L and Wilberg C. Enprostil, a synthetic prostaglandin E_2 analog does not affect oral contraceptive bioavailability. Gastroenterology (1988) 94, A500.

Oral contraceptives + Fluconazole

Abstract/Summary

Two pregnancies and six cases of intermenstrual bleeding have been described in women using oral contraceptives, attributed to the use of fluconazole. This interaction (if such it is) is rare.

Clinical evidence

Two pregnancies have been reported, despite the use of oral contraceptives, attributed to an interaction with single 150 mg doses of fluconazole. Intermenstrual bleeding has also been described in six other women on oral contraceptives when given a single 150 mg dose of fluconazole. No withdrawal bleeding was reported in one other patient.[1,2]

In contrast to these reports, a study in 10 women taking combined oral contraceptives found no evidence that a single 50 mg dose of fluconazole or 50 mg fluconazole daily for 10 days had significant effects on the pharmacokinetics of an oral contraceptive (30 μg ethinyloestradiol and 150 μg leveonorgestrel).[3] During clinical trials in which single 150 mg doses of fluconazole were used by over 700 women taking oral contraceptives, no evidence of an interaction was seen.[4]

Mechanism

Not understood. Unlike ketoconazole, fluconazole appears to have little effect on liver enzyme activity (P450-cytochrome mediated reactions).

Importance and management

Although the contraceptive failures and intermenstrual bleeding cited here have been attributed to the use of fluconazole, this interaction is not clearly established. The weight of evidence suggests that contraceptive failure is very unlikely if fluconazole is given, however spotting and breakthrough bleeding are possible signs of diminished contraceptive effectiveness and the ultracautious might consider advising the additional use of a barrier method of contraception if pregnancy is to be avoided more certainly.

References

1 Pfizer Ltd. Summary of unpublished reports: Female reproductive disorders possibly associated with Diflucan. Data on file (Ref DIFLU:diflu41.1) (1990).

2 West Midlands Centre for Adverse Drug Reaction Reporting January (1990), 30.

3 Pfizer Ltd. An open study to examine the effect of fluconazole on the metabolism of an oral contraceptive in healthy female volunteers. Unpublished data on file (ref 29/VG) (1990).

4 Dodd GJ (Pfizer Ltd). Personal communication (1990).

Oral contraceptives + Griseofulvin

Abstract/Summary

The effects of the oral contraceptives may possibly be disturbed (either intermenstrual bleeding or amenorrhoea) if griseofulvin is taken concurrently. A woman taking an oral contraceptive became pregnant while taking griseofulvin and two others on oral contraceptives became pregnant while taking griseofulvin and a sulphonamide.

Clinical evidence

15 out of 22 women experienced transient intermenstrual bleeding and five had amenorrhoea during the first or second cycle after starting to take griseofulvin (0.5—1.0 g daily). Four of the 22 (two with intermenstrual bleeding and two with amenorrhoea) developed their original reactions when rechallenged with griseofulvin. Two other women on the pill are reported to have become pregnant while taking griseofulvin and a sulphonamide (co-trimoxazole in one instance and an unknown sulphonamide in the other)[1].

Oligomenorrhoea and irregular menses have been described in a woman on an oral contraceptive when given griseofulvin (250–500 mg daily). When the oral contraceptive was substituted by another with 57% more oestrogen, the menstrual flow became normal again.[2] Break-through

337

bleeding has also been seen in three other women on the pill given griseofulvin[3] and one case of contraceptive failure has been reported.[4]

Mechanism

Not understood. Griseofulvin may possibly stimulate the activity of the liver enzymes concerned with the metabolism of the contraceptive steroids, thereby reducing their effects. This might explain the cases of break-through bleeding, but not those involving oligomenorrhoea and amenorrhoea. Contraceptive failure attributed to co-trimoxazole has also been reported (see 'Oral contraceptives + Co-trimoxazole').

Importance and management

Information about this interaction seems to be limited to these reports.[1–4] The risk of total contraceptive failure is uncertain but probably very small. It would now seem prudent for prescribers to warn women on oral contraceptives who are given griseofulvin that menstrual disturbances may possibly be signs of contraceptive unreliability, and that additional contraceptive precautions should be taken. For maximal contraceptive protection a barrier method should be used.

References

1 Van Dijke CPH and Weber JCP. Interaction between oral contraceptives and griseofulvin. Br Med J (1984) 288, 1125–6.
2 McDaniel PA and Caldroney RD. Oral contraceptives and griseofulvin interaction. Drug Intell Clin Pharm (1986) 20, 384.
3 Beeley L and Stewart P. Bulletin of the West Midlands Centre for Adverse Drug Reaction Reporting. (1987) 25, 23.
4 Back DJ, Grimmer FM, Orme L'E, Proudlove C, Mann RD and Breckenridge AM. Evaluation of Committee on Safety of Medicines yellow card reports on oral contraceptive-drug interactions with anticonvulsants and antibiotics. Br J clin Pharmac (1988) 25, 527–32.

Oral contraceptives + Isotretinoin

Abstract/Summary

There seems to be no evidence that the reliability of the combined oral contraceptives is affected by isotretinoin.

Clinical evidence, mechanism, importance and management

A study in nine women taking a combined oral contraceptive showed that the plasma concentrations of ethinyloestradiol and levonorgestrel were not significantly changed by the use of 0.5 mg/kg isotretinoin for severe pustular acne.[1] The authors conclude that oral contraceptives remain reliable during concurrent use, and they say that it seems unlikely that an interaction would occur with 1.0 mg/kg which is the dose commonly recommended in the USA.

Reference

1 Orme M, Back DJ, Shaw MA, Allen WL, Tjia J, Cunliffe WJ and Jones DH. Isotretinoin and contraception. Lancet (1984) ii, 752–3.

Oral contraceptives + Ketoconazole

Abstract/Summary

Ketoconazole can reduce the effectiveness of the oral contraceptives and cause intermenstrual bleeding. So far no pregnancies have been reported.

Clinical evidence, mechanism, importance and management

Seven out of 147 women taking low dose oral contraceptives (*Ovidon, Rigevidon, Anteovin*) experienced break-through bleeding or spotting within 2–5 days of starting a five-day course of ketoconazole, 400 mg daily. No pregnancies occurred.[1] The reason for this reaction is not understood. Its incidence is low (about 5%), its general importance is uncertain and information seems to be limited to this single report. However intermenstrual bleeding is a sign of a decrease in the effectiveness of the oral contraceptives so that the precautions suggested when taking antibiotics such as the penicillins (use an additional barrier contraceptive) would seem to be a wise precaution if pregnancy is be avoided with certainty (see 'Oral contraceptives + Penicillins').

Reference

1 Kovacs L, Somos P and Hamori M. Examination of the potential interaction between ketoconazole (Nizoral) and oral contraceptives with special regard to products of low hormone content (*Rigevidon, Anteovin*). Ther Hung (1986) 34, 167.

Oral contraceptives + Penicillins

Abstract/Summary

It is now accepted that very infrequently and unpredictably the penicillins can cause the combined oral contraceptives to fail. Rare failures of the progestogen-only oral contraceptives have also been attributed to the use of a penicillin, but cause-and-effect has not been established.

Clinical evidence

A woman is reported to have had two unwanted pregnancies while taking *Minovlar* (ethinyloestradiol + norethisterone). She had also been treated with wide-spectrum antibiotics, particularly ampicillin. Another woman on *Minovlar* for five years, with no history of break-through bleeding, lost a quantity of blood similar to a normal period loss within a day of starting to take ampicillin, one capsule four times a day. There was no evidence of diarrhoea or vomiting in either case.[1,2]

The British Committee on the Safety of Medicines (CSM) in the UK has on record 32 further cases of contraceptive failure over the 1968–84 period attributed to penicillin antibiotics: ampicillin, ampicillin with either fusidic acid, tetracycline or flucloxacillin, amoxycillin, talampicillin, phenoxymethylpenicillin (one also taking oxytetracycline) and 'penicillin'.[8,13] Another survey records contraceptive failures due to amoxycillin (16 cases), flucloxacillin, phenoxymethylpenicillin, pivampicillin (five cases) and amoxycillin with phenoxymethylpenicillin (two cases).[12] Yet another report describes 17 cases with amoxycillin and five cases with 'penicillin'.[14] Further cases attributed to oxacillin and *Triplopen* (benethamine, procaine and benzyl penicillins) are reported elsewhere.[9,11]

Mechanism

Not understood. The oestrogen component of the contraceptive is cycled in the entero-hepatic shunt (i.e. it is repeatedly secreted in the bile as steroid conjugates which are then hydrolysed by the gut bacteria before reabsorption). It is thought that if these bacteria are decimated by the use of an antibiotic, the steroid conjugates fail to undergo bacterial hydrolysis and are very poorly reabsorbed, resulting in lower-than-normal concentrations of circulating oestrogen in a very small number of women and in an inadequate suppression of ovulation.[7] However, although the penicillins reduce urinary oestriol secretion in pregnant women,[3–5] no marked changes in serum oestrogen levels in most women on contraceptives have been found.[6,8] The progestogens do not take part in the entero-hepatic shunt.

Importance and management

An established interaction. The incidence is not known but it is probably very low indeed. The oral contraceptives and the penicillins have been very widely used for many years, yet relatively speaking there are few reports of contraceptive failure. Most women do not appear to be at risk, but as yet there seems to be no way of identifying those likely to be affected. Spotting and break-through bleeding are possible signs of diminished contraceptive effectiveness. For maximal protection a barrier contraceptive method should be used routinely while taking a short course of a penicillin, and for at least seven days afterwards, possibly until the beginning of the next cycle. It has been suggested that those on long-term antibiotics for acne need only take extra precautions for the first two weeks because after that the gut flora becomes resistant to the antibiotic,[10] but this remains to be confirmed. Four contraceptive failures attributed to a progestogen-only contraceptive/pencillin interaction occur in the CSM records, but no definite link has been established.

References

1 Dossetor EJ. Drug interactions with oral contraceptives. Br Med J (1975) 4, 467.
2 Dossetor EJ. Personal communication (1976).
3 Willman K and Pulkkinen MO. Reduced maternal plasma and urinary oestriol during ampicillin treatment. Amer J Obstet Gyn (1971) 109, 893.
4 Tikkanen MJ, Aldercreutz H and Pulkinnen MO. Effect of antibiotics on oestrogen metabolism. Br Med J (1973) 1, 369.
5 Pulkinnen MO and Willeman K. Maternal oestrogen levels during penicillin treatment. Br Med J (1971) 4, 48.
6 Friedman CJ, Huneke AL, Kim MH and Powell J. The effect of ampicillin on oral contraceptive effectiveness. Obst Gynec (1980) 55, 33.
7 Back DJ, Breckenridge AM, Crawford FE, MacIver M, Orme L and Rowe PH. Interindividual variation and drug interactions with hormonal steroid contraceptives. Drugs (1981) 21, 46.
8 Back DJ, Breckenridge AM, MacIver M, Orme M, Rowe PH, Staiger Ch, Thomas E and Tjia A. The effect of ampicillin on oral contraceptive steroids in women. Br J clin Pharmac (1982) 14, 43–8.
9 Silber TJ. Apparent oral contraceptive failure associated with antibiotic administration. J Adolesc Health Care (1983) 4, 287–9.
10 Szarewski A and Guillebaud J. Hormonal contraception. In 'Update Postgraduate Centre Series. Contraception', McFadzean W (ed). Update-Siebert Publications, Guildford (1988) p 9–18.
11 Bainton R. Interaction between antibiotic therapy and contraceptive medication. Oral Surgery, Oral Medicine, Oral Pathology (1986) 61, 453–5.
12 Sparrow MJ. Pill method failures. NZ Med J (1987) 100, 102–5.
13 Back DJ, Grimmer FM, Orme L'E, Proudlove C, Mann RD and Breckenridge AM. Evaluation of Committee on Safety of Medicines yellow card reports on oral contraceptive-drug interactions with anticonvulsants and antibiotics. Br J clin Pharmac (1988) 25, 527–32.
14 Kovacs GT, Riddoch G, Duncombe P, Welberry L, Chick P, Weisberg E, Leavesley GM, Baker G. Inadvertent pregnancies in oral contraceptive users. Med J Aust (1989) 150, 549–51

Oral contraceptives + Rifampicin

Abstract/Summary

Oral contraceptives are unreliable during concurrent treatment with rifampicin. Intermediate break-through bleeding and spotting frequently take place and conception may not be prevented.

Clinical evidence

62 out of 88 women on oral contraceptives are described in a report as having developed menstrual cycle disorders of various kinds when treated with rifampicin. Five pregnancies in women taking both drugs are also mentioned.[1,2]

Since the first report[3] in 1971 describing a very marked increase in the frequency of intermenstrual break-through bleeding in women on oral contraceptives and rifampicin, other reports have confirmed this interaction and at least 15 pregnancies have been reported.[4–8,14] Contraceptive failure in a woman given rifampicin, streptomycin and isoniazid has also been described.[13]

Mechanism

Rifampicin acts as a potent liver enzyme inducing agent which markedly increases the metabolism and clearance of the oral contraceptive steroids from the body, thereby reducing their effects. 600 mg rifampicin daily for only six days has been found to increase the aromatic hydroxylation of ethinyloestradiol fourfold[9,10] and a significant reduction in serum norethisterone levels also occurs.[12] Mestranol is probably similarly affected.[11] These reduced steroid levels may be insufficient to prevent the re-establishment of a normal menstrual cycle and this would explain the break-through bleeding and pregnancies which can occur. The trend towards low-dose oestrogen contraceptives would seem to increase its likelihood.

Importance and management

The oestrogen/progestogen + rifampicin interaction is well-documented and established. There is no detailed information about the failure rate but a reported[1,2] menstrual cycle disturbance of 70% suggests that women undergoing treatment with rifampicin should use an alternative or additional form of contraception if pregnancy is to be avoided with certainty. No failures due to rifampicin have been reported with the progestogen-only contraceptives, but their reliability in the presence of rifampicin is doubtful.[12]

References

1 Reimers D, Nocke-Finck L and Breuer H. Rifampicin causes a lowering in efficacy of oral contraceptives by influencing oestrogen excretion. Reports on Rifampicin: XII International Tuberculosis Conference, Tokyo, September 1974.
2 Reimers D, Nocke-Finck L and Breuer H. Rifampicin, 'pill' do not go well together. J Amer Med Ass (1974) 227, 608.
3 Reimers D and Jezek A. Rifampicin und andere Antituberkulotika bei gleichzeitiger oraler Kontrazeption. Prax Pneumol (1971) 25, 255.
4 Kropp R. Rifampicin und Ovulationshemmer. Prax Pneumol (1974) 28, 270.
5 Bessot J-C, Vandevenne A, Petitjean R and Burghard G. Effets opposes de la rifampicine et de l'isoniazide sur le metabolisme des contraceptifs oraux? Nouv Presse med (1977) 6, 1568.
6 Hirsch A. Pilules endormies. Nouv Presse Med (1973) 2, 2957.
7 Piguet B, Muglioni JF and Chaline G. Contraception orale et rifampicine. Nouv Presse med (1975) 4, 115.
8 Skolnik JL, Stoler BS, Katz DB and Anderson WH. Rifampicin, oral contraceptives and pregnancy. J Amer Med Ass (1976) 236, 1382.
9 Bolt HM, Kappus H and Bolt M. Rifampicin and oral contraception. Lancet (1974) i, 1280.
10 Bolt HM, Kappus H and Bolt M. Effect of rifampicin treatment on the metabolism of oestradiol and 17 alpha-ethinyloestradiol by human liver microsomes. Europ J Clin Pharmacol (1975) 8, 301.
11 Bolt HM and Bolt WH. Pharmacokinetics of mestranol in man in relation to its oestrogenic activity. Europ J Clin Pharmacol (1974) 7, 295.
12 Back DJ, Breckenridge AM, Crawford F, MacIver M, Orme ML'E, Park BK, Rowe PH and Smith E. The effect of rifampicin on norethisterone pharmacokinetics. Europ J clin Pharmacol (1974) 15, 193.
13 Back DJ, Breckenridge AM, Crawford FE, MacIver M, Orme L'E and Rowe P. Interindividual variation and drug interactions with hormonal steroid contraceptives. Drugs (1981) 21, 46.
14 Gupta KC and Ali MY. Failure of oral contraceptive with rifampicin. Med J Zambia (1980/81) 15, 23.

Oral contraceptives + Tobacco smoking

Abstract/Summary

The risk of thromboembolic disease in women on oral contraceptives is increased if they smoke.

Clinical evidence, mechanism, importance and management

A study in women in the 40–41 age group on oral contraceptives who smoked showed that they had a lower level of high-density lipoprotein in their serum than women who neither smoked nor took the pill.[1] The significance of this finding is that low levels are a major risk factor in the development of coronary heart disease and related thrombotic diseases. This is borne out by epidemiological studies which show that the incidence of thromboembolic diseases in women on the pill increases both with age and if the subjects smoke.[2,3] Just another good reason why smoking should be discouraged.

References

1 Arntzenius AC, van Gent CM, van der Voort H, Stegerhoek C and Styblo K. Reduced high-density lipoprotein in women aged 40–41 using oral contraceptives. Lancet (1978) i, 1221.
2 Fredriksen H and Ravenholt RT. Thromboembolism, oral contraceptives and cigarettes. Public Health Rep (1970) 85, 197.
3 Collaborative Group for the study of stroke in young women. J Amer Med Ass (1975) 231, 718.

Oral contraceptives + Triacetyloleandomycin

Abstract/Summary

Severe pruritis and jaundice have been observed in women taking oral contraceptives shortly after commencing treatment with triacetyloleandomycin.

Clinical evidence

A report describes 10 cases of cholestatic jaundice and pruritis in women taking oral contraceptives and triacetyloleandomycin. All had been using the contraceptive for 7–48 months and were given the antibiotic in 250 or 500 mg doses four times a day. The pruritis was intense, lasting 2–24 days, and preceded the jaundice which in eight of the patients persisted for over a month.[1]

There are numerous other reports of this adverse reaction,[2–12] one of which describes 24 cases.[5,6]

Mechanism

Uncertain. Hepatotoxicity has been associated with the use of both types of drug. The reaction suggests that their damaging effects on the liver may be additive or supra-additive.

Importance and management

An established, well-documented and important interaction. The incidence is unknown. Concurrent use should be avoided.

References

1 Miguet JP, Monange C, Vuitton D, Allemand H, Hirsch JP, Carayon P and Gisselbrecht H. Ictere cholestatique survenu apres administration de triacetyloleandomycine: interference avec les contraceptifs oraux? Dix observations. Nouv Presse med (1978) 7, 4304.
2 Perol R, Hincky J and Desnos M. Hepatites cholestatiques lors de la prise de troleandomycine chez deux femmes prenant des estrogenes. Nouv Presse med (1978) 7, 4302.
3 Goldfain D, Cauveinc L, Guillan J and Verudron J. Ictere cholestatique chez des femmes prenant simultanement de triacetyloleandomycine et des contraceptifs oraux. Nouv Presse med (1979) 8, 1099.

4 Rollux R, Plottin F, Mingat J and Bessard G. Ictere apres association estroprogestatif-troleandomycine. Trois observations. Nouv Presse med (1979) 8, 1694.

5 Miguet J-P, Vuitton D, Pessayre D, Allemand H, Metreau J-M, Poupon R, Capron JP and Blanc F. Jaundice from troleandomycin and oral contraceptives. Ann Intern Med (1980) 92, 434.

6 Miguet JP, Vuitton D, Allemand H, Pessayre D, Monange C, Hirsch J-P, Metreau J-M, Poupon R, Capron J-P and Blanc F. Une epidemie d'icteres due a l'association troleandomycine-contraceptifs oraux. Gastroenterol Clin Biol (1980) 4, 420.

7 Haber I and Hubens H. Cholestatic jaundice after triacetyloleandomycin and oral contraceptives. Acta Gastro-Enterol Belg (1980) 43, 475.

8 Claudel S, Euvrard P, Bory R, Chaivallon A and Paliard P. Cholestase intrahepatique apres association triacetyloleandomycine-estroprogestatif. Nouv Presse med (1979) 8, 1182.

9 Descotes J, Evreux J Cl, Fouatier N, Gaumer R, Girard D and Savoye B. Trois nouvelles observations d'ictere apres estroprogestatifs et troleandomycine. Nouv Presse med (1979) 8, 1182.

10 Anon. Levertoxiciteit van troleandomycine en oestrogen. Fol Pharmaceutica (Brussels) (1979) 6, 64.

11 Dellas JA, Hugues FC, Roussel G and Marche J. Contraception orale et troleandomycine. Un nouveau cas d'ictere. Therapie (1982) 37, 443–6.

12 Girard D, Pillon M, Bal A, Petigny A and Savoye B. Hepatite au decours d'un traitment au TAO chez les jeunes femmes sous oestroprogestatifs. LL M Medecine Sud Est (1980) 16, 2335–44.

Oral contraceptives + Vitamins

Abstract/Summary

The oral contraceptives are reported to raise serum levels of vitamin A, and lower levels of ascorbic acid, cyanocobalamin, folic acid and pyridoxine. Ascorbic acid can raise serum ethinyloestradiol levels and pyridoxine may relieve depression in women on oral contraceptives, but the general clinical importance of concurrent treatment with these vitamins is uncertain.

Clinical evidence, mechanism, importance and management

There is evidence that the use of oral contraceptives can cause a biochemical deficiency of several vitamins, but clinical deficiency does not necessarily manifest itself. Serum levels of cyanocobalamin can be lowered,[1] folate deficiency with anaemia can occur,[2,3] and reduced levels of ascorbic acid[3,4] and pyridoxine[6,7] have been described. Treatment of pyridoxine deficiency has been shown to improve the mood of depressed women on oral contraceptives.[11] Raised levels of vitamin A has also been reported.[8] These changes in vitamin requirements induced by the oral contraceptives are reviewed in detail elsewhere.[9]

A study has shown that 1 g ascorbic acid can substantially raise serum ethinyloestradiol levels (+48% measured at 24 h) in women taking oral contraceptives,[14] and a single case report describes a woman on *Logynon* who experienced heavy break-through bleeding within 2–3 days of stopping her self-administered 1 g daily dose of ascorbic acid.[14]

Routine prophylactic treatment with vitamins in women on oral contraceptives has been advised by some,[10] but ques-

tioned by others[12,13] because an increased intake of some vitamins in some circumstances may be harmful. For example, in areas of the world where protein malnutrition is rife, a pyridoxine supplement might lead to an undesirable increase in amino-acid catabolism in those on a low daily intake of protein.[12] One author's comment on the indiscriminate supplementation of the diet with multivitamin preparations in women on oral contraceptives is that it can hardly be justified.[13]

References

1 Wertalik LF, Metz EN, LoBuglio AF and Balcerzak SP. Decreased serum B$_{12}$ levels with oral contraceptive use. J Amer Med Ass (1972) 221, 1371.

2 Streiff RR. Folate deficiency and oral contraceptives. Ibid (1970) 214, 214.

3 Meguid MM and Loebl WY. Megaloblastic anaemia associated with the oral contraceptive pill. Postgrad Med J (1974) 60, 470.

4 Harris AB, Pillay M and Hussein S. Vitamins and oral contraceptives. Lancet (1975) ii, 82.

5 Briggs M and Briggs M. Vitamin C requirements and oral contraceptives. Nature (1972) 238, 277.

6 Bennick HJTC and Schreurs WHP. Disturbance of tryptophan metabolism and its correction during hormonal contraception. Contraception (1972) 9, 347.

7 Doberenz AR, van Miller JP, Green JR and Beaton JR. Vitamin B6 depletion in women using oral contraceptives as determined by erythrocyte glutamic-pyruvic transaminase activities. Proc Soc Exp Biol Med (1971) 137, 1100.

8 Wild J, Schorah CJ and Smithells RW. Vitamin A, pregnancy and oral contraceptives. Br Med J (1974) 1, 57.

9 Larsson-Cohn U. Oral contraceptives and vitamins. A review. Amer J Obst Gynec (1975) 121, 84.

10 Briggs M and Briggs M. Oral contraceptives and vitamin requirements. Med J Aust (1975) 1, 407.

11 Adams PW, Wynn V, Seed M and Foklhard J. Vitamin B6, depression and oral contraception. Lancet (1974) ii, 515.

12 Adams PW, Wynn V, Rose DP, Folkhard J, Seed M and Strong R. Effect of pyridoxine hydrochloride (vitamin B6) upon depression associated with oral contraception. Lancet (1973) i, 897.

13 Back DJ, Breckenridge AM, MacIver M, Orme ML'E, Purba H and Rowe PH. Interaction of ethinyloestradiol with ascorbic acid in man. Br Med J (1981) 282, 1516.

14 Morris JC, Beeley L and Ballantine N. Interaction of ethinyloestradiol with ascorbic acid in man. Br Med J (1981) 283, 503.

Intrauterine Contraceptive Devices (IUD's) + Anti-inflammatory Agents

Abstract/Summary

There is some evidence that the very occasional failure of an IDU to prevent pregnancy may have been due to the concurrent use of a steroidal or non-steroidal anti-inflammatory agent.

Clinical evidence, mechanism, importance and management.

Two women out of a total of about 1000 fitted with *Multiload 250* (an IUD) became pregnant. One had taken aspirin, and the other mefenamic acid during the month when conception occurred. Another woman using a *Lippes C* conceived during the month when she took *Veganin* (aspirin, codeine, paracetamol).[1] A report[2] describes four women who, despite being fitted with IUD's, twice became pregnant. Two were taking corticosteroids regularly and the other two often took aspirin for migraine. Unwanted pregnancies have also been reported elsewhere in women with IUD's treated with corticosteroids.[3,4]

The evidence for this possible interaction is very slim and inconclusive, but the suggestion that drugs which affect prostaglandins might possibly affect the actions of the IUD's bears further investigation.

References

1 Dossetor J. Personal communication (1983).
2 Buhler M and Papiernik E. Successive pregnancies in women fitted with intrauterine devices who take anti-inflammatory drugs. Lancet (1983) 1, 483.
3 Inkeles DM and Hansen RI. Unexpected pregnancy in women using an intrauterine device and receiving steroid therapy. Ann Ophthalmol (1982) 14, 975.
4 Zerner J, Miller AB, and Festino MJ. Failure of an intrauterine device concurrent with administration of corticosteroids. Fertil Steril (1976) 27, 1467.

Medroxyprogesterone + Aminoglutethimide

Abstract/Summary

Aminoglutethimide markedly reduces the serum levels of medroxprogesterone.

Clinical evidence, mechanism, importance and management

A study in six postmenopausal women with breast cancer given 1500 mg medroxyprogesterone acetate daily showed that the concurrent use of aminoglutethimide (500–1000 mg daily) halved the plasma levels of the medroxyprogesterone.[1] A probable reason is that the aminoglutethimide acts as an enzyme inducing agent and increases the metabolism of the medroxyprogesterone by the liver. Monitor the effects of concurrent use and be alert for the need to increase the dosage of the medroxyprogesterone. The effects of aminoglutethimide on other steroids used in oral contraceptives seem not to have been studied.

Reference

1 Van Deijk WA, Blijhan GH, Mellink WAM and Meulenberg PMM. Influence of aminoglutethimide on plasma levels of medroxyprogesterone acetate: its correlation with serum cortisol. Cancer Treat Rep (1985) 69, 85–90.

13

CYTOTOXIC DRUG INTERACTIONS

The cytotoxic drugs (antineoplastics, cytostatics) are used in the treatment of malignant disease in conjunction with radiotherapy, surgery and immunosuppressants such as the corticosteroids and lymphocytic antisera. They also find application in the treatment of skin conditions such as psoriasis and a few are used with other immunosuppressant drugs (cyclosporin, corticosteroids) to prevent transplant rejection. These other immunosuppressant drugs are dealt with in Chapter 16.

Of all the drugs discussed in this book, the cytotoxic drugs are amongst the most toxic and have a low therapeutic index. This means that a quite small increase in their activity can lead to the development of serious and life-threatening toxicity. A list of the cytotoxic agents which are featured appears in Table 13.1. Unlike most of the other interaction synopses in this book, some of the information on the cytotoxic drugs is derived from animal experiments and still requires confirmation in man. The reason for including this data is that the drugs in this group generally do not lend themselves readily to the kind of clinical studies which can be undertaken with other drugs, and there would seem to be justification in this instance for including indirect evidence. The aim is not to make definite predictions, but to warn users of the interaction possibilities.

Table 13.1 Cytotoxic drugs

Non-proprietary names	Proprietary names
Aclarubicin (aclacinomycin A)	Aclacin
Actinomycin (dactinomycin)	Cosmegen, Lyovac
Aminoglutethimide	Cytraden, Orimeten, Orimeten
Azathioprine	Azamune, Azanin, Azapress, Imuran, Imurek, Imurek, Imurel, Thioprine
Bleomycin	Blenoxane, Bleo-oil, Bleo-s, Blocamicina, Verbublen
Carmofur	Mifurol, Yamaful
Carmustine (BCNU)	Becenun, BiCNU, Carmubris, Citrumon
Chlorambucil	Leukeran, Linfolysin
Chlorozotocin	
Cis-platin (CPDD)	Cisplatyl, Citoplatino, Neoplatin, Placis, Platamine, Platiblastin, Platinex, Platinol, Platistin, Platosin
Colaspase (asparaginase)	Crasnitin(e), Elspar, Erwinase, Kidrolase, Leucogen, Leunase, Laspar
Cyclophosphamide	Carloxan, Cycloblastin, Cyclostin(e), Cytoxan, Endoxan(a), Enduxan, Genoxal, Neosar, Procytox, Sendoxan
Cytarabine (cytosine arabinoside)	Alexan, Arabitin, Aracytin(e), Erpalfa, Iretin
Daunorubicin (daunomycin, rubidomycin)	Cerubidin(e), Daunoblastin(a)

343

Table 13.1 *continued*

Non-proprietary names	Proprietary names
Doxorubicin (adriamycin)	*Adriacin, Adriblastina, Farmiblastina,*
Etoposide	*Etopol, Vepesid*
Fluorouracil (5-FU)	*Adrucil, Arumel, Effluderm, Efudex, Efudix, Fluoroplex, Fluoroblastin(e), Timazin*
Hexamethylmelamine	*Hexastat, Hexinawas*
Hydroxyurea	*Hydrea, Litalir, Onco-Carbide*
Ifosfamide	*Holoxan, Mitoxana, Tronoxal*
Lomustine (CCNU)	*Belustine, Cecenu, CeeNU, CiNU, Lucostrine,*
Melphalan	*Alkeran(a)*
Mercaptopurine	*Ismipur, Purinethol*
Methotrexate (amethopterin)	*Emtexate, Emthexat(e), Farmotrex, Folex, Ledertrexate, Maxtrex, Methotrexat, Metotraxato, Metrexan, Mexate, Tremetex*
Meturedepa	*Turloc*
Misonidazole	
Mitomycin (mitomycin C)	*Ametycine, Mitomycine-C, Mutamycin*
Mithramycin	*Mithracin*
Mitotane	*Lysodren*
Mustine (methchlormthamine, Nitrogen mustard)	*Caryolysine, Cloramin, Mustargen*
Procarbazine	*Matulane, Natulan(ar)*
Streptozocin (streptozotocin)	*Zanosar*
Tamoxifen	*Istubol, Kessar, Noltam, Nolvadex, Tamaxin, Tamofen, Tamoxasta, Zitazonium*
Thioguanine	*Lanvis*
Thiotepa	*Ledertepa, Onco-Tiotepa, Tifosyl*
Vinblastine	*Velban, Velbe*
Vincristine	*Kyocristine, Onconvin, Pericristine*
Vindesine	*Eldesine, Enison*

Aclarubicin and Cytotoxic drugs

Abstract/Summary

The bone marrow depressant effects of aclarubicin can be increased by previous treatment with nitrosoureas or mitomycin.

Clinical evidence, mechanism, importance and management

Myelosuppression is among the adverse effects of aclarubicin (aclacinomycin A). The makers warn that the concurrent use of other drugs with similar myelosuppressant actions may be expected to have additive effects and dosage reductions should be considered.[3] Prior treatment with nitrosoureas (not specifically named) or mitomycin has been shown to increase the severity of the myelosuppression.[1,2]

References

1   Van Echo DA, Whitacre MY, Aisner J, Applefeld MM and Wiernik PH. Phase I trial of aclacinomycin A. Cancer Treat Rep (1982) 66, 1127–32.
2   Bedikian AY, Karlin D, Stoehlein J, Valdivieso M, Korinek J and Bodey G. Phase II evaluation of aclacinomycin A (ACM-A, NSC 208734) in patients with metastatic colorectal cancer. Am J Clin Oncol (CCT) (1983) 6, 187–190.
3   Aclacin (aclarubicin hydrochloride) data sheet. Lundbeck (Feb 1990).

Aminoglutethimide + Bendroflumethiazide

Abstract/Summary

A single case report describes the severe loss of sodium in a patient after 10 months treatment with both drugs.

Clinical evidence, mechanism, importance and management

A woman who for several years had been taking four tablets daily of bendroflumethiazide (2.5 mg) and potassium chloride (578 mg) for hypertension and mild cardiac incompensation, was additionally treated with aminoglutethimide, 1 g daily, and hydrocortisone, 60 mg daily, for breast cancer. After 10 months' treatment she was hospitalized with severe hyponatremia due, apparently, to the combined inhibitory effects of the aminoglutethimide on aldosterone production (which normally retains sodium in the body) and the diuretic. The serum sodium levels were subsequently kept normal by the addition of fludrocortisone (0.1 mg daily).[1]

Reference

1   Bork E and Hansen M. Severe hyponatremia following simultaneous administration of aminoglutethimide and diuretics. Cancer Treat Rep (1986) 70, 689–90.

Azathioprine/Mercaptopurine + Allopurinol

Abstract/Summary

The effects of azathioprine and mercaptopurine are markedly increased by the concurrent use of allopurinol when the cytotoxic agent is given orally. The dosage of the cytotoxic drug should be reduced to a third or a quarter if toxicity is to be avoided. No interaction appears to occur if these cytotoxic drugs are given intravenously.

Clinical evidence

(a) Azathioprine + allopurinol

A patient treated with 300 mg allopurinol daily developed pancytopenia when additionally treated with 150 mg azathioprine daily.[3]

Reversible bone marrow damage associated with anaemia, leucocytopenia and thrombocytopenia has also been described in two renal transplant recipients and in two other patients (one with myasthenia) who were given both drugs.[4–6]

(b) Mercaptopurine + allopurinol

A study in seven patients with chronic granulocytic leukaemia, treated with 50 mg mercaptopurine daily, showed that when additionally given 400 mg allopurinol daily their granulocyte counts fell by amounts equivalent to that expected with four to five times the dose of mercaptopurine.[1]

Profound pancytopenia developed in three children under treatment with mercaptopurine 2.5 mg/kg/day and allopurinol 10 mg/kg/day, but when the mercaptopurine dosage was halved no untoward effects were seen.[2] A pharmacokinetic study showed that allopurinol caused a five-fold increase in peak plasma mercaptopurine concentrations and AUC when the mercaptopurine was given orally, and the bioavailability increased from 12 to 59%.[7] This did not occur when the mercaptopurine was given intravenously.[7,8]

Mechanism

Azathioprine is firstly metabolized in the liver to mercaptopurine and then enzymatically oxidized in the liver and intestinal wall by xanthine oxidase to an inactive compound (6-thiouric acid) which is excreted. Allopurinol inhibits this latter enzyme (inhibition of first-pass metabolism) so that the mercaptopurine accumulates, blood levels rise and its toxic effects develop (leucopenia, thrombocytopenia etc). In effect the patient suffers a gross overdose.

Importance and management

A well-documented, well-established and clinically important interaction. The dosages of azathioprine and mercaptopurine should be reduced to about a third or a quarter when given orally to prevent the development of toxicity. On the basis of two studies[7,8] it would seem that this precaution may not be necessary if mercaptopurine is given intravenously.

References

1 Rundles RW, Wyngaarden JB, Hitchings GH, Elion GB and Silberman HR. Effects of xanthine oxidase inhibitor on thiopurine metabolism, hyperuricaemia and gout. Trans Assoc Am Phys (1963) 76, 126.
2 Levine AS, Sharpt HL, Mitchell J, Krivit W and Nesbit M. Combination therapy with 6-mercaptopurine (NSC-755) and allopurinol (NSC 1390) during induction and maintenance of remission of acute leukaemia in children. Cancer Chemother Rep (1969) 53, 53.
3 Glogner P and Heni N. Panzytopenie nach kombinationsbehandlung mit allopurinol und azathioprin. Med Welt (1976) 27, 1545.
4 Brooks RJ, Dorr RT and Durie BGM. Interaction of allopurinol with 6-mercaptopurine and azathioprine. Biomedicine (1982) 36, 217–22.
5 Klugkist H and Lincke HO. Panzytopenie unter Behandlung mit Azathioprin durch Interaktion mit Allopurinol bei Myasthenia gravis. Akt Neurol (1987) 14, 165–7.
6 Zazgornik J, Kopsa H, Schmidt P, Pils P, Kuschan K and Deutch E. Increased danger of bone marrow damage in simultaneous azathioprine-allopurinol therapy. Int J Clin Pharmacol Ther Toxicol (1981) 19, 96.
7 Zimm S, Collins JM, O'Neill D, Chabner BA and Poplak DG. Inhibition of first-pass metabolism in cancer chemotherapy: interaction of 6-mercaptopurine and allopurinol. Clin Pharmacol Ther (1983) 34, 810–17.
8 Coffey JJ, White CA, Lesk AB, Rogers WI and Serpick AA. The effect of allopurinol on the pharmacokinetics of 6-mercaptopurine in cancer patients. Cancer Res (1972) 32, 1283–9.

dition, impaired renal function may allow co-trimoxazole levels to become elevated, and haemodialysis may deplete folate levels which could exacerbate the anti-folate effects of the co-trimoxazole.

Importance and management

Information appears to be limited to the studies cited, but the interaction would seem to be established. The use of co-trimoxazole or trimethoprim in renal transplant patients may clearly be hazardous and potentially life-threatening. An as yet untested suggestion by the authors of the first study[1] is that folinic acid might be an effective treatment for bone marrow suppression without affecting the antimicrobial effects of the co-trimoxazole. A similar interaction would be expected with mercaptopurine. More study is needed.

References

1 Bradley PP, Warfen GD, Maxwell JG and Rothstein G. Neutropenia and thrombocytopenia in renal allograft recipients treated with trimethoprim-sulfamethoxazole. Ann Intern Med (1980) 93, 560.
2 Bailey RR. Leukopenia due to a trimethoprim-azathioprine interaction. NZ Med J (1984) 97, 739.

Azathioprine/Mercaptopurine + Co-Trimoxazole or Trimethoprim

Abstract/Summary

The risk of potentially life-threatening haematological toxicity may be increased in renal transplant patients taking azathioprine if they are treated with co-trimoxazole or trimethoprim, particularly if given for extended periods. The same interaction would be expected with mercaptopurine.

Clinical evidence

The observation that haematological toxicity often seemed to occur in renal transplant patients given azathioprine and co-trimoxazole, prompted a retrospective survey of the records of 40 patients. It was found that there was no difference in the incidence of thrombocytopenia and neutropenia in those given azathioprine alone or with co-trimoxazole (160–20 mg trimethoprim + 800–1600 mg sulphamethoxazole daily) for a short time (6–16 days), but a significant increase occurred in the incidence and duration of these cytopenias if both drugs were given together for 22 days or more.[1]

A marked fall in white cell counts in renal transplant recipients during concurrent treatment with either co-trimoxazole (described as frequent) or trimethoprim (three cases) has been reported elsewhere.[2] In one case the fall occurred within five days and was treated by temporarily withdrawing the azathioprine and reducing the trimethoprim dosage from 300 to 100 mg daily.[2]

Mechanism

Not understood. It seems possible that the bone marrow depressant effects of all three drugs may be additive. In ad-

Azathioprine/Mercaptopurine + Doxorubicin (Adriamycin)

Abstract/Summary

The heptatoxicity of mercaptopurine and probably azathioprine can be increased by doxorubicin.

Clinical evidence, mechanism, importance and management

A study on 11 patients showed that liver damage induced by treatment with mercaptopurine was increased by the concurrent use of doxorubicin.[1] Since azathioprine is converted to mercaptopurine within the body, it would seem probable that increased hepatotoxicity will also be seen with this drug and doxorubicin.

Reference

1 Minow RA, Stern MH and Casey JH. Clinico-pathological correlation of liver damage in patients treated with 6-mercaptopurine. Cancer (1976) 38, 1524.

Bleomycin + Cisplatin

Abstract/Summary

Cisplatin can increase the pulmonary toxicity of bleomycin by reducing its renal excretion.

Clinical evidence

A study[2] in 18 patients given both drugs for the treatment of disseminated testicular non-seminoma showed that the cisplatin-induced reduction in renal function was paralleled by an increase in bleomycin-induced pulmonary toxicity. Two patients developed pneumonitis.

A man with unrecognized acute renal failure due to cisplatin treatment died from pulmonary toxicity when he was given bleomycin.[4] A study[1] in patients showed that the total clearance of bleomycin was halved (from 39 to 18 ml/min/m²) when concurrently treated with cisplatin in doses exceeding 300 mg/m² and the renal clearance in one patient fell from 30 to 8.2 ml/min/m². There was no evidence of severe bleomycin toxicity in these patients. Renal dysfunction alone has also been reported in some instances to cause bleomycin toxicity.[3]

Mechanism

Excretion by the kidney accounts for almost half of the total body clearance of bleomycin. Cisplatin is nephrotoxic and reduces the glomerular filtration rate so that the clearance of the bleomycin is reduced.

Importance and management

An established interaction with a potentially serious, sometimes fatal, outcome. Concurrent use should be very closely monitored and renal function should be checked. It may be necessary to reduce the dosage of the bleomycin.

References

1 Yee GC, Crom WR, Champion JE, Brodeur GM and Evans WE. Cisplatin-induced changes in bleomycin elimination. Cancer Treat Rep (1983) 67, 587–9.
2 van Barneveld PWC, Sleijfer D Th, van der Mark Th W, Mulder NH, Donker AJM, Meijer S, Schraffordt Koops H, Sluiter HJ and Peset R. Influence of platinum-induced pulmonary toxicity in patients with disseminated testicular carcinoma. Oncology (1984) 41, 4–7.
3 Perry DJ, Weiss RB and Taylor HG. Enhanced bleomycin toxicity during acute renal failure. Cancer Treat Rep (1982) 66, 592–3.
4 Bennett WM, Pastore L and Houghton DC. Fatal pulmonary toxicity in cis-platin-induced renal failure. Cancer Treat Rep (1980) 64, 921–4.

Bleomycin + Oxygen

Abstract/Summary

Serious and potentially fatal pulmonary toxicity can develop in patients treated with bleomycin who are exposed to conventional oxygen concentrations during anaesthesia.

Clinical evidence

Five patients under treatment with bleomycin, exposed to oxygen concentrations of 39% during and immediately following anaesthesia, developed a severe respiratory distress syndrome and died. Bleomycin-induced pneumonitis and lung fibrosis were diagnosed at post-mortem. Another group of 12 matched patients who underwent the same procedures but with lower oxygen concentrations (22–25%) recovered uneventfully.[1]

Another comparative study similarly demonstrated that adult respiratory distress syndrome (ARDS) in patients on bleomycin was reduced by the use of lower oxygen concentrations (22–30%).[3] Bleomycin-induced pulmonary toxicity in man apparently related to oxygen concentrations has been described in other reports,[2,4,10,12,13] and has also been demonstrated in mice,[5] rats[6] and hamsters.[7] Other reports however found no obvious increase in pulmonary complications in patients on bleomycin exposed to oxygen in concentrations above 30%.[8,9]

Mechanism

Not understood. One suggestion is that bleomycin-injured lung tissue is less able to scavenge free oxygen radicals which may be present and damage occurs as a result.[2]

Importance and management

An established, well-documented, serious and potentially fatal interaction. It is advised that any patient on bleomycin undergoing general anaesthesia should have their inspired oxygen concentrations limited to less than 30% and the fluid replacement should be carefully monitored to minimize the crystalloid load. This is clearly very effective because having used these precautions Dr Goldiner writes that '...since ...1978 we have operated on more than 700 bleomycin treated patients....we have seen no postoperative pulmonary failure in this group of patients.'[11] It has also been suggested that reduced oxygen levels should be continued during the recovery period and at any time during hospitalization.[2] If an oxygen concentration equal or greater than 30% has to be used, short term prophylactic corticosteroid administration should be considered. Intravenous corticosteroids should be given at once if bleomycin toxicity is suspected.[2]

References

1 Goldiner PL, Carlon CG, Cvitkovic E, Schweizer O and Howland WS. Factors influencing postoperative morbidity and mortality in patients treated with bleomycin. Br Med J (1978) 1, 1664.
2 Gilson AJ and Sahn SA. Reactivation of bleomycin lung toxicity following oxygen administration. A second response to corticosteroids. Chest (1985) 88, 304–6.
3 El-Baz N, Ivankovich AD, Faber LP and Logas WG. The incidence of bleomycin lung toxicity after anesthesia for pulmonary lung resection: a comparison between HFV and IPPV. Anesthesiology (1984) 61, A107.
4 Cersosimo RJ, Matthews SJ and Hong WK. Bleomycin pneumonitis potentiated by oxygen administration. Drug Intell Clin Pharm (1985) 19, 921–3.
5 Toledo CH, Ross WE and Block ER. Potentiation of bleomycin toxicity by oxygen. Cancer Treat Rep (1982) 66, 359–62.
6 Berend N. The effect of bleomycin and oxygen on rat lung. Pathology (1984) 16, 136–9.
7 Rinaldo J, Goldstein RH and Snider GL. Modification of oxygen toxicity after lung injury by bleomycin in hamsters. Am Rev Resp Dis (1982) 126, 1030–3.
8 Douglas MJ and Coppin CML. Bleomycin and subsequent anesthesia: a retrospective study at Vancouver General Hospital. Can Anaesth Soc J (1980) 27, 449–52.

9   Mandelbaum I, Willaims SD and Einhorn LH. Aggressive surgical management of testicular carcinoma metastatic to lungs and mediastinum. Ann Thorac Surg (1980) 30, 224–9.

10   Hulbert JC, Grossman JE and Cummings KB. Risk factors of anesthesia and surgery in bleomycin-treated patients. J Urol (1983) 130, 163–4.

11   Goldiner PL. Editorial comment. J Urol (1983) 130, 164.

12   Allen SC, Riddell GS and Butchart EG. Bleomycin therapy and anaesthesia. The possible hazards of oxygen administration to patients after treatment with bleomycin. Anesthesia (1981) 36, 60–3.

13   Donohue JP and Rowland RG. Complications of retroperitoneal lymph node dissection. J Urol (1981) 125, 338–40.

Bleomycin + Various cytotoxic regimens

Abstract/Summary

There is evidence that the concurrent use of other cytotoxic drugs can increase the occurrence of bleomycin-induced pulmonary reactions.

Clinical evidence, mechanism, importance and management

A study showed that 18% (15 of 83) of the patients treated for non-Hodgkin's lymphomas with bleomycin (mean total dose 36 units) in conjunction with other cytotoxic drugs (M-BACOD methotrexate, bleomycin, adriamycin, cyclophosphamide, onconvin, dexamethasone), developed acute but completely reversible pulmonary reactions. This is high compared with the 3–10% incidence reported in those receiving bleomycin alone. Patients should be closely monitored. See also 'Bleomycin + Cisplatin.'

Reference

1   Bauer KA, Skarin AT, Balikina JP, Garnick MB, Rosenthal DS and Canellos GP. Pulmonary complications associated with combination chemotherapy program containing bleomycin. Am J Med (1983) 74, 557–63.

Carmofur + Alcohol

Abstract/Summary

A disulfiram-like reaction occurred in a patient on carmofur when given coeliac plexus blockade with alcohol

Clinical evidence, mechanism, importance and management

A man with pancreatic carcinoma treated with 500 mg carmofur daily for 25 days experienced a disulfiram-like reaction (facial flushing, diaphoresis, hypotension—BP 60/30 mm Hg, and tachycardia—128 bpm) within 30 min of being given coeliac plexus alcohol blockade for pain relief. Blood acetaldehyde levels were found to have risen sharply supporting the belief that the underlying mechanism is similar to the disulfiram-alcohol interaction (see 'Disulfiram + Alcohol'). It is suggested that alcohol blockade should be avoided for seven days after treatment with carmofur.[1]

Reference

1   Noda J, Umeda S, Mori K, Fukunaga T and Mizoi Y. Disulfiram-like reaction associated with carmofur after celiac plexus alcohol block. Anesthesiology (1987) 76, 908.

Carmustine (BCNU) + Cimetidine

Abstract/Summary

The bone marrow depressant effects of carmustine can be increased by the concurrent use of cimetidine and the fall in neutrophil and thrombocyte counts may become serious.

Clinical evidence

Six out of eight patients treated with carmustine, 80 mg/m^2 daily, for three days, cimetidine, 300 mg six-hourly, and steroids demonstrated marked leucopenia and thrombocytopenia after the first administrations. Biopsy confirmed the marked decrease in granulocytic elements. In comparison only six out of 40 patients treated similarly but without cimetidine showed comparable white cell and platelet depression.[1]

This increased myelotoxicity with marked falls in neutrophil counts has been described in another report.[2]

Mechanism

Cimetidine alone occasionally causes a marked fall in neutrophil numbers[3] and in some way, as yet not understood, it can augment the bone marrow depressant effects of carmustine.

Importance and management

Information appears to be limited to the reports cited, but it seems to be an established reaction. Patients given both drugs should be closely monitored for changes in neutrophil and platelet counts because the neutropenia may be life-threatening.

References

1   Selker RG, Moore P and LoDolce D. Bone-marrow depression with cimetidine plus carmustine. N Engl J Med (1978) 299, 834.

2   Volkin A, Shadduck RK, Winkelstein A, Zeigler ZR and Selker G. Potentiation of carmustine-cranial irradiation-induced myelosuppression by cimetidine. Arch Intern Med (1982) 142, 243–5.

3   Klotz S and Kay B. Cimetidine and agranulocytosis. Ann Intern Med (1978) 88, 579.

Cisplatin + Aminoglycoside antibiotics

Abstract/Summary

Acute and possibly life-threatening renal failure can occur in patients treated concurrently with cisplatin and aminoglycoside antibiotics such as gentamicin and tobramycin.

Clinical evidence

Four patients treated with cisplatin in dosages ranging from low to very high (eight doses of 0.5 to 5 mg/kg) and who were subsequently given gentamicin/cephalothin developed acute and fatal renal failure. Autopsy revealed extensive renal tubular necrosis.[1]

Two similar cases of severe renal toxicity attributed to the concurrent use of cisplatin with gentamicin/cephalothin are described elsewhere.[2,3] A very marked reduction in kidney function (as measured by a fall in creatinine clearance) has been described in three patients on cisplatin when they were subsequently treated with gentamicin or tobramycin.[5] Enhanced renal toxicity and ototoxicity have been reported in guinea pigs concurrently treated with cisplatin and kanamycin.[8] A comparative study on 17 patients given cisplatin and gentamicin confirmed that the incidence of nephrotoxicity was increased by concurrent use, but the renal insufficiency was described as usually mild and not clinically significant.[4] There is also evidence from studies in children to show that the half-life of gentamicin is approximately doubled by the presence of cisplatin.[6] Both cisplatin and the aminoglycosides can cause the excessive loss of magnesium and combined use increases this loss.[7]

Mechanism

Cisplatin is nephrotoxic and it would appear that its damaging effects on the kidney are additive with the nephrotoxic and possibly the ototoxic effects of the aminoglycoside antibiotics. The magnesium-losing effects of both also seem to be additive.

Importance and management

An established and potentially serious interaction. It has been recommended that these antibiotics should only be given with caution, or probably not at all, to patients under treatment with cisplatin,[1,2] although one report describing the use of gentamicin without cephalothin claims that concurrent use can be relatively safe.[4] The magnesium status should also be monitored.

References

1 Gonzalez-Vitale JC, Hayes DM, Cvitkovic E and Sternberg SS. Acute renal failure after cis-Dichlorodiammineplatinum (II) and gentamicin-cephalothin therapies. Cancer Treat Rep (1978) 62, 693.

2 Salem PA, Jabboury KW and Khalil MF. Severe nephrotoxicity: a probable complication of cis-dichorodiammineplatinum (II) and cephalothin-gentamicin therapy. Oncology (1982) 39, 31–2.

3 Leite JBF, De Campelo Gentil F, Burchenal J, Marques A, Teixeira MIC and Abrao FA. Insuficienza renal aguda apos o uso de cis-diaminodicloroplatina, gentamicina e cefalosporina. Rev Paul Med (1981) 97, 75–7.

4 Haas A, Anderson L and Lad T. The influence of aminoglycosides on the nephrotoxicity of cis-Diamminedichloroplatinum in cancer patients. J Infect Dis (1983) 147, 363.

5 Dentino M, Luft FC, Yum MN, Williams SD and Eihorn LH. Long term effect of cis-diamminedichloride platinum (CDDP) on renal functions and structure in man. Cancer (1978) 41, 1274–81.

6 Stewart CF, Christensen ML, Crom WR and Evans WE. The effect of cisplatin therapy on gentamicin pharmacokinetics. Drug Intell Clin Pharm (1984) 18, 512.

7 Flombaum CD. Hypomagnesiemia associated with cisplatin combination chemotherapy. Arch Intern Med (1984) 144, 2336–7.

8 Schweitzer VG, Hawkins JE, Lilly DJ, Litterst CJ, Abrams G, Davis JA and Christy M. Ototoxic and nephrotoxic effects of combined treatment with cis-diamminedichloroplatinum and kanamycin in the guinea pig. Otolaryngol (1984) 92, 38–49.

Cisplatin + Antihypertensive agents

Abstract/Summary

A single report describes the development of kidney failure in a patient whose cisplatin-induced hypertension was treated with frusemide, hydralazine, diazoxide and propranolol.

Clinical evidence, mechanism, importance and management

Three hours after receiving cisplatin intravenously (70 mg/m^2 body surface area) a patient experienced severe nausea and vomiting and his blood pressure rose from 150/90 to 248/140 mm Hg. This was treated with frusemide (40 mg IV), hydrallazine (10 mg IM), diazoxide (300 mg IV) and propranolol (40 mg orally for two days). Nine days later the patient showed evidence of renal failure which resolved within three weeks. The patient was subsequently similarly treated on two occasions with cisplatin and again developed hypertension, but no treatment was given and there was no evidence of kidney dysfunction.[1] The reasons for the kidney failure are not known, but studies in dogs[2] and rats[3] indicate that kidney damage may possibly be related to the concentrations of cisplatin and that frusemide can increase cisplatin levels in the kidney.

Information seems to be limited to the reports cited and its general clinical importance is uncertain, however the authors of the clinical report '...advise caution in treating hypertension or altering in any way renal hemodynamics in a patient receiving cisplatin.'[1]

References

1 Markman M and Trump DL. Nephrotoxicity with cisplatin and antihypertensive medications. Ann Intern Med (1982) 96, 257.

2 Cvitkovic E, Spaulding J, Bethune V. Improvement of cis-dichlorodiammineplatinum (NSC 119875): therapeutic index in an animal model. Cancer (1977) 39, 1357–61.

3 Pera MF, Zook BC and Harder HC. Effects of mannitol or furosemide diuresis on the nephrotoxicity and physiological disposition of cis-dichlordiammineplatinum (II) in rats. Cancer Res (1979) 39, 1269–79.

Cisplatin + Ethacrynic acid

Abstract/Summary

Animal studies show that the damaging effects of cisplatin on the ear can be markedly increased by the concurrent use of ethacrynic acid. It seems possible that this could also occur in man.

Clinical evidence, mechanism, importance and management

Both cisplatin and ethacrynic acid given alone can be ototoxic in man. A study[1] carried out on guinea pigs showed that when cisplatin (7 mg/kg) or ethacrynic acid (50 mg/kg) were given alone their ototoxic effects were reversible, but when given together the damaging effects on the ear were '...profound, and prolonged, if not permanent.' Although this adverse interaction has not yet been reported in man, in the light of this study and what is already known about the ototoxicity of these two drugs in man, it seems possible that this may be a clinically important interaction. Audiometric tests should be carried out if these drugs are used concurrently.

Reference

1 Komune S and Snow JB. Potentiating effects of cisplatinum and ethacrynic acid in ototoxicity. Arch Otolaryngol (1981) 107, 594–7.

Cisplatin + Methotrexate

Abstract/Summary

The risk of fatal methotrexate toxicity appears to be markedly increased by previous treatment with cisplatin.

Clinical evidence, mechanism, importance and management

Six out of 106 patients died with clinical signs of methotrexate toxicity 6–13 days after receiving 20–50 mg/m^2 in the absence of the usual signs of renal dysfunction and despite having previously been treated with methotrexate without serious toxicity. All had had prior treatment with cisplatin. Four of the patients were regarded as good-risk.[1] A study in children and adolescents suggested that the cumulative dose of cisplatin received appears to increase the risk of methotrexate toxicity.[2] Another study indicated that the sequential use of cisplatin and high-dose methotrexate was nephrotoxic and decreased the amount of methotrexate which could be given.[3] A report on 14 patients on high dose methotrexate indicated that prior treatment with one course of cisplatin sharply increased their serum levels of methotrexate, and after two courses the increase was even more marked (an eightfold rise).[4]

The picture is not totally clear but it seems possible that prior treatment with cisplatin causes kidney damage which may not necessarily be detectable with the usual creatinine clearance tests. The effect is to cause a marked reduction in the clearance of the methotrexate. The serum methotrexate levels of these patients should be closely monitored so that any delay in its clearance is detected early and appropriate measures taken.[2]

References

1 Haim N, Kedar A and Robinson E. Methotrexate-related deaths in patients previously treated with cis-diamminedichloride platinum. Cancer Chemother Pharmacol (1984) 13, 223–5.
2 Crom WR, Pratt CB, Green AA, Champion JE, Crom DB, Stewart CF and Evans WE. The effect of prior cisplatin therapy on the pharmacokinetics of high-dose methotrexate. J Clin Oncol (1984) 2, 655–661.
3 Pitman SW, Mino DR and Papac R. Sequential methotrexate-leucovorin (MTX-LCV) and cis-platinum (CDDP) in head and neck cancer. Proc AACR/ASCO (1979) 21, 166.
4 Crom WR, Teresi ME, Meyer WH, Green AA and Evans WE. The intrapatient effect of cisplatin therapy on the pharmacokinetics of high-dose methotrexate. Drug Intell Clin Pharm (1985) 19, 467.

Cisplatin + Probenecid

Abstract/Summary

On the basis of studies in animals it is uncertain whether the nephrotoxicity of cisplatin is increased or reduced by probenecid.

Clinical evidence, mechanism, importance and management

One study[1] in rats showed that probenecid could reduce cisplatin-induced nephrotoxicity, but other studies[2] found the complete opposite. The combination of cisplatin and probenecid was decidedly more toxic that cisplatin alone. Until this interaction has been more thoroughly studied this drug combination should be used with great care.

References

1 Ross DA, Gale GR. Reduction of renal toxicity of ci-dichlordiammineplatinum (II) by probenecid. Cancer Treat Rep (1979) 63, 781–7.
2 Daley-Yates PT, McBrien DCH. Enhancement of cisplatin nephrotoxicity by probenecid. Cancer Treat Rep (1984) 68, 445–6.

Cyclophosphamide + Allopurinol

Abstract/Summary

There is evidence that the incidence of serious bone marrow depression caused by cyclophosphamide can be markedly increased by the concurrent use of allopurinol, but this was not confirmed in one study.

Clinical evidence

A retrospective epidemiological survey of patients in four hospitals who, over a four-year period, had been treated with cyclophosphamide showed that the incidence of serious bone marrow depression was 57.7% in 26 patients who had also received allopurinol, and 18.8% in 32 patients who had not. A threefold increase.[2]

A study in nine patients with malignant disease and two normal subjects showed that while taking 200 mg allopurinol daily the concentration of the cytotoxic metabolites of cyclophosphamide increased by an average of 37.5% (range −1.5 to +109%).[2] Agranulocytosis has been reported in another patient.[5] However another study,[4] designed as a follow-up to the study cited above[1] involving cytotoxic regimens which contained cyclophosphamide, failed to confirm that allopurinol increased the toxicity in patients with Hodgkin's or non-Hodgkin's lymphoma.

Mechanism

Not fully resolved. Cyclophosphamide itself is inactive, but it is converted in the liver into metabolites which are cytotoxic. Allopurinol possibly increases the activity of the liver enzymes concerned with the production of these metabolites.[2] Another idea is that it inhibits their loss from the kidneys.[2] Since the toxicity is related to the concentration of the metabolites,[3] the increased incidence of bone marrow depression is explained.

Importance and management

This interaction is not established with any certainty. The authors of the survey[1] cited write that '...there seem to be good grounds for re-evaluating the routine practice of administering allopurinol [with cyclophosphamide] prophylactically.' This does not forbid concurrent use, but introduces a strong note of caution.

References

1 Boston Collaborative Drug Surveillance Programme. Allopurinol and cytotoxic drugs. Interaction in relation to bone marrow depression. J Amer Med Ass (1974) 227, 1036.
2 Witten J, Fredericksen PL and Mouridsen HT. The pharmacokinetics of cyclophosphamide in man after treatment with allopurinol. Acta pharmacol et toxicol (1980) 46, 392.
3 Mouridsen HT, Witten J, Fredericksen PL and Hulsbaek I. Studies on the correlation between rate of biotransformation and haematological toxicity of cyclophosphamide. Acta pharmacol et toxicol (1978) 42, 81.
4 Stolbach L, Begg C, Bennett JM, Silverstein M, Falkson G, Harris DT and Glick J. Evaluation of bone marrow toxic reaction in patients treated with allopurinol. J Amer Med Ass (1982) 247, 334–6.
5 Beeley L, Daly M and Steward P. Bulletin of the W Midlands Centre for Adverse Drug Reaction Reporting (1987) 24, 26.

Cyclophosphamide + Barbiturates

Abstract/Summary

Despite some animal data, the evidence from studies in man suggests that neither the toxicity nor the therapeutic effects of cyclophosphamide are significantly affected by the concurrent use of the barbiturates.

Clinical evidence, mechanism, importance and management

There is evidence from a number of animal studies that the barbiturates and other potent liver enzyme-inducing agents can affect the activity of cyclophosphamide,[1,2] but studies undertaken in man indicate that although some changes in the pharmacokinetics of cyclophosphamide occur, neither the toxicity nor the therapeutic effects of cyclophosphamide are significantly altered.[3–5] No special precautions seem to be necessary.

References

1 Donelli MG, Colombo T and Garattini S. Effect of cyclophosphamide on the activity and distribution of pentobarbital in rats. Biochem Pharmacol (1973) 22, 2609.
2 Alberts DS and Van Daalen Wetters T. The effect of phenobarbital on cyclophosphamide antitumour acitivity. Cancer Res (1976) 36, 2785.
3 Bagley CM, Bostick FW and De Vita VT. Clinical pharmacology of cyclophosphamide. Cancer Res (1973) 33, 226.
4 Jao JY, Jusko WJ and Cohen JL. Phenobarbital effects on cyclophosphamide pharmacokinetics in man. Cancer Res (1972) 32, 2761.
5 Mellett LB. Chemistry and metabolism of cyclophosphamide: in Vancil (Ed) 'Immunosuppressive Properties of Cyclophosphamide', Mead Johnson and Co, Indiana. (1971) pp 6–34.

Cyclophosphamide + Benzodiazepines

Abstract/Summary

Animal studies suggest that the benzodiazepines may possibly increase the toxicity of cyclophosphamide.

Clinical evidence, mechanism, importance and management

Studies in *mice* indicate that 3 days' treatment with benzodiazepines (chlordiazepoxide, diazepam, oxazepam) increased the lethality of the cyclophosphamide (without improving its effectiveness against Ehrlich solid tumour).[1] This may be due, it is suggested, to the induction of the liver enzymes concerned with the metabolism of cyclophosphamide to its active cytotoxic products. The importance of this possible interaction in man is uncertain, but the possibility should be borne in mind during concurrent use.

Reference

1 Sasaki K-I, Furusawa S and Takayanagi G. Effects of chlordiazepoxide, diazepam and oxazepam on the antitumour activity, the lethality and the blood level of active metabolites of cyclophosphamide and cyclophosphamide oxidase activity in mice. J Pharm Dyn (1983) 6, 767–72.

Cyclophosphamide + Chloramphenicol

Abstract/Summary

Some limited evidence suggests that chloramphenicol may reduce the production of the therapeutically active metabolites of cyclophosphamide, thereby reducing its activity.

Clinical evidence, mechanism, importance and management

Cyclophosphamide itself is inactive, but after administration it is metabolized within the body to active alkylating metabolites. Animal studies[1] have shown that pretreatment with chloramphenicol reduces the activity (lethality) of cyclophosphamide because, it is believed, the antibiotic inhibits its conversion to these active metabolites. Studies[2] in four patients showed that 2 g chloramphenicol daily for 12 days prolonged the mean half-life of cyclophosphamide from 7.5 to 11.5 h and the production of the active metabolites fell. So it seems possible that a reduction in the activity of cyclophosphamide may also occur in man, but the extent to which this affects treatment with cyclophosphamide is uncertain. Concurrent use need not be avoided, but be on the watch for evidence of a reduced response. More study is needed.

References

1 Dixon RL. Effect of chloramphenicol on the metabolism and lethality of cyclophosphamide in rats. Proc Soc Exp Biol Med (1968) 127, 1151–5
2 Faber OK, Mouridson HT and Skovsted L. The effect of chloramphenicol and sulphaphenazole on the biotransformation of cyclophosphamide in man. Br J Clin Pharmac (1975) 2, 281–5.

Cyclophosphamide + Corticosteroids

Abstract/Summary

There is evidence that single doses of prednisone can reduce the activity of cyclophosphamide, but longer term treatment may increase its activity.

Clinical evidence and mechanism

Cyclophosphamide itself is inactive, but after administration it is metabolized in the body to active metabolites. Single doses of prednisone have been shown to inhibit the activation of cyclophosphamide in man[1] (and animals[2]), probably due to competition for the drug-metabolizing enzymes in the liver. Longer-term treatment on the other hand (50 mg daily for 1–2 weeks) has been shown in man to have the opposite effect and increases the rate of activation of the cyclophosphamide, probably due to the induction of the liver enzymes.

Importance and management

The documentation is very limited and the interaction is poorly established, but changes in the activity of the cyclosphosphamide should be watched for during concurrent use. Whether other corticosteroids behave in the same way as prednisone is uncertain. More study is needed.

References

1 Faber OK and Mouridsen HT. Cyclophosphamide activation and corticosteroids. N Engl J Med (1974) 291, 211.
2 Sladek NE. Therapeutic efficacy of cyclophosphamide as a function of inhibition of its metabolism. Cancer Res (1972) 32, 1848.

Cyclophosphamide + Dapsone

Abstract/Summary

Some extremely limited evidence suggests that dapsone might be capable of reducing the activity of cyclophosphamide.

Clinical evidence, mechanism, importance and management

An unexplained and undetailed report has described patients with leprosy on dapsone and cyclophosphamide who showed inhibition of the leucopenia normally associated with cyclophosphamide treatment.[1] Whether this indicates a reduction in the effects of cyclophosphamide is uncertain, but it would seem prudent to be on the alert for signs of a depressed therapeutic response to cyclophosphamide during concurrent treatment. More study is needed.

Reference

1 Quoted by Warren RD and Bender RA. Drug interactions with antineoplastic agents. Cancer Treat Rep (1977) 61, 1231.

Cyclophosphamide + Doxorubicin (Adriamycin)

Abstract/Summary

A single case report suggests that the damaging effects of cyclophosphamide and doxorubicin on the bladder may be additive.

Clinical evidence, mechanism, importance and management

A woman was treated with cyclophosphamide (100–150 mg daily orally) for three years for the treatment of breast cancer. The cyclophosphamide was withdrawn and replaced by doxorubicin (30 mg weekly IV). After five doses she developed a severe haemorrhagic cystitis and bladder biopsy showed that the cyclophosphamide had caused chronic subclinical bladder damage which apparently was further damaged by the doxorubicin. The authors recommend that patients given doxorubicin should be carefully examined for microscopic haematuria, particularly if they have previously had cyclophosphamide or pelvic irradiation.[1]

Reference

1 Ershler WB, Gilchrist KW and Citrin DL. Adriamycin enhancement of cyclophosphamide-induced bladder injury. J Urol (1980) 123, 121–2.

Cyclophosphamide or Mustine + Morphine or Pethidine

Abstract/Summary

Animal studies indicate that the toxicity of cyclophosphamide and mustine is increased by morphine or pethidine.

Clinical evidence, mechanism, importance and management

Studies in mice[1] have shown that morphine in doses of 5–25 mg/kg increases sublethal doses of cyclophosphamide (300 mg/kg) and mustine (5 mg/kg) into maximally lethal doses. The effect of pethidine (meperidine) was less marked. This work suggests that there may be a need to re-evaluate the concurrent use of these drugs in man.

Reference

1 Akintonawa A. Potentiation of nitrogen mustard toxicity by narcotic analgesic. Clin Toxicol (1981) 18, 451–8.

Cyclophosphamide + Sulphaphenazole

Abstract/Summary

Some very limited evidence suggests that sulphaphenazole may increase or decrease the activity of cyclophosphamide, but the clinical importance of this is uncertain.

Clinical evidence, mechanism, importance and management

A study[1] in seven subjects on a 50 g dose of cyclophosphamide given 2 g sulphaphenazole daily for 9–14 days showed that the half-life of the cyclophosphamide was unchanged in three, longer in two and shorter in the remaining two. The reasons are not clear. Whether this has any practical importance or not is uncertain, but it would seem prudent to be on the watch for changes in the response to cyclophosphamide if sulphaphenazole is given concurrently. More study is needed. Information about other sulphonamides appears to be lacking.

Reference

1 Faber OK, Mouridson HT and Skovsted L. The effect of chloramphenicol and sulphaphenazole on the biotransformation of cyclophosphamide in man. Br J clin Pharmac (1975) 2, 281.

Cytotoxics + Calcium channel blockers

Abstract/Summary

Verapamil can increase the efficacy of doxorubicin both in tissue culture systems and in patients. It raises serum doxorubicin levels. The absorption of verapamil can be reduced by COPP and VAC cytotoxic drug regimens.

Clinical evidence, mechanism, importance and management

(a) The effect of calcium channel blockers on cytotoxics

The efficacy of doxorubicin can be increased by verapamil and nicardipine in doxorubicin-resistant tissue culture systems[1] and its pharmacokinetics can also be changed by verapamil. A study[2] in five patients with small cell lung cancer given doxorubicin, vincristine and cyclophosphamide showed that when given verapamil (240–480 mg daily) the AUC (area under the curve) of the doxorubicin was doubled, peak serum levels were raised and the clearance was reduced. No increased toxicity was seen in this study or in two others,[3,4] but be alert for this possibility if both drugs are used.

(b) The effect of cytotoxics on calcium channel blockers

A study in nine patients with a variety of malignant diseases showed that treatment with cytotoxic drugs reduced the absorption of 160 mg verapamil given orally. The AUC in eight patients was reduced by 40% (range 7–58%). One patient showed a 26% increase. Five patients received a modified COPP regimen (cyclophosphamide, onconvin, procarbazine, prednisone) and four VAC (vindesine, adriamycin, cisplatin).[5] It is believed that these cytotoxics damage the lining of the upper part of the small intestine which impairs the absorption of verapamil. Patients should be monitored for signs of a reduced response to verapamil during concurrent treatment.

References

1 Ramu A, Spanier R, Rahamimoff H and Fuks Z. Restoration of doxorubicin responsiveness in doxorubicin-resistant P388 murine leukaemia cells. Br J Cancer (1984) 50, 501–7.

2 Kerr DJ, Graham J, Cummings J, Morrison JG, Thompson GG, Brodie MJ and Kaye SB. The effect of verapamil on the pharmacokinetics of adriamycin. Cancer Chemother Pharmacol (1986) 18, 32.

3 Ozols RF, Rogan AM, Hamilton TC, Klecker R and Young RC. Verapamil plus adriamycin in refractory ovarian cancer: design of a clinical trial on basis of reversal of adriamycin resistance in human ovarian cancer cell lines. AACR (1986) Abstract 1186.

4 Presant CA, Kennedy P, Wiseman C, Gala K and Wyres M. Verapamil plus adriamycin—a phase I-II clinical study. Proc Am Soc Clin Oncol (1984) 3, 1–124.

5 Kuhlmann J, Woodcock B, Wilke J and Rietbrock N. Verapamil plasma concentrations during treatment with cytostatic drugs. J Cardiovasc Pharmacol (1985) 7, 1003–6.

Cytotoxics + Food

Abstract/Summary

The absorption of methotrexate and melphalan can be reduced by food, but etoposide is unaffected.

Clinical evidence, mechanism, importance and management

(a) Etoposide

The plasma etoposide concentrations of 11 patients with extensive small cell lung carcinoma given 100 mg oral doses were unaffected when taken with breakfast (milk, cornflakes, sugar, egg, sausage, bread, magarine, marmalade, coffee or tea). Also no changes were seen when the etoposide was taken with cyclophosphamide (100 mg/m²), methotrexate (12.5 mg/m²) or procarbazine (60 mg/m²) given orally.[3]

(b) Melphalan

A study in five patients with multiple myeloma showed that the half-life of melphalan (5 mg/m²) was unaffected when taken with a standardized breakfast, but the area under the curve was reduced to an average of 43% (range 0–78%). In one patient no melphalan was detectable when given with food.[2]

(c) Methotrexate

The peak serum methotrexate levels (measured at 1.5 h) of 10 children, following an oral dose, were reduced about 40% when taken with a milky meal (milk cornflakes, sugar, white bread and butter). The area under the 4 h concentration/time curve was reduced about 25%. A smaller reduction was seen after a 'citrus meal' (orange juice, fresh orange, white bread, butter and jam).[1] The reasons are not understood.

References

1 Pinkerton CR, Welshman SG, Glasgow JFT and Bridges JM. Can food influence the absorption of methotrexate in children with acute lymphoblastic leukaemia? Lancet (1980) 2, 944–5.

2 Kotasek D, Dale BM, Morris RG, Reece PA and Sage RE. Food reduces melphalan absorption. Aust NZ J Med (1985) 15 (Suppl 1) 120.

3 Harvey VJ, Slevin ML, Joel SP, Johnston A and Wrigley PFM. The effect of food and concurrent chemotherapy on the bioavailability of oral etoposide. Br J Cancer (1985) 52, 363–7.

Cytotoxics + Gentamicin

Abstract/Summary

There is evidence that the use of gentamicin with daunorubicin, thioguanine and cytarabine may cause hypomagnesaemia.

Clinical evidence, mechanism, importance and management

The observation of hypomagnesaemia in two patients given gentamicin (with lincomycin or mezlocillin) during induction therapy for non-lymphoblastic leukaemia prompted further study in another nine patients. They were all treated with the same cytotoxic regimen: daunorubicin 50 mg/m² IV day 1, thioguanine 100 mg/m² twice daily orally on days 1–5, and cytarabine 100 mg/m² twice daily IV on days 1–5. Six out of 11 patients demonstrated hypomagnesaemia.[1] The reasons are not known but suggestions include a direct nephrotoxic action of the cytotoxic drugs, or the cytotoxics may sensitize the kidneys to the actions of gentamicin. Concurrent use should be well monitored.

Reference

1 Davey P, Gozzard D, Goodall M and Leyland MJ. Hypomagnesaemia: an underdiagnosed interaction between gentamicin and cytotoxic chemotherapy for acute non-lymphoblastic leukaemia. J Antimicrob Chemother (1985) 15, 623–8.

Cytotoxic drugs + Vaccines

Abstract/Summary

The immune response of the body is suppressed by cytotoxic drugs. The effectiveness of the vaccine may be poor and generalized infection may occur in patients immunized with live vaccines.

Clinical evidence, mechanism, importance and management

Since the cytotoxic drugs are immunosuppressants, the response of the body to immunization is reduced. A study[1] in 53 patients with Hodgkins disease showed that chemotherapy reduced the antibody response 60% when measured three weeks after immunization with a pneumococcal vaccine. The patients were treated with mustine, vincristine, prednisone and procarbazine. A few of them also had bleomycin, vinblastine or cyclophosphamide. Subtotal radiotherapy reduced the response a further 15%. The response to influenza immunization in children with various malignancies was also found to be markedly suppressed by chemotherapy. The cytotoxic drugs used were mercaptopurine, methotrexate, vincristine and prednisone. Some of them were also treated with vincristine, actinomycin and cyclophosphamide.[2]

Immunization with live vaccines may result in a potentially life-threatening infection. For example, a woman who was under treatment with 15 mg methotrexate daily for psoriasis and who was vaccinated against smallpox, developed a generalized vaccinial infection.[3] Studies in animals given smallpox vaccine confirmed that they were more susceptible to infection if treated with methotrexate, mercaptopurine or cyclophosphamide.[4] Smallpox is no longer a problem, but other live vaccines such as rubella, measles, mumps and others continue to be used. Extreme care should therefore be exercised in immunizing patients with live vaccines who are receiving cytotoxics or other immunosuppressive treatment (see also 'Corticosteroids + Live vaccines').

References

1 Siber GR, Weitzman SA, Aisenberg AC, Weinstein HJ and Schiffman A. Impaired antibody response to pneumococcal vaccine after treatment for Hodgkins disease. N Engl J Med (1978) 299, 442–8.
2 Gross PA, Lee H, Wolff JA, Hall CB, Minnefore AB and Lazicki ME. Influenza immunization in immunosuppressed children. J Pediatr (1978) 92, 30–5.
3 Allison J. Methotrexate and smallpox vaccination. Lancet (1968) ii, 1250.
4 Rosenbaum EH, Cohen RA and Glatstein HR. Vaccination of a patient receiving immunosuppresive therapy for lymphosarcoma. J Amer Med Ass (1966) 198, 737.

Doxorubicin (Adriamycin) + Actinomycin + Plicamycin (Mithramycin)

Abstract/Summary

A case of fatal cardiomyopathy attributed to the concurrent use of doxorubicin (adriamycin), actinomycin-D and plicamycin (mithramycin) has been described.

Clinical evidence, mechanism, importance and management

A patient developed fatal cardiomyopathy apparently due to the use of doxorubicin, actinomycin-D and plicamycin. The general importance of this is uncertain, but it would seem prudent to be on the alert for changes in cardiac function in patients treated with these drugs.[1]

Reference

1 Kushner JP, Hansen VL and Hammar SP. Cardiomyopathy after widely separated courses of adriamycin exacerbated by actinomycin-D and mithramycin. Cancer (1975) 36, 1577.

Doxorubicin (Adriamycin) + Barbiturates

Abstract/Summary

The effects of doxorubicin may be reduced by the concurrent use of barbiturates.

Clinical evidence, mechanism, importance and management

A comparative study in patients treated with doxorubicin showed that those concurrently taking barbiturates had a plasma clearance which was 50% higher than those who were not (318 compared with 202 ml/min).[1] This clinical study confirms previous studies in mice.[2] A possible explanation is that the barbiturate increases the metabolism of the doxorubicin. It seems likely that the dosage of doxorubicin will need to be increased in barbiturate-treated patients to achieve maximal therapeutic effects.

References

1 Riggs CE, Engel S, Wesley M, Wiernik PH and Bachur NR. Doxorubicin pharmacokinetics, prochlorperazine and barbiturate effects. Clin Pharmacol Ther (1982) 31, 263.
2 Reich SD and Bachur NR. Alterations in adriamycin efficacy by phenobarbital. Cancer (1976) 36, 3803.

Doxorubicin (Adriamycin) + Beta-blockers

Abstract/Summary

Animal data suggest that additive cardiotoxicity may occur with doxorubicin and propranolol. This awaits clinical confirmation.

Clinical evidence, mechanism, importance and management

A very well recognized problem with doxorubicin is its cardiotoxicity and cardiomyopathy. Studies in mice[1] showed that mortality was significantly increased when doxorubicin (18 and 23 mg/kg) and propranolol (1 and 10 mg/kg) were given concurrently, possibly because both drugs can inhibit the activity of two cardiac CoQ_{10} enzymes (succinoxidase, NADH oxidase) which are essential for mitochondrial respiration. There is no clinical confirmation of this interaction in man, but the authors of this animal study suggest that concurrent use may be contraindicated.

Reference

1 Choe JY, Combs AB and Folkers K. Potentiation of the toxicity of adriamycin by propranolol. Res Comm Chem Pathol Pharmacol (1978) 21, 577.

5-Fluorouracil + Aminoglycosides

Abstract/Summary

Neomycin can delay the gastrointestinal absorption of 5-fluorouracil, but the clinical importance of this is uncertain.

Clinical evidence, mechanism, importance and management

Some preliminary information from a study in 12 patients under treatment for adenocarcinoma showed that treatment with oral neomycin (2 g daily for a week) delayed the absorption of 5-fluorouracil, but the effects were generally too small to reduce the therapeutic response, except possibly in one patient.[1] It seems probable that this interaction occurs because neomycin can induce a malabsorbtion syndrome. If neomycin, paromomycin or kanamycin are used in patients on 5-fluorouracil, the possibility of this interaction should be borne in mind.

Reference

1 Bruckner HW and Creasey WA. The administration of 5-fluorouracil by mouth. Cancer (1974) 33, 14.

5-Fluorouracil + Cimetidine

Abstract/Summary

Serum 5-fluorouracil levels are increased about 75% by the concurrent use of cimetidine for a month.

Clinical evidence

A study in six patients with carcinoma under treatment with 5-fluorouracil (15 mg/kg daily for five days, repeated every four weeks) showed that treatment with 1 g cimetidine daily for four weeks increased peak plasma 5-FU concentrations by 74% and the area under the curve (AUC) by 72% when given orally. When given intravenously the AUC was increased by 27%. The total body clearance was reduced by 28%.[1] The pharmacokinetics of 5-FU were unaltered by the use of cimetidine for only a week.

Mechanism

Uncertain. It is probably a combination of a reduction in the metabolism of the 5-FU caused by the cimetidine (a well-known enzyme inhibitor) and a reduction in blood flow through the liver.

Importance and management

Direct information appears to be limited to this study, but the interaction would seem to be established. Concurrent treatment should be undertaken with particular care because of the risks of 5-FU overdosage. A reduction in the dosage may be necessary.

Reference

1 Harvey VJ, Slevin ML, Dilloway MR, Clark PI, Johnston A and Lant AF. The influence of cimetidine on the pharmacokinetics of 5-fluorouracil. Br J clin Pharmac (1984) 18, 421–30.

Hexamethylmelamine + Antidepressants

Abstract/Summary

Severe orthostatic hypotension has been described in patients concurrently treated with hexamethylmelamine and either phenelzine, amitriptyline or imipramine.

Clinical evidence, mechanism, importance and management

Five patients experienced very severe (described by the authors as potentially life-threatening) orthostatic hypotension when concurrently treated with hexamethylmelamine (150–250 mg/m²) and either phenelzine (60 mg), amitriptyline (50–150 mg) or imipramine (50 mg).[1] They experienced incapacitating dizziness, severe lightheadedness and/or fainting within a few days of taking both drugs concurrently. Standing blood pressures as low as 50/30 and 60/40 mm Hg were recorded. The reasons are not known. One of the patients had no problems when imipramine was replaced by nortriptyline (50 mg). The incidence of this interaction is unknown but it is clear that the concurrent use of these drugs should be closely monitored.

Reference

1 Bruckner HW and Schleifer SJ. Orthostatic hypotension as a complication of hexamethylmelamine antidepressant interaction. Cancer Treat Rep (1983) 67, 516.

Hydroxyurea + CNS depressants

Abstract/Summary

Increased CNS depression may occur.

Clinical evidence, mechanism, importance and management

Hydroxyurea has CNS-depressant effects and can cause drowsiness. This may be expected to be increased by other drugs which can also cause drowsiness (e.g. alcohol, anti-emetics, antihistamines, barbiturates, cough and cold remedies, phenothiazines, narcotic analgesics, tranquillizers, some tricyclic antidepressants, etc.)

Ifosfamide + Barbiturates

Abstract/Summary

Encephalopathy developed in a girl on phenobarbitone when given a single first dose of ifosfamide/mesna.

Clinical evidence

A 15-year-old girl who had been taking phenobarbitone for epilepsy since infancy developed confusion and gradually became unconscious 6 h after being given a first dose of ifosfamide for metastatic rhabdomyosarcoma. She was treated with ifosfamide (3 g/m²), mesna (3.6 g/m²) vincristine (2 mg) and actinomycin D (1000 μg). An ECG revealed signs of severe diffuse encephalopathy. She remained unconscious for 24 h but was asymptomatic after 48 h.

Mechanism

Encephalopathy due to ifosfamide has been seen in other patients and apparently results from the alteration in the balance of dechloroethylation of ifosfamide and the clearance of chloracetaldehyde.[2–4] The doses used were greater than in the case cited (<3.5 g/m² daily) and repeated. The reason for the encephalopathy in this case is not understood but the authors of the report suggest that the enzyme induction caused by the phenobarbitone might have resulted in increased activation of the single dose of ifosfamide, resulting in increased toxicity. The vincristine may also have had additive effects.[1]

Importance and management

The relationship between this encephalopathy and the use of phenobarbitone is not established, but this case serves to emphasize the need for particular caution and good monitoring if concurrent use is undertaken. More study is needed.

References

1 Ghosn M, Carde P, Leclerq B, Flamant F, Friedman S, Droz JP and Hayat M. Ifosfamide/mesna related encephalopathy: a case report with a possible role of phenobarbital in enhancing neurotoxicity. Bull Cancer (1988) 75, 391–2.
2 Cantwell BMJ and Harris AL. Ifosfamide/mesna and encephalopathy. Lancet (1985) i, 752.
3 Goren MP, Wright RK, Pratd CB and Pell FR. Dechloroethylation of ifosfamide and neurotoxicity. Lancet (1986) ii, 1219–20.
4 Salloum E, Flamant F, Ghosn M, Taleb N and Akatcherian C. Irreversible encephalopathy with ifosfamide/mesna. J Clin Oncol (1987) 5, 1303–4.

Ifosfamide + Cisplatin

Abstract/Summary

Ifosfamide toxicity is more common in those who have had prior treatment with cisplatin.

Clinical evidence

A comparative study in 36 children with malignant solid tumours who were treated with a range of drugs including some known to be potentially nephrotoxic (high dose methotrexate, aminoglycosides, cyclophosphamide) indicated that if they had previously been treated with cisplatin, their susceptibility to ifosfamide toxicity (neurotoxicity, severe leucopenia or acute tubular damage) was increased.[1]

This confirms other studies in which pretreatment with cisplatin appeared to increase the nephrotoxicity of ifosfamide,[2,3] but not another study which suggested that no such interaction occurs.[4]

Mechanism

It is thought that prior treatment with cisplatin damages the kidney tubules so that the clearance of the ifosfamide metabolites from the body is reduced and their toxic effects are thereby increased. Damaged kidney tubules may also be less capable of converting mesna to its active kidney-protecting form.

Importance and management

This interaction appears to be established. It should be borne in mind if ifosfamide is used. The authors of the paper cited[1] point out that the majority of patients who develop toxicity as a result of this interaction have persistently high urinary NAG concentrations, even though serum creatinine levels remain within the acceptable range for ifosfamide treatment. They suggest that evidence of subclinical tubular damage should be sought for by monitoring the excretion of urinary NAG.

References

1 Goren MP, Wright RK, Pratt CB, Horowitz ME, Dodge RK, Viar MJ and Kovnar EH. Potentiation of ifosfamide neurotoxicity, hematoxicity, and tubular nephrotoxicity by prior cis-diamminedichloroplatinum(II) therapy. Cancer Res (1987) 47, 1457 60.
2 Wheeler BM, Loehrer PJ, Williams SD and Einhorn LH. Ifosfamide in refractory male germ cell tumors. J Clin Oncol (1986) 4, 28–34.
3 Niederle N, Scheulen ME, Cremer M, Schutte J, Schmidt CG and Seeber S. Ifosfamide in combination chemotherapy for sarcomas and testicular carcinomas. Cancer Treat Rev (1983) 10 (Suppl A) 129–35.
4 Hacke M, Schmoll H-J, Alt JM, Bauman K and Stolte H. Nephrotoxicity of cis-diamminedichloroplatinum with or without ifosfamide in cancer treatment. Clin Physiol Biochem (1983) 1, 17–26.

Lomustine (CCNU) + Theophylline

Abstract/Summary

A single case report describes thrombocytopenia and bleeding attributed to the concurrent use of lomustine and theophylline.

Clinical evidence, mechanism, importance and management

An asthmatic woman taking theophylline and under treatment for medulloblastoma with lomustine, prednisone and vincristine, developed severe nose bleeding and thrombocytopenia three weeks after the third cycle of chemotherapy.[1] This was attributed to the concurrent use of the lomustine and theophylline. It is suggested that the theophylline inhibited the activity of phosphodiesterase within the blood platelets, thereby increasing cyclic AMP levels and disrupting normal platelet function. This theory seems to be supported by an experimental study.[2] What is known is far too limited to act as more than a warning of the possibility of increased thrombopathia and myelotoxicity during the concurrent use of theophylline and lomustine.

References

1 Zeltzer PM and Feig SA. Theophylline-induced lomustine toxicity. Lancet (1979) ii, 960.
2 DeWys WD and Bathina S. Synergistic anti-tumour effect of cyclic AMP elevation (induced by theophylline) and cytotoxic drug treatment. Proc Am Assoc Cancer Res (1978) 19, 104.

Melphalan + Cimetidine

Abstract/Summary

Cimetidine reduces the bioavailability of melphalan.

Clinical evidence, mechanism, importance and management

A study in eight patients with multiple myeloma or monoclonal gammopathy showed that pretreatment with 1 g cimetidine daily for six days reduced the bioavailability of a 10 mg oral dose of melphalan by 30%.[1] The melphalan half-life was reduced from 1.94 to 1.57 h. The reasons for this reaction and its clinical importance await assessment.

Reference

1 Sviland L, Robinson A, Proctor SJ and Bateman DN. Interaction of cimetidine with oral melphalan. Cancer Chemother Pharmacol (1987) 20, 173–5.

Mercaptopurine + Food

Abstract/Summary

Food reduces and delays the absorption of mercaptopurine.

Clinical evidence

A study in 17 children with acute lymphoblastic leukaemia showed that the absorption of 6-mercaptopurine (75 mg/m²) was markedly reduced if given 15 min after a standard breakfast (250 ml of milk and 50 g biscuits) compared with the situation when fasting. The area under the time-concentration curve (AUC) was reduced by 26% (from 143 to 105 μM min). The maximum serum concentration was reduced 36% (from 0.98 to 0.63 μM) and delayed from 1.2 to 2.3 h.[1] Some individuals showed more marked effects than others. One subject showed a 2.6-fold decrease in AUC and a sixfold decrease in maximum serum levels.[1]

This study confirms the findings of another study on two patients.[2]

Mechanism

Not understood. Delayed gastric emptying is a suggested reason.[1]

Importance and management

The documentation is small but this interaction appears to be established and of clinical importance. Mercaptopurine should be taken while fasting to optimize its absorption.

References

1 Riccardi R, Balis FM, Ferrara P, Lasorella A, Poplak DG and Mastrangelo R. Influence of food intake on bioavailability of oral 6-mercaptopurine in children with acute lymphoblastic leukaemia. Paed Haematol Oncol (1986) 3, 319–24.
2 Burton NK, Aherne GW and Marks VA. Novel method for the quantitation of 6-mercaptopurine in human plasma using high-peformance liquid chromatography with fluorescent detection. J Chromatogr (1984) 309, 409–14.

Methotrexate + Alcohol

Abstract/Summary

There is some inconclusive evidence that the consumption of alcohol may increase the risk of methotrexate-induced hepatic cirrhosis and fibrosis.

Clinical evidence, mechanism, importance and management

It has been claimed that alcohol can increase the hepatotoxic effects of methotrexate.[2] Two studies indicate that this may be so, in one of which three out of five patients with methotrexate-induced cirrhosis were reported to have taken alcohol concurrently,[1,3] but the evidence is by no means conclusive and no direct causal relationship has been established. The manufacturers of methotrexate (Lederle) advise the avoidance of drugs, including alcohol, which have hepatotoxic potentialities.

References

1 Tobias H and Auerbach R. Hepatotoxicity of long-term methotrexate therapy. Arch Intern Med (1973) 132, 391.
2 Pai SH, Werthamer S and Zak FG. Severe liver damage caused by treatment of psoriasis with methotrexate. NY State J Med (1973) 73, 2585.
3 Almeyda J, Barnardo D and Baker H. Drug reactions XV. Methotrexate, psoriasis and the liver. Br J Dermatol (1971) 85, 302–5.

Methotrexate + Amiodarone

Abstract/Summary

An isolated case report tentatively attributes the development of methotrexate toxicity to additional treatment with amiodarone.

Clinical evidence, mechanism, importance and management

An elderly woman, effectively treated for two years with methotrexate for psoriasis, developed ulceration of the psoriatic plaques within two weeks of starting treatment with amiodarone. The reason is not understood. A modest increase in the dosage of frusemide is a suggested contributory factor because it might have interfered with the excretion of the methotrexate.[1]

Reference

1 Reynolds NJ, Jones SK, Crossley J and Harman RRM. Methotrexate induced skin necrosis: a drug interaction with amiodarone? Br Med J (1989) 299, 980–1.

Methotrexate + Aminoglycoside antibiotics

Abstract/Summary

There is evidence that the gastrointestinal absorption of methotrexate can be reduced by paromomycin, neomycin and possibly other oral aminoglycosides, but increased by kanamycin.

Clinical evidence

A study in 10 patients with small cell bronchogenic carcinoma, under treatment with methotrexate, showed that when concurrently treated with a range of oral antibiotics (paromomycin, vancomycin, polymyxin B, nystatin) the gastrointestinal absorption of the methotrexate was reduced by over one third (from 69 to 44%).[1] The paromomycin was believed to have been responsible. In another study the concurrent use of neomycin (500 mg four times a day for three days) reduced the methotrexate area under the curve and the 72-hour culmulative excretion by 50%.[2] In contrast, the same report suggests that kanamycin can increase the absorption of methotrexate, but no details are given.

Mechanism

Paromomycin[3] and neomycin, in common with other oral aminoglycosides, can cause a malabsorption syndrome which reduces drug absorption. Kanamycin may possibly be different because it causes less malabsorption. It also reduces the activity of the gut flora which metabolize methotrexate so that more is available for absorption.

Importance and management

The documentation of these interactions is sparse, but it would seem prudent to be on the alert for a reduction in the response to methotrexate if patients are given oral aminoglycosides such as paromomycin or neomycin. An increased response may possibly occur with kanamycin. No interaction would be expected if the aminoglycosides are given parenterally.

References

1 Cohen MH, Creaven PJ, Fossieck BE, Johnston AV and Williams CL. Effect of oral prophylactic broad spectrum nonabsorbable antibiotics on the gastrointestinal absorption of nutrients and methotrexate in small cell bronchogenic carcinoma patients. Cancer (1976) 38, 1556.
2 Shen DD and Azarnoff D. Clinical pharmacokinetics of methotrexate. Clin Pharmacokinetics (1978) 3, 1–13.
3 Keusch GT, Troneale FJ and Buchanan RD. Malabsorption due to paromomycin. Arch Intern Med (1970) 125, 273.

Methotrexate + Ascorbic acid (Vitamin C)

Abstract/Summary

The urinary excretion of methotrexate is not significantly changed by the concurrent ingestion of large amounts of vitamin C (1–3 g daily) and it may possibly relieve the nausea of chemotherapy.

Clinical evidence, mechanism, importance and management

A patient with breast cancer, treated with methotrexate and cyclophosphamide, and who was also taking propranolol, amitriptyline, perphenazine and prochlorperazine said that the nausea caused by the cytotoxic therapy was relieved by large daily doses of vitamin C. A study on this patient showed that the concurrent ingestion of 1–3 g vitamin C daily had little effect on the excretion of methotrexate in the urine.[1]

Reference

1 Sketris IS, Farmer PS and Fraser A. Effect of vitamin C on the excretion of methotrexate. Cancer Treat Rep (1984) 68, 446–7.

Methotrexate + Barbiturates

Abstract/Summary

Animal studies suggest that phenobarbitone may possibly enhance the alopecia caused by methotrexate.

Clinical evidence, mechanism, importance and management

A study in rats showed that severe alopecia could be induced by the concurrent use of methotrexate and phenobarbitone in dosages which when given alone failed to cause any hair loss.[1] Whether this occurs in man is uncertain.

Reference

1 Basu TK, Williams DC and Raven RW. Methotrexate and alopecia. Lancet (1973) ii, 331.

Methotrexate + Chloramphenicol, PAS, Sodium salicylate, Sulphamethoxypyridazine, Tetracycline, Tolbutamide

Abstract/Summary

Animal studies suggested that the toxicity of methotrexate might be increased by the use of these drugs, but confirmation of this in man has only been seen with the salicylates, sulphonamides and tetracycline.

Clinical evidence, mechanism, importance and management

Some lists, reviews and books on interactions say that the drugs listed above interact with methotrexate, apparently based largely on a study in which male mice were treated for five days with each of four doses of methotrexate (1.53–12.25 mg/kg IV) and immediately afterwards with non-toxic intraperitoneal doses of the drugs listed. These drugs '...appeared to be capable of decreasing the lethal dose and/or decreasing the median survival time of the mice.'[1] That is to say, the toxicity of the methotrexate was increased. The reasons are not understood, but it is suggested that displacement of the methotrexate from its plasma protein binding sites could result in a rise in the levels of unbound and active methotrexate, and in the case of sodium salicylate to a decrease in renal clearance.

These animal studies were done in 1968. Since then the clinical importance of the interaction with salicylates has been confirmed, there are three cases involving another sulphonamide (sulphamethoxazole in the form of co-trimoxazole) and there is an isolated case report of an interaction with tetracycline (see appropriate synopsis), but there appears to be no direct clinical evidence of interactions between methotrexate and any of the other drugs. The results of animal experiments cannot be applied directly and uncritically to man and it now seems probable that some of these suggested or alleged interactions are more theoretical than real.

Reference

1 Dixon RL. The interaction between various drugs and methotrexate. Toxicol Appl Pharmacol (1968) 12, 308.

Methotrexate + Cholestyramine

Abstract/Summary

The serum methotrexate levels of two patients (methotrexate given by infusion) were markedly reduced by the concurrent use of cholestyramine.

Clinical evidence

A girl of 11 with osteosarcoma who developed colitis when treated with high dose intravenous methotrexate, was subsequently treated with 2 g cholestyramine six hourly from 6 to 48 h after the methotrexate. Serum methotrexate concentrations at 24 h were approximately halved. A marked fall in serum methotrexate levels were seen in another patient similarly treated.[1] *In vitro* studies showed that methotrexate becomes totally bound to cholestyramine.[1]

Mechanism

Methotrexate (whether given orally or by infusion) takes part in the entero-hepatic cycle, that is to say it is excreted into the gut in the bile and re-absorbed further along the gut. If cholestyramine is given orally, it can bind strongly to the methotrexate in the gut, thereby preventing its reabsorbtion and, as a result, the serum levels fall.

Importance and management

The documentation seems to be limited to this study.[1] In this instance the cholestyramine was deliberately used to reduce serum methotrexate levels, but in some circumstances it might represent an unwanted interaction. Since methotrexate is excreted into the gut in the bile, separating the oral dosages of the cholestyramine and methotrexate would not be expected to prevent their coming into contact and interacting together.

Reference

1 Erttmann R and Landbeck G. Effect of oral cholestyramine on the elimination of high-dose methotrexate. J Cancer Res Clin Oncol (1985) 110, 48.

Methotrexate + Corticosteroids

Abstract/Summary

There is evidence that the corticosteroids may possibly increase the toxicity of methotrexate. The efficacy of methotrexate may also possibly be reduced by hydrocortisone with cephalothin.

Clinical evidence, mechanism, importance and management

Although methotrexate and the corticosteroids have been used together successfully (for example in the treatment of psoriatic arthritis where a 50% reduction in the corticosteroid dosage was possible[2,3]), a number of serious reactions have been reported.

Two patients being treated for psoriasis with methotrexate (5 mg daily for 5–7 days) and who were on long-term corticosteroid therapy, died apparently from severe bone marrow depression. One was also on chloramphenicol.[1] Another patient taking 30 mg prednisone daily for psoriasis and who was given 50 mg, 100 mg and 150 mg methotrexate by injection at 10-day intervals, developed severe leucopenia and thrombocytopenia.[2] Yet another patient, debilitated from arthritis and prolonged corticosteroid therapy, died of generalized systemic moniliasis after two doses of methotrexate. She had no haematological abnormalities.[4]

In vitro experiments with blast cells from seven patients with acute myelogenous leukaemia indicated that the intracellular uptake of methotrexate is reduced by the presence of cephalothin (21 μg/ml) and hydrocortisone (20 μg/ml) which are normal achievable clinical serum concentrations.[5]

These cases suggest that particular care should be exercised during concurrent use to confirm that the clinical outcome is, as intended, advantageous.

References

1 Haim S and Alrey G. Methotrexate in psoriasis. Lancet (1967) i, 1156.
2 Black RL, O'Brien WM, Van Scott EJ, Auerbach R, Eisen AZ and Bunim JJ. Methotrexate therapy in psoriatic arthritis. J Amer Med Ass (1964) 189, 743.
3 Schewach-Millet M and Ziprkowski L. Methotrexate in psoriasis. Br J Derm (1968) 80, 535.
4 Roenigk HH, Fowler-Bergfeld W and Curtis GH. Methotrexate for psoriasis in weekly oral doses. Arch Derm (1969) 99, 86.
5 Bender AR, Bleyer WA, Frisby SA and Oliverio VJ. Alterations in methotrexate uptake in human leukaemia cells by other agents. Cancer Res (1975) 35, 1305–8.

Methotrexate + Co-trimoxazole or Trimethoprim

Abstract/Summary

Five cases of bone marrow depression have been reported, one of them fatal, caused by the concurrent use of methotrexate and co-trimoxazole or trimethoprim.

Clinical evidence

A 61-year-old patient with rheumatoid arthritis, taking 7.5 mg methotrexate daily, developed generalized bone marrow hypoplasia over two months after a 10-day course of treatment with co-trimoxazole for a urinary tract infection. She had taken a total of 775 mg methotrexate when the hypoplasia appeared.[1]

Two cases of megaloblastic pancytopenia, one of them fatal, have been described in patients on methotrexate who were given co-trimoxazole concurrently or sequentially.[2,3] Skin ulceration and marked pancytopenia occurred in a woman on methotrexate and naproxen when given trimethoprim.[6] Pancytopenia also occurred in another patient on methotrexate given co-trimoxazole.[7] A study[4] in children with acute lymphoblastic leukaemia showed that the concurrent use of co-trimoxazole had no effect on the pharmacokinetics of methotrexate.

Mechanism

Uncertain. Both drugs can suppress the activity of dihydrofolate reductase and it seems possible that the methotrexate and co-trimoxazole acted additively to produce folate deficiency, which lead to the bone marrow changes seen. Another sulphonamide, sulphafurazole (sulfisoxazole),[5] has been found to cause a small reduction in the clearance of methotrexate by kidney, but it is doubtful if this mechanism had any part to play in the interactions cited.

Importance and management

Information seems to be limited to the reports cited. If these drugs are given, either concurrently or sequentially, the haematological picture should be very closely monitored because the outcome can be serious.

References

1 Thomas MH and Gutterman LA. Methotrexate toxicity in a patient receiving trimethoprim-sulfamethoxazole. J Rheumatol (1986) 13, 440–1.
2 Dan M and Shapira I. Possible role of methotrexate in trimethoprim-sulphamethoxazole-induced acute megaloblastic anemia. Isr J Med Sci (1984) 20, 262–3.
3 Kobrinsky NL and Ramsay NKC. Acute megaloblastic anaemia induced by high dose trimethoprim-sulfamethoxazole. Ann Intern Med (1981) 94, 780–1.
4 Beach BJ, Woods WG and Howell SB. Influence of cotrimoxazole on methotrexate pharmacokinetics in children with acute lymphoblastic leukaemia. Am J Pediatr Hematol Oncol (1981) 3, 115–9.
5 Liegler DG, Henderson ES, Hahn MA and Oliverio VT. The effect of organic acids on renal clearance of methotrexate in man. Clin Pharmacol Ther (1969) 10, 849–57.
6 Ng HWK, MacFarlane AW, Graham RM and Verbov JL. Near fatal drug interactions with methotrexate given for psoriasis. Br Med J (1987) 295, 752–3.
7 Therenet JP, Ristori JM, Cure H, Mizony MH and Bussiere JL. Pancytopenie au cours due traitement d'une polyarthrite rheumatoide par methotrexate apres administration de trimethoprime-sulphmethoxazole. La Presse Med (1987) 16, 1487.

Methotrexate + Diuretics

Abstract/Summary

There is some unconfirmed evidence that bone marrow suppression may possibly be increased by concurrent use.

Clinical evidence, mechanism, importance and management

A study in nine patients showed that neither frusemide nor hydroflumethiazide had any effect on the clearance of methotrexate in the urine.[1] However a study in women with breast cancer and under treatment with methotrexate, cyclophosphamide and 5-fluorouracil showed that the concurrent use of a thiazide diuretic appeared to increase the myelosuppressant effects.[2] It is uncertain which of the cytotoxic drugs was responsible. Concurrent use should clearly be undertaken with caution.

References

1 Krisensen LO, Weismann K and Hutters L. Renal function and the rate of disappearance of methotrexate from serum. Eur J Clin Pharmacol (1975) 8, 439–44.
2 Orr LE. Potentiation of myelosuppression from cancer chemotherapy and thiazide diuretics. Drug Intell Clin Pharm (1981) 15, 967.

Methotrexate + 5-Fluorouracil (5-FU)

Abstract/Summary

In vitro *and animal data suggest that the cytotoxic effects of methotrexate and 5-fluorouracil (5-FU) may possibly be reduced by concurrent use, but this has yet to be confirmed in man.*

Evidence, mechanism, importance and management

5-FU and another compound, 5-fluorodeoxyuridine (FldUrd), are metabolized in the body to a third compound, FldUrd monophosphate which is the active cytotoxic agent. This acts by inhibiting an enzyme (thymidilate synthetase) which takes part in the biosynthesis of DNA so that DNA production is reduced. In this way 5-FU and FldUrd impair tumour growth.[4,5] Tests on tumour cells in culture indicate that methotrexate interferes with and reduces the activity of FldUrd.[1] In vitro studies in the L1210 cells system, Friend leukaemia system and in human bone marrow have similarly shown that in the presence of methotrexate the activity of 5-FU is also suppressed.[2] The likely reason is that the methotrexate inhibits a co-factor (5,10,methylenetetrahydrofolic acid) which is required by the FldUrd in order to allow it to bind to thymidilate synthetase. Thus the activity of the FldUrd is weakened (and by implication 5-FU as well) which would explain the antagonistic effects of methotrexate.

One cannot uncritically extrapolate tissue culture or animal experiments to man, moreover there is already considerable debate about the time-scheduling of administration[3] and whether combinations of methotrexate and 5-FU are antagonistic or even additive.[6] However the evidence (if it does nothing else) emphasises that these two drugs should not be given concurrently without a full awareness that they may possibly be less effective than each drug given alone.

References

1 Maugh TH. Cancer chemotherapy: an unexpected drug interaction. Science (1976) 194, 310.
2 Waxman S and Bruckner H. Antitumour drug interactions: additional data. Science (1976) 194, 672.
3 Bertino J, Sawicki WL, Lindquist CA and Gupta VS. Schedule-dependent antitumour effects of methotrexate and 5-fluorouracil. Cancer Res (1977) 37, 327.
4 Tattersall MNH, Jackson RC, Connors TA and Harrap KR. Combination chemotherapy: the interaction of methotrexate and 5-fluorouracil. Eur J Cancer (1973) 9, 733.
5 Waxman S, Rubinoff M, Greenspan E and Bruckner H. Interaction of methotrexate (MTX) and 5-fluorouracil (5-FU): effect on de novo DNA synthesis. Proc Am Assoc Cancer Res (1976) 17, 157.
6 Brown I and Ward HWC. Therapeutic consequences of antitumour drug interactions: methotrexate and 5-fluorouracil in the chemotherapy of C3H mice with transplanted mammary adenocarcinoma. Cancer Letters (1978) 5, 291.

Methotrexate + Nitrous oxide

Abstract/Summary

Methotrexate-induced stomatitis and other toxic effects may possibly be increased by the use of nitrous oxide.

Clinical evidence, mechanism, importance and management

Studies in which intravenous methotrexate, cyclophosphamide and 5-fluorouracil were used after mastectomy suggested that the stomatitis which can develop may be caused by a toxic interaction between methotroxate and nitrous oxide used during anaesthesia. A possible reason is that the effects of methotrexate on tetrahydrofolate metabolism are increased by nitrous oxide. It was found that the incidence of stomatitis, severe leucopenia, thrombocytopenia, and of severe systemic and local infections could be reduced by giving calcium folinate (leucovorin), intravenous hydration and withdrawal of the drugs where necessary.[1]

Reference

1 Goldhirsch A, Gelber RD, Tattersall MNH, Rudenstam C-M and Cavalli F. Methotrexate/nitrous oxide toxic interaction in perioperative chemotherapy for early breast cancer. Lancet (1987) ii, 151.

Methotrexate + Non-steroidal anti-inflammatory drugs (NSAID's)

Abstract/Summary

Rises in serum methotrexate levels accompanied by life-threatening increases in methotrexate toxicity can occur if aspirin, salicylates or ketoprofen are given concurrently. Acute toxicity (sometimes lethal) has also been associated in a handful of cases with the concurrent use of azapropazone, diclofenac, ibuprofen, indomethacin, naproxen and phenylbutazone.

Clinical evidence

(a) Methotrexate + aspirin and other salicylates

Prompted by the development of lethal pancytopenia in two patients given methotrexate and aspirin, a retrospective survey was carried out on the records of other patients treated with intra-arterial infusions of methotrexate (50 mg daily for 10 days) for epidermoid carcinoma of the oral cavity. Six out of seven who developed a rapid and serious pancytopenia were found to have had aspirin or other salicylates.[1] Similar results were observed in experiments on mice.[1]

There are other case reports[2,3] of methotrexate toxicity in patients taking salicylates but whether a causal relationship exists is uncertain. A study in four patients showed that the renal clearance of methotrexate was reduced by 35% when they received an infusion of sodium salicylate (2 g initially, then 33 mg/min). It has been suggested that pneumonitis in patients on low-dose methotrexate may have resulted from the concurrent use of 4–5 g aspirin daily.[6]

(b) Methotrexate + azapropazone

A woman given methotrexate (25 mg weekly for four years) for psoriasis showed acute toxicity (oral and genital ulceration, bone marrow failure) shortly after starting to take azapropazone (1.2 g daily). She was also taking 300 mg aspirin daily.[5]

(c) Methotrexate + ibuprofen

A patient on methotrexate who was given ibuprofen required leucovorin rescue because the clearance of methotrexate had fallen by two-thirds.[12]

(d) Methotrexate + indomethacin

Two patients on sequential intermediate dose methotrexate and 5-fluorouracil who were concurrently taking indomethacin (75–100 mg daily) died from acute drug toxicity which the authors of the report attributed to indomethacin-associated renal failure.[7]

Another case of acute renal failure has been described[10] and toxicity was seen in a patient given methotrexate and indomethacin,[8] but not in four other patients on methotrexate given either paracetamol or indomethacin.[3]

(e) Methotrexate + ketoprofen or diclofenac

A retrospective study[8] of 118 cycles of high-dose methotrexate treatment in 36 patients showed that four out the nine patients who developed severe methotrexate toxicity (800–8300 mg/m²; mean 3200 mg/m²) had also taken ketoprofen (150–200 mg daily for 2–15 days). Three of them died. A marked and prolonged rise in serum methotrexate levels were observed. Another patient who showed toxicity had been given diclofenac (150 mg in one day).

(f) Methotrexate + naproxen

A woman died of gross methotrexate toxicity apparently exacerbated by the concurrent use of naproxen.[11]

(g) Methotrexate + phenylbutazone

Two patients on methotrexate for psoriasis developed methotrexate toxicity and skin ulceration shortly after starting to take phenylbutazone (200–600 mg daily). One of them died from septicaemia following bone marrow depression.[9]

Mechanisms

Methotrexate is largely cleared unchanged from the body by renal excretion. The NSAID's as a group inhibit the synthesis of the prostaglandins (PGE_2) resulting in a fall in renal perfusion which would lead to a rise in serum methotrexate levels, accompanied by increased toxicity. In addition, salicylates and phenylbutazone competitively inhibit the tubular secretion of methotrexate which would further reduce its clearance.[4] Phenylbutazone and indomethacin can also cause renal failure which would allow the methotrexate to accumulate. Both phenylbutazone and methotrexate cause bone marrow depression which could be additive. Protein binding displacement of the major extracellular metabolite of methotrexate (7-hydroxy-methotrexate) has also been suggested as a possible additional mechanism because it is highly bound to plasma proteins.[14]

Importance and management

None of these interactions is very well-documented, but they should be regarded seriously because the outcome of concurrent use in some instances can be potentially life-threatening. The incidence of serious reactions is uncertain, but it is probably not large. For example, a study of 87 patients on long-term treatment with methotrexate (mean weekly dose 8.19 mg), most of whom were also taking unspecified NSAID's, found that the majority (72%) experienced no untoward effects and in the rest they were only relatively mild.[13] So concurrent use can be uneventful. The risks must therefore be balanced against the possible benefits. Patients particularly at risk are those on high dose methotrexate and those with reduced renal function due to age, disease or other drugs.

Aspirin and other salicylates should be avoided. The authors of the report cited[1] state that ketoprofen should not be given at the same time as methotrexate, but it is safe to give it 12–24 h after high dose methotrexate because 50% of the methotrexate is excreted by the kidneys within 6–12 h. This was tried in two patients without ill-effects.

The evidence against phenylbutazone, azapropazone, ibuprofen, naproxen, indomethacin and diclofenac is much thinner, and there appears to be no direct evidence against any other NSAID's, nevertheless it seems possible that all of them will impair the renal clearance of methotrexate to some extent (by inhibition of renal prostaglandin synthesis) quite apart from any other toxic effects they may have. If concurrent use is thought appropriate, it should be closely monitored.

References

1 Zuik M and Mandel MA. Methotrexate-salicylate interaction: a clinical and experimental study. Surg For (1975) 26, 567.
2 Dubin HV and Harrell RE. Liver disease associated with methotrexate treatment of psoriatic patients. Arch Dermatol (1970) 102, 498–503.
3 Baker H. Intermittent high dose oral methotrexate therapy in psoriasis. Br J Derm (1970) 82, 65.
4 Liegler DG, Henderson ES, Hahn MA and Oliverio VT. The effect of organic acids on renal clearance of methotrexate in man. Clin Pharmacol Ther (1969) 10, 849–57.
5 Daly HM, Scott GL, Boyle J and Roberts CJC. Methotrexate toxicity precipitated by azapropazone. Br J Dermatol (1986) 114, 733–35.
6 Maier WP, Leon-Perez R and Miller SB. Pneumonitis during low-dose methotrexate therapy. Arch Intern Med (1986) 146, 602–3.
7 Ellison NM and Servi RJ. Acute renal failure and death following sequential intermediate-dose methotrexate and 5-FU: a possible adverse effect due to concomitant indomethacin administration. Cancer Treat Rep (1985) 69, 342–3.
8 Thyss A, Milano G, Kubar J, Namer M and Schneider M. Clinical and pharmacokinetic evidence of a life-threatening interaction between methotrexate and ketoprofen. Lancet (1986) i, 256–8.
9 Adams JD and Hunter GA. Drug interaction in psoriasis. Aust J Derm (1976) 17, 39.
10 Maiche AG. Acute renal failure due to concomitant action of methotrexate and indomethacin. Lancet (1986) i, 1390.
11 Singh RR, Malaviya AN, Pandey JN and Guleria JS. Fatal interaction between methotrexate and naproxen. Lancet (1986) i, 1390.
12 Bloom EJ, Ignoffo RJ, Reis CA and Cadman E. Delayed clearance (CL) of methotrexate (MTX) associated with antibiotics and antiinflammatory agents (abstract). Clin Res (1986) 34, 560A.
13 Wilke WS, Calabrese LH and Segal AM. Incidence of untoward reactions in patients with rheumatoid arthritis treated with methotrexate. Arthritis Rheum (1983) 26 (Suppl) S56.
14 Slordal L, Sager G and Aarbakke J. Pharmacokinetic interactions with methotrexate: is 7-hydroxy-methotrexate the culprit? Lancet (1988) i, 591–2.

Methotrexate + Penicillins

Abstract/Summary

The loss of methotrexate from the body can be markedly reduced by the concurrent use of penicillins. There is a considerable risk of methotrexate toxicity.

Clinical evidence

Four patients treated with methotrexate showed a marked reduction in its clearance when concurrently treated with different penicillins: with penicillin a 35% reduction; with piperacillin 66%; with ticarcillin 40%; and with dicloxacillin and indomethacin 93%. Prolonged use of leucovorin rescue was necessary. They were given the methotrexate as an intravenous bolus (15–60 mg/m^2) and then 15–60 mg by infusion over 36 h.[1]

A patient under treatment with 50 mg methotrexate (weekly, given intravenously) diethylstilboestrol, prednisone and frusemide, developed severe methotrexate toxicity within a week of starting to take 250 mg penicillin every other day.[2] Increased methotrexate plasma levels and decreased excretion, attributed to the use of 30 mg carbenicillin daily, and necessitating an increase in the folinic acid dosage, is described in another patient.[3]

Mechanism

It is thought that weak acids such as the penicillins can successfully compete with methotrexate in the kidney tubules for excretion so that the methotrexate is retained.

Importance and management

Information is limited but the interaction appears to be established. The authors of the very brief report cited[1] suggest that concurrent use should be avoided if possible. If not, the plasma methotrexate levels should be closely monitored.

References

1 Bloom EJ, Ignoffo RJ, Reis CA and Cadman E. Delayed clearance (CL) of methotrexate (MTX) associated with antibiotics and antiinflammatory agents. Clin Res (1986) 34, 560A.
2 Nierenberg DW and Mamelok RD. Toxic reaction to methotrexate in a patient receiving penicillin and furosemide: a possible interaction. Arch Dermatol (1983) 119, 449–50.
3 Gibson DL, Bleyer AW and Savitch JL. Carbenicillin potentiation of methotrexate plasma concentration during high dose methotrexate therapy. Am Soc Hosp Pharm. Mid year clinical meeting abstracts, New Orleans, Dec 6–10 (1981) p 111.

Methotrexate + Probenecid

Abstract/Summary

Serum methotrexate levels are markedly increased (3–4-fold) by the concurrent use of probenecid. The dosage of methotrexate may need to be reduced to avoid the development of toxicity.

Clinical evidence

A study in four patients showed that the concurrent use of probenecid (500–1000 mg) and methotrexate (200 mg/m^2 intravenous bolus injection) resulted in serum methotrexate levels which were four times higher at 24 h than in four other patients who had not received probenecid (0.4 compared with 0.09 mg/l).[1]

In another study on four other patients the methotrexate serum levels were raised threefold at 24 h when probenecid was given concurrently.[2]

Mechanism

Studies in rats have shown that probenecid inhibits the excretion of methotrexate by the kidney and in the bile. A similar effect on renal excretion has been seen in monkeys.[3,4] This is also probably the mechanism in man. Changes in the protein binding of methotrexate may have some part to play.[5]

Importance and management

An established interaction although the information is limited. The increased methotrexate toxicity seen in rats almost certainly occurs in man as well. If both drugs are given concurrently the dosage of the methotrexate will need to be reduced. Some evidence from animal studies suggests that despite the rise in methotrexate levels caused by the probenecid, the clinically useful cytotoxic (antitumour) effects of the methotrexate may actually be reduced by the presence of probenecid.[6]

References

1 Aherne GW, Piall E, Marks V, Mould G and White WF. Prolongation and enhancement of serum methotrexate concentrations by probenecid. Brit Med J (1978) 1, 1097–99.
2 Howell SB, Olshen RA and Rice JA. Effect of probenecid on cerebrospinal fluild methotrexate kinetics. Clin Pharmacol Ther (1979) 26, 641–6.
3 Bourke RS, Chhada G, Bremer A, Watanabe O and Tower DB. Inhibition of renal tubular transport of methotrexate by probenecid. Cancer Res (1975) 35, 110–6.
4 Kates RE, Tozer TN and Sorby DL. Increased methotrexate toxicity due to concurrent probenecid administration. Biochem Pharmacol (1976) 25, 1485–8.
5 Paxton JW. Interaction of probenecid with the protein binding of methotrexate. Pharmacology (1984) 28, 86–9.
6 Gangji D, Ross WE, Bleyer WA, Poplak DG and Glaubiger DL. Probenecid inhibition of methotrexate toxicity in mouse L1210 leukaemia cells. Cancer Treat Rep (1984) 68, 521–5.

Methotrexate + Retinoids

Abstract/Summary

Although concurrent use can be successful, the serum levels of methotrexate are increased by etretinate and the incidence of severe toxic hepatitis appears to be considerably increased.

Clinical evidence

A study in a man with chronic discoid psoriasis being treated weekly with methotrexate (infusion of 10 mg over 48 h) found that when given 30 mg (0.05 mg/kg) etretinate daily his serum methotrexate levels were almost doubled. Concentrations at 12 and 24 h during the infusion were 0.11 mmol/l compared with 0.07 and 0.05 mmol/l before the etretinate.[1]

Other reports describe severe toxic hepatitis in other patients when these drugs were used concurrently.[2,3,7] It may take several months to develop.[7]

Mechanism

Uncertain. The increased incidence of toxic hepatitis probably relates to the increased methotrexate serum levels.

Importance and management

Although both drugs have apparently been used concurrently with success for psoriasis, pityriasis rubra pilaris and Reiter's disease,[4–6] the risk of severe drug-induced hepatitis seems to be considerably increased. One author states that hepatitis developed in two of 10 patients given both drugs, but none in 531 patients on methotrexate alone and none in 110 patients on etretinate alone.[2] He says that he has decided not to use this combination in future.[2] Concurrent use should clearly be undertaken with great care.

References

1 Harrison PV, Peat M, James R and Orrell D. Methotrexate and retinoids in combination for psoriasis. Lancet (1987) i, 512.
2 Zachariae H. Danger of methotrexate/etretinate combination therapy. Lancet (1988) i, 422.
3 Zachariae H. Methotrexate and etretinate as concurrent therapies in the treatment of psoriasis. Arch Dermatol (1984) 120, 155.
4 van der Veen E, Ellis C, Cambell J. Methotrexate and etretinate as concurrent therapies in severe psoriasis. Arch Dermatol (1982) 118, 660.
5 Adams J. Concurrent methotrexate and etretinate therapy for psoriasis. Arch Dermatol (1983) 119, 793.
6 Rosenbaum M and Roenigk H. Treatment of generalised pustular psoriasis with etretinate (RO-10-9359) and methotrexate. J Am Acad Dermatol (1984) 10, 357–61.
7 Beck H-I and Foged EK. Toxic hepatitis due to combination therapy with methotrexate and etretinate in psoriasis. Dermatologica (1983) 167, 94–6.

Methotrexate + Tetracycline

Abstract/Summary

An isolated case report describes the development of methotrexate toxicity in a patient when additionally given tetracycline.

Clinical evidence, mechanism, importance and management

A man being successfully and uneventfully treated for psoriasis with methotrexate (25 mg weekly) was additionally started on 2 g tetracycline daily for a mycoplasmal infection. Within five days he developed recurrent fever, ulcerative stomatitis and diarrhoea, and he was found to have a white cell count of 1000 and a platelet count of 30,000—all signs of methotrexate toxicity. The problem resolved when the methotrexate was withdrawn, but the psoriasis returned.[1] This interaction has also been observed in mice.[2] It may possibly be due to displacement of the methotrexate from its binding sites.

This appears to be the only clinical report of this interaction on record. Concurrent treatment should be well monitored.

References

1 Turck M. Successful psoriasis treatment then sudden 'cytotoxicity'. Hosp Pract (1984) 19, 175–6.
2 Dixon RL. The interaction between various drugs and methotrexate. Toxicol Appl Pharmacol (1968) 12, 308.

Methotrexate + Urinary alkalinizers

Abstract/Summary

Alkalinization increases the solubility of the methotrexate in the urine but also increases its excretion.

Clinical evidence, mechanism, importance and management

Methotrexate is much more soluble in alkaline than in acid fluids. For this reason urinary alkalinizers (and ample fluids) have been given to patients on high dose methotrexate therapy to prevent the precipitation of methotrexate in the kidney tubules which would cause damage. However alkalinization also increases the loss of methotrexate in the urine because at high pH values more of the drug exists in the ionized form which is not readily reabsorbed by the tubules. This increased loss was clearly shown in a very large number of patients (69–75) in whom alkalinization of the urine (pH 7+) with sodium bicarbonate and hydration reduced the serum methotrexate concentrations at 24 h by 40%, at 48 h by 73% and at 72 h by 77%.[1] In this instance the interaction was being exploited therapeutically to avoid toxicity. This interaction has also been shown by others.[2] Its possible consequences should be recognized if concurrent use is undertaken.

References

1 Nirenberg A, Mosende C, Mehta BM, Gisolfi AL and Rosen G. High dose methotrexate with citrovorum factor rescue: predictive value of serum methotrexate concentrations and corrective measures to avert toxicity. Cancer Treat Rep (1977) 61, 779–83.
2 Sand TE and Jacobsen S. Effect of urine pH and flow on renal clearance of methotrexate. Eur J Clin Pharmacol (1981) 19, 453–6.

Misonidazole + Cimetidine

Abstract/Summary

There is evidence that cimetidine does not interact with misonidazole.

Clinical evidence, mechanism, importance and management

Cimetidine increases the half-life and area under the curve of misonidazole in mice,[2] but 1 g cimetidine daily given to six normal human subjects for nine days had no effect on the pharmacokinetics of misonidazole.[1] Even so it would be prudent to monitor the effects to confirm that cimetidine used for longer periods does not interact.

References

1 Workman P, Donaldson J and Smith NC. Effects of cimetidine, antipyrine and pregnenolone carbonitrile on misonidazole pharmacokinetics. Cancer Treat Rep (1983) 67, 723–5.

2 Begg EJ, Williams KM, Wade DN and O'Shea KF. No significant effect of cimetidine on the pharmacokinetics of misonidazole in man. Br J clin Pharmac (1983) 15, 575–6.

Misonidazole + Miscellaneous drugs

Abstract/Summary

Phenytoin, phenobarbitone and dexamethasone increase the clearance of misonidazole from the body. Dexamethasone appears to reduce the neurotoxicity of misonidazole without reducing its radiosensitizing effects, but this does not seem to be true for phenytoin and phenobarbitone. Metoclopramide does not interact with misonidazole.

Clinical evidence, mechanism, importance and management

A study in patients suggests that the use of corticosteroids confers some protection against the peripheral neuropathy which can occur with misonidazole,[5] a possible explanation being provided by another study which showed that dexamethasone increased the clearance of misonidazole and reduced the plasma area under the curve.[6]

A study in normal subjects showed that after taking phenytoin (300 mg daily for a week) or phenobarbitone (200 mg daily for a week) the half-life of misonidazole was decreased by 27 and 23% respectively. The clearance increased by 42 and 31%.[1] This confirms previous human studies in which phenytoin shortened the misonidazole half-life by 31%[2] and 30–40%.[4] Both phenytoin and phenobarbitone were found to reduce plasma misonidazole concentrations.[3] It seems probable that this interaction results from an increase in the metabolism of the misonidazole caused by these two enzyme-inducing drugs. Whether concurrent use helps to reduce the neurotoxicity of misonidazole is uncertain although this was not apparent in two studies.[3,8] Peak plasma concentrations of misonidazole are not affected so that its radiosensitizing effects may not be reduced.[1]

A study in six normal subjects indicates that metoclopramide has no significant effect on the pharmacokinetics of misonidazole.[7]

References

1 Williams K, Begg E, Wade D and O'Shea K. Effects of phenytoin, phenobarbital and ascorbic acid on misonidazole elimination. Clin Pharmacol Ther (1983) 33, 314–21.
2 Workman P, Bleehen NM and Wiltshire CR. Phenytoin shortens the half-life of the hypoxic cell radiosensitizer misonidazole in man: implications for possible reduced toxicity. Br J Cancer (1980) 41, 302–4.
3 Walker MD and Strike TA. Misonidazole peripheral neuropathy. Its relationship to plasma concentration and other drugs. Cancer Clin Trials (1980) 3, 105–9.
4 Moore JL, Paterson ICM, Dawes PJD K and Henk JM. Misonidazole in patients receiving radical radiotherapy: pharmacokinetic effects of phenytoin tumor response and neurotoxicity. Int J Radiation Oncology Biol Phys (1982) 8, 361–4.
5 Walker MD and Strike TA. Misonidazole peripheral neuropathy. Its relationship to plasma concentration and other drugs. Cancer Clin Trials (1980) 3, 105–9.

6 Jones DH, Bleehen P, Workman P and Walton MI. The role of dex-amethasone in the modification of misonidazole pharmacokinetics. Br J Cancer (1983) 48, 553–7.
7 Williams KM, Begg EJ, Wade DN and O'Shea K. No significant effect of metoclopramide on misonidazole elimination in man. Br J clin Pharmac (1983) 15, 390–1.
8 Jones DH, Bleehen NM, Workman P and Smith NC. The role of microsomal enzyme inducers in the reduction of misonidazole neurotoxicity. Br J Radiol (1983) 56, 865–70.

Mitomycin + Chlorozotocin

Abstract/Summary

Pneumonitis developed in a patient concurrently treated with mitomycin and chlorozotocin.

Clinical evidence, mechanism, importance and management

A woman with pancreatic cancer developed acute interstitial pneumonitis (characterized by increasing dyspnoea and a dry cough) after receiving modest doses of mitomycin and chlorozotocin in combination with 5-fluorouracil and dox-orubicin (FAM-chlorozotocin). Mitomycin and chlorozotocin rarely cause lung damage at low doses and it is concluded that when given concurrently they may act synergistically or additively to cause lung damage. The problem responded rapidly to treatment with prednisone.[1]

Reference

1 Godert JJ, Smith FP, Tsou E and Weiss RB. Combination chemotherapy pneumonitis: a case report of possible synergistic toxicity. Med Paed Oncol (1983) 11, 116–18.

Mitomycin + Frusemide (Furosemide)

Abstract/Summary

Frusemide does not interact with mitomycin C.

Clinical evidence, mechanism, importance and management

A study in five patients with advanced solid tumours treated with mitomycin C (10 mg/m²) showed that frusemide given as a 40 mg IV bolus either 120 or 200 min after the mitomycin had no effect on its pharmacokinetics.[1]

Reference

1 Verweij J, Kerpel-Fronius S, Stuurman M, de Vries J and Pinedo HM. Absence of interaction between furosemide and mitomycin C. Cancer Chemother Pharmacol (1987) 19, 84–6.

Procarbazine + CNS depressants or Antihypertensives

Abstract/Summary

The effects of drugs which can cause CNS depression or lower blood pressure may possibly be increased by the presence of procarbazine

Clinical evidence, mechanisms, importance and management

Procarbazine can cause CNS depression ranging from mild drowsiness to profound stupor. The incidence is variously reported as being 31%, 14% and 8%.[1–3] Additive CNS depression may therefore be expected if other drugs possessing CNS-depressant activity are given concurrently.

Orthostatic hypotension has been described in four out of 48 patients on procarbazine.[3] Elsewhere a patient with hypertension and Hodgkin's disease has been reported whose blood pressure returned to normal when treated with procarbazine.[4] Additive hypotensive effects may therefore be seen with the concurrent use of antihypertensive drugs.

References

1 Brunner KW and Young CW. A methylhydrazine derivative in Hodgkin's disease and other malignant neoplasms: therapeutic and toxic effects studies in 51 patients. Ann Intern Med (1965) 63, 69.
2 Stolinsky DC, Solomon J, Pugh RP, Jacobs EM, Irwin LE, Wood DA, Steinfeld JL and Bateman JR. Clinical experience with procarbazine in Hodgkin's disease, reticulum cell sarcoma and lymphosarcoma. Cancer (1970) 26, 984.
3 Samuels ML, Leary WB, Alexanian R, Howe CD and Frei E. Clinical trials with N-isopropyl-alpha-(2-methylhydrazino)-p-toluamide hydrochloride in malignant lymphoma and other disseminated neoplasia. Cancer (1967) 20. 1187.
4 Frei E. Quoted as a personal communication by De Vita VT, Hahn MA and Oliverio VT in Monoamine oxidase inhibition by a new carcino-static agent, N-isopropyl-α-(2-methylhydrazino)-p-toluamide (MIH). Proc Soc Exp Biol Med (1965) 120, 561.

Procarbazine + Mustine (Mechlorethamine, Nitrogen mustard)

Abstract/Summary

A report on two patients suggests that the concurrent use of high doses of procarbazine with mustine may result in neurological toxicity.

Clinical evidence, mechanism, importance and management

Two patients with acute myelogenous leukaemia admitted to hospital for marrow transplantation and who were given high doses of procarbazine (12.5/15 mg/kg) and mustine (0.75/1.0 mg/kg) on the same day became lethargic, somnolent and disorientated for about a week. Although no interaction has been proved, the authors suggest that the mustine may have enhanced the neurotoxic effects of the procarbazine, and advise that it would be prudent to avoid high-dose administration of these drugs on the same day.[1]

Reference

1 Weiss GB, Weiden PL and Thomas ED. Central nervous system disturbances after combined administration of procarbazine and mechlorethamine. Cancer Treat Rep (1977) 61, 1713.

Procarbazine + Tyramine-containing foods and Sympathomimetic amines

Abstract/Summary

It seems doubtful whether the weak MAO-inhibitory properties of procarbazine can normally cause a hypertensive reaction with tyramine or other sympathomimetic amines. An itching skin reaction attributed to an interaction with cheese has been described in one patient.

Clinical evidence, mechanism, importance and management

The manufacturers of procarbazine state that it '... is a weak MAO inhibitor and therefore interactions with certain foodstuffs and drugs, although very rare, must be borne in mind.' This is apparently based on the results of animal experiments which show that the monoamine oxidase inhibitory properties of procarbazine are weaker than pheniprazine.[1] There seem to be no formal reports of a hypertensive reaction in patients on procarbazine who have eaten tyramine-containing foods (e.g. cheese) or after using indirectly-acting sympathomimetic amines (e.g. phenylpropanolamine, amphetamines, etc.). The only account I have been able to trace is purely anecdotal and unconfirmed: '...I recall one patient who described vividly reactions to wine and chicken livers which had occurred while he was taking MOPP chemotherapy several years earlier. Since he had not been forewarned, the reactions had been a frightening experience.'[3] An itching skin eruption observed after the ingestion of cheese has been attributed to the MAO-inhibitory properties of procarbazine.[2]

A practical way of dealing with this interaction problem has been suggested by a practitioner in an Oncology unit:[3] patients on procarbazine should ideally be given a list of the potentially interacting foodstuffs (see 'Tyramine-rich foods + MAOI'), with a warning about the nature of the possible reaction but also with the advice that it very rarely occurs. The foods may continue to be eaten, but patients should start with small quantities to ensure that they still agree with them. Those taking MOPP should also be told that any reaction is most likely to occur during the second week while on a 14 day treatment with procarbazine, and during the week following when not taking it.

References

1 De Vita VT, Hahn MA and Oliverio VT. Monoamine oxidase inhibition by a new carciostatic agent. N-isopropyl-alpha(2-methylhydrazino)-p-toluamide (MIH). Proc Soc Exp Biol Med (NY) (1965) 120, 561.
2 Cooper IA, Madigan RC, Motteran R, Maritz JS and Turner C. Combination chemotherapy (MOPP) in the management of advanced Hodgkin's disease. A progress report on 55 patients. Med J Aust (1972) 1, 41.
3 Maxwell MB. Re-examining the dietary restrictions with procarbazine (an MAOI). Cancer Nursing (1980) December, 451-7.

Streptozocin + Phenytoin

Abstract/Summary

A single case report indicates that phenytoin can reduce or abolish the cytotoxic effects of streptozocin (streptozotocin).

Clinical evidence, mechanism, importance and management

A patient with an organic hypoglycaemic syndrome, due to a metastatic apud cell carcinoma of the pancreas, and who was treated with 2 g streptozocin daily for four days together with 400 mg phenytoin, failed to show the expected response until the phenytoin was withdrawn.[1] It would seem that the phenytoin protected the beta-cells of the pancreas from the cytotoxic effects of the streptozocin by some mechanism as yet unknown. Although this is an isolated case report its authors recommend that concurrent use should be avoided.

Reference

1 Koranyi L and Gero L. Influence of diphenylhydantoin on the effect of streptozotocin. Brit Med J (1979) 1, 127.

Vinblastine + Bleomycin + Cisplatin

Abstract/Summary

This drug combination appears to cause serious life-threatening cardiovascular toxicity.

Clinical evidence, mechanism, importance and management

A report describes five patients (aged 23, 24, 33, 42 and 58) under treatment for germ cell tumours who died from acute life-threatening vascular events (myocardial infarction, rectal infarction, cerebrovascular accident) following VBP therapy (vinblastine, bleomycin, cisplatin). A survey of the literature by the authors of this paper revealed 14 other cases of both acute and long-term cardiovascular problems (myocardial infarction, coronary heart disease, cerebrovascular accident) in patients given VBP therapy. Reynaud's phenomenon is common (37%) in those treated with vinblastine and bleomycin or VBP and there is evidence that blood vessels are pathologically altered. This drug combination is very effective in the treatment of testicular carcinoma but its potential toxicity is serious.[1]

Reference

1 Samuels BL, Vogelzang NJ and Kennedy BJ. Severe vascular toxicity associated with vinblastine, bleomycin and cisplatin chemotherapy. Cancer Chemother Pharmacol (1987) 19, 253–6.

Vinca alkaloids + Mitomycin

Abstract/Summary

Vinblastine and vindesine can increase the pulmonary toxicity of mitomycin. Severe and life-threatening bronchospasm has been described.

Clinical evidence, mechanism, importance and management

There are now several reports describing an increase in lung disease in patients treated with mitomycin and vinca alkaloids. Diffuse lung damage characterized by interstitial infiltrates and pleural effusions resulting in respiratory distress and cough have been described after treatment with vinblastine.[1–3] Severe and life-threatening bronchospasm has also been described when vindesine sulphate was given after treatment with mitomycin.[4] The potential hazards of combining these drugs should be recognized.

References

1 Konits PH, Aisner J, Sutherland JC and Wiernik PH. Possible

pulmonary toxicity secondary to vinblastine. Cancer (1982) 50, 2771–4.

2 Gunstream SR, Seidenfeld JJ, Sobonya RE and McMahon LJ. Mitomycin-associated lung disease. Cancer Treat Rep (1983) 67, 301–4.

3 Ozols RF, Hogan WM, Ostchega T and Young RC. MVP (mitomycin, vinblastine, progesterone): a second-line regimen in ovarian cancer with a high incidence of pulmonary toxicity. Cancer Treat Rep (1983) 67, 721–2.

4 Dyke RW. Acute bronchospasm after a vinca alkaloid in patients previously treated with mitomycin. N Engl J Med (1984) 310, 389.

Vincristine + Colaspase, Isoniazid and Pyridoxine

Abstract/Summary

Some limited evidence suggests that vincristine neurotoxicity may possibly be increased by the concurrent use of these drugs.

Clinical evidence, mechanism, importance and management

Severe neurotoxicity has been described in three patients who were under treatment with vincristine. One of them was also taking colaspase and the other two were concurrently receiving isoniazid and pyridoxine.[1] A definite link between the use of these drugs and this serious toxicity has not been established, but the evidence suggests that particular care should be exercised if given concurrently.

Reference

1 Hildebrand J and Kenis Y. Vincristine neurotoxicity. N Engl J Med (1972) 287, 517.

14
DIGITALIS GLYCOSIDE DRUG INTERACTIONS

Plant extracts containing cardiac glycosides have been in use for thousands of years. The ancient Egyptians were familar with squill, as were the Romans who used it as a heart tonic and diuretic. The foxglove was mentioned in the writings of Welsh physicians in the thirteenth century and features in 'An Account of the Foxglove and some of its Medical Uses', published by William Withering in 1785, in which he described its application in the treatment of 'dropsy' or the oedema which results from heart failure.

The most commonly used cardiac glycosides are those obtained from the members of the foxglove family, *Digitalis purpurea* and *Digitalis lanata*. The leaves of these two plants are the source of a number of purified glycosides (digoxin, digitoxin, gitoxin, lanatoside C and others), of gitalin (an amorphous mixture largely composed of digitoxin and digoxin), and of powdered whole leaf digitalis. Occasionally ouabain or strophanthin (also of plant origin) are used for particular situations, while for a number of years the Russians have exploited cardiac glycosides from lily of the valley. All of these cardiac glycosides have similar actions, but they differ in their potency and in their rates of elimination from the body, and this determines how much is given and how often. Table 14.1 lists many of the cardiac glycosides in use.

Digitalization

The cardiac glycosides have two main actions and two main applications: for the treatment of cardiac arrhythmias and fibrillation, and to a much lesser extent these days, for congestive heart failure. Because the most commonly used glycosides are derived from digitalis, the achievement of the desired therapeutic serum concentration of any cardiac glycoside is usually referred to as 'digitalization'. The digitalis glycosides are said to have a 'positive inotropic effect' on the heart muscle, meaning that the force of contraction of the heart muscle is increased.

It is usual to start treatment with a large 'loading dose' so that the therapeutic concentrations are achieved reasonably quickly, but once this has been reached the amount is reduced to a maintenance dose which is intended to keep a nice balance between drug intake and drug loss. This has to be done carefully because there is a relatively narrow gap between serum concentrations which are therapeutic and those which are toxic. Normal therapeutic levels are about one third of those which are fatal, and serious toxic arrhythmias begin at about two thirds of the fatal levels. If a patient is over-digitalized, he will demonstrate signs of intoxication: he may first lose his appetite, then begin to be nauseated, and vomit. Visual disturbances may also be experienced, headache, drowsiness, occasionally diarrhoea, and the pulse rate can fall as low as 40 beats per minute. Death can take place from cardiac arrhythmias which are associated with total AV block. Patients under treatment for cardiac arrhythmias can therefore demonstrate arrhythmias when they are both under- as well as over-digitalized, which may complicate the decision to increase or reduce the dosage.

Interactions of the cardiac glycosides

The pharmacological actions of these glycosides are very similar, but their rates and degree of absorption, metabolism and clearance are different and this determines the dosages used. For example, the half-life of digoxin is 30–40 h compared with 4–6 days for digitoxin, and this is reflected in their daily maintenance doses of 0.125–0.5 mg and 0.15 mg respectively. It is therefore most important not to extrapolate an interaction seen with one glycoside and apply it uncritically to any other.

Because the therapeutic ratio of the cardiac glycosides is low, a quite small change in serum levels may lead to inadequate digitalization or to toxicity. For this reason interactions which have a relatively modest effect on serum levels may sometimes have serious consequences.

Table 14.1 Cardiac glycosides

Non-proprietary names	Proprietary names
Acetyldigitoxin	Acetil Digitoxina, Acylanid(e)
Acetyldigoxin	Agolanid, Allocor, Cardioreg, Cedigocin(a)(e), Cedigossina, Ceverin, Decardil, Digisistabil, Digostada, Digostab, Dioxanin, Kardiamed, Lanadigin, Longidox, Novodigal, Sandolanid, Stillacor
Acetylstrophanthidin	
Convallaria	
Cymarin	Alvonal MR
Delanoside	Cedilanid, Desace, Desaci
Digitalin	
Digitalis leaf	
Prepared digitalis	Augentonicum, Digifortis, Digiglusin, Digiplex, Digitalysat, Pil-digis
Digitoxin	Asthensilo, Coramedan, Crystodigin, Digicor,Digilong, Digimed, Digimerck, Digipural, Digitalina-Bescansa, -Mialhe, -Nativelle, Digitasid, Digitox, Digitoxina Simes, Digitoxine, Digitrin, Ditaven, Mono-Glycocard, Purodigin, Tardigal
Digoxin	Allocor, Cardigox(in), Cardioreg, Cardiox, Coragoxine, Digacin, Digazolan, Digivern, Digomal, Dixina, Eudigox, Lanacordin, Lanacrist, Lanorale, Lanoxicaps, Lanoxin(e), Lenoxin, Natigoxin, Novodigal, Prodigox, Purgoxin
Gitalin	Cistaloxine, Formigitalin, Gitalide, Gitaligin, Verodigeno
Gitoformate	Dynocard, Formiloxine
Lanatoside C	Cedilanid(e), Celenat(e), Dilanosid-C, Lanatosid, Lanimerck, Lanocide
Medigoxin	Cardiolan, Lanirapid, Lanitop, Metidi, Miopat
Meproscillarin	Clift
Ouabain (Stophanthin-G)	g-Strofantin, Ouabaine Aguettant, Arnaud, Purostrophan, Strodival, Strophoperm
Pengitoxin	Carnacid-Cor, Cordoval
Proscillaridin	Caradrin, Proscillan, Sandoscill, Stelarid, Sucblorin, Talucard, Talusin, Tradenal, Urgilan, Wirnesin
Strophanthin-K	Estrofosid, Kombetin, Myokombin, Strofopan, Strophosid, Trauphantin

Digitalis glycosides + ACE inhibitors

Abstract/Summary

Some studies have found that serum digoxin levels rise by about 20–25% if captopril is used concurrently, but another found no significant changes. Enalapril, lisinopril and ramipril appear not to interact.

Clinical evidence

(a) Digoxin + captopril

A study in 20 patients with severe chronic congestive heart failure showed that while taking captopril (averaging 93.7 mg daily) their serum digoxin levels rose by 26% (from 1.38 to 1.74 nmol/l). Three of the patients had serum digoxin levels above the therapeutic range (2.6 nmol/l) but no toxicity was seen.[1]

A later study by the same workers showed that captopril increased serum digoxin levels by about 21%.[6] However another controlled study in 31 patients with stable congestive heart failure, given 25 mg captopril three times daily, found no significant changes in serum digoxin levels over a six-month period.[7]

(b) Digoxin + enalapril, lisinopril and ramipril

A study in seven patients with congestive heart failure on 0.25 mg digoxin daily showed that the concurrent use of 20 mg enalapril daily for 30 days did not significantly change the pharmacokinetics of digoxin.[4] A double-blind placebo controlled study in 14 patients on digoxin showed that the concurrent use of 5 mg lisinopril daily over a four-week period had no significant effect on serum digoxin levels.[2] This confirms the findings of a previous single dose study.[3] A study in 12 normal subjects given 0.5 mg digoxin daily showed that the concurrent use of 5 mg ramipril daily for 14 days had no effect on the serum levels of the digoxin.[5]

Mechanism

The mechanism of the digoxin–captopril interaction is not fully understood. Both glomerular filtration and tubular secretion of the digoxin are reduced (possibly related to aldosterone inhibition), but other mechanisms may have some part to play.[6]

Importance and management

Information about digoxin and captopril is limited and not consistent. If any interaction occurs it would seem that the increase in serum digoxin levels is relatively modest (20–25%) and therefore probably of little or only moderate clinical importance except for those patients with serum levels already at the top end of the therapeutic range. However it would be prudent to monitor concurrent use. Enalapril, lisinopril and ramipril appear to be non-interacting alternatives.

References

1 Cleland JGF, Dargie HJ, Hodsman GP, Robertson IS and Ball SG. Interaction of digoxin and captopril. Br J clin Pharmac (1984) 17, 214P.
2 Vandenburg MJ, Kelly JG, Wiseman HT, Mannering D, Long C and Glover DR. The effect of lisinopril on digoxin pharmacokinetics in patients with congestive heart failure. Br J clin Pharmac (1988) 21, 657P.
3 Morris FP, Tamrazian S, Marks C, Kelly J, Stephens JD and Vandenberg MJ. An acute pharmacokinetic study of the potential interaction of lisinopril and digoxin in normal volunteers. Br J clin Pharmac (1985) 20, 281–2P.
4 Douste-Blazy Ph, Blanc M, Montastruc JL, Conte D, Cotonat J and Galinier F. Is there any interaction between digoxin and enalapril? Br J clin Pharmac (1986) 22, 752.
5 Doering W, Maass L, Irmisch R and Konig E. Pharmacokinetic interaction study with ramipril and digoxin in healthy volunteers. Am J Cardiol (1987) 59, 60–4D.
6 Cleland JGF, Dargie HJ, Pettigrew A, Gillen C and Robertson JLS. The effects of captopril on serum digoxin and urinary urea and digoxin clearances in patients with congestive heart failure. Amer Heart J (1986) 112, 130–5.
7 Magelli C, Bassein L, Ribani MA, Liberatore S, Ambrosioni E and Magnani B. Lack of effect of captopril on serum digoxin in congestive heart failure. Eur J Clin Pharmacol (1989) 36, 99–100.

Digitalis glycosides + Acipimox

Abstract/Summary

Acipimox does not interact with digoxin.

Clinical evidence, mechanism, importance and management

A study in six elderly patients on digoxin showed that the concurrent use of 250 mg acipimox three times daily for a week had no significant effect on their serum digoxin levels, clinical condition, ECG's, plasma urea or electrolyte levels.[1] No special precautions during concurrent use would seem necessary.

Reference

1 Chijioke PC, Pearson RM, Johnston A and Blackett A. Effect of acipimox on plasma digoxin levels in elderly patient volunteers. Br J clin Pharmac (1987) 25, 102–3P.

Digitalis glycosides + Allopurinol

Abstract/Summary

Allopurinol has been shown not to affect serum digoxin levels.

Clinical evidence, mechanism, importance and management

Five normal subjects, digitalized with digoxin, showed no significant changes in their serum digoxin levels over a seven-day period while taking 300 mg allopurinol daily.[1] No special precautions would appear to be necessary.

Reference

1 Havelund T, Abildtrup N, Birkebaek N, Breddam E and Rosager AM. Allopurinols effekt pa koncentrationen af digoksin i serum. Ugeskr Laeger (1984) 146, 1209–11.

Digitalis glycosides + Amiloride

Abstract/Summary

Amiloride has little effect on blood digoxin levels in normal subjects, but it reduces the contractility of the heart. In patients with renal impairment it possibly raises serum digoxin levels.

Clinical evidence, mechanism, importance and management

A study[1] in six healthy subjects of a possible interaction between these drugs showed that amiloride (10 mg daily for eight days) virtually doubled the renal clearance of digoxin (from 1.3 to 2.4 ml/kg/min) but almost blocked the extra-renal clearance (from 2.1 to 0.2 ml/kg/min). The balance of the two effects was to cause a small fall in total body clearance and a small rise in serum digoxin levels. The positive inotropic effects of digoxin were reduced, but whether this is clinically important or not is uncertain. Studies in patients with congestive heart failure are needed. Patients with poor kidney function would be expected to show a rise in digoxin levels but the clinical importance of this also awaits confirmation. The effects of concurrent use should be well monitored.

Reference

1 Waldorff S, Hansten PB, Kjaergard H, Buch J, Egeblad H and Steiness E. Amiloride-induced changes in digoxin dynamics and kinetics: abolition of digoxin-induced inotropism with amiloride. Clin Pharmacol Ther (1980) 30, 1981.

Digitalis glycosides + Aminoglutethimide

Abstract/Summary

The clearance of digitoxin is markedly increased by the concurrent use of aminoglutethimide and a reduction in its effects would be expected.

Clinical evidence, mechanism, importance and management

A study[1] in six patients on digitoxin showed that while receiving aminoglutethimide, 250 mg four times a day, the clearance of digitoxin was increased by 109%. The likely reason is that the aminoglutethimide increases the metabolism of the digitoxin by the liver. This would be expected to be clinically important, but it appears not to have been assessed. Check that patients do not become under-digitalized during concurrent treatment. No interaction would be expected with digoxin because it is largely excreted unchanged in the urine and metabolism by the liver has little part to play in its clearance.

Reference

1 Lonning PE, Kvinnsland S and Bakke OM. Effect of aminoglutethimide on antipyrine, theophylline and digitoxin disposition in breast cancer. Clin Pharmacol Ther (1984) 36, 796–802.

Digitalis glycosides + Aminosalicylic acid (PAS)

Abstract/Summary

Blood levels of digoxin can be reduced by the concurrent use of neomycin

Clinical evidence

Studies in normal subjects showed that neomycin (1–3 g orally) depressed and delayed the absorption of digoxin by the gut.[1,2] The area under the concentration/time curve was reduced as much as 50%. Absorption was affected even when the neomycin was given 3–6 h before the digoxin. The probable reason is that neomycin can cause a general but reversible malabsorption syndrome which affects the absorption of several drugs. The extent of this is probably offset in some patients because the neomycin depresses the destruction of the digoxin by the bacteria in the gut.[3] Information is limited but it appears to be an established interaction. Patients on digoxin should be monitored for reduced effects if neomycin is given and suitable dosage adjustments made if necessary. Separating the dosages of the two drugs does not prevent this interaction. Kanamycin and paromomycin possibly interact similarly, but this requires confirmation. There seems to be no information about other aminoglycosides.

References

1 Lindenbaum J, Maulitz RM, Saha JR and Butler VP. Impairment of digoxin absorption by neomycin. Clin Res (1972) 20, 410.
2 Lindenbaum J, Maulitz RM and Butler V. Inhibition of digoxin absorption by neomycin. Gastroenterology (1976) 71, 399.
3 Lindenbaum J, Tse-Eng D, Butler BV and Rund DG. Urinary excretion of reduced metabolites of digoxin. Amer J Med (1981) 71, 67.

Digitalis glycosides + (Para)-Aminosalicylic acid (PAS)

Abstract/Summary

Blood levels of digoxin in normal subjects are reduced to a small extent by p-aminosalicyclic acid, but the importance of this in patients is uncertain.

Clinical evidence, mechanism, importance and management

10 normal subjects showed a 20% reduction in the absorption of a single 0.75 mg dose of digoxin (using urinary excretion as a measure) when concurrently treated with 8 g p-aminosalicylic acid (PAS) daily for two weeks.[1] This seems to be just another aspect of the general malabsorption caused by aminosalicylic acid. The importance of this interaction in patients is not known (it is probably small) but it would be prudent to monitor concurrent use.

Reference

1 Brown DD, Juhl RP and Warner SL. Decreased bioavailability of digoxin due to hypocholesterolemic interventions. Circulation (1978) 58, 164.

Digitalis glycosides + Amiodarone

Abstract/Summary

Blood levels of digoxin can be doubled by the concurrent use of amiodarone. Some individuals may show even greater increases. Digitalis intoxication will occur if the dosage of digoxin is not reduced appropriately.

Clinical evidence

The observation[1] that patients on digoxin developed intoxication and unexpectedly high digoxin blood levels when given amiodarone prompted study of this interaction. Seven patients on constant daily doses of digoxin for 14 days showed a mean rise in serum digoxin levels of 69% (from 1.17 to 1.98 μg/ml) when given 600 mg amiodarone daily. Two other patients similarly treated also showed this interaction.

Numerous studies in large numbers of patients have confirmed this interaction with reported increases in serum digoxin levels of 75%,[9] 90%,[7] 95%[11] and 104%.[12] The occasional patient may show three- to fourfold increases, whereas others may show little or no change.[7,14] Children seem particularly sensitive with two- to threefold rises, and even as much as eightfold.[13] Other reports confirm that the digoxin levels are markedly increased or roughly doubled, and intoxication occurs.[4-6,8,14,15,19,20] In contrast, one group of workers state that they observed no change in serum digoxin levels in five patients given amiodarone.[2,3]

Mechanism

Not fully understood. Amiodarone reduces both the renal and non-renal excretion of digoxin,[10] and amiodarone-induced changes in thyroid function may also have some part to play in this interaction.[18] Displacement of digoxin from its binding sites has been suggested.[16,17] One study suggests that increased absorption from the gut is responsible.[21]

Importance and management

A well-documented and well-established interaction of considerable clinical importance. It occurs in most patients. It is clearly evident after a few days and develops over the course of 1–4 weeks.[11] If no account is taken of this interaction the patient may develop digitalis intoxication. Reduce the digoxin dosage by a third to a half when amiodarone is added[1,9,8,21] with further adjustment of the dosage after a week or two, and possibly a month or more, as necessary.[8] Children may show much larger rises in digoxin levels than adults so that particular care is needed. Amiodarone is lost from the body very slowly so that the effects of this interaction will persist for several weeks after its withdrawal.

References

1 Moysey JO, Jaggarao NSV, Grundy EN and Chamberlain DA. Amiodarone increases plasma digoxin concentrations. Br Med J (1981) 282, 272.

2 Achilli A and Serra N. Amiodarone increases plasma digoxin concentrations. Br Med J (1981) 282, 1630.

3 Achilli A, Giacci M, Capezzuto A, de Luca F, Guerra R and Serra N. Interazione digossina-chinida e digossina-amiodarone. G Ital Cardiol (1981) 11, 918–25.

4 Nademance K, Kannan R and Hendrikson JA, Burbham M, Kay I and Singh BN. Amiodarone digoxin interaction during treatment of resistant cardiac arrhythmias. Am J Cardiol (1982) 49, 1026.

5 McQueen EG. New Zealand Committee on Adverse Drug Reactions. 17th Annual Report 1982. NZ J Med (1983) 96, 95–9.

6 McGovern B, Garan H, Kelly E and Ruskin JN. Adverse reactions during treatment with amiodarone hydrochloride. Br Med J (1983) 287, 175–80.

7 Oetgen WJ, Sobol SM, Tri TB, Heydorn WH, Davia JE and Rakita L. Amiodarone-digoxin interaction. Clinical and experimental observations. Chest (1984) 86, 75–9.

8 Marcus FI and Fenster PE. Drug therapy. Digoxin interactions with other cardiac drugs. J Cardiovasc Med (1983) 8, 25–8.

9 Fornaro G, Rossi P, Padrini R, Piovan D, Ferrari M, Fortina A, Tomassini G and Aquili C. Ricerca farmacologico-clinica sull'interazione digitale-amiodarone in pazienti cardiopatici con insufficiencza cardiaca di vario grado. G Ital Cardiol (1984) 14, 990–8.

10 Fenster PE, White NW and Hanson CD. Pharmacokinetic evaluation of the digoxin-amiodarone interaction. J Am Coll Cardiol (1985) 5, 108–12.

11 Vitale P, Jacono A, Gonzales y Reyero E and Zeuli L. Effect of amiodarone on serum digoxin levels in patients with atrial fibrillation. Clin Trial J (1984) 21, 199–206.

12 Nademanee K, Kannan R, Hendrickson J, Ookhtens M, Kay I and Singh BN. Amiodarone-digoxin interaction: clinical significance, time course of development, potential pharmacokinetic mechanisms and therapeutic implications. J Amer Coll Cardiol (1984) 4, 111–16.

13 Koren G, Hesslein PS and MacLeod SM. Digoxin toxicity associated with amiodarone therapy in children. J Pediatr (1984) 104, 467–70.

14 Nager F and Nager G. Interaktion zwischen Amiodaron und Digoxin. Schweiz med Wsch (1983) 113, 1727–30.

15 Strocchi E, Malini PL, Graziani A, Ambrosioni E and Magnani B. L'interazione tra digossina e amiodarone. G Ital Cardiol (1984) 14, 12–15.

16 Douste-Blazy Ph, Montastruc JL, Bonnet B, Auriol P, Conte D and Bernadet P. Influence of amiodarone on plasma and urine digoxin concentrations. Lancet (1984) i, 905.

17 Mingardi G. Amiodarone and plasma digoxin levels. Lancet (1984) i, 1238.

18 Ben-Chetrit E, Ackerman Z and Eliakim M. Case-report: Amiodarone-associated hypothyroidism—a possible cause of digoxin intoxication. Amer J Med Sci (1985) 289, 114–16.

19 Robinson KC, Walker S, Johnston A, Mulrow JP, McKenna WJ and Holt DW. The digoxin-amiodarone interaction. Circulation (1986) 74, II-225.

20 Johnston A, Walker S, Robinson KC, McKenna WJ and Holt DW. The

digoxin-amiodarone interaction. Br J clin Pharmac (1987) 24, 253P.

21 Santostasi G, Fantin M, Marango I, Gaion RM, Basadonna O, Dalla-Volta S. Effects of amiodarone on oral and intravenous digoxin kinetics in healthy subjects. J Cardiovasc Pharmacol (1987) 9, 385–90.

Digitalis glycosides + Amphotericin

Abstract/Summary

Amphotericin causes potassium loss which could lead to the development of digitalis toxicity.

Clinical evidence, mechanism, importance and management

Among the well-recognized adverse effects of amphotericin treatment is increased potassium loss.[1–3] The hypokalaemia can be severe. Although there seem to be no reports of adverse interactions, it would be logical to expect that digitalis toxicity could develop in patients given both drugs if the potassium levels were allowed to fall unchecked. Concurrent treatment should be well monitored and any potassium deficiency made good.

References

1 Holeman CW and Einstein H. The toxic effects of amphotericin B in man. Californ Med (1963) 99, 290.

2 Butler WT, Bennett JE, Hill GJ, Szwed CF and Cotlove E. Electrocardiographic and electrolyte abnormalities caused by amphotericin B in dog and man. Proc Soc Exp Biol Med (1964) 116, 857.

3 Miller RP and Bates JH. Amphotericin B toxicity. A follow-up report of 53 patients. Ann Intern Med (1969) 71, 1089.

Digitalis glycosides + Antacids

Abstract/Summary

Although the bioavailability of digoxin is reduced by some antacids, the clinical importance of this is uncertain. It may be advisable to separate the dosages by 1–2 h to avoid admixture in the gut. This is effective with digitoxin.

Clinical evidence

(a) Digoxin

(i) Evidence of an interaction with digoxin

A study in 10 normal subjects given 0.75 mg digoxin (*Lanoxin*) with 60 ml of either 4% aluminium hydroxide gel, 8% magnesium hydroxide gel or magnesium trisilicate showed that the cumulative six-day urinary excretion expressed as a percentage of the original dose was as follows: control 40%; aluminium hydroxide 31%; magnesium hydroxide 27%.[1]

Other studies describe reductions in digoxin absorption of 11% with aluminium hydroxide, 15% with bismuth carbonate and light magnesium carbonate, and 99.5% with magnesium trisilicate.[2] *In vitro* studies with digitoxin suggest that it may possibly interact similarly,[3] but lanatoside C probably does not.[4]

(ii) Evidence of no interaction

A study on four patients chronically treated with 250–500 μg digoxin daily showed that concurrent treatment with either 10 ml aluminium hydroxide mixture BP or magnesium trisilicate mixture BP, three times a day, did not reduce the bioavailability of the digoxin and none of the patients showed any reduction in the control of their symptoms.[5]

Other bioavailability studies failed to show a significant interaction between digoxin (in capsule but not tablet form)[7] or beta-acetyldigoxin[6] and magnesium-aluminium hydroxide.

(b) Digitoxin

Evidence of no interaction

A study in 10 patients with heart failure showed that their steady-state serum digitoxin levels were slightly but not significantly raised (from 13.6 to 15.1 ng/ml) while taking 20 ml aluminium-magnesium hydroxide gel three or four times a day, separated from the digitoxin dosage by at least 1–2 h.[8]

Mechanism

Not established. One suggestion is that the digoxin can become adsorbed onto the antacids and therefore unavailable for absorption.[1,3]

Importance and management

The digoxin–antacid interactions are moderately well documented but their clinical importance is not established. Watch for any evidence of a reduced response to digoxin if given concurrently. Raise the digoxin dosage if necessary. Alternatively, separate the dosages by 1–2 h to minimize admixture in the gut. This is effective with digitoxin and many other drugs which interact within the gut.

References

1 Brown DD, Juhl RP, Lewis K, Schrott M and Bartels B. Decreased bioavailability of digoxin due to antacids and kaolin-pectin. N Engl J Med (1976) 295, 1034.

2 McElnay JC, Harron DWG, D'Arcy PF and Eagle MRG. Interaction of digoxin with antacid constituents. Br Med J (1978) i, 1554.

3 Khalil SAH. The uptake of digoxin and digitoxin by some antacids. J Pharm Pharmac (1974) 26, 961.

4 Aldous S and Thomas R. Absorption and metabolism of lanatoside. Clin Pharmacol Ther (1977) 21, 647.

5 Cooke J and Smith JA. Absence of interaction of digoxin with antacids under clinical conditions. Br Med J (1978) 2, 1166.

6 Bonelli J, Hruby K, Magometschigg D, Hitzenberger G and Kaik G. The bioavailability of beta-acetyldigoxin alone and combined with aluminium hydroxide and magnesium hydroxide. Int J Clin Pharmacol (1977) 15, 337.

7 Allen MD, Greenblatt DJ, Harmatz JS and Smith TW. Effect of magnesium-aluminium hydroxide and kaolin-pectin on the absorption of digoxin from tablets and capsules (1981) 21, 26.

8 Kuhlmann J. Plasmaspiegel und renale Elimination von Digitoxin bei

Langzeittherapie mit Aluminium-Magnesium-Hydroxide-Gel. Dtsch med Wsch (1984) 109, 59–61.

Digitalis glycosides + Aspirin

Abstract/Summary

Aspirin does not interact with digoxin.

Clinical evidence, mechanism, importance and management

Although aspirin can double the serum concentrations of digoxin in dogs, a study in eight normal subjects demonstrated no interaction in man, even when taking high doses (975 mg three times a day).[1] This finding is in line with common experience.

Reference

1 Fenster PE, Comess KA, Hanson CD and Finley PR. Kinetics of digoxin-aspirin combination. Clin Pharmacol Ther (1982) 32, 428–30.

Digitalis glycosides + Azaproprazone

Abstract/Summary

Azapropazone appears not to interact with digitoxin in most patients, but the occasional patient may possibly show a small rise in serum levels. The importance of this is uncertain.

Clinical evidence, mechanism, importance and management

A cross-over study[1] in eight arthritic patients showed that 900 mg azapropazone daily did not significantly alter the mean half-life of a single intravenous dose of digitoxin or the area under the plasma concentration/time curves, although two patients showed individual half-life increases of almost a third and a half. This suggests that concurrent use is normally likely to be uneventful, but the possibility of an interaction in the occasional patient cannot be dismissed. Information about digoxin appears to be lacking.

Reference

1 Faust-Tinnefeldt G and Gilfrich HJ. Digitoxin-Kinetik und der antirheumatischer Therapie mit Azapropazon. Arzneim-Forsch./Drug Res (1977) 27, 2009.

Digitalis glycosides + Barbiturates

Abstract/Summary

Blood levels of digitoxin can be halved by the concurrent use of phenobarbitone, and its effects may be expected to be reduced accordingly.

Clinical evidence

A study in patients taking digitoxin (0.1 mg daily) showed that when concurrently treated with 180 mg phenobarbitone daily for 12 weeks their steady-state serum digitoxin levels fell by 50%. In associated studies the half-life of digitoxin decreased from eight to five days during phenobarbitone treatment.[1,2]

In another study[1] the rate of conversion of digitoxin to digoxin in one patient increased from 4% to 27% while taking 96 mg phenobarbitone daily for 13 days. In contrast,[4] a study in 10 normal subjects given digitoxin (0.4 mg), digoxin (1 mg) or acetyldigitoxin (0.8 mg) daily failed to find changes in the serum concentrations of any of these glycosides while concurrently taking 100 mg phenobarbitone daily for 7–9 days.

Mechanism

Phenobarbitone and other barbiturates are well known as potent liver enzyme inducing agents which, it would seem, increase the metabolism and conversion of digitoxin to digoxin.[1,2,3] The failure of one study[4] to demonstrate this interaction may possibly have been because the barbiturate was taken for a relatively short time.

Importance and management

An established interaction, although its clinical importance is somewhat uncertain because there seem to be few reports of the effects of concurrent use or of problems in practice. Nevertheless, patients taking both drugs should be monitored for expected underdigitalization and the dosage of digitoxin increased if necessary. The result of this interaction is an increase in the levels of digoxin, but as its duration of action is considerably shorter than digitoxin, a much larger dose is needed to achieve the same degree of digitalization. Thus an increased conversion of digitoxin to digoxin means a reduction in the total activity of the two glycosides. It seems likely that digoxin itself will not be affected by the barbiturates because it is largely excreted unchanged in the urine. Other barbiturates would be expected to behave like phenobarbitone.

References

1 Jelliffe RW and Blankenhorn DH. Effect of phenobarbital on digitoxin metabolism. Clin Res (1966) 14, 160.
2 Solomon HM, Reich S, Gaul Z, Pocelinko R and Abrams WB. Induction of the metabolism of digitoxin in man by phenobarbital. Clin Res (1971) 19, 356.
3 Solomon HM and Abrams WB. Interactions between digitoxin and other drugs in man. Amer Heart J (1972) 83, 277.
4 Kaldor A, Somogyi GY, Debreczeni LA and Gachalyi B. Interaction of heart glycosides and phenobarbital. Int J Clin Pharmacol (1975) 12, 403.

Digitalis glycosides + Benoxaprofen

Abstract/Summary

Benoxaprofen does not interact with digoxin

Clinical evidence, mechanism, importance and management

A study[1] in 12 patients with rheumatic disease showed that over a four-week period the concurrent use of benoxaprofen, 600 mg daily, had no effect on their serum digoxin levels. Benoxaprofen has been withdrawn from general use in most countries because of its adverse side effects.

Reference

1 Zoller B, Engel HJ, Faust-Tinnefeldt G, Geissler HE, Gilfrich HJ and Zimmer M. An interaction study between benoxaprofen and digoxin. Eur J Rheumatol Inflamm (1982) 5, 82–6.

Digitalis glycosides + Benzodiazepines

Abstract/Summary

An isolated case report describes digoxin intoxication in a patient when given alprazolam but a later trial in normal subjects found no significant changes in the loss of digoxin from the body while on alprazolam. A reduction in the urinary clearance of digoxin has been described during the use of diazepam.

Clinical Evidence

An elderly woman on maprotiline, isosorbide dinitrate, frusemide, potassium chloride and digoxin, and with a serum digoxin concentration of 1.6–1.8 ng/ml, was additionally given 1 mg alprazolam daily. During the second week she began to demonstrate signs of digitalis intoxication and on admission to hospital her serum digoxin levels were found to have risen by about 300% (to 4.3 ng/ml). The apparent oral clearance had fallen from 126.3 to 49.8 l/day[1].

However a two-way crossover study in eight normal subjects found no changes in the clearance of digoxin while taking 1.5 mg alprazolam daily.[3] The observation[2] that three patients showed raised digoxin levels while taking diazepam prompted a further study in seven normal subjects. After taking 5 mg diazepam with a single 0.5 mg dose of digoxin, and another 5 mg diazepam 12 h later, all of them were said to have a 'substantial reduction in urinary excretion' and five of them showed a 'modest increase in the digoxin half-life'. No further details were given.[2]

Mechanism

Uncertain. The suggestion is that diazepam may possibly alter the extent of the protein binding of digoxin within the plasma, which may have some influence on the renal tubular excretion.[2] The reason for the digoxin–alprazolam interaction in the patient described is not understood.

Importance and management

The adverse interaction cited above is an isolated report and it was not confirmed by a later study. Both digoxin and the benzodiazepines have been used for a very considerable time and these reports appear to be among the few on record. There would therefore seem to be no good reason for avoiding concurrent use but the effects should be monitored. More study is needed.

References

1 Tollefson G, Lesar T, Grothe D and Garvey M. Alprazolam-related digoxin toxicity. Am J Psychiatry (1984) 141, 1612–14.
2 Castillo-Ferrando JR, Garcia M and Carmona J. Digoxin levels and diazepam. Lancet (1980) ii, 368.
3 Ochs HR, Greenblatt DJ and Verburg-Ochs B. Effect of alprazolam on digoxin kinetics and creatinine clearance. Clin Pharmacol Ther (1985) 38, 595–8.

Digitalis glycosides + Beta-blockers

Abstract/Summary

Concurrent use is common but controversial. Excessive and potentially fatal bradycardia can occur if beta-blockers are used to control digitalis-induced arrhythmias unless appropriate precautions are taken.

Clinical evidence, mechanism, importance and management

Digitalis glycosides and beta-blockers are commonly used together, but such use is controversial. Some claim that it is beneficial[2] whereas others say that it is not.[1]

Cardiac arrhythmias and cardiac flutter which can occur in digitalis intoxication can be controlled with propranolol, but under these circumstances patients appear to be particularly sensitive to the actions of propranolol and show marked bradycardia.[3] There have been fatalities. It has been suggested that if propranolol is used in this situation, it would be wise to give the patient a test dose of 5 mg or less before giving the full dose, or to combine the full dose with a protective dose of atropine.[4] Atropine can be used in this way because it blocks the normal parasympathetic (heart slowing) activity which, if not adequately balanced by sympathetic (heart accelerating) activity, results in further bradycardia. The pharmacokinetics of digoxin has been shown to be unaffected by the concurrent use of acebutolol[5] or esmolol.[6] The pharmacodynamics of digoxin are also unaffected by esmolol and no significant changes in heart rate or blood pressure occur.[6,7]

References

1 O'Reilly M, Goldberg E and Chaithiraphan S. Propranolol and digitalis. Lancet (1974) i, 138.
2 Crawford MH, LeWinter M, Karliner JS and O'Rourke RA. Propranolol and digitalis. Lancet (1974) i, 458.
3 Turner JRB. Propranolol in the treatment of digitalis-induced and digitalis resistant tachycardias. Amer J Cardiol (1966) 18, 450.
4 Watt DAL. Sensitivity to propranolol after digoxin intoxication. Br J Med (1968) 3, 413.
5 Ryan JR. Clinical pharmacology of acebutolol. Am Heart J (1985) 109, 1131–6.
6 Lowenthal DT, Porter RS, Conry K, Bies C, Laddu A, Turlapaty P and Hulse JD. Digoxin-esmolol drug interaction. Clin Pharmacol Ther (1985) 37, 209.
7 Lowenthal DT, Porter RS, Achari R, Turlapaty P, Laddu AR and Matier WL. Esmolol-digoxin drug interaction. J Clin Pharmacol (1987) 27, 561–6.

Digitalis glycosides + Calcium channel blockers

Abstract/Summary

Concurrent use can be valuable, but tiapamil may cause an approximately 50% and bepridil a 33% rise in serum digoxin levels which may possibly cause toxicity if the digoxin dosage is not reduced. Gallopamil, nicardipine and nisoldipine cause a small but normally clinically unimportant increase (about 15%), whereas amlodipine, felodipine, isradipine and nimodipine appear not to affect serum digoxin levels. The situation with nitrendipine is uncertain but it possibly only causes a small rise. The interactions of digoxin with diltiazem, nifedipine and verapamil are dealt with individually elsewhere.

Clinical evidence

(a) Digoxin + amlodipine

A study in 21 normal subjects showed that over a 14 day period while receiving digoxin (0.375 mg daily) the concurrent use of amlodipine (5 mg daily) had no significant effect on serum digoxin levels nor on its renal clearance.[6,17]

(b) Digoxin + bepridil

A study[1] in 12 normal subjects taking 0.375 mg digoxin daily, showed that the concurrent use of 300 mg bepridil daily for a week raised serum digoxin levels by 34% (from 0.93 to 1.25 ng/ml).[1] Five of the subjects experienced mild headache, nausea and dizziness for 1–3 days shortly after concurrent use started. The heart-slowing effects of the two were found to be additive, while the negative inotropic effects of the bepridil and the positive inotropism of the increased serum digoxin levels were almost balanced.[7,8]

In another study 23 subjects were given 0.25 mg digoxin and 300 mg bepridil daily for 14 days. Peak serum digoxin levels rose by 48% (from 1.49 to 2.2 ng/ml) and the AUC rose by 21% (from 18.7 to 22.6 ng/h/ml).[9]

(c) Digoxin + gallopamil

A study in 12 normal subjects on 0.375 mg digoxin daily showed that while taking 150 mg gallopamil daily for two weeks their serum digoxin levels rose by 16% (from 0.57 to 0.67 ng/ml).[10]

(d) Digoxin + felodipine

A trial in 14 patients with congestive heart failure with steady-state serum digoxin levels showed that these were not significantly changed by the concurrent use of 10 mg felodipine daily for a week, either as a plain or slow-release tablet formulation.[13]

(e) Digoxin + isradipine

A study in 24 normal subjects showed that isradipine (5–15 mg daily) for 10 days did not interact significantly with digoxin given as an intravenous infusion.[5] Another study in 19 normal subjects showed that isradipine (15 mg daily) for seven days had no significant effect on the absorption or on the steady-state serum levels of digoxin.[15]

(f) Digoxin + nicardipine

A study[11] in 10 patients on digoxin (0.13–0.25 mg daily) showed that the concurrent use of nicardipine (20 mg three times a day) for 14 days increased the mean serum digoxin levels by about 15%, but the increase was said not to be statistically significant.

(g) Digoxin + nimodipine

A study in 12 normal subjects found that 30 mg nisoldipine twice daily caused no change in the pharmacokinetics or haemodynamic effects of digoxin.[16]

(h) Digoxin + nisoldipine

A double blind study in 10 patients with heart failure treated with digoxin showed that the concurrent use of 20 mg nisoldipine daily increased serum trough digoxin levels by about 15%.[4,12,14]

A study in eight normal subjects found that 10 mg nisoldipine twice daily caused no change in the pharmacokinetics or haemodynamic effects of digoxin.[16]

(i) Digoxin + nitrendipine

A study in eight normal subjects who had been taking 0.5 mg digoxin daily for two weeks showed that the concurrent use of 10 mg nitrendipine daily caused a slight but insignificant rise in plasma digoxin levels. 20 mg nitrendipine daily increased the digoxin AUC (area under the curve) by 15% (from 9.7 to 11.2 ng/ml) and maximum plasma digoxin levels rose from 1.34 to 2.10 ng/ml. Clearance fell by 13% (from 315.1 to 274.5 ml/min). One subject dropped out of the study because of dizziness, nausea, palpitation, insomnia and nervousness.[1–3]

Another study found that plasma digoxin levels were approximately doubled when nitrendipine was given,[12] but two others in 12 normal subjects and eight patients found that 20 mg nisoldipine twice daily caused no change in the pharmacokinetics or haemodynamic effects of digoxin.[16,18]

(j) Digoxin + tiapamil

Eight patients on digoxin who were given tiapamil (200 mg three times a day) for 14 days showed an approximately mean 50% rise in serum digoxin levels. No signs of digitalis toxicity occurred.[11]

Mechanism

Where an interaction occurs it is probably due to changes in the renal excretion of the digoxin.

Importance and management

Information about the effects of using digoxin and these calcium channel blockers together is limited. Concurrent use can be therapeutically valuable but what is known indicates that the effects of bepridil or tiapamil should be monitored to ensure that digoxin serum levels do not rise excessively. Reduce the digoxin dosage as necessary. The other calcium channel blockers listed here (gallopamil, nicardipine, nisoldipine) either cause only minimal increases which are unlikely to be clinically important in most patients or do not interact at all (amlodipine, felodipine, isradipine, nimodipine). The situation with nitrendipine needs clarification. The interactions of digoxin with diltiazem, nifedipine and verapamil are detailed in individual synopses.

References

1 Kirch W, Logemann C, Heidemann H, Santos SR and Ohnhaus EE. Effect of two different doses of nitrendipine on steady-state plasma digoxin levels and systolic time intervals. Eur J Clin Pharmacol (1986) 31, 391–5.
2 Kirch W, Logemann C, Santos SR and Ohnhaus EE. Influence of different doses of nitrendipine on digoxin plasma concentrations. Br J clin Pharmacol (1986) 23, 111–2P.
3 Kirch W, Logemann C, Santos SR and Ohnhaus EE. Nitrendipine increases digoxin plasma levels dose dependently. J Clin Pharmacol (1986) 26, 553.
4 Kirch W, Stenzel J, Dylewicz P, Hutt HJ, Santos SR and Ohnhaus EE. Influence of nisoldipine on haemodynamic effects and plasma levels of digoxin. Br J clin Pharmac (1986) 22, 155–9.
5 Johnson BF, Wilson J, Marwaha R, Hoch K and Johnson J. The comparative effects of verapamil and a new dihydropyridine calcium channel blocker on digoxin pharmacokinetics. Clin Pharmacol Ther (1987) 42, 66–7.
6 Schwartz JB. Amlodipine does not affect serum digoxin concentrations or renal clearance. Clin Res (1987) 35, 380A.
7 Belz GG, Wistuba S and Matthews JH. Digoxin and bepridil: pharmacokinetic and pharmacodynamic interactions. Clin Pharmacol Ther (1986) 39, 65–71.
8 Fenzl E, Toburen D, Wistuba S, Stern HC and Belz GG. Pharmacodynamic interactions between digoxin and bepridil. J Mol Cell Cardiol (1984) 16, (Suppl 3, no. 12).
9 Doose DR, Wallen S, Nayak RK and Minn FL. Pharmacokinetic interaction of bepridil and digoxin in steady-state. Clin Pharmacol Ther (1987) 42, 204.
10 Belz GG, Doering W, Munkes R and Matthews J. Interaction between digoxin and calcium antagonists and antiarrhythmic drugs. Clin Pharmacol Ther (1983) 33, 410–17.
11 Lessem J and Bellinetto A. Interaction between digoxin and the calcium antagonists nicardipine and tiapamil. Clin Therapeutics (1983) 5, 595–602.
12 Kirsch W, Hutt HJ, Heidemann H, Ramsch K, Janisch HD and Ohnhaus EE. Drug interactions with nitrendipine. J Cardiovasc Pharmacol (1984) 6, S982–5.
13 Kirsch W, Laskowski M and Ohnhaus EE. The felodipine/digoxin interaction. A placebo-controlled study in patients with heart failure. Br J clin Pharmac (1988) 26, 644P.
14 Kirsch W, Stenzel J, Santos SR and Ohnhaus EE. Nisolidipine, a new calcium channel antagonist, elevates plasma levels of digoxin. Arch Toxicol (1987) Suppl, 11, 310–12.
15 Rodin SM, Johnson BF, Wilson J, Ritchie P and Johnson J. Comparative effects of verapamil and isradipine on steady-state digoxin levels. Clin Pharmacol Ther (1988) 43, 668–72.
16 Ziegler R, Horstmann R, Wingender W, Kuhlmann J. Do dihydropyridines influence pharmacokinetic and hemodynamic parameters of digoxin? J Clin Pharmacol (1987) 27, 712.
17 Schwartz JB. Effects of amlodipine on steady-state digoxin concentrations and renal digoxin clearance. J Cardiovasc Pharmacol (1988) 12, 1–5.
18 Debbas NMG, Johnston A, Jackson SHD, Banim SO, Camm AJ, Turner P. The effect of nitrendipine on predose digoxin serum concentration. Br J clin Pharmac (1988) 19, 151P.

Digitalis glycosides + Calcium preparations

Abstract/Summary

The effects of digitalis can be increased by increases in blood calcium levels, and the administration of intravenous calcium may result in the development of potentially life-threatening digitalis-induced heart arrhythmias.

Clinical evidence

Two patients developed heart arrhythmias and died after being given digitalis intramuscularly and either calcium chloride or gluconate intravenously. No absolutely certain causative relationship was established.[1]

There is other evidence that increases or decreases in blood calcium levels can increase or decrease respectively the effects of digitalis. A patient with congestive heart failure and atrial fibrillation was resistant to the actions of digoxin in the usual therapeutic range (1.5–3.0 ng/ml) until his serum calcium levels were raised from 6.7 to about 8.5 mg% by the administration of calcium and oral vitamin D.[2] Disodium edetate[3–5] and sodium and potassium citrate,[6] which lower ionic blood calcium levels, have been used successfully in the treatment of digitalis intoxication.

Mechanism

The actions of the cardiac glycosides (even now not fully understood) are closely tied up with movement of calcium ions into heart muscle cells. Increased concentrations of calcium outside these cells increase the inflow of calcium and this enhances the activity of the glycosides. This can lead to effective over-digitalization and even potentially life-threatening arrhythmias.

Importance and management

The report cited[1] (published in 1936) seems to be the only direct clinical evidence of a serious adverse interaction, although there is plenty of less direct evidence that an interaction is possible. Intravenous calcium should be avoided in patients on cardiac glycosides. If that is not possible, it has been suggested[7] that it should be given slowly or only in small amounts in order to avoid transient serum calcium levels higher than 15 mEq/l.

References

1 Bower JO and Mengle HAK. The additive effects of calcium and digitalis. A warning with a report of two deaths. J Amer Med Ass (1936) 106, 1151.
2 Chopra D, Janson P and Sawin CT. Insensitivity to digoxin associated with hypocalcaemia. N Engl J Med (1977) 296, 917.
3 Jick S and Karsh R. The effect of calcium chelation on cardiac arrhythmias and conduction disturbances. Amer J Cardiol (1959) 43, 287.
4 Szekely P and Wynne NA. Effects of calcium chelation on digitalis induced cardiac arrhythmias. Br Heart J (1963) 25, 589.
5 Rosenbaum JL, Mason D and Seven M. The effect of disodium EDTA on digitalis intoxication. Amer J Med Sci (1960) 240, 77.
6 Barbieri FF, Gold H, Lang TW, Bernstein H and Corday E. Sodium and potassium citrate salts for the treatment of digitalis toxicity. Amer J Cardiol (1964) 14, 650.
7 Nola GT, Pope S and Harrison DC. Assessment of the synergistic relationship between serum calcium and digitalis. Amer Heart J (1970) 79, 499.

Digitalis glycosides + Carbamazepine

Abstract/Summary

One report attributes an increase in digitalis-induced bradycardia to the use of carbamazepine.

Clinical evidence, importance and management

Bradycardia seen in patients on digitalis and carbamazepine was tentatively attributed to their concurrent use[1], but as yet this has not been confirmed by other observations. No special precautions seem to be necessary.

Reference

1 Killian JM and Fromm GH. Carbamazepine in the treatment of neuralgia. Use and side-effects. Arch Neurol (1968) 19, 129.

Digitalis glycosides + Carbenoxolone

Abstract/Summary

Carbenoxolone can raise blood pressure, cause fluid retention and reduce serum potassium levels. It is generally regarded as contraindicated in those using digitalis for congestive heart failure.

Clinical evidence, mechanism, importance and management

The side-effects of carbenoxolone treatment include an increase in blood pressure (both systolic and diastolic), fluid retention and reduced serum potassium levels. The incidence of these side-effects is said in some reports to be as high as 50%. Others quote lower figures, nevertheless it is clear that they are not an uncommon occurrence. Hypertension and fluid retention occur early in carbenoxolone treatment, whereas the hypokalaemia develops later and may occur in the absence of the other two side-effects.[1–4] The hypokalaemia may be exacerbated if thiazide diuretics are used to control the fluid retention without the use of suitable potassium supplements. For example, severe hypokalaemia has been described in a patient taking carbenoxolone and chlorthalidone without potassium supplementation.[5] For all these reasons carbenoxolone is unsuitable for patients with congestive heart failure who are taking digitalis glycosides.

References

1 Geismar P, Mosebech J and Myren J. A double-blind study of the effect of carbenoxolone sodium in the treatment of gastric ulcer. Scand J Gastroenterol (1973) 8, 251.
2 Turpie AGG and Thomson TJ. Carbenoxolone sodium in the treatment of gastric ulcer with special reference to side-effects. Gut (1965) 6, 591.
3 Langman MJS, Knapp DR and Wakley E. Treatment of chronic gastric ulcer with carbenoxolone and gefarnate; a comparative trial. Br Med J (1973) 3, 84.
4 Davis GJ, Rhodes J and Calcraft BJ. Complications of carbenoxolone therapy (1974) 3, 400.
5 Descamps C. Rhabdomycosis and acute tubular necrosis associated with carbenoxolone and diuretic treatment. Br Med J (1977) 1, 272.

Digitalis glycosides + Cholestyramine

Abstract/Summary

The blood levels of both digoxin and digitoxin can be reduced by the concurrent use of cholestyramine, but the clinical importance of this is uncertain. Minimize the possible effects of this interaction by giving the cholestyramine not less than one-and-a-half hours after the cardiac glycoside.

Clinical evidence

(a) Digitalis glycoside serum levels unaffected

10 patients on long-term treatment with either digoxin (0.125–0.25 mg daily) or digitoxin (0.1–0.2 mg daily) were concurrently treated for a year with 12 g cholestyramine or a placebo taken 1.5 h after the digitalis. Their serum digitalis levels were not significantly altered by the cholestyramine.[6]

The half-life of digitoxin is reported to have remained unchanged when cholestyramine was used.[10]

(b) Digitalis glycoside serum levels reduced

A study carried out with 12 subjects given 0.75 mg digoxin showed that the cumulative six-day recovery of the digoxin from the urine was reduced almost 20% (from 40.5 to 33.1%) when 4 g cholestyramine was given concurrently.[1]

Other reports describe a fall in serum digoxin levels during the concurrent use of cholestyramine[2,9,11] and an increase in the loss of digoxin and its metabolites in the faeces during concurrent long-term use.[3] A reduction by cholestyramine of the half-life of digitoxin of 35 to 40% has been described.[4,5,8]

Mechanism

Not totally understood. Cholestyramine appears to bind with digitoxin in the gut, thereby reducing its bioavailability and interfering with the enterohepatic cycle so that its half-life is shortened. Just how digoxin interacts is uncertain.[3]

Importance and management

The overall picture is far from clear. Some interaction seems possible but the extent to which it impairs the treatment of patients on these glycosides is uncertain. Be alert for any evidence of under-digitalization if digoxin or more particularly digitoxin are given with cholestyramine. Give the cholestyramine not less than 1.5–2 h after the digitalis to minimize the possibility of an interaction.[6] An alternative is to use beta-methyldigoxin which one study suggests may be minimally affected by cholestyramine.[7] Another study showed that giving digoxin as a solution in a capsule also reduced the effects of this interaction.[11]

References

1 Brown DD, Juhl RP and Warner SL. Decreased bioavailability of digoxin produced by dietary fibre and cholestyramine. Amer J Cardiol (1977) 39, 297.
2 Smith TW. New approaches to the management of digitalis intoxication. In 'Symposium on Digitalis' Glydendal Norsk Forlag, Oslo (1977) 39, 312.
3 Hall WH, Shappell SD and Doherty JE. Effect of cholestyramine on digoxin absorption and excretion in man. Amer J Cardiol (1977) 39, 213.
4 Caldwell JH and Greenberger NJ. Cholestyramine enhances digitalis excretion and protects against lethal intoxication. Clin Invest (1970) 49, 16a.
5 Caldwell JH, Bush CA and Greenberger NJ. Interruption of the enterohepatic circulation of digitoxin by cholestyramine. J Clin Invest (1971) 50, 2638.
6 Bazzano G and Bazzano GS. Effects of digitalis binding resins on cardiac glycoside plasma levels. Clin Res (1972) 20, 24.
7 Hahn K-J and Weber E. Effect of cholestyramine on absorption of drugs. In 'Frontiers of Internal Medicine' 12th Int Cong Int Med, Tel Aviv 1974. Karger, Basel (1975) p. 409.
8 Carruthers SG and Dujovne CA. Cholestyramine and spironolactone and their combination in digitoxin elimination. Clin Pharmacol Ther (1980) 27, 184.
9 Brown DD, Juhl RP and Warner SL. Decreased bioavailability of digoxin due to hypocholesterolemic interventions. Circulation (1978) 58, 164.
10 Pabst J, Leopold D, Schad W and Meub R. Bioavailability of digitoxin during chronic administration and influence of food and cholestyramine on the bioavailability after a single dose. Nauyenschmiedbergs Arch Pharmacol (1979) 307, R70.
11 Brown DD, Schmidt J, Long RA and Hull JH. A steady-state evaluation of the effects of propanthenline bromide and cholestyramine on the bioavailability of digoxin when administered as tablets or capsules. J Clin Pharmacol (1985) 25, 360–4.

Digitalis glycosides + Cibenzolone

Abstract/Summary

Cibenzoline does not interact with digoxin.

Clinical evidence, mechanism, importance and management

A study in 12 normal subjects taking 0.25–0.375 mg digoxin daily showed that the concurrent use of 160 mg cibenzoline twice daily for seven days had no effect on the pharmacokinetics of the digoxin.[1]

Reference

1 Khoo K-c, Givens SV, Parsonnet M and Massarella JW. Effect of oral cibenzoline on steady-state concentrations in healthy volunteers. J Clin Pharmacol (1988) 28, 29–35.

Digitalis glycosides + Cicletanine

Abstract/Summary

Cicletanine appears not to affect serum digoxin levels.

Clinical evidence, mechanism, importance and management

Single 50 mg and 100 mg doses of cicletanine were found to have no effect on the serum digoxin levels of six patients stabilized on long term treatment (0.125–0.25 mg digoxin daily).[1] This absence of an interaction needs further confirmation.

Reference

1 Clement DL, Teirlynck O and Belpaire F. Lack of effect of cicletanine on plasma digoxin levels. Int J Clin Pharm Res (1988) VIII, 9–11.

Digitalis glycosides + Cimetidine

Abstract/Summary

Changes in serum digoxin levels, both rises and falls, have been seen in patients given cimetidine, but these do not appear to be of clinical importance.

Clinical evidence, mechanism, importance and management

A study[1] on 11 patients on digoxin for congestive heart failure showed that while taking 600–1200 mg cimetidine daily their steady-state serum digoxin levels fell on average by 25% (from 2.0 to 1.5 ng/ml), but none of them showed any ECG changes or signs that their condition had worsened.

Three single dose studies on 11 and eight normal subjects respectively and six patients with duodenal ulcers[5] showed that cimetidine (600–1200 mg) had no significant effect on the absorption[2] or the kinetics[3,5] of digoxin. Another study found a small increase in digoxin levels in normal subjects, but only a small statistically insignificant rise (0.02 ng/ml) in the steady-state levels of 11 patients given 1600 mg cimetidine daily.[4] No interaction of clinical importance has been established and no special precautions would seem to be necessary.

References

1 Fraley DS, Britton HL, Schwinghammer TL and Kalla R. Effect of cimetidine on steady-state serum digoxin concentrations. Clin Pharm (1983) 2, 163–5.
2 Ochs HR, Gugler R, Guthoff T and Greenblatt DJ. Effect of cimetidine on digoxin kinetics and creatinine clearance. Amer Heart J (1984) 107, 170–2.
3 Jordaens L, Hoegaerts J and Belpaire F. Non-interaction of cimetidine with digoxin absorption. Acta Clin Belg (1981) 36, 109.
4 Crome P, Curl B, Holt D, Volans GN, Bennett PN and Cole DS. Digoxin and cimetidine: investigation of the potential for a drug interaction. Human Toxicol (1985) 4, 391–9.
5 Garty M, Perry G, Shmueli H, Illfield D, Boner G, Pitlik S and Rosenfeld J. Effect of cimetidine on digoxin disposition in peptic ulcer patients. Eur J Clin Pharmacol (1986) 30, 489–91.

Digitalis glycosides + Cisapride

Abstract/Summary

Cisapride causes a small but probably clinically unimportant fall in the absorption of digoxin.

Clinical evidence, mechanism, importance and management

A study in six normal subjects taking 0.75–1.0 mg digoxin daily showed that the concurrent use of 10 mg cisapride three times a day reduced the digoxin AUC (area under the curve) and the peak serum concentrations by 12–13%.[1] This is probably too small normally to be of much if any clinical importance.

Reference

1 Kirsch W, Janisch HD, Santos SR, Duhrsen U, Dylewicz P and Ohnhaus EE. Effect of cisapride and metoclopramide on digoxin bioavailability. Eur J Drug Metab Pharmacokinet (1986) 11, 249–50.

Digitalis glycosides + Clovoxamine or Fluvoxamine

Abstract/Summary

Neither clovoxamine nor fluvoxamine appear to interact with digoxin.

Clinical evidence, mechanism, importance and management

A study in eight normal subjects found that after taking 150 mg clovoxamine or 100 mg fluvoxamine daily for 15 days, the pharmacokinetics (distribution, elimination or clearance) of a single intravenous dose of 1.25 mg digoxin were unchanged.[1] It seems unlikely therefore that either of these drugs will affect the steady-state serum levels of digoxin in patients, but this needs confirmation.

Reference

1 Ochs HR, Greenblatt DJ, Verburg-Ochs B and Labedski L. Chronic treatment with fluvoxamine, clovoxamine and placebo: interaction with digoxin and effects on sleep and alertness. J Clin Pharmacol (1989) 29, 91–95.

Digitalis glycosides + Colestipol

Abstract/Summary

Colestipol appears not to interfere with the absorption of either digoxin or digitoxin if it is given at least 1.5 h after the glycoside. It can be used to reduce serum digitoxin or digoxin levels if intoxication occurs.

Clinical evidence

(a) Digitoxin and digoxin levels reduced in intoxication

Four patients intoxicated with digitoxin were given 10 g colestipol at once and 5 g every 6–8 h to reduce their digitoxin serum levels. The average digitoxin half-life fell to 2.75 days compared with an untreated control patient in whom the digitoxin half-life was 9.3 days. Another patient intoxicated with digoxin was similarly treated. His digoxin half-life was 16 h compared with 1.8–2.0 days in two other control patients.[2]

(b) Digitoxin and digoxin levels unaffected

10 patients on long-term treatment with either digoxin (0.125–0.25 mg daily) or digitoxin (0.1–0.2 mg daily) were concurrently treated for a year with 15 g colestipol daily or a placebo, taken 1.5 h after the digitalis. Their serum digitalis levels were not significantly altered by the colestipol.[3]

A comparative study in 11 patients with serum digitoxin levels above the therapeutic range (> 40 ng/ml) showed that giving 5 g colestipol four times daily before meals and stopping the digitoxin immediately did not affect the digitoxin half-life (6.3 days) when compared with 11 other patients not given colestipol (6.8 days).[1]

Mechanism

Colestipol is an ion-exchange resin which can bind to digitalis glycosides.[2] It can apparently interfere with the enterohepatic circulation and increase the loss during intoxication.

Importance and management

This interaction is neither well established nor apparently of great clinical importance. Giving either digoxin or digitoxin followed by the colestipol at least 1.5 h later appears to avoid any possible interaction in the gut.[3] In cases of intoxication it may possibly reduce serum digitalis levels because under these circumstances the excretion of digitalis in the bile increases and more becomes available for binding in the gut.[3]

References

1 Van Bever RJ, Duchateau AMJ A, Pluym BFM and Merkus FWHM. The effect of colestipol on digitoxin serum levels. Arzneimittel Forsch (1976) 26, 1891–3.
2 Bazzano G and Bazzano GS. Digitalis intoxication. Treatment with a new steroid-binding resin. J Amer Med Ass (1972) 220, 828.
3 Bazzano G and Bazzano GS. Effect of digitalis-binding resins on cardiac glycosides plasma levels. Clin Res (1972) 20, 24.

Digitalis glycosides + Cyclosporin(e)

Abstract/Summary

A report describes kidney dysfunction and marked rises in serum digoxin levels in patients concurrently treated with cyclosporin.

Clinical evidence

Four patients on digoxin developed kidney dysfunction and elevated serum digoxin levels when given cyclosporin before receiving heart transplants. Two of them on 0.375 mg digoxin daily showed four-fold rises (from 1.5 to 5.7 nmol/l, and 2.6 to 10.6 nmol/l respectively) within 2–3 days of starting to take 400 mg cyclosporin twice daily. Marked rises in creatinine levels occurred (a reflection of kidney dysfunction). A subsequent study on four other patients given both drugs found that serum creatinine levels rose sharply and in two of them plasma digoxin clearances fell by 58 and 47%.[1] The apparent volume of distribution of the digoxin also decreased markedly.

Mechanism

Not understood.

Importance and management

Information seems to be limited to the study cited. If concurrent use is thought appropriate, the effects should be very closely monitored and the digoxin dosage should be substantially lowered if necessary.

Reference

1 Dorian P, Cardella C, Strauss M, David T, East S and Ogilvie R. Cyclosporine nephrotoxicity and cyclosporine-digoxin interaction prior to heart transplantation. Transplant Proc (1987) 19, 1825–7.

Digitalis glycosides + Cytotoxic (Antineoplastic) agents

Abstract/Summary

Treatment with radiation and/or cytotoxic agents can damage the lining of the intestine so that digoxin is much less readily absorbed when given in tablet form. This can be overcome by giving the digoxin in liquid or liquid-in-capsule form, or by substituting digitoxin.

Clinical evidence

A study[4] in 13 patients with various forms of neoplastic disease showed that radiation therapy and/or various high dose cytotoxic regimens (including carmustine (BCNU), cyclophosphamide, melphalan, cytarabine and methotrexate) reduced the absorption of digoxin from tablets (*Lanoxin*) by almost 46%, but the reduction was not significant (15%) when the digoxin was given in capsule form (*Lanoxicaps*).

Other studies in patients confirm a 50% reduction in serum digoxin levels (using beta-acetyldigoxin) while using drug regimens of cyclophosphamide, onconvin, procarbazine and prednisone (COPP); cyclophosphamide, onconvin and prednisone (COP); cyclophosphamide, onconvin, cytarabine and prednisone (COAP); and adriamycin, bleomycin and prednisone (ABP). These effects disappeared about a week after withdrawal.[2] Radiation has a smaller effect.[3] Digitoxin absorption is not affected.[5]

Mechanism

The reduced absorption is thought to result from damage to the intestinal epithelium caused by the cytotoxic agents.[1]

Importance and management

The interaction appears to be established. Patients on digoxin and receiving treatment with cytotoxic drugs should be monitored for signs of under-digitalization. The problem can be overcome by replacing digoxin tablets with digoxin in liquid form or in solution inside a capsule. The effects of the interaction are short-lived so that a downward readjustment may be necessary about a week after treatment is withdrawn. An alternative is to use digitoxin which is not affected.

References

1 Jusko WB, Conti DR, Molson A, Kuritzky P, Giller J and Schultz. Digoxin absorption from tablets and elixir: the effect of radiation-induced malabsorption. J Amer Med Ass (1974) 230, 1554–5
2 Kuhlmann J, Zilly W and Wilke J. Effects of cytostatic drugs on plasma levels and renal excretion of beta-acetyldigoxin. Clin Pharmacol Ther (1981) 30, 518–27.
3 Sokol GH, Greenblatt DJ, Lloyd BL, Georgotas A, Allen MD, Harmatz JS, Smith TW and Shader RI. Effect of abdominal radiation therapy on drug absorption in humans. J Clin Pharmacol (1978) 18, 388–96.
4 Bjornsson TD, Huang AT, Roth P, Jacob SS and Christenson R. Effects of high-dose cancer chemotherapy on the absorption of digoxin in two different formulations. Clin Pharmacol Ther (1986) 39, 25–8.
5 Kuhlmann J, Wilke J, and Rietbrock N. Cytostatic drugs are without significant effect on digitoxin plasma level and renal excretion. Clin Pharmacol Ther (1982) 32, 646–51.

Digitalis glycosides + Dietary fibre (bran) and Laxatives

Abstract/Summary

Large amounts of dietary fibre and neither of two bulk-forming laxatives containing isphagula (psyllium) appear to have a significant effect on the absorption of digoxin from the gut.

Clinical evidence

(a) Digoxin + fibre (bran)

A study on 12 patients on digoxin (0.125–0.25 mg daily taken 15–30 min before breakfast) showed that over a 10-day period, while on a diet supplemented each day with 22 g dietary fibre, their serum digoxin levels were not changed. The fibre was given in this way to simulate the conditions which might be encountered clinically, for example to reduce the symptoms of diverticular disease.[1]

Another study in 16 geriatric patients showed that 7.5 g wheat bran twice daily caused a small reduction (10%) in serum digoxin levels after two weeks, but no significant change after four weeks.[7] A study in 16 normal subjects found that 11 g bran fibre caused a 6–7% reduction in the absorption and the steady-state serum levels of digoxin.[9] Two single dose studies in normal subjects showed that the cumulative urinary recovery of an oral dose of digoxin was reduced almost 20% by 5 g and 15 g fibre respectively, whereas a normal amount of fibre (0.75 g) had no effect.[2,3]

(b) Digoxin + bulk laxatives

A study in 16 geriatric patients on digoxin showed that an ispaghula formulation (*Vi-Siblin S*) had no significant effect on serum digoxin levels.[7]

The same lack of effect was seen in another study in 15 patients given 3.6 g psyllium (*Metamucil*) three times a day.[8]

Mechanism

Not established. Digoxin can bind to some extent to fibre within the gut[5] and *in vitro* studies show that the cellulose component is probably responsible.[4] However other *in vitro* studies (with bran, pectin, sodium pectinate, xylan and carboxymethylcellulose) have shown that most of the binding is reversible.[6]

Importance and management

Information seems to be limited to the reports cited. Neither dietary fibre (bran) nor the two bulk-forming laxatives (*Vi-Siblin, Metamucil*) have a clinically important effect on serum digoxin levels. No special precautions would appear to be necessary.

References

1 Woods MN and Ingelfinger JA. Lack of effect of bran on digoxin absorption. Clin Pharmacol Ther (1979) 26, 21.

2 Brown DD, Juhl RP and Warner SL. Decreased bioavailability of digoxin produced by dietary fibre and cholestyramine. Amer J Cardiol (1977) 39, 297.

3 Brown DD, Juhl RP and Warner SL. Decreased bioavailability of digoxin due to hypocholesterolemic interventions. Circulation (1978) 78, 164.

4 Spector R, Vernick R and Lorenzo AV. Effects of pressure on the plasma binding of digoxin and ouabain in an ultrafiltration apparatus. Biochem Pharmacol (1973) 22, 2485.

5 Floyd RA, Greenberg WM and Caldwell C. *In vitro* interaction between digoxin and bran. Presented at the 12th Annual ASHP Midyear Clinical Meeting, Atlanta, Georgia, December 1977.

6 Hamamura J, Burros BC, Clemens RA and Smith CH. Dietary fiber and digoxin. Fed Proc (1985) 44, 759.

7 Nordstrom M, Melander A, Robertsson E and Steen B. Influence of wheat bran and of a bulk-forming isphaghula cathartic on the bioavailability of digoxin in geriatric in-patients. Drug-Nutrient Interactions (1987) 5, 67–9.

8 Walan A, Bergdahl B and Skoog M-L. Study of digoxin bioavailability during treatment with a bulk forming laxative (*Metamucil*). Scand J Gastroenterol (1977) 12 (Suppl) 45, 111.

9 Johnson BF, Rodin SM, Hoch K and Shekar V. The effect of dietary fiber on the bioavailability of digoxin in capsules. J Clin Pharmacol (1987) 27, 487–90.

Digitalis glycosides + Diltiazem

Abstract/Summary

Serum digoxin levels are reported in a number of studies to be unchanged by the concurrent use of diltiazem, but others describe increases ranging from 20 to 85%. An approximately 20% rise in serum digitoxin levels has also been described.

Clinical evidence

(a) Digoxin

(i) Evidence of no interaction

A study in nine patients treated chronically for heart disease with digoxin (0.25 mg daily) showed that the concurrent use of 120 or 240 mg diltiazem daily had no significant effect on serum digoxin levels.[1]

Other studies in 12 patients,[3] and nine, five, seven and eight normal subjects[2,7,8,13,14] given 120–360 mg diltiazem daily confirm the absence of an interaction.

(ii) Evidence of an interaction

A study in 17 Japanese patients, some with rheumatic valvular disease, and taking either digoxin or medigoxin showed that the concurrent use of 180 mg diltiazem daily for two weeks increased their serum digoxin levels measured at 24 h by 36 and 51% respectively.[6]

Other studies in European and American patients have shown rises of 20–85% in plasma digoxin levels while taking diltiazem concurrently.[4,9,10,12,15–17]

(b) Digitoxin

Five out of 10 patients on digitoxin showed a 6–31% (mean 21%) rise in serum digitoxin levels while taking 180 mg diltiazem daily for 4–6 weeks.[11]

Mechanism

Uncertain. Falls in total digoxin clearance of about 25% have been described.[5,10]

Importance and management

The effects of the concurrent use of digoxin and diltiazem have been thoroughly investigated, but there is no clear explanation for the inconsistent results. All patients on digoxin given diltiazem should be well monitored for signs of over-digitalization and dosage reductions should be made if necessary. Those most at risk are patients with digoxin levels near the top end of the range. Similar precautions would appear to be necessary with digitoxin, although the documentation of this interaction is very limited.

References

1 Elkayam U, Parikh K, Torkan B, Weber L, Cohen JL and Rahimtoola SH. Effect of diltiazem on renal clearance and serum concentration of digoxin in patients with cardiac disease. Am J Cardiol (1985) 55, 1393–5.
2 Boden WE, More G, Sharma S, Bough EW, Korr KS and Shulman RS, Does high-dose diltiazem increase serum digoxin levels? J Am Coll Cardiol (1985) 5, 419.
3 Schrager BR, Pina I, Frangi M, Applewhite S, Sequeira R and Chahine RA. Diltiazem, digoxin interaction? Circulation (1983) 68, Suppl III-368.
4 Gallet M, Aupetit JF, Manchon M, Manchon J, Lopez M and Leizorovicz A. Effet du diltiazem sur la concentration serique de digoxine. La Presse Med (1984) 13, 2455–6.
5 Yoshida A, Fujita M, Kurosawa N, Nioka M, Shichinohe T, Asrakawa M, Fukuda R, Owada E and Ito K. Effects of diltiazem on plasma level and urinary excretion of digoxin in healthy subjects. Clin Pharmacol Ther (1984) 35, 681–5.
6 Oyama Y, Fujii S, Kanda K, Akino E, Kawasaki H, Nagata M and Goto K. Digoxin-diltiazem interaction. Am J Cardiol (1984) 53, 1480–1.
7 Beltrami TR, May JJ and Bertino JS. Lack of effects of diltiazem on digoxin pharmacokinetics. J Clin Pharmacol (1985) 25, 390–392.
8 Young PM, Boden WE, and More G. Lack of effect of high dose diltiazem on serum digoxin levels. Clin Pharmacol Ther (1985) 37, 239.
9 Kuhlmann J St M and Frank KH. Effects of nifedipine and diltiazem on the pharmacokinetics of digoxin. Naunyn-Schmiedberg Arch Pharmacol (1983) 324 (Suppl) R81.
10 Rameis H, Magometschnigg D and Ganzinger U. The diltiazem-digoxin interaction. Clin Pharmacol Ther (1984) 36, 183–9.
11 Kuhlmann J. Effects of verapamil, diltiazem, and nifedipine on plasma levels and renal excretion of digitoxin. Clin Pharmacol Ther (1985) 38, 667–73.
12 North DS, Mattern AL and Hiser WW. The influence of diltiazem hydrochloride on trough serum digoxin levels. Drug Intell Clin Pharm (1986) 20, 500–3.
13 Boden WE, More G, Sharma S, Bough EW, Korr KS, Young PM and Shulman RS. No increase in serum digoxin concentrations with high dose diltiazem. Am J Med (1986) 81, 425–8.
14 Jones WN, Kern KB, Rindone JP, Mayersohn M, Bliss M and Goldman S. Digoxin-diltiazem interaction: a pharmacokinetic evaluation. Eur J Clin Pharmacol (1986) 31, 351–3.
15 Gallet M, Aupetit JF, Lopez M, Manchon J, Lestaevel M and Lefrancois JJ. Interaction diltiazem-digoxine. Evolution de la digoxinemie et de parametres electocardiographique chez le sujet sain. Arch Mal Coeur (1986) 79, 1216–20.
16 Andrejak M, Hary L, Andrjak M-Th and Lesbre J Ph. Diltiazem increases steady state digoxin serum levels in patients with cardiac disease. J Clin Pharmacol (1987) 27, 967–70.
17 Larman RC. A pharmacokinetic evaluation of the digoxin-diltiazem interaction. J Pharm Sci (1987) 76, S79.

Digitalis glycosides + Disopyramide or Procainamide

Abstract/Summary

Neither disopyramide nor procainamide cause a significant change in serum digoxin levels.

Clinical evidence, mechanism, importance and management

(a) Disopyramide

A number of studies have clearly shown that disopyramide causes only a very small increase or no increase at all in the serum concentrations of digoxin.[1–5,7] A small but insignificant reduction in systolic time intervals has been seen[6] but the weight of evidence suggests that no adverse interaction occurs if these drugs are used together.

(b) Procainamide

A study in 26 patients who had been taking digoxin for at least seven days showed that while taking procainamide the serum digoxin levels remained unaltered.[2,8]

References

1 Doering W. Digoxin-quinidine interaction. N Engl J Med (1979) 301, 400–5.
2 Leahey EB, Reiffel JA, Giardina E-G and Bigger JT. The effect of quinidine and other oral antiarrhythmic drugs on serum digoxin: a prospective study. Ann Intern Med (1980) 92, 605–8.
3 Manolas EG, Hunt D and Sloman G. Effects of quinidine and disopyramide on serum digoxin concentrations. Aust NZ J Med (1980) 10, 426–9.
4 Wellens HJ, Gorgels AP, Breat SJ, Vanagt EJ and Phaf B. Effect of oral disopyramide on serum digoxin levels. A prospective study. Am Heart J (1981) 100, 934–5.
5 Risler T, Burk M, Peters U, Grabensee B and Seipel L. On the interaction between digoxin and disopyramide. Clin Pharmacol Ther (1983) 34, 176–80.
6 Elliott HL, Kelman AW, Sumner DJ, Bryson SM, Campbell BC, Hillis WS and Whiting B. Pharmacodynamic and pharmacokinetic evaluation of the interaction between digoxin and disopyramide. Br J Clin Pharmac (1982) 14, 141P.
7 Garcia-Barreto D, Groning E, Gonzalez-Gomera A, Perez A, Hernandez-Canero A and Toruncha A. Enhancement of the antiarrhythmic action of disopyramide by digoxin. J Cardiovasc Pharmacol (1981) 3, 1236–42.
8 Leahey EB, Giardina EGV, Reiffel JA and Bigger JT. Serum digoxin concentrations during administration of oral antiarrhythmic drugs. Clin Res (1986) 25, 602A.

Digitalis glycosides + Diuretics, potassium depleting

Abstract/Summary

It is generally believed, but not unequivocally established, that the potassium loss caused by these diuretics increases the toxicity of the digitalis glycosides. It is common practice to give these diuretics with potassium supplements or potassium-sparing diuretics.

Table 14.2 Potassium-depleting Diuretics

Carbonic anhydrase inhibitors:
Acetazolamide, dichlorphenamide, ethoxzolamide, methazolamide.

Loop diuretics:
Ethacrynic acid, frusemide, bumetanide.

Organomercurials:
Chlormerodrin, meraluride, mercaptomerin.

Thiazides and related diuretics:
Bendrofluazide, benzthiazide, chlorothiazide, chlorthalidone, clopamide, clorexolone, cyclopenthiazide, cyclothiazide, hydrochlorothiazide, hydroflumethiazide, mefruside, metolazone, polythiazide, quinethazone, trichlormethiazide.

Clinical evidence

(a) Evidence of an interaction

An extensive study[1] of the medical records of 418 patients on digitalis over the 1950–52 period, and of 679 patients over the period 1964–66, showed that the incidence of digitalis toxicity had more than doubled. 8.6% of the earlier group showed toxicity (58% on diuretics, mainly of the organomercurial type) compared with 17.17% of the latter group (81% taking diuretics, mainly the chlorothiazides, frusemide, ethacrynic acid, chlorthalidone), the conclusion being that the increased toxicity was related to the increased usage of potassium-depleting diuretics.

A retrospective study[2] of a large number of patients on digoxin showed that almost one in five had some toxic reactions attributable to the use of the glycoside. Of these, 16% had demonstrable hypokalaemia (less than 3.5 mEq/l). Almost half of the patients who showed toxicity were taking potassium-depleting diuretics, notably hydrochlorothiazide or frusemide. Similar results were found in other studies[3–9] on a considerable number of patients. There are other reports not listed here. In addition there is also some evidence that frusemide may raise serum digoxin levels.[13]

(b) Evidence of no interaction

A retrospective study of 191 patients who developed digitalis toxicity showed that the likelihood of its development in those with potassium levels below 3.5 mEq/l was no greater than those with normal potassium levels.[10]

Two other studies on a total of almost 200 patients failed to detect any association between the development of digitalis toxicity and the use of diuretics or changes in potassium levels.[11,12]

Mechanism

Not fully understood. The cardiac glycosides inhibit sodium-potassium ATP-ase which is concerned with the transport of sodium and potassium ions across the membranes of the myocardial cells, and this is associated with an increase in the availability of calcium ions concerned with the contraction of the cells. Potassium loss caused by these diuretics exacerbates the potassium loss from the myocardial cells, thereby increasing the activity and the toxicity of the digitalis. Some loss of magnesium may also have a part to play. The mechanism of this interaction is still being debated.

Importance and management

A direct link between the use of these diuretics and the development of digitalis toxicity is not established beyond doubt, but the weight of evidence favours the belief that concurrent use can result in digitalis intoxication. Because it is only a short step from effective therapy with digitalis to a state of intoxication, those given potassium-depleting diuretics should be well monitored for signs of toxicity. Ideally serum potassium (normal range 3.8 to 5.0 mEq/l) and magnesium levels should be monitored. One of the problems is that serum potassium levels and body stores of potassium are not uniformly correlated. If necessary potassium supplements should be given. It may be possible to do this with foods which are high in potassium but low in sodium (citrus fruits, bananas, peaches, dates, wheat germ, potatoes). An alternative is to use a potassium-sparing diuretic such as triamterene or spironolactone.

References

1 Jorgenson AW and Sorensen OH. Digitalis intoxication: a comparative study on the incidence of digitalis intoxication during the periods 1950–1952 and 1964–1966. Acta Med Scand (1970) 188, 179.
2 Shapiro S, Slone D, Lewis GP and Jick H. The epidemiology of digoxin. A study in three Boston Hospitals. J Chron Dis (1969) 22, 361.
3 Tawakkol AA, Nutter DO and Massumi RA. A prospective study of digitalis toxicity in a large city hospital. Med Ann D C (1967) 36, 402.
4 Soffer A. The changing clinical picture of digitalis intoxication. Arch Int Med (1961) 107, 681.
5 Rodensky PL and Wasserman F. Observation on digitalis intoxication. Arch Int Med (1961) 108, 171.
6 Steiness E and Olesen KH. Cardiac arrhythmias induced by hypokalaemia and potassium loss during maintenance digoxin therapy. Br Heart J (1976) 38, 167.
7 Binnion PE. Hypokalaemia and digoxin-induced arrhythmias. Lancet (1975) i, 343.
8 Poole-Wilson PA, Hall R and Cameron IR. Hypokalaemia, digitalis and arrhythmias. Lancet (1975) i, 575.
9 Shapiro W and Taubert K. Hypokalaemia and digoxin induced arrhythmias. Lancet (1975) ii, 604.
10 Ogilvie RI and Ruedy J. An educational program in digitalis therapy. J Amer Med Ass (1972) 222, 50.
11 Smith TW and Haber E. Digoxin intoxication: the relationship of clinical presentation to serum digoxin concentration. J Clin Invest (1970) 49, 2377.
12 Beller GA, Smith TW, Abelmann WH, Haber E and Hood WB. Digitalis intoxication: a prospective clinical study with serum level correlations. N Engl J Med (1971) 284, 989.

13 Tsutsumi E, Fujiki H, Takeda H and Fukushima H. Effect of furosemide on serum clearance and renal excretion of digoxin. J Clin Pharmacol (1979) 200.

Digitalis glycosides + Edrophonium

Abstract/Summary

Excessive bradycardia and AV-block may occur in patients on digitalis glycosides given edrophonium.

Clinical evidence, mechanism, importance and management

The rapid IV injection of 10 mg edrophonium has proved to be useful in the differentiation of cardiac arrhythmias, but it has been recommended that it should not be given to patients with auricular flutter or tachycardia who are taking digitalis glycosides because of the risk of producing AV-block due to the additive heart slowing effects.[1] This recommendation is reinforced by the case of an elderly woman who developed bradycardia, AV block and asystole following concurrent use.[2]

References

1 Reddy RCV, Gould L and Gomprecht RF. Use of edrophonium (Tensilon) in the evaluation of cardiac arrhythmias. Amer Heart J (1971) 82, 742.
2 Gould L, Zahir M and Gomprecht RF. Cardiac arrest during edrophonium administration. Amer Heart J (1971) 81, 437.

Digitalis glycosides + Encainide

Abstract/Summary

Digoxin and encainide do not interact adversely.

Clinical evidence, mechanism, importance and management

A study in 17 patients on digoxin showed that no significant changes occurred in serum digoxin levels when concurrently taking 100–200 mg encainide daily. A further study in 10 patients with severe congestive heart failure confirmed these findings. The efficacy of neither drug was changed.[1]

Reference

1 Quart BD, Gallo DG, Sami MH and Wood AJJ. Drug interaction studies and encainide use in renal and hepatic impairment. Am J Cardiol (1986) 58, 104–13C.

Digitalis glycosides + Enoximone

Abstract/Summary

Enoximone does not affect the serum levels of either digoxin or digitoxin.

Clinical evidence, mechanism, importance and management

A study in 23 patients on long-term treatment with digitalis glycosides (18 on digoxin and five on digitoxin) showed that the concurrent use of enoximone, 100 mg three times daily for a week, had no significant effect on the serum levels of either of these glycosides.[1]

Reference

1 Glauner T, Winkelmann FHB, Dieterich HA, Trenk D and Jaehnchen E. Lack of effect of enoximone on steady-state plasma concentrations of digoxin and digitoxin. Eur Heart J (1988) 9 (Suppl 1) 151.

Digitalis glycosides + Enprostil or Rioprostil

Abstract/Summary

Neither enprostil nor rioprostil interact with digoxin.

Clinical evidence, mechanism, importance and management

A study in 12 normal subjects taking 0.25 mg digoxin daily showed that while taking 35 μg enprostil daily for six days the pharmacokinetics of the digoxin were not significantly changed.[1] Another study in nine normal subjects on digoxin showed that 600 μg rioprostil daily decreased the rate of absorption of digoxin but not its extent, and did not significantly change the steady-state levels of digoxin.[2]

References

1 Winters L, Windle S, Cohen A and Wolbach R. Enprostil does not interact with steady state digoxin. Gastroenterology (1988) 94, A500.
2 Demol P, Wingender W, Weihrauch TR and Kuhlmann J. Effect of rioprostil, a synthetic prostaglandin E1 on the bioavailability of digoxin. Gastroenterology (1988) 92, 1368.

Digitalis glycosides + Erythromycin, Tetracycline or other antibiotics

Abstract/Summary

Blood digoxin levels may be approximately doubled in about 10% of patients treated with erythromycin. Digitalis intoxication has been seen. A smaller increase may occur with tetracycline. No interaction normally occurs with cefazolin or rokitamycin. No important interaction occurs between ampicillin and digitoxin.

Clinical evidence

An elderly woman with a prosthetic heart valve was under treatment for left ventricular dysfunction with warfarin, frusemide, hydralazine, isosorbide and digoxin, to which was added erythromycin. Four days later her serum digoxin levels were found to have risen to 2.6 ng/ml from a normal steady-state range of 1.4–1.7 ng/ml, and she showed evidence of digitalis intoxication.[1]

This report is in line with a previous report describing two patients on 0.5 mg digoxin daily whose serum digoxin levels roughly doubled after five days of erythromycin (1–2 g daily).[2] A patient on digoxin developed signs of toxicity (nausea, vomiting, cardiac arrhythmias) within four days of starting to take 500 mg erythromycin three times daily. Her serum digoxin levels were elevated. This patient recalled having similar problems during a previous course of erythromycin.[7] Another patient on tetracycline (2 g daily) for five days showed a rise in digoxin levels of about 30%. A marked fall in the excretion of digoxin metabolites from the gut (see Mechanism) in the presence of erythromycin and tetracycline is confirmed in another brief report, but not with cefazolin and only occasionally with penicillin.[4] A later report found that ampicillin did not have a significant effect on digitoxin serum levels.[6] Rokitamycin also does not interact.[5]

Mechanism

About 10% of patients on oral digoxin excrete it in substantial amounts in the faeces and urine as inactive metabolites. This metabolism seems to be the responsibility of the gut flora.[2,3] In the presence of antibiotics which decimate these bacteria, much more digoxin is available for absorption which results in a marked rise in serum levels. At the same time the inactive metabolites derived from the gut disappear.[3]

Importance and management

Evidence is very limited and this is not a well established interaction. Only a small proportion (about 10%) of patients is likely to be at risk, but it is usually not known if a particular patient falls into the 'excretor' category. Monitor patients for signs of increased digoxin effects if they are given antibiotics which reduce the activity of the gut flora, reducing the digoxin dosage as necessary. So far only erythromycin[1,2] and tetracycline[2] have been implicated. There is unconfirmed evidence that it does not occur with cefazolin, only occasionally with penicillin,[4] and no changes in digoxin levels occur if rokitamycin is given.[5] Ampicillin does not interact significantly with digitoxin.[6]

References

1 Friedman HS and Bonventre MV. Erythromycin-induced toxicity. Chest (1982) 82, 202.
2 Lindenbaum J, Rund DG, Butler VP, Tse-Eng D and Saha JR. Inactivation of digoxin by the gut flora: reversal of antibiotic therapy. N Engl J Med (1981) 305, 789–94.
3 Lindenbaum J, Tse-Eng D, Butler VP and Rund DG. Urinary excretion of reduced metabolites of digoxin. Am J Med (1981) 71, 67.
4 Dobkin JF, Saha JR, Butler VP and Lindenbaum J. Effects of antibiotic therapy on digoxin metabolism. Clin Res (1982) 30, 517A.
5 Ishioka T. Effect of a new macrolide antibiotic 3'-O-propionyl-leucomycin A5 (Rotikamycin) on serum concentrations of theophylline and digoxin in the elderly. Acta Therapeutica (1987) 13, 17–23.
6 Lucena MI, Moreno A, Fernandez MC, Garcia-Morillas M and Andrade R. Digitoxin elimination in healthy subjects taking ampicillin. Int J Clin Pharm Res (1987) VII, 33–7.
7 Maxwell DL, Gilmour-White SK, Hall MR. Digoxin toxicity due to interaction of digoxin with erythromycin. Br Med J (1989) 298, 572.

Digitalis glycosides + Fenoldopam

Abstract/Summary

Fenoldopam appears to cause a small and clinically unimportant reduction in serum digoxin levels in most patients, but more marked changes may occur in a few individuals.

Clinical evidence, mechanism, importance and management

10 patients with congestive heart failure on chronic digoxin treatment (doses not stated) were additionally given 100 mg fenoldopam three times daily for nine days. The mean AUC (area under the concentration-time curve) and steady-state digoxin levels were reduced about 20%. The steady-state serum levels of two patients fell by 48% (from 1.36 to 0.71 ng/ml) and 68% (from 1.36 to 0.71 ng/ml), and rose by 45% (from 1.03 to 1.49 ng/ml) in another.[1] Most patients appear therefore not to show marked changes in serum digoxin levels, but a few individuals may possibly need some dosage adjustment. Monitor the effects of concurrent use.

Reference

1 Strocchi E, Tartagni F, Malini PL, Valtancoli G, Ambrosioni E, Pasinelli F, Riva E and Fuccella LM. Interaction study of fenoldopam-digoxin in congestive heart failure. Eur J Clin Pharmacol (1989) 37, 395–7.

Digitalis glycosides + Flecainide

Abstract/Summary

Serum digoxin levels are unaltered or only modestly increased by the use of flecainide, but this is not likely to be important in most patients.

Clinical evidence

A study in five patients with congestive heart failure showed that while taking 100–200 mg flecainide twice daily for seven days their serum digoxin levels remained unaltered. The same result was seen in four patients over a four-week period.[3]

In contrast, a study in 15 normal subjects showed that, while taking 200 mg flecanide twice daily, their serum digoxin levels measured just before and six hours after taking their daily dose of digoxin (0.25 mg) rose by 24% and 13% respectively.[1] The changes observed in vital signs were not clinically significant. In a single dose study the steady-state digoxin levels were predicted to rise about 15% while taking 200 mg flecainide twice daily.[2]

Mechanism

Uncertain. It is suggested that any changes may be due to alterations in the volume of distribution.[2]

Importance and management

Documentation is limited but what is known suggests that either no interaction occurs or any changes are small and unlikely to be clinically important in most patients. However the authors of one of the reports[1] suggest that patients with high drug levels, atrioventricular nodal dysfunction, or both, should be monitored during concurrent treatment.

References

1 Weeks CE, Conard GJ, Kvam DC, Fox JM, Chang SF, Paone RP and Lewis GP. The effect of flecainide acetate, a new antiarrhythmic, on plasma digoxin levels. J Clin Pharmacol (1986) 26, 27–31.
2 Tjandramaga TB, Verbesselt R, van Hecken A, Mullie A and De Schepper PJ. Oral digoxin pharmacokinetics during multiple-dose flecainide treatment. Arch Int Pharmacodyn (1982) 260, 302–3.
3 McQuinn RL, Kvam DC, Parrish SL, Fox TL, Miller AM and Franciosa JA. Digoxin levels in patients with congestive heart failure are not altered by flecainide. Clin Pharmacol Ther (1988) 44, 150.

Digitalis glycosides + Guanethidine and Related drugs

Abstract/Summary

Guanadrel does not affect the pharmacokinetics of digoxin.

Clinical evidence, mechanism, importance and management

No change in the pharmacokinetics of a single intravenous dose of digoxin occurred in 13 normal subjects after taking 10 mg guanadrel sulphate orally every 12 h for three days. One subject experienced a 10 min episode of asymptomatic second degree heart block (Wenckebach) 3 h after the dose of digoxin, the reason for which was not clear.[1] There seem to be no reports of adverse interactions between the digitalis glycosides and any of the guanethidine-like antihypertensive drugs.

Reference

1 Wright CE and Andreadis NA. Digoxin pharmacokinetics when administered concurrently with guanadrel sulfate. Drug Intell Clin Pharm (1986) 20, 465.

Digitalis glycosides + Hydroxychloroquine and Chloroquine

Abstract/Summary

The blood levels of digoxin were found to be markedly increased (+70%) in two elderly patients while they were treated with hydroxychloroquine. A similar increase has been seen with chloroquine in dogs.

Clinical evidence, mechanism, importance and management

Two women of 65 and 68 who had been taking digoxin (0.25 mg daily) for 2–3 years for heart arrhythmias were concurrently treated with hydroxychloroquine (0.25 g twice daily) for rheumatoid arthritis. When the hydroxychloroquine was withdrawn the serum digoxin levels of both women fell by 70–75% (from 3.0 to 0.7 nmol/l and from 3.1 to 0.9 nmol/l respectively). Neither showed any evidence of intoxication during concurrent use, and one of them claimed that the regularity of her heart rhythm had been improved.[1] The reason for this apparent interaction is not understood. It would now seem prudent to check on the effects of adding or withdrawing hydroxychloroquine in any patient on digoxin. No interaction between digoxin and chloroquine has been described in man, but increases (+77%) in peak serum digoxin levels have been seen in dogs.[2]

References

1 Leden I. Digoxin-hydroxychloroquine interaction? Acta Med Scand (1982) 211, 411–12.
2 McElnay JC, Sidahmed AM, D'Arcy PF and McQuale RD. Chloroquine-digoxin interaction. Int J Pharmaceut (1985) 26, 267–74.

Digitalis glycosides + Ibuprofen

Abstract/Summary

There is some unconfirmed evidence that serum digoxin levels may be increased by ibuprofen during early concurrent treatment.

Clinical evidence

The serum digoxin levels of 12 patients rose by about 60% after being treated with 1600 mg ibuprofen daily for a week, but after a month of concurrent treatment the serum digoxin concentrations had fallen to their former levels.[1] The reason is not understood, but it seems possible that ibuprofen may reduce the renal clearance. This interaction is not well established because half of the patients were not satisfactorily compliant and other reports of this interaction are lacking. Nevertheless it would now seem reasonable to monitor patients for changes in the effects of digoxin if ibuprofen is started or stopped.

Reference

1 Quattrocchi FP, Robinson JD, Curry RW, Grieco ML and Schulman SG. The effect of ibuprofen on serum digoxin concentrations. Drug Intell Clin Pharm (1983) 17, 286.

Digitalis glycosides + Indomethacin

Abstract/Summary

Serum digoxin levels in premature babies can be raised up to 40% by the use of indomethacin. Toxicity can occur if the digoxin dosage is not reduced appropriately. There seem to be no reports of this interaction in adults, and evidence that it is not likely to occur.

Clinical evidence, mechanism, importance and management

A study[1] in 11 preterm babies (25–33 weeks) given digoxin showed that when four days later they were given indomethacin (mean total dose of 0.32 mg/kg) for the treatment of patient ductus arteriosus, their mean serum digoxin levels rose on average by 40%. The digoxin was stopped in five of the patients because serum concentrations were potentially toxic.

This confirms the observation of digitalis toxicity in three other preterm babies when treated similarly,[2] and of toxic serum digoxin concentrations in another.[3] A single dose study in six normal subjects suggests that no interaction occurs in adults[4] and this was confirmed in another study in six normal subjects who had digoxin by infusion over 4 h.[5]

Mechanism

Indomethacin reduces the clearance of digoxin by the kidney, thereby allowing it to accumulate in the body.[1,3] The digoxin half-life can be doubled.[1]

Importance and management

Documentation is limited but the interaction appears to be established. It has been suggested that the digoxin dosage should be halved if indomethacin is given to preterm infants and the serum digoxin levels and urinary output monitored. No special precautions seem necessary in adults.

References

1 Koren G, Zarfin Y, Perlman M and MacLeod SM. Effects of indomethacin on digoxin pharmacokinetics in preterm babies. Ped Pharmacol (1984) 4, 25–30.
2 Mayes LC and Boerth RC. Digoxin-indomethacin interaction. Pediatric Res (1980) 14, 469.
3 Schimmel MS, Inwood RL, Eidelman AI and Eilath U. Toxic digitalis levels associated with indomethacin therapy in a neonate. Clin Pediatr (1980) 19, 768–9.
4 Finch MB, Johnston GD, Kelly JG and McDevitt DG. Pharmacokinetics of digoxin alone and in the presence of indomethacin therapy. Br J clin Pharmac (1984) 17, 353–5.

5 Sziegoleit W, Weimss M, Fah A and Forster W. Are serum levels and cardiac effects of digoxin influenced by indomethacin? Pharmazie (1986) 41, 340.

Digitalis glycosides + Isoxicam and Piroxicam

Abstract/Summary

Isoxicam and piroxicam do not interact with digoxin.

Clinical evidence, mechanism, importance and management

A study[1] in 12 normal subjects on beta-acetyldigoxin showed that their steady-state serum digoxin levels were not affected by the concurrent use of 200 mg isoxicam daily. This confirms the findings of a previous study.[2] A study in 10 patients taking digoxin for mild cardiac failure similarly showed that the concurrent administration of 10 or 20 mg piroxicam daily for 15 days had no effect on steady-state digoxin levels nor were consistent effects seen on the pharmacokinetics of digoxin.[3] No special precautions would seem necessary.

References

1 Zoller B, Engel HJ, Faust-Tinnefeldt G, Gilfrich HJ and Zimmer M. Untersuchungen zur Wechselwirkung von Isoxicam und Digoxin. Z. Rheumatol (1984) 43, 182–4.
2 Chlud K. Zur Frage der Interaktionen in der Rheumatherapie: Untersuchungen von Isoxicam und Glibenclamid bei Diabetien mit rheumatischen Enkrankungen. Tempo Medical (1983) 12A, 15–18.
3 Rau R. Interaction study of piroxicam with digoxin. In 'Piroxicam: A New Non-steroidal Anti-inflammatory Agent.' Proc IXth Eur Cong Rheumatol, Wiesbaden, September 1979, pp 41–6. Academy Professional Information Services, NY.

Digitalis glycosides + Kaolin-pectin

Abstract/Summary

Serum digoxin levels can be reduced by kaolin-pectin, but the reduction is small and probably of minimal clinical importance. The interaction can be avoided by taking the two drugs 2 h apart, or by giving the digoxin in liquid or capsule form.

Clinical evidence

A study on seven patients taking digoxin showed that when given digoxin and a kaolin-pectin suspension together, peak serum digoxin levels were reduced 36% while the area under the 24 h concentration/time curve was reduced by 15%. When two doses of kaolin-pectin were taken, one 2 h before and the other 2 h after the digoxin, no significant changes were seen.[1]

Single dose studies have found 42% and 62% reductions in

the bioavailability of digoxin caused by kaolin-pectin.[2,3] Another study showed an interaction with digoxin tablets but not with digoxin capsules.[4]

Mechanism

Not understood. The digoxin may possibly become adsorbed onto the kaolin so that less is available for absorption. Another possibility is that the kaolin reduces the motility of the gut which normally increases mixing and brings the digoxin into contact with the absorbing surface.

Importance and management

Steady-state studies reflect the every-day situation much more closely than single dose studies, and the one cited above[1] indicates that the total reduction in digoxin absorption is small (15%). This is unlikely to be of clinical importance, however the interaction can be avoided by separating the dosages (in any order) by 2 h or by giving the digoxin in capsule or liquid form.

References

1 Albert KS, Elliott WJ, Abbott RD, Gilbertson TJ and Data JL. Influence of kaolin-pectin on steady-state digoxin levels. J Clin Pharmacol (1981) 21, 449–55.
2 Brown DD, Juhl RP, Lewis K, Schrott M and Bartels B. Decreased bioavailability of digoxin due to antacids and kaolin-pectin. N Engl J Med (1976) 295, 1034.
3 Albert KS, Ayres JW, Disanto AR, Weidler DJ, Sakmar E, Hallmark MR, Stoll RG, Desante KA and Wagner JG. Influence of kaolin-pectin suspension on digoxin bioavailability. J Pharm Sci (1978) 67, 1582.
4 Allen MD, Greenblatt DJ, Harmatz JS and Smith TW. Effect of magnesium aluminium hydroxide and kaolin-pectin on absorption of digoxin from tablets and capsules. J Clin Pharmacol (1981) 21, 26.

Digitalis glycosides + Ketanserin

Abstract/Summary

Experimental evidence suggests that ketanserin is unlikely to affect the serum levels of either digoxin or digitoxin.

Clinical evidence, mechanism, importance and management

A pharmacokinetic study in 10 normal subjects showed that 80 mg ketanserin daily did not cause significant changes in the pharmacokinetics of single doses of either digoxin or digitoxin, and it is concluded that ketanserin is unlikely to alter serum concentrations of either glycoside during clinical use.[1]

Reference

1 Ochs HR, Verburg-Ochs B, Holler M and Greenblatt DJ. Effect of ketanserin on the kinetics of digoxin and digitoxin. J Cardiovasc Pharmacol (1985) 7, 205–7.

Digitalis glycosides + Lithium carbonate

Abstract/Summary

Lithium carbonate appears not to interact with digoxin.

Clinical evidence, mechanism, importance and management

A study in six normal subjects taking lithium carbonate (mean steady-state serum levels 0.76 mmol/l, range 0.4–1.0 mmol/l) showed that the pharmacokinetics of digoxin given intravenously were unchanged, and no significant effects on sodium pump activity or electrolyte concentrations were found.[1] No special precautions would seem necessary during concurrent use.

Reference

1 Cooper SJ, Kelly JG, Johnston GD, Copeland S, King DJ and McDevitt DG. Pharmacodynamics and pharmacokinetics of digoxin in the presence of lithium. Br J clin Pharmac (1984) 18, 21–5.

Digitalis glycosides + Methyldopa

Abstract/Summary

Methyldopa does not affect serum digoxin levels, but marked bradycardia has been seen in two elderly women when given both drugs.

Clinical evidence

(a) Serum digoxin levels unchanged

A study in eight normal subjects given 0.25 mg digoxin daily for a week showed that the concurrent use of 250 mg methyldopa daily had no effect on their steady-state serum digoxin levels.[1]

(b) Bradycardia

Two elderly women with hypertension and left ventricular failure developed marked bradycardia when given digoxin and methyldopa (375 or 750 mg daily) but not with digoxin alone. Average and minimum heart rates of 50 and 32, and 48 and 38 beats per min respectively were recorded. They were subsequently discharged on digoxin and hydralazine with heart rates within the normal range.[2]

Mechanism

Uncertain. Both digoxin and methyldopa can cause some bradycardia but these effects seem to have been more than simply the sum of the two.

Importance and management

Information is limited but it would seem that concurrent use need not be avoided, but monitor the effects for any evidence of excessive heart slowing.

References

1 May CA, Vlasses PH, Rocci ML, Rotmensch HH, Swanson BN, Tannenbaum RP, Ferguson RK and Abrams WB. Methyldopa does not alter the disposition of digoxin. J Clin Pharmacol (1984) 24, 386–9.
2 Davis JC, Reiffel JA and Bigger JT. Sinus node dysfunction caused by methyldopa and digoxin. J Amer Med Ass (1981) 245, 1241.
3 Lund-Johansen P. Hemodynamic changes on long term alpha-methyldopa therapy of essential hypertension. Acta Med Scand (1972) 192, 221.

Digitalis glycosides + Metoclopramide

Abstract/Summary

The serum levels of digoxin may be reduced by about a third if metoclopramide and slowly dissolving forms of digoxin are given concurrently. No interaction is likely with digoxin in liquid form or in fast dissolving preparations.

Clinical evidence

A study on 11 patients taking a slowly dissolving digoxin formulation showed that concurrent treatment with metoclopramide (10 mg three times a day for 10 days) reduced the the serum digoxin levels by 36% (from 0.72 to 0.46 ng/ml).[1] The digoxin concentrations rose to their former levels when the metoclopramide was withdrawn.

Another study in normal subjects found a 19% reduction in AUC (area under the curve) and a 27% reduction in peak serum digoxin levels while taking digoxin in an un-named formulation.[6] Yet another study clearly showed that an interaction occurred between metoclopramide and digoxin tablets but not in capsule form.[7]

Mechanism

It would seem[3–5] that the metoclopramide increases the motility of the gut to such an extent that full dissolution and absorption of the digoxin is unfinished by the time it is lost in the faeces. Another idea[2] is that the metoclopramide stimulates the excretion of digoxin in the bile.

Importance and management

Information is very limited, but the interaction seems to be established. It is not likely to occur with solid form, fast-dissolving digoxin preparations or digoxin in liquid form, but only those preparations which are slowly dissolving. A reduction in digoxin levels of a third could result in under-digitalization. There is no information about digitoxin.

References

1 Manninen V, Apajalahti A, Melin J and Kavesoja M. Altered absorption of digoxin in patients given propantheline and metoclopramide. Lancet (1973) i, 398.
2 Thompson WG. Altered absorption of digoxin in patients given propantheline and metoclopramide. Lancet (1973) i, 783.
3 Manninen V, Apajalahti A, Simonen H and Reissell P. Effect of propantheline and metoclopramide on the absorption of digoxin. Lancet (1973) i, 1118.
4 Medin S and Nyberg L. Effect of propantheline and metoclopramide on the absorption of digoxin. Lancet (1973) i, 1393.
5 Fraser EJ, Leach RH, Poston JW, Bold AM, Culank LS and Lipede AB. Dissolution rates and bioavailability of digoxin tablets. Lancet (1973) i, 1393.
6 Kirsch W, Janish HD, Santos SR, Duhrsen U, Dylewicz P and Ohnhaus EE. Effect of cisapride and metoclopramide on digoxin bioavailability. Eur J Drug Metab Pharmacokinet (1986) 11, 249–50.
7 Johnson BF, Bustrack JA, Urbach DR, Hull JH and Marawaha R. Effect of metoclopramide on digoxin absorption from tablets and capsules. Clin Pharmacol Ther (1984) 36, 724–30.

Digitalis glycosides + Mexiletine

Abstract/Summary

Serum digoxin levels are not significantly altered by mexiletine.

Clinical evidence, mechanism, importance and management

A study[1,2] in 10 normal subjects taking 0.25 mg digoxin daily showed that their steady-state serum digoxin levels were slightly but not significantly altered while concurrently taking 600 mg mexiletine daily for four days (a fall from 0.32 to 0.27 ng/ml). When the mexiletine was given with 30 ml of an aluminium magnesium hydroxide antacid the area under the digoxin time/concentration curve was approximately halved (from a range of 4.1–15.6 to 2.6–8.5 ng/ml h). This is in line with other studies showing that antacids can reduce serum digoxin levels (see 'Digitalis glycosides+Antacids'). The serum mexiletine levels were not significantly altered by the antacid. Another study on nine patients confirmed that mexiletine does not significantly affect serum digoxin levels.[3]

References

1 Affrime MB, Lowenthal DT and Saris S. Drug interaction study of oral mexiletine and digoxin. Drug Intell Clin Pharm (1982) 16, 469.
2 Saris SD, Lowenthal DT and Affrime MB. Steady-state digoxin concentration during oral mexiletine administration. Ther Res (1983) 34, 662–66.
3 Leahey EB, Reiffel JA, Giardina E-GV and Bigger T. The effect of quinidine and other oral antiarrhythmic drugs on serum digoxin. Ann Intern Med (1980) 92, 605–8.

Digitalis glycosides + Moricizine (Ethmozine)

Abstract/Summary

Serum digoxin levels are not significantly increased by the concurrent use of moricizine in patients with normal renal function.

Clinical evidence

13 patients on digoxin (0.125–0.25 mg daily) showed a non-significant rise in their serum digoxin levels of 10–15% when concurrently treated with moricizine (10 mg/kg) for two weeks. Nine patients concurrently treated for 1–6 months showed no significant changes in their serum digoxin levels.[1]

No changes in the pharmacokinetics of digoxin were seen in a single dose study of digoxin and moricizine[2] nor in another study in patients over a 13-day period.[3]

Importance and management

No clinically important adverse interaction occurs if digoxin and moricizine are used concurrently in patients with normal renal function. However the authors of the report cited[1] point out that the renal clearance of moricizine is reduced in patients with renal insufficiency and that this might possibly cause a clinically significant rise in serum digoxin levels.

References

1 Kennedy HL, Sprague MK, Redd RM, Wiens RD, Blum RI and Buckingham TA. Serum digoxin concentrations during ethmozine antiarrhythmic therapy. Am Heart J (1986) 111, 667–72.
2 MacFarland RT, Moeller VR, Pieniaszek HJ, Whitney CC and Marcus FI. Assessment of the potential pharmacokinetic interaction between digoxin and ethmozine. J Clin Pharmacol (1985) 25, 138–43.
3 Antman EM, Arnold JM, Friedman PL, White H, Bosak M and Smith TW. Drug interactions with cardiac glycosides: evaluation of a possible digoxin-ethmozine pharmacokinetic interaction. J Cardiovasc Pharmacol (1987) 9, 622–7.

Digitalis glycosides + Neuromuscular blockers

Abstract/Summary

Serious cardiac arrhythmias can develop in patients receiving digitalis glycosides who are given suxamethonium (succinylcholine) or pancuronium.

Clinical evidence

Eight out of 17 digitalized patients (anaesthetized with sodium thiamylal and then maintained with nitrous oxide and oxygen) developed serious ventricular arrhythmias following the intravenous injection of 40–100 mg suxamethonium. Three of the others had immediate and definite ST/T wave changes, and the remaining six showed frequent multifocal premature ventricular contractions.[1]

There are other reports of this interaction.[2,3] Another report describes sinus tachycardia and atrial flutter in six out of 18 patients on digoxin when given pancuronium.[4] In contrast, five out of eight patients with ventricular arrhythmias returned to normal rhythm when given 15–30 mg tubocurarine, and one patient returned to a regular nodal rhythm from ventricular tachycardia.[1]

Mechanism

Not understood. One possibility is that the suxamethonium may cause the rapid removal of potassium from the myocardial cells. Another idea is that it affects catecholamine-releasing cholinergic receptors.

Importance and management

Information is limited but the interaction appears to be established. Suxamethonium should be avoided, or used with great caution, in patients taking digitalis glycosides. Similar caution would seem appropriate with pancuronium.

References

1 Dowdy EG and Fabian LW. Ventricular arrhythmias induced by succinylcholine in digitalized patients. A preliminary report. Anesth Analg (1963) 42, 501.
2 Perez HR. Cardiac arrhythmia after succinylcholine. Anesth Analg (1970) 49, 33.
3 Smith RB and Petrusack J. Succinylcholine, digitalis and hypercalcaemia; a case report. Anesth Analg (1972) 51, 202.
4 Bartolone RS and Rao TLK. Dysrhythmia following muscle relaxant administration in patients receiving digitalis. Anesthesiology (1983) 58, 567.

Digitalis glycosides + Nifedipine

Abstract/Summary

Serum digoxin levels are normally unchanged or only modestly increased by the concurrent use of nifedipine. One unexplained and conflicting study indicated that a 45% rise could occur. Digitoxin appears not to interact.

Clinical evidence

(a) Digoxin

(i) Serum digoxin levels unchanged

Studies on 14 patients[4], 10 patients[7,11] and 28 subjects[5,6,15] showed that serum digoxin levels were not significantly altered while taking 30–60 mg nifedipine daily. Similarly no significant changes in the pharmacokinetics of digoxin were found in six patients[8] or eight subjects[9] on 60–90 mg nifedipine daily when given a single intravenous dose of digoxin. No changes in the pharmacokinetics of nifedipine were seen.[8]

(ii) Serum digoxin levels increased

A study in 12 normal subjects taking 0.375 mg digoxin daily showed that over a period of 14 days while concurrently taking 30 mg nifedipine daily their serum digoxin levels rose by 45% (from 0.505 to 0.734 ng/ml).[1]

A study[2] in nine patients chronically treated with digoxin showed that 20 mg nifedipine daily increased steady-state serum digoxin levels by 15% (from 0.87 to 1.04 ng/ml). A 15% increase was also seen in a study[3,16] in seven subjects given 15–60 mg nifedipine daily.

(b) Digitoxin

A study in eight and 10 normal subjects showed that 40–60 mg nifedipine daily had no significant effect on their steady-state serum digitoxin levels over a six-week period.[17]

Mechanism

Not understood. Changes and lack of changes in both renal and non-renal excretion of digoxin have been reported.

Importance and management

The digoxin-nifedipine interaction is well documented but the findings are inconsistent. The weight of evidence appears to be that serum digoxin levels are normally unchanged or only very moderately increased by nifedipine. Concurrent use appears normally to be safe and effective,[10,12,13] but it would clearly be prudent to monitor the response. One report suggests that nifedipine has some attenuating effect on the digoxin-induced inotropism.[14] Another[3] points out that under some circumstances (renal insufficiency or pre-existing digoxin overdosage) some risk of an undesirable interaction still exists. Nifedipine appears not to interact with digitoxin significantly.

References

1 Belz GG, Doering W, Munkes R and Matthews J. Interaction between digoxin and calcium antagonists and antiarrhythmic drugs. Clin Pharmacol Ther (1983) 33, 410–17.
2 Kleinbloesem CH, van Brummelen P, Hillers J, Moolenaar AJ and Breimer DD. Interaction between digoxin and nifedipine at steady state in patients with atrial fibrillation. Ther Drug Monit (1985) 7, 372–6.
3 Kirch W, Hutt HJ, Dylewicz P, Graf KJ and Ohnhaus EE. Dose-dependence of the nifedipine-digoxin interaction? Clin Pharmacol Ther (1986) 39, 35–9.
4 Schwartz JB, Raizner A and Akers S. The effect of nifedipine on serum digoxin concentrations in patients. Am Heart J (1984) 107, 669–73.
5 Schwartz JB and Migliore PJ. Nifedipine does not alter digoxin level or clearance. J Am Coll Cardiol (1984) 3, 478.
6 Schwartz JB and Migliore PJ. Effect of nifedipine on serum digoxin concentration and renal digoxin clearance. Clin Pharmacol Ther (1984) 36, 19–24.
7 Kuhlmann J, Marcin S, and Frank KH. Effects of nifedipine and diltiazem on the pharmacokinetics of digoxin. Naunyn-Schmied Arch Pharmacol (1983) 324 (Suppl) R81.
8 Garty M, Shamir E, Ilfield D, Pilik S and Rosenfeld JB. Non-interaction of digoxin and nifedipine in cardiac patients. J Clin Pharmacol (1986) 26, 304–5.
9 Koren G, Zylber-Katz E, Granit L and Levy M. Pharmacokinetic studies of nifedipine and digoxin co-administration. Int J Clin Pharmacol Ther Toxicol (1986) 24, 39–42.
10 Pedersen KE, Dorph-Pedersen A, Hvidt S, Klitgaard NA, Kjaer K and

Nielsen-Kudsk F. Effect of nifedipine on digoxin kinetics in healthy subjects. Clin Pharmacol Ther (1982) 32, 562–5.
11 Kuhlmann J. Effects of nifedipine and diltiazem on levels and renal excretion of beta-acetyldigoxin. Clin Pharmacol Ther (1985) 37, 150–6.
12 Belz GG, Aust PE and Munkes R. Digoxin concentrations and nifedipine. Lancet (1981) i, 844.
13 Cantelli I, Pavesi PC, Parchi C, Naccarella F and Bracchetti D. Acute hemodynamic effects of combined therapy with digoxin and nifedipine in patients with chronic heart failure. Am Heart J (1983) 106, 308–15.
14 Hansen PB, Buch J, Rasmussen OO, Waldorff S and Steiness E. Influence of atenolol and nifedipine on digoxin-induced inotropism in humans. Br J clin Pharmac (1984) 18, 817–22.
15 Pedersen KE, Madsen JL, Klitgaard NA, Kjoer K and Hvidt S. Non-interaction between nifedipine and digoxin. Dan Med Bull (1986) 33, 109–10.
16 Hutt HJ, Kirsch W, Dylewicz P and Ohnhaus EE. Dose-dependence of the nifepidine/digoxin interaction? Arch Toxicol (1986) Suppl 9, 209–12.
17 Kuhlmann J. Effects of quinidine, verapamil and nifedipine on the pharmacokinetics and pharmacodynamics of digitoxin during steady-state conditions. Arzneim-Forsch/Drug Res (1987) 37, 545–8.

Digitalis glycosides + Penicillamine

Abstract/Summary

Serum digoxin levels can be reduced by the concurrent use of penicillamine.

Clinical evidence

A study in 10 patients showed that while taking 1 g penicillamine daily 2 h after taking digoxin orally, their serum digoxin levels measured 2, 4 and 6 h later were reduced by 13, 20 and 39% respectively. In 10 other patients similarly treated but given digoxin intravenously, the serum digoxin levels measured 4 and 6 h later were reduced by 23 and 64% respectively.[1]

This interaction is reported by the same authors to occur in children.[2]

Mechanism

Unknown

Importance and management

The reasons for this reaction are not understood and information seems to be limited to the reports cited. Patients on digoxin should be checked for signs of under-digitalization if penicillamine is given concurrently. Information about digitoxin appears to be lacking.

References

1 Moezzi B, Fatourechi V, Khozain R and Eslami B. The effect of penicillamine on serum digoxin levels. Jpn Heart J (1978) 19, 366–70.
2 Moezzi B, Khozein R, Pooymeh F and Shakibi JG. Reversal of digoxin-induced changes in erythrocyte electrolyte concentrations by penicillamine in children. Jpn Heart J (1980) 21, 335–9.

Digitalis glycosides + Phenylbutazone

Abstract/Summary

Serum digitoxin levels can be approximately halved by the concurrent use of phenylbutazone.

Clinical evidence

A study in six patients taking 0.1 mg digitoxin daily showed that on two occasions when concurrently taking 200 or 400 mg phenylbutazone daily, their serum digitoxin levels were approximately halved within 8–10 days, and returned to their former values within roughly the same period of time following its withdrawal.[1]

A similar response has been described elsewhere in one patient.[2]

Mechanism

Not understood. One suggestion is that the phenylbutazone increases the rate of metabolism of the digitoxin by the liver.[1]

Importance and management

Information is limited but the interaction appears to be established. The dosage of digitoxin will need to be increased to avoid under-digitalization if phenylbutazone is added to established treatment. Phenylbutazone may be inappropriate for some patients because it can cause sodium retention and oedema.

References

1 Wirth KE. Arzneimittelinteraktionen bei der Anwendung herzwirksamer Glykoside. Med Welt (1981) 32, 234.
2 Solomon HM, Reich S, Spirt N and Abrams WB. Interactions between digitoxin and other drugs *in vitro* and *in vivo*. Ann NY Acad Sci (1971) 179, 362.

Digitalis glycosides + Phenytoin

Abstract/Summary

Phenytoin is of proven value in the treatment of digitalis-induced heart arrhythmias but sudden cardiac arrest has been reported. Phenytoin reduces serum digoxin levels and a marked fall in serum digitoxin levels has also been seen. There is a single case report of marked bradycardia.

Clinical evidence

(a) Bradycardia and cardiac arrest

A patient with digitalis-induced heart arrhythmias died following the intravenous injection of phenytoin.[1] Sudden cardiac arrest has also been seen in dogs.[5] Marked bradycardia (34 beats/min) and complete heart block has been described in a mongol patient taking 0.25 mg digoxin daily for mitral insufficiency when he was given 200 mg phenytoin daily.[7]

(b) Reduced serum digoxin levels

A study in six normal subjects showed that after taking 400 mg phenytoin daily for a week the half-life of digoxin was reduced by 30% (from 33.9 to 23.7 h) and the AUC by 23% (from 31.6 to 24.4 ng/ml/h). Total clearance increased by 27% (from 258.6 to 328.3 ml/min).[8]

(c) Reduced serum digitoxin levels

The serum digitoxin levels of a man were observed to fall on three occasions when he was concurrently treated with phenytoin. On the third occasion while taking 0.2 mg digitoxin daily, the addition of 900 mg phenytoin daily caused a 60% fall (from 25 to 10 μg/ml) over a 7–10 day period.[6]

Mechanisms

Phenytoin has a stabilizing effect on the responsiveness of the myocardial cells to stimulation so that the toxic threshold at which arrhythmias occurs is raised. But the heart-slowing effects of the digitalis are not opposed and the lethal dose is unaltered, so that the cardiac arrest would appear to be the result of the excessive bradycardia. It seems possible that the fall in serum digitoxin levels may have been due to a phenytoin-induced increase in the metabolism of the digitoxin by the liver. The reduction in serum digoxin levels by phenytoin is not understood.

Importance and management

The value of phenytoin in the treatment of digitalis-induced arrhythmias is well established.[2-5] The authors of one report[5] warn that phenytoin should not be used in patients with a high degree of heart block or marked bradycardia because of the risk that cardiac arrest may occur. This is confirmed by the reports cited.[1,5,7] Information about the effects of phenytoin on serum digitoxin seems to be confined to these single reports, but it would now be prudent to check that patients on digoxin or digitoxin who are subsequently given phenytoin do not become under-digitalized.

References

1 Zoneraich S, Zoneraich O and Siegel J. Sudden death following intravenous sodium diphenylhydantoin. Am Heart J (1976) 91, 375.
2 Helfant RH, Seuffert GW, Patton RD, Stein E and Damato AN. The clinical use of diphenylhydantoin (Dilantin) in the treatment and prevention of cardiac arrhythmias. Am Heart J (1969) 77, 315.
3 Lang TW, Bernstein H, Barbieri F, Gold H and Corday E. Digitalis toxicity. Treatment with diphenylhydantoin. Arch Intern Med (1965) 116, 573.
4 Karliner JS. Intravenous diphenylhydantoin sodium (Dilantin) in cardiac arrhythmias. Dis Chest (1967) 51, 256.
5 Rosen MR, Lisak R and Rubin IL. Diphenylhydantoin in cardiac arrhythmias. Am J Cardiol (1967) 20, 674.
6 Solomon HM, Reich S, Spirt N and Abrams WB. Interactions between digitoxin and other drugs *in vitro* and *in vivo*. Ann NY Acad Sci (1971) 179, 362.

7 Vlukari NMA and Aho K. Digoxin-phenytoin interaction. Br Med J (1970) 2, 51.

8 Rameis H. On the interaction between phenytoin and digoxin. Eur J Clin Pharmacol (1985) 292, 49–53.

Digitalis glycosides + Pinaverium bromide

Abstract/Summary

Serum digoxin levels are not affected by the concurrent use of pinaverium bromide in patients taking either beta-acetyl or beta-methyl digoxin.

Clinical evidence, mechanism, importance and management

A double-blind study[1] on 25 patients, taking either beta-acetyl digoxin or beta-methyl digoxin for congestive heart failure, showed that the concurrent use of pinaverium bromide (50 mg three times a day) for 12 days had no significant effect on their serum digoxin levels. No special precautions would appear to be necessary.

Reference

1 Weitzel O, Seidel G, Engelbert S, Berksoy M, Eberhardt G and Bode R. Investigation of possible interaction between pinaverium bromide and digoxin.Curr Med Res Op (1983) 8, 600–2.

Digitalis glycosides + Prazosin

Abstract/Summary

A rapid and marked rise in serum digoxin levels occurs if prazosin is given.

Clinical evidence

A study in 20 patients with steady-state serum digoxin levels of 0.30–1.80 ng/ml showed that when given 5 mg prazosin for a day their serum plasma digoxin rose by 43% (to 1.34 ng/ml) and after three days by 60% (to 1.51 ng/ml). Three days after the prazosin was stopped the serum digoxin levels had fallen to their previous values.[1] The reason for this response is not understood. Serum digoxin levels should be closely monitored and appropriate dosage reductions made if prazosin is added. More study is needed.

Reference

1 Copur S, Tokgozoglu L, Oto A, Oram E and Ugurlu S. Effects of oral prazosin on total plasma digoxin levels. Fundam Clin Pharmacol (1988) 2, 13–17.

Digitalis glycosides + Probenecid

Abstract/Summary

Some limited evidence suggests that probenecid has no clinically significant effects on serum digoxin levels.

Clinical evidence, mechanism, importance and management

A study[1] over a 16 day period on two normal subjects taking 0.25 mg digoxin daily showed that while concurrently taking two daily doses of *Colbenemid* (probenecid 500 mg+colchicine 0.5 mg) for three days their serum digoxin levels were slightly but not significantly raised (from 0.67 to 0.70 ng/ml, and from 0.60 to 0.67 ng/ml respectively). More study is needed to confirm this finding.

Reference

1 Jaillon P, Weissenburger J, Cheymol G, Graves P and Marcus F. Les effets de probenecide sur la concentration plasmatique a l'equilibre de digoxine. Therapie (1980) 35, 635.

Digitalis glycosides + Propafenone

Abstract/Summary

Propafenone can increase serum digoxin levels by 30–90% or even more. A digoxin dosage reduction may be necessary.

Clinical evidence

A study[3] in five patients on digoxin (0.125–0.25 mg daily) showed that after taking 900 mg propafenone daily for three days their mean serum digoxin levels had risen by 83%. Three patients continued with concurrent treatment for six months and showed a 63% rise. No digitalis toxicity was seen.

Studies[1,2] in 12 normal subjects showed that 450 mg propafenone daily increased their plasma digoxin levels on average by about 35% (from 0.58 to 0.78 ng/ml) and the cardiac effects were increased accordingly. 600 mg propafenone daily increased the serum digoxin levels of nine patients by 90% (from 0.97 to 1.54 ng/ml) and two of them showed symptoms of intoxication (nausea, vomiting).[6,7] A pharmacokinetic study found a 24 h AUC increase of about 25%.[4] Another found a steady-state increase of 28%.[5]

Mechanism

Not understood. One suggestion is that propafenone increases the bioavailability of the digoxin.[4] Another is that the volume of distribution and non-renal clearance of digoxin are changed by the propafenone.[8]

Importance and management

An established interaction of clinical importance. Monitor the effects of concurrent use and reduce the digoxin dosage appropriately in order to avoid toxicity. Most patients appear to be affected[6] and dosage reductions in the range 13–79% were found necessary in one of the studies cited.[6,7] The data available suggests that the extent of the rise may possibly depend on the dose of propafenone used.[8]

References

1 Belz GG, Matthews J, Doering W and Belz G. Digoxin-antiarrhythmics: pharmacodynamic and pharmacokinetic studies with quinidine, propafenone and verapamil. Clin Pharmacol Ther (1982) 31, 202.

2 Belz GG, Doering W, Munkes R and Matthews J. Interaction between digoxin and calcium antagonists and antiarrhythmic drugs. Clin Pharmacol Ther (1983) 33, 410–17.

3 Salerno DM, Granrud G, Sharkey P, Asinger R and Hodges M. A controlled trial of propafenone for treatment of frequent and repetitive ventricular premature complexes. Am J Cardiol (1984) 53, 77–83.

4 Cardaioli P, Compostella L, De Domenico R, Papalia D, Zeppellini R, Libardoni M, Pulido E and Cucchini F. Influenza del propafenone sulla farmacocinetica della digossina somministrata per via orale: studio su volontari sani. G Ital Cardiol (1986) 16, 237–40.

5 Nolan PE, Marcus FI, Erstad BL, Hoyer GK, Furman C and Kirsten EB. Pharmacokinetic interaction between propafenone and digoxin. J Amer Coll Cardiol (1988) 11, 168A.

6 Calvo MV, Martin-Suarez A, Avila MC, Luengo CM. Interaccion digoxina-propafenona. Medicina Clinica (1987) 89, 171–2.

7 Calvo MV, Martin-Suarez A, Luengo CM, Avila C, Cascon M, Hurle AD-G. Interaction between digoxin and propafenone. Ther Drug Monit (1989) 11, 10–15.

8 Nolan PE, Marcus FI, Erstad BL, Hoyer GK, Furman C and Kirsten E. Effects of coadministration of propafenone on the pharmacokinetics of digoxin in healthy subjects. J Clin Pharmacol (1989) 29, 46–52.

form when propantheline is given is confirmed by another study.[4]

Mechanism

Propantheline is an anticholinergic agent which reduces gut motility. This allows the slowly-dissolving formulations of digoxin more time to pass into solution so that more is available for absorption. Propantheline may also reduce the excretion of digoxin in the bile.[3]

Importance and management

An established interaction, but only of importance if slowly-dissolving digoxin formulations are used. No interaction is likely with liquid or soft gelatine capsule forms of digoxin, or with fast-dissolving tablets such as Lanoxin which fulfill BP or USP standards. With slowly dissolving forms of digoxin it may be necessary to reduce the digoxin dosage. No interaction seems likely with digitoxin because it is better absorbed from the gut than digoxin, but this requires confirmation.

References

1 Manninen V, Apajalahti A, Melin J and Kavesoja M. Altered absorption of digoxin in patients given propantheline and metoclopramide. Lancet (1973) i, 398.

2 Manninen V. Effect of propantheline and metoclopramide on absorption of digoxin. Lancet (1973) i, 1118.

3 Thompson WG. Altered absorption of digoxin in patients given propantheline and metoclopramide. Lancet (1973) i, 783.

4 Brown DD, Schmidt J, Long RA and Hull JH. A steady-state evaluation of the effects of propantheline bromide and cholestyramine on the bioavailability of digoxin when administered as tablets or capsules. J Clin Pharmacol (1985) 25, 360–4.

Digitalis glycosides + Propantheline

Abstract/Summary

Serum digoxin levels may be increased by a third or more if propantheline and slowly-dissolving forms of digoxin are given concurrently. No interaction is likely with digoxin given as a liquid or in soft-gelatine capsules or in the form of fast-dissolving tablets such as Lanoxin.

Clinical evidence

The serum digoxin levels of nine out of 13 patients rose by 30% (from 1.02 to 1.33 ng/ml) while taking a slowly dissolving formulation of digoxin with 15 mg propantheline daily for 10 days. Serum levels stayed the same in three patients and fell slightly in one. An associated study in four normal subjects given digoxin in liquid form, with and without propantheline, showed that serum digoxin levels were higher than those when given digoxin in tablet form, and they remained unaffected by propantheline.[1]

Another study by the same workers showed that propantheline only increased digoxin serum levels (by 40%) with slowly dissolving formulations but not with fast dissolving preparations.[2] Increased bioavailability of digoxin in capsule

Digitalis glycosides + Quinidine

Abstract/Summary

The serum levels of digoxin in most patients are doubled within five days if quinidine is added. The digoxin dosage will need to be halved if intoxication is to be avoided. Digitoxin levels are also increased but it occurs more slowly and the extent may be less.

Clinical evidence

(a) Digoxin + quinidine

Arising out of the observation that quinidine appeared to increase serum digoxin levels, a retrospective study of patient records revealed that 25 out 27 patients on digoxin had shown a significant rise (from 1.4 to 3.2 ng/ml) in serum digoxin levels when given quinidine. 16 showed typical signs of intoxication (nausea, vomiting, anorexia) which resolved in 10 of them when the digoxin dosage was reduced or withdrawn, and in five when the quinidine was reduced.[1]

This is one of the first reports published in 1978 (two other groups independently reported it the same year[2,6]) which clearly describe this interaction, although hints of its existence can be found in papers published over the previous 50 years. Since then very considerable numbers of research reports, both retrospective and prospective, and case studies on very considerable numbers of patients have confirmed and established the extent (a 100% increase in serum digoxin levels) and incidence (+90%) of this interaction beyond doubt. I have on file almost 150 reports and reviews, only a selection of which are listed here for economy of space. Two reviews published in 1982 and 1983 contain extensive and valuable bibliographies.[13,16]

(b) Digitoxin + quinidine

A study in eight normal subjects showed that their steady-state serum digitoxin levels rose by 45% (from 13.6 to 19.7 ng/ml) over 32 days while taking 750 mg quinidine daily.[17]

Another study over only 10 days found a 31% increase in serum digitoxin levels,[18] whereas yet another found a 115% increase.[19] A study in five subjects found that quinidine reduced the total body clearance of digitoxin by 63% and the serum digitoxin levels were raised.[7]

Mechanisms

Quinidine reduces the excretion of digoxin by the kidney by 40–50%, and it also appears to have some effects on non-renal clearance which includes an approximately 50% reduction in its excretion in the bile.[14] It displaces digoxin from tissue binding sites and significant changes in the volume of distribution occur. There is also some limited evidence that changes in the rate and extent of absorption of digoxin from the gut may have a small part to play.[9] Digoxin also appears to cause a small reduction in the renal clearance of quinidine.[15] Quinidine appears to increase digitoxin serum levels by reducing the non-renal clearance.

Importance and management

The digoxin-quinidine interaction is overwhelming well-documented, well-established and of clinical importance. Since serum digoxin levels are usually roughly doubled (up to a five-fold increases have been seen[8]) and most (90%+) patients are affected, digitalis toxicity will develop unless the dosage of digoxin is reduced appropriately (approximately halved).[1,3,4,8] A suggested rule-of-thumb is that if serum digoxin levels are no greater than 0.9 ng/ml the addition of quinidine is unlikely to cause cardiotoxic digoxin levels (if serum potassium levels are normal) whereas with levels of 1.0 ng/ml toxic concentrations may develop.[12] Monitor the effects and readjust the dosage as necessary. Significant effects occur within a day of taking the quinidine and reach a maximum after about 3–6 days (quicker or slower in some patients), but it will only stabilize when the quinidine has reached steady-state and that depends on whether a loading dose is given. The effects are to some extent dose-related but the correlation is not good: less than 400–500 mg quinidine daily have minimal effects, and increasing doses up to 1200 mg having greater effects.[3,5] After withdrawing the quinidine about five days are needed before serum digoxin levels fall to their former levels. It has been recommended that patients with chronic renal failure should have their

digoxin dosage reduced to a half or a third.[10,11,20] An appropriate upward readjustment will be necessary if the quinidine is subsequently withdrawn.

Far less is known about the digitoxin-quinidine interaction but the same precautions should be taken. It develops much more slowly.

Alternative non-interacting antiarrhythmics include disopyramide, mexiletine, procainamide and possibly flecainide.

References

1 Leahey EB, Reiffel JA, Drusin RE, Heisenbuttel RH, Lovejoy WP and Bigger JT. Interaction between quinidine and digoxin. J Amer Med Ass (1978) 240, 533.
2 Ejvinsson G. Effect of quinidine on plasma concentrations of digoxin. Br Med J (1978) 1, 279.
3 Doering W. Quinidine-digoxin interaction: pharmacokinetics, underlying mechanism and clinical implications. N Engl J Med (1979) 301, 400–4.
4 Leahey EB, Reiffel JA, Heissenbuttel RH, Drusin RE, Lovejoy WP and Bigger JT. Enhanced cardiac effect of digoxin during quinidine treatment. Arch Intern Med (1979) 139, 519–21.
5 Fenster PE, Powell JR, Hager WD, Graves PE, Conrad K and Goldman S. Onset and dose dependence of digoxin-quinidine interaction. Amer J Cardiol (1980) 45, 413.
6 Reid PR and Meek AG. Digoxin-quinidine interaction. Johns Hopkins Med J (1979) 145, 227–9.
7 Garty M, Sood P and Rollins DE. Digitoxin elimination reduced during quinidine therapy. Ann Intern Med (1981) 94, 35–7.
8 Bigger JT and Leahey EB. Quinidine and digoxin. An important interaction. Drugs (1982) 24, 229–39.
9 Pedersen KE, Christiansen BD, Klitgaard NA and Nielsen-Kudsk F. Effect of quinidine on digoxin bioavailability. Eur J Clin Pharmacol (1983) 24, 41–7.
10 Fichtl B, Doering W and Seidel H. The quinidine-digoxin interaction in patients with impaired renal function. Int J Clin Pharmacol Ther Toxicol (1983) 21, 229–33.
11 Fenster PE, Hager WD, Perrier D, Powell JR, Graves PE and Michael UF. Digoxin-quinidine interaction in patients with chronic renal failure. Circulation (1982) 66, 1277–80.
12 Friedman HS and Chen T-S. Use of control steady-state digoxin levels for predicting serum digoxin concentration after quinidine administration. Am Heart J (1983) 104, 72–6.
13 Bigger JT and Leahey EB. Quinidine and digoxin. An important drug interaction. Drugs (1982) 24, 229–39.
14 Schenck-Gustafsson K, Angelin B, Hedman A, Arvidsson A and Dahlqvist R. Quinidine-induced reduction of the biliary excretion of digoxin in patients. Circulation (1985) 72, Suppl III-19.
15 Rameis H. Quinidine-digoxin interaction: are the pharmacokinetics of both drugs altered? Int J Clin Pharmacol Ther Toxicol (1985) 23, 145–53.
16 Fichtl B and Doering W. The quinidine-digoxin interaction in perspective. Clin Pharmacokinet (1983) 8, 137–54.
17 Kuhlmann J, Dohrmann M and Marcin S. Effects of quinidine on pharmacokinetics and pharmacodynamics of digitoxin achieving steady-state conditions. Clin Pharmacol Ther (1986) 39, 288–94.
18 Peters U, Risler T, Graben see B, Falkstein U and Kroukou J. Interaktion von Chinidin und Digitoxin beim Menschen. Dtsch Med Wsch (1980) 105, 438–42.
19 Kreutz G, Keller F, Gast D and Prokein E. Digitoxin-quinidine interaction achieving steady-state conditions for both drugs. Naunyn-Schmied Arch Toxicol (1982) 319, R82.
20 Woodcock BG and Rietbrock N. Digitalis-quinidine interactions. TIPS (1982) 3, 118–22.

Digitalis + Quinidine + Pentobarbitone

Abstract/Summary

Digitalis toxicity arising from the digoxin–quinidine interaction only manifested itself in an elderly woman when the enzyme-inducing effects of pentobarbitone were removed.

Clinical evidence, mechanism, importance and management

A woman in her nineties who had been taking 100 mg pentobarbitone at bedtime for at least a year was given digoxin and quinidine to control paroxysmal atrial fibrillation. Her serum quinidine levels remained below the therapeutic range and its half-life was unusually short (1.6 h compared with the normal 10 h) until the pentobarbitone was withdrawn, whereupon both the quinidine and the digoxin levels rose, accompanied by signs of digoxin toxicity.[1] It seems that the pentobarbitone (an enzyme-inducer) kept the quinidine levels depressed by allowing rapid liver metabolism, as a result of which the normal digoxin–quinidine interaction was minimal. Once the enzyme-inducing agent was withdrawn, the quinidine serum levels climbed and the digoxin-quinidine interaction (see 'Digitalis glycosides+Quinidine') which results in elevated digoxin levels was able to manifest itself fully. An interaction involving the interplay of three drugs like this is fairly unusual.

Reference

1 Chapron DJ, Mumford D and Pitegoff GJ. Apparent quinidine-induced digoxin toxicity after withdrawal of pentobarbital. A case of sequential drug interactions. Arch Int Med (1979) 139, 363.

Digitalis glycosides + Quinine

Abstract/Summary

Some but not all patients may show a marked rise (+60%) in serum digoxin levels if given quinine.

Clinical evidence

A study in four normal subjects taking 0.25 mg digoxin daily showed that their steady-state digoxin levels rose by 63% (from 0.63 to 1.03 nmol/l) after taking 300 mg quinine four times daily for a day. After taking the quinine for a further three days the digoxin levels rose another 11% (to 1.10 nmol/l). Digoxin renal clearance fell by 20% (from 2.32 to 1.86 ml/min/kg).[1]

A later study in seven normal subjects found that 250 mg daily for seven days increased the mean serum digoxin levels by 25% (from 0.64 to 0.80 ng/ml). When given 750 mg quinine daily there was a further 8% rise. Considerable individual differences were seen, one subject demonstrating a 92% rise.[4] In contrast another study in 17 patients given 750 mg

quinine daily found only a small and statistically insignificant rise in serum digoxin levels (from 0.80 to 0.91 ng/ml). Serum levels were virtually unaltered in 11 patients, decreased in two and markedly increased (amount not stated) in four.[3] Another study found that quinine reduced the total body clearance of digoxin by 26%.[2]

Mechanism

Not fully understood. A reduction in non-renal clearance is apparently largely responsible for the rise in serum digoxin levels.[2,4] This is possibly due to changes in digoxin metabolism or in its biliary excretion.[2]

Importance and management

An established interaction of clinical importance but only moderately documented compared with digoxin+quinidine. Monitor the effects of concurrent use and reduce the digoxin dosage where necessary. Some patients may show a substantial increase in serum digoxin levels whereas others will show only small or moderate rise. There appear to be no case reports of digoxin intoxication because of concurrent use.

References

1 Aronson JK and Carver JG. Interaction of digoxin with quinine. Lancet (1981) i, 1418.

2 Wandell M, Powell JR, Hager WD, Fenster PE, Graves PE, Conrad KA and Goldman S. Effect of quinine on digoxin kinetics. Clin Pharmacol Ther (1980) 28, 425–30.

3 Doering W. Is there a clinically relevant interaction between quinine and digoxin in human beings? Am J Cardiol (1981) 48, 975–6.

4 Pedersen KE, Madsen JL, Klitgaard NA, Kjaer K and Hvidt S. Effect of quinine on plasma digoxin concentration and renal digoxin clearance. Acta Med Scand (1985) 218, 229–32.

Digitalis glycosides + Rauwolfia alkaloids

Abstract/Summary

Concurrent use is not uncommon and usually uneventful, but the incidence of arrhythmias appears to be increased, particularly in those with atrial fibrillation. Excessive bradycardia and hypotension have also been described.

Clinical evidence

(a) Increased cardiac arrhythmias

Three patients on digoxin and either reserpine or whole root Rauwolfia serpentina developed arrhythmias: atrial tachycardia with 4:1 Wenckebach irregular block; ventricular bigeminy and tachycardia; and atrial fibrillation. A large number of other patients received both drugs without problems.[1]

The incidence of premature ventricular systoles was roughly doubled (seven out of 15) in patients taking both drugs compared with a similar group taking only rauwolfia.[2] Reserpine reduced the tolerated dose of acetyl strophanthidin in 15 patients with congestive heart failure; eight out of nine with atrial fibrillation showed advanced toxic rhythms during acute digitalization compared with only one who responded in this way without reserpine.[3]

(b) Excessive bradycardia and syncope

A man on digoxin (0.25 and 0.375 mg alternate days) and reserpine (0.25 mg daily) developed a very slow heart rate, sinus bradycardia and carotid sinus supersensitivity. He was hospitalized because of syncope which remitted when the reserpine was withdrawn.[4]

Mechanism

Not understood. A possible explanation is that the rauwolfia alkaloids deplete the sympathetic nerve supply (i.e. accelerator) to the heart of its neurotransmitter which allows the parasympathetic vagal supply (i.e. heart slowing) to have full rein. Digitalis also causes heart slowing, so that the total additive bradycardia becomes excessive. In this situation the rate could become so slow that ectopic foci which would normally be swamped by a faster, more normal beat, begin to fire, leading to the development of arrhythmias. Syncope could also result from the combination of bradycardia and the hypotensive effects of reserpine elsewhere in the cardiovascular system.

Importance and management

Concurrent use is not unusual, but some caution is advisable. One group of authors who, despite having described the adverse reactions cited above,[1] conclude that '...time has proven the safety of the combination.' However they continue with the proviso that '... the development of arrhythmias must be anticipated and appropriate steps taken at their appearance...'. Particular risk of arrhythmias seems to occur with patients with atrial fibrillation (eight out of nine in the report cited[3]), and with digitalized patients given reserpine parenterally because of the sudden release of catecholamines which takes place.[4]

References

1 Dick HLH, McCawley EL and Fisher WA. Reserpine-digitalis toxicity. Arch Intern Med (1962) 109, 49.
2 Schreader CJ and Etzel MM. Premature ventricular contractions due to rauwolfia therapy. J Amer Med Ass (1956) 162, 1256.
3 Lown B, Ehrlich L, Lipschultz B and Blake J. Effect of digitalis in patients receiving reserpine. Circulation (1961) 24, 1185.
4 Bigger JT and Strauss HC. Digitalis toxicity: drug interactions prompting toxicity and the management of toxicity. Seminars in Drug Treatment (1972) 2, 147.

Digitalis glycosides + Rifampicin (Rifampin)

Abstract/Summary

The serum levels of digitoxin can be halved by the concurrent use of rifampicin. Digoxin serum levels may be similarly affected in patients with kidney failure, but it is unlikely to occur in those with normal kidney function.

Clinical evidence

(a) Digitoxin

A comparative study[1] on 21 tuberculous patients and 19 normal subjects taking 0.1 mg digitoxin daily showed that the serum digitoxin levels of the patients on rifampicin were approximately 50% of those not on rifampicin (18.4 compared with 39.1 ng/ml). The half-life of digitoxin was found to be reduced by the rifampicin from 8.2 to 4.5 days.

There are case reports confirming that rifampicin can markedly reduce serum digitoxin levels.[2,4]

(b) Digoxin

A woman, hospitalized for endocarditis and under treatment with digoxin (0.25–0.375 mg daily), frusemide, aspirin, isosorbide and potassium chloride, showed a marked fall (about 80%) in her serum digoxin levels when given 600 mg rifampicin daily. The serum digoxin climbed to its former levels when the rifampicin was withdrawn.[3] She had only moderate renal impairment (serum creatinine 2.5 mg/dl).

Another report describes two patients on renal dialysis whose digoxin dosage needed to be doubled while taking rifampicin, and similarly reduced when the rifampicin was withdrawn.[5] This confirms an earlier report.[7]

Mechanism

Rifampicin is a potent liver enzyme inducing agent which can increase the normal metabolism of digitoxin (and reduce its half-life[1,6]) thereby hastening its clearance. Digoxin on the other hand is largely excreted unchanged in the urine, so that a similar increase in its metabolism would not be expected to increase its clearance except in patients with poor kidney function. However the case cited[3] would suggest that non-renal clearance may sometimes account for a considerable amount of the total body clearance.

Importance and management

The digitoxin–rifampicin interaction is established and clinically important. Under-digitalization may occur unless the digitoxin dosage is increased appropriately (approximately doubled). An interaction of the same magnitude can occur with digoxin in patients with renal failure,[5] and sometimes in those with only moderate renal impairment,[3] but a digoxin–rifampicin interaction is unlikely in patients with normal kidney function in whom most of the digoxin is eliminated unchanged in the urine. Nevertheless it would seem prudent to be on the alert for signs of under-digitalization in all patients on digoxin.

References

1 Peters U, Hausmen T-U and Gross-Brockhoff F. Einfluss von Tuberkulostatika auf die Pharmakokinetik des Digitoxins. Deut Med Wchsch (1974) 99, 2381.

2 Boman G, Eliasson K and Odarcederlof I. Acute cardiac failure during treatment with digitoxin—an interaction with rifampicin. Br J clin Pharmacol (1980) 10, 89.
3 Bussey HI, Merritt GJ and Hill EG. The influence of rifampin on quinidine and digoxin. Arch Intern Med (1984) 144, 1021–3.
4 Poor DM, Self TH and Davis HL. Interaction of rifampin and digoxin. Arch Intern Med (1983) 143, 599.
5 Gault H, Longerich L, Dawe M and Fine A. Digoxin-rifampin interaction. Clin Pharmacol Ther (1984) 35, 750–4.
6 Zilly W, Breimer DD and Richter E. Pharmacokinetic interactions with rifampicin. Clin Pharmacokinetics (1977) 2, 61.
7 Novi C, Bissoli F, Simonati V, Volpini T, Baroli A and Vignati G. Rifampin and digoxin: possible drug interaction in a dialysis patient. J Amer Med Ass (1980) 244, 2522–3.

Digitalis glycosides + Spironolactone

Abstract/Summary

The available evidence suggests that serum digoxin levels may be increased 25% by spironolactone, but as spironolactone can interfere with some digoxin assay methods, the evaluation of this interaction is difficult. The effects of digitoxin are reported to be both increased and decreased by spironolactone.

Clinical evidence

(a) Digoxin

A study[1] on nine patients on chronic digoxin treatment indicated that the serum levels were increased about 20% (from 0.85 to 1.0 ng/ml) when given 200 mg spironolactone daily. One patient showed a 3–4-fold rise.

Another study on four patients and four subjects showed that the clearance of digoxin after single 0.75 mg intravenous doses was reduced about 25% following five days treatment with 200 mg spironolactone daily.[2] A marked fall in serum digoxin was reported in an elderly patient when spironolactone was withdrawn[6] but the accuracy of the assay method used is uncertain. One study found that no clinically important reduction in digoxin clearance occurred when *Aldactazide* (spironolactone-hydrochlothiazide) was used.[5]

(b) Digitoxin

A study[3] in six normal subjects who had been taking 0.1 or 0.15 mg digitoxin daily for 30 days showed that the concurrent use of 300 mg spironolactone daily increased the digitoxin half-life by a third (from 141 to 192 h).

Other studies however found that the digitoxin half-life was *reduced* (from 256 to 204 h).[4]

Mechanism

Not fully understood. Spironolactone inhibits the excretion of digoxin by the kidney and probably causes a reduction in the volume of distribution.

Importance and management

The digoxin–spironolactone interaction appears to be established. What is known suggests a rise of about 25% in serum digoxin levels, although much greater increases can apparently occur.[1] It would be prudent to monitor concurrent use carefully for signs of over-digitalization. The reports cited here appear to be reliable, but the total picture of this interaction is confused by a number of other reports (not cited) of doubtful reliability. The latter are based on the results of digoxin assays which are believed to give falsely high digoxin values due to the interference by spironolactone with the assay method. This means that the monitoring of concurrent use is difficult unless the digoxin assay method is known to be reliable. The situation with digitoxin is even more confusing because the reports are contradictory. Concurrent use should be monitored, but the effects are uncertain.

References

1 Steiness E. Renal tubular secretion of digoxin. Circulation (1974) 50. 103.
2 Waldorff S, Andersen JD, Heeboll-Nielsen N, Nielsen OG, Moltke E and Steiness E. Spironolactone-induced changes in digoxin kinetics. Clin Pharmacol Ther (1978) 24, 162.
3 Carruthers SG and Dujovne CA. Cholestyramine and spironolactone and their combination in digitoxin elimination. Clin Pharmacol Ther (1980) 27, 184.
4 Wirth KE, Frohlich JC, Hollifield JW, Falkner FC, Sweetman BS and Oates JA. Metabolism of digitoxin in man and its modification by spironolactone. Europ J Clin Pharmacol (1976) 9, 345.
5 Finnegan TP, Spence JD and Cape R. Potassium-sparing diuretics: interaction with digoxin in elderly men. J Amer Ger Soc (1984) 32, 129–31.
6 Paladino JA, Davidson KH and McCall BB. Influence of spironolactone on serum digoxin concentration. J Amer Med Ass (1984) 251, 470–1.

Digitalis glycosides + Sucralfate

Abstract/Summary

Sucralfate causes a small, probably clinically unimportant, reduction in the absorption of digoxin.

Clinical evidence, mechanism, importance and management

1 g sucralfate four times daily for two days given to 12 normal subjects had no effect on most of the pharmacokinetic parameters of single 0.75 mg doses of digoxin except that the AUC (area under the concentration-time curve) was reduced by 19% (from 41.85 to 39.47 ng/ml.h) and the amount eliminated in the urine was reduced by 12%. It was also absorbed faster.[1] Nobody seems to have looked at the effects of sucralfate on steady-state serum digoxin levels in patients but on the basis of this study it seems unlikely that it will have much effect. This needs confirmation. No interaction occurred when the digoxin was given 2 h before the sucralfate.[1] There seems to be nothing documented about other digitalis glycosides.

Reference

1 Giesing DH, Lamman RC, Dimmitt DC and Runser DJ. Lack of effect of sucralfate on digoxin pharmacokinetics. Gastroenterology (1983) 84, 1165.

Digitalis glycosides + Sulphasalazine

Abstract/Summary

Serum digoxin levels can be reduced by the concurrent use of sulphasalazine.

Clinical evidence

The observation that a patient taking 8 g sulphasalazine daily had low serum digoxin levels, prompted a cross-over study in 10 normal subjects given 0.5 mg digoxin alone and later after six days' treatment with 2–6 g sulphasalazine daily. Digoxin absorption was reduced, ranging from 50% to virtually nothing, depending on the dosage of sulphasalazine used.[1] Serum digoxin levels were depressed accordingly.

Mechanism

Not understood.

Importance and management

Documentation is limited to this report, but the interaction appears to be established. Concurrent use need not be avoided, but serum digoxin levels should be monitored and/ or the patient checked for signs of under-digitalization. In one patient examined, separating the dosages appeared not to prevent this interaction.

Reference

1 Juhl RP, Summers RW, Guillory JK, Blaug SM, Cheng FH and Brown DD. Effect of sulfasalazine on digoxin availability. Clin Pharmacol Ther (1976) 20, 387.

Digitalis glycosides + Tiaprofenic acid

Abstract/Summary

Serum digoxin levels are slightly but not significantly increased by the concurrent use of tiaprofenic acid.

Clinical evidence, mechanism, importance and management

A study[1] in 12 normal subjects showed that the concurrent use of 600 mg tiaprofenic acid daily for 10 days caused a non-significant rise (from 0.97 to 1.12 ng/ml, i.e. about 15%) in serum digoxin levels. No particular precautions would seem to be necessary.

Reference

1 Doering Von W and Isbary J. Der Einfluss von Tiaprofensaure auf die Digoxin-Konzentration im Serum. Arzneim-Forsch/Drug Res (1983) 33, 167–8.

Digitalis glycosides + Ticlopidine

Abstract/Summary

Ticlopidine causes a small reduction in serum digoxin levels.

Clinical evidence, mechanism, importance and management

A study in 15 normal subjects taking 0.125–0.5 mg digoxin daily showed that the concurrent use of ticlopidine, 250 mg twice daily for 10 days, reduced the peak serum digoxin concentrations by 11% and the AUC (area under the curve) by 9%.[1] These reductions are small and likely to be of minimal clinical importance.

Reference

1 Vargas R, Reitman M, Teitelbaum P, Ryan JR, McMahon FG, Jain AK, Ryan M and Regel G. Study of the effect of ticlopidine (T) on digoxin (D) blood levels. Clin Pharmacol Ther (1988) 43, 146.

Digitalis glycosides + Trapidil

Abstract/Summary

Trapidil does not alter serum digoxin levels.

Clinical evidence, mechanism, importance and management

A study in 10 normal subjects taking digoxin (0.375 mg daily) showed that the concurrent use of trapidil (400 mg daily) for eight days had no effect on their steady-state serum digoxin levels. It was noted that trapidil opposed the negative chronotropic effect of digoxin to a small extent.[1]

Reference

1 Sziegoleit W, Weiss M, Fah A and Scharfe S. Trapidil does not affect serum levels and cardiotonic action of digoxin in healthy humans. Jap Circ J (1987) 51, 1305–9.

Digitalis glycosides + Trazodone

Abstract/Summary

A rise in serum digoxin levels, accompanied by intoxication in one instance, has been seen in two patients on digoxin when treated with trazodone.

Clinical evidence, mechanism, importance and management

An elderly woman stabilized on digoxin (and also taking quinidine, clonidine and a triamterene-hydrochlorthiazide diuretic) complained of nausea and vomiting within a fortnight of starting to take trazodone (50–300 mg daily for 11 days). Her serum digoxin levels had risen more than threefold (from 0.8 to 2.8 ng/ml). The digoxin was stopped and then restarted at half the original dosage which maintained therapeutic levels.[1] The patient had poor renal function, but this did not change significantly during this incident. Another case has been reported.[2] Even though direct information seems to be limited to these two reports, and a study in dogs failed to confirm this interaction,[3] it would now seem prudent to monitor the effects of concurrent use.

References

1 Rauch PK and Jenike MA. Digoxin toxicity possibly precipitated by trazodone. Psychosomatics (1984) 25, 334–5.
2 Knapp JE. Mead Johnson Pharmaceutical Newsletter, 1983.
3 Dec GW, Jenike MA and Stern TA. Trazodone-digoxin interaction in an animal model. J Clin Psychopharmacol (1984) 4, 153–5.

Digitalis glycosides + Trimethoprim

Abstract/Summary

Serum digoxin levels can be increased about 25% or more by trimethoprim but some individuals may show a much greater rise.

Clinical evidence

A study[1,2] in nine patients on digoxin showed that after taking 400 mg trimethoprim daily for 14 days their mean serum digoxin levels had risen by an average of 22% (from 1.17 to 1.50 nmol/l). One patient showed a 75% rise. When the trimethoprim was withdrawn, the serum digoxin levels fell once again.

Mechanism

It is suggested that the trimethoprim reduces the renal excretion of digoxin and may also reduce the liver metabolism as well.[1,2]

Importance and management

Information seems to be limited to the reports cited, but the interaction appears to be established. More study is needed to confirm the observations. Normally the serum digoxin rise is modest, but monitor the effects because some individuals can apparently experience a marked rise. Reduce the digoxin dosage if necessary. Trimethoprim is contained in co-trimoxazole, but the dosage is relatively small (80 mg per tablet). It is uncertain therefore whether co-trimoxazole will also interact.

References

1 Kastrup J, Bartram R, Petersen P and Hansen JM. Trimethoprims indvirkning pa serum-digoksin og serum-kreatinin. Ugeskr Laeger (1983) 145, 2286–8.
2 Petersen P, Kastrup J, Bartram R and Hansen JM. Digoxin-trimethoprim interaction. Acta Med Scand (1985) 217, 423–7.

Digitalis glycosides + Vasodilators

Abstract/Summary

A reduction in serum digoxin levels can occur during the concurrent use of sodium nitroprusside or hydralazine, but the importance of this is as yet uncertain.

Clinical evidence, mechanism, importance and management

An experimental study[1] on eight patients with congestive heart failure showed that when they were given either sodium nitroprusside by infusion (7–425 μg/min) or hydralazine by injection (5 mg every 10–20 min), their total renal digoxin clearance went up by 50% and their serum digoxin levels fell by 20% and 11% respectively. It is not known whether these changes would be sustained during chronic concurrent treatment, or the extent to which the digoxin dosage might need to be increased. More study is needed to find out if this interaction is of practical importance.

Reference

1 Cogan JJ, Humphreys MH, Carlson CJ, Benowitz NL and Rapaport E. Acute vasodilator therapy increases renal clearance of digoxin in patients with congestive heart failure. Circulation (1981) 64, 973–6.

Digitalis glycosides + Verapamil

Abstract/Summary

Serum digoxin levels are increased about 40% by the concurrent use of 160 mg verapamil daily, and about 70% by 240 mg verapamil or more daily. Digoxin toxicity may develop if the dosage is not reduced. Deaths have occurred. A rise of about 35% occurs with digitoxin.

Clinical evidence

(a) Digoxin

A study in 49 patients with chronic atrial fibrillation and receiving digoxin found that after two weeks concurrent treatment with 240 mg verapamil daily their mean serum digoxin levels had risen by 72%. It was seen in most patients. Most (90%) of this rise occurred within the first seven days. The rise was less with a smaller dose of verapamil (160 mg). Some of the patients showed signs of digoxin toxicity.[1]

Reports on nine and 12 normal subjects,[8,9] and on 41 and seven patients[3,6] taking digoxin describe rises of 53%, 69%, 70% and 96% (range 44–147%) respectively when given 240–360 mg verapamil daily. A 40% rise was seen with 160 mg verapamil daily.[14] Similar rises are reported elsewhere.[12–15] Toxicity[20] and a fatality occurred in patients whose digoxin levels became markedly increased by verapamil,[2] and asystole has been described.[16] Nine normal subjects on digoxin showed a 53% rise while taking 240 mg verapamil daily for a fortnight which increased to a total of 155% when additionally given 480 mg quinidine daily.[8] Sinus arrest has also been seen.[21] A single dose study indicated that cirrhosis magnifies the extent of this interaction.[22]

(b) Digitoxin

Eight out of 10 patients showed a mean 35% rise (range 14–97%) in serum digitoxin levels over a 4–6 week period while taking 240 mg verapamil daily. Two patients showed no changes, and no changes in the pharmacokinetics of a single dose digitoxin were found in three normal subjects.[18,19]

Mechanism

The rise in serum digoxin levels is due to reductions in both renal and extra-renal clearance; a diminution in the volume of distribution also takes place.[3,4,7,12,14] Impaired extra-renal excretion is suggested as the reason for the rise in serum digitoxin levels.[18]

Importance and management

The digoxin–verapamil interaction is well documented and well established. It occurs in most patients.[11,12] Serum digoxin levels should be well monitored and downward dosage adjustments made to avoid digoxin toxicity (deaths have occurred[2]). A 33–50% dosage reduction has been recommended.[10,17] The interaction develops within 2–7 days, approaching or reaching a maximum within 14 days or so.[1,6] The magnitude of the rise is dose-dependent[5] with a significant increase if the verapamil dosage is increased from 160 to 240 mg daily,[1] but with no further increase if the dose is raised any higher.[9] The mean response to 160 mg daily is about 40%, and with 240 mg verapamil or more it is about 60–80%, but the response is variable. Some patients may show rises of up to 150% while others show only a modest increase. One study found that serum digoxin levels which had risen by 60% within a week had fallen to about 30% five weeks later.[12] Regular monitoring and dosage adjustments would seem to be necessary.

The documentation of the digitoxin–verapamil interaction is limited, but the interaction appears to be established. The incidence was 80% in the study cited.[18] Downward dosage adjustment may be necessary, particularly in some patients. Serum digitoxin levels rise less than digoxin levels and more slowly so that they are easier to control. It has been suggested therefore that digitoxin is a valuable alternative to digoxin in this situation.[18] For alternative non-interacting calcium-channel blockers see 'Digitalis + Calcium channel blockers' and 'Digitalis + Nifedipine'.

References

1 Klein HO, Lang R, Weiss E, Segni ED, Libhaber C, Guerrero J and Kaplinsky E. The influence of verapamil on serum digoxin concentrations. Circulation (1982) 65, 998–1003.

2 Zatuchni J. Verapamil-digoxin interaction. Am Heart J (1984) 108, 412–3.

3 Klein HO, Lang R, Di Segni E and Kaplinsky E. Verapamil-digoxin interaction. N Engl J Med (1980) 303, 160.

4 Pedersen KE, Dorph-Pedersen A, Hvidt S, Litgaard NA and Nielsen-Kudsk F. Digoxin-verapamil interaction. Clin Pharmacol Ther (1981) 30, 311.

5 Schwartz JB, Keefe D, Kates RE, Kirsten E and Harrison DC. Acute and chronic pharmacodynamic interaction of verapamil and digoxin in atrial fibrillation. Circulation (1982) 65, 1163.

6 Merola P, Badin A, Paleari DC, De Petris A and Maragno I. Influenza del verapamile sui livelli plasmatici di digossina nell'uomo. Cardiologia (1984) 27, 683–7.

7 Pedersen KE et al. Digoxin-verapamil interaction. Acta Med Scand (1982) 211 (Suppl 655) 37.

8 Doering W. Effect of co-administration of verapamil and quinidine on serum digoxin concentration. Eur J Clin Pharmacol (1983) 25, 517–21.

9 Belz GG, Doering W, Munkes R and Matthews J. Interaction between digoxin and calcium antagonists and antiarrhythmic drugs. Clin Pharmacol Ther (1983) 33, 410–17.

10 Marcus FI. Pharmacokinetic interactions between digoxin and other drugs. J Amer Coll Cardiol (1985) 5, 82–90A.

11 Belz GG, Aust PE and Munkes R. Digoxin plasma concentrations and nifedipine. Lancet (1981) i, 844.

12 Pedersen KE, Dorph-Pedersen A, Hvidt S, Klitgaard NA and Pedersen KK. The long term effect of verapamil on plasma digoxin concentrations and renal digoxin clearance in healthy subjects. Eur J Clin Pharmacol (1982) 22, 123–7.

13 Klein HO, Saba K, Lang R, Di Segni E, Sareli P, David D and Kaplinsky E. Oral verapamil versus digoxin in the management of chronic atrial fibrillation. Chest (1980) 78, 524.

14 Lang R, Klein HO, Saba K, Weiss E, Libhaber C and Kaplinsky E. Effect of verapamil on digoxin blood levels and clearance. Chest (1980) 78, 525.

15 Schwartz JB, Keefe D, Kates RE and Harrison DC. Verapamil and digoxin. Another drug-drug interaction. Clin Res (1981) 29, 501A.

16 Kounis NG. Asystole after verapamil and digoxin. Brit J Clin Prac (1980) 34, 57.

17 Klein HO and Kaplinsky E. Verapamil and digoxin: their respective effects on atrial fibrillation and their interaction. Am J Cardiol (1982) 50, 894–902.

18 Kuhlmann J and Marcin S. Effects of verapamil on pharmacokinetics and pharmacodynamics of digitoxin in patients. Am Heart J (1985) 110, 1245–50.

19 Kuhlmann J. Effects of verapamil, diltiazem, and nifedipine on plasma levels and renal excretion of digitoxin. Clin Pharmacol Ther (1985) 38, 667–73.

20 Gordon M and Goldenberg LMC. Clinical digoxin toxicity in the aged in association with co-administered verapamil. A report of two cases and a review of the literature. J Am Geriatr Soc (1986) 34, 659–62.

21 Kounis NG and Mallioris C. Interactions with cardioactive drugs. Br J Clin Prac (1986) 40, 537–8.

22 Maragno I, Gianotti C, Tropeano PF, Rodighiero V, Gaion RM, Paleari C, Prandoni R and Menozzi L. Verapamil-induced changes in digoxin kinetics in cirrhosis. Eur J Clin Pharmacol (1987) 32, 309–11.

15

HYPOGLYCAEMIC AGENT DRUG INTERACTIONS

The hypoglycaemic agents are used to control diabetes mellitus, a disease in which there is total or partial failure of the beta-cells within the pancreas to secrete into the circulation enough insulin, one of the hormones concerned with the handling of glucose. In some cases there is evidence to show that the disease results from the presence of factors which oppose the activity of insulin.

With insufficient insulin, the body tissues are unable to take up and utilize the glucose which is in circulation in the blood. Because of this, the glucose which is derived largely from the digestion of food and which would normally be removed and stored in tissues throughout the body, accumulates and boosts the glucose in the blood to such grossly elevated proportions that the kidney is unable to cope with such a load and glucose appears in the urine. Raised blood sugar levels (hyperglycaemia) with glucose and ketone bodies in the urine (glycosuria and ketonuria) are among the manifestations of a serious disturbance in the metabolic chemistry of the body which, if untreated, can lead on to the development of diabetic coma and death.

There are two main types of diabetes: one develops early in life and occurs when the ability of the pancreas suddenly, and often almost totally, fails to produce insulin. The first is called Type I, Juvenile or insulin-dependent diabetes (IDDM). The other form of diabetes is the maturity-onset type and is most often seen in those over 40. This occurs when the pancreas gradually loses the ability to produce insulin over a period of months or years. It is often associated with being over-weight and can sometimes be satisfactorily controlled simply by losing weight and adhering to an appropriate diet. Its alternative names are Type II or non-insulin dependent diabetes mellitus (NIDDM).

The modes of action of the hypoglycaemic agents

Insulin

Insulin extracted from the pancreatic tissue of pigs and cattle is so similar to human insulin that it can be used as a replacement. Human insulin is also increasingly being used because it can now be made by micro-organisms which have been modified by genetic engineering. It is given, not by mouth, but by injection in order to bypass the enzymes of the gut which would digest and destroy it like any other protein. There are now many formulations of insulin, some of them designed to delay absorption from the subcutaneous or intramuscular tissue into which the injection is made so that repeated daily injections can be avoided, but all of them sooner or later release insulin into the circulation where it acts to replace or top-up the insulin from the human pancreas.

Sulphonylurea and biguanide oral hypoglycaemic agents

The sulphonylurea and other sulphonamide-related compounds such as chlorpropamide and tolbutamide were the first synthetic compounds used in medicine as hypoglycaemic agents which had the advantage of being given by mouth. Among their actions they stimulate the remaining beta-cells of the pancreas to grow and secrete insulin which, with a restricted diet, controls blood sugar levels and permits normal metabolism to occur. Clearly they can only be effective in those diabetics whose pancreas still has the capacity to produce some insulin, so their use is confined to the maturity-onset, type II, non-insulin dependent diabetics.

The mode of action of the other synthetic oral hypoglycaemic agents, the biguanides such as metformin, is obscure, but they do not stimulate the pancreas like the sulphonylureas to release insulin, but appear to facilitate the uptake and utilization of glucose by the cells in some way. Their use is restricted to maturity-onset diabetics because they are not effective unless insulin is also present.

Other oral hypoglycaemic agents

Outside orthodox Western medicine, there are herbal preparations which are used to treat diabetes and which can be given by mouth. Blueberries were traditionally used by the Alpine peasants, and bitter gourd or karela (*Momordica charantia*) is an established

part of herbal treatment in the Indian subcontinent and elswhere. The Chinese herbals also contain remedies for diabetes. As yet it is not known how these herbal remedies act and their efficacy awaits formal clinical evaluation.

Interactions

The commonest interactions are those which result in a rise or fall in blood glucose levels, thereby disturbing the control of diabetes. These are detailed in this chapter. Other interactions where the hypoglycaemic agent is the affecting agent are described elsewhere. A full listing is to be found in the Index.

Table 15.1 Hypoglycaemic agents

Approved or generic names	Proprietary names
Biguanides	
Buformin	*Diabrin, Silubin Retard, Sindiatil*
Metformin	*Diabex, Diaberit, Diabetosan, Diabexyl, Glufagos, Glucadal, Glucophage, Islotin, Metiguanide, Orabet, Stagid, Mellitin*
Phenformin	*Cronoformin, DBI, Diabenide, Dibotin, Dipar, Glucopostin, Insoral (also used for carbutamide), Meltrol*
Sulph(f)onylureas	
Acetohexamide	*Dimelor, Dymelor, Gamadiabet, Metaglucina, Ordimel*
Carbutamide (glybutamide)	*Biouren, Carbutil, Diabetin, Diabetoplex, Diabutan, Dia-Tablinen, Dibefanil, Dicarbul, Glucidoral, Glucofren, Insoral (see also phenformin), Invenol, Nadisan*
Chlorpropamide	*Bioglumin, Clordiabet, Clordiasan, Cloro-Hipoglucina, Diabet, Glucosulfina, Catanil, Diabetasi, Diabexan, Diatron, Gliconorm, Melisar, Normoglig, Chloromide, Chloronase, Diabenal, Diabetal, Diabinese, Diabines, Diabetoral, Diabinese, Glymese, Insulase, Melitase, Mellinese, Nogluc, Novopropamide, Promide*
Glibenclamide (glyburide)	*Adiab, Daonil, Diabeta, Euglucan, Euglucon, Gilemal, Glidiabet, Glucolon, Gliben*
Glibornuride	*Glutril, Giltrim, Gluborid, Glutrid*
Gliclazide	*Diamicron, Dramion*
Glipizide	*Glibenese, Minodiab, Minidiab*
Gliquidone	*Glurenorm, Glurenor*
Glisoxepide	*Glisepin, Glucoben, Pro-Diaban*
Glybuzole	*Gludease*
Glycopyramide	*Deamelin-S*
Glycyclamide	*Diaborate*
Metahexamide	*Isodiane*
Tolazamide	*Diabewas, Norglycin, Tolinase, Tolanase*
Tolbutamide	*Aglicem, Aglycid, Arcosal, Artosin, Chembutamide, Diaben, Diabeton, Diasulfon, Dolipol, Fordex, Guabeta N, Insilange-D, Mellitol, Metilato, Mobenol, Neo-Insoral, Nigloid, Neo-Dibetic, Novobutamide, Oramide, Oribetic, Orinase, Pramidex, Proinsul, Rastinon, Tolbutone*
Sulph(f)onamide-related compounds	
Gliflumide	—
Glymidine (glycodiazine)	*Glyconormal, Gondafon, Lycanol, Redul*

Hypoglycaemic agents + ACE inhibitors

Abstract/Summary

Hypoglycaemia has been seen in a few diabetics treated with captopril and enalapril, but concurrent use normally appears to be uneventful.

Clinical evidence, mechanism, importance and management

A study, prompted by three unexplained cases of hypoglycaemia in insulin-dependent diabetics on captopril, failed to find any evidence of an interaction.[1] Another report describes two diabetics who experienced recurrent hypoglycaemia when treated with enalapril.[2] The insulin requirements of one of them fell, and the sulphonylurea was withdrawn from the other. Two other diabetic patients treated with glibenclamide and meformin developed marked hypoglycaemia (2.2 and 2.9 mmol/l) within 24–48 h of starting to take captopril.[6] However further studies in diabetics (on insulin or sulphonylureas and/or metformin) given enalapril (20–40 mg daily) or captopril (37.5–100 mg daily)[3,4] failed to find any evidence of an interaction. It is not understood why this interaction occurs or why it only affects a few individuals.

Concurrent use need not be avoided but it would be prudent to warn patients that excessive hypoglycaemia has very occasionally been seen and it may be necessary to modify the dosage of the hypoglycaemic agent. A false positive urine ketone test can also occur with captopril when using the alkaline-nitroprusside test (Keto-diastix, Ames).[5]

References

1 Ferriere M, Lachkar H, Richard J-L, Bringer J, Orsetti A and Mirouze J. Captopril and insulin sensitivity. Ann Intern Med (1985) 102, 134–5.

2 McMurray J and Fraser DM. Captopril, enalapril and blood glucose. Lancet (1986) i, 1035.

3 Passa Ph, Marre M and Leblanc H. Enalapril, captopril and blood glucose. Lancet (1986) i, 1447.

4 Geissler C and Horton T. Captopril and blood glucose. Lancet (1986) ii, 461.

5 Warren SE. False-positive urine ketone test with captopril. N Engl J Med (1980) 303, 1003–4.

6 Rett K, Wicklmayr M and Dietz GJ. Hypoglycemia in hypertensive diabetic patients treated with sulfonylureas, biguanides and captopril. N Engl J Med (1988) 319, 1609.

Hypoglycaemic agents + Alcohol

Abstract/Summary

Diabetics on insulin or oral hypoglycaemic agents or simply using a controlled diet need not avoid alcohol altogether, but they should only drink in moderation and accompanied by food. Alcohol makes the signs of hypoglycaemia less clear and delayed hypoglycaemia can occur. The CNS depressant effects of alcohol plus hypoglycaemia can make driving or the operation of dangerous machinery much more hazardous. A flushing reaction is common in patients on chlorpropamide who drink, but is rare with other sulphonylureas. Alcoholic patients may require above-average doses of tolbutamide.

Clinical evidence

(a) Hypoglycaemic agents in general + alcohol

The blood glucose levels of diabetics may be reduced or may remain unchanged by alcohol. In one study, two out of seven diabetics using insulin became severely hypoglycaemic after drinking the equivalent of about three measures of spirits.[2] In a hospital study over a three-year period, five insulin-dependent diabetics were hospitalized with severe hypoglycaemia after going on the binge. Two of them died without recovery from the initial coma and the other three suffered permanent damage to the nervous system.[3] In another study it was found that alcohol was involved in 4% of hypoglycaemic episodes requiring hospitalization.[4] In contrast to these alcohol-induced hypoglycaemic episodes, it was found in two other studies[5,6] that either pure alcohol or dry wine had little effect on blood glucose levels.

(b) Sulphonylureas + alcohol

About one third of those on chlorpropamide who drink alcohol, even in quite small amounts, experience a warm, tingling or burning sensation of the face, and sometimes the neck and arms as well. It may also involve the conjunctivae. This can begin within 5–20 min of drinking, reaching a peak within 30–40 min, and may persist for 1–2 h. Very occasionally headache occurs, and lightheadedness, palpitations, wheezing and breathlessness have also been experienced.[11]

This flushing reaction has been described in numerous reports (far too many to list here) involving large numbers of patients on chlorpropamide and these reports have been extensively reviewed.[7–10] A similar reaction can occur, but only very rarely, with other sulphonylureas (glipizide,[11] glibenclamide,[11,12] tolbutamide,[13–15] tolazamide[16]). A comparative study showed that the mean half-life of tolbutamide in alcoholics was reduced about a third (from 384 to 232 min).[17] Alcohol is also reported to prolong but not increase the hypoglycaemic effects of glipizide.[30]

(c) Biguanides + alcohol

A controlled study in five ketosis-resistant type II diabetics taking 50–100 mg phenformin daily showed that the equivalent of 3 oz whiskey markedly raised their blood lactate and lactate-pyruvate levels. Two of them attained blood-lactate levels of more than 50 mg%, and one of these patients had previously experienced nausea, weakness and malaise while taking phenformin and alcohol.[18] The ingestion of alcohol is described in other reports as having preceded the onset of phenformin-induced lactic-acidosis[19–23] or a rise in blood lactate levels. Some patients have complained that alcohol tastes metallic. Phenformin has been withdrawn because of the high incidence of lactic acidosis.

Mechanism

The exacerbation of hypoglycaemia by alcohol is not fully understood. However it is known that if hypoglycaemia occurs when liver glycogen stores are low, the liver turns to the formation of new glucose from amino acids (neoglucogenesis) which is released into the circulation. Neoglucogenesis is inhibited by the presence of alcohol so that blood glucose levels may then continue to fall, and a full-scale hypoglycaemic coma may result. The chlorpropamide-alcohol flush (CPAF) reaction has been extensively studied, but it is by no means fully understood. It seems to be related to the disulfiram-alcohol reaction and is accompanied by a rise in blood-acetaldehyde levels (see 'Alcohol+Disulfiram'). It also appears to be genetically determined[11] and may involve both the prostaglandins and the endogenous opioids.[24] The decreased half-life of tolbutamide in alcoholics is probably due to the inducing effects of alcohol on liver microsomal enzymes.[17,25,26]

The reasons for the raised blood lactate levels seen during the concurrent use of phenformin and alcohol are not clear, but one suggestion is that it may possibly be related to the competitive demands for NAD by the reactions which convert alcohol to acetaldehyde, and lactate to pyruvate.[18]

Importance and management

The documentation of the hypoglycaemic agent-alcohol interactions is surprisingly patchy (with the exception of chlorpropamide and alcohol) but they are of recognized clinical importance. The following contains the main recommendations of The British Diabetic Association based on a review of what is currently known.[1]

General comments

Most diabetics need not avoid alcohol totally, but they are advised not to exceed three drinks daily, and the fewer the drinks the better. 'A drink' is defined as either half a pint (300 ml) beer, a single measure of spirits (one-sixth of a gill or 25 ml) or one small glass of sherry or wine. Drinks with a high carbohydrate content (sweet sherries, sweet wines and most liqueurs) should be avoided. Diabetics should not drink on an empty stomach but should avoid the simultaneous use of readily absorbed carbohydrates, and they should know that the warning signs of hypoglycaemia may possibly be obscured by the effects of the alcohol. Diabetics should not drink if they intend to drive or handle dangerous machinery because the CNS depressant effects of alcohol plus hypoglycaemia can be particularly hazardous. They should also be warned of the risks of hypoglycaemia occurring several hours after drinking. Those with peripheral neuropathy should be warned that alcohol may aggravate the condition and they should not have more than one drink daily. Provided drinking is restricted as suggested and drinks containing a lot of carbohydrate are avoided, there is no need to include the drink in the dietary allowance. However diabetics on a weight-reducing diet should not exceed one drink daily and it should be included in their daily calorie allowance.

Additional comments about the oral hypoglycaemic agents

The chlorpropamide-alcohol interaction (flushing reaction) is very well documented, but of minimal importance. It is a nuisance and may be socially embarrassing but normally requires no treatment. Patients should be warned. The incidence is said to lie between 13 and 33%[27,28] although one study claims that it may be as low as 4%.[29] Since it can be provoked by quite small amounts of alcohol (half a glass of sherry or wine) it is virtually impossible for sensitive patients to avoid it if they drink. Most manufacturers give a warning about the possibility of this reaction with other sulphonylureas, but it is rarely seen and can therefore almost always be avoided by exchanging chlorpropamide for another sulphonylurea. Alcoholic subjects may need above-average doses of tolbutamide.

Metformin does not carry the same risk of lactic acidosis seen with phenformin (now withdrawn) and in the paper[1] prepared for and approved by the British Diabetic Association it is suggested that one or two drinks a day are unlikely to be harmful, however it should not be given to alcoholic patients because of the possibility of liver damage.

References

1 Connor H and Marks V. Alcohol and diabetes. A position paper prepared by the Nutrition Subcommittee of the British Diabetic Association's Medical Advisory Committee and approved by the Executive Council of the British Diabetic Association. Human Nutr: Appl Nutr (1985) 39A, 393–9.
2 Walsh CH and O'Sullivan DJ. Effect of moderate alcohol intake on control of diabetes. Diabetes (1974) 23, 440–2.
3 Arky RA, Veverbrandts E and Abramson EA. Irreversible hypoglycaemia. J Amer Med Ass (1968) 206, 575–8.
4 Potter J, Clarke P, Gale EAM, Dave SH and Tattersall RB. Insulin induced hypoglycaemia in an accident and emergency department: the tip of an iceberg? Br Med J (1982) 285, 1180–2.
5 McMonagle J and Felig P. Effects of ethanol ingestion on glucose tolerance and insulin secretion in normal and diabetic subjects. Metabolism (1975) 24, 625–32.
6 Lolli G, Balboni C and Ballatore C. Wine in the diets of diabetic patients. QJ Stud Alcohol (1963) 24, 412–6.
7 Johnston C, Wiles PG and Pyke DA. Chlorpropamide-alcohol flush: the case in favour. Diabetologia (1984) 26, 1–5.
8 Hillson RM and Hockaday TDR. Chlorpropamide-alcohol flush: a critical appraisal. Diabetologia (1984) 26, 6–11.
9 Waldhäusl W. To flush or not to flush? Comments on the chlorpropamide-alcohol flush. Diabetologia (1984) 26, 12–14.
10 Groop L, Erksson CJP, Huupponen R, Ylikahri R and Pelkonen R. Roles of chlorpropamide, alcohol and acetaldehyde in determining the chlorpropamide-alcohol flush. Diabetologia (1984) 26, 34–38.
11 Leslie RDG and Pyke DA. Chlorpropamide-alcohol flushing: a dominantly inherited trait associated with diabetes. Br Med J (1978) 2, 1519.
12 Stowers JM. Alcohol and glibenclamide. Br Med J (1971) 3, 533.
13 Doger H. Experience with the tolbutamide treatment of 500 cases of diabetes on an ambulatory basis. Ann NY Acad Sci (1957) 71, 275.
14 Signorelli S. Tolerance for alcohol in patients on chlorpropamide. Ann NY Acad Sci (1959) 74, 900.
15 Buttner H. Athanolunvertraglichkeit beim Menschen nach Sulfonylharnstoffen. Dtsch Arch Klin Med (1961) 207, 1.
16 McKendry JBR and Gfeller KF. Clinical experience with the oral antidiabetic compound tolazamide. Can Med Ass J (1967) 96, 531.
17 Carulli N, Manenti F, Gallo M and Salvioli GF. Alcohol-drugs interaction in man: alcohol and tolbutamide. Eur J clin Invest (1971) 1, 421.
18 Johnson HK and Waterhouse C. Relationship of alcohol and hyperlactatemia in diabetic subjects treated with phenformin. Am J Med (1968) 45, 98.
19 Davidson MB, Bozarth WR, Challoner DR and Goodner CJ. Phenfor

min hypoglycaemia and lactic acidosis. Report of an attempted suicide. N Engl J Med (1966) 275, 886.

20 Gottlieb A, Duberstein J and Geller A. Phenformin acidosis. N Engl J Med (1962) 267, 806.

21 Maclachlan MJ and Rodman GP. Effects of food, fast and alcohol on serum uric acid and acute attacks of gout. Am J Med (1967) 42, 38.

22 Dubas TC and Johnson WJ. Metformin-induced lactic acidosis: potentiation by ethanol. Res Comm Chem Pathol Pharmacol (1981) 33, 21.

23 Schaffalitzky de Muckadell OB, Koster A and Jensen SL. Fenformin-alkohol interaktion. Ugeskr Laeg (1973) 135, 925.

24 Johnston C, Wiles PG, Medbak S, Bowcock S, Cooke ED, Pyke DA and Rees LH. The role of endogenous opioids in the chlorpropamide alcohol flush. Clin Endocrinol (1984) 21, 489–97.

25 Kater RMH, Roggin G, Tobon F, Zieve P and Iber FL. Increased rate of clearance of drugs from the circulation of alcoholics. Amer J Med Sci (1969) 258, 35.

26 Kater RMH, Tobon F and Iber FL. Increased rate of tolbutamide metabolism in alcoholic patients. J Amer Med Ass (1969) 207, 363.

27 Fitzgerald MG, Gaddie R, Malins JM and O'Sullivan DJ. Alcohol sensitivity in diabetics receiving chlorpropamide. Diabetes (1962) 11, 40.

28 Daeppen JP, Hofstetter JR, Curchod B and Saudan Y. Traitment oral du diabete par un nouvel hypoglycemiant, le P 607 ou Diabinese. Schweiz med Woch (1959) 89, 817.

29 De Silva NE, Tunbridge WMG and Alberti KGMM. Low incidence of chlorpropamide-alcohol flushing in diet-treated, non-insulin-dependent diabetics. Lancet (1981) i, 128–31.

30 Hartling SG, Faber OK, Wegmann M-L, Wahlin-Boll E and Melander A. Interaction of ethanol and glipizide in humans. Diabetes Care (1987) 10, 683–6.

Hypoglycaemic agents + Allopurinol

Abstract/Summary

An increase in the half-life of chlorpropamide, and a decrease in the half-life of tolbutamide during treatment with allopurinol have been described. The effect of these changes on the hypoglycaemic response of patients to these drugs is uncertain.

Clinical evidence

(a) Chlorpropamide + allopurinol

A brief report describes seven patients given chlorpropamide and allopurinol concurrently. The half-life of chlorpropamide in one patient with gout but normal renal function exceeded 200 h (normal 36 h) after 10 days' treatment with allopurinol. In two others the half-life was extended to 44 and 55 h. The other three patients were given allopurinol for only one or two days and the half-life of chlorpropamide remained unaltered.[1]

(b) Tolbutamide + allopurinol

A study in 10 normal subjects showed that after 15 days treatment with allopurinol (2.5 mg/kg twice daily) the half-life of tolbutamide given intravenously was reduced about 25% (from 360 to 267 m).[2,3]

Mechanism

Not understood. In the case of chlorpropamide it has been suggested that it possibly involves some competition for renal tubular mechanisms.[1]

Importance and management

Information is very limited. There seem to be no reports of either grossly enhanced hypoglycaemia in the case of chlorpropamide, or reduced hypoglycaemia with tolbutamide. More study is needed to find out whether these interactions have any clinical importance. Information about other hypoglycaemic agents seems to be lacking.

References

1 Petitpierre B, Perrin L, Rudhardt M, Herrera A and Fabre J. Behaviour of chlorpropamide in renal insufficiency and under the effects of associated drug therapy. Int J clin Pharmacol (1972) 6, 120.

2 Gentile S, Porcellini M, Loguercio C, Foglia F and Coltorti M. Modificazione della depurazione plasmatica di tolbutamide e rifampicina-SV indotte del trattamento con allopurinolo in volontari sono. Il Progresso Medico (Roma) (1979) 35, 637.

3 Gentile S, Porcellini M, Foglia F, Loguercio C and Coltorti M. Influenza di allopurinolo sull'emivita plasmatica di tolbutamide e rifampicina-SV in soggetti sono. Boll Soc Ital Sper (1979) 55, 345.

Hypoglycaemic agents + Amiloride

Abstract/Summary

There is some limited evidence that diabetic patients may possibly be predisposed to the development of amiloride-induced hyperkalaemia.

Clinical evidence, mechanism, importance and management

Two cases of hyperkalaemia (6.5 mEq/l or more) occurred in four hypertensive diabetic patients treated with amiloride. One of them died. It is suggested that diabetics may have some electrolyte abnormality which predisposes them to this condition during the use of potassium-retaining diuretics. Merck Sharp and Dohme who manufacture amiloride issue the warning that the renal status of diabetics should be determined before giving amiloride, and that the diuretic should be discontinued for at least three days before giving glucose tolerance tests. However there is also evidence that concurrent use can be uneventful.[1] Strictly speaking this is not an interaction but an adverse response to amiloride in patients who need hypoglycaemic agents.

Reference

1 Lowenthal DT, Gould A, Shirk J, Mazzella J, Affrine MB, Walker F, Onesti G. Effects of amiloride on oral glucose loading, serum potassium, renin, and aldosterone in diet-controlled diabetics. Clin Pharmacol Ther (1980) 27, 671.

Hypoglycaemic agents + Anabolic steroids

Abstract/Summary

Nandrolone, methandienone (methandrostenolone), testosterone and stanozolol can enhance the blood sugar reducing effects of insulin. The dosage of the hypoglycaemic agent may need to be lowered.

Clinical evidence

In a study in 54 diabetics under treatment with 25 mg nandrolone (norandrostenolone) phenylpropionate given weekly or 50 mg decanoate given 3-weekly it was found necessary to reduce the insulin dosage by an average of 36% (reduction range of 4 to 56 U).[1]

Other reports similarly describe this response in diabetics treated with insulin and nandrolone,[2,3] methandienone (methandrostenolone),[4] testosterone propionate[7] or stanozolol.[6] A reduction in blood sugar levels has also been seen in normal subjects given testosterone propionate.[5] No changes were seen when ethyloestrenol was used.[1,2]

Mechanism

Uncertain.

Importance and management

An established interaction. The total picture is incomplete because not all the anabolic steroids appear to have been studied and they may not necessarily behave identically. A fall in the dosage requirements of insulin (an 'insulin-sparing' effect) may be expected in many patients with the steroids cited. An average reduction of a third is reported.[1] Whether this is also true for other anabolic steroids with oral hypoglycaemic agents appears not to have been documented.

References

1 Houtsmuller AJ. The therapeutic applications of anabolic steroids in ophthalmology: biochemical results. Acta Endocrinol (1961) 39 (Suppl 63) 154.
2 Dardenne U. The therapeutic applications of anabolic steroids in ophthalmology. Acta Endocrinol (1961) 39 (Suppl 63) 143–53.
3 Weissel W. Anaboles Hormon bei malignem oder kompliziertem Diabetes mellitus. Wien Klin Wsch (1962) 74, 234.
4 Landon J, Wynn V, Samois E and Bilkus D. The effect of anabolic steroids on blood sugar and plasma insulin levels in man. Metabolism (1963) 12, 924–5.
5 Talaat M, Habib YA and Habib M. The effect of testosterone on the carbohydrate metabolism in normal subjects. Arch int pharmacodyn (1957) 61, 215–26.
6 Pergola F. El estanozolol, nuevo anabolico. La Prensa Med Argent (1962) 49, 274–90.
7 Veil WH and Lippross O. 'Unspezifische' wirkungen der Mannlichen keimdrusenhormone. Klin Wchnsch (1938) 19, 655–8.

Hypoglycaemic agents + Anaesthetics

Abstract/Summary

Halothane and thiopentone-nitrous oxide appear to have relatively unimportant effects on blood sugar and insulin levels. A change from oral antidiabetic treatment to insulin may be advisable if the surgical procedures are very extensive.

Clinical evidence

The table summarizes the findings of 10 studies carried out on a large number of patients:

Mechanism

Extremely complex and by no means fully understood.

Table 15.2. The effects of anaesthetics on blood sugar & insulin levels (after Hagan & Kendall[9]).

Anaesthetic	Patient no's	Glucose load	Insulin levels ($\mu U/ml$)		Glucose levels (mg%)		Refs
			Before	After	Before	After	
Ether-N$_2$O	10	-	16	25 at 30' 28 at 60'	83	118 at 60'	1
Ether-N$_2$O	19	-	38	30 at 60' 30 at 45'	85	124 at 45'	7
Halothane-N$_2$O	8	-	17	14 at 60'	80	88 at 60'	1
Halothane-N$_2$O	20	-	11	10 at 45'	83	93 at 45'	2
Halothane-N$_2$O	5	-	16	15 at 30'	78	102 at 30'	3
Halothane-N$_2$O	4	-	18	14 at 20'	84	94 at 20'	4
Thiopentone-N$_2$O	20	-	12	12 at 45'	92	135 at 45'	5
Methoxyflur.-N$_2$O	5	-	8	8 at 30'	84	103 at 30'	3
Methoxyflur.-N$_2$O	20	-	23	19 at 45'	99	108 at 45'	8
Droperidol-N$_2$O	25	+	16	24 at 45'	102	169 at 30'	6

Importance and management

Among the work summarized in the table, halothane[2] or nitrous oxide-thiopentone[1] have been recommended as anaesthetics for diabetics because they neither increase the blood sugar or growth hormone levels significantly nor do they decrease insulin levels. A change from oral hypoglycaemics to insulin before anaesthesia has been a not uncommon practice, but it would seem that there is now an increasing tendency to leave the patient's antidiabetic treatment unchanged,[9,10] although one recommendation is that those undergoing extensive and prolonged procedures should be switched to insulin.[11]

References

1 Yoshimura N, Kodama K and Yoshitake J. Carbohydrate metabolism and insulin release during ether and halothane anaesthesia. Br J Anaesth (1971) 43, 1022.

2 Oyama T and Takasawa T. Effect of halothane anaesthesia and surgery on human growth hormone and insulin levels in plasma. Br J Anaesth (1971) 43, 573.

3 Merin RG, Samuelson PN and Schalch DS. Major inhalation anaesthetics and carbohydrate metabolism. Anaesth Analg (Curr Res) (1971) 50, 625.

4 Allison SP, Tomblin PJ and Chamberlain MJ. Some effects of anaesthesia and surgery on carbohydrate and fat metabolism. Br J Anaesth (1969) 41, 588.

5 Oyama T, Takiguchi M and Kudo T. Metabolic effects of anaesthesia: effect of thiopentone-nitrous oxide anesthesia on human growth hormone and insulin levels in plasma. Can Anaesth Soc J (1971) 18, 442.

6 Oyama T and Takiguchi M. Effects of neuroleptanaesthesia on plasma levels of growth hormone and insulin. Br J Anesth (1970) 42, 1105.

7 Oyama T and Takasawa T. Effects of diethyl ether anaesthesia and surgery on carbohydrate and fat metabolism in man. Can Anaesth Soc J (1971) 18, 51.

8 Oyama T and Takasawa T. Effect of methoxyflurane anaesthesia and surgery on human growth hormone and insulin levels in plasma. Can Anaesth Soc J (1970) 17, 347.

9 Hagan JJ and Kendall CHG. Insulin and oral antidiabetic drugs. Int Anesthesiol Clinics (1975) 13, 127.

10 Fletcher J, Langman MJS and Kelloch TD. Effects of surgery on blood sugar levels in diabetes mellitus. Lancet (1965) 22, 52.

11 Stehling L. Clinical Anaesthesia: Pharmacology of adjuvant drugs. Philadelphia (1973) vol 10, 219.

Hypoglycaemic agents + Anticoagulants

Abstract/Summary

Dicoumarol and tolbutamide mutually interact. This can result in increased hypoglycaemia (possibly coma) and increased anticoagulant effects (possibly bleeding). Dicoumarol can also increase the hypoglycaemic effects of chlorpropamide and this has also been seen in one patient given acencoumarol (nicoumalone). An isolated report describes increased warfarin effects in a patient given glibenclamide. The effects of phenprocoumon are reduced by metformin but bleeding was seen in another patient on warfarin given phenformin. Other anticoagulants and hypoglycaemic agents seem not to interact together.

Clinical evidence

Effect of anticoagulants on hypoglycaemic agents

(a) Tolbutamide + dicoumarol or phenindione

Dicoumarol can increase the serum levels of tolbutamide, prolong its half-life (more than three-fold), and reduce blood sugar levels in both diabetics[1] and normal subjects.[1,2] The hypoglycaemic effects are increased. This may become excessive in a few patients and coma has been described.[1,3,6,8] Phenindione does not affect the half-life of tolbutamide.[1]

(b) Chlorpropamide + dicoumarol or nicoumalone (acenocoumarol)

The observation of severe hypoglycaemia in a patient on chlorpropamide while taking dicoumarol prompted further study in three other patients and two non-diabetics. Dicoumarol doubled the serum chlorpropamide levels within 3–4 days and the half-life was more than doubled.[9] A woman with normal kidney function showed an increase in the half-life of chlorpropamide to 88 h (normally about 36 h) when treated with acenocoumarol.[13]

(c) Glibenclamide, glibornuride, glymidine, tolbutamide + phenprocoumon

Phenprocoumon has been found to cause a slight increase in the half-life of glibornuride,[11] but the pharmacokinetics of glibenclamide[12] and the hypoglycaemic effects of tolbutamide remained unchanged. The half-life of glymidine is increased.

Effect of hypoglycaemic agents on anticoagulants

(a) Dicoumarol + tolbutamide

Two patients on dicoumarol showed marked increases in prothrombin times (a rise from 33 to 60 s) within two days of starting tolbutamide but no bleeding occurred. Increases were seen in three other patients.[5] Another patient on dicoumarol showed a similar increase in his prothrombin time and bled (haematuria, purpura) within five days of starting tolbutamide.[6] The half-life of dicoumarol was approximately halved in two out of four normal subjects given tolbutamide, but the hypoprothrombinaemic effects were unchanged.[14] A retrospective study on 15 patients treated concurrently found no evidence that the anticoagulant effects of the dicoumarol were altered by tolbutamide but the form of the study may possibly have obscured evidence of an interaction.[7] No change in overall anticoagulant control was seen in another study.[4]

(b) Phenprocoumon and warfarin + metformin

The observation that a woman diabetic needed more phenprocoumon while taking metformin prompted further study in 13 diabetics. It was found that those taking 1.0–4.0 g metformin daily were less well anticoagulated than those taking only 0.4–1.0 g, even though the phenprocoumon dosage of the former was slightly higher.[1] The half-life of phenprocoumon is reduced about a third (from 123 to 85 h) while taking 1700 mg metformin daily.[17]

Haematuria occurred in a patient on warfarin three months after concurrent treatment with phenformin was started. Her prothrombin values were normal.[16] The phenformin may have increased fibrinolysis to the point where it was additive with the effects of the warfarin.

(c) Other anticoagulants + hypoglycaemic agents

Treatment of diabetic patients and normal subjects for a week with glibenclamide, glibornuride, tolbutamide or insulin had no effect on the plasma levels or half-life of single doses of phenprocoumon.[10] A retrospective study of 24 patients given dicoumarol and 54 given warfarin suggested that insulin did not alter their anticoagulant effects; similarly tolbutamide is said not to have altered the anticoagulant effects of warfarin taken by 42 patients.[7] However what is not clear is whether this study would have revealed an interaction because the patients were already taking the hypoglycaemic agent and would have been routinely stabilized on the anticoagulant. An isolated report describes increased warfarin effects in a patient given glibenclamide.[15]

Mechanisms

Dicoumarol appears to increase the effects of tolbutamide by inhibiting its metabolism by the liver.[1,2] This may also be true for chlorpropamide.[9] The increase in the anticoagulant effects of dicoumarol by tolbutamide may in part be due to a plasma protein binding interaction. In the case of phenprocoumon there seem to be several different mutually opposing processes going on which cancel each other out and produce a 'silent' interaction.[4] Metformin possibly reduces the effects of phenprocoumon by altering blood flow to the liver and interfering with the enterohepatic circulation. There is no clear explanation for most of these interactions.

Importance and management

Information is patchy and incomplete. Dicoumarol with tolbutamide has been most thoroughly investigated and the interactions are clinically important. Increased hypoglycaemic effects may be expected if dicoumarol is given to patients taking tolbutamide and there is a risk of coma. If tolbutamide is given to those taking dicoumarol an increase in prothrombin times and possibly bleeding will occur. Avoid concurrent use unless the outcome can be well monitored and dosage adjustments made. The same precautions should be taken with dicoumarol and chlorpropamide, but what is known is limited to one study.[9] Some caution is appropriate with nicoumalone (acenocoumarol) and chlorpropamide, and warfarin with glibenclamide although information seems to be limited to two single observations.[13,17] A small increase in the dosage of phenprocoumon may be necessary if metformin is given. There appears to be no other information about interactions between any other hypoglycaemic agent and anticoagulant.

The 'Clinical Evidence' section lists those which seem to be free from interactions: tolbutamide + phenindione; glibornuride + phenprocoumon; dicoumarol or warfarin + tolbutamide; phenprocoumon + glibenclamide, glibornuride, tolbutamide or insulin; warfarin + tolbutamide. Warfarin and phenprocoumon seem to be safer than dicoumarol, nevertheless

be alert for any evidence of changes in the anticoagulant or hypoglycaemic effects if either is given with any hypoglycaemic agent.

References

1 Kristensen M and Hansen JM. Potentiation of the tolbutamide effect by dicoumarol. Diabetes (1967) 16, 211–14.
2 Solomon HM and Schrogie JJ. Effect of phenyramidol and bishydroxycoumarin on the metabolism of tolbutamide in human subjects. Metabolism (1967) 16, 1029–33.
3 Spurney OM, Wolf JW and Devins GS. Protracted tolbutamide-induced hypoglycaemia. Arch Intern med (1965) 115, 53.
4 Jahnchen E, Meinertz T, Gilfrich H-J and Groth U. Pharmacokinetic analysis of the interaction between dicoumarol and tolbutamide in man. Eur J clin Pharmacol (1976) 10, 349–56.
5 Chaplin H and Cassell M. Studies on the possible relationship of tolbutamide to dicoumarol in anticoagulant therapy. Am J Med Sci (1958) 235, 706–15.
6 Schwartz JF. Tolbutamide-induced hypoglycaemia in Parkinson's disease. A case report. J Amer Med Ass (1961) 176, 106–9.
7 Poucher RL and Vecchio TJ. Absence of tolbutamide effect on anticoagulant therapy. J Amer Med Ass (1966) 197, 1069–70.
8 Fontana G, Addavil F and Peta G. Su di uno casa di coma ipoglicemico in corso di terapie con tolbutamide e dicumarolici. G Clin Med (1968) 49, 849.
9 Kristensen M and Hansen JM. Accumulation of chlorpropamide caused by dicoumarol. Acta Med Scand (1968) 183, 83–6.
10 Heine P, Kewitz H and Wiegboldt K-A. The influence of hypoglycaemic sulphonylureas on elimination and efficacy of phenprocoumon following a single oral dose in diabetic patients. Eur J clin Pharmacol (1976) 10, 31–6.
11 Eckhardt W, Rudolph R, Sauer H, Schuber WR and Undeutsch D. Zur pharmacologischen Interferenz von Glibornurid mit Sulfaphenazol, Phenylbutazon und phenprocoumon beim Menschen. Arzneim-Forsch (1972) 22, 2212.
12 Schulz E and Schmidt FH. Uber den Einfluss von Sulphaphenazol, Phenylbutazon und Phenprocoumarol auf die Elimination von Glibenclamid beim Menschen. Vern Dtsch Ges Inn Med (1970) 76, 435.
13 Petitpierre B, Perrin L, Rudhardt M, Herrera A and Fabre J. Behaviour of chlorpropamide in renal insufficiency and under the effect of associated drug therapy. Int J Clin Pharmacol (1972) 6, 120.
14 Jahnchen E, Gilfrich HJ, Groth U and Meinertz T. Pharmacokinetic analysis of the dicoumarol-tolbutamide interaction in man. Naunyn-Schmied Arch Pharmacol (1975) 287 (Suppl) R88.
15 Beeley L, Stewart P and Hickey FM. Bull W Midlands Centre for Adverse Drug Reaction Reporting. (1988) 26, 27.
16 Hamblin TJ. Interaction between warfarin and phenformin. Lancet (1971) ii, 1323.
17 Ohnhaus EE, Berger W, Duckert F and Oesch F. The influence of dimethylbiguanide on phenprocoumon elimination and its mode of action. Klin Wchsch (1983) 61, 851–8.

Hypoglycaemic agents + Azapropazone

Abstract/Summary

Two case reports and a study in three normal subjects show that azapropazone can increase the effects of tolbutamide and cause severe hypoglycaemia.

Clinical evidence

A diabetic woman, well controlled for three years on 500 mg tolbutamide daily, became confused and semi-comatose four days after starting to take 900 mg azapropazone daily. She complained of having felt agitated since starting the azapropazone so it was withdrawn on suspicion of causing hypoglycaemia. Later that evening she became semicomatose and had a plasma glucose level of 2.0 mmol/l.[1] A subsequent study in three normal subjects showed that the same dosage of azapropazone increased the serum half-life of tolbutamide threefold (from 7.7 to 25.2 h) and reduced its clearance accordingly.[1]

Acute hypoglycaemia occurred in a patient on tolbutamide 5.5 h after taking a single 600 mg dose of azapropazone.[2]

Mechanism

The clinical study suggests that azapropazone can inhibit the liver enzymes concerned with the metabolism of the tolbutamide, thereby prolonging its stay in the body and increasing its effects.[1] The rapidity of the second case suggests that displacement from plasma protein binding may also occur.[2]

Importance and management

The cases cited and the associated clinical study appear to be all that is on record about this interaction so far. It would be prudent to avoid concurrent use. Information about other sulphonylurea hypoglycaemic agents seems to be lacking.

References

1 Andreasen PB, Simonsen K, Brocks K, Dimo B and Bouchelouche P. Hypoglycaemia induced by azapropazone-tolbutamide. Br J Clin Pharmac (1980) 12, 581.
2 Waller DG and Waller D. Hypoglycaemia due to azapropazone-tolbutamide interaction. Brit J Rheumatol (1984) 23, 24–5.

Hypoglycaemic agents + Benzodiazepines

Abstract/Summary

No adverse interaction normally occurs between these drugs but an isolated case of hyperglycaemia has been seen in an insulin-treated diabetic associated with the use of chlordiazepoxide.

Clinical evidence, mechanism, importance and management

A woman with maturity-onset diabetes of 27 years' duration, controlled on 45 U isophane insulin suspension daily, showed a fasting blood sugar rise from 200 to 400 mg/100 ml during a three-week period while taking 40 mg chlordiazepoxide daily. Four other diabetics, two controlled on diet alone and the other two on tolbutamide, showed no changes in blood sugar levels while taking chlordiazepoxide.[1] No change in the half-life of chlorpropamide is reported to have occurred in another study when diazepam was used concurrently.[2] There seems to be nothing in the literature to suggest that an adverse interaction normally takes place between the hypoglycaemic agents and the benzodiazepines. No special precautions would appear necessary.

References

1 Zumoff B and Hellman L. Aggravation of diabetic hyperglycemia by chlordiazepoxide. J Amer Med Ass (1977) 237, 1960.
2 Petitpierre B, Perrin L, Rudhardt M, Herrera A and Fabre J. Behaviour of chlorpropamide in renal insufficiency and under the effect of associated drug therapy. Int J Clin Pharmacol (1972) 6, 120.

Hypoglycaemic agents + Barbiturates

Abstract/Summary

The hypoglycaemic effects of glymidine are reported not to be affected by phenobarbitone. There appear to be no reports of adverse hypoglycaemic agent-barbiturate interactions.

Clinical evidence, mechanism, importance and management

A study in man showed that the hypoglycaemic effects of glymidine were unaffected by the concurrent use of phenobarbitone.[1] There seems to be nothing in the literature to suggest that an adverse interaction takes place between any of the hypoglycaemic agents and barbiturates. No special precautions would appear necessary.

Reference

1 Gerhards E, Kolb KH and Schulz PE. Uber 2-Benzolsulfonylamino- 5-(beta-methoxy-athoxy)-pyrimidin (Glycodiazin). V. *In vitro-* und *in vivo-*Versuche zum Einfluss von Phenylathylbarbitursaure (Luminal) auf en Stoffwechsel und die blutzuckersendkende Wirkung des Glycodiazins. Naunyn-Schmied Arch Pharmak u exp Path (1966) 255, 200.

Hypoglycaemic agents + Beta-blockers

Abstract/Summary

(A) Propranolol can impair to some extent the normal recovery reaction (a rise in blood sugar levels) if hypoglycaemia occurs in diabetics using insulin, but serious and severe hypoglycaemia has only been seen in a few patients. A sharp rise in blood pressure may also occur if hypoglycaemia develops. Other beta-blockers normally interact to a lesser extent or not at all. (B) The hypoglycaemic effects of the sulphonylureas may possibly be reduced by the beta-blockers. Whether using insulin, the sulphonylureas or the biguanides, some of the familiar warning signs of hypoglycaemia (tachycardia, tremor) may not occur, although sweating may be increased.

Clinical evidence

Insulin + beta-blockers (Insulin-dependent, Type I) diabetics

(i) Hypoglycaemia

Although propranolol has occasionally been associated with spontaneous episodes of hypoglycaemia in non-diabetics,[1] and a number of studies in patients[4] and normal subjects[5-8] have shown that propranolol impairs the normal blood sugar rebound which should follow if blood sugar levels fall too low, there appear to be few reports of severe hypoglycaemia or coma in diabetics on insulin given propranolol. Marked hypoglycaemia and/or coma occurred in five diabetic patients on insulin due to the use of propranolol,[1-3] pindolol,[3] and timolol eye-drops.[13] Other contributory factors (fasting, haemodialysis, etc.) probably had some part to play.[3] Metoprolol interacts like propranolol but to a lesser extent,[5,7,20] whereas the other beta-blockers examined (acebutalol,[4,7] alprenolol[9], atenolol,[10,12] oxprenolol,[20] penbutolol,[8] pindolol[11]) were found to to interact minimally or not at all. The situation with pindolol is therefore not clear.

(ii) Hypertension

Marked increases in blood pressure (systolic and diastolic) and bradycardia may develop if hypoglycaemia occurs in diabetics on insulin and beta-blockers.[15] Systolic/diastolic pressure rises of $+38.8/+14.3$ mm Hg with propranolol, $+27.9/0$ mm Hg with atenolol and $+15.6/-9.2$ mm Hg with placebo were seen in one study in insulin-treated diabetics.[16] In another study rises of $+27/+14$ mm Hg were seen with alprenolol but no rise with metoprolol.[17] A report describes a pressure rise to 258/144 mm Hg in a patient within two days of starting propranolol.[2] Another patient on metoprolol experienced a rise from 190/96 to 230/112 mm Hg during a hypoglycaemic episode.[16]

Oral hypoglycaemic agents + beta-blockers (non-insulin dependent, type II, maturity-onset diabetics)

(i) Hyperglycaemia

The sulphonylurea-induced insulin-release from the pancreas can be inhibited by beta-blockers so that the hypoglycaemic effects are opposed to some extent. The effects of glibenclamide,[22] chlorpropamide[18] and tolbutamide[19] have been shown to be inhibited by propranolol. Acebutalol affects glibenclamide about the same as propranolol but has fewer unwanted haemodynamic effects[22] and has no effect on tolbutamide.[23] However one study failed to find an interaction between tolbutamide and either propranolol or metoprolol.[21,24] An isolated report describes hyperosmolar non-ketotic coma in a patient on tolbutamide and propranolol.[14]

Mechanism

Among other mechanisms, the normal physiological response to a fall in blood sugar levels is the mobilization of glucose from the liver under the stimulation of adrenaline (epinephrine) from the adrenals. This sugar mobilization is blocked by non-selective beta-blockers (such as propranolol) so that recovery from hypoglycaemia is delayed and may even proceed into a full-scale episode in a hypoglycaemia-prone diabetic. Normally the adrenaline would also increase the heart rate, but with the beta-receptors in the heart already blocked this fails to occur. A rise in blood pressure occurs because the stimulant effects of adrenaline on the beta-2 receptors (vasodilators) are blocked leaving the alpha (vasoconstrictor) effects unopposed. Non-selective beta-blockers can also block beta-2 receptors in the pancreas concerned with insulin-release, so that the effects of the sulphonylureas may be blocked.

Importance and management

Extremely well-studied interactions. Concurrent use can be uneventful but there are some risks. The overall picture is as follows:

(A) Diabetics on insulin may have (i) a prolonged or delayed recovery response to hypoglycaemia while on beta-blockers, but very severe hypoglycaemia and/or coma is rare. (ii) If hypoglycaemia occurs it may be accompanied by a sharp rise in blood pressure. The risk is greatest with propranolol and possibly other non-selective blockers and least with the cardio-selective blockers (e.g. metoprolol, etc.). Monitor the effects of concurrent use well, avoid the non-selective blockers, and check for any evidence that the insulin dosage needs some adjustment. Warn all patients that some of the normal pre-monitory signs of 'going hypo' may not appear, in particular tachycardia and tremors, whereas the hunger, irritability and nausea signs may be unaffected and sweating may even be increased.

(B) Diabetics taking oral sulphonylureas rarely seem to have serious hypoglycaemic episodes caused by beta-blockers, and reductions in the hypoglycaemic effects of the sulphonylureas normally appear to be of little clinical importance. However, monitor concurrent use well to confirm that diabetic control is maintained (increase the dosage if necessary), and warn all patients (as above) that some of the premonitory signs of hypoglycaemia may not occur.

Direct information about biguanide oral hypoglycaemic agents and beta-blockers seems to be lacking, but patients on these drugs should also be warned that the premonitory signs of hypoglycaemia will be obscured. There is also a hint from one report that the peripheral vasoconstrictive effects of non-selective beta-blockers and the poor peripheral circulation in diabetics could be additive.[2] Another good reason for avoiding this type of beta-blocker.

References

1 Kotler MN, Berman L and Rubenstein AH. Hypoglycaemia precipitated by propranolol. Br Med J (1966) 1, 1389.
2 McMurty RJ. Propranolol, hypoglycemia, and hypertensive crisis. Ann Intern Med (1974) 80, 669–70.
3 Samii K, Ciancioni C, Rottembourg J, Bisseliches F and Jacobs C. Severe hypoglycaemia due to beta-blocking drugs in haemodialysis patients. Lancet (1976) i, 545–6.
4 Deacon SP, Karunanayake A and Barnett D. Acebutalol, atenolol, and propranolol and metabolic response to acute hypoglycaemia in diabetics. Br Med J (1977) 2, 1255–7.
5 Davidson NM, Corrall RJM and Shaw TRD. Observations in man of hypoglycaemia during selective and non-selective beta-blockade. Scott Med J (1976) 22, 69–72.
6 Abramson EA, Arky RA, Woeber KA. Effects of propranolol on the hormonal and metabolic responses to insulin-induced hypoglycaemia. Lancet (1966) i, 1386–9.
7 Newman RJ. Comparison of propranolol, metoprolol and acebutalol on insulin-induced hypoglycaemia. Br Med J (1976) 2, 447–9.
8 Sharma SD, Vakil BJ, Samuel MR et al. Comparison of penbutolol and propranolol during insulin-induced hypoglycaemia. Curr Ther Res (1979) 26, 252–9.

9 Eisalo A, Heino A and Munter J. The effect of alprenolol in elderly patients with raised blood pressure. Acta Med Scand (1974) Suppl, 554, 32–31.

10 Deacon SP, and Barnett D. Comparison of atenolol and propranolol during insulin-induced hypoglycaemia. Br Med J (1976) 2, 272–3.

11 Patsch W, Patsch JR and Sailer S. Untersuchung zur Wirkung von Pindolol auf Kohlehydrat- und Fettstoffwechsel bei Diabetes Mellitus. Int J Clin Pharmacol Biopharm (1977) 15, 394–6.

12 Waal-Manning HJ. Atenolol and three non-selective beta-blockers in hypertension. Clin Pharmacol Ther (1979) 25, 8–18.

13 Angelo-Nielsen K. Timolol topically and diabetes mellitus. J Amer Med Ass (1980) 244, 2263.

14 Podolsky S and Pattavina CG. Hyperosmolar non-ketotic diabetic coma. A complication of propranolol therapy. Metabolism (1973) 22, 685–93.

15 Shepherd AMM, Lin M-S and Keeton TK. Hypoglycaemia-induced hypertension in a diabetic patient on metoprolol. Ann Intern Med (1981) 94, 357–8.

16 Ryan JR, Lacorte W, Jain A and McMahon FG. Response of diabetics treated with atenolol or propranolol to insulin-induced hypoglycaemia. Drugs (1983) 25 (Suppl) 256–7.

17 Ostman J, Arner P, Haglund K, Juhlin-Dannfelt A, Nowak J and Wennlund A. Effect of metoprolol and alprenolol on the metabolic, hormonal and haemodynamic response to insulin-induced hypoglycaemia in hypertensive, insulin-dependent diabetics. Acta Med Scand (1982) 211, 381–8.

18 Holt RJ and Gaskins JD. Hyperglycaemia associated with propranolol and chlorpropamide administration. Drug Intell Clin Pharm (1981) 15, 599–600.

19 Massara F, Stumia E, Camanni E and Mollnatti GM. Depressed tolbutamide-induced insulin response in subjects treated with propranolol. Diabetalogia (1971) 7, 287–9.

20 Vibert GC, Stimmler M and Kein H. The effect of oxprenolol and metoprolol on the hypoglycaemic response to insulin in normals and insulin-dependent diabetics. Diabetalogia (1978) 15, 278.

21 Groop L, Totterman KJ, Harna K and Gordin A. Influence of beta-blocking drugs on glucose metabolism in patients with non-insulin dependent diabetes. Acta Med Scand (1982) 211, 7–12.

22 Zaman R, Kendall MJ and Biggs PI. The effect of acebutalol and propranolol on the hypoglycaemic action of glibenclamide. Br J clin Pharmac (1982) 13, 507–12.

23 Ryan JR. Clinical pharmacology of acebutalol. Amer Heart J (1985) 109, 1131–6.

24 Totterman KJ and Groop LC. No effect of propranolol and metoprolol on the tolbutamide-stimulated insulin-secretion in hypertensive diabetic and non-diabetic patients. Ann Clin Res (1982) 14, 190–3.

Hypoglycaemic agents + Calcium channel blockers

Abstract/Summary

Calcium channel blockers are known to have effects on insulin secretion and glucose regulation but significant disturbances in the control of diabetes are uncommon. A report describes a patient whose diabetes worsened and who needed more insulin when treated with diltiazem. Another patient needed a 30% increase in insulin while taking nifedipine.

Clinical evidence

(a) Diltiazem

An insulin-dependent diabetic developed worsening and intractable hyperglycaemia (mean serum glucose levels above 13 mmol) when given 90 mg diltiazem six-hourly. Her insulin requirements dropped when the diltiazem was withdrawn. When restarted on 30 mg diltiazem six-hourly her blood sugar levels were still high, but she needed less insulin than when taking the higher diltiazem dosage.[14]

A study in normal subjects showed that 60 mg diltiazem three times daily had no effect on the secretion of insulin or glucagon, or on plasma glucose levels.[12]

(b) Nifedipine and nicardipine

A study in 20 non-insulin dependent diabetics (five on metformin and 15 diet-controlled) showed that neither nifedipine (10 mg eight-hourly) nor nicardipine (30 mg eight-hourly) for four weeks had any effect on glucose tolerance tests and no effect on the control of the diabetes, but significant reductions in blood pressures occurred (4–7 mm Hg diastolic and systolic).[1] Another study on eight non-diabetics and eight diabetics (three on chlorpropamide, one on glipizide and four on diet alone) showed that the use of 30 mg nifedipine daily for a month did not significantly alter their glucose tolerance tests.[2] No important changes occurred in seven diabetic patients taking glibenclamide when chronically treated for 12–75 weeks with 20–60 mg nifedipine daily.[8] Another study on six diabetics showed that single 20 mg doses of nifedipine had no effect on the pharmacokinetics or actions of glipizide (5–20 mg daily).[7] This confirms other studies with nifedipine[3] and nicardipine.[4] There are however other reports of a deterioration in glucose tolerance during the use of nifedipine,[5,6] and the need to increase insulin dosage by 30%.[15]

(c) Verapamil

A study in 23 type II diabetics, seven of whom were taking glibenclamide, showed that verapamil improved the oral glucose tolerance test but did not increase the hypoglycaemic effects of the glibenclamide.[9] Two studies in type II diabetics found that verapamil improved glucose tolerance tests,[10,11] but no alterations in the hypoglycaemic effects of glibenclamide were found in another study.[10] A study in normal subjects found that verapamil raised serum glibenclamide levels but plasma glucose levels were unchanged.[13]

Mechanism

The changes which occur are not fully understood. Suggestions include inhibition of insulin secretion by the calcium channel blockers and inhibition of glucagon secretion by glucose; changes in glucose uptake by liver and other cells; blood glucose rises following catecholamine release after vasodilation, and changes in glucose metabolism.

Importance and management

Very extensively studied but many reports describe single dose studies or multiple dose studies in normal subjects (only a few are cited here) which give no clear picture of what may be expected in diabetic patients. Those studies which have concentrated on diabetics indicate that the control of the diabetes is not usually adversely affected by concurrent use although isolated cases with diltiazem and nifedipine have been reported.[13,15] No particular precautions normally seem to be necessary, nevertheless be alert for any signs of a worsening control of the diabetes. More study in diabetic patients is needed.

References

1. Collins WCJ, Cullen MJ and Feeley J. Calcium channel blocker drugs and diabetic control. Clin Pharmacol Ther (1987) 42, 420–3.
2. Donnelly T and Harrower ADB. Effect of nifedipine on glucose tolerance and insulin secretion in diabetic and non-diabetic patients. Curr Ther Res Opin (1980) 6, 690–3.
3. Abadia E and Passa PH. Diabetogenic effects of nifedipine. Br Med J (1984) 289, 438.
4. Sakta S and Miura K. Effect of nicardipine in a hypertensive patient with diabetes mellitus. Clin Therap (1984) 6, 600–2.
5. Guigliano D, Torella R, Cacciapuoti F, Gentile S, Kerza M and Varricchio M. Impairment of insulin secretion in man by nifedipine. Eur J Clin Pharmacol (1980) 18, 395–8.
6. Bhatnagar SK, Amin MMA and Al-Yusuf AR. Diabetogenic effects of nifedipine. Br Med J (1984) 289, 19.
7. Connacher AA, El Debani AH and Stevenson IH. A study of the influence of nifedipine on the disposition and hypoglycaemic action of glipizide. Brit J clin Pharmac (1986) 22, 240 P.
8. Kantatsuna T, Nakano K, Mori H, Kano Y, Nishioka H, Kajiyama S, Kitagawa Y, Yoshida T, Kondo M, Nakamura N and Aochi O. Effects of nifedipine on insulin secretion and glucose metabolism in rats and hypertensive type two (non-insulin dependent) diabetes. Arzneim Forsch (1985) 35, 514.
9. Rojdmark S and Andersson DEH. Influence of verapamil on human glucose tolerance. Am J Cardiol (1986) 57, 39–43D.
10. Rojdmark S and Andersson DEH. Influence of verapamil on glucose tolerance. Acta Med Scand (1984) Suppl 681, 37–42.
11. Andersson DEH and Rojdmark S. Improvement of glucose tolerance by verapamil in patients with non-insulin-dependent diabetes mellitus. Acta Med Scand (1981) 210, 27–33.
12. Segrestaa JM, Caulin C, Dahan R, Houlbert D, Thiercelin JF, Herman P and Sauvanet JP. Effect of diltiazem on plasma glucose, insulin and glucagon during an oral glucose tolerance test in healthy volunteers. Eur J clin Pharmacol (1984) 26, 481–3.
13. Semple CG, Omile C, Buchanan KD, Beastall GH and Paterson KR. Effect of oral verapamil on glibenclamide stimulated insulin secretion. Br J clin Pharmac (1986) 22, 187–90.
14. Pershadsingh HA, Grant N and McDonald JM. Association of diltiazem therapy with increased insulin resistance in a patient with type one diabetes mellitus. J Am Med Ass (1987) 257, 930–1.
15. Heyman SN, Heyman A and Halperin I. Diabetogenic effect of nifedipine. DICP Ann Pharmacother (1989) 23, 236–7.

Hypoglycaemic agents + Chloramphenicol

Abstract/Summary

The hypoglycaemic effects of tolbutamide and chlorpropamide can be increased by the concurrent use of chloramphenicol. Acute hypoglycaemia can occur.

Clinical evidence

While taking 2 g chloramphenicol daily, a man was additionally started on a course of 2 g tolbutamide daily. Three days later he had a typical hypoglycaemic collapse and was found to have serum tolbutamide levels 3–4-fold higher than expected.[1]

Studies in diabetics have shown that 2 g daily doses of chloramphenicol can approximately double the half-lives of tolbutamide[2] and chlorpropamide,[3] and double the serum levels of tolbutamide.[3] Other studies using 1 g daily doses of chloramphenicol similarly showed that serum levels of tolbutamide could be doubled, and blood sugar levels reduced 25–30%.[4,5] Hypoglycaemia, acute in one case, developed in two other patients on tolbutamide given chloramphenicol.[6,7]

Mechanism

Chloramphenicol inhibits the liver enzymes concerned with the metabolism of tolbutamide, and probably chlorpropamide as well, leading to their accumulation in the body. This is reflected in prolonged half-lives, reduced blood sugar levels and occasionally acute hypoglycaemia.[1–6]

Importance and management

The tolbutamide–chloramphenicol interaction is well-established and of clinical importance. The incidence is uncertain, but an increased hypoglycaemic response should be expected if concurrent use is undertaken. The chlorpropamide–chloramphenicol interaction is less well documented. The dosage of both sulphonylureas should be reduced appropriately. Some patients may show a particularly exaggerated response. The manufacturers of other sulphonylureas often list chloramphenicol as an interacting drug, based on its interactions with tolbutamide and chlorpropamide, but direct information of an interaction appears not to be available.

References

1. Hansen JM and Kristensen M. Tolbutamide in the treatment of Parkinson's disease. Dan Med Bull (1965) 12, 181.
2. Christensen LK and Skovsted L. Inhibition of drug metabolism by chloramphenicol. Lancet (1969) ii, 1397.
3. Petitpierre B, Perrin L, Rudhardt M, Herrera A and Fabre J. Behaviour of chlorpropamide in renal insufficiency and under associated drug therap. Int J Clin Pharmacol (1972) 6, 120.
4. Brunova E, Slabachova Z and Platilova H. Influencing the effect of dirastan (tolbutamide). Simultaneous administration of chloramphenicol in patients with diabetes and bacterial urinary tract inflammation. Cas Lek ces (1974) 113, 72.
5. Brunova E, Slabachova Z, Platilova H, Pavlik F, Grafnetterova J and Dvoracek K. Interaction of tolbutamide and chloramphenicol in diabetic patients. Int J Clin Pharmacol (1977) 15, 7.
6. Ziegelasch H-J. Extreme Hypoglykamie unter kombinierter Behandlung mit Tolbutamid, n-1-Butylbiguanidhydrochlorid und Chloramphenikol. Z Gesamte inn Med (1972) 27, 63.
7. Soeldner JS and Steinke J. Hypoglycemia in tolbutamide-treated diabetes. J Amer Med Ass (1965) 193, 398–9.

Hypoglycaemic agents + Chlorpromazine

Abstract/Summary

Chlorpromazine can raise blood sugar levels, particularly in daily doses of 100 mg or more, and disturb the control of diabetes. It may be necessary to increase the dosage of the hypoglycaemic agent.

Clinical evidence

A long-term study over the period 1955–1966 on a large number of women treated for a year or more with chlorpromazine in daily doses of 100 mg or more, showed that about 25% developed hyperglycaemia accompanied by glycosuria, compared with only about 9% in the control group who were not taking phenothazines of any kind. Of those given chlorpromazine, about a quarter showed complete remission of the symptoms when the chlorpromazine was withdrawn or the dosage reduced.[2]

There are numerous other reports of this response.[1,3–12,14,15] A single report is out of step in claiming that chlorpromazine has no effect at all on blood sugar levels.[13] Chlorpromazine in doses of less than 100 mg daily (50–70 mg) does not affect blood sugar levels significantly.[15]

Mechanism

It seems that chlorpromazine can inhibit the release of insulin, and possibly cause adrenaline (epinephrine) release from the adrenals, both of which could result in a rise in blood sugar levels.

Importance and management

A well-documented and long-established reaction first recognized in the early 1950's. The incidence is about 25% with daily doses of chlorpromazine of 100 mg or more. Increases in the dosage requirements of the hypoglycaemic agent should be anticipated during concurrent use. Smaller daily doses (50–70 mg) do not apparently cause hyperglycaemia. There seems to be no clinical evidence that other phenothiazines significantly disturb blood sugar levels in diabetics.

References

1 Hiles BH. Hyperglycaemia and glycosuria following chlorpromazine therapy. J Amer Med Ass (1956) 162, 1651.
2 Thonnard-Neumann E. Phenothazines and diabetes in hospitalized women. Am J Psychiat (1968) 124, 978.
3 Dobkin A, Lamoreux R and Gilbert RGB. Some studies with largactil. Can Med Ass J (1954) 2, 565.
4 Lancaster NP and Jones DH. Chlorpromazine and insulin in psychiatry. Br Med J (1954) 2, 565.
5 Glacobini F and Lassenius B. Chlorpromazine therapy in psychiatric practice: secondary effects and complications. Nord Med (1954) 52, 1693.
6 Moyer J, Kinross-Wright V and Finney RM. Chlorpromazine as a therapeutic agent in clinical medicine. Arch Int Med (1955) 95, 202.
7 Celice J, Porcher P and Plas S. Action de la chlorpromazine sur la vesicule biliare et le clon droit. Therapie (1955) 10, 30.
8 Charatan F and Bartlett N. The effect of chlorpromazine ('Largactil') on glucose tolerance. J Ment Sci (1955) 101, 351.
9 Cooperberg AA and Eidlow S. Haemolytic anaemia, jaundice and diabetes mellitus following chlorpromazine therapy. Can Med Ass J (1956) 75, 746.
10 Blair D and Brady DM. Recent advances in the treatment of schizophrenia: group training and tranquillizers. J Ment Sci (1958) 104. 625.
11 Amidsen A. Diabetes mellitus as a side-effect of treatment with tricyclic neuroleptics. Acta Psychiat Scand (1964) 40 (Suppl 180) 411.
12 Arneson G. Phenothiazine derivatives and glucose metabolism. J Neuropsychiatr (1964) 5, 181.
13 Schwarz L and Munoz R. Blood sugar levels in patients treated with chlorpromazine. Amer J Psychiat (1968) 125, 253.
14 Korenyl C and Lowenstein B. Chlorpromazine induced diabetes. Dis Ner Syst (1971) 32, 777.
15 Erle G, Basso M, Federspil G, Sicolo N and Scandellari C. Effect of chlorpromazine on blood glucose and plasma insulin in man. Eur J clin Pharmacol (1977) 11, 15.

Hypoglycaemic agents + Cimetidine or Ranitidine

Abstract/Summary

(i) Cimetidine can increase the hypoglycaemic effects of glipizide, gliclazide and possibly glibenclamide in diabetics and there is the risk of excessive hypoglycaemia. Ranitidine appears to behave similarly. The clinical relevance of other studies in normal subjects is uncertain: some report that no significant interactions occur in normal subjects with tolbutamide, glibenclamide, chlorpropamide or glipizide and cimetidine, whereas one says that the effects of glibenclamide are reduced by cimetidine and ranitidine. (ii) Cimetidine increases the serum levels of metformin.

Clinical evidence

(i:a) Studies in diabetic patients given sulphonylureas

Six diabetics were given 400 mg cimetidine 1 h before taking a dose of glipizide (average 5.7 mg dose) and then 3 h later they were given a standard meal with 200 mg of cimetidine. The expected rise in blood sugar levels after the meal was reduced by 40% and in three of the patients it fell to less than 3 mmol/l.[6] In another report an elderly diabetic taking 160 mg glipizide daily developed very low blood sugar levels (1 mmol/l) after starting treatment with 800 mg cimetidine daily.[7] A study in diabetics indicated that ranitidine can also increase the effects of glipizide.[8] Marked hypoglycaemia was seen in a patient on glibenclamide when treated with ranitidine.[10]

(i:b) Studies in normal subjects given sulphonylureas

A study in seven subjects, given 250 mg tolbutamide daily for four days, showed that when additionally given 800 mg cimetidine daily for a further four days the pharmacokinetics of the tolbutamide were not significantly changed.[3] Another study found no interaction between tolbutamide and cimetidine.[2] Other studies in normal subjects showed that 800 mg cimetidine daily for seven days had no significant effect on the serum levels or the pharmacokinetics of tolbutamide or chlorpropamide.[4] The hypoglycaemic activities of tolbutamide, chlorpropamide, glibenclamide and glipizide remained unaltered.[5] In contrast in another study the AUC of tolbutamide was found to be increased by 20% and the elimination half-life decreased by 17% by 1200 mg cimetidine, but plasma glucose levels were not significantly changed. Ranitidine had no effect.[1] Yet another study reported that the hypoglycaemic effects of glibenclamide were reduced by cimetidine and ranitidine.[9]

800 mg cimetidine daily was found to reduce the renal clearance of metformin in seven normal subjects by 27% and increase the AUC by 50%.[11]

Mechanism

If an interaction occurs[1] it may be because the cimetidine inhibits the metabolism of the sulphonylurea by the liver, thereby increasing its effects. Cimetidine appears to inhibit the excretion of metformin by the kidneys.[11]

Importance and management

(i) Information is limited and difficult to assess because of the differences between the sulphonylureas and between normal subjects and diabetics. Cimetidine and ranitidine are probably best avoided in diabetics taking glibenclamide, glipizide or gliclazide because of the risk of excessive hypoglycaemia unless the effects can be well monitored. Whether this is equally true for other sulphonylureas is less clear but certainly diabetics should be warned to watch for any evidence of hypoglycaemia or hyperglycaemia if cimetidine or ranitidine is added or withdrawn. More study is needed.

(ii) The metformin dosage may need to be reduced if cimetidine is used, bearing in mind the possibility of lactic acidosis if levels become too high. It is uncertain whether other H_2-blockers interact similarly.

References

1 Case EW, Rogers JF and Powell JR. Inhibition of tolbutamide elimination by cimetidine but not ranitidine. J Clin Pharmacol (1986) 26, 372–7.
2 Dey NG, Castleden CM, Ward J, Cornhill J and McBurney A. The effect of cimetidine on tolbutamide kinetics. Br J Clin Pharmacol (1983) 16, 438–440.
3 Stockley C, Keal J, Rolan P, Bochner F and Somogyi A. Lack of inhibition of tolbutamide hydroxylation by cimetidine in man. Eur J Clin Pharmacol (1986) 31, 235–7.
4 Shah GF, Ghandi TP, Patel PR, Patel MR, Gilbert RN and Shridhar PA. Tolbutamide and chlorpropamide kinetics in the presence of cimetidine in human volunteers. Indian Drugs (1985) 22, 455–8.
5 Shah GF, Ghandi TP, Patel PR, Patel MR, Gilbert RN and Shridhar PA. The effect of cimetidine on the hypoglycaemic activity of four commonly used sulphonylurea drugs. Indian Drugs (1985) 22, 570–2.
6 Feeley J and Peden N. Enhancement of sulphonylurea-induced hypoglycaemia with cimetidine. Br J Clin Pharmacol (1983) 15, 607.
7 Archambeaud-Mouveroux F, Nouaille Y, Nadalon S, Treves R and Merles L. Interaction between gliclazide and cimetidine. Eur J Clin Pharmacol (1987) 31, 631.
8 MacWalter RS, El Debani AH, Feeley J and Stevenson IH. Potentiation by ranitidine of the hypoglycaemic response to glipizide in diabetic patients. Br J clin Pharmac (1985) 21, 121–2P.
9 Kubacka RT, Antal EJ and Juhl RP. The paradoxical effects of cimetidine and ranitidine on glibenclamide pharmacokinetics and pharmacodynamics. Br J clin Pharmac (1987) 23, 743–51.
10 Leek K, Mize R and Lowenstein SR. Glyburide-induced hypoglycaemia and ranitidine. Ann Intern Med (1987) 107, 261–2.
11 Somogyi A, Stockley C, Keal J, Rolan P and Bochner F. Reduction of metformin renal tubular secretion by cimetidine in man. Br J clin Pharmac (1987) 23, 545–51.

Hypoglycaemic agents + Clofibrate

Abstract/Summary

(a) The effects of the sulphonylurea hypoglycaemic agents can be enhanced by clofibrate in some patients, possibly advantageously in those with poorly controlled diabetes. A reduction in the dosage of the hypoglycaemic agent may be necessary. (b) The antidiuretic effects of clofibrate in the treatment of diabetes insipidus are opposed by glibenclamide, and the diuretic effects of glibenclamide are opposed by carbamazepine and desmopressin.

Clinical evidence

(a) Increased hypoglycaemic effects

A study in 13 maturity-onset diabetics on various sulphonylureas (names not stated) showed that, over a five day period while taking 2 g clofibrate daily, the control of the diabetes was improved in six patients. Hypoglycaemia (blood glucose levels of 30–40 mg per 100 ml) was seen in four patients.[1]

Other studies confirm that some, but not all, patients show a fall in blood glucose levels while taking clofibrate and the control of the diabetes can improve.[2,3,4–6,8–11] One study showed that the clofibrate increased the half-life of chlorpropamide from 38 to 47 h.[1]

(b) Reduced antidiuretic effects

A study on 11 patients with pituitary diabetes insipidus showed that clofibrate reduced the volume of urine excreted, but when given with glibenclamide the volume increased once again. For example, one patient without treatment excreted 5.8 litre urine daily, but only 2.3 litre while taking 2 g clofibrate. Whereas with glibenclamide and clofibrate he excreted 3.61 litre daily. The action of glibenclamide was also found to be inhibited by carbamazepine and desmopressin (DDAVP).[12]

Mechanism

(a) Not understood. Among the suggestions are the displacement of the sulphonylureas from their plasma protein binding sites,[5] alterations in their renal excretion,[1] and a decrease in insulin resistance.[4,7] Clofibrate has also been shown to have a hypoglycaemic action of its own which improves the glucose tolerance of diabetics.[11] It seems possible that any or all of these mechanisms might contribute towards the enhanced hypoglycaemia which is seen.

(b) Not understood.

Importance and management

(a) The sulphonylurea–clofibrate interaction is established and well documented. The incidence is uncertain, but what is known suggests that between about a third and a half may be affected. Concurrent use need not be avoided, but patients should be monitored for excessive hypoglycaemia. Reduce the dosage of the hypoglycaemic agent if necessary. (b) Information about reduced diuretic effects is limited. It would seem prudent to avoid the concurrent use of drugs with actions which are antagonistic rather than additive.

References

1 Petitpierre B, Perrin L, Rudhardt M, Herrera A and Fabre J. Behaviour of chlorpropamide in renal insufficiency and under the effect of associated drug therapy. Int J Clin Pharmacol (1972) 6, 120.
2 Jain AK, Ryan JR and McMahon FG. Potentiation of hypoglycaemic effect of sulphonylureas by halofenate. N Engl J Med (1975) 293, 1284.
3 Daubresse J-C, Luyckx AS and Lefebrve P. Potentiation of hypoglycaemic effect of sulphonylureas by clofibrate. N Engl J Med (1976) 294, 613.
4 Ferrari C, Frezzati S, Testori GP and Bertazzoni A. Potentiation of hypoglycaemic response to intravenous tolbutamide by clofibrate. N Engl J Med (1976) 294, 1184.
5 Jain AK, Ryan JR and McMahon FG. Potentiation of hypoglycaemic effect of sulphonylureas by clofibrate. N Engl J Med (1976) 294, 613.
6 Daubresse J-C, Daigneux D, Bruwler M, Luyckx A and Lefebrve PJ. Clofibrate and diabetes control in patients treated with oral hypoglycaemic agents. Br J clin Pharmac (1979) 7, 599.
7 Ferrari C, Frezzati S, Romussi M, Bertazzoni A, Testori GP, Antonini S and Paracchi A. Effect of short-term clofibrate administration on glucose tolerance and insulin secretion in patients with chemical diabetes or hypertriglyceridaemia. Metabolism (1977) 26, 129.
8 Miller RD. Atromid in the treatment of post-climacteric diabetes. J Atheroscler Res (1963) 3, 694.
9 Csogor SI and Bornemisza P. The effect of clofibrate (Atromid) on intravenous tolbutamide, oral and intravenous glucose tolerance tests. Clin Trials J (1977) 14, 15.
10 Herriott SC, Percy-Robb IW, Strong JA and Thompson CG. The effect of Atromid on serum cholesterol and glucose tolerance in diabetes mellitus. J Atheroscler Res (1963) 3, 679.
11 Barnett D, Craig JG, Robinson DS and Rogers MP. Effect of clofibrate on glucose tolerance in maturity-onset diabetics. Br J clin Pharmac (1977) 4, 455.
12 Rado JP, Szende L, Marosi J, Juhos E, Sawinsky I and Tako J. Inhibition of the diuretic action of glibenclamide by clofibrate, carbamazepine and 1-deamino-8-D-arginine-vasopressin (DDAVP) in patients with pituitary diabetes insipidus. Acta diabet lat (1974) 11, 179.

Hypoglycaemic agents + Clonidine

Abstract/Summary

There is evidence that clonidine may possibly suppress the signs and symptoms of hypoglycaemia in diabetic patients

Clinical evidence, mechanism, importance and management

Studies in normal subjects and patients with hypertension showed that their normal response to hypoglycaemia (tachycardia, palpitations, perspiration) caused by a dose of insulin was markedly reduced when they were taking 0.45–0.9 mg clonidine daily.[1,2] The reason is that clonidine depresses the output of the catecholamines (adrenaline, noradrenaline) which are secreted in an effort to raise blood sugar levels and which are also responsible for these signs. It seems possible that clonidine will similarly suppress the signs and symptoms of hypoglycaemia which can occur in diabetics, but this appears not to have been reported. Nevertheless diabetic patients should be warned.

References

1 Hedeland H, Dymling J-F and Hokfelt A. The effect of insulin induced hypoglycaemia on plasma renin activity and urinary catecholamines before and following clonidine (Catapresan) in man. Acta Endocrinol (1972) 71, 321–33.
2 Hedeland H, Dymling J-F and Hokfelt A. Pharmacological inhibition of adrenaline secretion following insulin-induced hypoglycaemia in man: the effect of Catapresan. Acta Endocrinol (1971) 67, 97–103.

Hypoglycaemic agents + Contraceptives (oral)

Abstract/Summary

Some diabetics may require small increases or decreases in their dosage of hypoglycaemic agent while taking oral contraceptives, but it is unusual for the control of diabetes to be seriously disturbed.

Clinical evidence

More than half of a group of 30 menopausal diabetics showed abnormal tolerance when given an oral contraceptive (norethynodrel 5 mg+mestranol 0.075 mg) but the changes in their requirements of insulin or oral hypoglycaemic agent were '...few, scattered and slight in magnitude.'[1]

34% of a group[2] of 179 diabetic women needed an increase in insulin and 7% a decrease when given a variety of oral contraceptives, whereas in another group of 38 insulin dependent diabetics it was found that progestogen-only and combined oral contraceptives had little effect on the control of diabetes.[8] Another report[3] about women on *Orthonovin* (norethisterone + mestranol) stated that no insulin changes were necessary. In contrast there are a few scattered reports of individual diabetics who experienced a marked disturbance of their diabetic control when given an oral contraceptive.[4–6]

Mechanism

Not understood. Many mechanisms have been considered including changes in cortisol secretion, alterations in tissue glucose utilization, production of excesssive amounts of growth hormone, alterations in liver function, and others.[7]

Importance and management

Moderately well documented. Concurrent use need not be avoided, but because some patients need a small adjustment in their dosage of hypoglycaemic agent (increases or decreases) and because very occasionally serious disturbances occur, the diabetic response should be monitored.

References

1 Cochran B and Pote WWH. C-19 nor-steroid effects on plasma lipid and diabetic control of postmenopausal women. Diabetes (1963) 12, 366.
2 Zeller WJ, Brehm H, Schoffling K and Melzer H. Vertraglichkeit von

hormonalen Ovulationshemmern bei Diabetikerinnen. Arzneim-Forsch (1974) 24, 351.

3 Tyler ET, Olsen HJ, Gotlib M, Levin M and Behne D. Long term usage of norethindrone with mestranol preparations in the control of human fertility. Clin Med (1964) 71, 997.

4 Kopera H, Dukes NG and Ijzerman GL. Critical evaluation of clinical data on Lyndiol. Int J Fertil (1964) 9, 69.

5 Peterson WF, Stell MW and Coyne RY. Analysis of the effect of ovulatory suppressants on glucose tolerance. Amer J Obst Gyn (1966) 95, 484.

6 Reder JA and Tulgan H. Impairment of diabetic control by norethynodrel with mestranol. NY State J Med (1967) 67, 1073.

7 Spellacy WN. A review of carbohydrate metabolism and the oral contraceptives. Amer J Obst Gynecol (1969) 104, 448.

8 Radberg T, Gustafson A, Skryten A and Karlsson K. Oral contraception in diabetic women. Diabetes control, serum and high density lipoprotein lipids during low-dose progestogen, combined oestrogen/progestogen and non-hormonal contraception. Acta Endocrinol (1981) 98, 246–51.

Hypoglycaemic agents + Corticosteroids

Abstract/Summary

The blood sugar lowering effects of the hypoglycaemic agents are opposed by the concurrent use of corticosteroids with glucocorticoid (hyperglycaemic) activity. It may be necessary to raise the dosage of the hypoglycaemic agent appropriately.

Clinical evidence, mechanism, importance and management

Corticosteroids with glucocorticoid activity can raise blood sugar levels and induce diabetes.[1] This can oppose the blood sugar lowering effects of the hypoglycaemic agents used in the treatment of diabetes mellitus. For example, a study in five diabetics showed that a single 200 mg dose of cortisone modified their glucose tolerance curves while taking an unstated amount of chlorpropamide. The blood glucose levels of four of them rose (three showed an initial fall), whereas in a previous test with chlorpropamide alone the blood sugar levels of four of them had fallen.[2] This almost certainly reflects a direct antagonism between the pharmacological effects of the two drugs, and this would seem to be confirmed by a study in normal subjects which showed that another glucocorticoid corticosteroid, prednisone, had no significant effect on the metabolism or clearance of tolbutamide.[3]

There are very few studies of this interaction, probably because the hyperglycaemic activity of the corticosteroids has been known for such a long time that the outcome of concurrent use is self-evident. The effects of corticosteroid treatment in diabetics (using insulin or oral hypoglycaemic agents) should be closely monitored and the dosage of the hyperglycaemic agent raised as necessary. Hypoglycaemic agents are sometimes deliberately given to non-diabetic patients taking corticosteroids to reduce blood sugar levels.

References

1 David DS, Cheigh JS, Braun DW, Fotino M, Stenzel KH and Rubin AL. HLA-A28 and steroid-induced diabetes in renal transplant patients. J Amer Med Ass (1980) 423, 532–3.

2 Danowski TS, Mateer FM and Moses C. Cortisone enhancement of peripheral utilization of glucose and the effects of chlorpropamide. Ann NY Acad Sci (1959) 74, 988.

3 Breimer DD, Zilly W and Richter E. Influence of corticosteroids on hexobarbital and tolbutamide disposition. Clin Pharmacol Ther (1978) 24, 208.

Hypoglycaemic agents + Cytotoxics

Abstract/Summary

Colaspase (L-asparaginase) sometimes induces diabetes mellitus. Changes in the hypoglycaemic agent dosage requirements seems a possibility in some diabetic patients. There is also evidence that the control of diabetes can also be severely disturbed in patients given cyclophosphamide.

Clinical evidence, mechanisms

Colaspase (L-asparaginase)

Three patients with acute lymphocytic leukaemia developed diabetes after treatment with colaspase (asparaginase): two of them two and four days after a single dose of colaspase, and another patient two days after the fourth dose. Plasma insulin was undetectable. A normal insulin reponse returned in one patient after 23 days, whereas the other two showed a suboptimal reponse two weeks and nine months afterwards.[1] In another study, five out of 39 patients developed hyperglycaemia and glycosuria after treatment with colaspase.[2] The reasons are not understood but suggestions include inhibition of insulin synthesis,[5] direct damage to the Islets of Langerhans,[1] and reduced insulin binding.[5]

Cyclophosphamide

Acute hypoglycaemia has been described in two diabetic patients under treatment with insulin and carbutamide who were concurrently treated with cyclophosphamide.[3] Three cases of diabetes, apparently induced by the use of cyclophosphamide, have also been reported.[4] The reasons are not understood.

Importance and management

Strictly speaking none of these reactions is probably an interaction, but they serve to underline the importance of monitoring the diabetic control of patients receiving either colaspase or cyclophosphamide.

References

1 Gailani S, Nussbaum A, Takao O and Freeman A. Diabetes in patients treated with asparaginase. Clin Pharmacol Ther (1971) 12, 487.

2 Ohnuma T, Holland JF, Freeman A and Sinks L. Biochemical and pharmacological studies with asparaginase in man. Cancer Res (1970) 30, 2297.

3 Kruger H-U. Blutzuckersenkende Wirkung von Cyclophosphamid bei Diabetikern. Med Klin (1966) 61, 1462.
4 Pengelly CR. Diabetes mellitus and cyclophosphamide. Br Med J (1965) 1, 1312.
5 Burghen G, Pui C-H, Yasuda K and Kitabchi AE. Decreased insulin binding and production: probable mechanism for hyperglycaemia due to therapy with prednisone (PRED) and l-asparaginase (ASP). Ped Res (1981) 15, 626.

Hypoglycaemic agents + Dextropropoxyphene

Abstract/Summary

Dextropropoxyphene does not interact with tolbutamide.

Clinical evidence, mechanism, importance and management

A study in six normal subjects showed that after taking 65 mg dextropropoxyphene eight-hourly for four days the clearance of tolbutamide (500 mg given IV) was not affected.[1] There would seem to be no reason for avoiding concurrent use or for taking particular precautions. There seems to be no evidence of an interaction between dextropropoxyphene and any other hypoglycaemic agent.

Reference

1 Robson RA, Miners JO, Whitehead AG and Birkett DJ. Specificity of the inhibitory effect of dextropropoxyphene on oxidative drug metabolism in man: effects on theophylline and tolbutamide disposition. Br J clin Pharmac (1987) 23, 772–5.

Hypoglycaemic agents + Disulfiram

Abstract/Summary

Disulfiram does not interact with tolbutamide and there appears to be no evidence that it interacts with any other hypoglycaemic agent.

Clinical evidence, mechanism, importance and management

Studies on 10 normal subjects showed that disulfiram (first day 400 mg three times; second day 400 mg; third and fourth days 200 mg) had no significant effect on the half-life or clearance of tolbutamide given intravenously.[1]

Reference

1 Svendsen TL, Kristensen MB, Hansen JM and Skovsted L. The influence of disulfiram on the half-life and metabolic clearance rate of diphenylhydantoin and tolbutamide in man. Eur J clin Pharmacol (1976) 9, 439.

Hypoglycaemic agents + Ethacrynic acid

Abstract/Summary

Ethacrynic acid can raise blood sugar levels in diabetics which opposes to some extent the effects of the hypoglycaemic agents, but the clinical importance of this seems to be small.

Clinical evidence and mechanism

A double-blind study on 24 hypertensive patients, one third of whom were diabetics, showed that daily treatment with 200 mg ethacrynic acid over a 6-week period impaired their glucose tolerance and raised the blood sugar levels of those who were diabetic to the same extent as those taking hydrochlorothiazide.[1] In another study[2] no changes in carbohydrate metabolism was seen in six diabetics given 150 mg ethacrynic acid daily for a week. The reasons are not understood.

Importance and management

Information is very limited indeed. Some impairment of the glucose tolerance may possibly occur, but there seems to be a singular lack of evidence in the literature to show that normally ethacrynic acid has much effect on the control of diabetes in most patients. Nevertheless it would be prudent to monitor the effects of concurrent use.

References

1 Russell RP, Lindeman RD and Prescott LF. Metabolic and hypotensive effects of ethacrynic acid. Comparative study with hydrochlorothiazide. J Amer Med Ass (1968) 205, 81.
2 Dige-Petersen H. Ethacrynic acid and carbohydrate metabolism. Nord Med (1966) 75, 123–5.

Hypoglycaemic agents + Fenfluramine

Abstract/Summary

Fenfluramine has inherent hypoglycaemic activity which can add to, or in some instances replace, the effects of conventional hypoglycaemic agents.

Clinical evidence, mechanism, importance and management

A study in a group of obese maturity-onset diabetics who were given either fenfluramine (initially 40 mg daily increased over four weeks to 160 mg) or a placebo showed that four of the six were better controlled than when previously taking a biguanide hypoglycaemic agent.[1] The hypoglycaemic effects of fenfluramine are described elsewhere.[2,4] It seems that fenfluramine increases the uptake of glucose into skeletal muscle, thereby lowering blood glucose levels.[3,4]

This is a well established and, on the whole, an advantageous rather than an adverse reaction, but it would be prudent to check on the extent of the response if fenfluramine is added or withdrawn from the treatment being received by diabetics.

References

1 Jackson WPU. Fenfluramine trials in a diabetic clinic. S Afr med J (1971) (Suppl), 29.
2 Turtle JR and Burgess JA. Hypoglycaemic effect of fenfluramine in diabetes mellitus. Diabetes (1973) 22, 858.
3 Kirby MJ and Turner P. Effect of amphetamine, fenfluramine and norfenfluramine on glucose uptake into human isolated skeletal muscle. Fr J clin Pharmac (1974) 1, 340P.
4 Dykes JRW. The effect of a low-calorie diet with and without fenfluramine, and fenfluramine alone on the glucose tolerance and insulin secretion of overweight non-diabetics. Postgrad med J (1973) 49, 314.

Hypoglycaemic agents + Frusemide

Abstract/Summary

The control of diabetes is not usually disturbed by the concurrent use of frusemide, although there are a few reports showing that it can sometimes raise blood sugar levels.

Clinical evidence, mechanism, importance and management

Although frusemide can elevate blood sugar levels[1] (but to a much lesser extent than the thiazide diuretics), worsen glucose tolerance tests[5] and occasionally cause glycosuria and even acute diabetes in individual patients,[2] the general picture is that the control of diabetes is not usually affected by the use of frusemide.[3] It has been described as the 'diuretic of choice for the diabetic patient.'[4] Even so, prescribers should be aware of its hyperglycaemic potentialities.

References

1 Hutcheon DE and Leonard G. Diuretic and antihypertensive action of frusemide. J Clin Pharmac (1967) 7, 26.
2 Toivnonen S and Mustala O. Diabetogenic action of frusemide. Br Med J (1966) 1, 920.
3 Bencomo L, Fyvolent J, Kahana S and Kahana L. Clinical experience with a new diuretic, furosemide. Curr Ther Res (1965) 7, 339.
4 Malins JM. Diuretics in diabetes mellitus. Practitioner (1968) 201, 529.
5 Breckenridge A, Welborn TA, Dollery CT and Frazer R. Glucose tolerance in hypertensive patients on long-term diuretic therapy. Lancet (1967) i, 61–4.

Hypoglycaemic agents + Gemfibrozil

Abstract/Summary

Gemfibrozil does not cause a significant change in the control of diabetes treated with oral hypoglycaemic agents or insulin.

Clinical evidence, mechanism, importance and management

A study in diabetic patients treated with insulin (1), acetohexamide (4), chlorpropamide (6) or glipizide (1) found that the control of their diabetes was not impaired and even slightly improved when concurrently treated with gemfibrozil (800 mg daily initially, reduced later to 400–600 mg daily).[1] A later study found that a slight increase in the oral hypoglycaemic agent dosage was needed.[2] Neither of these studies nor any other report suggests that an interaction of clinical importance occurs.

References

1 De Salcedo I, Gorringe JAL, Silva JL and Santos JA. Gemfibrozil in a group of diabetics. Proc Roy Soc Med (1976) 69, Suppl 2, 64–70.
2 Kontinnen A, Kuisma I, Ralli R, Pohjola S and Ojala K. The effect of gemfibrozil on serum lipids in diabetic patients. Ann Clin Res (1979) 11, 240–5.

Hypoglycaemic agents + Guanethidine and related drugs

Abstract/Summary

Guanethidine has hypoglycaemic activity which may possibly add to the effects of conventional hypoglycaemic agents. Soluble insulin may also exaggerate the hypotensive effects of debrisoquine.

Clinical evidence, mechanism

(a) Hypoglycaemia increased

A diabetic needed an insulin increase from 70 to 94 units daily when guanethidine was withdrawn.[1] A later study on three maturity-onset diabetics showed that guanethidine in daily doses of 50–90 mg caused a significant improvement in their glucose tolerance.[2] Other reports also describe the hypoglycaemic effects of guanethidine in man.[3,4] A suggested reason is that guanethidine can impair the homeostatic mechanism concerned with raising blood sugar levels by affecting the release of catecholamines. The balance of the system thus impaired tends to be tipped in favour of a reduced blood sugar level, resulting in a reduction in hypoglycaemic agent needs.

(b) Hypotension increased

An insulin-dependent man taking debrisoquine (20 mg twice daily) developed severe postural hypotension within an hour of using a short-acting insulin (28 units soluble insulin + 20 units isophane insulin). He became dizzy and was found to have a standing blood pressure of 97/72 mm Hg. The postural fall in systolic pressure was 65 mm Hg. He had no evidence of hypoglycaemia and no hypotension when using 48 units of isophane insulin.[4] Insulin can cause hypotension but this is only seen in those with an impaired reflex control of blood pressure.[5]

Importance and management

Information about the guanethidine-insulin interaction is limited, the case cited being the only one describing an adverse response. Check on the dosage requirements of the hypoglycaemic agent if guanethidine or related drugs (bethanidine, guanadrel, debrisoquine, etc.) are started or stopped. Also check patients given debrisoquine and insulin, particularly if they are taking vasodilators, to ensure that excessive hypotension does not develop.

References

1 Gupta KK and Lillicrap CA. Guanethidine and diabetes. Br Med J (1968) 2, 697.
2 Gupta KK. The antidiabetic action of guanethidine. Postgrad Med J (1969) 45, 455.
3 Kansal PC, Buse J and Durling FC. Effect of guanethidine and reserpine on glucose tolerance. Curr Ther Res (1971) 13, 517.
4 Woeber KA, Arky R and Braverman LE. Reversal by guanethidine of abnormal oral glucose tolerance in thyrotoxicosis. Lancet (1966) i, 895.
5 Hume L. Potentiation of hypotensive effect of debrisoquine by insulin. Diabetic Medicine (1985) 2, 390–1.

Hypoglycaemic agents + Halofenate

Abstract/Summary

Halofenate can enhance the blood sugar lowering effects of chlorpropamide, tolbutamide, tolazamide and phenformin in some patients. The dosage of the hypoglycaemic agent may need to be reduced to avoid excessive hypoglycaemia.

Clinical evidence

A double-blind trial over 48 weeks on diabetics with type IV hyperlipoproteinaemia showed that halofenate (0.5 to 1.5 g) enhanced the effects of the sulphonylureas and biguanides in some patients. The reductions in the dosage of the hypoglycaemic agents were as follows: chlorpropamide 80% (four patients), tolazamide 46% (four patients), phenformin 33% (five patients). No change was needed in two patients taking insulin. Some of the patients taking the sulphonylureas were also given phenformin. A study in 12 normal subjects also showed that halofenate increased serum tolbutamide levels and decreased blood sugar levels.[1]

Similar results have been described in another study.[2]

Mechanism

Not understood. One suggestion is that the halofenate displaces the sulphonylureas from their protein binding sites in the plasma, thereby increasing the biological activity.[1] As a full explanation this seems unlikely because the full effects take up to a month to develop.

Importance and management

An established interaction. Concurrent use need not be avoided. The dosage of the hypoglycaemic agent can be reduced with full control of the diabetes, but the interaction may take 2–4 weeks to develop fully. Not all patients may show this interaction.[1,2] Excessive hypoglycaemia has not been reported, but the possibility should be borne in mind. Information about other hypoglycaemic agents appears to be lacking.

References

1 Jain AK, Ryan JR and McMahon FG. Potentiation of hypoglycaemic effect of sulphonylureas by halofenate. N Engl J Med (1975) 293, 1283–6.
2 Kudzma DJ and Friedenberg SJ. Potentiation of hypoglycaemic effect of chlorpropamide and phenformin by halofenate. Diabetes (1977) 26, 291.

Hypoglycaemic agents + Heparin

Abstract/Summary

Two reports describe hypoglycaemia in a diabetic on glipizide and another on glibenclamide attributed to concurrent treatment with heparin.

Clinical evidence, mechanism, importance and management

A diabetic, treated for six months with glipizide with fair control, experienced recurring episodes of hypoglycaemia over a period of four days after a single 5 mg dose of glipizide while hospitalized for the treatment of peripheral vascular disease. It was suggested that this might possibly have been due to an interaction with subcutaneous heparin calcium (5000 U every 12 h) which, it is postulated, might have displaced the glipizide from its protein binding sites.[1] The patient was also treated with diamorphine. Another very brief report describes hypoglycaemia in a patient treated with glibenclamide and heparin.[2] Concurrent use should be monitored.

References

1 McKillop G, Fallon M and Slater SD. Possible interaction between heparin and a sulphonylurea: a cause of prolonged hypoglycaemia? Brit Med J (1986) 293, 1073,
2 Beeley L, Daly M and Stewart P. Bulletin of the West Midlands Centre for Adverse Drug Reaction Reporting. (1987) 24, 24.

Hypoglycaemic agents + Isoniazid

Abstract/Summary

Some reports state that isoniazid can raise blood sugar levels in diabetics, whereas one describes a fall. The outcome of concurrent use is uncertain. The dosage of the hypoglycaemic agent may possibly need to be adjusted to control the diabetes adequately.

Clinical evidence

A study on six diabetics taking insulin showed that while taking 250–400 mg isoniazid daily their fasting blood sugar levels were raised 40% (from an average of 255 to 357 mg%), and their glucose tolerance curves rose and returned to normal levels more slowly. After six days treatment the average rise was only 20%. Two other patients needed an increased dosage of insulin while taking 200 mg isoniazid daily, but a reduction when the isoniazid was withdrawn.[1]

Another report describes glycosuria and the development of frank diabetes in three out of 50 patients given 300 mg isoniazid daily,[2] and hyperglycaemia has been seen in cases of isoniazid poisoning.[3]

In contrast, a study in six out of eight diabetics[4] showed that isoniazid can have a hypoglycaemic effect. A 500 mg dose of isoniazid caused an 18% (range 5–34%) reduction in blood sugar levels after 4 h; 3 mg tolbutamide caused a 28% (19–43%) reduction, and together they caused a 35% (17–57%) reduction. One patient however showed a 10% increase after isoniazid, a 41% decrease after tolbutamide, and a 30% decrease after taking both. The other diabetic responded to neither drug.

Mechanism

Not understood.

Importance and management

The major documentation for these reactions dates back to the 1950's, since when the literature has been virtually (and perhaps significantly?) silent. The outcome of concurrent use is therefore somewhat uncertain. Nevertheless it would be prudent for diabetics given isoniazid to be monitored for changes in the control of the diabetes. Appropriate dosage adjustments (up or down?) of the hypoglycaemic agent should be made where necessary.

References

1 Luntz GRWN and Smith SG. Effect of isoniazid on carbohydrate metabolism in controls and diabetics. Br Med J (1953) 1, 296.
2 Dickson I. Glycosuria and diabetes mellitus following INAH therapy. Med J Aust (1962) 49, 325.
3 Tovarys A and Siler Z. Diabetic syndrome and intoxication with INH. Prakt Lekar (1968) 48, 286; quoted in Int Pharm Abs (1968) 5, 286.
4 Seggara FO, Sherman DS and Charif BS. Experiences with tolbutamide and chlorpropamide in tuberculous diabetic patients. Ann NY Acad Sci (1959) 74, 656.

Hypoglycaemic agents + Lithium carbonate

Abstract/Summary

Lithium carbonate can raise blood sugar levels and in some instances cause the development of diabetes mellitus, but there is little or no evidence that its use normally disturbs the control of diabetes significantly.

Clinical evidence, mechanism, importance and management

A study in 10 psychiatric patients showed that when treated with lithium carbonate for two weeks their blood glucose levels were raised and their glucose tolerance tests impaired.[1] Other reports describe the development of hyperglycaemia and frank diabetes mellitus in patients treated with lithium carbonate.[2–4]

Although there appear to be no reports of disturbed diabetic control in diabetics treated with lithium carbonate (any marked effect might be expected to have been reported by now), it would seem prudent to monitor the response if lithium is added to the treatment being received by diabetic patients.

References

1 Shopsin B, Stern S and Gershon S. Altered carbohydrate metabolism during treatment with lithium carbonate. Arch Gen Psychiat (1972) 26, 566–71.
2 Craig J, Abu-Saleh M, Smith B and Evans I. Diabetes mellitus in patients on lithium. Lancet (1977) ii, 1028.
3 Johnstone BB. Diabetes mellitus in patients on lithium. Lancet (1977) ii, 935.
4 Martinez-Maldone M and Terrell J. Lithium carbonate-induced nephrogenic diabetes insipidus and glucose intolerance. Arch Intern Med (1973) 132, 881–4.

Hypoglycaemic agents + Methysergide

Abstract/Summary

A preliminary study indicates that methysergide may enhance the activity of tolbutamide.

Clinical evidence, mechanism, importance and management

A study of eight maturity-onset diabetics showed that two days' pretreatment with methysergide (2 mg six-hourly) increased the amount of insulin secreted in response to 1 g tolbutamide given intravenously by almost 40%.[1] Whether in practice the addition or withdrawal of methysergide adversely affects the control of diabetes is uncertain, but prescribers should be aware of this reaction.

Reference

1 Baldridge JA, Quickel KE, Feldman JM and Lebovitz HE. Potentiation of tolbutamide-mediated insulin release in adult onset diabetics by methysergide maleate. Diabetes (1974) 23, 21.

Hypoglycaemic agents + Mianserin

Abstract/Summary

The control of diabetes appears to be unaffected by the use of mianserin.

Clinical evidence, mechanism, importance and management

Although there is some evidence of a change in glucose metabolism during treatment with mianserin,[1,2,4] the alteration failed to affect the control of diabetes in 10 subjects under study and there appear to be no reports of adverse effects caused by concurrent use.[3]

References

1 Fell PJ, Quantock DC and van der Burg WJ. The human pharmacology of GB94—a new psychotropic agent. Eur J clin Pharmac (1973) 5, 166.
2 Peet M and Behagel H. Mianserin: a decade of scientific development. Br J clin Pharmac (1978) 5, 5S.
3 Weinges A. Unpublished data quoted in ref. 2.
4 Moonie J. Unpublished data quoted by Brogden RN, Heel RC, Speight TM and Avery GS. Mianserin: a review of its pharmacological properties and therapeutic efficacy in depressive illness. Drugs (1978) 16, 273.

Hypoglycaemic agents + Miconazole

Abstract/Summary

Hypoglycaemia has been seen in diabetics taking tolbutamide, glibenclamide or gliclazide when they were concurrently treated with miconazole.

Clinical evidence, mechanism, importance and management

A diabetic patient taking tolbutamide was hospitalized with severe hypoglycaemia about 10 days after starting to take miconazole.[1] The French Commission Nationale de Pharmacovigilance has on record six reports of diabetics on sulphonylureas who also developed hypoglycaemia within 2–6 days of beginning treatment with miconazole.[1] Five occurred with gliclazide and one with glibenclamide. Three other cases (two on gliclazide and one on glibenclamide) are reported elsewhere in patients given miconazole (250–1250 mg daily).[2] The mechanism of this interaction is not understood.

Information is limited to these reports. Concurrent use should be avoided unless the outcome can be monitored and the dosage of the sulphonylurea reduced as necessary. Information about other sulphonylureas is lacking but it seems possible that they may interact similarly.

References

1 Meurice JC, Lecomte P, Renard JP and Girard JJ. Interaction miconazole et sulfamides hypoglycemiants. La Presse Medicale. (1983) 12, 1670.
2 Loupi E, Descotes J, Lery N and Evreux JCl. Interactions medicamenteuses et miconazole. A propos de 10 observations. Therapie (1982) 37, 437–41.

Hypoglycaemic agents + Monoamine oxidase inhibitors (MAOI)

Abstract/Summary

The hypoglycaemic effects of insulin and the oral hypoglycaemic agents can be increased by the concurrent use of the MAOI. This may improve the control of blood sugar levels in most diabetics, but in a few it may cause undesirable hypoglycaemia which can be controlled by reducing the dosage of the hypoglycaemic agent.

Clinical evidence

A woman diabetic, stabilized on insulin-zinc suspension, exhibited hypoglycaemic sopors and postural syncope when treated with 15–25 mg mebanazine daily. She required a 30% reduction in the dosage of insulin (from 48 to 35 units daily) to achieve restabilization. Her insulin requirements rose once again when the mebanazine was withdrawn.[1]

Other reports on diabetics showed that the concurrent use of mebanazine increased the hypoglycaemic activity of insulin, tolbutamide or chlorpropamide, and improved the control of their diabetes.[2–5]

Mechanism

Not fully understood. A reduction in blood sugar levels has been demonstrated in man in the absence of conventional hypoglycaemic agents with mebanazine,[3] iproniazid,[6] isocarboxazid,[7] and phenelzine,[3] possibly due to some direct action by the MAOI on the pancreas which causes the release of insulin.[8] It would seem that this can be additive with the effects of the conventional hypoglycaemics.

Importance and management

An established interaction, of only moderate clinical importance. It can benefit the control of diabetes in many patients, but some individuals may need a reduction in their hypoglycaemic agent dosage to avoid excessive hypoglycaemia. The effects of concurrent use should be monitored. Only a few MAOI-hypoglycaemic agent combinations appear to have been examined, but this interaction would seem possible with any of them. This requires confirmation.

References

1 Cooper AJ and Keddie KMG. Hypotensive collapse and hypoglycaemia after mebanazine—a monoamine oxidase inhibitor. Lancet (1964) i, 1133.
2 Wickstrom L and Pettersson K. Treatment of diabetics with monoamine oxidase inhibitors. Lancet (1964) ii, 995.
3 Adnitt PI. Hypoglycaemic actions of monoamine oxidase inhibitors (MAOI's). Diabetes (1968) 17, 628.
4 Cooper AJ. The action of mebanazine, a monoamine oxidase inhibitor antidepressant drug in diabetes—part II. Int J Neuropsychiatry (1966) 2, 342.
5 Adnitt PI, Oleesky S and Schneiden H. The hypoglycaemic action of monoamine oxidase inhibitors (MAOI's). Diabetologia (1968) 4, 379.
6 Weiss J, Weiss J and Weiss B. Effects of iproniazid and similar compounds on the gastrointestinal tract. Ann NY Acad Sci (1959) 80, 854.
7 Van Praag HM and Leijnse B. The influence of some antidepressives of the hydrazine type on the glucose metabolism in depressed patients. Clin Chim Acta (1963) 8, 466.
8 Bressler R, Vargas-Cordon M and Lebovitz HE. Tranylcypromine: a potent insulin secretagogue and hypoglycaemic agent. Diabetes (1968) 17, 617.

Hypoglycaemic agents + Non-steroidal anti-inflammatory drugs (NSAID's)

Abstract/Summary

No adverse interactions have been shown to occur between chlorpropamide or tolbutamide and ibuprofen; glibenclamide and acemetacin, diclofenac or tolmetin; glipizide or tolbutamide and indoprofen; or between tolbutamide and diflunisal or sulindac. A report describes severe hypoglycaemia in a patient given fenclofenac with chlorpropamide and metformin. Indobufen increases the effects of glipizide. See the Index for interactions with azapropazone, phenylbutazone, oxyphenbutazone and the salicylates.

Clinical evidence

(a) Chlorpropamide or tolbutamide + ibuprofen

1200 mg ibuprofen had no significant effect on the blood sugar levels of diabetic patients taking 62.5–375 mg chlorpropamide daily.[7] In other patients on tolbutamide it was found that ibuprofen lowered fasting blood sugar levels, but not below the normal lower limits.[8]

(b) Chlorpropamide + fenclofenac or flurbiprofen

A woman diabetic, well controlled on 500 mg chlorpropamide and 850 mg metformin daily, developed hypoglycaemia within two days of exchanging flurbiprofen plus indomethacin for 1200 mg fenclofenac daily. The hypoglycaemic agents were withdrawn the next day, but later in the evening she went into a hypoglycaemic coma. The reasons for this are not understood.[5]

(c) Glibenclamide + acemetacin, diclofenac or tolmetin

The blood sugar levels of 12 glibenclamide-treated diabetics with rheumatic diseases remained unchanged when they were concurrently treated with 150 mg diclofenac daily for four days,[2] nor were any changes seen in the blood sugar levels of 40 other diabetics given 1200 mg tolmetin daily for five days.[6] No changes in the control of diabetes was seen in 20 patients on glibenclamide when concurrently treated with 60 mg acemetacin three times daily.[12]

(d) Glipizide + indobufen

Six normal subjects showed a rise in serum glipizide levels when treated with 200 mg indobufen for 15 days and blood sugar levels were lowered.[11]

(e) Glipizide or tolbutamide + indoprofen

No important changes in blood sugar levels occurred in 24 diabetic patients on tolbutamide or glipizide when given 600 mg indoprofen daily for five days.[10] A single dose study showed that although 200 mg indoprofen lowered the plasma levels of 5 mg glipizide, the blood sugar levels remained unaffected.[9]

(f) Tolbutamide + diflunisal or sulindac

A brief report states that no changes in serum tolbutamide or in fasting blood glucose levels were seen in diabetics given 375 mg diflunisal twice daily.[3,4] 12 maturity-onset tolbutamide-treated diabetics demonstrated no changes in tolbutamide half-life, serum levels, time-to-peak or AUC when given 400 mg sulindac daily. An unimportant reduction in fasting blood sugar levels was seen.[1]

Importance and management

Information is limited. No adverse interaction appears to occur between the oral hypoglycaemic agents and most of the NSAID's cited here. The general silence in the literature would suggest that this is true for many NSAID's, but this requires confirmation. Some caution is needed with fenclofenac and indobufen. However adverse interactions can certainly occur between hypoglycaemic agents and azapropazone, phenylbutazone, oxyphenbutazone and salicylates, details of which are given in the appropriate synopses.

References

1 Ryan JR, Jain MD, McMahon FG and Vargas R. On the question of an interaction between sulindac and tolbutamide in the treatment of diabetes. Clin Pharmacol Ther (1976) 21, 231.
2 Chlud K, von. Untersuchungen zur Wechselwirkung von Diclofenac und Glibenclamid. Zeit Rheumatologie (1976) 35, 377.
3 Tempero KF, Cirillo VJ and Steelman SL. Diflunisal: a review of the pharmacokinetic and pharmacodynamic properties, drug interactions, and special tolerability studies in human. Br J Clin Pharmac (1977) 4, 31S.
4 McMahon FG and Ryan JR. Unpublished observations quoted in ref. 3.
5 Allen PA and Taylor RT. Fenclofenac and thyroid function tests. Brit Med J (1980) 281, 1642.
6 Chlud K and Kaik B. Clinical studies of the interaction between tolmetin and glibenclamide. J Clin Pharmacol (1977) 15, 409.
7 Shah SJ, Bhandarkar SD and Satoskar RS. Drug interaction between

chlorpropamide and non-steroidal anti-inflammatory drugs, ibuprofen and phenylbutazone. Int J Clin Pharmacol Ther Toxicol (1984) 22, 470–2.

8 Andersen LA. Ibuprofen and tolbutamide drug interaction study. Br J Clin Pract (1980) 34 (Suppl 6) 10.

9 Melander A and Wahlin-Boll E. Interaction of glipizide and indoprofen. Eur J Rheum Inflamm (1981) 4, 22–5.

10 Pedrazzi F, Bommartini F, Freddo J and Emanueli A. A study of the possible interaction of indoprofen with hypoglycemic sulphonylureas in diabetic patients. Eur J Rheum Inflamm (1981) 4, 26–31.

11 Elvander-Stahl E, Melander A and Wahlin-Boll E. Indobufen interacts with the sulphonylurea, glipizide, but not with the beta-adrenergic receptor antagonists, propranolol and atenolol. Br J clin Pharmac (1984) 18, 773–8.

12 Haupt E, Hoppe FK, Rechziegler H, Zundorf P. Zur Frage der Interaktionen von nichtsteroidalen Antirheumatika mit oralen Antidiabetika: Acemetacin—Glibenclamid. Z. Rheumatol (1987) 46, 170–3.

Hypoglycaemic agents + Phenylbutazone or Oxyphenbutazone

Abstract/Summary

The hypoglycaemic effects of tolbutamide, acetohexamide, chlorpropamide, carbutamide, glymidine and glibenclamide can be increased by the concurrent use of phenylbutazone. Severe hypoglycaemia has occurred in a few patients. Oxyphenbutazone may be expected to behave similarly.

Clinical evidence

A diabetic man under treatment with tolbutamide experienced an acute hypoglycaemic episode four days after beginning to take 200 mg phenylbutazone three times a day, although there was no change in his diet or in the dosage of tolbutamide. He was able to control the hypoglycaemia by eating a large bar of chocolate.[1]

There are numerous other case reports and studies of this interaction involving phenylbutazone with tolbutamide,[2,4,5,8,10,11,17] carbutamide,[3] acetohexamide,[6] chlorpropamide,[11,20] glibenclamide,[12] and glymidine,[18,19] some of which describe acute hypoglycaemic episodes.[2,5,6,10] There is a report suggesting that the glibornuride-phenylbutazone may not be clinically important.[7] Oxyphenbutazone has been shown to interact with glymidine[13] and tolbutamide.[15,16] In contrast to these reports, a single study describes a paradoxical rise in blood sugar levels in three negro patients while receiving tolbutamide and phenylbutazone.[14]

Mechanism

Not fully resolved. Some evidence shows that phenylbutazone can inhibit the renal excretion of glibenclamide,[12] tolbutamide,[8] and the active metabolite of acetohexamide[6] so that they are retained in the body longer and their hypoglycaemic effects are increased and prolonged. It has also been shown that phenylbutazone can inhibit the metabolism of the sulphonylureas[15] as well as causing their displacement from protein binding sites.[9]

Importance and management

Well-documented and potentially clinically important interactions. Blood sugar levels may be lowered, but the number of reports of acute hypoglycaemic episodes seems to be small. Concurrent use should therefore be well monitored. A reduction in the dosage of the sulphonylurea may be necessary if excessive hypoglycaemia is to be avoided. Not all sulphonylureas have been shown to interact (glibornuride probably does not) but it would be prudent to assume that they all do until the contrary is proved. Oxyphenbutazone may be expected to interact similarly (it is the metabolite of phenylbutazone).

References

1 Mahfouz M, Abdel-Maguid R and El-Dakhakhny M. Potentiation of the hypoglycaemic action of tolbutamide by different drugs. Arzneim-Forsch (1970) 20, 120.

2 Dalgas M, Christiansen I and Kjerulf K. Fenylbutazoninduceret hypoglykaemitilfaelde hos klorpropamidbehandlet diabetiker. Ugeskr Laeg (1965) 127, 834.

3 Kaindl F, Kretschy A, Puxkandl H and Wutte J. Zur steigerung des Wirkundseffektes peroraler Antidiabetika durch Pyrazolonderivate. Wien Klin Wcsch (1961) 73, 79.

4 Gulbrandsen R. Okt tolbutamid-effekt ved hjelp av fenylbutazon? Tidskr Norsk Laeg (1959) 79, 1127.

5 Tannenbaum H, Anderson LG and Soeldner JS. Phenylbutazone-tolbutamide drug interaction. N Engl J Med (1974) 290, 344.

6 Field JB, Ohata M, Boyle C and Remer A. Potentiation of acetohexamide hypoglycaemia by phenylbutazone. N Engl J Med (1967) 277, 889.

7 Eckhardt W, Rudolph R, Sauer H, Schubert WR and Undeutsch D. Zur pharmackologischen Interferenz von Glibornurid mit Sulfaphenazol, Phenylbutazon und Phenprocoumon beim Menschen. Arzneim-Forsch (1972) 22, 2212.

8 Ober K-F. Mechanism of interaction of tolbutamide and phenylbutazone in diabetic patients. Europ J clin Pharmacol (1974) 7, 291.

9 Hellman B. Potentiating effects of drugs on the binding of glibenclamide to pancreatic beta cells. Metabolism (1974) 23, 839.

10 Dent LA and Jue SG. Tolbutamide + phenylbutazone: a dangerous and predictable interaction. Drug Intell Clin Pharm (1976) 10, 711.

11 Schulz E. Severe hypoglycaemic reactions after tolbutamide, carbutamide and chlorpropamide. Arch Klin Med (1968) 214, 135.

12 Schulz E, Koch K and Schmidt FH. Ursachen der Potenzierung der hypoglykämischen Wirkung von Sulfonylharnstoffderivaten durch Medikamente. II. Pharmakokinetik und Metabolismus von Glibenclamid (HN 419) in Gegenwart von Phenylbutazon. Eur J Clin Pharmacol (1971) 4, 32.

13 Held H, Scheible G, von Olderhausen HF. Uber Stoffwechsel unter Interferenz von Arzneimitteln bei Gesunden und Leberkranken. Kongress fur Innere Medizin (Wiesbaden) (1970) 76, 1153.

14 Owasu SK and Ocran K. Paradoxical behaviour of phenylbutazone in African diabetics. Lancet (1972) i, 440.

15 Pond SM, Birkett J and Wade DN. Mechanisms of inhibition of tolbutamide metabolism: phenylbutazone, oxyphenbutazone, sulfafenazole. Clin Pharmacol Ther (1977) 22, 573.

16 Kristensen M and Christensen LK. Modificazioni dell'effeto ipoglicemizzante dal farmaci ipoglicemizzsanti indotte da altri farmaci. Acta diabet lat (Milan) (1969) six (Suppl 1) 116.

17 Christensen LK, Hansen JM and Kristensen M. Sulphaphenazole-induced hypoglycaemic attacks in tolbutamide-treated diabetics. Lancet (1963) ii, 1298.

18 Held H, Kaminski B and von Olderhausen HF. Die beeinflussung der Elimination von Glycodiazin durch Leber und Nierenfunktionsstorungen und durch eine Behandlung mit Phenylbutazon, Phenprocoumarol und Doxycyclin. Diabetolgia (1970) 6, 386.

19 Held von H and Scheible G. Interaktion von Phenylbutazon und Oxyphenbutazon mit glymidine. Arzneim-Forschd/Drug Res. (1981) 31, 1036–8.

20 Shah SJ, Bhandarkar SD and Satoskar RS. Drug interaction between

chlorpropamide and non-steroidal anti-inflammatory drugs, ibuprofen and phenylbutazone. Int J Clin Pharmacol Ther Toxicol (1984) 22, 470–2.

Hypoglycaemic agents + Phenylephrine

Abstract/Summary

Insulin-dependent diabetics can develop elevated blood pressures if treated with phenylephrine eye-drops.

Clinical evidence, mechanism, importance and management

A comparative study of 14 insulin-dependent diabetics who over a period of 2 h before ocular surgery were given phenylephine eye-drops (a total of four doses of one or two drops of 10%), showed that they demonstrated an average blood pressure rise of 34/17 mm Hg, whereas another 176 non-diabetic patients similarly treated showed no increases in blood pressure.[1] The reason for this 'supersensitivity' reaction is not understood but clearly enough phenylephrine was absorbed systemically to stimulate the adrenoceptors of the sympathetic system which innervates the cardiovascular system. The authors of this report say that they readily controlled these hypertensive reactions with halothane and by neuroleptanalgesia accompanying regional block with anesthesia standby. Strictly speaking this is not a drug interaction, but a drug-disease reaction. The mydriatic dosage of phenylephrine should be reduced in insulin-dependent diabetics but whether this is also true for non insulin-dependent diabetics is uncertain.

Reference

1 Kim JM, Stevenson CE and Mathewson HS. Hypertensive reactions to phenylephrine eyedrops in patients with sympathetic denervation. Am J Ophthalmol (1978) 85, 862–8.

Hypoglycaemic agents + Phenyramidol

Abstract/Summary

The hypoglycaemic effects of tolbutamide are increased by phenyramidol but the clinical importance of this is uncertain.

Clinical evidence, mechanism, importance and management

The half-life of tolbutamide was increased from 7 to 18 h and serum tolbutamide levels raised in three normal subjects after taking 1200 mg phenyramidol daily for four days because (so it is suggested) the phenyramidol inhibits the metabolism of the tolbutamide by the liver, thereby prolonging its stay in the body.[1] A reduction in the dosage of tolbutamide may be nec-

essary to avoid excessive hypoglycaemia, but this requires confirmation. Information about other sulphonylureas is lacking.

Reference

1 Solomon HM and Schrogie JJ. Effect of phenyramidol and bishydroxy-coumarin on the metabolism of tolbutamide in human subjects. Metabolism (1967) 16, 1029.

Hypoglycaemic agents + Probenecid

Abstract/Summary

The clearance of chlorpropamide from the body is prolonged by probenecid, but the clinical importance of this is uncertain.

Clinical evidence, mechanism, importance and management

A study in six patients given single oral doses of chlorpropamide showed that the concurrent use of probenecid (1–2 g daily) increased its half-life from about 36 to 50 h.[1] It seems that the probenecid reduces the renal excretion of chlorpropamide. Another report claimed that the half-life of tolbutamide was also prolonged by probenecid,[2] but this was not confirmed by another properly controlled study.[3]

Information is very limited. It may possibly be necessary to reduce the dosage of the chlorpropamide in the presence of probenecid. Information about other sulphonylureas (with the exception of tolbutamide) appears to be lacking.

References

1 Petitpierre B, Perrin L, Rudhardt M, Herrera A and Fabre J. Behaviour of chlorpropamide in renal insufficiency and under the effect of associated drug therapy. Int J clin Pharmacol (1972) 6, 120.
2 Stowers JM, Mahler RF and Hunter RB. Pharmacology and mode of action of the sulphonylureas in man. Lancet (1958) i, 278.
3 Brook R, Schrogie JJ and Solomon HM. Failure of probenecid to inhibit the rate of metabolism of tolbutamide in man. Clin Pharmacol Ther (1968) 9, 314.

Hypoglycaemic agents + Quinine or Quinidine

Abstract/Summary

Patients with falciparum malaria who are treated with quinine or quinidine may show very severe hypoglycaemia. The impact of this on the control of diabetes has yet to be determined.

Clinical evidence, mechanism, importance and management

Patients with severe faciparum malaria who are treated with quinine may develop severe and life-threatening hypoglycaemia.[1,2] The reasons are not fully understood but it seems that in these patients the quinine causes the release of large amounts of insulin from the pancreas, although other factors may also be involved. Quinidine has been shown to have a similar effect.[3] Whether these changes can also occur in patients with malaria and diabetes, despite their pancreatic beta cell impairment, seems not to have been studied, but any interpretation of disturbances in the control of the diabetes should take into account these possible effects of quinine or quinidine. Chloroquine, amodiaquine, mefloquine and halofantrine do not apparently stimulate the release of insulin.[3]

References

1 White NJ, Warrell DA, Chanthavanich P, Looareesuwan S, Warrell MJ, Krishna S, Williamson DH and Turner RC. Severe hypoglycaemia and hyperinsulinemia in falciparum malaria. N Engl J Med (1983) 309, 61–6.
2 Looareesuwan S, Phillips RE, White NJ, Kietinun S, Karbwang J, Rackow C, Turner RC and Warrell DA. Quinine and severe falciparum malaria in late pregnancy. Lancet (1985) ii, 4–8.
3 Phillips RE, Looaressuwan S, White NJ, Chanthavanich P, Karbwang J, Supanaranond W, Turner RC and Warrell DA. Hypoglycaemia and antimalarial drugs: quinidine and release of insulin. Br Med J (1986) 292, 1319–21.

Hypoglycaemic agents + Rifampicin

Abstract/Summary

Rifampicin reduces the serum levels of tolbutamide, glycodiazine and chlorpropamide (single case). A reduction in the hypoglycaemic effects of these sulphonylureas would be expected.

Clinical evidence

A study in a group of nine patients with tuberculosis who were receiving tolbutamide showed that after four weeks' treatment with rifampicin the half-life of tolbutamide was reduced by 43%, and the serum concentrations measured at 6 h were halved compared with other patients not taking rifampicin.[1]

Similar results have been found in other studies in patients with cirrhosis or cholestasis,[2] in normal subjects[3] and in other patients.[6] The half-life of glymidine in man is also approximately halved by the concurrent use of rifampicin.[4] A single case report describes a diabetic man who needed an increase in his daily dosage of chlorpropamide from 250 to 400 mg daily when he was given 600 mg rifampicin daily, and a reduction 12 months later when the rifampicin was withdrawn.[5]

Mechanism

Rifampicin is a potent inducer of the liver microsomal enzymes concerned with the metabolism of tolbutamide and other drugs, which hastens their clearance from the body.[1–3]

Importance and management

The tolbutamide–rifampicin interaction is established. Patients taking tolbutamide may need an increase in the dosage while taking rifampicin (possibly roughly doubled, but this needs confirmation). This also seems to be true for glymidine and possibly chlorpropamide, but the documentation for these two drugs is much more limited. Information about other hypoglycaemic agents does not seem to be available.

References

1 Syvalahti EKG, Pihlajamaki KK and Ilsalo EJ. Rifampicin and drug metabolism. Lancet (1974) i, 232.
2 Zilly W, Breimer DD and Richter E. Stimulation of drug metabolism by rifampicin in patients with cirrhosis or cholestasis measured by increased hexobarbital and tolbutamide clearance. Eur J clin Pharmacol (1977) 11, 287.
3 Zilly W, Breimer DD and Richter E. Induction of drug metabolism in man after rifampicin treatment measured by hexobarbital and tolbutamide clearance. Eur J clin Pharmacol (1975) 9, 219.
4 Held HK, Schoene B, Laar HJ and Fleischmann R. Die Aktivitat der Benzpyrenhydroxylaze im Leberpunktat des Menschen in vitro und ihre Beziehung zur Eliminations-geschwindigkeit von Glycodiazin in vivo. Verhandhlungen der Deutschen Gesellschaft fur Innere Medizin (1974) 80, 501.
5 Self TH and Morris T. Interaction of rifampin and chlorpropamide. Chest (1980) 77, 800–1.
6 Sylvalahti E, Pihlajamki K and Iisalo E. Effect of tuberculostatic agents on the response of serum growth hormone and immunoreactive insulin to intravenous tolbutamide, and on the half-life of tolbutamide. Int J Clin Pharmacol (1976) 13, 83–9.

Hypoglycaemic agents + Salicylates

Abstract/Summary

Aspirin and other salicylates can lower blood sugar levels, but small analgesic doses do not normally have an adverse effect on patients taking hypoglycaemic agents. Some reduction in the dosage of the hypoglycaemic agent may be appropriate if large doses of salicylate are used.

Clinical evidence

(a) Insulin

12 juvenile diabetics treated with insulin showed a reduction in blood glucose levels averaging 15% (from 188 to 159 mg%) when additionally given either 1200 mg daily doses of aspirin (patients under 60 lb) or 2400 mg (patients over 60 lb) daily for a week. No significant changes in insulin requirements were necessary.[1]

Eight patients on 12–48 U insulin zinc suspension daily required no insulin when treated for 2–3 weeks with aspirin in doses large enough to give blood concentrations of 350–450 µg/ml. Six other patients were able to reduce their insulin requirements by about a half (from 22–112 to 10–72 U).[5]

(b) Chlorpropamide

A study in five normal subjects showed that the blood glucose lowering effects of chlorpropamide and sodium salicylate were additive; a further study on six subjects showed that 100 mg chlorpropamide with 1.5 g sodium salicylate lowered blood sugar levels the same amount as either 200 mg chlorpropamide or 3 g sodium salicylate.[6]

The blood glucose levels of a patient on 500 mg chlorpropamide daily were lowered about two-thirds by aspirin in doses sufficient to give serum salicylate levels of 26 mg%.[2]

Mechanism

Aspirin and salicylates have hypoglycaemic properties and in relatively large doses have been used on their own in the treatment of diabetes.[3,4] The most likely explanation for this interaction is that the blood sugar lowering effects are simply additive.[6] In addition there is some evidence that aspirin can raise serum chlorpropamide levels so that its effects are increased, possibly by interfering with renal tubular excretion.[2]

Importance and management

An established interaction but of limited importance. Considering the extremely wide use of aspirin it might reasonably be expected that any generally serious interaction would have come to light by now. The data available, coupled with the common experence of diabetics,[7] is that excessive and unwanted hypoglycaemia is very unlikely with small analgesic doses. Some downward readjustment of the dosage of the hypoglycaemic agent may be appropriate if large doses of salicylates are used. Information about other hypoglycaemic agents and salicylates appears to be lacking, but they may be expected to behave similarly

References

1 Kay R, Athreya BH, Kunzman EE and Baker L. Antipyretics in patients with juvenile diabetes mellitus. Amer J Dis Child (1966) 112, 52.
2 Stowers JM, Constable LW and Hunter RB. A clinical and pharmacological comparison of chlorpropamide and other sulfonylureas. Ann NY Acad Sci (1959) 74, 689.
3 Gilgore SG and Rupp JJ. The long-term response of diabetes mellitus to salicylate therapy. Report of a case. J Amer Med Ass (1962) 180, 65.
4 Reid J, Macdougall AI and Andrews MM. Aspirin and diabetes mellitus. Br Med J (1957) 2, 1071.
5 Reid J and Lightbody TD. The insulin equivalence of salicylate. Br Med J (1959) 1, 897.
6 Richardson T, Foster J and Mawer GE. Enhancement by sodium salicylate of the blood glucose lowering effect of chlorpropamide—drug interaction or summation of similar effects? Br J clin Pharmac (1986) 22, 43–48.
7 Logie AW, Galloway DB and Petrie JC. Drug interactions and long-term diabetic treatment. Br J clin Pharmac (1976) 3, 1027–32.

Hypoglycaemic agents + Sucralfate

Abstract/Summary

Sucralfate appears not to interact significantly with chlorpropamide.

Clinical evidence, mechanism, importance and management

A two-way cross-over study in 12 normal subjects showed that 1 g sucralfate four times a day 1 h before meals had no effect on the pharmacokinetics of a single 250 mg dose of chlorpropamide, except for a small but statistically significant change in the zero to infinity AUC.[1] This seems unlikely to be clinically important, but it needs confirmation. There seems to be no information about the effects of sucralfate on other hypoglycaemic agents.

Reference

1 Letendre PW, Carlson JD, Siefert RD, Dietz AJ and Dimmit D. Effect of sucralfate on the absorption and pharmacokinetics of chlorpropamide. J Clin Pharmacol (1986) 26, 622–5.

Hypoglycaemic agents + Sugar-containing pharmaceuticals

Abstract/Summary

Some pharmaceutical preparations such as cough linctuses, liquid antibiotics, bulk laxatives and others can contain significant amounts of sugar. Diabetics should be warned.

Clinical evidence, mechanism, importance and management

Many pharmaceuticals contain sugar in considerable amounts. Some liquid oral antibiotic preparations may contain up to 70% sucrose (e.g. *Broxil*, 7 g/10 ml, *Erythroped Pi*, 6.8 g/10 ml) and the sugar-content of many elixirs and linctuses (e.g. *Phensedyl*, 3.36 g per 5 ml dose) also may be high. The extent to which the administration of preparations like these will affect the control of diabetes clearly depends upon the amounts ingested, but the problem is by no means merely theoretical. One report[1] describes a significant loss of control in a woman diabetic with diverticulitis when she was prescribed a psyllium effervescent powder (*Metamucil instant-mix*) which contains sugar. The range of other sugar-containing preparations is far too extensive to be listed here, but diabetics should be made aware that sugar is present in a variety of pharmaceuticals in unsuspected guises and disguises. Unfortunately package labels are not always as informative as they might be. The National Pharmaceutical Association has published two very useful lists[2,3] of the sugar content of prescribed and over-the-counter medicines available in the UK, one of them drawn up in collaboration with the British Diabetic Association.[3] Another valuable list appeared more recently in the Pharmaceutical Journal.[4]

References

1 Catellani J and Collins RJ. Drug labelling. Lancet (1978) ii, 98.
2 The NPA notes for proprietors. Sugar content of medicines. Published by the National Pharmaceutical Association, Mallinson House, 40–42 St Peters Street, St Albans, Herts, England. December (1986).
3 Carbohydrate content of proprietary medicines available without prescription. Published by the National Pharmaceutical Association (address above) and the British Diabetic Association, 10 Queen Anne St, London W1M 0BD. April (1987).
4 Greenwood J. Sugar content of liquid prescription medicines. Pharm J (1989) 243, 553–7.

Hypoglycaemic agents + Sulphinpyrazone

Abstract/Summary

Sulphinpyrazone has no effect on the insulin requirements of diabetics, nor does it affect the control of patients taking glibenclamide. There is good evidence that excessive hypoglycaemia might occur with tolbutamide, but as yet there appear to be no case reports of this interaction, nor of any adverse interactions with other hypoglycaemic agents.

Clinical evidence

(a) Insulin + sulphinpyrazone

A double blind study, extending over 12 months, on 41 adult diabetics, showed that the daily administration of 600–800 mg sulphinpyrazone had no clinically significant effects on their insulin requirements.[1]

(b) Glibenclamide + sulphinpyrazone

A study of 19 type II diabetics taking glibenclamide showed that 800 mg sulphinpyrazone daily did not affect the control of their diabetes.[3]

(c) Tolbutamide + sulphinpyrazone

A detailed study of the pharmacokinetics of tolbutamide in six normal subjects showed that after taking 200mg sulphinpyrazone every 6 h for a week, the half-life of tolbutamide was almost doubled (from 7.3 to 13.2 h) and the plasma clearance reduced by 40%.[2]

Mechanism

The available evidence suggests that the tolbutamide/sulphinpyrazone interaction occurs because the sulphinpyrazone inhibits the metabolism of tolbutamide by the liver.[2]

Importance and management

Information about the tolbutamide/sulphinpyrazone interaction appears to be limited to the report cited. So far there appear to be no reports of adverse interactions in patients, but what is known suggests that excessive hypoglycaemia could occur if the dosage of tolbutamide is not reduced. Such an interaction has been described with phenylbutazone with which sulphinpyrazone has a close structural similarity (see appropriate synopsis). There seems to be nothing documented about any other clinically important hypoglycaemic agent/sulphinpyrazone interaction.

References

1 Pannebakker MAG, den Ottolander JH and ten Pas, JG. Insulin requirements in diabetic patients treated with sulphinpyrazone. J Int Med Res (1979) 7, 328.
2 Miners JO, Foenander T, Wanwimolruk S, Gallus AS and Birkett DJ. The effect of sulphinpyrazone on oxidative drug metabolism in man: inhibition of tolbutamide elimination. Eur J Clin Pharmacol (1982) 22, 321.
3 Kritz H, Najemnik C and Irsigler K. Interaktionsstudie mit Sulfinpyrazon (Anturan) und Glibenclamid (Euglucon) bei Typ-II-Diabetikern. Wien Med Wchsch (1983) 133, 237–43.

Hypoglycaemic agents + Sulphonamides

Abstract/Summary

The hypoglycaemic effects of chlorpropamide, glibenclamide and tolbutamide can be increased by some sulphonamides and a few cases of acute hypoglycaemia have been reported. Some sulphonylurea/sulphonamide pairs do not interact. There appear to be no reports of adverse insulin/sulphonamide interactions.

Clinical evidence

The table summarizes the information I have been able to trace on the hypoglycaemic agent/sulphonamide interactions.

Table 15.3 Hypoglycaemic agent/Sulphonamede interactions

Drugs	Information documented	Refs.
Chlorpropamide		
+sulphafurazole (sulfisoxazole)	1 case of acute hypoglycaemia	7
+sulphamethizole	1 case of acute hypoglycaemia	8
+co-trimoxazole	2 cases of acute hypoglycaemia	9,14
Glibenclamide		
+co-trimoxazole	11% incidence of hypoglycaemia.	15
	Stated to be no pharmacokinetic interaction.	17
Glibornuride		
+sulphaphenazole	Stated to be no interaction	10
Tolbutamide		
+co-trimoxazole	Clearance reduced 25%, half-life increased 30%	16
+sulphafurazole (sulfisoxazole)	3 cases of severe hypoglycaemia	1,2
	2 reports state no interaction	6,11

Table 15.3 *continued*

Drugs	Information documented	Refs.
Tolbutamide (cont.)		
+sulphamethizole	Half-life of tolbutamide increased 60%. Metabolic clearance reduced 40%	3,4
+sulphaphenazole	1 case of severe hypoglycaemia	5,11
	Half-life of tolbutamide increased × 4–6	
+sulphadiazine	Half-life of tolbutamide increased 50%	5
+sulphadimethoxine	Stated to be no interaction	6
+sulphamethoxy-pyridazine	Stated to be no interaction	6
+sulphamethoxazole	Clearance reduced 14%, half-life increased 20%	16
Un-named sulphonylurea +co-trimoxazole	1 case of acute hypoglycaemia	13

Mechanism

Not fully understood. The sulphonamides may inhibit the metabolism of the sulphonylureas so that they accumulate in the body, in this way their serum levels and effects are enhanced.[3,5,6,12] There is also evidence that the sulphonamides can displace the sulphonylureas from their protein binding sites.

Importance and management

The documentation of these interactions is too variable and their incidence is also too uncertain for firm predictions to be made about what will and what will not interact, or how clinically important any interactions may prove to be, nevertheless the table can be used as a general guide.

Avoid any of the sulphonylurea-sulphonamide pairs where an adverse interaction is known to have occurred. If, nevertheless, concurrent use is undertaken the patient should be clearly warned that increased hypoglycaemia, sometimes excessive, can occur. Some prescribers may feel it prudent to give some warning even when giving sulphonylurea/sulphonamide pairs not reported to interact. There appear to be no reports of adverse interactions in patients given insulin and a sulphonamide.

References

1 Soeldner JS and Steinke J. Hypoglycaemia in tolbutamide-treated diabetes. J Amer Med Ass (1965) 193, 148.
2 Robinson DS. The application of basic principles of drug interaction to clinical practice. J Urology (1975) 113, 100.
3 Lumholtz B, Siersbaek-Nielsen K, Skovsted L, Kampmann J and Hansen JM. Sulphamethizole-induced inhibition of diphenylhydantoin, tolbutamide, and warfarin metabolism. Clin Pharmacol Ther (1975) 17, 731.
4 Siersbaek-Nielsen K, Hansen JM, Skovsted L, Lumholtz B and Kampmann J. Sulphamethizole-induced inhbition of diphenylhydantoin and tolbutamide metabolism in man. Clin Pharmacol Ther (1973) 14, 148.
5 Kristensen M and Christensen LK. Drug induced changes of blood glucose lowering effect of oral hypoglycaemic agents. Acta diabet lat (1969) six (Suppl 1) 116.
6 Christensen IK, Hansen JM and Kristensen M. Sulphaphenazole-induced hypoglycaemic attacks in tolbutamide-treated diabetics. Lancet (1963) ii, 1298.
7 Tucker HSG and Hirsch JI. Sulphonamide-sulphonylurea interaction. N Eng J Med (1972) 286, 110.
8 Dall JLC, Conway H and McAlpine SG. Hypoglycaemia due to chlorpropamide. Scot Med J (1967) 12, 403.
9 Ek I. Langvarigt klorpropamidutlost hypoglykemitillstand Lakemedelsinteraktion? Lakartidningen (1974) 71, 2597.
10 Eckhardt W, Rudolph R, Sauer H, Schubert WR and Undeutsch D. Zur pharmakologischen Interferenz von Glibornurid mit Sulfaphenazol, Phenylbutazon und Phenprocoumon beim Menschen. Artzneim-Forsch (1972) 22, 2212.
11 Dubach UC, Buckert A and Raaflaub J. Einfluss von Sulfonamiden auf die blutzuckersenkende Wirkung oraler Antidiabetica. Schweiz med Wsch (1966) 96, 1483.
12 Hellman B. Potentiating effects of drugs on the binding of glibenclamide to pancreatic beta cells. Metabolism (1974) 23, 839.
13 Baciewicz AM and Swafford WB. Hypoglycaemia induced by the interaction of chlorpropamide and co-trimoxazole. Drug Intell Clin Pharm (1984) 181, 3093–3110.
14 Mihic M, Mautner LS, Feness JZ and Grant K. Effect of trimethoprim-sulphamethoxazole on blood insulin and glucose concentrations of diabetics. Can Med Assoc J (1975), 112, 80s.
15 Sjoberg S, Widholm BE, Gunnarsson R, Emilsson H, Thunberg E, Christenson I and Ostman J. No evidence for pharmacokinetic interaction between glibenclamide and trimethoprim-sulfametoxazole. Diabetes Res Clin Prac (1985) (Suppl 1) S 522.
16 Wing LMH and Miners JO. Co-trimoxazole as an inhibitor of oxidative drug metabolism effects of trimethoprim and sulfamethoxazole separately and combined on tolbutamide disposition. Br J Clin Pharmacol (1985) 20, 482–5.
17 Sjoberg S, Wiholm BE, Gunnarsson R, Emilsson H, Thunberg E, Christenson I, Ostman J. Lack of pharmacokinetic interaction between glibenclamide and trimethoprim-sulphamethoxazole. Diabet Med (1987) 4, 245–7.

Hypoglycaemic agents + Tetracyclines

Abstract/Summary

A few scattered reports indicate that the hypoglycaemic effects of insulin and the sulphonylureas may sometimes be increased by oxytetracycline, and limited evidence suggests that this may also occur with doxycycline.

Clinical evidence

(a) Insulin or sulphonylureas + tetracyclines

A diabetic, poorly controlled on insulin, needed a marked reduction in his dosage of insulin (from 104 to 62 units daily) in order to control the hypoglycaemia which developed when he was also given 250 mg oxytetracyline four times a day. This reaction was also seen in another patient.[1]

Another report[2] describes marked hypoglycaemia in an elderly patient on tolbutamide when given oxytetracycline. Another study in diabetic subjects similarly showed that oxytetracycline can reduce blood sugar levels.[11] The hypogly-caemic effects of oxytetracyline has also been demonstrated in dogs.[2] A very brief report describes hypoglycaemia in a patient on insulin when given doxycycline.[3] The half-life of glymidine in man has been shown to be prolonged from 4.6 to 7.6 h by doxycycline,[4] whereas a brief comment in another report suggests that demeclocycline may not affect chlorpropamide.[5]

(b) Biguanides + tetracyclines

There are now at least six cases on record of lactic-acidosis in patients on phenformin which was apparently precipitated by the concurrent use of tetracycline.[6–10]

Mechanisms

Not understood.

Importance and management

Information about the interaction between the sulphonylureas or insulin and the tetracyclines is very limited indeed. Concurrent use need not be avoided, but it would be prudent to be on the alert for any signs of hypoglycaemia, particularly with oxytetracycline and doxycycline. Reduce the dosage of the hypoglycaemic agent if necessary. Phenformin has been withdrawn because of the high incidence of lactic acidosis but there is nothing to suggest that there is an increased risk if tetracyclines are given with metformin.

References

1 Miller JB. Hypoglycaemic effect of oxytetracycline. Brit Med J (1966) 2, 1007.
2 Hiatt N and Bonorris G. Insulin response in pancreatectomised dogs treated with oxytetracycline. Diabetes (1970) 19, 307–10.
3 New Zealand Committee on Adverse Drug Reactions. Ninth Annual Report. NZ Dent J (1975) 71, 28.
4 Held H, Kaminski B and von Olderhausen HF. Die beeinflussung der Elimination von Glycodiazin durch Leber- und Nierenfunc-tionssorungen und durch eine Behandlung mit Phenylbutazon, Phen-procoumarol und Doxycyclin. Diabetologica (1970) 6, 386.
5 Petitpierre B, Perrin L, Rudhardt M, Herrera A and Fabre J. Behaviour of chlorpropamide in renal insufficiency and under the effect of associated drug therapy. Int J clin Pharmacol (1972) 6, 120.
6 Aro A, Korhonen T and Halinen M. Phenformin-induced lactic acidosis precipitated by tetracycline. Lancet (1978) 1, 673.
7 Tashima CK. Phenformin, tetracycline and lactic acidosis. Brit Med J (1971) 4, 557.
8 Blumenthal SA and Streeten DHP. Phenformin-related lactic acidosis in a 30-year old man. Ann Interm Med (1976) 84, 55.
9 Korhonen T, Idanpaan-Heikkila JE and Aro A. Unpublished data quoted in reference 6.
10 Philips PJ and Pain RW. Phenformin, tetracycline and lactic acidosis. Ann Intern Med (1977) 86, 111.
11 Sen S and Mukerjee AB. Hypoglycaemic action of oxytetracycline. A preliminary study. J Indian Med Ass (1969) 52, 366–9.

Hypoglycaemic agents + Thiazides, Chlorthalidone or related diuretics

Abstract/Summary

(a) By raising blood sugar levels the thiazide diuretics, chlorthalidone and other related diuretics can reduce the effects of the hypoglycaemic agents and impair the control of diabetes. Some, but by no means all, patients will require a modest increase in the dosage of their hypoglycaemic agent. (b) Hypo-natraemia also occurs occasionally.

Clinical evidence

(a) Reduced hypoglycaemic effects

Chlorothiazide, the first of the thiazide diuretics, was found within a year of its introduction in 1958 to have hyper-glycaemic effects.[1] Since then a very large number of reports have described this same effect with other thiazides, the precipitation of diabetes in prediabetics, and the disturbance of blood sugar control in diabetics. One example from many:

A long-term study on 53 diabetics showed that treatment with chlorothiazide (0.5 or 1 g daily) or trichlormethiazole (4 or 8 mg daily) caused a mean rise in blood sugar levels from 120 to 140 mg%. Only seven patients needed a change in their treatment: four required more of their oral agent, two an increase in insulin, and one was transferred from tolbut-amide to insulin. The oral agents used included tolbutamide, chlorpropamide, acetohexamide and phenformin.[2]

A rise in blood sugar levels has been observed with ben-drofluazide,[10] benzthiazide,[3] hydrochlorothiazide,[5] dihydro-flumethiazide,[5] and chlorthalidone.[6]

(b) Hyponatraemia

A hospital report describes eight cases of low serum sodium concentrations observed over a five-year period in patients taking chlorpropamide and *Moduretic* (hydrocholothiazide 50 mg + amiloride 5 mg).[11]

Mechanisms

(a) Not understood. One study suggested that the hyper-glycaemia is due to some inhibition of insulin release by the pancreas.[9] Another is that the peripheral action of insulin is affected in some way.[8] There is also evidence that it may be related in part to potassium depletion.[7] (b) The hypo-natraemia appears to be due to the additive sodium-losing effects of the chlorpropamide, thiazide and amiloride.

Importance and management

(a) The reduction in hypoglycaemia is extremely well-documented (a full list of references is not given here for the sake of economy of space) but of only moderate practical importance. The report of the study cited above[2] stated that '...it is not of serious degree...and in no patient was a dramatic deterioration of diabetic control observed.' The incidence is said to lie between 10 and 30%.[2,4] Concurrent use need not be avoided but the effects should be monitored. There is evidence that the full effects may take many months to develop in some patients.[10] Most patients respond to a modest increase in the dosage of the hypoglycaemic agent, or to a change from an oral drug to insulin. The adverse hyperglycaemic effects can also be reversed significantly by the use of potassium supplements.[7]

In addition to the thiazides already named, the interaction may be expected to occur with the other thiazides in common use (cyclopenthiazide, cyclothiazide, methyclothiazide, polythiazide) and related diuretics such as clopamide, clorexolone, metolazone, quinethazone, etc. This requires confirmation.

(b) Hyponatraemia seems to be uncommon but be aware that it can occur during concurrent use.

References

1 Wilkins RW. New drugs for the treatment of hypertension. Ann Intern Med (1959) 50, 1.
2 Kansal PC, Buse J and Buse MG. Thiazide diuretics and control of diabetes mellitus. S Med J (1969) 62, 1374.
3 Runyan JW. Influence of thiazide diuretics on carbohydrate metabolism in patients with mild diabetes. N Engl J Med (1961) 267, 541.
4 Wolff FW, Parmley WW, White KW and Okun RJ. Drug-induced diabetes. Diabetogenic activity of long-term administration of benzothiadiazines. J Amer Med Ass (1963) 185, 568.
5 Goldner MG, Zarowitz H and Akgun S. Hyperglycaemia and glycosuria due to thiazide derivatives administered in diabetes mellitus. N Engl J Med (1960) 262, 403.
6 Carliner NH, Schelling J-L, Russell RP, Okun R and Davis M. Thiazide- and phthalimidine-induced hyperglycaemia in hypertensive patients. J Amer Med Ass (1965) 191, 535.
7 Rapoport MI and Hurd HF. Thiazide-induced glucose intolerance treated with potassium. Arch Intern Med (1964) 113, 405.
8 Remenchik AP, Hoover C and Talso PJ. Insulin secretion by hypersensitive patients receiving hydrochlorothiazide. J Amer Med Ass (1970) 212, 869.
9 Fajans SS, Floyd JC, Knopf RF, Rull J, Guntsche EM and Conn JW. Benzothiazide suppression of insulin release from normal and abnormal islet tissue in man. J Clin Invest (1966) 45, 481.
10 Lewis PJ, Kohner EM, Petrie A and Dollery CT. Deterioration of glucose tolerance in hypertensive patients on prolonged diuretic treatment. Lancet (1976) i, 564–6.
11 Zalin AM, Hutchinson CE, Jong M and Matthews K. Hyponatraemia during treatment with chlorpropamide and Moduretic (amiloride plus hydrochlorothiazide). Br Med J (1984) 289, 659.

Hypoglycaemic agents + Tobacco smoking

Abstract/Summary

Diabetics who smoke need more insulin than those who do not.

Clinical evidence, mechanism, importance and management

Two studies[1,2] carried out on large numbers of insulin-dependent smokers showed that on average they needed 15–20% more insulin than non-smokers, and up to 30% more if they smoked heavily. This is apparently because smoking causes a significant rise (40–120%) in the levels of the hormones which oppose the actions of insulin.[3] A consequence of this interaction is that diabetics who give up smoking may need a downward adjustment of their insulin dosage.

References

1 Klemp P, Staberg B, Madsbad S and Kolendorf K. Smoking reduces insulin absorption from subcutaneous tissue. Brit Med J (1982) 284, 237.
2 Madsbad S, McNair P, Christensen MS, Christiansen C, Faber OK, Binder C and Transbol I. Influence of smoking on insulin requirement and metabolic status in diabetes mellitus. Diabetes Care (1980) 3, 41–3.
3 Helve E, Yki-Jarvinen H and Koivisto VA. Smoking and insulin sensitivity in type I diabetes. Diabetes Res Clin Prac (1985) (Suppl 1) S 232.

Hypoglycaemic agents + Tricyclic antidepressants

Abstract/Summary

Two isolated reports describe hypoglycaemia in two patients, one on tolazamide and the other on chlorpropamide shortly after starting treatment with doxepin and nortriptyline respectively.

Clinical evidence, mechanism, importance and management

There are two cases of apparent interactions on record: a patient on tolazamide became hypoglycaemic 11 days after starting to take 75 mg doxepin daily, and another on chlorpropamide developed marked hypoglycaemia three days after starting 125 mg nortriptyline daily.[2] The reasons are not understood. An earlier study suggested that no interaction was likely: four patients given nine days' treatment with 25 mg amitriptyline daily showed no change in the half-life of a single 500 mg dose of tolbutamide.[1] Apart from these two cases the literature seems to be silent about interactions between the sulphonylureas and the tricyclic antidepressants. Bearing in mind the length of time these two groups of drugs have been available, the risk of a clinically important interaction would seem to be small, nevertheless be alert for any evidence of an increase in hypoglycaemia if both are given. The patient on doxepin was eventually stabilized on a daily dose of tolazamide which was only 10% of that used before the doxepin was given.[2]

References

1 Pond SM, Graham GG, Birkett DJ and Wade DN. Effects of tricyclic antidepressants on drug metabolism. Clin Pharmacol Ther (1975) 18, 191.
2 True BL, Perry PJ and Burns EA. Profound hypoglycemia with the addition of a tricyclic antidepressant to maintenance sulfonylurea therapy. Am J Psychiatry (1987) 144, 1220–1.

Hypoglycaemic agents + Urinary alkalinizers and Acidifiers

Abstract/Summary

On theoretical grounds the response to chlorpropamide may be decreased if the urine is made alkaline, and increased if urine is acidified, but so far no adverse interactions appear to have been reported.

Clinical evidence, mechanism, importance and management

A study in six normal subjects given 250 mg oral doses of chlorpropamide showed that when their urinary pH was raised from 7.1 to 8.2 with sodium bicarbonate, the half-life of the chlorpropamide was reduced from 50 to 13 h, and the 72 h clearance was increased fourfold. In contrast, when their urinary pH was lowered from 5.5 to 4.7 with ammonium chloride, the chlorpropamide half-life was increased from 50 to 69 h and the 72 h urinary clearance was decreased to one-twentieth.[1] Another study showed that the renal clearance was almost 100 times greater at pH 7 than at pH 5.[2] The reasons are that changes in urinary pH affect the ionization of the chlorpropamide, and this affects the ability of the kidney to reabsorb it from the kidney filtrate (see more details of this interaction mechanism in the introductory chapter.)

There appear to be no reports of adverse interactions between chlorpropamide and drugs which can alter urinary pH, but prescribers should be aware of the possibilities: a reduced response if the pH is raised significantly (e.g. with sodium bicarbonate, acetazolamide, some antacids); an increased response if the pH is made more acid than usual (e.g. with ammonium chloride).

References

1 Neuvonen PJ and Karkkainen S. Effects of charcoal, sodium bicarbonate and ammonium chloride on chlorpropamide kinetics. Clin Pharmacol Ther (1983) 33, 386–93.
2 Neuvonen PJ, Karkkainen S and Lehtovaara R. Pharmacokinetics of chlorpropamide in epileptic patients: effects of enzyme induction and urine pH on chlorpropamide elimination. Eur J Clin Pharmacol (1987) 32, 297–301.

16

IMMUNOSUPPRESSANT DRUG INTERACTIONS

The immunosuppressant drugs dealt with in this chapter are the corticosteroids and cyclosporin. Other drugs which are also used for immunosuppression (e.g. azathioprine and methotrexate) are to be found in Chapter 13 which deals with the cytotoxic drugs. When any of these drugs acts as the interacting agent the relevant synopsis is categorized in the chapter dealing with the drug whose effects are changed. A list of the agents which are featured appears in Table 16.1.

Table 16.1

Non-proprietary names	Proprietary names
Cyclosporin A (Cyclosporin(e))	Sandimunn
Corticosteroids	
Cloprednol	
Dexamethasone	
Hydrocortisone	
Fludrocortisone	
Methylprednisolone	
Prednisolone	
Prednisone	

Corticosteroids + Aminoglutethimide

Abstract/Summary

The effects of dexamethasone but not hydrocortisone can be reduced or abolished by the concurrent use of aminoglutethimide.

Clinical evidence

A study in six patients showed that when given 500–750 mg aminoglutethimide daily the half-life of dexamethasone (1 g daily) was reduced from 264 to 120 min. In another 22 patients it was found that increasing the dexamethasone dosage to 1.5–3.0 mg daily compensated for the increased dexamethasone metabolism and complete adrenal suppression was achieved over a prolonged period.[1]

A patient, dependent on dexamethasone due to brain oedema caused by a tumour, deteriorated rapidly with headache and lethargy when additionally treated with aminoglutethimide.[2] The problem was solved by withdrawing the aminoglutethimide and temporarily increasing the dexamethasone dosage.

Mechanism

Aminoglutethimide is an enzyme inducing agent and it seems probable that it interacts by increasing the metabolism and clearance of the steroids by the liver.[4]

Importance and management

Information is limited but the interaction appears to be established. The reduction in the serum corticosteroid levels can be enough to reduce or even abolish intended adrenal suppression[1] or to cause loss of control of a disease condition.[2] The former situation has been successfully accommodated by increasing the dosage of the corticosteroid or by increasing the dosage of both.[1] An alternative is to use hydrocortisone which appears not to be affected by aminoglutethimide.[3] A standard fixed dose regimen of 1 g aminoglutethimide and 40 mg hydrocortisone daily has been shown to block adrenal steroid synthesis effectively without the 'adrenal escape phenomenon'.[3]

References

1 Santen RJ, Lipton A and Kendall J. Successful medical adrenalectomy with aminoglutethimide. Role of altered drug metabolism. J Amer Med Ass (1974) 230, 1661–5.
2 Halpern J, Catane R and Baerwald H. A call for caution in the use of aminoglutethimide: negative interactions with dexamethasone and beta blocker treatment. Journal of Medicine (1984) 15, 59–63.
3 Santen RJ, Wells SA, Runic S, Gupta C, Kendall J, Ruby EB and Samojlik E. Adrenal suppression with aminoglutethimide. I. Differential effects of aminoglutethimide on glucocorticoid metabolism as a rationale for the use of hydrocortisone. J Clin Endocrinol Metab (1977) 45, 469–79.
4 Santen RJ and Brodie AMH. Suppression of oestrogen production as treatment of breast carcinoma: pharmacological and clinical studies with aromatase inhibitors. Clinics in Oncology (1982) 1, 77–130.

Corticosteroids + Antacids

Abstract/Summary

The absorption of prednisone can be reduced by large, but not small, doses of aluminium and magnesium hydroxide antacids. Prednisolone probably behaves similarly. Dexamethasone absorption is reduced by magnesium trisilicate. Phosphate-depletion caused by antacids can confuse the diagnostic picture.

Clinical evidence

(a) Prednisone or prednisolone

A study on five patients with neurological disorders and two normal subjects given single 10 or 20 mg doses of prednisone showed that 20 ml *Gastrogel* (aluminium hydroxide, magnesium hydroxide and trisilicate) had no significant effect on serum levels, half-life or corticosteroid AUC's.[1]

Other studies in eight normal subjects given 20 mg doses of prednisolone showed that 30 ml Magnesium Trisilicate Mixture BP or *Aludrox* (aluminium hydroxide gel) caused small but not statistically significant changes in peak prednisolone levels and absorption, however one subject given magnesium trisilicate had considerably reduced levels.[2] Aluminium phosphate has also been found not to affect prednisolone absorption.[6,7] In contrast, another study in normal subjects and patients given 60 ml of *Aldrox* or *Melox* (both containing aluminium hydroxide and magnesium hydroxide) found that the bioavailability of 10 mg prednisone was reduced on average by 30%, and even 40% in some individuals.[5]

(b) Dexamethasone

5 g magnesium trisilicate in 100 ml of water considerably reduced the bioavailability of single 1 mg oral doses of dexamethasone given to six subjects. Using the urinary excretion of 11-hydroxycorticosteroids as a measure, the reduction was about 75%.[4]

Mechanism

The reduction in dexamethasone absorption is attributed to adsorption onto the surface of the magnesium trisilicate.[4,8]

Importance and management

Information seems to be limited to these studies. The indication is that large doses of some antacids can reduce bioavailability, but small doses do not. More study is needed to confirm this. Concurrent use should be monitored to confirm that the therapeutic response is adequate. Also be alert for evidence of a phosphate-depletion syndrome which can mimic steroid-induced side-effects and confuse the diagnostic picture.[3] This has been reported in a prednisolone-dependent asthmatic man given *Maalox* and *Mylanta*, both of which are phosphate-binding antacids.[1]

References

1 Tanner AR, Caffin JA, Halliday JW and Powell LW. Concurrent administration of antacids and prednisone: effect on serum levels of prednisolone. Br J clin Pharmac (1979) 7, 397.

2 Lee DAH, Taylor GM, Walker JG and James VHT. The effect of concurrent administration of antacids on prednisolone absorption. Br J clin Pharmac (1979) 8, 92.

3 Goodman M, Solomons CC and Miller PD. Distinction between the common symptoms of the phosphate-depletion syndrome and glucocorticoid-induced disease. Am J Med (1978) 65, 868.

4 Naggar VF, Khalil SA and Gouda MW. Effect of concomitant administration of magnesium trisilicate on GI absorption of dexamethasone in humans. J Pharm Sci (1978) 67, 1029.

5 Uribe M, Casian C, Rojas S, Sierra JG, Go VLW, Munoz RM and Gil S. Decreased bioavailability of prednisone due to antacids in patients with chronic active liver disease and in healthy subjects. Gastroenterology (1981) 80, 661.

6 Albin H, Vincon G, Demotes-Mainard F, Begaud B and Bedjauoi A. Effects of aluminium phosphate on bioavailability of cimetidine and prednisolone. Eur J Clin Pharmacol (1984) 26, 271–3.

7 Albin H, Vincon G, Pehourcq F, Lecorre C, Fleury B and Conri C. Influence d'un anti-acide sur la biodisponibilite de la prednisolone. Therapie (1983) 38, 61–5.

8 Prakash A and Verma RK. In vitro adsorption of dexamethasone and betamethasone on antacids. Ind J Pharm Sci (1984) Jan-Feb, 55–6.

Corticosteroids + Anti-infective agents

Abstract/Summary

Because the corticosteroids can suppress the normal responses of the body to attack by micro-organisms, it is important to ensure that any anti-infective 'cover' is sufficient to prevent generalized and potentially life-threatening infections.

Clinical evidence

A patient with severe cystic acne vulgaris who had been treated with low dose oral tetracyline, 500 mg daily, and betamethasone, 2 mg daily, for seven months became toxaemic and pyrexic with severe acne and cellulitis of the face due to the emergence of a gram-negative organism not susceptible to the antibiotic.[1]

Mechanism

The corticosteroids reduce inflammation and impair antibody formation which increases the susceptibility of the body to infection. In the case cited an organism emerged which was not controlled by the tetracycline, and in the presence of some adrenal insufficiency induced by the corticosteroid, became disseminated throughout the body.

Importance and management

Not, strictly speaking, an interaction, but the case cited amply illustrates the importance of monitoring concurrent use. The author of the report points out that '. . . it appears that if oral corticoids or combined therapy are ever warranted, they should be very carefully policed because of the risk of turning a benign disease into one that is potentially fatal.'

Reference

1 Paver K. Complications from combined oral tetracycline and oral corticoid therapy on acne vulgaris. Med J Aust (1970) 1, 509.

Corticosteroids + Barbiturates

Abstract/Summary

The therapeutic effects of systemically administered corticosteroids (dexamethasone, hydrocortisone, methylprednisolone, prednisone and prednisolone) are decreased by the concurrent use of phenobarbitone (and probably other barbiturates as well) because the loss of these corticosteroids from the body is increased. An increase in the corticosteroid dosage may be needed.

Clinical evidence

(a) Asthmatic patients on prednisone, prednisolone, methylprednisolone

Three prednisone-dependent patients with bronchial asthma taking 10–40 mg prednisone daily showed a marked worsening of their symptoms within a few days of starting to take 120 mg phenobarbitone daily. There was a deterioration in their pulmonary function tests (FEV1, degree of bronchospasm) and a rise in eosinophil counts, all of which improved when the phenobarbitone was stopped. The prednisone clearance increased while taking the phenobarbitone.[1]

A study in asthmatic children found that phenobarbitone increased the clearance of prednisolone by 41% and of methylprednisolone by 209%.[8] In contrast another study in children on prednisone found that their corticosteroid requirements were unaltered while taking a compound preparation containing 24 mg phenobarbitone daily.[3]

(b) Kidney transplant patients on prednisone

A study indicated that the survival of kidney transplants in a group of 75 children being given azathioprine and prednisone as immunosuppressants was reduced in those given anticonvulsant treatment with 60–120 mg phenobarbitone daily. Two of the 11 epileptic children were also taking 100 mg phenytoin daily.[4]

(c) Patients with rheumatoid arthritis on prednisolone

Nine patients with rheumatoid arthritis on 8–15 mg prednisolone daily showed strong evidence of clinical deterioration (worsening joint tenderness, pain, morning stiffness, fall in grip strength) when treated with phenobarbitone for two weeks (plasma concentrations 0–2 mg%). The prednisolone half-life fell by 25%.[6]

Mechanism

Phenobarbitone is a recognized potent liver enzyme inducing agent which increases the metabolism and loss from the body of administered corticosteroids, thereby reducing their effects. Pharmacokinetic studies in man have shown that phenobarbitone reduces the half-lives of these corticosteroids and increases their clearances by 90–209%.[1,5,8]

Importance and management

A well-documented and well-established interaction of clinical importance. Concurrent use need not be avoided but the outcome should be well monitored and the corticosteroid dosage increased as necessary. Dexamethasone,[1] hydrocortisone,[2] methylprednisolone,[5,8] prednisone[1,4] and prednisolone[6,8] are all known to be affected. Prednisone and prednisolone appear to be less affected than methylprednisolone and may be preferred.[8] Be alert for the same interaction with other corticosteroids and other barbiturates (which also are enzyme-inducing agents) although direct evidence seems to be lacking. The dexamethasone adrenal suppression test may be expected to be unreliable in those taking phenobarbitone, however 50 mg hydrocortisone instead of dexamethasone gives reliable results in the presence of phenytoin,[7] another potent enzyme inducer, and might also be considered for those on barbiturates (see 'Corticosteroids + Phenytoin').

References

1 Brooks SM, Werk EE, Ackerman SJ, Sullivan I and Thrasher K. Adverse effects of phenobarbital on corticosteroid metabolism in patients with bronchial asthma. N Engl J Med (1972) 286, 1125.
2 Burstein S and Klaiber EL. Phenobarbital-induced increase in 6-beta-hydroxycortisol excretion: clue to its significance in human urine. J Clin Endocrinol Metab (1965) 25, 293.
3 Falliers CJ. Corticosteroids and phenobarbital in asthma. N Engl J Med (1972) 287, 201.
4 Wassner SJ, Pennisi AJ, Malekzadeh MH and Fine RN. The adverse effect of anticonvulsant therapy on renal allograft survival. J Pediat (1976) 88, 134.
5 Stjernholm MR and Katz FH. Effects of diphenylhydantoin, phenobarbital and diazepam on the metabolism of methylprednisolone and its sodium succinate. J Clin Endocrinol Metab (1975) 41, 887.
6 Brooks PM, Buchanan WW, Grove M and Downie WW. Effects of enzyme induction on metabolism of prednisolone. Clinical and laboratory study. Ann Rheum Dis (1975) 35, 339.
7 Meikle AW, Stanchfield JB, West CD and Tyler FH. Hydrocortisone suppression test for Cushings syndrome: therapy with anticonvulsants. Arch Intern Med (1974) 134, 1068.
8 Bartoszek M, Brenner AM, Szefler SJ. Prednisolone and methylprednisolone kinetics in children receiving anticonvulsant therapy. Clin Pharmacol Ther (1987) 42, 424–32.

Corticosteroids + Caffeine

Abstract/Summary

The results of the dexamethasone suppression test can be falsified by the ingestion of substantial amounts of caffeine.

Clinical evidence, mechanism, importance and management

A study in 22 normal subjects and six depressed patients showed that when they were given a single 480 mg dose of caffeine at 2.0 pm following a single 1 mg dose of dexamethasone at 11.0 am, cortisol levels taken at 4.0 pm were increased from 2.3 to 5.3 μg/dl, but at 8.0 am they were unaffected.[1] Thus the equivalent of about 4–5 cups of coffee can effectively falsify the results of the dexamethasone suppression test.

Reference

1 Unde TW, Bieren LM and Post RM. Caffeine-induced escape from dexamethasone suppression. Arch Gen Psychiatry (1985) 42, 737–8.

Corticosteroids + Carbamazepine

Abstract/Summary

The loss of dexamethasone, methylprednisolone and prednisolone from the body is increased in patients taking carbamazepine and a dosage increase will be needed. The results of the dexamethasone suppression test may be invalid.

Clinical evidence

A study in eight patients on long-term treatment with carbamazepine showed that the elimination half-life of prednisolone was 27% shorter (1.98 compared with 2.73 h) and the clearance was 42% higher (4.2 versus 2.96 ml/min/kg) than in nine normal subjects.[1]

A study in asthmatic children found that carbamazepine increased the clearance of prednisolone by 97% and of methylprednisolone by 342%.[4] A study in eight normal subjects found that while taking 800 mg carbamazepine daily the dosage of dexamethasone needed to suppress cortisol secretion (as part of the dexamethasone adrenal suppression test) was increased 2–4-fold.[2] A further study found that it took 2–13 days for false-positive results to occur and 3–12 days to recover when the carbamazepine was stopped.[3]

Mechanism

The almost certain reason is that the carbamazepine stimulates the liver enzymes to metabolize the corticosteroids much faster.

Importance and management

Information is limited but the interaction appears to be established. Patients taking carbamazepine will need increased doses of dexamethasone, methylprednisolone or prednisolone. Prednisolone is less affected than methylprednisolone and is probably preferred. The same interaction seems possible with other corticosteroids but more study is needed to confirm this.

References

1 Olivesi A. Modified elimination of prednisolone in epileptic patients on carbmazepine monotherapy, and in women using low-dose oral contraceptives. Biomed and Pharmacother (1986) 40, 301–8.
2 Kobberling J and v zur Muhlen A. The influence of diphenylhydantoin and carbamazepine on the circadian rhythm of free urinary corticoids and on the suppressibility of the basal and the 'impulsive' activity of dexamethasone. Acta Endocrinologica (1973) 72, 303–18.
3 Privitera MR, Greden JF, Gardner RW, Ritchie JC and Carroll BJ. Interference by carbamazepine with the dexamethasone suppression test. Biol Psychiat (1982) 17, 611–20.
4 Bartoszek M, Brenner AM, Szefler SJ. Prednisolone and methylprednisolone kinetics in children receiving anticonvulsant therapy. Clin Pharmacol Ther (1987) 42, 424–32.

Corticosteroids + Carbimazole or Methimazole

Abstract/Summary

The loss of prednisolone from the body is increased by the use of carbimazole or methimazole. Its dosage may therefore need to be increased.

Clinical evidence

A comparative study was taken of (a) eight women taking thyroxine and under treatment with 2.5 mg methimazole or 5 mg carbimazole daily for Grave's ophthalmology, (b) six women on thyroxine who had had subtotal thyroidectomy, and (c) six other normal women. All were euthyroid. It was found that the clearance of a single 0.54 mg/kg prednisolone (IV) in those taking the methimazole or carbimazole was much greater than in the other two groups (0.37, 0.24. 0.20 l/h.kg respectively). After 6 h the plasma prednisolone levels in methimazole/carbimazole group were only about 10% of those in the normal women and none was detectable after 8 h, whereas total and unbound prednisolone levels were much higher and measurable over the 10 hour study period in the two control groups. In another group of previously hyperthyroidic patients, now euthyroid because of carbimazole treatment, the total prednisolone clearance was 0.40 l/h.[1]

Mechanism

Not established. It seems possible that the methimazole and carbimazole increase the metabolism of the prednisolone by the liver microsomal enzymes, thereby increasing its loss from the body.

Importance and management

Direct information seems to be limited to this study although the authors point out that there is a clinical impression that higher doses of prednisolone are needed in patients with Graves' disease. Be alert for the need to use higher doses of prednisolone in patients taking either methimazole or carbimazole.

Reference

1 Legler UF. Impairment of prednisolone disposition in patients with Graves disease taking methimazole. J Clin Endocrinol Metab (1988) 66, 221–3.

Corticosteroids + Cimetidine or Ranitidine

Abstract/Summary

Cimetidine does not interact with prednisolone, prednisone or dexamethasone, nor ranitidine with prednisone.

Clinical evidence, mechanism, importance and management

Prednisone is a pro-drug which must be converted to prednisolone within the body to become active. A double-blind cross-over study in nine normal subjects showed that after taking either cimetidine (300 mg six-hourly) or ranitidine (150 mg twice daily) for four days the pharmacokinetics of the prednisolone after a single 40 mg oral dose of prednisone were little changed.[1] Another double-blind cross-over study also showed that 1 g cimetidine daily only caused minor changes in plasma prednisolone levels following the administration of 10 mg of enteric-coated prednisolone.[2] Yet another study found that seven days' treatment with 1200 mg cimetidine daily had no effect on the pharmacokinetics of a single 8 mg IV dose of dexamethasone sodium phosphate.[3] There would seem to be no reason for avoiding concurrent use. Information about other corticosteroids appears to be lacking.

References

1 Sirgo MA, Rocci ML, Ferguson RK, Eshleman FN and Vlasses PH. Effects of cimetidine and ranitidine on the conversion of prednisone to prednisolone. Clin Pharmacol Ther (1985) 37, 534–8.
2 Morrison PJ, Rogers HJ, Bradbrook ID and Parsons C. Concurrent administration of cimetidine and enteric-coated prednisolone: effect on plasma levels of prednisolone. Br J clin Pharmac (1980) 10, 87.
3 Peden NR, Rewhorn I, Champion MC, Mussani R and Ooi TC. Cortisol and dexamethasone elimination during treatment with cimetidine. Br J clin Pharmac (1984) 18, 101–3.

Corticosteroids + Contraceptives (oral)

Abstract/Summary

The serum levels of prednisone, prednisolone, cloprednol and possibly other corticosteroids are considerably increased in those taking oral contraceptives. Both the therapeutic and toxic effects may be expected to be increased accordingly. Fluocortolone is not affected.

440

Clinical evidence

A comparative pharmacokinetic study on six women showed that, while taking an oral contraceptive, the plasma clearance of a single dose of prednisolone was decreased by a factor of 2.5, the area under the plasma concentration time curve was increased by 6, and the half-life increased by 2.5.[1]

This is in broad agreement with the results of other studies,[2,3,5–8] in one of which[2] the plasma clearance of prednisolone was roughly halved and the area under the plasma concentration time curve approximately doubled in eight women taking an oral contraceptive. A marked increase in plasma cloprednol levels has also been reported.[9] In another study in women with skin diseases, the use of oestrogens (chlorotrianisene or hexestrol) markedly increased the anti-inflammatory effects of prednisone or hydrocortisone given by mouth[4] and increased the concentration of serum corticosteroids by a factor of 3.

In contrast, a study in seven women showed that the pharmacokinetics of fluocortolone were unaffected by the concurrent use of oral contraceptives.[10]

Mechanism

Not understood. The possibilities include a change in the metabolism of the corticosteroids, or in their binding to serum protein.[6]

Importance and management

An established interaction. Concurrent use should be monitored. Both the therapeutic and the toxic effects of the corticosteroid would be expected to be increased but there seem to be no clinical reports of adverse reactions. A dosage reduction may be necessary to avoid corticosteroid overdosage. Only prednisone, prednisolone, cloprednol and hydrocortisone have been reported to interact but other corticosteroids possibly behave similarly, the exception being fluocortolone.

References

1 Legler UF and Benet LZ. Marked alterations in prednisolone elimination for women taking oral contraceptives. Clin Pharmacol Ther (1982) 31, 243.
2 Boekenoogen SJ, Szefler SJ, and Jusko WJ. Prednisolone disposition and protein binding in oral contraceptive users. J Clin Endocrinol Metab (1983) 56, 702–9.
3 Kozower M, Veatch L and Kaplan MM. Decreased clearance of prednisolone, a factor in the development of corticosteroid side effects. J Clin Endocrinol Metab (1974) 38, 407–12.
4 Spangler AS, Antoniades HN, Sotman SL and Inderbitizin TM. Enhancement of the anti-inflammatory action of hydrocortisone by estrogen. J Clin Endocrinol Metab (1969) 29, 650–5.
5 Legler UF and Benet LZ. Marked alterations in dose-dependent prednisolone kinetics in women taking oral contraceptives. Clin Pharmacol Ther (1986) 39, 425–9.
6 Frey BM, Schaad HJ and Frey FL. Pharmacokinetic interaction of contraceptive steroids with prednisone and prednisolone. Eur J Clin Pharmacol (1984) 26, 505–11.
7 Meffin PJ, Wing LMH, Sallustio BC and Brooks PM. Alterations in prednisolone disposition as a result of oral contraceptive use and dose. Br J clin Pharmacol (1984) 17, 655–64.
8 Olivesi A. Modified elimination of prednisolone in epileptic patients
on carbamazepine monotherapy, and in women using low-dose oral contraceptives. Biomed Pharmacother (1986) 40, 301–8.
9 Legler UF. Altered cloprednol disposition in oral contraceptive users. Clin Pharmacol Ther (1987) 41, 237.
10 Legler UF. Lack of impairment of fluocortolone disposition in oral contraceptive users. Eur J Clin Pharmacol (1988) 35, 101–3.

Corticosteroids + Diuretics, potassium-losing

Abstract/Summary

Since both of these groups of drugs cause potassium to be lost from the body, an excessive loss of potassium may occur if these drugs are used concurrently, possibly leading to severe depletion. The intake of potassium may need to be increased to balance this loss.

Clinical evidence, mechanism, importance and management

Some corticosteroids and some diuretics can cause a significant loss of potassium from the body. This is very well documented. Additive effects would therefore be expected if taken together and severe potassium depletion is possible, but there seem to be no formal clinical trials describing the extent of the depletion during concurrent use. The effects should be monitored and the intake of potassium increased as necessary to balance this loss if members of both groups of drugs are used together.

The corticosteroids which cause the greatest potassium loss are those which are naturally occurring. These include cortisone and hydrocortisone. Fludrocortisone also causes potassium loss. Corticotrophin (ACTH) which is a pituitary hormone and tetracosactrin (a synthetic polypeptide) stimulate corticosteroid secretion by the adrenal cortex and can thereby indirectly cause potassium loss. The synthetic corticosteroids (glucocorticoids) have a much less marked potassium-losing effect and are less likely to cause problems. These include prednisone, prednisolone, dexamethasone, betamethasone and triamcinolone.

The potassium-losing diuretics include bumetanide, frusemide, ethacrynic acid, piretanide and the thiazides and related diuretics (bendrofluazide, benzthiazide, chlorothiazide, clopamide, cyclopenthiazide, hydrochlorothiazide, hydroflumethiazide, indapamide, mefruside, methyclothiazide, metolazone, polythiazide, xipamide).

Corticosteroids + Ephedrine and Theophylline

Abstract/Summary

Ephedrine increases the loss of dexamethasone from the body, but theophylline appears not to interact.

441

Clinical evidence, mechanism, importance and management

Nine asthmatic patients showed a 40% increase in the clearance of the dexamethasone when concurrently given 100 mg ephedrine daily for three weeks.[1] This would be expected to reduce the overall control of asthma, but this requires confirmation. Theophylline appeared not to interact.[1] It is not clear whether other corticosteroids behave similarly.

Reference

1 Brooks SM, Sholiton LJ, Werk EE and Altenau P. The effects of ephedrine and theophylline on dexamethasone metabolism in bronchial asthma. J Clin Pharmacol (1977) 17, 308.

Corticosteroids + Ketoconazole

Abstract/Summary

Ketoconazole reduces the metabolism and loss of prednisone, prednisolone and methylprednisolone from the body. Reduce the corticosteroid dosage.

Clinical evidence

(a) Methylprednisolone

A study in six normal subjects showed that 200 mg ketoconazole daily for six days increased the mean AUC (area under the concentration-time curve) of a single 20 mg dose of methylprednisolone by 135% and decreased the clearance by 60%. The 24 h cortisol AUC was reduced by 44%.[1]

These findings are confirmed by the results of another study by the same group of workers.[2]

(b) Prednisone and prednisolone

A study in 10 normal subjects found that 200 mg ketoconazole daily for 6–7 days caused a 50% rise in the total and unbound prednisolone serum levels following oral prednisone or intravenous prednisolone.[3]

Mechanism

Ketoconazole inhibits cytochrome P-450 dependent enzymes in the liver so that the metabolism of the corticosteroids and endogenous cortisol is reduced, thereby reducing their loss from the body and increasing their effects.

Importance and management

An established and adequately documented interaction. A 50% reduction in the corticosteroid dosage is recommended in one study.[2] It has been pointed out that increased corticosteroid serum levels have an increased immunosuppressive effect which may be undesirable in those with a fungal infection needing treatment with ketoconazole.[3]

References

1 Glynn AM, Slaughter RL, Brass C, D'Ambrosio R and Jusko WJ. Effects of ketoconazole on methylprednisolone pharmacokinetics and cortisol secretion. Clin Pharmacol Ther (1986) 39, 654–9.
2 Kandrotas RJ, Slaughter RL, Brass C and Jusko WJ. Ketoconazole effects on methylprednisolone disposition and their joint suppression of endogenous cortisol. Clin Pharmacol Ther (1987) 42, 465–70.
3 Zurcher RM, Frey BM and Frey FJ. Impact of ketoconazole on the metabolism of prednisolone. Clin Pharmacol Ther (1989) 45, 366–72.

Corticosteroids + Macrolide antibiotics

Abstract/Summary

Triacetyloleandomycin and to a lesser extent erythromycin can reduce the loss of methylprednisolone from the body, thereby increasing both its therapeutic and toxic effects. Prednisolone appears not to be affected except in those taking enzyme-inducing agents such as phenytoin and phenobarbitone. Other corticosteroids are probably not affected.

Clinical evidence

(a) Methylprednisolone + erythromycin

A study in nine adolescent patients aged 9–18 with asthma showed that after taking 250 mg erythromycin four times a day for a week, the clearance of methylprednisolone was decreased by 46% (range 28–61%) and the half-life was increased by 51% (from 2.34 to 3.45 h).[4]

(b) Methylprednisolone and prednisolone + triacetyloleandomycin

A pharmacokinetic study in four children and six adults who were steroid-dependent asthmatics showed that one week's treatment with 14 mg/kg triacetyloleandomycin daily increased the half-life of methylprednisolone by 90% (from 2.46 to 4.63 h) and reduced the total body clearance by 44% (from 406 to 146 ml/min/1.73 m²). All 10 showed cushingoid symptoms (cushingoid facies and weight gain) which resolved when the methylprednisolone dosage was reduced, without any loss in the control of the asthma.[1]

A later study by the same group of workers confirmed these findings but they also found that prednisolone clearance was not affected except in those who were also taking phenytoin or phenobarbitone which are enzyme inducers.[2,3]

A number of other reports confirm that triacetyloleandomycin can act as a 'steroid-sparing' agent.[5–7] One of them reported a 50% reduction in steroid clearance.[7]

Mechanism

What is known suggests that these macrolide antibiotics inhibit the metabolism of methylprednisolone, thereby reducing its loss from the body and increasing its effects. The volume of distribution is also decreased.[1–4]

Importance and management

Information about the erythromycin–methylprednisolone interaction is much more limited than the triacetyloleandomycin–methylprednisolone interaction, but both appear to be established and of clinical importance. This 'steroid-sparing' effect should be taken into account during concurrent use and appropriate dosage reductions made to avoid the development of the side-effects of corticosteroid overdosage. One study suggests that this reduction should be '...empirical and based primarily on clinical symptomatology.'[1] Triacetyloleandomycin appears to have a larger effect than erythromycin. Prednisolone seems not to interact with triacetyloleandomycin and is a non-interacting alternative except in those taking enzyme-inducing drugs (e.g. phenytoin, phenobarbitone). The general silence in the literature suggests that these macrolide antibiotics do not interact with other corticosteroids but be on the alert for any changes until this is confirmed. There also seems to be no information about other macrolide antibiotics.

References

1 Szefler SJ, Rose JQ, Ellis EF, Spector SL, Green AW and Jusko WJ. The effect of troleandomycin on methylprednisolone elimination. J Allergy Clin Immunol (1980) 66, 447–51.

2 Szefler SJ, Ellis EF, Brenner M, Rose JQ, Spector SL, Yurchak A, Andrews F and Jusko WJ. Steroid-specific and anticonvulsant interaction aspects of triacetyloleandomycin-steroid therapy. J Allergy Clin Immunol (1982) 69, 455–60.

3 Szefler SJ, Brenner M, Jusko WJ, Spector SL, Flesher KA and Ellis EF. Dose- and time-related effects of troleandomycin on methylprednisolone elimination. Clin Pharmacol Ther (1982) 32, 166–171.

4 Laforce CF, Szefler SJ, Miller MF, Ebling W and Brenner M. Inhibition of methylprednisolone elimination in the presence of erythromycin. J Allergy Clin Immunol (1983) 72, 34–9.

5 Fox JL. Infectious asthma treated with triacetyloleandomycin. Penn Med J (1961) 64, 634–5.

6 Itkin IH and Menzel M. The use of macrolide antibiotic substances in the treatment of asthma. J Allergy (1970) 45, 146–62.

7 Ball BD, Hill M, Brenner M, Sanks R and Szefler SJ. Critical assessment of troleandomycin in severe steroid-requiring asthmatic children. Ann Allergy (1988) 60, 155.

Corticosteroids + Non-steroidal anti-inflammatory drugs (NSAID's)

Abstract/Summary

Concurrent use increases the incidence of gastro-intestinal bleeding and probably ulceration. Indomethacin and naproxen can have a 'steroid sparing' effect.

Clinical evidence, mechanism, importance and management

(a) Gastrointestinal bleeding and ulceration

A retrospective study of more than 20,000 patients who had had corticosteroids showed that the incidence of upper gastrointestinal bleeding was no greater than in the control group who had not had corticosteroids (95 compared with 91). However there was found to be an increased risk of bleeding if the patients were also taking aspirin or other non-steroidal anti-inflammatory drugs.[1] This is consistent with the results of another study on patients taking prednisone and indomethacin,[2] and gives support to the widely held belief that concurrent use of the NSAID's (well-known as gastric irritants) can cause bleeding and ulceration. Concurrent use should be very well monitored. See also 'Aspirin and Salicylates + Corticosteroids'.

(b) Steroid-sparing effect

A study in 11 patients with stable rheumatoid disease on regular corticosteroid therapy showed that when given either 75 mg indomethacin or 250 mg naproxen twice daily for two weeks the total serum levels of a single 7.5 mg dose of prednisolone remained unchanged but the amount of unbound (free) prednisolone increased by 30–60%.[3] The probable reason is that these NSAID's displace prednisolone and endogenous corticosteroids from their plasma protein binding sites. It should therefore be possible to reduce the corticosteroid dosage while maintaining the therapeutic effects.

References

1 Carson JL, Strom BL, Schinnar R, Sim E, Maislin G and Morse ML. Do corticosteroids really cause upper GI bleeding? Clin Res (1987) 35, 340A.

2 Emmanuel JH and Montgomery RD. Gastric ulcer and anti-arthritic drugs. Postgrad Med J (1971) 47, 227.

3 Rae SA, Williams IA, English J and Baylis EM. Alteration of plasma prednisolone levels by indomethacin and naproxen. Br J clin Pharmac (1982) 14, 459–61.

Corticosteroids + Phenytoin

Abstract/Summary

(a) The therapeutic effects of dexamethasone, prednisone, prednisolone, methylprednisolone (probably other glucocorticoids) and fludrocortisone can be markedly reduced by the concurrent use of phenytoin. (b) The results of the dexamethasone adrenal suppression test may prove to be unreliable, and (c) serum phenytoin levels may be changed by dexamethasone.

Clinical evidence

(a) Reduced corticosteroid levels

A comparative pharmacokinetic study in six neurological or neurosurgical patients taking dexamethasone (orally) and phenytoin showed that the average amount of dexamethasone which reached the general circulation was a quarter of that observed in nine other patients taking only dexamethasone (mean oral bioavailability fractions of 0.21 and 0.84 respectively).[1]

Other patients have been described who needed increased doses of dexamethasone while taking phenytoin.[2] The fludrocortisone dosages of two patients required marked increases (fourfold in one patient and 10–20 times in the

Table 16.2. A comparison of the effects of phenytoin on the kinetics of different glucocorticoids (after Petereit and colleagues[3])

			Corticosteroid		
	Daily dosage of phenytoin (mg)	Half-life without phenytoin (min)	Decreased half life with phenytoin (%)	Increased mean clearance rate with phenytoin (%)	Reference
Hydrocortisone	300–400	60–90	−15	+25	11
Methylprednisolone	300	165	−56	+130	12
Prednisone	Prednisolone is the biologically active metabolite of prednisone so that the values for prednisone and prednisolone should be similar.				13
Prednisolone	300	190–240	−45	+77	7,8
Dexamethasone	300	250	−51	+140	14, 15

other) while taking phenytoin.[17] Renal allograft survival is decreased in patients on prednisone taking phenytoin due (it is believed) to reduced immunosuppressant effects.[8] The effects of phenytoin on the half-lives and clearance rates of other corticosteroids are shown in Table 16.2.

(b) Interference with the dexamethasone adrenal suppression test

A study on seven patients showed that while taking 300–400 mg phenytoin daily their plasma cortisol levels were only reduced by dexamethasone from 22 to 19 μg% compared with a reduction from 18 to 4 μg% in the absence of phenytoin.[4]

Other studies confirm that plasma cortisol and urinary 17-hydroxycorticosteroid levels are suppressed far less than might be expected with small doses of dexamethasone (0.5 mg six-hourly for eight doses), but with larger doses (2.0 mg six-hourly for eight doses) suppression was normal.[5]

(c) Serum phenytoin levels increased or decreased

A post-traumatic epilepsy prophylaxis study showed that the serum phenytoin levels in those taking dexamethasone (16–150 mg: mean 63.6 mg) was 40% higher than those on phenytoin alone (17.7 compared with 12.5 μg/ml). The phenytoin was given as a loading dose of 11 mg/kg IV and then 13 mg/kg IM.[6]

A retrospective study of 40 patient records indicated that dexamethasone reduced serum phenytoin levels. The serum phenytoin levels of six patients on fixed doses of phenytoin were halved by the presence of dexamethasone.[7]

Mechanism

Phenytoin is a potent liver enzyme inducing agent which increases the metabolism of the corticosteroids so that they are cleared from the body more quickly, reducing both their therapeutic and adrenal suppressant effects

Importance and management

(a) The fall in serum corticosteroid levels is established and of clinical importance where treatment depends upon transport by the circulation (e.g. in immunosuppression), but it seems unlikely to affect the response to steroids ad-

ministered topically or by inhalation, intra-articular injection or enema.[3] The interaction can be accommodated in several ways: (i) Increase the corticosteroid dosage proportionately to the increase in clearance (see Table 16.2). With prednisolone an average increase of 100% (range 58–260% in five individuals) proved effective.[3] A fourfold increase may be necessary with dexamethasone,[1] and much greater increases have been required with fludrocortisone.[17] (ii) Exchange the corticosteroid for another which is less affected (see Table 16.2). A switch from dexamethasone to equivalent doses of methylprednisolone has been reported to be effective[9] but another report found that methylprednisolone was affected more than prednisolone.[18] In another case the exchange of 16 mg dexamethasone daily for 100 mg prednisone was successful.[10] (iii) Exchange the phenytoin for another anticonvulsant: Barbiturates, and to some extent primidone[16] and carbamazepine, are also enzyme-inducing agents, but sodium valproate is a successful non-interacting alternative.[2]

(b) The effects on the dexamethasone adrenal suppression test can apparently be accommodated by using larger than usual doses of dexamethasone (2 mg every 6 h for eight doses)[5] or by using an overnight test using 50 mg hydrocortisone.[9]

(c) The reports on the changes in serum phenytoin levels are inconsistent (rises and falls). The effects of concurrent use should be monitored.

References

1 Chalk JB, Ridgeway K, Brophy TrO'R, Yelland JDN and Eadie MJ. Phenytoin impairs the bioavailability of dexamethasone in neurological and neurosurgical patients. J Neurol Neurosurg Psychiatry (1984) 47, 1087–90.
2 McLelland J and Jack W. Phenytoin/dexamethasone interaction: a clinical problem. Lancet (1978) i, 1096.
3 Petereit LB and Meikle AW. Effectiveness of prednisolone during phenytoin therapy. Clin Pharmacol Ther (1977) 22, 912.
4 Werk EE, Choi Y, Sholiton L, Olinger C and Haque N. Interference in the effect of dexamethasone by diphenylhydantoin. N Engl J Med (1969) 281, 32.
5 Jubiz W, Meikle AW, Levinson RA, Mizutani S, West CD and Tyler FH. Effect of diphenylhydantoin on the metabolism of dexamethasone. N Engl J Med (1970) 283, 11.
6 Lawson LA, Blouin RA, Smith RB, Rapp RP and Young AB. Phenytoin-dexamethasone interaction: a previously unreported observation. Surg Neurol (1981) 16, 23.
7 Wong DD, Longenecker RG, Liepman M, Baker S and LaVergne M.

Phenytoin-dexamethasone: a possible drug-drug interaction. J Amer Med Ass (1985) 254, 2062–3.

8 Wassner SJ, Pennisi AJ, Malekzadeh MH and Fine RN. The adverse effect of anticonvulsant therapy on renal allograft survival. J Pediat (1976) 88, 134–7.

9 Meikle AW, Stanchfield JB, West CD and Tyler FH. Hydrocortisone suppression test for Cushing syndrome: therapy with anticonvulsants. Arch Intern Med (1974) 134, 1068.

10 Boyland JJ, Owen DS and Chin JB. Phenytoin interference with dexamethasone. J Amer Med Ass (1976) 235, 802.

11 Choi Y, Thrasher K, Werk EE, Sholiton LJ and Ollinger C. Effect of diphenylhydantoin on cortisol kinetics in humans. J Pharmacol Exp Ther (1971) 176, 27.

12 Stjernholm MR and Katz FH. Effects of diphenylhydantoin, phenobarbitone and diazepam on the metabolism of methylprednisolone and its hemisuccinate. J Clin Endocrinol Metab (1975) 41, 887.

13 Meikle AW. Weed JA and Tyler FH. Kinetics and interconversion of prednisolone and prednisone studies with new radio-immunoassays. J Clin Endocrinol Metab (1975) 41, 717.

14 Brooks SM, Werk EE, Ackerman S, Sullivan I and Thrasher K. Adverse effects of phenobarbital on corticosteroid metabolism in patients with bronchial asthmas. N Engl J Med (1972) 286, 1125.

15 Haque N, Thrasher K, Werk EE, Knowles HC and Sholiton LJ. Studies of dexamethasone metabolism in man. Effect of diphenylhydantoin. J Clin Endocrinol Metab (1972) 34, 44.

16 Hancock KW and Levell MJ. Primidone/dexamethasone interaction. Lancet (1978) i, 97.

17 Keilholz U and Guthrie GP. Case report: adverse effect of phenytoin on mineralocorticoid replacement with fludrocortisone in adrenal insufficiency. Amer J Med Sci (1986) 291, 280–3.

18 Bartoszek M, Brenner AM and Szefler SJ. Prednisolone and methylprednisolone kinetics in children receiving anticonvulsant therapy. Clin Pharmacol Ther (1987) 42, 424–32.

Corticosteroids + Primidone

Abstract/Summary

A case report describes a reduction in the effects of dexamethasone due to the concurrent use of primidone. Primidone may also possibly invalidate the results of the dexamethasone adrenal suppression tests.

Clinical evidence, mechanism, importance and management

Direct evidence of an interaction seems to be limited to a letter describing a reduction in the effects of dexamethasone in a woman with congenital adrenal hyperplasia when treated with primidone for petit mal.[1] The probable reason for this reaction is that primidone is metabolized to phenobarbitone which is a potent liver enzyme inducing agent. This would be expected to increase the metabolism of the dexamethasone by the liver, thereby hastening its loss from the body and reducing its effects. For the same reason the results of the dexamethasone adrenal suppression test should be viewed with caution in patients taking primidone. See also 'Corticosteroids + Barbiturates'.

Reference

1 Hancock KW and Leveli A. Primidone/dexamethasone interaction. Lancet (1978) ii, 97.

Corticosteroids + Rifampicin (Rifampin)

Abstract/Summary

The effects of the corticosteroids can be markedly reduced by the concurrent use of rifampicin.

Clinical evidence

A child with nephrotic syndrome on prednisolone, accidentally given BCG vaccine, was treated with rifampicin and isoniazid to prevent possible dissemination of the vaccine. When the nephrotic condition failed to respond, the prednisolone dosage was raised from 2 to 3 mg/kg daily without any evidence of corticosteroid overdosage. Later when the rifampicin and isoniazid were withdrawn, remission of the nephrotic condition was achieved with the original dosage of prednisolone.[3]

A number of other reports describe a reduction in the response to corticosteroids (prednisone, prednisolone, methylprednisolone) in patients when given rifampicin, including a number who had had renal transplants.[2,3–5,7,8,11] A patient with Addison's disease stabilized on cortisone and fludrocortisol showed typical signs of corticosteroid overdosage when the rifampicin he was taking was replaced by ethambutol.[1] A pharmacokinetic study in patients with TB showed that the AUC of prednisolone was reduced 66% by rifampicin.[7] Another study found a 48% reduction and a decrease in the elimination half-life from 3.72 to 2.11 h.[9]

Mechanism

Rifampicin is a potent liver enzyme inducing agent which increases the metabolism of the corticosteroids by the liver,[4,6] thereby increasing their loss from the body and reducing their effects.

Importance and management

An established, well documented and clinically important interaction. The need to increase the dosage of cortisone, hydrocortisone, fludrocortisone, prednisone, prednisolone and methylprednisolone should be expected if rifampicin is given. A number of workers suggest that as a first approximation the dosage should be increased 2–3-fold, and reduced proportionately if the rifampicin is withdrawn.[4,7,9,10] There seems to be no direct information about other corticosteroids but be on the alert for them to be similarly affected.

References

1 Edwards OM, Courtnay-Evans RJ, Galley JM, Hunter J and Tait AD. Changes in cortisol metabolism following rifampicin therapy. Lancet (1974) ii, 549.

2 Hendrickse W, McKiernan J, Pickup M and Lowe J. Rifampicin-induced non-responsiveness to corticosteroid treatment in nephrotic syndrome. Br Med J (1979) 1, 306.

3 Van Marle W, Woods KL and Beeley L. Concurrent steroid and rifampicin therapy. Br Med J (1979) 1, 1020.

4 Buffington GA, Dominguez JH, Piering WF, Hebert LA, Kaufmann HM and Lemann J. Interaction of rifampin and glucocorticoids. J Amer Med Ass (1976) 236, 1958.

5 Mendez-Picon G, Murai M and Pierce JC. Tuberculosis in transplant patients: two possible cases of rifampin renal toxicity. Read before the 8th Annual Meeting of the American Society of Nephrology, Washington 1975.

6 Sotianemi EA, Medzihradsky F and Eliasson G. Glutaric acid as an indicator of use of enzyme-inducing drugs. Clin Pharmacol Ther (1974) 15, 417.

7 McAllister WAC, Thompson PJ, Al-Habet SM and Rogers HJ. Rifampicin reduces effectiveness and bioavailability of prednisolone. Br Med J (1983) 286, 923–5.

8 Powell-Jackson A, Gray BJ, Heaton RW, Costello JF, Williams R and English J. Adverse effect of rifampicin administration on steroid-dependent asthma. Am Rev Resp Dis (1983) 128, 307–10.

9 Bergram H and Refvan OK. Altered prednisolone pharmacokinetics in patients treated with rifampicin. Acta Med Scand (1983) 213, 339–43.

10 Lofhahl C-G, Mellstrand T, Svedmyr N and Wahlen P. Increased metabolism of prednisolone and rifampicin after rifampicin treatment. Am Rev Resp Dis (1984) 129, A201.

11 Bitaudeau Ph, Clement S, Chartier JPh, Papapietro PM, Bonnafoux A, Arnaud M, Treves R and Desproges-Gotteron R. Interaction rifampicine-prednisolone. A propos de deux cas au cours d'une maladie de Horton. Rev Rhumatisme (1989) 56, 87–8.

Corticosteroids + Sucralfate

Abstract/Summary

Sucralfate appears not to interact with prednisone.

Clinical evidence, mechanism, importance and management

A cross-over study in 12 normal subjects showed that the concurrent use of 1 g sucralfate every 6 h had no effect on the pharmacokinetics of a single 20 mg dose of prednisone, except that the peak serum levels were delayed by about three-quarters of an hour when given at the same time, but not when the sucralfate was given 2 h after the prednisone.[1] Information about other corticosteroids is lacking.

Reference

1 Gambertoglio JG, Romac DR, Yong C-L, Birnbaum J, Lizak P and Amend WJ C. Lack of effect of sucralfate on prednisone bioavailability. Amer J Gastroenterology (1987) 82, 42–5.

Corticosteroids + Live vaccines

Abstract/Summary

Patients who are immunized with live virus vaccines while receiving immunosuppressive doses of corticosteroids may develop a generalized, possibly life-threatening, infection.

Clinical evidence, mechanism, importance and management

The administration of the corticosteroids can reduce the number of circulating lymphocytes and suppress the normal immune response so that concurrent immunization with live vaccines can lead to generalized infection. It is considered that prednisone in doses greater than 10–15 mg daily will suppress the immune response, whereas 40–60 mg doses of prednisone on alternate days probably do not.[4] A patient with lymphosarcoma and hypogammaglobulinaemia, taking 15 mg prednisone daily, developed a generalized vaccinial infection when she was vaccinated.[1] A fatal vaccinial infection developed in another patient treated with cortisone.[2] This problem can be controlled by giving immunoglobulin to give cover against a general infection while immunity develops, and this has been successfully used in steroid-dependent patients needing smallpox vaccination.[3]

Smallpox vaccination is no longer necessary but other live attenuated vaccines (measles, mumps, rubella, poliomyelitis, BCG) are still used and the principles relevant for smallpox are probably generally applicable, but no studies seem to have been done to establish what is safe.[4] These are some of the published warnings: '...extreme caution must be observed in administering live virus vaccine to any patient receiving steroid therapy...' and '...it seems unwise to administer live virus vaccines to any person receiving steroids for a systemic effect in any dosage.'[4] There would seem to be no problem with topical or inhalation steroids in normal dosages because the amounts absorbed are small.[4]

References

1 Rosenbaum EH, Cohen RA and Glatstein HR. Vaccination of a patient receiving immunosuppressive therapy for lymphosarcoma. J Amer Med Ass (1966) 198, 737–40.

2 Olansky S, Smith JG and Hansen OC E. Fatal vaccinia associated with cortisone therapy. J Amer Med Ass (1956) 162, 887–8.

3 Joseph MR. Vaccination of patients on steroid therapy. Med J Aust (1974) 2, 181.

4 Shapiro L. Questions and Answers. Live virus vaccine and corticosteroid therapy. J Amer Med Ass (1981) 246, 2075–6. Answered by Fauci AS, Bellanti JA, Polk IJ and Cherry JD.

Cyclosporin(e) + Aminoglycoside antibiotics

Abstract/Summary

Both animal and human studies indicate that kidney toxicity may be increased by concurrent use of cyclosporin and gentamicin, tobramycin, framycetin or possibly other aminoglycosides.

Clinical evidence, mechanism, importance and management

A comparative study in patients given 30 mg gentamicin with lincomycin just prior to transplantation showed that the concurrent use of cyclosporin increased the incidence of nephrotoxicity from 5% to 67%.[1] When ampicillin, ceftazidime and lincomycin were used instead the incidence of nephrotoxicity was 10%.[1] Three other reports describe increased nephrotoxicity associated with the concurrent use of cyclosporin and gentamicin,[6] tobramycin[2,3] or framycetin.[2] This interaction has also been well demonstrated in animals.[4,5] Information from human studies is limited but what is known suggests that aminoglycosides and cyclosporin can have additive nephrotoxic effects and should therefore probably be avoided or only used with great caution. Ceftazidime has also been implicated in an increase in serum cyclosporin levels.[7]

References

1 Termeer A, Hoitsma AJ and Koene RAP. Severe nephrotoxicity caused by the combined use of gentamicin and cyclosporine in renal allograft recipients. Transplantation (1986) 42, 220–1.
2 Hows JM, Chipping PM, Fairhead S, Smith J, Baughan A and Gordon-Smith EC. Nephrotoxicity in bone marrow transplant recipients treated with cyclosporin A. Br J Haematol (1983) 54, 69–78.
3 Hows JM, Palmer S, Want S, Dearden C and Gordon-Smith EC. Serum levels of cyclosporin A and nephrotoxicity in bone marrow transplant patients. Lancet (1981) ii, 145–6.
4 Whiting PH and Simpson JG. The enhancement of cyclosporin A-induced nephrotoxicity by gentamicin. Biochem Pharmacol (1983) 32, 2025–8.
5 Ryffel B, Muller AM and Mihatsch MJ. Experimental cyclosporine nephrotoxicity: risk of concomitant chemotherapy. Clin Nephrol (1986) 25, Suppl 1, S121–5.
6 Morales JM, Andres A, Prieto C, Rolon JAD and Rodicio JL. Reversible acute renal toxicity by toxic synergic effect between gentamicin and cyclosporine. Clin Nephrol (1988) 29, 272.
7 Cockburn I. Cyclosporin A: a clinical evaluation of drug interactions. Transplantation Proc (1986) 18, (Suppl 5), 50–5.

Cyclosporin(e) + Amphotericin (B)

Abstract/Summary

Kidney toxicity is increased if cyclosporin and amphotericin are used concurrently.

Clinical evidence

A comparative study in 47 patients with bone marrow transplants showed that the concurrent use of amphotericin B increased the incidence of kidney toxicity. Out of a total of 10 patients who had had both drugs, five doubled and three tripled their serum creatinine levels within five days. In contrast only 8 out of 21 (38%) on cyclosporin alone and 3 out of 16 (19%) on methotrexate and amphotericin B doubled their serum creatinine within 14–30 and 5 days respectively.[1]

Another study in patients on cyclosporin with bone marrow transplants found that amphotericin B contributed significantly to renal failure.[2] It can apparently develop even after the amphotericin has been withdrawn.

Mechanism

Not understood.

Importance and management

An established and clinically important interaction. The authors of the study cited[1] point out that if amphotericin must be given and where withdrawal of the cyclosporin may be dangerous if creatinine levels rise because graft rejection or graft-versus-host-disease may develop acutely, they suggest witholding cyclosporin until serum levels are less than about 150 ng/ml. This may reduce the renal toxicity without losing the immunosuppressive effect.

References

1 Kennedy MS, Deeg HJ, Siegel M, Crowley JJ, Storb R and Thomas ED. Acute renal toxicity with combined use of amphotericin B and cyclosporine after bone marrow transplantation. Transplantation (1983) 35, 211–15.
2 Tutschka PJ, Beschorner WE, Hess AD and Santos GW. Cyclosporin-A to prevent graft-versus-host-disease: a pilot study in 22 patients receiving allogeneic marrow transplants. Blood (1983) 61, 318–25.

Cyclosporin(e) + Anticoagulants

Abstract/Summary

The cyclosporin levels of a patient fell when given warfarin. When the cyclosporin dosage was increased an increase in the warfarin dosage was needed. Another report describes a rise in serum cyclosporin levels when an un-named anticoagulant was given. Yet another describes increased nicoumalone effects while receiving cyclosporin.

Clinical evidence, mechanism, importance and management

A man with erythrocyte aplasia effectively treated with cyclosporin for 18 months, relapsed within a week of starting warfarin. His cyclosporin levels had fallen from a range of 300–350 to 170 ng/ml. He responded well when the cyclosporin dosage was increased from 3 to 7 mg/kg daily, but his prothrombin activity rose from 17% of control to 64% and he needed an increase in the warfarin dosage to achieve satisfactory anticoagulation. The patient was also taking phenobarbitone.[1] Another patient on nicoumalone (acenocoumarol) showed the opposite effect. His anticoagulant dosage needed to be approximately halved when he was started on cyclosporin following a kidney transplant.[3] The reasons are not understood. Another report briefly says that serum cyclosporin levels rose in a patient when given a warfarin derivative.[2] These reports serve to emphasize the need to monitor concurrent use. The outcome is uncertain.

447

References

1 Snyder DS. Interaction between cyclosporine and warfarin. Ann Intern Med (1988) 108, 311.

2 Cockburn I (Sandoz, Basel). Cyclosporin A: a clinical evaluation of drug interactions. Transplantation Proc (1986) 18, (Suppl 5) 50–5.

3 Campistol JM, Maragall D and Andreu J. Interaction between cyclosporin A and sintrom. Nephron (1989) 53, 291–2

Cyclosporin(e) + Anticonvulsants

Abstract/Summary

Serum cyclosporin levels are markedly reduced by the concurrent use of carbamazepine, phenobarbitone and phenytoin. The dosage of cyclosporin may need to be increased 2–3-fold to maintain adequate immunosuppression. Valproic acid appears not to affect cyclosporin levels but it may possibly damage renal grafts.

Clinical evidence

(a) Cyclosporin + carbamazepine

A report describes a kidney transplant patient on cyclosporin whose serum levels fell from 346 to 64 ng/ml within three days of starting to take 200 mg carbamazepine three times daily. A week later serum levels were down to 37 ng/ml. They rose again when the carbamazepine was stopped but fell once more when it was restarted. The cyclosporin dosage was increased to keep the levels within the therapeutic range.[3]

Two other patients have shown this interaction. One needed her cyclosporin dosage to be doubled in order to maintain adequate serum levels while taking 800 mg carbamazepine daily. When the carbamazepine was replaced by sodium valproate in both patients, the cyclosporin dosages became normal again.[4]

(b) Cyclosporin + phenobarbitone

A 4-year-old child on phenobarbitone (50 mg twice daily) with a bone marrow transplant had serum cyclosporin levels of less than 60 ng/ml even after raising the dosage to 18 mg/kg daily. When the phenobarbitone dosage was halved and later halved again the trough serum cyclosporin levels rose to 205 ng/ml.[5]

A threefold increase in cyclosporin clearance was seen in another child with a kidney transplant while on phenobarbitone (12.6 compared with 3.8 ml/min/kg).[6] Reductions in cyclosporin levels due to phenobarbitone have been described in other patients.[8,11,12]

(c) Cyclosporin + phenytoin

The observation of five patients on cyclosporin who needed dosage increases while taking phenytoin prompted a further study in six normal subjects. It was found that while taking 300–400 mg phenytoin daily the maximal serum cyclosporin levels and the AUC (area under the curve) following a single 15 mg/kg dose were reduced by 37% (from 1325 to 831 μg/l) and 47% (10.4 to 5.5 mg l^{-1} h) respectively.[1,13]

Another report by the same authors describes six patients whose serum cyclosporin levels were more than halved while treated with phenytoin (750–1000 mg daily orally and intravenously) despite an almost twofold increase in the cyclosporin dosage. It persisted for about a week after the phenytoin was stopped.[2] 2–4-fold increases in cyclosporin dosages were needed in nine heart transplant patients when given phenytoin,[9] and increases were also needed in an 11-year-old boy with a bone marrow transplant.[10]

Mechanisms

Not fully resolved. It is thought that phenytoin,[1,2] carbamazepine[3] and phenobarbitone[5,12] increase the metabolism of the cyclosporin by the liver (hepatic P450 oxygenase system) thereby increasing its loss from the body and lowering the serum levels accordingly. Phenytoin also possibly reduces the absorption of the cyclosporin.[7]

Importance and management

None of these interactions is extensively documented but all appear to be established and of clinical importance. Serum cyclosporin levels should be well monitored if carbamazepine, phenobarbitone or phenytoin are given concurrently and the cyclosporin dosage increased appropriately (by a factor of two or even more). The effects of the interaction may persist for a week or more after the anticonvulsant is withdrawn. Sodium valproate seems to be a non-interacting anticonvulsant,[4] however interstitial nephritis was suspected in one patient with a renal graft.[8]

References

1 Freeman DJ, Laupacis A, Keown PA, Stiller CR and Carruthers SG. Evaluation of cyclosporin-phenytoin interaction with observations on cyclosporin metabolites. Br J clin Pharmac (1984) 18, 887–93.

2 Keown PA, Laupacis A, Carruthers G, Stawecki M, Koegler J, McKenzie FN, Wall W and Stiller CR. Interaction between phenytoin and cyclosporine following organ transplantation. Transplantation (1984) 38, 304–6.

3 Lele P, Peterson P, Yang S, Jarell B and Burke JF. Cyclosporine and tegretol—another drug interaction. Kidney Int (1985) 27, 344.

4 Hillebrand G, Castro LA, van Scheidt W, Beukelmann D, Land W and Schmidt D. Valproate for epilepsy in renal transplant recipients receiving cyclosporine. Transplantation (1987) 43, 915–16.

5 Carstenen H, Jacobsen N and Dieperink H. Interaction between cyclosporin A and phenobarbitone. Br J clin Pharmac (1986) 21, 550–1.

6 Burckart GJ, Venkataramanan R, Starz T, Ptachcinski J, Gartner JC and Rosenthal T. Cyclosporine clearance in children following organ transplantation. J Clin Pharmacol (1984) 24, 412.

7 Rowland M and Gupta SK. Cyclosporin-phenytoin interaction: re-evaluation using metabolite data. Br J clin Pharmac (1987) 24, 329–34.

8 Kramer G, Dillmann U and Tettenborn B. Cyclosporine-phenobarbital interaction. Epilepsia (1989) 30, 701.

9 Grigg-Damberger MM, Costanzo-Nordin R, Kelly MA, Bahamon-Dussan JE, Silver M, Zucker MJ and Celesia GG. Phenytoin may compromise efficacy of cyclosporine immunosuppresion in cardiac transplant patients. Epilepsia (1988) 29, 693.

10 Schmidt H, Naumann R, Jaschonek K, Einsele H, Dopfer R and Ehn-

inger G. Drug interaction between cyclosporin and phenytoin in allogeneic bone marrow transplantation. Bone Marrow Transplantation (1989) 4, 212–13.

11 Kramer G, DillmR M, Frey BM and Frey FJ. Impact of ketoconazole on the metabolism of prednisolone. Clin Pharmacol Ther (1989) 45, 366–72.

12 Beierle FA and Bailey L. Cyclosporine metabolism impeded/blocked by co-administration of phenobarbitol. Clin Chem (1989) 35, 1160.

13 Freeman DJ, Laupacis A, Keown P, Stiller C and Carruthers G. The effects of agents that alter drug metabolizing enzyme activity on the pharmaokinetics of cyclosporin. Ann Roy Coll Phys Can (1984) 17, 301.

Cyclosporin(e) + Calcium channel blockers

Abstract/Summary

Diltiazem, nicardipine and verapamil raise serum cyclosporin levels but also appear to possess kidney-tissue protective and increased immunosuppressive effects which can improve the viability of transplanted kidneys. Nifedipine appears not to raise serum cyclosporin levels.

Clinical evidence

(a) Cyclosporin + diltiazem

Diltiazem raises cyclosporin levels. One study found that 65 kidney transplant patients on cyclosporin and diltiazem needed less cyclosporin than 63 control patients not given diltiazem (7.3 compared with 9 mg/kg/day). There were considerable individual differences.[18]

A number of other studies clearly confirm that diltiazem can raise cyclosporin serum levels.[1,2,12,15] In some cases the serum cyclosporin levels were not only controlled by reducing the cyclosporin dosage by about one-third but it appeared that diltiazem had a kidney protective role (fewer rejection episodes and haemodialyses).[5,17] Other studies also found increased serum cyclosporin levels but lowered nephrotoxicity when diltiazem was used.[6,7]

(b) Cyclosporin + nicardipine

A review of nine patients on cyclosporin showed that when given 20 mg nicardipine three times a day their serum cyclosporin levels rose by 110% (from 226 to 430 ng/ml—range 24 to 341%) and their serum creatinine levels rose from 135 to 147 μmol/l).[3]

Other studies have found increases in serum cyclosporin levels, in some cases as much as 2–3-fold, when nicardipine was used concurrently.[10,14,23,24]

(c) Cyclosporin + nifedipine

Five out of nine patients who showed an interaction with nicardipine showed no increase in serum cyclosporin levels when given nifedipine.[3] Yet another study found that nifedipine appeared to protect patients against the nephrotoxicity of cyclosporin,[8] however there is some evidence that

the side effects of nifedipine (flushing, rash) may be increased by the concurrent use of cyclosporin.[16] No changes in cyclosporin levels were seen in two other studies.[17,25]

(d) Cyclosporin + verapamil

A study in 22 kidney transplant patients on cyclosporin and verapamil found that although the same daily dosages were given, the serum cyclosporin levels were 50–70% higher than in 18 other patients not given verapamil but serum creatinine levels were lower. Moreover only three of the 22 had rejection episodes within four weeks compared with 10 out of 18 not given verapamil.[21]

Other studies have demonstrated that 120–320 mg verapamil daily can double or even triple serum cyclosporin levels in individual patients with kidney or heart transplants.[4,11,13,22]

Importance and management

The cyclosporin/diltiazem,/nicardipine/verapamil interactions are established and relatively well documented. Concurrent use need not be avoided but cyclosporin levels should be well monitored and dosage reductions made as necessary. Even though cyclosporin serum levels are increased, these calcium channel blockers appear both to have a kidney-protective effect and to improve immunosuppression. One study found that '...calcium channel blockers lead to an alteration of the cyclosporin pharmacokinetics by increasing cyclosporin blood levels...this interference, however, is of no harm to the patient, since no change in kidney function was observed despite drastic elevation of cyclosporin levels.'[19] With diltiazem and verapamil the cyclosporin dosage can apparently be reduced by about a quarter to a third but larger reductions are probably necessary with nicardipine. Nifedipine appears not to raise serum cyclosporin levels but may possibly have a kidney-protective effect. More study is needed to find out what happens with other calcium channel blockers.

References

1 Pochet JM and Pirson Y. Cyclosporin-diltiazem interaction. Lancet (1986) i, 979.

2 Grino JM, Sabate I, Castelao AM and Alsina J. Influence of diltiazem on cyclosporin clearance. Lancet (1986) i, 1387.

3 Bourbigot B, Guiserix J, Airiau J, Bressollette L, Morin JF and Cledes J. Nicardipine increases cyclosporin blood levels. Lancet (1986) i, 1447.

4 Lindholm A and Henricsson S. Verapamil inhibits cyclosporin metabolism. I. Lancet (1987)1, 1262-3

5 Neumayer H-H and Wagner K. Diltiazem and economic use of cyclosporin. Lancet (1986) ii, 523.

6 Wagner K, Albrecht S and Neumayer H-H. Prevention of delayed graft function in cadaveric kidney transplantation by a calcium antagonist. Preliminary results of two prospective randomized trials. Transplant Proc (1986) 18, 510–15.

7 Wagner K, Albrecht S and Neumayer H-H. Prevention of delayed graft function by a calcium antagonist—a randomized trial in renal graft recipients on cyclosporin A. Transplant Proc (1986) 18, 1269–71.

8 Feehally J, Walls J, Mistry N, Horsburgh T, Taylor J, Veitch PS and Bell PRF. Does nifedipine ameliorate cyclosporin A nephrotoxicity ? Br Med J (1987) 295, 310.

9 Hampton EM, Stewart CF, Herrod HG and Valenski WR. Augmentation of *in vitro* immunosuppressive effects of cyclosporin by verapamil. Clin Pharmacol Ther (1987) 41, 169.

10 Cantarovich M, Hiesse C, Lockiec F, Charpentier B and Fries D. Confirmation of the interaction between cyclosporine and the calcium channel blocker nicardipine in renal transplant patients. Clin Nephrol (1987) 28, 190–3.

11 Robson RA, Fraenkel M, Barratt LJ and Birkett DJ. Cyclosporin-verapamil interaction. Br J clin Pharmac (1988) 25, 402–3.

12 Brockmoller J, Wagner K, Neumayer HH and Heinemeyer G. Interaction of ciclosporine and diltiazem. Naunyn-Schmied Arch Pharmakol (1988) 337, Suppl R126.

13 Angermann CE, Spes CH, Anthuber M, Kemkes BM and Theisen K. Verapamil increases cyclosporin-A blood trough levels in cardiac recipients. J Amer Coll Cardiol (1988) 11, 206A.

14 Kessler M, Renoult E, Jonon B, Vigneron T, Huu C and Netter P. Interaction ciclosporine-nicardipine chez le transplante renal. Therapie (1987) 42, 273–5.

15 Kunzerdorf G, Walz G, Neumayer H-H, Wagner K, Keller F and Offermann G. Einfluss von Diltiazem auf die Ciclosporin-Blutspiegel. Klin Wschr (1987) 65, 1101–3.

16 McFadden JP, Pontin JE, Powles AV, Fry L and Idle JR. Cyclosporin decreases nifedipine metabolism. Br Med J (1989) 299, 1224.

17 Wagner K, Philipp Th, Heinemeyer G, Brockmuller F, Roots I and Neumayer HH. Interaction of cyclosporin and calcium antagonists. Transplant Proc (1989) 1453–6.

18 Kohlhaw K, Wonigeit K, Frei U, Oldhafer K, Neumann K and Pichlmayr R. Effect of calcium channel blocker diltiazem on cyclosporin A blood levels and dose requirements. Transplant Proc (1988) XX Suppl 2, 572–4.

19 Wagner K, Henkel M, Heinemeyer G and Neumayer H-H. Interaction of calcium blockers and cyclosporine. Transplant Proc (1988) XX, Suppl 2, 561–8.

20 Sabate I, Grino JM, Castelao AM, Huguet J, Seron D and Blanco A. Cyclosporin-diltiazem interaction: comparison of cyclosporin levels measured with two monoclonal antibodies. Transplant Proc (1989) 21, 1460–1. Lancet (1987) i, 1262–3.

21 Dawidson I, Rooth P, Fry WR, Sandor Z, Willms C, Coorpender L, Alway C and Reisch J. Prevention of acute cyclosporin induced renal blood flow inhibition and improved immunosuppression with verapamil. Transplantation (1989) 484, 4 575–80.

22 Sabate I, Grino JM, Castelao AM and Ortloa J. Evaluation of cyclosporin–verapamil interaction, with observations on parent cyclosporin and metabolites. Clin Chem (1989) 34, 2151–2.

23 Deray G, Aupeptit B, Martinez F, Baumelou A, Worcel A, Benhmikda M, Lagrand JC and Jacobs C. Cyclosporin–nicardipine interaction. Am J Nephrol (1989) 9, 349.

24 Kessler M, Netter P, Renoult E, Jonon B, Mur JM, Trechot P and Dousset B. Influence of nicardipine on renal function and plasma cyclosporin in renal transplant patients. Eur J Clin Pharmacol (19899) 36, 637–8.

25 McNally P, Mistry N, Idle J, Walls J and Freehally J. Calcium channel blockers and cyclosporin metabolism. Transplantation (1989) 48, 1071.

Cyclosporin(e) + Cholestyramine and Food

Abstract/Summary

Cholestyramine and different drinks can have an effect on the absorption of cyclosporin.

Clinical evidence, mechanism, importance and management

A study in four patients with transplants and receiving cyclosporin and prednisolone showed that the concurrent use of cholestyramine for a week caused only a very small average change (+6%) in the AUC (area under the curve) of the cyclosporin, but one patient had a 55% increase and another a

23% decrease.[1] Patients taking cyclosporin with milk had a 39% higher AUC after food and 23% higher when fasting compared with others taking cyclosporin with orange juice.[1] The general clinical importance of these changes is uncertain.

Reference

1 Keogh A, Day R, Critchley L, Duggin G and Baron D. The effect of food and cholestyramine on the absorption of cyclosporine in cardiac transplant patients. Transplant Proc (1988) 20, 27–30.

Cyclosporin(e) + Cimetidine and Ranitidine

Abstract/Summary

Cimetidine and ranitidine appear not to affect serum cyclosporin levels but a deterioration in kidney function may possibly occur. Cases of thrombocytopenia and hepatotoxicity have been seen.

Clinical evidence

A study in seven patients with kidney transplants treated with cyclosporin showed that the concurrent use of either cimetidine or ranitidine increased their mean serum creatinine levels by 62% (from 2.28 to 3.22 mg/dl). All of them showed a rise, whereas only two out of five other patients with heart transplants showed a serum creatinine level rise when given either cimetidine or ranitidine, nevertheless the mean rise was 37% (from 1.72 to 2.36 mg/dl). No changes in serum cyclosporin levels were seen.[1]

Elevated serum cyclosporin levels have been seen in another patient when treated with cimetidine and metronidazole.[6] A further report claimed that ranitidine does not alter serum cyclosporin levels[4], and elsewhere cimetidine is stated not to affect the pharmacokinetics of cyclosporin in normal subjects.[7] A report describes thrombocytopenia in a man with a kidney transplant on cyclosporin when given ranitidine.[2] Another patient experienced hepatotoxicity while taking cyclosporin when given ranitidine.[3]

Mechanisms

Not understood. In a study in which azathioprine and prednisone were used for immunosuppression in patients with kidney transplants, no changes in serum creatinine levels were found when cimetidine was used for six weeks.[5] This suggests that the rise in serum creatinine levels described in the study cited results from a cyclosporin-H_2 antagonist interaction.

Importance and management

Information is very limited indeed. Monitor concurrent use for any evidence of kidney function deterioration.

References

1 Jarowenko MV, Van Buren CT, Kramer WG, Lorber MI, Flechner SM and Kahan BD. Ranitidine, cimetidine and the cyclosporin-treated recipient. Transplantation (1986) 42, 311–12.

2 Bailey RR, Walker RJ and Swainson CP. Some new problems with cyclosporin A? NZ Med J (1985) 98, 915–6.

3 Hiesse C, Cantarovich M, Santelli C, Francais P, Charpentier B and Fries D. Ranitidine heptatotoxicity in renal transplant patient. Lancet (1985) i, 1280.

4 Zazgornik J, Schindler J, Gremmel F, Balcke P, Kopsoa H, Derfler K and Minar E. Ranitidine does not influence the blood cyclosporin levels in renal transplant patients (RTP). Kidney Int (1985) 28, 410.

5 Garvin PJ, Carney K, Castenada M and Codd JE. Peptic ulcer disease following transplantation: the role of cimetidine. Am J Surg (1982) 114, 545.

6 Zylber-Katz E, Rubinger D and Berlatsky Y. Cyclosporine interactions with metronidazole and cimetidine. Drug Intell Clin Pharm (1988) 22, 504.

7 Freeman DJ, Laupacis A, Keown P, Stiller C and Carruthers G. The effect of agents that alter drug metabolyzing enzyme activity on the pharmacokinetics of cyclosporin. Ann Roy Coll Phys Surg Can (1984) 17, 301.

Cyclosporin(e) + Corticosteroids

Abstract/Summary

Concurrent use is very common. Some evidence suggests that cyclosporin serum levels are raised but other evidence suggests the opposite (possibly an artefact of one assay method used?) Cyclosporin can reduce the loss of the corticosteroids from the body and corticosteroid overdosage may occur. Convulsions have also been described during concurrent use.

Clinical evidence

(a) Corticosteroid levels increased

A pharmacokinetic study in 40 patients showed that the clearance of prednisolone was reduced about 30% in those on cyclosporin when compared with those on azathioprine (1.9 compared with 2.6 ml/min/kg).[2]

Another study by the same group of workers reported a 25% reduction in clearance of prednisolone in the presence of cyclosporin in patients with kidney transplants.[6] Other studies[1,5] confirm that cyclosporin reduces the clearance of prednisolone from the body, as a result some patients develop signs of overdosage (cushingoid symptoms such as steroid diabetes, osteonecrosis of the hip joints).[1] These studies have all been questioned in another study which found that the metabolism of prednisolone was not affected by cyclosporin.[8]

(b) Cyclosporin levels increased or reduced

The serum cyclosporin levels of 22 out of 33 patients were reported to be more than doubled when given intravenous prednisolone. The cyclosporin dosage was reduced in six patients.[1,3] Another study found that high doses of methylprednisolone more than doubled serum cyclosporin levels.[11] However a later study suggested quite the opposite:

that the clearance of cyclosporin is increased by high dose steroids,[7] a possible explanation being that Radioimmunoassay (RIA) may give results which are different from those obtained with High Pressure Liquid Chromatography (HPLC) assay methods. There is other evidence that low-dose steroids do not increase the immunosuppression of cyclosporin, but they can reduce the nephrotoxicity.[10]

(c) Convulsions

A report describes four young patients (aged 10, 12, 13 and 18) who had had bone marrow transplants for severe aplastic anaemia and who developed convulsions while treated with high dose methylprednisolone (5–20 mg/kg/day) and cyclosporin.[4]

Another report describes convulsions in a woman of 25 when treated with cyclosporin and high dose methylprednisolone.[9]

Mechanisms

One suggestion is that the cyclosporin reduces the metabolism of the corticosteroids by the liver thereby reducing their loss from the body.[5]

Importance and management

None of these adverse interactions is well established. Concurrent use is common and advantageous but be alert for any evidence of increased cyclosporin and corticosteroid effects. It is not clear whether high dose corticosteroids cause a rise in serum cyclosporin levels or not. Assay results should be interpreted with caution. The authors of one report point out that this interaction could possibly lead to a misinterpretation of clinical data. In patients with kidney transplants a rise in serum creatinine levels is assumed to be due to rejection, unless proved otherwise. If a corticosteroid is then given, this could lead to increased cyclosporin levels which might be interpreted as cyclosporin nephrotoxicity.[3]

References

1 Ost L, Klintmalm G and Ringden O. Mutual interaction between prednisolone and cyclosporine in renal transplant patients. Transplant Proc (1985) 17, 1252–5.

2 Langhoff E, Madsen S, Olgaard K and Ladefoged J. Clinical results and cyclosporin effect on prednisolone metabolism. Kidney Int (1984) 26, 642.

3 Klintmalm G and Sawe J. High dose methylprednisolone increases plasma cyclosporin levels in renal transplant recipients. Lancet (1984) i, 731.

4 Durrant S, Chipping PM, Palmer S and Gordon-Smith EC. Cyclosporin A, methylprednisolone and convulsions. Lancet (1982) ii, 829–30.

5 Ost L. Effects of cyclosporin on prednisolone metabolism. Lancet (1984) i, 451.

6 Langhoff E, Madsen S, Flachs H, Olgaard K, Ladefoged J and Hvidberg EF. Inhibition of prednisolone metabolism by cyclosporine in kidney-transplanted patients. Transplantation (1985) 39, 107–9.

7 Ptachcinski RJ, Venkataramanan R, Burckart GJ, Hakal TR, Rosenthal JT, Carpenter BJ and Taylor RJ. Cyclosporine—high dose steroid interaction in renal transplant recipients: assessment by HPLC. Transplant Proc (1987) 19, 1728–9.

8 Frey FJ, Schnetzer A, Horber FF and Frey BM. Evidence that cyclosporine does not affect the metabolism of prednisolone after renal transplantation. Transplantation (1987) 43, 494–8.

9 Boogaerts MA, Zachee P and Verwilghen RL. Cyclosporin, methylprednisolone and convulsions. Lancet (1982) ii, 1216–17.

10 Nott D, Griffin PJA and Salaman JR. Low-dose steroids do not augment cyclosporine immunosuppression but do diminish cyclosporine nephrotoxicity. Transplant Proc (1985) 17, 1289–90.

11 Klintmalm G, Sawe J, Ringden O, Von Bah C and Magnusson A. Cyclosporine plasma levels in renal transplant patients. Association with renal toxicity and allograft rejection. Transplantation (1985) 39, 132–7.

Cyclosporin(e) + Diuretics

Abstract/Summary

Nephrotoxicity has been described in three patients on cyclosporin when given either amiloride-chlorothiazide, metolazone or mannitol. Animal studies suggest that there may be a risk with frusemide (furosemide).

Clinical evidence, mechanism, importance and management

A 39-year-old man on cyclosporin whose second kidney transplant functioned subnormally and who required treatment of hypertension with atenolol and minoxidil, developed ankle oedema which was resistant to increasing doses of frusemide (up to 750 mg daily). When metolazone (2.5 mg daily) was added for two weeks his serum creatinine levels more than doubled (from 193 to 449 μmol/l). When it was stopped the creatinine levels fell again. Cyclosporin serum levels were unchanged and neither graft rejection nor hypovolaemia occurred.[1] The kidney transplant of another patient on cyclosporin almost ceased to function when mannitol was used, and biopsy indicated severe cyclosporin nephrotoxicity. Transplant function recovered when the mannitol was stopped.[2] The same reaction was demonstrated in rats.[2] A woman showed a rise in serum creatinine levels from 121 to 171 μmol/l three weeks after starting to take *Moduretic* (amiloride+chlorothiazide). Trough serum cyclosporin levels were unchanged.[4] There is also some evidence from animal studies that the nephrotoxicity of cyclosporin may be increased by frusemide, but this interaction has yet to be reported in man.[3]

References

1 Christensen P and Leski M. Nephrotoxic drug interaction between metolazone and cyclosporin. Br Med J (1987) 294, 578.

2 Brunner FP, Hermle M, Mihatsch MJ and Thiel G. Mannitol potentiates cyclosporine nephrotoxicity. Clin Nephrol (1986) 25 (Suppl 1) S130–6.

3 Whiting PH, Cunningham C, Thompson AW and Simpson JG. Enhancement of high dose cyclosporin A toxicity by frusemide. Biochem Pharmacol (1984) 7, 1075–9.

4 Deray G, Baumelou B, Le Hoang P, Aupetit B, Girard B, Baumelou A. Legrand JC and Jacobs C. Enhancement of cyclosporin nephrotoxicity by diuretic therapy. Clin Nephrol (1989) 32, 47.

Cyclosporin(e) + Etoposide

Abstract/Summary

A single report describes their effective use in the treatment of leukaemia, but the side-effects are severe.

Clinical evidence, mechanism, importance and management

The leukaemic cells in the bone marrow of a patient with acute T-lymphocyte leukaemia were totally cleared by the concurrent use of cyclosporin (8.3 mg/kg orally twice daily) and etoposide (100–300 mg daily for 2–5 days), but the side-effects were severe (mental confusion, renal and hepatic toxicity).[1] The patient died from respiratory failure.

Reference

1 Kloke O and Isieka R. Interaction of cyclosporin A and antineoplastic agents. Klin Wsch (1985) 63, 1081–2.

Cyclosporin(e) + Fluconazole, Itraconazole, Ketoconazole

Abstract/Summary

A very marked and rapid rise (up to 5–10-fold) in serum cyclosporin levels can occur if ketoconazole is given concurrently. This drug combination should be avoided unless the dosage is markedly reduced because of the risk of nephrotoxicity. A rise in cyclosporin serum levels has been seen in some but not all patients when given fluconazole or itraconazole.

Clinical evidence

(a) Cyclosporin + fluconazole

The serum cyclosporin levels of a woman with a kidney transplant doubled within six days of starting additional treatment with 100 mg fluconazole daily. Her drug regimen consisted of daily doses of 10 mg prednisone, 25 mg azathioprine and 100 mg cyclosporin. No cyclosporin toxicity developed.[13]

Another report describes the rapid development of kidney toxicity (creatinine levels of 400 mmol/l) in a patient on 400 mg cyclosporin and 17.5 mg prednisone daily when additionally given 200 mg fluconazole daily. The problem resolved with a small reduction (unspecified) in the cyclosporin dosage and a halving of the fluconazole dosage.[14] In contrast, other reports claim that a group of 10 patients on cyclosporin given 100 mg fluconazole daily for 14 days, and another group of 20 given 200 mg daily for 100 days showed no changes in their cyclosporin levels.[15,17]

(b) Cyclosporin + itraconazole

A woman of 48 who had successfully had a kidney graft two years previously was maintained on prednisolone, atenolol, nifedipine, hydralazine and 90 mg cyclosporin twice daily. When itraconazole (100 mg twice daily) was added for a six-week period her serum cyclosporin levels doubled (from 376 to 850 ng/ml) and fell once again when the itraconazole was withdrawn.[11]

A threefold increase in trough serum cyclosporin was seen in a heart transplant patient treated with cyclosporin, azathioprine and prednisone when treated with 200 mg itraconazole daily for six weeks.[12] The cyclosporin serum levels were kept within the therapeutic range (400–800ng/ml) by reducing the cyclosporin dosage. The raised levels persisted for more than four weeks after the itraconazole was stopped.

These reports contrast with another describing 14 patients given bone marrow transplants taking cyclosporin. Those given 100 mg itraconazole twice daily showed no significant changes in cyclosporin or creatinine serum levels.[18]

(c) Cyclosporin + ketoconazole

A renal transplant patient taking 12 mg/kg cyclosporin daily showed a marked rise in serum cyclosporin levels when concurrently treated with 400 mg ketoconazole daily. Even though the cyclosporin dosage was reduced from 900 to 850 mg, and later to 800 mg daily, the trough serum level of cyclosporin climbed from 149–185 ng/ml to 2828 ng/ml after nine days concurrent treatment. The cyclosporin levels fell when the ketoconazole was withdrawn.[1]

Other reports[2,3,5,8,16] describe essentially the same dramatic rise in serum cyclosporin levels during concurrent treatment with ketoconazole. One of the patients showed a rise from 335–385 to 2450 ng/ml within five days of starting to take 200 mg ketoconazole daily.[2] A hint of the existence of an interaction occurs in an earlier report.[7]

Mechanism

The interactions with fluconazole and itraconazole are not understood. Ketoconazole does not appear to inhibit liver enzyme metabolism in man[4] although this may be the mechanism in animals.[9] It has been suggested that the interaction may possibly be due to a change in the volume of distribution caused by the ketoconazole or to some change in protein binding.[4,6]

Importance and management

The cyclosporin–ketoconazole interaction is established and clinically important. The extent and rapidity of the rise in serum cyclosporin levels is very considerable and the risk of nephrotoxicity accordingly great. This interaction has been successfully managed by close monitoring of serum cyclosporin levels and marked dosage reductions.[3,10,16] One report describes the successful exploitation of this interaction in 18 kidney transplant patients to save money. The cyclosporin dosage was reduced by 68–89% (reducing the cost

by 75%) over a 13-month period without any change in kidney or liver function or in immunosuppressive activity. The overall cost saving was about 65% because of the need to follow up more frequently and the cost of the ketoconazole.[16] Ketoconazole may possibly have a kidney-protective effect.[16]

Information about cyclosporin with fluconazole or itraconazole is more limited. Because an interaction can apparently occur unpredictably in few patients, monitor cyclosporin serum levels and kidney function during concurrent use and take appropriate action where necessary.

References

1 Ferguson RM, Sutherland DE, Simmonds RL and Najarian JS. Ketoconazole-cyclosporin metabolism and renal transplantation. Lancet (1982) ii, 882–3

2 Morgenstern GR, Powles R, Robinson BL and McElwain TJ. Cyclosporin interaction with ketoconazole and melphalan. Lancet (1982) ii, 1342–3

3 Dieperink H and Moller J. Ketoconazole and cyclosporin A. Lancet (1982) ii, 1217

4 Daneshmend TK. Ketoconazole-cyclosporin interaction. Lancet (1982) ii, 1342–4

5 Lokjec F. Pharmacokinetic monitoring during graft-versus-host disease treatment following bone marrow transplantation. International Symposium on Cyclosporin A (Trinity Hall, Cambridge. September 16–18, 1981). Quoted in reference 3.

6 Smith JM, Hows JM, Gordon-Smith EC, Baughan A and Gooldman JM. Interaction of CyA and ketoconazole. Clin Sci (1983) 64, 67–8P.

7 Gluckman E, Devergie A, Lokiec F, Poirier O and Baumelon A. Nephrotoxicity of cyclosporin in bone marrow transplantation. Lancet (1981) ii, 144–5.

8 Shepard JH, Canafax DM, Simmons RL and Najarian JS. Cyclosporin-ketoconazole: a potentially dangerous drug-drug interaction. Clin Pharm (1986) 5, 468.

9 Gumbleton M, Brown JE, Hawksworth G and Whiting PH. The possible relationship between hepatic drug metabolism and ketoconazole enhancement of cyclosporin nephrotoxicity. Transplantation (1985) 40, 454–5.

10 Schroeder TJ, Melvin DB, Clardy CW, Myre SA, Reising JM, Wolf RK, Collins JA, Pesce AJ and First MR. The use of cyclosporine and ketoconazole without nephrotoxicity in two heart transplant recipients. J Heart Transplantation (1986) 5, 391.

11 Kwan JT C, Foxall PJD, Davidson DGC, Bending MR and Eisinger AJ. Interaction of cyclosporin and itraconazole. Lancet (1987) ii, 282.

12 Trenk D, Brett W, Jahnchen E and Birnbaum D. Time course of cyclosporin/itraconazole interaction. Lancet (1987) ii, 1335–6.

13 Sugar AM, Saunders C, Idelson BA and Bernard DB. Interaction of fluconazole and cyclosporine. Ann Intern Med (1989) 110, 844.

14 Collignon P, Hurley B and Mitchell D. Interaction of fluconazole with cyclosporin. Lancet (1989) ii, 1262.

15 Ehninger G, Jaschonek K, Schuler U and Kruger HU. Interaction of fluconazole with cyclosporin. Lancet (1989) ii, 104–5.

16 First MR, Schroeder TJ, Weiskittel P, Myre SA, Alexander JW and Pesce AJ. Concomitant administration of cyclosporin and ketoconazole in renal transplant patients. Lancet (1989) ii, 1198–1201.

17 Kruger HU, Schuler U, Zimmerman R and Ehninger G. Absence of significant interaction of fluconazole with cyclosporin. J Antimicrob Chemother (1989) 24, 781–6.

18 Novakova I, Donnelly P, de Witte T, de Pauw B, Boezeman J and Veltman G. Itraconazole and cyclosporin nephrotoxicity. Lancet (1987) ii, 920–1.

Cyclosporin(e) + Macrolide and related antibiotics

Abstract/Summary

Cyclosporin levels can be markedly raised by the concurrent use of erythromycin. Cyclosporin toxicity will occur if the dosage of cyclosporin is not reduced. Josamycin and pristinamycin appear to interact similarly but no interaction is seen with spiramycin.

Clinical evidence

(a) Cyclosporin + erythromycin

A study in nine patients with transplants on cyclosporin showed that when treated with erythromycin the mean trough serum levels of the three patients with kidney transplants rose sevenfold (from 147 to 1125 ng/ml) and in the six patients with heart transplants 4–5-fold (from 185 to 815 ng/ml). Acute nephrotoxicity occurred in all nine patients and seven showed mild to severe liver toxicity caused by the increased cyclosporin serum levels.[1]

Markedly raised serum cyclosporin levels and/or toxicity have been described in a number of other studies and case reports with erythromycin given orally or intravenously in more than 30 other patients[2–13] and demonstrated in normal subjects.[14]

(b) Cyclosporin + josamycin

A man with a renal transplant treated with azathioprine, prednisone and cyclosporin (330 mg daily) showed a marked rise in his serum cyclosporin levels (from about 90 to 600 ng/ml) when treated with 2 g josamycin daily for five days. He responded in the same way when later rechallenged with josamycin. Another patient reacted in the same way.[15]

(c) Cyclosporin + pristinamycin

A patient with a kidney transplant showed a 10-fold rise in serum cyclosporin levels (from 30 to 290 ng/ml) after being given 2 g pristinamycin daily for eight days. Blood creatinine levels rose from 75 to 120 μmol/l. Another patient given 1.25 g pristinamycin showed a rise in cyclosporin levels from 78 to 855 ng/ml after six days. Cyclosporin and creatinine levels fell to normal levels within two days of stopping both drugs.[18]

A study in 10 patients on cyclosporin found that pristinamycin raised serum cyclosporin levels by 65% (from 560 to 925 ng/ml) when given 50 mg/kg pristinamycin daily.[22] Cyclosporin levels fell when the pristinamycin was stopped. Within five days of starting to take 4 g pristinamycin daily the cyclosporin levels of another patient more than doubled. His serum creatinine levels also rose. Both fell back to baseline levels within three days of stopping the antibiotic.[19]

(d) Cyclosporin + spiramycin

A study in six patients with heart transplants and receiving steroids, azathioprine and cyclosporin for immunosuppression showed that when given three MIU of spiramycin twice daily for 10 days their cyclosporin serum levels remained unchanged.[16]

The same absence of an interaction was found in other studies in patients with renal transplants.[17,20,21]

Mechanism

Not fully understood. One suggestion is that erythromycin reduces the metabolism of cyclosporin by the liver,[7] but later work indicates that erythromycin possibly increases the absorption of cyclosporin from the gut.[13] The mechanisms of interaction of the other antibiotics is uncertain.

Importance and management

The cyclosporin–erythromycin interaction is well documented, well established and potentially serious. If concurrent use is thought appropriate, monitor the cyclosporin serum levels closely and reduce the dosage appropriately. The dosage should be increased again when the erythromycin is stopped to maintain adequate immunosuppression. A possible alternative is to give the cyclosporin intravenously which by-passes the effects of erythromycin on the absorption of cyclosporin from the gut.[13] Information about the interactions with josamycin and pristinamycin seem to be limited to the reports cited but they appear to behave like erythromycin. Spiramycin does not interact. There seems to be nothing documented about an interaction with the other macrolide antibiotics (triacetyloleandomycin, midecamycin) but be on the alert if they are used.

References

1   Jensen CWB, Flechner SM, Van Buren CT, Frazier OH, Cooley DA, Lorber MI and Kahan BD. Exacerbation of cyclosporin toxicity by concomitant administration of erythromycin. Transplantation (1987) 43, 263–70.
2   Kohan DE. Possible interaction between cyclosporin and erythromycin. N Eng J Med (1986), 314, 448.
3   Hourmant M, Le Bigot JF, Vernillet L, Sagniez G, Remi JP and Soulilou JP. Coadministration of erythromycin results in an increase of blood cyclosporine to toxic levels. Transplant Proc (1985) 17, 2723–7.
4   Wadhawa NK, Schroeder TJ, O'Flaherty E, Pesce AJ, Myre SA, Munda R and First FR. Interaction between erythromycin and cyclosporine in a kidney and pancreas allograft recipient. Ther Drug Monitor (1987) 9, 123–5.
5   Murray BM, Edwards L, Morse GD, Kohli RR and Venuto RC. Clinically important interaction of cyclosporin and erythromycin. Transplantation (1987) 43, 602–4.
6   Grino JM, Sabate I, Castelao AM, Guardia M, Seron D and Alsina J. Erythromycin and cyclosporine. Ann Intern Med (1986) 105, 467–8.
7   Gonwa TA, Nghiem DD, Schulak JA and Corry RJ. Erythromycin and cyclosporine. Transplantation (1986) 41, 797–9.
8   Harnett JD, Parfrey PS, Paul MD and Gault MH. Erythromycin-cyclosporine interaction in renal transplant patients. Transplantation (1987) 43, 316–18.
9   Kessler M, Louis J, Renoult E, Vigneron B and Netter P. Interaction between cyclosporin and erythromycin in a kidney transplant patients. Eur J Clin Pharmacol (1986) 30. 633–4.
10 Godin JRP, Sketris IS and Belitsky P. Erythromycin-cyclosporin interaction. Drug Intell Clin Pharm (1986) 20, 504–5.

11 Martell R, Heinrichs D, Stiller CR, Jenner M, Keown PA and Dupre J. The effects of erythromycin in patients treated with cyclosporin. Ann Intern Med (1986) 104, 660–1.

12 Ptachcinski PJ, Carpenter BJ, Burckart GJ, Venkataramana R and Rosenthal JT. Effect of erythromycin on cyclosporine levels. N Engl J Med (1985) 22, 1416–17.

13 Gupta SK, Bakran A, Johnson RWG and Rowland M. Erythromycin enhances the absorption of cyclosporin. Br J clin Pharmac (1988) 25, 401–2.

14 Freeman DJ, Martell R, Carruthers SG, Heinrichs D, Keown PA and Stiller CR. Cyclosporin-erythromycin interaction in normal subjects. Br J Clin Pharmac (1987) 23, 776–8.

15 Kreft-Jais C, Billaud EM, Gaudry C and Bedrossan J. Effect of josamycin on plasma cyclosporine levels. Eur J Clin Pharmacol (1987) 32, 327–8.

16 Guillemain R, Billaud E, Dreyfus G, Amrein C, Kitzis M, Jebara VA and Kreft-Jais C. The effects of spiramycin on plasma cyclosporin A concentrations in heart transplant patients. Eur J Clin Pharmacol (1989) 36, 97–8.

17 Kessler M, Netter P, Zerrouki M, Renoult E, Trechot P, Dousset B, Jonon B and Mur JM. Spiramycin does not increase plasma cyclosporin concentrations in renal transplant. Eur J Clin Pharmacol (1988) 35, 331–2.

18 Gagnadoux MF, Loirat C, Pillion G, Bertheleme JP, Pouliquen M, Guest G and Broyer M. Nephrotoxicite due a l'interaction pristinamycine-cyclosporine chez le transplante renal. La Presse Med (1987) 16, 1761.

19 Garraffo R, Monnier B, Lapalus P, Duplay H. Pristinamycin increases cyclosporin blood levels. Med Sci Res (1987) 15, 461.

20 Vernillet L, Bertault-Peres P, Berland Y, Barradas J, Durand A, Olmer M. Lack of effect of spiramycin on cyclosporin pharmacokinetics. Br J Clin Pharmacol (1989) 27, 789–94.

21 Birmele B, Lebranchu Y, Beliveauu F, Rateau H, Furet Y, Nivet H and Bagros PH. Absence of interaction between cyclosporine and spiramycin. Transplantation (1989) 47, 927–8.

22 Herbrecht R, Garcia J-J, Bergerat J-P and Oberling F. Effect of pristinamycin on cyclosporin levels in bone marrow transplant recipients. Bone Marrow Transplant (1989) 4, 457–8.

Cyclosporin(e) + Melphalan

Abstract/Summary

Melphalan appears to increase the nephrotoxic effects of cyclosporin.

Clinical evidence, mechanism, importance and management

A comparative study showed that 13 out of 17 patients receiving bone marrow transplants given cyclosporin (12.5 mg/kg daily) and high-dose melphalan (single injection of 140–250 mg/m²) developed kidney failure, compared with no cases of kidney failure in seven other patients given melphalan but no cyclosporin.[1] In another study one out of four patients given both drugs developed nephrotoxicity.[2] The reasons are not understood. The effects of concurrent use on kidney function should be very closely monitored.

References

1 Morgenstern GR, Powles R, Robinson B and McElwain TJ. Cyclosporin interaction with ketoconazole and melphalan. Lancet (1982) ii, 1342.

2 Dale BM, Sage RE, Norman JE, Barber S and Kotasek D. Bone marrow transplantation following treatment with high-dose melphalan. Transplantation Proc (1985) 17, 1711–12.

Cyclosporin(e) + Metoclopramide

Abstract/Summary

Metoclopramide increases the absorption of cyclosporin and raises the serum levels.

Clinical evidence, mechanism, importance and management

A study in 14 kidney transplant patients showed that when given metoclopramide and cyclosporin concurrently their peak serum cyclosporin levels were increased by 46% (from 388 to 567 ng/ml) and the AUC (area under the concentration-time curve) was increased by 29% (from 3370 to 4120 ng.h/ml).[1] The probable reason is that the metoclopramide hastens gastric emptying. Cyclosporin is largely absorbed by the small intestine. The clinical importance of this interaction is uncertain but it has been suggested that it could be used to save money because it might be possible to give smaller doses of the expensive cyclosporin. Concurrent use should be well monitored to ensure that cyclosporin levels do not rise to toxic levels.

Reference

1 Wadhwa NK, Schroeder TJ, O'Flaherty E, Pesce AJ, Myre SA and First MR. The effect of oral metoclopramide on the absorption of cyclosporin. Transplant Proc (1987) 18, 1730–3.

Cyclosporin(e) + Miscellaneous drugs

Abstract/Summary

Isolated and unconfirmed interactions have been reported with acetazolamide, acyclovir, captopril, cephalosporins, disopyramide, doxycycline, imipenem/cilastatin, nafcillin and sulphinpyrazone.

Clinical evidence, mechanism, importance and management

The Drug Monitoring Centre of Sandoz (the manufacturers of cyclosporin) in Basel has on record a number of previously unpublished spontaneous and isolated reports of interactions between cyclosporin and other drugs.[1] There are also other isolated case reports of interactions involving cyclosporin:

A man with a heart transplant demonstrated increased serum cyclosporin levels, marked renal impairment and neurotoxicity when given oral acetazolamide for raised intra-ocular pressure secondary to panuveitis.[2] An increase in serum creatinine levels and in acyclovir levels accompanied by reversible acute tubular necrosis has been noted during the concurrent use of cyclosporin and acyclovir.[1] Transient oliguria was seen in a patient given cyclosporin and captopril.[1] Increased serum cyclosporin levels have been reported with moxalactam (latamoxef).[1] A woman treated with cyclosporin with a year old kidney transplant rapidly developed

455

nephrotoxicity shortly after starting to take 100 mg disopyramide three times daily. She also experienced the anticholinergic side-effects of disopyramide (mouth dryness, dysuria).[3] A patient showed an increase in serum creatinine levels when treated with doxycycline.[1] A woman with a kidney transplant and on cyclosporin developed a urinary tract infection for which 500 mg imipenem/cilastatin intravenously 12-hourly was given. 20 min after the second dose she became confused, disorientated, and agitated and developed motor aphasia and intense tremor. This was interpreted as being a combination of the adverse central nervous effects of both drugs. The imipenem/cilastatin was not given again and these adverse effects subsided over the next few days. However it was noted that the cyclosporin serum levels climbed over the next four days from about 400 to 1000 ng/ml.[5] Reduced serum cyclosporin levels following the use of imipenem/cilastin have been seen in rats.[6] A kidney transplant patient on cyclosporin and prednisone experienced a marked fall in her serum cyclosporin levels on two occasions when treated with nafcillin (2 g 6-hourly). Trough serum levels fell from 229 to 119 and then to 68 ng/ml after three and seven days of nafcillin, before climbing again when the nafcillin was stopped. On the second occasion levels fell from 272 to 42 ng/ml after nine days treatment with nafcillin.[4] Increased serum cyclosporin levels have been reported with sulphinpyrazone, although there is the possibility that this may be an artefact due to interference with the assay method.[1]

All of these reports need to be viewed in perspective because most of them are isolated and unconfirmed, and in some instances both drugs have been used uneventfully on a number of occasions. However it should also be appreciated that many now well-recognized interactions first came to light because someone took the trouble to make a report, even though it involved only one patient. Monitor the concurrent use of any of these drugs carefully.

References

1 Cockburn I, (Sandoz, Basel). Cyclosporin A: a clinical evaluation of drug interactions. Transplantation Proc (1986) 18, (Suppl 5) 50–5.
2 Keogh A, Esmore D, Spratt P, Savdie E and McClusky P. Acetazolamide and cyclosporine. Transplantation (1988) 46, 478–9.
3 Nanni G, Magalini SC, Serino F and Castagneto M. Effect of disopyramide in a cyclosporine-treated patient. Transplantation (1988) 45, 257.
4 Veremis SA, Maddux MS, Pollak R and Mozes MF. Subtherapeutic cyclosporine concentrations during nafcillin therapy. Transplantation (1987) 43, 913–5.
5 Zazgornik J, Schein W, Heimberger K, Shaheen FAM and Stockenhuber F. Potentiation of neurotoxic side effects by coadministration of imipenem to cyclosporine therapy in a kidney transplant recipient—synergism or side effects or drug interaction? Clin Nephrol (1986) 26, 265–6.
6 Mraz W, Sido B, Knedel M and Hammer C. Concomitant immunosuppressive and antibiotic therapy—reduction of cyclosporin A blood levels due to treatment with imipenem/cilastin. Transplantation Proc (1987) 19, 4017–20.

Cyclosporin(e) + Non-steroidal anti-inflammatory drugs (NSAID's)

Abstract/Summary

There is limited evidence that some NSAID's (diclofenac, ketoprofen, piroxicam and possibly sulindac) can increase the nephrotoxicity of cyclosporin which is reflected in serum creatinine level rises and changes in cyclosporin levels.

Clinical evidence

A man with a kidney transplant and treated with cyclosporin, prednisolone, digoxin, frusemide and spironolactone showed a marked rise in serum creatinine levels immediately after starting to take 25 mg diclofenac three times daily. A fall in serum cyclosporin levels (from 409 to 285 ng/ml) also occurred. Another patient with a kidney transplant also showed a rise in serum creatinine levels when sulindac was used. Serum cyclosporin levels fell and rose again when the sulindac was stopped.[1] Another report states that the cyclosporin levels of a woman with a kidney transplant more than doubled within three days of starting to take 150 mg sulindac twice daily.[2] Increased nephrotoxicity was seen in a patient when given 150 mg diclofenac daily.[3] Yet another report describes increased serum creatinine levels in a patient with rheumatoid arthritis when treated with ketoprofen, but not when given sulindac. Piroxicam increased serum creatinine levels in another patient.[5]

Mechanism

Uncertain. One idea is that intact kidney prostacyclin synthesis is needed to maintain the glomerular filtration rate and renal blood flow in patients given cyclosporin which possibly may protect the kidney from the development of cyclosporin-induced nephrotoxicity. If NSAID's are used which inhibit prostaglandin production in the kidney, the nephrotoxic effects of the cyclosporin manifest themselves, independently of changes in serum cyclosporin levels.[1] A study in rats showed that indomethacin and cyclosporin together can cause rises in serum creatinine levels which are much greater than with either drug alone.[4]

Importance and management

Direct information is very limited (involving only diclofenac, ketoprofen, piroxicam and sulindac) so the general importance of these reactions is uncertain, but it has been suggested that all NSAID's should be given to patients with caution, and only if kidney function can be well monitored.[1]

References

1 Harris KP, Jenkins D and Walls J. Nonsteroidal antiinflammatory drugs and cyclosporine. A potentially serious adverse interaction. Transplantation (1988) 46, 598–9.
2 Sesin GP, O'Keefe E and Roberto P. Sulindac-induced elevation of serum cyclosporin concentration. Clin Pharm (1989) 8, 445–6.
3 Deray G, Le Hoang P, Aupetit B, Achour A, Rottembourg J and Baumelou A. Enhancement of cyclosporine A nephrotoxicity by diclofenac. Clin Nephrol (1987) 27, 213.
4 Whiting PH, Burke MD and Thomson AW. Drug interactions with cyclosporine. Implications from animal studies. Transplant Proc (1986) XVIII Suppl 5, 56–70.

5 Ludwin D, Bennett KJ, Grace EM, Buchanan WA, Bensen W, Bombardier C and Tugwell PX. Nephrotoxicity in patients with rheumatoid arthritis treated with cyclosporine. Transplant Proc (1988) XX Suppl 4, 367–70.

Cyclosporin(e) + Octreotide

Abstract/Summary

Octreotide causes a marked fall in the serum levels of cyclosporin and inadequate immunosuppression may result.

Clinical evidence

A diabetic man with kidney and pancreatic segment transplants was successfully immunosuppressed with azathioprine, methylprednisolone and cyclosporin. When he was additionally treated twice daily, subcutaneously, with 100 µg octreotide (a long-acting somatostatin analogue) to reduce fluid collection around the pancreatic graft, his trough serum cyclosporin levels fell below the assay detection limit of 50 ng/ml. Nine other diabetics similarly treated with octreotide for peripancreatic fluid collection and fistulas after pancreatic transplantation also showed significant falls in their serum cyclosporin levels within 24–48 hr, in three patients to undetectable levels.[1]

A similar interaction was seen in another patient.[2]

Mechanism

Uncertain. A suggestion is that the octreotide reduces the intestinal absorption of the cyclosporin.[1,2]

Importance and management

An established and clinically important interaction, although the documentation is limited. The authors of the report cited recommend that before giving octreotide the oral dosage of cyclosporin should be increased on average by 50% and the serum levels monitored daily.[1]

References

1 Landgraf R, Landgraf-Leurs MMC, Nusser J, Hillebrand G, Illner WD, Abendroth D and Land W. Effect of somatostatin analogue (SMS 201–995) on cyclosporin levels. Transplantation (1987) 44, 724–5.
2 Rosenberg L, Dafoe DC, Schwartz R and Campbell DA. Administration of somatostatin analog (SMS 201–995) in the treatment of fistula occurring after pancreas transplantation. Transplantation (1987) 43, 764–6.

Cyclosporin(e) + Probucol

Abstract/Summary

Probucol reduces blood cyclosporin levels.

Clinical evidence

A study in heart transplant patients (number not stated) taking 2.44 mg/kg cyclosporin 12-hourly daily showed that the concurrent use of 500 mg probucol 12-hourly decreased whole blood cyclosporin levels and the area under the curve. The clearance and volume of distribution were increased. Comparative whole blood cyclosporin levels in ng/ml before and while taking the probucol were as follows: 1034 v 786 (1 h), 1272 v 933 (3 h), 958 v 728 (5 h), 5995 v 413 (11 h).[1]

Mechanism

Not understood.

Importance and management

Information appears to be limited to this study, but the conclusion to be drawn is that the cyclosporin dosage will need to be increased if probucol is added. Monitor the effects and adjust the dosage appropriately.

Reference

1 Corder CN, Sundarajan V, Liguori C, Cooper DKC, Muchmore J, Zuhdi N, Novitzky D, Barbi G, Larscheid P and Manion CV. Interference with steady state cyclosporine levels by probucol in heart transplant patients. Clin Pharmacol Ther (1990) 47, 204.

Cyclosporin(e) + Quinolone antibiotics

Abstract/Summary

No changes in the pharmacokinetics of cyclosporin were seen in studies in normal subjects or patients given cyclosporin and ciprofloxacin but two other reports describe nephrotoxicity in two patients. A single report describes a rise in cyclosporin levels with norfloxacin but another states than no difficulties occurred. Ofloxacin appears not to interact.

Clinical evidence

(a) Ciprofloxacin

A single dose study in 10 normal subjects showed that after taking 500 mg ciprofloxacin twice daily for seven days the pharmacokinetics of oral cyclosporin (5 mg/kg) were unchanged.[1] Another study in 10 renal transplant patients also found no changes after taking 750 mg ciprofloxacin twice daily for 13 days.[6] However two cases of nephrotoxicity have been reported. A heart transplant patient developed acute renal failure within four days of being given ciprofloxacin (750 mg eight-hourly).[4] Another patient who had had a kidney transplant developed reversible nephrotoxicity.[2] The authors of this latter report advocate caution if ciprofloxacin in doses greater than 250 mg 12-hourly are used.[2]

(b) Norfloxacin

Six renal transplant patients showed no changes in serum cyclosporin levels when given 400 mg norfloxacin twice daily for 3–23 days for urinary tract infections,[7] however a single case report describes a marked rise in serum cyclosporin levels in a heart transplant patient when given norfloxacin.[3]

(c) Ofloxacin

39 patients with kidney transplants under treatment with cyclosporin and prednisolone showed no evidence of nephrotoxicity nor any other interaction when concurrently treated with 100–400 mg ofloxacin daily for periods of 3–500 days.[5]

Mechanism

Not understood.

Importance and management

Information seems to be limited to these reports. They suggest that while concurrent use it usually uneventful, toxicity can occur occasionally, for which reason the outcome should be well monitored. There seem to be no reports of problems with ofloxacin.

References

1 Tan KKC, Trull AK and Shawket S. Study of the potential pharmacokinetic interaction between ciprofloxacin and cyclosporin in man. Br J clin Pharmacol (1988) 26, 644P.
2 Elston RA and Taylor J. Possible interaction of ciprofloxacin with cyclosporin A. J Antimicrob Chemother (1988) 29, 679–80.
3 Thomson DJ, Menkis AH and McKenzie FN. Norfloxacin-cyclosporine interaction. Transplantation (1988) 46, 312–13.
4 Advent CK, Krinsky JK, Bourge RC and Figg WD. Synergistic nephrotoxicity due to ciprofloxacin and cyclosporine. Am J Med (1988) 85, 452.
5 Vogt P, Schorn T and Frei U. Ofloxacin in the treatment of urinary tract infection in renal transplant recipients. Infection (1988) 16, 175–8.
6 Lang J, Finaz de Villaine J, Garraffo R and Touraine J-L. Cyclosporine (cyclosporin A) pharmacokinetics in renal transplant patients receiving ciprofloxacin. Am J Med (1989) 87 (Suppl 5A) 82–85S.
7 Jadoul M, Pirson Y and van Ypersele de Strihou C. Norfloxacin and cyclosporine—a safe combination. Transplantation (1989) 47, 747–8.

Cyclosporin(e) + Rifampicin (Rifampin)

Abstract/Summary

Cyclosporin serum levels are markedly reduced by the concurrent use of rifampicin unless the dosage is raised (2–3-fold). Transplant rejection can rapidly develop if the cyclosporin dosage is not increased.

Clinical evidence

A patient with a heart transplant and on cyclosporin was started on 600 mg rifampicin daily in addition to amphotericin B for the treatment of an *Aspergillus fumigatus*f infection. Within 11 days her serum cyclosporin levels had fallen from 473 to less than 31 ng/ml and severe acute graft rejection occurred. The dosage of cyclosporin was increased stepwise and the levels climbed to a plateau before suddenly falling again. The dosage had to be increased to more than 30 mg/kg daily to achieve serum levels in the range 100–300 ng/ml.[1]

A number of other reports about individual patients confirm that a very marked fall in serum cyclosporin levels occurs (often to undetectable levels), accompanied by transplantation rejection in many instances, if rifampicin is given.[2–13] Levels can rise to toxic proportions within two weeks of stopping the rifampicin unless the cyclosporin dosage is very much reduced.[2,4]

Mechanism

The evidence suggests that rifampicin (well recognized as a potent liver enzyme inducing agent) stimulates the metabolism of the cyclosporin by the liver resulting in a marked increase in its loss from the body, accompanied by a fall in its serum levels. Its immunosuppressant effects are thereby markedly reduced.

Importance and management

A well documented, well established and clinically important interaction. If concurrent use is undertaken the serum cyclosporin levels should be very closely monitored. A very large increase (threefold) in the dosage of cyclosporin may be needed to accommodate this interaction in order to prevent the risk of transplant rejection.[5] Effective alternative tuberculostatic drugs which are reported not to interact with cyclosporin include pyrazinamide (25 mg/kg)[4] and isoniazid,[10] however there is a case report describing a patient who showed a gradual rise in serum cyclosporin levels when isoniazid and ethambutol were stopped.[12] Another alternative if using rifampicin is to replace the cyclosporin with azathioprine and low-dose prednisolone for immunosuppression.[11]

References

1 Modry DL, Stinson EB, Oyer PE, Jamieson SW, Baldwin JC and Shumway NE. Acute rejection and massive cyclosporine requirements in heart transplant recipients treated with rifampin. Transplantation (1985) 39, 313–14.
2 Langhoff E and Madsen S. Rapid metabolism of cyclosporin and prednisone in kidney transplant patients on tuberculostatic treatment. Lancet (1983) ii, 1303.
3 Cassidy MJD, Van Zyl-Smit R, Pascoe MD, Swanepoel CR and Jacobson JE. Effect of rifampicin on cyclosporin A blood levels in a renal transplant recipient. Nephron (1985) 41, 207–8.
4 Coward RA, Raferty AT and Brown CB. Cyclosporin and antituberculous therapy. Lancet (1985) i, 1342–3.
5 Howard P, Bixler TJ and Gill B. Cyclosporine-rifampin drug interaction. Drug Intell Clin Pharm (1985) 19, 763–4.
6 Van Buren D, Wideman CA, Reid M, Gibbons S, Van Buren CT, Jarowenko M, Flechner SM, Frazier OH, Cooley DA and Kahan BD.

The antagonistic effect of rifampin upon cyclosporine bioavailability. Transplant Proc (1984) 16, 1642–5.

7 Allen RDM, Hunnisett AG and Morris PJ. Cyclosporin and rifampicin in renal transplantation. Lancet (1985) i, 980.

8 Langhoff E and Madsen S. Rapid metabolism of cyclosporin and prednisone in kidney transplant patient receiving tuberculostatic treatment. Lancet (1983) ii, 1031.

9 Offermann G, Keller F and Molzahn M. Low cyclosporin A blood levels and acute graft rejection in a renal transplant recipient during rifampin treatment. Am J Nephrol (1985) 5, 385–7.

10 Jurewicz WA, Gunson BK, Ismail T, Angrisani L and McMaster P. Cyclosporin and antituberculous therapy. Lancet (1985) i, 1343.

11 Daniels NJ, Dover JS and Schachter RK. Interaction between cyclosporin and rifampicin. Lancet (1984) ii, 639.

12 Leimenstoll G, Schlegelberger T, Fulde R and Niedermayer W. Interaktion von Ciclosporin und Ethambutol-Isoniazid. Dtsch med Wsch (1988) 113, 514–15.

13 Prado A, Ramirez M, Aguirre EC, Martin RS and Zucchini A. Interaccion entre ciclopsorina y rifampicina en un caso de transplante renal. Medicina (Buenos Aires) (1987) 47, 521–4.

Cyclosporin(e) + Sex hormones and Related Drugs

Abstract/Summary

Hepatotoxicity has been described in two patients when concurrently treated with cyclosporin and oral contraceptives. Rises in serum cyclosporin levels can also occur. Marked increases in serum cyclosporin levels have been seen in three patients taking danazol and one taking methyltestosterone.

Clinical evidence

(a) Cyclosporin + contraceptives (oral)

A woman treated for uveitis with cyclosporin (5 mg/kg daily) showed an increase in trough serum cyclosporin levels (very roughly doubled) on two occasions when given an oral contraceptive (levonorgestrel 150 μg + ethinyloestradiol 30 μg). She also experienced nausea, vomiting and heptalgia, and showed evidence of severe hepatotoxicity (very marked increases in aspartate and alanine aminotransferases, and rises in serum bilirubin and alkaline phosphatase).[4]

Another report describes hepatotoxicity in a patient when concurrently treated with cyclosporin and an oral contraceptive (desogestrel 150 μg + ethinyloestradiol 30 μg). Rises in serum cyclosporin levels were also seen.[5]

(b) Cyclosporin + danazol

A 15-year-old girl who had had a kidney transplant for a year and taking cyclosporin and prednisone, showed a marked rise in serum cyclosporin levels over about two weeks (from a range of 250–325 to 700–850 μmol/l) when given 200 mg danazol twice daily, even though the cyclosporin dosage was reduced from 350 to 250 mg daily.[1]

Similar rises in cyclosporin levels (from about 400 to 600 ng/ml, and from 150 to about 450 ng/ml) were seen in another patient on two occasions over about a six-week period when given 400 mg and later 600 mg danazol daily.[2]

A marked rise in serum cyclosporin levels has been described in another patient when given 200 mg danazol four times daily.[6]

(c) Cyclosporin + methyltestosterone

A man with a kidney transplant was given methyltestosterone a few days before an attempt was made to change his immunosuppressive treatment from azathioprine and prednisone to cyclosporin. Although the cyclosporin dosage was initially only 15 mg daily and later considerably less, the serum cyclosporin levels were more than 2000 ng/ml and severe cyclosporin toxicity was seen (raised serum creatinine, bilirubin and alanine aminotransferase levels).[3]

(d) Cyclosporin + norethisterone

The 15-year-old girl on cyclosporin who had shown a marked increase in serum cyclosporin levels when given danazol (referred to above) continued to have elevated levels, but not as high, when the danazol was replaced by norethisterone, 5 mg three times daily, and the levels fell once again when the norethisterone was stopped.[1] No changes in cyclosporin levels were seen in another patient when treated with norethisterone intermittently.[6]

Mechanism

Uncertain. It seems possible that these compounds inhibit the metabolism of the cyclosporin by the liver, thereby reducing its loss from the body and leading to an increase in its serum levels.

Importance and management

Information is very limited indeed but what is known suggests that concurrent use of any of these drugs and cyclosporin should be well monitored and dosage reductions made if cyclosporin toxicity is to be avoided. There also seems to be the risk of heptatoxicity if oral contraceptives are given.

References

1 Ross WB, Roberts D, Griffin PJA and Salaman JR. Cyclosporin interaction with danazol and norethisterone. Lancet (1986) i, 330.

2 Schroder O, Schmitz N, Kayser W, Euler HH and Loffler H. Erhohte Ciclosporin-A-Spiegel bei gleichzeitiger Therapie mit Danazol. Dtsch med Wsch (1986) 111, 602–3.

3 Moller BB and Ekelund B. Toxicity of cyclosporin during treatment with androgens. N Engl J Med (1985) 313, 1416.

4 Deray G, Le Hoang P, Cacoub P, Assogba U, Grippon P and Baumelou A. Oral contraceptive interaction with cyclosporin. Lancet (1987) i, 158–9.

5 Leimenstoll G, Jessen P, Zabel P and Niedermayer W. Arzneimittelschadigungder Leber bei Kombination von Cyclosporin A und einem Antikonzeptivum. Dtsch med Wsch (1984) 109, 1989.

6 Koneru B, Hartner C, Iwatsuki S, Starzl TE. Effect of danazol on cyclosporine pharmacokinetics. Transplantation (1988) 45, 1001.

Cyclosporin + Sulphonamides, Trimethoprim or Co-trimoxazole

Abstract/Summary

Evidence of a deterioration in renal function may occur in patients treated with cyclosporin and these other drugs. A dramatic fall in serum cyclosporin levels may also occur if trimethoprim and sulphadimidine are given intravenously. The immunosuppression may become inadequate as a result.

Clinical evidence

(a) Evidence of renal deterioration

Seven renal transplant patients on cyclosporin (12.5–20 mg/kg daily) were additionally treated with either 200 mg trimethoprim daily or 960 mg co-trimoxazole twice daily for urinary or respiratory tract infections. Six showed a rise in serum creatinine levels suggesting a deterioration in renal function, and a fall when the anti-infective agent was stopped. There was no clinical evidence of transplant rejection.[1]

Other reports similarly describe apparent nephrotoxicity in patients on cyclosporin attributed to the concurrent use of trimethoprim[2] or co-trimoxazole (trimethoprim + sulfamethoxazole).[5,6]

(b) Reduced serum cyclosporin levels

A man with a heart transplant treated with cyclosporin and prednisolone was found to have unmeasurably low serum cyclosporin levels seven days after starting intravenous treatment with sulphadimidine (2 g four times daily) and trimethoprim (300–500 mg twice daily). Doubling the cyclosporin dosage had little effect and evidence of transplant rejection was seen. Within 10 days of starting to take the anti-infective agents orally instead of intravenously the serum cyclosporin levels climbed to approximately their former levels and the rejection problem disappeared.[3]

Another report by some of the same authors describes a similar marked fall in in serum cyclosporin levels in five patients (one of them the same as the report already cited[3]) when given sulphadimidine and trimethoprim intravenously.[4]

Mechanisms

(a) Cyclosporin, trimethoprim and co-trimoxazole are all nephrotoxic to a greater or lesser degree and it seems possible that their effects are additive. (b) The reduction in serum cyclosporin levels is not understood.

Importance and management

Neither of these effects is well established nor well documented, but there is enough evidence to take them seriously. If concurrent use is undertaken it should be realized that intravenous (but not oral) administration of some sulphonamides can result in a marked reduction in serum cyclosporin levels and inadequate immunosuppression may result. It should also be appreciated that rises in serum creatinine levels during concurrent use may be drug-induced (due to cyclosporin, sulphonamide, trimethoprim) and not necessarily evidence of transplant rejection.[1] It has been suggested that as transplanted kidneys seem to be especially sensitive to the combined nephrotoxic effects of cyclosporin and co-trimoxazole, this drug combination should be avoided.[5]

References

1 Thompson JF, Chalmers DHJ, Hunnisett AGW, Wood RFM and Morris PJ. Nephrotoxicity of trimethoprim and cotrimoxazole in renal allograft recipients treated with cyclosporin. Transplantation (1983) 36, 204–6.

2 Nyberg G, Gabel H, Althoff P, Bjork S, Herlitz H and Brynger H. Adverse effect of trimethoprim on kidney function in renal transplant patients. Lancet (1984) i, 394–5.

3 Wallwork J, McGregor CGA, Wells FC, Cory-Pearce R and English TAH. Cyclosporin and intravenous sulphadimidine and trimethoprim therapy. Lancet (1983) i, 336–7.

4 Jones DK, Hakim M, Wallwork J, Higgenbottam TW and White DJG. Serious interaction between cyclosporin A and sulphadimidine. Br Med J (1986) 292, 728–9.

5 Ringden O, Myrenfors P, Klintmalm G, Tyden G and Ost L. Nephrotoxicity by co-trimoxazole and cyclosporin in transplanted patients. Lancet (1984) i, 1016–7.

6 Klintmalm G, Sawe J, Ringden O, von Bah C and Magnusson A. Cyclosporine plasma levels in renal transplant patients. Association with renal toxicity and allograft rejection. Transplantation (1985) 39, 132–7.

Cyclosporin(e) + Vaccines

Abstract/Summary

Cyclosporin reduces the ability of the body to develop immunity when given influenza vaccine. Whether this is equally true for other vaccines is as yet uncertain.

Clinical evidence

(a) Cyclosporin + influenza vaccine

A comparative study in 59 patients who had had kidney transplants showed that those who were on cyclosporin and prednisone (21 patients) had a significantly lower immune response to influenza vaccine (inactivated trivalent) than those on azathioprine and prednisone (38 patients) or normal subjects taking no drugs (29). All of the immune response measurements made (mean antibody levels, fourfold titre rise, seroconversion to protective titres, the effects of booster immunization in those who responded poorly to the first vaccination) were reduced 20–30% in those on cyclosporin.[1]

Confirmation of the practical importance of this is described in a case report of a heart transplant patient on cyclosporin who twice failed to respond to influenza vaccination while receiving cyclosporin and prednisone.[2]

(b) Cyclosporin + other vaccines

Since the effectiveness of influenza vaccination is reduced by cyclosporin it seems logical to expect that other vaccines will be similarly affected, however there seems to be no direct evidence confirming that this is so. It has even been suggested that because cyclosporin can induce tolerance to antigens, this could lead to a situation where the patient becomes more (instead of less) susceptible to the infections against which one is trying to provide protection.[3]

Mechanism

Immunosuppression by cyclosporin diminishes the ability of the body to respond immunologically both to transplants and to influenza vaccination.

Importance and management

An established and clinically important interaction. The effectiveness of influenza vaccination may be reduced or abolished if cyclosporin is being used. One suggestion is that if patients remain unprotected after a single vaccination and a booster dose also fails to be effective, amantadine should be given during an influenza epidemic. It will protect against influenza A but not B infection. 200 mg daily is reported to be well tolerated.[2] It is not clear whether immunization with other vaccines is adversely affected by cyclosporin.

References

1 Versluis DJ, Beyer WEP, Masurel N, Wenting GJ and Weimar W. Impairment of the immune response to influenza vaccination in renal transplant recipients by cyclosporine, but not azathioprine. Transplantation (1986) 42, 376–9.

2 Beyer WEP, Diepersloot RJA, Masurel N, Simoons ML and Weimar W. Double failure of influenza vaccination in a heart transplant patient. Transplantation (1987) 43, 319.

3 Grabenstein JD and Baker JR. Comment: cyclosporine and vaccination. Drug Intell Clin Pharm (1985) 19, 679–80.

17
LITHIUM DRUG INTERACTIONS

Lithium carbonate is used in the treatment of manic depression and depression and is given in doses of up to 2 g daily, the dosages being adjusted to give plasma concentrations of 0.6 to 1.2 mEq/l. It should only be given under close supervision when the blood concentrations can be monitored regularly—initially at least once a week—because there is a narrow margin between therapeutic concentrations and those which are toxic.

Side-effects which are not usually considered serious include nausea, weakness, fine tremor, mild polydipsia and polyuria. If blood concentrations exceed about 1.5 mEq/l, more serious side-effects which amount to intoxication are seen: the gastrointestinal symptoms include abdominal pain, nausea, vomiting, diarrhoea, anorexia and thirst. Neurological symptoms include drowsiness, giddiness with ataxia, coarse tremor, slurred speech, blurred vision and muscular twitching. If concentrations rise as high as 3 mEq/l, life-threatening epileptic seizures, coma, hyperextension of the limbs, syncope and circulatory failure may occur. In addition to these side-effects, lithium can induce diabetes insipidus and hypothyroidism in some patients, and is contraindicated in those with renal or cardiac insufficiency. Just how lithium exerts its beneficial effects is not known, but it may compete with sodium ions in various parts of the body and its alters the electrolyte composition of body fluids.

Most of the interactions involving lithium are discussed in this chapter but a few are found elsewhere in this book. The index should be consulted for a full listing. Virtually all the reports are concerned with the carbonate, but sometimes lithium is given as the acetate, aspartate, chloride, citrate, gluconate, orotate or sulphate instead. There is no reason to believe that these lithium salts will not interact just like lithium carbonate.

Table 17.1. Lithium salts: generic and proprietary names

Non-proprietary names	Proprietary names
Lithium acetate	*Quilonium, Quilonorm*
Lithium carbonate	*Camcolit, Carbolith, Ceglution, Eskalith, Hypnorex, Lentolith, Lithane, Lithicarb, Lithiobid, Litilent, Lithizine, Lithonate, Lithotabs, Lithuril, Manialith, Maniprex, Phasal, Plenur, Priadel, Quilonium Retard, Quilonorm-Retard, Teralithe*
Lithium chloride	
Lithium citrate	
Lithium gluconate	*Lithium Oligosol, Microplex Lithium, Neurolithium*
Lithium orotate	*Lithium Rotat*
Lithium sulphate	*Lithiofor, Lithionit, Lithium-Duriles*

Lithium carbonate + ACE inhibitors

Abstract/Summary

Isolated cases of lithium toxicity in patients treated with captopril and enalapril have been reported.

Clinical evidence, mechanism, importance and management

A woman developed signs of lithium intoxication (ataxia, dysarthria, tremor, confusion, etc.) within 2–3 weeks of starting to take 20 mg enalapril daily. When admitted to hospital after five weeks her serum lithium levels were found to have risen from 0.88 to 3.3 mmol/l.[1] No toxicity occurred when the enalapril was later replaced by nifedipine. Lithium intoxication was seen in another patient when given 20 mg enalapril daily.[3] Another patient developed a serum lithium level of 2.35 mmol/l and intoxication (tremor, dysarthria, digestive problems) within 10 days of starting to take 50 mg captopril daily. He was restabilized on half the former dose of lithium.[2] The reasons for this reaction are not understood. Information is very limited but it would seem prudent to monitor the lithium serum levels closely if ACE inhibitors are given. More study is needed.

References

1 Douste-Blazy Ph, Rostin M, Livarek B, Tordjman E, Montastruc JL and Galinier F. Angiotensin converting enzyme inhibitors and lithium treatment. Lancet (1986) i, 1448.
2 Pulik M and Lida H. Interaction lithium-inhibiteurs de l'enzyme de conversion. La Presse Med (1988) 17, 755.
3 Mahieu M, Houvenagel E, Leduc JJ and Choteau Ph. Lithium-inhibiteurs de conversion: une association a eviter? La Presse Med (1988) 17, 281.

Lithium carbonate + Acetazolamide, Chlormerodrin, Spironolactone, Triamterene

Abstract/Summary

There is evidence that the excretion of lithium can be increased by triamterene and acetazolamide, but a case of lithium intoxication has also been seen. Chlormerodrin does not interact whereas serum lithium levels may rise if spironolactone is used.

Clinical evidence, mechanism, importance and management

There is very little information about the possible interactions of any of these diuretics with lithium. A short-term study[1] on six subjects given lithium and acetazolamide demonstrated a 27–31% increase in the urinary excretion of lithium, and an increased clearance was found in another study.[5] A woman was successfully treated for a toxic overdose of lithium with acetazolamide, IV fluids, sodium bicarbonate, potassium chloride and mannitol,[4] but paradoxically lithium intoxication (a rise in serum levels from 0.8 to 5 mmol/l) occurred in another patient after treatment for a month with acetazolamide.[6] Chlormerodrin was found not to interact.[1] The same study[1] found that spironolactone had no effect on the excretion of lithium, whereas in another report[2] the use of spironolactone was accompanied by a rise in serum lithium levels. Triamterene, administered to two patients taking lithium while on a salt restricted diet, is said to have led to a strong lithium diuresis.[3]

None of these reports gives a clear indication of the outcome of using these diuretics in patients on lithium, but they emphasize the need to monitor the response to concurrent use carefully.

References

1 Thomsen K and Schou M. Renal lithium excretion in man. Amer J Physiol (1968) 215, 823.
2 Baer L, Platman SR, Kassir S and Fieve RR. Mechanism of renal lithium handling and their relationship to mineralocorticoids: a dissociation between sodium and lithium ions. J Psychiat Res (1971) 8, 91–105.
3 Baer L, Platman S and Fieve RR. Lithium metabolism: its electrolyte actions and relationship to aldosterone. Recent Advances in the Psychobiology of the Depresssive Illnesses. Williams, Katz and Shield (eds) DHEW Publications, Washington DC (1972). p 49.
4 Horowitz LC and Fisher GU. Acute lithium toxicity. N Engl J Med (1969) 281, 1369.
5 Steele TH. Treatment of lithium intoxication with diuretics. In 'Clinical Chemistry and Chemical Toxicology of Metals.' (Ed SS Brown). Elsevier/North Holland (1977) p 289–93.
6 Gay C, Plas J, Granger B, Olie JP and Loo H. Intoxication au lithium. Deux interaction inedites: l'acetazolamide et l'acide niflumique. L'Encephale (1985) 11, 261–2.

Lithium carbonate + Baclofen

Abstract/Summary

Two patients with Huntington's chorea showed an aggravation of their hyperkinetic symptoms within a few days of starting concurrent treatment.

Clinical evidence, mechanism, importance and management

A patient with Huntington's chorea and under treatment with lithium and haloperidol, was additionally given baclofen. Another patient being treated with imipramine, clopenthixol, chlorpromazine and baclofen was additionally given lithium. Within a few days both patients showed a severe aggravation of their hyperkinetic symptoms which disappeared within three days of withdrawing the baclofen.[1] It is uncertain whether this is an interaction, but on the basis of this very limited evidence it would now seem prudent to monitor the effects of concurrent use carefully.

Reference

1 Anden N-E, Dalen P and Johansson B. Baclofen and lithium in Huntington's chorea. Lancet (1973) ii, 93.

Lithium carbonate + Calcium channel blockers

Abstract/Summary

Increases in the effects and toxicity of lithium as well as decreases in serum lithium levels have been seen in a few patients given verapamil. Profound bradycardia occurred in two other patients on lithium when given verapamil. An acute parkinsonian syndrome developed in another patient on lithium and thiothixene when given diltiazem.

Clinical evidence

(a) Increased lithium effects

A 42-year-old on 900 mg lithium carbonate daily developed toxicity (nausea, vomiting, muscular weakness, ataxia and tinnitus) within nine days of starting to take 80 mg verapamil three times daily although her bipolar depressive disorder improved. Her serum lithium levels remained unchanged at 1.1 mEq/l. The toxicity disappeared within 48 h of stopping the verapamil but her disorder worsened. The same pattern was repeated when the verapamil was re-started and then withdrawn.[1] A 74-year-old woman on lithium experienced similar toxicity two weeks after starting 240 mg verapamil daily. Her serum lithium level remained stable at 0.9 mEq/l. She was later well controlled on half the dose of lithium with a serum level of 0.3–0.5 mEq/l.[3]

(b) Reduced lithium effects

A patient, well controlled on 900–1200 mg lithium daily for over eight years, showed a marked fall in serum lithium levels when given 320 mg verapamil daily. He was restabilized on approximately double the dose of lithium. Another patient showed an increased lithium clearance when given verapamil for three days, and a fall in serum lithium levels from 0.61 to 0.53 mEq/l.[4]

(c) Other toxic effects

An acute parkinsonism syndrome developed in a man of 58 within four days of adding 30 mg diltiazem three times daily to his treatment with lithium and thiothixene.[2] Two elderly patients on lithium developed profound bradycardia when given 320–480 mg verapamil daily. Fatal myocardial infarction followed in one case.[5]

Mechanisms

Not understood.

Importance and management

The adverse reactions cited above contrast with other reports describing uneventful concurrent use.[6,7] This unpredictability emphasises the need to monitor the effects closely where it is thought appropriate to give both drugs. It has been suggested that particular caution should be exercised in old patients and those with cardiovascular disease.[5]

References

1 Price WA and Giannini AJ. Neurotoxicity caused by lithium-verapamil. J Clin Pharmacol (1986) 26, 717–19.
2 Valdiserri EV. A possible interaction between lithium and diltiazem: case report. J Clin Psychiatry (1985) 46, 540–1.
3 Price WA and Shalley JE. Lithium-verapamil toxicity in the elderly. J Amer Geriatr Soc (1987) 35, 177–9.
4 Weinrauch LA, Belok S and D'Elia JA. Decreased serum lithium during verapamil therapy. Amer Heart J (1984) 108, 1378–9.
5 Dubovsky SL, Franks RD and Allen S. Verapamil: a new antimanic drug with potential interactions with lithium. J Clin Psychiatry (1987) 48, 371–2.
6 Brotman AW, Farhadi AM and Gelenberg AJ. Verapamil treatment of acute mania. J Clin Psychiatry (1986) 47, 136–8.
7 Gitlin MJ and Weiss J. Verapamil as maintenance treatment in bipolar illness: a case report. J Clin Psychopharmacol (1984) 4, 341–3.

Lithium carbonate + Carbamazepine

Abstract/Summary

Although the combination of lithium and carbamazepine is beneficial in some patients, severe neurotoxicity is reported to have developed in others.

Clinical evidence

A patient on 1800 mg lithium daily developed severe neurotoxicity (ataxia, truncal tremors, nystagmus, limb hyperreflexia, muscle fasciculation) within three days of starting to take 600 mg carbamazepine daily. Blood levels of both drugs remained within the therapeutic range. The symptoms resolved when each drug was withdrawn in turn and re-occurred within three days of restarting concurrent treatment.[1]

Five rapid-cycling manic patients developed similar neurotoxic symptoms (confusion, drowsiness, generalized weakness, lethargy, coarse tremor, hyperreflexia, cerebellar signs) when concurrently treated with lithium carbonate and carbamazepine (doses not stated). Plasma levels of both drugs remained within the accepted range.[7] Other reports describe adverse neurological effects during concurrent use which were also not accompanied by changes in drug serum levels.[2,5,8]

In contrast, combined treatment in other patients is said not only to have been well tolerated but beneficial.[3,4,6]

Mechanism

Not understood.

Importance and management

This interaction is established, but its incidence is not known. If concurrent use is undertaken, the outcome should be closely monitored. This is particularly important because neurotoxicity can develop even though the drug serum levels remain within the accepted therapeutic range. The authors of one paper suggest that '...the risk factors appear to be a history of neurotoxicity with lithium therapies and the presence of concurrent compromised medical or neurological functioning.'[7]

References

1 Ghose K. Interaction between lithium and carbamazepine. Br Med J (1980) 250, 112.
2 Chaudhry RP and Waters BGH. Lithium and carbamazepine interaction: possible neurotoxicity. J Clin Psychiatry (1983) 44, 30–1.
3 MacCallum WAG. Interaction of lithium and phenytoin. Br Med J (1980) 280, 610–11.
4 Lipinski JF and Pope HG. Possible synergistic action between carbamazepine and lithium carbonate in the treatment of three acutely manic patients. Am J Psychiatry (1982) 139, 948–9.
5 Andrus PF. Lithium and carbamazepine. J Clin Psychiatry (1984) 45, 525.
6 Moss GR and James CR. Carbamazepine and lithium carbonate synergism in mania. Arch Gen Psychiatry (1983) 40, 588.
7 Shukla S, Godwin CD, Long EB, and Miller MG. Lithium-carbamazepine neurotoxicity and risk factors. Am J Psychiatry (1984) 141, 1604–6.
8 Hassan MH, Thakar J, Weinberg AL and Grimes JD. Lithium-carbamazepine interaction: clinical and laboratory observations. Neurology (1987) 37 (Suppl 1) 172.

Lithium carbonate + Cisplatin

Abstract/Summary

A single case report describes a transient and clinically unimportant fall in serum lithium levels in a woman given cisplatin and a fluid load.

Clinical evidence, mechanism, importance and management

A woman, well controlled for several years on 1200 mg lithium carbonate daily, showed a fall in serum lithium levels from 1.0 to 0.3, and from 0.8 to 0.5 mEq/l on two occasions over periods of two days when given 100 mg/m² cisplatin IV over 2 h. Over the next 24 h she was also given one litre of normal saline over 4 h, 25 g sodium chloride and 20% mannitol over 4 h, and 5% dextrose in normal saline to prevent renal toxicity. Serum lithium levels returned to normal at the end of two days. No change in the control of the psychotic symptoms was seen.[1] It is not clear whether the fall in serum lithium levels was due to increased renal clearance caused by the cisplatin, the fluid-loading, or both.

Although the interaction was not clinically important, the authors point out that some regimens of cisplatin involve the use of higher doses (40 mg/m²) with a normal saline fluid load over five days, and under these circumstances it would be prudent to monitor the serum lithium levels carefully.

Reference

1 Pietruszka LJ, Biermann WA and Vlasses PH. Evaluation of cisplatin-lithium interaction. Drug Intell Clin Pharm (1985) 19, 31–2.

Lithium carbonate + Co-trixoxazole

Abstract/Summary

Two reports describe lithium intoxication in three patients given co-trimoxazole, paradoxically accompanied by a fall in serum lithium levels.

Clinical evidence, mechanism, importance and management

Two patients stabilized on lithium carbonate (serum levels 0.75 mmol/l) showed signs of lithium intoxication (tremor, muscular weakness and fasciculation, apathy) within a few days of being given co-trimoxazole (dose not stated), yet their serum lithium levels were found to have *fallen* to 0.3–0.4 mmol/l. Within 48 h of withdrawing the co-trimoxazole, the signs of intoxication had gone and their serum lithium concentrations had climbed to their former levels.[1] Another report[2] very briefly states that ataxia, tremor and diarrhoea developed in a patient on lithium and timolol when given co-trimoxazole. The reasons are not understood. The general importance of this interaction is uncertain but if concurrent use is undertaken it would clearly be prudent to monitor the clinical response closely because it would appear that serum level monitoring may not always be a reliable guide.

References

1 Desvilles M and Sevestre P. Effet paradoxal de l'association lithium et sulfamethoxazol-trimethoprime. Nouv Presse Med (1982) 11, 3267–8.
2 Edwards IR. Medicines Adverse Reactions Committee: eighteenth annual report, 1983. NZ Med J (1984) 97, 729–32.

Lithium carbonate + Diazepam

Abstract/Summary

An isolated case of serious hypothermia has been reported during concurrent treatment with lithium carbonate and diazepam.

Clinical evidence, mechanism, importance and managmement

A mentally retarded patient showed occasional hypothermic episodes (below 35°C) while taking lithium and diazepam, but not while on either drug alone. After taking both drugs for 17 days during a test (lithium 1 g and diazepam 30 mg daily) the patient experienced a temperature fall from 35.4 to 32°C over 2 h, and became comatose with reduced reflexes, dilated pupils, a systolic blood pressure of 40–60 mmHg, a pulse rate of 40 and no piloerector response.[1] The reasons are not known. This is an isolated case so that concurrent use need not be avoided, but be alert for any evidence of hypothermia. There seems to be no evidence of an adverse interaction with any of the other benzodiazepines.

Reference

1 Naylor GJ and McHarg A. Profound hypothermia on combined lithium carbonate and diazepam treatment. Br Med J (1977) 3, 22.

Lithium carbonate + Fluoxetine

Abstract/Summary

An isolated report describes lithium toxicity in a patient caused by the concurrent use of fluoxetine.

Clinical evidence, mechanism, importance and management

A woman with a bipolar affective disorder successfully maintained for 20 years on 1200 mg lithium carbonate daily, developed stiffness of her arms and legs, dizziness, unsteadiness in walking and speech difficulties within a few days of starting additional treatment with 20 mg fluoxetine daily. Her serum lithium levels had risen from a range of 0.75–1.15 meq/l to 1.70 meq/l. Her serum lithium levels fell and these toxic symptoms disappeared when the lithium dosage was reduced and the fluoxetine withdrawn. The reasons for this adverse reaction are not understood. The authors of the report suggest that concurrent use should be discouraged.[1]

Reference

1 Salama AA, Shafey M. A case of severe lithium toxicity induced by combined fluoxetine and lithium carbonate. Am J Psychiatry (1989) 146, 278.

Lithium carbonate + Frusemide or Bumetanide

Abstract/Summmary

The concurrent use of lithium carbonate and frusemide can be safe and uneventful, but serious lithium intoxication has been described in a few individuals. Bumetanide can interact similarly.

Clinical evidence

Six normal subjects stabilized on 900 mg lithium carbonate daily (mean serum levels 4.3 mEq/l) were given 40 mg frusemide daily for 14 days. Five experienced some minor side-effects, probably attributable to the frusemide, but one subject experienced such a marked increase in the toxic effects of lithium that she withdrew from the study after taking both drugs for only five days. Her serum lithium levels were found to have risen by over 60% (from 0.44 to 0.71 mEq/l).[1]

There are four case reports of individual patients who experienced serious lithium intoxication or other adverse reactions when given lithium and frusemide.[3–6] One of the patients was also on a salt-restricted diet.[3] In contrast, another study on six patients who had been stabilized on lithium for over six years found that no significant change took place in their serum lithium levels over a 12 week period while taking 20–80 mg frusemide daily.[2] Bumetanide has also been responsible for the development of lithium toxicity.[8]

Mechanism

Not fully understood. If and when a rise in serum lithium levels occurs, it may be related to the salt depletion which can accompany the use of frusemide. As with the thiazides, such an interaction would not be expected to be immediate but would take a few days to develop. This may explain why one study in subjects given a single dose of lithium failed to demonstrate any effect on the urinary excretion of lithium after the administration of frusemide.[7]

Importance and management

Information seems to be limited to the reports cited. The incidence of this interaction is uncertain and its development unpredictable. It would therefore be imprudent to give frusemide or bumetanide to patients stabilized on lithium unless the effects can be well monitored because the occasional patient may develop serious intoxication.

References

1 Jefferson JW and Kalin NH. Serum lithium levels and long term diuretic use. J Amer Med Ass (1979) 241, 1134–6
2 Saffer D and Coppen A. Frusemide: a safe diuretic during lithium therapy? J Affective Disorders (1983) 5, 289–92.
3 Hurtig HI and Dyson WL. Lithium toxicity enhanced by diuresis. N Eng J Med (1974) 290, 748–9
4 Oh TE. Frusemide and lithium toxicity. Anaesth Intens Care (1977) 5, 60–2.
5 Segura EG, Ogne P and Peral MF. Intoxicacion por sales de litio. Presentacion de uno caso. Med Clin (Barc) (1984) 83, 294–6.
6 Thornton WE and Pray BJ. Lithium intoxication: a report of two cases. Can Psychiat Ass (1975) 20, 281–2.
7 Thomsen K and Schou M. Renal lithium excretion in man. Amer J Physiol (1968) 215, 823–7.
8 Kerry RJ, Ludlow JM and Owen G. Diuretics are dangerous with lithium. Br Med J (1980) 281, 371.

Lithium carbonate + Haloperidol

Abstract/Summary

Although very serious adverse reactions have been described in some patients treated with lithium carbonate and haloperidol, there is ample evidence that concurrent use can be uneventful and therapeutically valuable.

Clinical evidence

(a) Adverse effects during concurrent use

Four patients with acute mania who were treated with 1500–1800 mg lithium carbonate daily and high doses of haloperidol (up to 45 mg per day), developed encephalopathic syndromes (lethargy, fever, tremulousness, confusion, extrapyramidal and cerebellar dysfunction) accompanied by leukocytosis and elevated levels of serum enzymes, blood urea nitrogen and fasting blood sugar.[1] Two of them suffered irreversible widespread brain damage and two others were left with persistent dyskinesias.

A woman patient was observed with neuromuscular symptoms, impaired consciousness and hyperthermia after 12 days treatment with 1500 mg lithium carbonate and 40 mg haloperidol daily. She recovered fully and uneventfully.[2] Three patients, two of them oligophrenic, who were given 1800 mg lithium carbonate with 10–20 mg haloperidol by injection for 10 days, 27 h and 24 h respectively, developed hypertonic-hypokinetic and extrapyramidal syndromes. All recovered.[3] There are other reports of adverse reactions including severe extrapyramidal symptoms and organic brain damage in individual patients when given both drugs.[5,6,8,9,11,15–17] Another report claims that measurable brain damage may have occurred in seven patients.[10] A small rise in serum lithium levels occurs in the presence of haloperidol, but it is almost certainly of little or no clinical significance.[12]

(b) Advantageous concurrent use

In contrast to the reports cited above, there are others describing successful and uneventful use.[7] Cohen and Cohen who first described the adverse interaction[1] have also written that '...at least 50 other patients have been similarly treated without reported adverse effects'.[1] They also say that '...a survey of the experiences of leading experts indicate that although hundreds of patients have been treated with various regimens of combined lithium carbonate/haloperidol, there have been no previous observations of substantial irreversible brain damage or persistent dyskinesia'. A retrospective search of Danish hospital records showed that 425 patients had been treated with both drugs and none of them had developed serious adverse reactions. There are other reports confirming that concurrent use can be useful and safe, involving 18 patients,[13] 59 patients[14] and 18 patients.[18]

Mechanism

Not understood. An unconfirmed suggestion is that the adverse effects are possibly due to the combined effects of lithium and haloperidol on basal striatal adenylate cyclase.[19]

Importance and management

The effects of concurrent use, both adverse and advantageous, are well documented. The Danish investigators offer the opinion that 'the combination of lithium and haloperidol is therapeutically useful when administered to diagnostically appropriate patients. To discourage or prohibit is use would, in our opinion, be injudicious, but treatment must be carried out under proper clinical control.'[4]. This implies very close monitoring to detect any signs of adverse reactions. At the moment there seems to be no way of identifying the apparently small number of patients who are particularly at risk, but possible likely factors include a previous history of extrapyramidal reactions with neuroleptics and the use of large doses of haloperidol.

References

1 Cohen WJ and Cohen NH. Lithium carbonate, haloperidol, and irreversible brain damage. J Amer Med Ass (1974) 230, 1283.
2 Thornton WE and Pray BJ. Lithium intoxication: a report of two cases. Canada Psychiat Ass J (1975) 20, 281.
3 Marhold J, Zimanova J, Lachman M, Kral J and Vojtechovsky M. To the incompatibility of haloperidol with lithium salts. Acta Nerv Super (Praha) (1974) 16, 199.
4 Baastrup PC, Hollnagel P, Sorensen R and Schou M. Adverse reactions in treatment with lithium carbonate and haloperidol. J Amer Med Ass (1976) 236, 2645.
5 Loudon JB and Waring H. Toxic reactions to lithium and haloperidol. Lancet (1976) ii, 1088.
6 Juhl RP, Tsuang MT and Perry PJ. Concomitant administration of haloperidol and lithium carbonate in acute mania. Dis Nerv Syst (1977) 38, 675.
7 Garfinkel PE, Stancer HC and Persad E. A comparison of haloperidol, lithium carbonate and their combination in the treatment of mania. J Affect Dis (1980) 2, 279.
8 Spring G and Frankel M. New data on lithium and haloperidol incompatibility. Amer J Psychiatry (1981) 138, 818–21.
9 Menes C, Burra P and Hoaken PCS. Untoward effects following combined neuroleptic-lithium therapy. Can J Psychiatry (1980) 25, 573.
10 Thomas C, Tatham A and Jakubowski S. Lithium/haloperidol combinations and brain damage. Lancet (1982) i, 626.
11 Keitner GI and Rahman S. Reversible neurotoxicity with combined lithium-haloperidol administration. J Clin Psychopharmacol (1984) 4, 104–5.
12 Schaffer CB, Batra K, Garvey MJ, Mungas DM and Schaffer LC. The effect of haloperidol on serum levels of lithium in adult manic patients. Biol Psychiatry (1984) 19, 1495–9.
13 Baptista T. Lithium-neuroleptic combination and irreversible brain damage. Acta Psychiatr Scand (1986) 73, 111.
14 Goldney RD and Spence ND. Safety of the combination of lithium and neuroleptic drugs. Am J Psychiatry (1986) 143, 882–4.
15 Kamlana SH, Kerry RJ and Khan IA. Lithium: some drug interactions. Practitioner (1980) 224, 1291–2.
16 Fetzer J, Kader G and Dahany S. Lithium encephalopathy: a clinical, psychiatric and EEG evaluation. Am J Psychiatry (1981) 138, 1622–3.
17 Thomas CJ. Brain damage with lithium/haloperidol. Br J Psychiatry (1979) 134, 552.
18 Biederman J, Lerner Y and Belmaker H. Combination of lithium and haloperidol in schizo-affective disorder. Arch Gen Psychiatry (1979) 36, 327.
19 Geisler A and Klysner R. Combined effect of lithium and flupenthixol on striatal adenylate cyclase. Lancet (1977) i, 430–1.

Lithium carbonate + Iodides

Abstract/Summary

The hypothyroidic and goitrogenic effects of lithium carbonate, potassium iodide and possibly other iodides may be additive if given concurrently.

Clinical evidence

A man with normal thyroid function showed evidence of hypothyroidism after three weeks' treatment with lithium carbonate (750—1500 mg daily). After two further weeks' treatment with potassium iodide as well, the hypothyroidism became even more marked, but resolved completely within a fortnight of the withdrawal of both drugs.[1]

A number of other reports describe the antithyroid effect of lithium when given on its own[1-3,7-10] as well as with potassium iodide.[4,5,11] There is also a case on record involving lithium, isopropamide iodide and haloperidol.[6]

Mechanism

Lithium accumulates in the thyroid gland and blocks the release of the thyroid hormones by thyroid-stimulating hormone. The mechanism is not well understood. Potassium iodide temporarily prevents the production of the thyroid hormones but, as time goes on, synthesis recommences. Thus, both lithium ions and iodide ions can depress the production or release of the hormones and, it would appear, thereby have additive hypothyroidic effects.

Importance and management

The incidence and clinical importance of this interaction are difficult to assess. Hypothyroidism due to lithium treatment is not infrequent (variously reported as 12 out of 33 patients,[2] two out of 56 men[9] and 20 out of 93 women[9]) but there are very few reports of hypothyroidism due to the concurrent use of these drugs. Nevertheless the outcome of concurrent use should be monitored. Only potassium iodide and isopropamide iodide have been implicated but it would seem possible with other iodides. It should be remembered that some over-the-counter preparations contain iodine.

References

1 Shopsin B, Shenkman L, Blum M and Hollander CS. Iodine and lithium-induced hypothyroidism. Documentation of synergism. Amer J Med (1973) 55, 695.
2 Schou M, Amidsen A, Jensen SE and Olsen T. Occurrence of goitre during lithium treatment. Br Med J (1968) 3, 710.
3 Shopsin B, Blum M and Gershon S. Lithium-induced thyroid disturbance: case report and review. Compr Psychiatry (1969) 10, 215.
4 Jorgensen JD. Lithium-carbonate-induced myxedema. J Amer Med Ass (1971) 220, 587.
5 Weiner JD. Lithium carbonate-induced myxedema. J Amer Med Ass (1971) 220, 587.
6 Luby ED, Schwartz D and Rosenbaum H. Lithium carbonate-induced myxedema. J Amer Med Ass (1971) 218, 1298.
7 Emerson CH, Dyson WL and Utiger RD. Serum thyrotropin and thyroxine concentrations in patients receiving lithium carbonate. J Clin Endocrinol Metab (1973) 36, 338.
8 Candy J. Severe hypothyroidism—an early complication of lithium therapy. Br Med J (1972) 3, 277.
9 Villeneuve A, Grantier J, Jus A and Perron D. Effect of lithium on thyroid in man. Lancet (1973) ii, 502.
10 Lloyde GG, Rosser RM and Crowe MJ. Effect of lithium on thyroid in man. Lancet (1973) ii, 619.
11 Spaulding SW, Burrow GN, Ramsey JN and Donabedian RK. Effect of increased iodide intake on thyroid function in subjects on chronic lithium therapy. Acta Endocrinol (1977) 84, 290—6.

Lithium carbonate + Ispaghula husk

Abstract/Summary

An isolated report describes reduced serum lithium levels attributed to the concurrent use of ispaghula.

Clinical evidence, mechanism, importance and management

A woman, recently started on lithium, showed a fall in her serum lithium levels from 0.53 to 0.4 mmol/l when she started to take one teaspoonful of isphagula husk in water twice daily, despite an increase in her lithium dosage. Four days after the ispaghula was stopped, her serum lithium levels rose to 0.76 mmol/l with no change in her lithium dosage.[1] The reasons are not understood. The author of the report suggests that the ispaghula may have reduced the absorption of the lithium from the gut. An alternative suggestion is that the ispaghula preparation in question (not specifically named) might have had a high sodium content which would result in an increase in the excretion of the lithium by the kidneys.

The general importance of this interaction is unknown, but it would now seem prudent to monitor the serum lithium levels in patients given ispaghula preparations.

Reference

1 Perlman BB. Interaction between lithium salts and ispaghula husk. Lancet (1990) 335, 416.

Lithium carbonate + Mazindol

Abstract/Summary

An isolated case report describes lithium intoxication caused by the concurrent use of mazindol.

Clinical evidence

A manic depressive woman, well controlled on lithium carbonate, showed signs of lithium intoxication within three days of starting to take 2 mg mazindol daily. After nine days concurrent treatment she developed twitching, limb rigidity and muscle fasciculation, and was both dehydrated and stuporose. Her serum lithium levels were found to have risen from 0.4–1.3 mmol/l to 3.2 mmol/l. She recovered when the mazindol was withdrawn.[1] The reason is not understood. This is an isolated case and its general importance is uncertain but the rapidity of onset and the potentially serious outcome are good reasons for not giving these drugs together unless the response can be well monitored.

Reference

1 Hendy MS, Dove AF and Arblaster PG. Mazindol-induced lithium toxicity. Br Med J (1980) 1, 684–5.

Lithium carbonate + Methyldopa

Abstract/Summary

Lithium intoxication has been described in four patients and three normal subjects when concurrently treated with methyldopa.

Clinical evidence

A manic-depressive woman, stabilized on lithium carbonate, rapidly developed signs of lithium intoxication (blurred vision, hand tremors, mild diarrhoea, confusion, and slurred speech) when additionally given 1 g methyldopa daily, although her serum lithium levels remained within the range 0.5–0.7 mEq/l.[1] Later the author of this report demonstrated this interaction on himself.[2] He found that within two days of starting to take 1 g methyldopa daily the signs of lithium intoxication had clearly developed, although his serum levels had risen only moderately, reaching a maximum of 0.9 mEq/l after only 4–5 days of concurrent use.

This interaction has been described in three other patients[3,4,6] and in three normal subjects.[5] In three cases the signs of intoxication developed although the serum lithium levels were within the normal therapeutic range.

Mechanism

Not understood.

Importance and management

Information appears to be limited to the reports cited, but the interaction would seem to be established. Avoid concurrent use whenever possible, but if not the effects should be closely monitored. Serum lithium measurements may not be a reliable guide because intoxication can occur even though the levels remain within the accepted therapeutic range.

References

1 Byrd GJ. Methyldopa and lithium carbonate: suspected interaction. J Amer Med Ass (1975) 233, 320.
2 Byrd GJ. Lithium carbonate and methyldopa: apparent interaction in man. Clin Toxicol (1977) 11, 1–4.
3 Osanloo E and Deglin JH. Interaction of lithium and methyldopa. Ann Int Med (1980) 92, 433.
4 O'Regan JB. Adverse interaction of lithium carbonate and methyldopa. Can Med Ass J (1976) 115, 385

5 Walker N, White K, Tornatore F, Boyd JL and Cohen JL. Lithium-methyldopa interactions in normal subjects. Drug Intell Clin Pharm (1980) 14, 638.
6 Yassa R. Lithium-methyldopa interaction. Can Med Ass J (1986) 134, 141–2.

Lithium carbonate + Metronidazole

Abstract/Summary

Three patients have been described whose serum lithium levels rose, to toxic concentrations in two of them, when concurrently treated with metronidazole.

Clinical evidence, mechanism, importance and management

A woman of 40 taking 1800 mg lithium carbonate, 0.15 mg thyroxine and 60 mg propranolol daily whose serum lithium level two weeks previously was 1.3 mEq/l, developed signs of lithium intoxication (ataxia, rigidity, poor cognitive function, impaired co-ordination etc) while completing a one-week course of metronidazole (500 mg twice daily). Her serum lithium levels had climbed by 46% (to 1.9 mEq/l).[1] Two other patients are described in another report whose serum lithium levels rose by 20% and 125% respectively 12–19 days after starting a one-week course of metronidazole (500–750 mg daily).[3] Both of these two patients showed evidence of kidney abnormalities possibly caused by the concurrent use of these drugs. One other patient at least is said to have taken both drugs together uneventfully.[2] There seem to be no strong reasons for avoiding concurrent use but the outcome should be well monitored. The authors of one of the reports also recommend frequent analysis of creatinine and electrolyte levels and urine osmolality in order to detect any renal problems.[3]

References

1 Brinkley JR. Quoted as personal communication by Ayd JF in Int Drug Ther Newsletter (1982) 17, 15–16.
2 Strathman I (GD Searle and Co). Quoted as personal communication by Ayd JF in Int Drug Ther Newsletter (1982) 17, 15.
3 Teicher MH, Altesman RI, Cole JO and Schatzberg AF. Possible nephrotoxic interaction of lithium and metronidazole. J Amer Med Ass (1987) 257, 3365–6.

Lithium carbonate + Non-steroidal anti-inflammatory drugs (NSAID's)

Abstract/Summary

A marked and rapid rise in serum lithium levels (+60%) may occur and intoxication may develop in patients given clometacin and indomethacin. A more moderate rise (+15–34%) occurs with diclofenac and ibuprofen. Increased serum lithium levels and/or intoxication has also been seen in a few patients when given ketoprofen, mefenamic acid, naproxen, niflumic acid, phenylbutazone and piroxicam. Sulindac is reported to reduce or have no effect on serum lithium levels. Aspirin, lysine acetylsalicylate and sodium salicylate do not interact.

Clinical evidence

(a) Aspirin and other salicylates

10 normal women stabilized on lithium sulphate showed a slight fall in serum lithium levels (from 0.63 to 0.61 mEq/l), and a slight rise in their renal excretion of lithium (from 22.0 to 23.3 ml/min) when given 4 g aspirin daily for seven days.[1]

Another report states that 2.4 g aspirin daily had no effect on the absorption or renal excretion of single doses of lithium carbonate given to six normal subjects,[2] and a further report[3] very briefly describes the absence of an interaction between lithium carbonate and lysine acetylsalicylate or sodium salicylate.[4]

(b) Clometacin

The observation of lithium intoxication in three patients on lithium when given clometacin, prompted further study of this interaction. Six women stabilized on lithium showed an almost 60% rise (from 0.64 to 1.01 mmol/l) in their serum lithium levels after receiving 450 mg clometacin daily for five days.[5] The clearance of lithium by the kidney was found to be reduced.

(c) Diclofenac

Five normal subjects[6,7] stabilized on lithium showed a 26% rise in serum lithium levels after taking 150 mg diclofenac daily for 7–10 days. Lithium excretion by the kidney fell by 23%.

(d) Ibuprofen

A clinical study showed that the serum lithium levels of a patient rose by 25% (from 0.8 to 1.0 mEq/l) over a seven-day period while taking 2400 mg ibuprofen daily.[8,9] He also experienced nausea and drowsiness. Two other patients in the study taking 1200–2400 mg ibuprofen daily did not show this interaction.

A study in 11 subjects showed that serum lithium levels were raised by 15% when given 1600 mg ibuprofen daily.[10] Another study in nine patients showed that 1800 mg ibuprofen daily for six days raised lithium levels by 34% (range 12–66%)[21] Toxicity occurred in another patient within 24 h.[28]

(e) Indomethacin

A single-blind study[9] on five subjects, stabilized on lithium carbonate (300–900 mg daily), showed that when concurrently treated with indomethacin (50 mg three times a day) their serum lithium levels climbed until, at the end of seven days, they had risen by 43%. Renal clearance fell by 31%.

Other studies have found rises of 59% and 61% in serum lithium levels in patients taking 150 mg indomethacin daily,[7,11] and lithium intoxication has been seen.[8,12] A similar rise in serum lithium levels was found in another study on 10 normal subjects taking lithium sulphate rather than carbonate.[1]

(f) Ketoprofen

A manic-depressive patient stablized on lithium carbonate showed a rise in his serum lithium levels from 0.9 to 1.32 mmol/l over a three-week period when treated with 400 mg ketoprofen daily.[3]

(g) Mefenamic acid

Acute lithium toxicity accompanied by a sharp deterioration in kidney function was seen in a patient when concurrently treated with lithium carbonate and 500 mg mefenamic acid three times daily.[25] Withdrawal of the drugs and subsequent re-challenge confirmed this interaction. Another case of toxicity was seen in a patient but renal function was impaired before both drugs were given.[26] Another extremely brief report also describes this interaction in a patient.[23]

(h) Naproxen

A study in seven patients showed that over a six day period while taking 760 mg naproxen daily their serum lithium levels rose by 16% (from 0.81 to 0.94 mEq/l). The range was 0–42% and four showed a rise of over 20%. One patient whose levels rose from 0.95 to 1.13 mEq/l developed signs of toxicity (staggering gait and tremors).[22]

(i) Niflumic acid

An isolated report describes lithium intoxication in a woman after taking niflumic acid (three capsules) and 1.5 g aspirin daily for five days. Her serum lithium levels rose from 0.8 to 1.6 mmol/l.[24]

(j) Phenylbutazone and oxyphenbutazone

The serum lithium levels of a manic depressive patient doubled (from 0.7 to 1.44 mEq/l), accompanied by signs of intoxication within three days of starting treatment with 750 mg phenylbutazone daily in the form of suppositories.[14] Renal clearance of the lithium was found to have halved (from 10 to 5 ml/min/1.73 m). The patient was also taking viloxazine, clorazepate, spironolactone, isosorbide and dipyridamole.

The same authors describe another patient who showed a sharp rise in serum lithium levels when given 500 mg oxyphenbutazone.[3]

(k) Piroxicam

A manic depressive woman, well controlled for over nine years on lithium, experienced lithium toxicity (unsteadiness, trembling, confusion) and was admitted to hospital on three occasions after taking piroxicam. Her serum levels on two occasions had risen to 2.7 and 1.6 mmol/l, although in the latter instance the lithium had been withdrawn the previous day. In a subsequent study her serum lithium levels when given 20 mg piroxicam daily rose by one-third (from 1.0 to 1.5 mmol/l) while continuing to take the same dose of lithium (250 mg three time a day).[15]

This interaction has also been described in three other patients.[16-19] Another report describes lithium intoxication in a man given 20 mg piroxicam daily which apparently took four months to develop completely.[2]

(l) Sulindac

A patient stabilized on lithium showed a marked fall in serum lithium levels (from 0.65 to 0.39 mEq/l) after two weeks concurrent treatment with sulindac, 200 mg daily. His serum lithium levels gradually climbed over the next six weeks to 0.71 mEq/l and restabilized without any change in the dosage of either lithium or sulindac. The serum lithium levels of another patient were approximately halved a week after his dosage of sulindac was doubled to 400 mg daily.[20] Control of depression was not entirely lost in either patient.

In contrast three other studies found that serum lithium levels in one, four and six patients were unaffected by the use of sulindac.[13,22,27]

Mechanism

One suggestion is that the interacting NSAID's do so by inhibiting the synthesis of the renal prostaglandins (PGE_2) so that the renal blood flow is reduced, thereby reducing the renal excretion of the lithium. However this fails to explain why aspirin which blocks renal prostaglandin synthesis by 65–70% does not affect serum lithium levels.[1]

Importance and management

The documentation of these interactions is variable and limited, but what is known indicates that clometacin and indomethacin should be avoided unless serum lithium levels can be very well monitored and the dosage reduced appropriately. The other NSAID's cited which increase serum lithium levels and/or cause intoxication (diclofenac, ibuprofen, ketoprofen, mefenamic acid, naproxen, niflumic acid, phenylbutazone, oxyphenbutazone, piroxicam) seem to be less risky, but they should not be given with lithium unless the outcome can be well monitored and serum lithium dosages reduced as necessary. Loss of control of depression seems a possibility with sulindac in some but not all patients. Aspirin, lysine acetylsalicylate and sodium salicylate appear to be non-interacting alternatives. There seems to be nothing docuented about other NSAID's but be alert for evidence of an interaction with any of them because they have similar pharmacological characteristics.

References

1 Reimann IW, Diener U and Frohlich JC. Indomethacin but not aspirin increases plasma lithium ion levels. Arch Gen Psychiatry (1983) 40, 283–6.
2 Bikin D, Conrad KA and Mayersohn M. Lack of influence of caffeine and aspirin on lithium elimination. Clin Res (1982) 30, 249A.
3 Singer L, Imbs JL, Danion JM, Singer P, Krieger-Finance F, Schmidt M and Schwartz J. Risque d'intoxication par le lithium en cas de traitement associe par les anti-inflammatoires non steroidiens. Therapie (1981) 36, 323–6.
4 Reimann IW, Golbs E, Fischer C and Frohlich JC. Influence of intravenous acetylsalicylic acid and sodium salicylate on human renal function and lithium clearance. Eur J Clin Pharmacol (1985) 29, 435–41.
5 Edou D, Godin M, Colonna L, Petit M and Fillastre JP. Interaction medicamenteuse: clometacin-lithium. La Presse Med (1983) 12, 1551.
6 Reimann IW and Frohlich JC. Effects of diclofenac on lithium kinetics. Clin Pharmacol Ther (1980) 30, 348–52.
7 Reimann IW. Risks of non-steroidal anti-inflammatory drug therapy in lithium treated patients. Naunyn-Schmiedbergs Arch Pharmacol (1980) 3ll, R75.
8 Ragheb M, Ban TA, Buchanan D and Frohlich JC. Interaction of indomethacin and ibuprofen with lithium in manic patients under a steady-state lithium level. J Clin Psychiatry (1980) 41, 397–8.
9 Leftwich RB, Walker LA, Ragheb M, Oates JA and Frohlich JC. Inhibition of prostaglandin synthesis increases plasma lithium levels. Clin Res (1978) 26, 291A.
10 Kristoff CA, Hayes PE, Barr WH, Small RE, Townsend RJ and Ettigi PG. Effect of ibuprofen on lithium plasma and red blood cell concentrations. Clin Pharm (1986) 5, 51–5.
11 Frohlich JC, Leftwich R, Ragheb M, Oates JA, Riemann I and Buchanan D. Indomethacin increases plasma lithium. Br Med J (1979) 2, 1115.
12 Herschberg SN and Sierles FS. Indomethacin-induced lithium toxicity. Am Fam Phys (1983) 28, 155–7.
13 Ragheb MA and Powell AL. Failure of sulindac to increase serum lithium levels. J Clin Psychiatry (1986) 47, 33–4.
14 Imbs JL, Schmidt M, Mack G, Sebban M and Danion JM. Baisse de la clearance renale du lithium sous l'effet de la phenylbutazone. L'Encephale (1978) IV, 33.
15 Kerry RJ, Owen G and Michaelson S. Possible interaction between lithium and piroxicam. Lancet (1983) i, 418–9.
16 Nadarajah J and Stein GS. Piroxicam induced lithium toxicity. Ann Rheum Dis (1985) 44, 502.
17 Walbridge DG and Bazire SR. An interaction between lithium carbonate and piroxicam presenting as lithium toxicity. Br J Psychiat (1985) 147, 206–7.
18 Harrison TM, Wynne Davies D and Norris CM. Lithium and Piroxicam. Brit J Psychiat (1986) 148, 124–5.
19 Shelley RK. Lithium and piroxicam. Brit J Psychiat (1986) 147, 343.
20 Furnell MM and Davies J. The effect of sulindac on lithium therapy. Drug Intell Clin Pharm (1986) 19, 374–6.
21 Ragheb M. Ibuprofen can increase serum lithium levels in lithium-treated patients. J Clin Psychiatry (1987) 48, 161–3.
22 Ragheb M and Powell AL. Lithium interaction with sulindac and naproxen. J Clin Psychopharmacol (1986) 6, 150–4.
23 Honey J. Lithium-mefenamic acid interaction. Pharmabulletin (1982) 59, 20. Quoted by Ayd FJ. in Int Drug Ther Newsletter (1982) 17, 16.
24 Gay C, Plas J, Granger B, Olie JP and Loo H. Intoxication au lithium. Deux interaction inedites: l'acetazolamide et l'acide niflumique. L'Encephale (1985) 11, 261–2.
25 MacDonald J and Neale TJ. Toxic interaction of lithium carbonate and mefenamic acid. Br Med J (1988) 297, 1339.
26 Shelley RK. Lithium toxicity and mefenamic acid: a possible interaction and the role of prostaglandin inhibition. Br J Psychiatry (1987) 151, 847–8.
27 Miller LG, Bowman RC, Bakht F. Sparing effect of sulindac on lithium levels. J Fam Prac (1989) 28, 592–3.
28 Bailey CE, Stewart JT, McElroy RA. Ibuprofen-induced lithium toxicity. S Med J (1989) 82, 1197.

Lithium carbonate + Phenytoin

Abstract/Summary

Signs of lithium intoxication have been seen in three patients concurrently treated with phenytoin. The serum lithium levels may remain the same.

Clinical evidence, mechanism, importance and management.

A patient with a long history of depression and convulsions was treated with increasing doses of lithium carbonate and phenytoin over a period of about 12 years. Although the serum levels of both drugs remained within the therapeutic range, he eventually began to manifest signs of lithium intoxication (thirst, polyuria, polydipsia and tremor) which disappeared when the phenytoin was replaced by carbamazepine. The patient claimed that he felt normal for the first time in years.[1] Another report[2] describes a man on phenytoin who became ataxic within three days of starting to take lithium. He had no other toxic symptoms and his serum lithium level was 2.0 mEq/l. A further report states that intoxication can develop during concurrent use even though the serum levels remain within the normally accepted therapeutic range.[3]

Information seems to be limited to these reports and none of them[1-3] presents a clear picture of the role of phenytoin in the reactions described.[1-3] The interaction is not well established. However it would be prudent to be alert for signs of intoxication during concurrent use, particularly because it seems that intoxication can develop even though serum levels are within the therapeutic range.

References

1 MacCallum WAG. Interaction of lithium and phenytoin. Br Med J (1980) 280, 10.
2 Salem RB, Director K and Muniz CE. Ataxia as the primary symptom of lithium toxicity. Drug Intell Clin Pharm (1980) 14, 622
3 Spiers J and Hirsch SR. Severe lithium toxicity with normal serum concentrations. Br Med J (1978) 1, 185.

Lithium carbonate + Sodium chloride or Bicarbonate

Abstract/Summary

Dietary salt restriction can cause a rise in serum lithium to toxic concentrations if not adequately controlled. Conversely, the ingestion of marked amounts of sodium as the chloride or bicarbonate can prevent the establishment or maintenance of adequate serum lithium levels.

Clinical evidence

(a) Lithium response reduced by the ingestion of sodium

A depressive man, initially given 250 mg lithium carbonate four times a day, achieved a serum lithium level of 0.5 mEq/l by the following morning. When the dosage frequency was progressively increased to five, and later six, times a day, his serum lithium levels failed to exceed 0.6 mEq/l because, unknown to his doctor, he was also taking sodium bicarbonate. In the words of the patient's wife: '...he's been taking soda bic for years for an ulcer, doctor, but since he started on that lithium he's been shovelling it in...'. When the sodium bicarbonate was stopped, relatively stable serum lithium levels of 0.8 mEq/l were achieved on the initial dosage of lithium carbonate.[1]

An investigation carried out to find out why a number of in-patients failed to reach, or maintain, adequate therapeutic serum lithium levels, revealed that a clinic nurse had been giving the patients doses of a proprietary saline drink (*Efferdex*), used for 'upset stomachs' and containing about 50% sodium bicarbonate, because the patients complained of nausea. The depression in the expected serum lithium levels was as much as 40% in some cases.[6]

Other studies confirm that serum lithium levels fall and the effectiveness of treatment can lessen if the intake of sodium is increased.[4,9,11]

(b) Lithium response increased by sodium restriction

A clinical study on four manic depressive patients on lithium showed that serum lithium levels rose more rapidly and to a higher peak when given during salt restriction than when taking a dietary salt supplement.[2]

Other studies and observations confirm that salt restriction can, if the effects are not monitored, lead to lithium intoxication.[5,7,11]

Mechanism

Not established. One suggested mechanism is as follows. Lithium is eliminated from the body almost exclusively in the urine. The proximal tubule does not readily distinguish between sodium and lithium ions and reabsorbs 60–70% of the filtered load. It seems possible that during sodium depletion, the extracellular volume of the body is contracted so that both ions are maximally reabsorbed, leading to an increased retention of the lithium. Conversely, when the sodium levels are high (e.g. when a salt supplement is used), the extracellular volume is expanded and both sodium and lithium are excreted rather than reabsorbed. Beyond the proximal tubule, lithium and sodium appear to be handled differently, but in any case lithium reabsorption is relatively small so that any interference by sodium is likely to be minimal.[3]

Importance and management

A well-established and important interaction. The establishment and maintenance of adequate serum lithium levels can be jeopardized if the intake of ionic sodium is not controlled. Patients should be warned about taking over-the-counter antacids or urinary alkalinizers without first seeking informed advice. Sodium bicarbonate comes in various guises and disguises (e.g. *Efferdex* (50%), *Eno's Fruit Salts* (56%), *Andrews Liver Salts* (22.6%), *Bismarex Antacid Powder* (65%), *BiSoDoL Powder* (58%)). Substantial amounts also occur in some urinary alkalinizing agents (e.g. *Citralka, Citravescent*).[12] There are many similar preparations available throughout the world. An antacid containing aluminium and magnesium hydroxides with simethicone has been found to have no effect on the bioavailability of lithium carbonate.[10]

Patients already stabilized on lithium should not begin to

limit their intake of salt unless their serum lithium levels can be monitored and suitable dosage adjustments made if necessary.

References

1 Arthur RK. Lithium levels and 'Soda Bic'. Med J Aust (1975) 2, 918.
2 Platman SF and Fieve RR. Lithium retention and excretion. Arch Gen Psychiat (1969) 20, 285.
3 Thomsen K and Schou M. Renal lithium excretion in man. Am J Physiol (1968) 215, 823.
4 Bleiweiss H. Salt supplements with lithium. Lancet (1970) i, 416.
5 Hurtig HI and Dyson WL. Lithium toxicity enhanced by diuresis. N Eng J Med (1974) 290, 748.
6 McSwiggan C. Interaction of lithium and bicarbonate. Med J Aust (1978) 1, 38.
7 Corcoran AC, Taylor RD and Page IH. Lithium poisoning from the use of salt substitutes. J Am Med Ass (1949) 139, 685.
8 Singer I and Rotenburg D. Mechanisms of lithium action. N Eng J Med (1973) 289, 254.
9 Demers RG and Heninger GR. Sodium intake and lithium treatment in man. Am J Psychiatry (1971) 128, 100–4.
10 Goode DL, Newton DW, Ueda CT, Wilson JE, Wulf BG and Kafonek D. Effect of antacid on the bioavailability of lithium carbonate. Clin Pharm (1984) 3, 284–7
11 Baer L, Platman SR, Kassir S and Fieve RR. Mechanisms of renal lithium handling and their relationship to mineralocorticoids: a dissociation between sodium and lithium ions. J Psychiat Res (1971) 8, 91–105.
12 Beard TC, Wilkinson SJ and Vial JH. Hazards of urinary alkalizing agents. Med J Aust (1988) 149, 723.

Lithium carbonate + Spectinomycin

Abstract/Summary

A single case report describes a patient who developed lithium intoxication when concurrently treated with spectinomycin.

Clinical evidence, mechanism, importance and management

A depressive woman[1] controlled on lithium developed intoxication (tremor, nausea, vomiting, ataxia and dysarthria) when given spectinomycin injections (dose not stated) for the treatment of gonorrhoea. Her serum lithium levels had climbed from a range of 0.8–1.1 mEq/l to 3.2 mEq/l. A likely explanation is that spectinomycin, particularly in multiple doses, decreases creatinine clearance, elevates BUN and reduces urine output which would be expected to reduce the excretion of lithium, resulting in a rise in serum levels. Information seems to be limited to this report, but it would now seem prudent to monitor the effects of concurrent use in any patient.

Reference

1 Conroy RW. Quoted as a personal communication by Ayd FJ. Possible adverse drug-drug interaction report. Int Drug Therapy Newsletter (1978) 13, 15.

Lithium carbonate + Tetracycline

Abstract/Summary

Concurrent use is normally uneventful, but an isolated report describes lithium intoxication in a woman attributed to the use of tetracycline.

Clinical evidence, mechanism, importance and management

An isolated report[1] describes a manic depressive woman, well stabilized on lithium for three years, with serum concentrations within the range 0.5–0.84 mmol/l. Within two days of starting to take a sustained-release form of tetracycline (Tetrabid—Organon) her serum lithium levels had risen to 1.7 mmol/l, and two days later they had climbed to 2.74 mmol/l. By then she showed clear signs of lithium intoxication (slight drowsiness, slurring of the speech, fine tremor and thirst). The suggested reason is that the tetracycline (known to have nephrotoxic potentialities) may have adversely affected the renal clearance of lithium from the body.

In contrast, a study in 14 normal subjects taking 450 mg lithium carbonate twice daily showed that the concurrent use of 1 g tetracycline hydrochloride for seven days caused a small reduction in serum lithium levels (from 0.51 to 0.47 mEq/l).[2] The incidence of adverse reactions remained largely unchanged except for a slight increase in CNS and gastrointestinal side-effects. Another report describes the uneventful use of lithium and tetracyclines in patients.[3]

There seems to be no reason for avoiding concurrent use nevertheless it would be prudent to monitor the effects.

References

1 McGennis AJ. Lithium carbonate and tetracycline interaction. Br Med J (1978) 2, 1183.
2 Fankhauser MP, Lindon JL, Connolly B and Healey WJ. Evaluation of lithium-tetracycline interaction. Clin Pharm (1988) 7, 314–17.
3 Jefferson JW. Lithium and tetracycline. Br J Dermatol (1982) 107, 370.

Lithium carbonate + Theophylline

Abstract/Summary

Serum lithium levels are reduced by 20–30% by the concurrent use of theophylline and patients may relapse as a result. The interaction can be accommodated by raising the dosage of lithium.

Clinical evidence

A study in 10 normal subjects given 900 mg lithium carbonate daily showed that when additionally given theophylline (400–800 mg daily) their serum lithium levels fell by 20–30%, and the urinary clearance increased by 30%.[1,2]

A case report described a manic patient on lithium who very rapidly relapsed when given theophylline. It was found necessary to raise the dosage in a stepwise manner as the dosage of theophylline was increased in order to maintain the serum lithium levels and to control the mania.[3] Theophylline has also been used to treat lithium intoxication.[4,5]

Mechanism

Uncertain. Theophylline has some effect on the renal clearance of lithium.

Importance and management

Information is limited but the interaction appears to be established. Depressive and manic relapses may occur if the dosage of lithium is not raised appropriately. Serum lithium levels should be monitored during concurrent use.

References

1 Perry PJ, Calloway RA, Cook BL and Smith RE. Theophylline precipitated alterations of lithium clearance. Acta Psychiatr Scand (1984) 69, 528–37.
2 Cook BL, Smith RE, Perry PJ and Calloway RA. Theophylline-lithium interation. J Clin Psychiatry (1985) 46, 278–9.
3 Sierles FS and Ossowski MG. Concurrent use of theophylline and lithium in a patient with chronic obstructive lung disease and bipolar disorder. Am J Psychiat (1982) 139, 117.
4 Thomsen K and Schou M. Renal lithium excretion in man. Amer J Physiol (1968) 215, 823.
5 Jefferson JW and Greist JH. A Primer of Lithium Therapy. Williams and Wilkins Co., Baltimore (1977) p 204.

Lithium carbonate + Thiazides or Related diuretics

Abstract/Summary

Serum lithium levels can be increased by the concurrent use of the thiazide diuretics or chlorthalidone. Lithium intoxication can develop. The interaction can be accommodated by reducing the dosage of lithium appropriately. It seems probable that the same interaction will occur with a number of related diuretics.

Clinical evidence

A patient being treated with lithium carbonate showed a rise in serum lithium concentrations from 1.3 to 2.0 mEq/l each time he was administered 500 mg chlorothiazide daily.[4]

A study carried out on 22 patients showed that long-term treatment with either hydroflumethiazide (25 mg daily) plus KCl (3.4 g daily) or bendrofluazide (2.5 mg daily) led to a 24% reduction in the urinary excretion of lithium.[2]

A fall in the urinary excretion of lithium due to the use of chlorothiazide has been described elsewhere.[6] Lithium toxicity arising from the use of thiazide diuretics either alone[10,11] with other diuretics has been seen with *Moduretic* (hydrochlorothiazide + amiloride),[1,2,13,14] *Aldactazide* (hydro-

chlorothiazide + spironolactone),[3] and chlorothiazide with spironolactone and amiloride,[3] or triamterene.[12] It seems almost certain that in each case the thiazide component was principally responsible for the interaction. Chlorthalidone[9] has also been responsible for the development of lithium toxicity.

Mechanism

Not fully understood. The interaction occurs even though the thiazides and similar diuretics exert their major actions in the distal part of the kidney tubule whereas lithium is reabsorbed in the proximal part. The reason for the interaction could be that thiazide diuresis is accompanied by sodium loss which, within a few days, is compensated by a retention of sodium, this time in the proximal part of the tubule. Since both sodium and lithium ions are treated virtually indistinguishably, the increased reabsorption of sodium would include lithium as well, hence a significant and measurable reduction in its excretion. This would seem to be a long-term rather than an immediate effect which might explain why a short-term single-dose study in man with bendrofluazide failed to show any effect on lithium excretion.[5]

Importance and management

An established, well-documented and potentially serious interaction. None of the thiazides or the related diuretics cited should be given to patients on lithium unless the serum lithium levels can be closely monitored and appropriate dosage adjustments made. Concurrent use under controlled conditions has been advocated for certain psychiatric conditions and for the control of lithium-induced nephrogenic diabetes insipidus. Himmelhoch and his colleagues[13] calculate that 500 mg chlorothiazide daily would increase the serum lithium levels by 40% so that an approximately 40% reduction in lithium dosage would be necessary. Reductions of 60–70% would be necessary if 750–1000 mg were used.[8,13] Quinethazone, metazolone, clorexolone, clopamide and several other diuretics are closely related to the thiazides and have similar actions. They may be expected to interact with lithium, but so far there are no reports confirming that they do so.

References

1 Macfie AC. Lithium poisoning precipitated by diuretics. Br Med J (1975) 1, 516.
2 Petersen V, Hvidt S, Thomsen K and Schou M. Effect of prolonged thiazide treatment on renal lithium excretion. Br Med J (1974) 2, 143.
3 Lutz EG. Lithium toxicity precipitated by diuretics. J Med Soc New Jersey (1975) 72, 439.
4 Levy ST, Forrest JN and Heninger GR. Lithium-induced diabetes insipidus: manic symptoms, brain and electrolyte correlates, and chlorothiazide treatment. Amer J Psychiat (1973) 130, 1014.
5 Thomsen K and Schou M. Renal lithium excretion in man. Amer J Physiol (1968) 215, 823.
6 Baer L, Platman S and Fieve RK. Lithium metabolism: its electrolyte actions and relationship to aldosterone. Recent Advances in the Psychobiology of the Depressive Illnesses. Williams, Katz and Shield (eds). DHEW Publications, Washington DC. (1972) p. 49.
7 Basdevant A, Beaufils M and Corvol P. Influence des diuretiques sur l'elimination renale du lithium. Nouv Presse Med (1976) 5, 2085.
8 Himmelhoch JM, Forrest J, Neil J and Detre TP. Thiazide-lithium synergy in refractory mood swings. Amer J Psychiat (1977) 134, 149.
9 Solomon JG. Lithium toxicity precipitated by a diuretic. Psycho

10 Kerry RJ, Ludlow JM and Owen G. Diuretics are dangerous with lithium. Br Med J (1980) 281, 371.

11 Konig P, Kufferle B and Lenz G. Ein fall von Lithium-toxikation bei therapeutischen Lithium dosaen infolge zusatzlicher Gabe eines Diuretikums. Wien Klin Wochensch (1978) 90, 380.

12 Mehta BR and Robinson BHB. Lithium toxicity induced by triamterene-hydrochlorothiazide. Postgrad Med J. (1980) 56, 783.

13 Himmelhoch JM, Proust RI and Malinger AG. Adjustment of lithium dosage during lithium-chlorothiazide therapy. Clin Pharmacol Ther (1977) 22, 225.

14 Dorevitch A, Baruch E. Lithium toxicity induced by combined amiloride hydrochloride-hydrochlorothiazide administration. Am J Psychiatry (1986) 143, 257–8.

18

MONOAMINE OXIDASE INHIBITOR (MAOI) DRUG INTERACTIONS

Drugs with monoamine oxidase inhibitory activity were first developed as antidepressants because it was noticed that patients with tuberculosis given isoniazid, and more particularly iproniazid, showed some degree of mood elevation. A further development occurred when postural hypotension was seen to be one of the side-effects of treatment with iproniazid and, as a result, pheniprazine and later pargyline were introduced as antihypertensive agents. Among the serious and unexpected problems with the older MAOI were the serious and potentially lethal interactions which occurred with the sympathomimetics found in some proprietary medicines and in some foodstuffs. Some of the newer and more recently developed MAOI used for the treatment of Parkinson's disease as well as depression are safer because they interact to a much lesser extent than the old ones. Table 18.1 is a list of the MAOI used for depression, hypertension and Parkinson's disease. Some of them are currently available, some are still undergoing trials and a few have been withdrawn.

Table 18.1 Monoamine Oxidase Inhibitors (MAOI)

Non-proprietary (generic) names	Proprietary names
Older MAOI	
Iproclozide	*Sursum*
Iproniazid	*Marsilid*
Isocarboxazid	*Marplan*
Mebanazine	*Actomol*
Nialamide	*Niamid(e)*
Phenelzine	*Nardil, Nardelzine*
Phenelzine with pentaerythritol tetranitrate	*Perfenil*
Tranylcypromine	*Parnate*
Tranylcypromine with trifluoperazine	*Parstelin*
Newer MAOI	
Amiflamine	
Bromfaromine	
Cimoxatone	
Moclobemide	*Auroxix*
Selegiline (Deprenyl)	*Eldepryl, Jumex, Jumexal, Movergan*
Toloxatone	*Humoryl, Perenum*

The Role of Monoamine Oxidase

The arrival of a nerve impulse at the end of a nerve causes the release of a small amount of chemical transmitter which, after rapidly diffusing across the gap (the synaptic cleft) separating it from the receptors of the next nerve or organ, stimulates a response. Adrenergic neurones use noradrenaline (nor-epinephrine) as the chemical transmitter and this is synthesised from tyrosine by a series of biochemical steps and stored in vesicles at the nerve endings. The enzyme MAO is found associated with this store of noradrenaline, its action being to limit the amount of transmitter present. To use a crude analogy, the synthesis of the transmitter represents a dripping tap with the MAO acting as an enzymic leak, so that a constant level of noradrenaline is maintained. MAO is found in other types of neurone in the brain which use dopamine or 5-HT as transmitters where its function is essentially the same.

MAO is also found in other parts of the body, and in particularly high concentrations in the gut and liver where it acts as a protective detoxifying enzyme against tyramine and possibly other potentially hazardous amines which exist in foods which have undergone bacterial degradation. For this reason MAO was originally called tyramine oxidase.

Mode of Action of the MAO-Inhibitor Drugs

Most of the MAOI inactivate MAO by forming a complex with the enzyme, the intended target of the antidepressant MAOI being the MAO within the brain. Since the synthesis of the noradrenaline (nor-epinephrine) continues unchecked while the enzymic 'leak' is blocked, the concentration of noradrenaline rises and it was originally thought that the mood-elevating or antidepressant activity of the MAOI was associated with this rise, although this idea is almost certainly too simplistic.

The effects of the MAOI are not however confined to the brain. The MAO in the gut and liver are also inactivated. So too is the MAO within the sympathetic nervous system so that large amounts of noradrenaline accumulate at adrenergic nerve endings throughout the body. These actions of the MAOI outside the brain account for the interactions which occur with the sympathomimetic amines. Some MAOI cause irreversible enzyme inhibition, resynthesis only taking place relatively slowly so that the beneficial effects as well as some of the interactions can still occur 2-3 weeks after the drug has been withdrawn. Tranylcypromine differs in being a reversible inhibitor of MAO so that the onset and disappearance of its actions are much quicker than the other MAOI.

In addition to the interactions of the MAO described in this chapter, there are others dealt with elsewhere. A full listing is to be found in the Index.

Monoamine oxidase inhibitors + Amantadine

Abstract/Summary

An isolated report describes a rise in blood pressure in a patient on amantadine when given phenelzine.

Clinical evidence, mechanism, importance and management

A woman of 49 was treated for Parkinson's disease with amantadine (200 mg daily), haloperidol (5 mg daily) and flurazepam (30 mg at night). Within 72 h of starting to take 30 mg phenelzine daily for depression her blood pressure rose from 140/90 to 160/110 mm Hg and it remained high for a further 72 h after the amantadine and haloperidol had been withdrawn.[1] The reason for this hypertensive reaction is not understood. Another woman is reported to have been given amantadine (200 mg daily) and phenelzine (43 mg daily) successfully and uneventfully.[2] If concurrent use is undertaken the effects should be well monitored.

References

1 Jack RA and Daniel DG. Possible interaction between phenelzine and amantadine. Arch Gen Psychiatry (1984) 41, 726.
2 Greenberg R and Meyers BS. Treatment of major depression and Parkinson's disease with combined phenelzine and amantadine. Am J Psychiatry (1985) 142, 273.

Monoamine oxidase inhibitors + Barbiturates

Abstract/Summary

Although the MAOI can enhance and prolong the activity of the barbiturates in animals, only a few isolated cases attributed to an interaction have been described in man.

Clinical evidence

Kline has stated, without giving details, that on three or four occasions patients of his taking an MAOI continued, without his knowledge, to take their usual barbiturate hypnotic and thereby '...unknowingly raised their dose of barbiturate by five to ten times, and as a consequence barely managed to stagger through the day.'[3]

A patient on tranylcypromine was inadvertently given 250 mg sodium amylobarbitone (amobarbital) intravenously for sedation. Within an hour she became ataxic, fell to the floor repeatedly hitting her head. After complaining of nausea and dizziness the patient became semicomatose and remained in that state for a further 36 h. To what extent the head trauma played a part is uncertain.[5]

Two other cases of coma attributed to concurrent use have been described.[6,7] In contrast, mebanazine is reported not to have enhanced the hypnotic activities of quinalbarbitone (secobarbital) or butobarbitone (butobarbital) in a number of patients, nor was there any evidence of a hangover effect.[8]

Mechanism

Not known. Animal studies[1,2,4] suggest that the MAOI have a general inhibitory action on the liver microsomal enzymes, thereby prolonging the activity of the barbiturates, but whether this also occasionally occurs in man is uncertain.

Importance and management

The evidence for this interaction seems to be confined to a few unconfirmed anecdotal reports. There is no well-documented evidence showing that concurrent use should be avoided, although some caution is clearly appropriate. Mebanazine appears not to interact with quinalbarbitone or butobarbitone.

References

1 Wulfsohn NL and Politzer WM. 5-Hydroxytryptamine in anaesthesia. Anaesthesia (1962) 17, 64.
2 Lechat P and Lemergnan A. Monoamine oxidase inhibitors and potentiation of experimental sleep. Biochem Pharmacol (1961) 8, 8.
3 Kline NS. Psychopharmaceuticals: effects and side-effects. Bull WHO (1959) 21, 397.
4 Buchel L and Levy J. Mecanisme des phenomenes de synergie due sommeil experimental. II. Etude des associations iproniazide-hypnotique, chez le rat et la souris. Arch Sci Rech Sci Physiol (1965) 19, 161.
5 Domino EF, Sullivan TS and Luby E. Barbiturate intoxication in a patient treated with a MAO inhibitor. Amer J Psychiat (1962) 118, 941.
6 Etherington L. Personal communication (1973).
7 MacLeod I. Fatal reaction to phenelzine. Br Med J (1965) 1, 1554.
8 Gilmour SJG. Clinical trial of mebanazine—a new monoamine oxidase inhibitor. Br J Psychiat (1965) 111, 899.

Monoamine oxidase inhibitors + Benzodiazepines

Abstract/Summary

The concurrent use of the MAOI and the benzodiazepines is usually safe and effective, but a very small number of adverse reactions (chorea, massive oedema, MAOI-toxicity) attributed to an interaction have been described.

Clinical evidence, mechanism, importance and management

A patient with depression responded well when given 15 mg phenelzine and 10 mg chlordiazepoxide three times a day, but 4–5 months later developed choreiform movements of moderate severity and slight dysarthria. These symptoms subsided when the drugs were withdrawn.[1] Two patients on chlordiazepoxide and either isocarboxazid or phenelzine developed severe oedema which was attributed to the use of both drugs.[2,3] A patient on 60 mg phenelzine daily developed MAOI toxicity (excessive sweating, postural hypotension) within 10 days of increasing his daily dosage of nitrazepam to 15 mg. The patient was a slow acetylator.[7] The reasons for the development of these reactions are unknown.

The general picture portrayed by the reports in the literature is that concurrent use is usually effective and uneventful.[4–6] The adverse interaction reports appear to be the exception, and it is by no means certain that all the responses were due to a drug interaction rather than to a reaction to one or other of the drugs.

References

1 MacLeod DM. Chorea induced by tranquillizers. Lancet (1964) i, 388.
2 Goonewardene A and Toghill PJ. Gross oedema occurring during treatment for depression. Br Med J (1977) 1, 879.
3 Pathak SK. Gross oedema during treatment for depression. Br Med J (1977) 1, 1220.
4 Frommer EA. Treatment of childhood depression with antidepressant drugs. Br Med J (1967) 1, 729.
5 Mans J and Sennes M. L'isocarboxazide, le RO 5–0690 et chlordiazepoxide, le RO-4-0403 derive des thixanthenes. Etude sur leur effect propres et leurs possibilites d'association. J Med Bord (1964) 141, 1909.
6 Suerinck A and Suerinck E. Etats depressifs en milieu sanatorial et inhibiteurs de la mono-amine oxydase. (Resultats therepeutiques par l'association d'iproclozide et de chlodiazepoxide.) A propos de 146 observations. J Med Lyon (1966) 47, 573.
7 Harris AL and McIntyre N. Interaction of phenelzine and nitrazepam in a slow acetylator. Br J clin Pharmac (1981) 12, 254–5.

Monoamine oxidase inhibitors + Chloral hydrate

Abstract/Summary

An isolated case of fatal hyperpyrexia and another of serious hypertension have been attributed to interactions between chloral and phenelzine.

Clinical evidence, mechanism, importance and management

A woman taking 45 mg phenelzine daily was found in bed deeply comatose with marked muscular rigidity, twitching down one side and a temperature of 41°C. She died without regaining consciousness. A postmortem failed to establish the cause of death, but it subsequently came to light that she had started drinking whiskey again (she had been treated for alcoholism), and she had access to chloral hydrate. She may have taken a fatal dose.[1] Another patient, also taking 45 mg phenelzine daily and chloral hydrate for sleeping, developed an excruciating headache followed by nausea, photophobia and a substantial rise in blood pressure.[2] This latter reaction is similar to the 'cheese reaction', but at the time the authors of the report were unaware of this type of reaction so that they failed to find out if any tyramine-rich foods had been eaten on the day of the attack.[2]

There is no clear evidence that either of these adverse reactions was due to an interaction between phenelzine and chloral, and no other reports to suggest that an interaction between these drugs is normally likely.

References

1 Howarth E. Possible synergistic effects of the new thymoleptics in connection with poisoning. J Ment Sci (1961) 107, 100.
2 Dillon H and Leopold RL. Acute cerebro-vascular symptoms produced by an antidepressant. J Psychiatry (1965) 121, 1012.

Monoamine oxidase inhibitors + Cyproheptadine

Abstract/Summary

An isolated report describes unexplained hallucinations which developed in a woman two months after cyproheptadine was added to her treatment with phenelzine.[1]

Reference

1 Kahn DA. Possible toxic interaction between cyproheptadine and phenelzine. Am J Psychiatry (1987) 144, 1242.

Monoamine oxidase inhibitors + Dextromethorphan

Abstract/Summary

Two fatal cases of hyperpyrexia and coma have occurred in patients on phenelzine who ingested dextromethorphan (in overdosage in one case). A serious but non-fatal reaction occurred in another on isocarboxazid.

Clinical evidence, mechanism, importance and management

A woman taking 60 mg phenelzine daily complained of nausea and dizziness before collapsing 30 min after drinking about 2 oz (55 ml) of a cough mixture containing 100 mg dextromethorphan. She remained hyperpyrexic (42°C), hypotensive (systolic pressure not above 70 mm Hg) and unconscious for 4 h before dying of cardiac arrest.[1] A 15-year-old girl taking 45 mg phenelzine daily (as well as thioridazine, procyclidine and metronidazole) took 13 capsules of *Romilar CF* (dextromethorphan 15 mg, phenylephrine 5 mg and acetaminophen 120 mg in each capsule). She became comatose, hyperpyrexic (103°F), had a blood pressure of 100/60 mm Hg, a pulse of 160 and later developed cardiac fibrillation which appeared to be the cause of her death.[2] Neither of these cases is easily understood, the latter being complicated by the overdosage and multiplicity of drugs present, particularly the phenylephrine. A woman taking 30 mg isocarboxazid daily ingested 1 mg diazepam and 10 ml *Robitussin DM* (15 mg dextromethophan+100 mg guaiaphensin). Within 20 min she was nauseated and dizzy and within 45 min she began to have a fine bilateral leg tremor and muscle spasms of the abdomen and lower back. These were followed by bilateral and persistent myoclonic jerks of legs, occasional choreoathetoid movements and marked urinary retention. These adverse effects persisted for about 19 h, gradually becoming less severe.[4] The authors of this report suggest that these effects may have been due to an increase in serotonin activity in the CNS. A reaction has been seen in rabbits treated with dextromethorphan with nialamide, phenelzine or pargyline[3] (hyperpyrexia, dilated pupils, hyperexcitability and motor restlessness) and there is some similarity to the MAOI–pethidine interaction.

Despite the very limited information available and our lack of understanding of why it can happen, the severity of the reaction suggests that patients on MAOI should avoid taking preparations containing dextromethorphan. Chlorpromazine opposes the development of this interaction in rabbits and has been used successfully in the clinical treatment of the MAOI–pethidine interaction, so it might also prove to be useful for this interaction. This needs confirmation.

References

1 Rivers N and Horner B. Possible lethal reaction between Nardil and dextromethorphan. Can Med Ass J (1970) 103, 85.
2 Shamsie JC and Barriga C. The hazards of use of monoamine oxidase inhibitors in disturbed adolescents. Can Med Ass J (1971) 104, 715.
3 Sinclair JG. Dextromethorphan-monoamine oxidase inhibitor interaction in rabbits. J Pharm Pharmac (1973) 25, 803.
4 Sovner R and Wolfe J. Interaction between detromethorphan and monoamine oxidase inhibitor therapy with isocarboxazid. N Eng J Med (1988) 319, 1671.

Monoamine oxidase inhibitors + Dextropropoxyphene

Abstract/Summary

An isolated report describes a marked increase in the sedative effects of dextropropoxyphene in a woman taking phenelzine.

Clinical evidence, mechanism, importance and management

A woman taking propranolol, an oestrogen and phenelzine became '. . . very sedated and groggy and had to lie down. . .' on two occasions within 2 h of taking dextropropoxyphene, 100 mg, and paracetamol (acetaminophen), 650 mg. She had had no problems with either paracetamol or dextropropoxphene-paracetamol before starting the phenelzine.[1] The mechanism of this interaction is not understood but the symptoms appear to be an increase in the effects of the dextropropoxyphene. Concurrent use need not be avoided but the effects should be checked.

Reference

1 Garbutt JC. Potentiation of propoxyphene by phenelzine. Am J Psychiatry (1987) 144, 251–2.

Monoamine oxidase inhibitors + Fenfluramine

Abstract/Summary

A confusing situation: the manufacturers advise against combined use, but it has also been claimed that concurrent use is effective.

Clinical evidence, mechanism, importance and management

The recommendation of the manufacturers is that fenfluramine should not be used in patients with a history of depression and during treatment with antidepressants (especially the MAOI's) and there should be an interval of three weeks between stopping the MAOI's and starting fenfluramine.[1] Acute confusional states have been described when fenfluramine was used with phenelzine,[2] but it has also been claimed that in some instances fenfluramine has been used effectively with an MAOI.[3]

References

1 ABPI Data Sheet Compendium, 1985–6 p 1400. Datapharm publications, London.
2 Brandon S. Unusual effect of fenfluramine. Br Med J (1969) 4, 557.
3 Mason EC. Servier Laboratories Ltd. Personal communication (1976).

Monoamine oxidase inhibitors + Ginseng

Abstract/Summary

Two patients have been reported who developed adverse effects when concurrently treated with phenelzine and ginseng.

Clinical evidence, mechanism, importance and management

A woman of 64 treated with phenelzine developed headache and tremulousness when ginseng was added.[1] Another depressed woman of 42 taking ginseng and bee pollen experienced a relief of her depression and became active and extremely optimistic when she was started on phenelzine (45 mg daily), but this was accompanied by insomnia, irritability, headaches and vague visual hallucinations. When the phenelzine was stopped and then re-started in the absence of the ginseng and bee pollen her depression was not relieved. It is thought unlikely that the bee pollen had any part to play in these reactions and suspicion therefore falls on the ginseng. It would seem that the psychoactive effects of the ginsenosides from the ginseng and the MAOI were additive in some way as yet not understood. Ginseng has stimulant effects but its adverse effects include sleeplessness, nervousness, hypertension and euphoria. These two cases once again illustrate that over-the-counter herbal or 'green' medicines are not necessarily problem-free if combined with orthodox drugs.

References

1 Shader RI and Greenblatt DJ. Phenelzine and the dream machine—ramblings and reflections. J Clin Psychopharmacol (1985) 5, 65.
2 Jones BD and Runikis AM. Interaction with ginseng. J Clin Psychopharmacol (1987) 7, 201–2.

Monoamine oxidase inhibitors + Lithium carbonate

Abstract/Summary

Four patients are reported to have been successfully and uneventfully treated with phenelzine and lithium carbonate.

Clinical evidence, mechanism, importance and management

Four severely depressed patients who had failed to respond to tricyclic antidepressants or to MAOI, did so when lithium was added to their MAOI treatment. Each of them was treated with relatively modest doses of phenelzine (30–60 mg daily) and lithium carbonate (600–900 mg daily). No adverse reactions were reported.[1]

Reference

1 Fein S, Paz V, Rao N and LaGrassa J. The combination of lithium carbonate and an MAOI in refractory depression. Am J Psychiatry (1988) 145, 249–50.

Monamine oxidase inhibitors + Mazindol

Abstract/Summary

An isolated report describes a marked rise in blood pressure in a patient on phenelzine when given a single dose of mazindol.

Clinical evidence, mechanism, importance and management

A woman on phenelzine (30 mg three times a day) showed a blood pressure rise from 110/60 to 200/100 mm Hg within 2 h of receiving a 10 mg test dose of mazindol. The blood pressure remained elevated for another hour, but had fallen again after another 3 h. The patient experienced no subjective symptoms.[1] It is uncertain whether this hypertensive reaction was a direct response to the mazindol (the dose was large compared with the manufacturers recommended dosage of 2 mg daily) or to an interaction. The general importance is uncertain, but it would seem wise to avoid mazindol in patients on MAOI. This is in line with the manufacturers recommendations.

Reference

1 Oliver RM. Interaction between phenelzine and mazindol. Personal communication (1981).

Monoamine oxidase inhibitors + Methyldopa

Abstract/Summary

The concurrent use of pargyline and methyldopa appears to be safe, although an isolated report describes the delayed development of hallucinosis. The order of administration may be important. The concurrent use of antidepressant MAOI and methyldopa may not be desirable because methyldopa can sometimes cause depression.

Clinical evidence, mechanism, importance and management

A number of reports describe no unusual reactions or toxic effects in man during the concurrent use of pargyline and methyldopa,[1-4] and the hypotensive response can be enhanced.[5] In contrast, a hypertensive woman on pargyline, 25 mg four times a day, developed hallucinosis about a month after starting to take 250 mg methyldopa daily, later increased to 500 mg.[5]

Concurrent use normally seems to be safe, but it has been suggested that the methyldopa should not be given after the pargyline to prevent the possibility of the sudden release by the methyldopa of the MAOI-accumulated stores of catecholamines.[6] There seems to be no documentation about the concurrent use of antidepressant MAOI's and methyldopa, but the potential depressant side-effects of methyldopa may make it an unsuitable drug for patients with depression.

References

1 Maronde RF, Haywood LJ, Feinstein D and Sobel C. The monoamine oxidase inhibitor, pargyline hydrochloride, and reserpine. J Amer Med Ass (1963) 184, 7.
2 Herting RL. Monoamine oxidase inhibitors. Lancet (1965) i, 1324.
3 Kinross-Wright J and Charolampous KD. Concurrent administration of dopa decarboxylase and monoamine oxidase inhibitors in man. Clin Res (1963) ii, 177.
4 Gillespsie L, Oates JA, Grout R and Sjoerdsma A. Clinical and chemical studies with alpha-methyldopa in patients with hypertension. Circulation (1962) 25, 281.
5 Paykel ES. Hallucinosis on combined methyldopa and pargyline. Br Med J (1966) 1, 803.
6 Natajaran S. Potential dangers of monoamine oxidase inhibitors and alpha-methyldopa. Lancet (1964) i, 1330.

Monoamine oxidase inhibitors + Miscellaneous drugs

Abstract/Summary

No adverse interactions between the MAOI and either anticholinergics, beta-blockers, carbamazepine or doxapram have been reported, although the possibility has been suggested. An isolated report suggests that the CNS stimulant effects of caffeine may possibly be increased by the MAOI.

Clinical evidence, mechanism, importance and management

Drug manufacturers often include warnings in their data sheets and package inserts about alleged interactions with the MAOI, despite the absence of direct evidence in man that an interaction can actually take place. It is usually suggested that three weeks should elapse between stopping the MAOI and starting the other drug. This prudent precaution protects both the health of patients and the legal liability of manufacturers, but it also means that patients may sometimes be denied the use of a drug which may be perfectly safe. If you telephone manufacturers many will freely admit that this is the case.

(a) MAOI + anticholinergics

Although some books and lists of drug interactions state that the effects of the anticholinergic drugs used in the treatment of Parkinson's disease are increased by the MAOI, there appears to be no documentary evidence of this in man, although a hyperthermic reaction has been reported in animals.[6]

(b) MAOI + beta-blockers

It has been claimed[1] that 'MAO inhibitors should be discontinued at least two weeks prior to the institution of propranolol therapy...', but studies in animals[2] using mebanazine as a representative MAOI failed to show '...any undesirable property of propranolol following MAO inhibition.' Bradycardia (46–53 bpm) has been described in two patients taking 40 mg nadolol or 150 mg metoprolol daily for hypertension within 8–11 days of starting 60 mg phenelzine daily. No noticeable ill effects were seen but the authors recommend careful monitoring particularly in the elderly who may tolerate bradycardia poorly.[9]

(c) MAOI + caffeine

It is claimed[4] that a patient who normally drank 10 or 12 cups of coffee daily, without adverse effects, experienced extreme jitteriness during treatment with an MAOI which subsided when the coffee consumption was reduced to two or three cups a day. The same reaction was also said to have occurred in other patients on MAOI who drank tea or some of the 'Cola' drinks which contain caffeine. Another patient claimed that a single cup of coffee taken in the morning kept him jittery all day and up the entire night as well, a reaction which occurred on three separate occasions. Apart from this report and another[5] stating that the effects of caffeine *in mice* are enhanced by MAOI, the literature appears otherwise to be silent about this alleged interaction. Whether this reflects its mildness and unimportance, or its rarity, is not clear.

(d) MAOI + doxapram

On the basis of animal studies which reportedly show that the actions of doxapram are potentiated by pretreatment with MAOI, the manufacturers[7] advise that concurrent use should be undertaken with great care. The adverse cardiovascular effects of doxapram (hypertension, tachycardia, arrhythmias) are said elsewhere[8] to be markedly increased in patients on MAOI, and it is also claimed that the pressor effects are enhanced[3] but no clinical data in support of these statements is cited.

References

1 Frieden J. Propranolol as an antiarrhythmic agent. Am Heart J (1967) 74, 283.

2 Barrett AM and Cullum VA. Lack of interaction between propranolol and mebanazine. J Pharm Pharmacol (1968) 20, 911.

3 Martindale's Extra Pharmacopoeia, 29th edn p 1442. Reynolds JEF (ed). Pharmaceutical Press, London (1989).

4 Kline NS. Psychopharmaceuticals: effects and side-effects. Bull WHO (1959) 21, 397.

5 Berkowitz BA, Spector S and Pool W. The interaction of caffeine, theophylline and theobromine with MAOI. Eur J Pharmacol (1971) 16, 315.

6 Pedersen V and Nielsen IM. Hyperthermia in rabbits caused by interaction between MAOI's, antiparkinson drugs and neuroleptics. Lancet (1975) i, 409.

7 ABPI Data Sheet Compendium 1985–6 p 1226. Datapharm Publications (1986).

8 Esplin DW and Zablocka-Esplin B. Central nervous stimulants. In 'The Pharmacological Basis of Therapeutics' 4th edn p 335. Goodman LS and Gillman A (eds). Macmillan NY (1970).

9 Reggev A and Vollhardt BR. Bradycardia induced by an interaction between phenelzine and beta-blockers. Psychosomatics (1989) 30, 106–8.

Monoamine oxidase inhibitors + Monoamine oxidase inhibitors

Abstract/Summary

Two patients suffered strokes (one fatal) and another experienced a hypertensive reaction when phenelzine or isocarboxazid were replaced by tranylcypromine.

Clinical evidence, mechanism, importance and management

A patient on 30 mg isocarboxazid daily was switched to 10 mg tranylcypromine, and on the following day to 30 mg daily. Later she complained of feeling 'funny', had difficulty in talking, a headache, was restless, flushed, sweating, a blood pressure of 210/110 mm Hg (normal for the patient) and a pulse rate of 130 bpm. She died the following day. The cause of death was either a subarachnoid haemorrhage or some other unidentified reaction.[1] Another patient, switched from 75 mg phenelzine daily to 10, 20, 30 and then 20 mg tranylcypromine daily, suffered a subcortical cerebral haemorrhage on the fourth day which resulted in total right-sided hemiplegia.[2,3] Another patient taking 45 mg phenelzine daily, followed by a two-day drug free period and then

20 mg tranylcypromine daily, experienced a rise in blood pressure to 240/130 mm Hg.[2]

The reasons for these reactions are not understood, but one idea is that the amphetamine-like properties of tranylcypromine may have had some part to play. Certainly there are cases of spontaneous rises in blood pressure and intracranial bleeding in patients given tranylcypromine, no other precipitating factor being known.[5] Not all patients experience adverse reactions when switched from one MAOI to another,[4] but until more is known it would seem prudent to have a drug-free wash-out interval when doing so, and to start dosing in a conservative and step-wise manner.

References

1 Bazire SR. Sudden death associated with switching monoamine oxidase inhibitors. Drug Intell Clin Pharm (1986) 20, 954–5.
2 Gelenberg AJ. Switching MAOI. Biol Ther Psychiatr (1984) 7, 36.
3 Gelenberg AJ. Switching MAOI. The sequel. Biol Ther Psychiatr (1985) 8, 41.
4 True BL, Alexander B and Carter BL. Comment: switching MAO inhibitors. Drug Intell Clin Pharm (1986) 20, 384.
5 Cooper AJ, Magnus RV and Rose MJ. A hypertensive syndrome with tranylcypromine medication. Lancet (1964) 1, 527–9.

Monoamine oxidase inhibitors + Morphine or Methadone

Abstract/Summary

No adverse interaction normally occurs in patients on MAOI given morphine, but there are two isolated and unexplained reports of patients on MAOI who showed hypotension, marked in one case and accompanied by unconsciousness. Some very limited evidence also suggests that no interaction occurs with methadone.

Clinical evidence

(a) MAOI + morphine

A patient taking 40 mg tranylcypromine and 20 mg trifluoperazine daily and undergoing a preoperative test with morphine, became unconscious and unresponsive to stimuli with pinpoint pupils and showed a systolic blood pressure fall from 160 to 40 mm Hg after receiving a total of 6 mg morphine. 2 min after being given 4 mg naloxone IV, the patient was awake and rational with a systolic blood pressure fully restored.[1] A moderate fall in blood pressure (from 140/90 to 90/60 mm Hg) was seen in another patient on an MAOI given morphine.[6] In contrast, a study in 15 patients who had been taking either phenelzine, isocarboxazid, iproniazid or tranylcypromine + trifluoperazine (*Parstelin*) for 3–8 weeks, showed no changes in blood pressure, pulse rate or state of awareness when given test doses of up to 4 mg morphine, or to test doses of up to 40 mg pethidine (meperidine).[7] Other patients on MAOI who reacted adversely to pethidine (meperidine), did not do so when given morphine.[3–5] Another study reported no adverse interaction in patients on MAOI given morphine.[8]

(b) MAOI + methadone

A patient on methadone maintenance therapy (30 mg daily) was successfully and uneventfully treated for depression with tranylcypromine, initially 10 mg gradually increased to 30 mg daily.[2]

Mechanism

Not understood.

Importance and management

The serious MAOI–pethidine interaction also cast a shadow over morphine, and this probably accounts for the appearance of morphine in a number of lists and charts of drugs which are said to interact with the MAOI, despite good evidence that patients on MAOI who had reacted adversely with pethidine did not do so when given morphine.[3–5] The hypotensive reactions cited here[1,6] are of a different character and appear to be rare. There seems to be no good reason for avoiding morphine in patients on MAOI, but some caution should be exercised. Naloxone proved to be a rapid and effective treatment in one of the cases cited.[1] The extremely limited evidence available suggests that methadone can be given to patients on MAOI, but a stepwise dosing would seem to be a prudent precaution.

References

1 Barry BJ. Adverse effects of MAO inhibitors with narcotics reversed with naloxone. Anaesth Intens Care (1979) 7, 194.
2 Mendelson G. Narcotics and monoamine oxidase inhibitors. Med J Aust (1979) 1, 400.
3 Palmer H. Potentiation of pethidine. Br Med J (1960) 2, 944.
4 Denton PH, Borelli VM and Edwards NV. Dangers of monoamine oxidase inhibitors. Br Med J (1962) 2, 1752.
5 Shee JC. Dangerous potentiation of pethidine by iproniazid and its treatment. Br Med J (1960) 2, 507.
6 Jenkins LC and Graves HB. Potential hazards of psychoactive drugs in association with anaesthesia. Can Anaesth Soc J (1965) 12, 121.
7 Evans-Prosser CDG. The use of pethidine and morphine in the presence of MAOI. Brit J Anaesth (1968) 40, 279–82.
8 El-Ganzouri A, Ivankovich AD, Braverman B and Land PC. Should MAOI be discontinued preoperatively? Anesthesiology (1983) 59, A384.

Monoamine oxidase inhibitors + Oxtriphylline

Summary

An isolated report describes the development of tachycardia and apprehension in a patient on phenelzine after taking a cough syrup containing oxytriphylline (choline theophyllinate).

Interaction

A woman with agorophobia which was successfully treated with 45 mg phenelzine daily, developed tachycardia, palpitations and apprehension lasting about 4 h after taking a cough syrup (*Bronchodon*) containing oxtriphylline and guiaphenesin. The symptoms recurred when she was given the syrup, and again when given oxtriphylline (*Choledyl*) alone, but not when given guiaphenesin.[1] The reasons are not understood. An adverse reaction with an MAOI has also been reported with caffeine which is another xanthine, but MAOI–xanthine interactions seem to be rare. It would seem prudent to check that patients given these drugs together are not experiencing any adverse effects, but there would not appear to be a general need to avoid the xanthine bronchodilators.

Reference

1   Shader RI and Greenblatt DJ. MAOI's and drug interactions—A proposal for a clearinghouse. J Clin Psychopharmacol (1985) 5, A17.

Monoamine oxidase inhibitors + Phenothiazines

Abstract/Summary

The concurrent use of the MAOI and phenothiazines is usually safe and effective. The exception appears to be methotrimeprazine which has been implicated in two fatal reactions attributed to interactions with pargyline and tranylcypromine.

Clinical evidence, mechanism, importance and management

Concurrent use of the MAOI and phenothiazines has been recommended,[1–3] and a fixed combination (tranylcypromine with trifluoperazine, *Parstelin*) is marketed. Tranylcypromine with chlorpromazine has been found valuable in the treatment of schizophrenia and it may possibly prevent the occurrence of extra-pyramidal symptoms.[9] Promazine has been used safely and effectively in the treatment of overdosage with tranylcypromine.[4] A single report[5] describing the development of a severe occipital headache in a woman on an MAOI as a result of taking 30 ml of a child's cough linctus, attributed this reaction by inference to an interaction with promethazine, but it is now known that the linctus in question contained phenylpropanolamine which is much more likely to have been the cause.[6] (see 'Indirectly-acting sympathomimetic amines+MAOI'). In addition, unexplained fatalities attributed to the concurrent use of methotrimeprazine with pargyline,[7] another with methotrimeprazine and tranylcypromine[8] and the third with an unnamed MAOI-phenothiazine combination have also been reported.[8]

No special precautions would normally seem to be necessary during the concurrent use of most MAOI's and phenothiazines, with the exception of methotrimeprazine which, because it has been implicated in two fatalities, should probably be regarded as contraindicated.

References

1   Winkelman NW. Three evaluations of an MAOI and phenothiazine (a methodological and clinical study). Dis Nerv Syst (1965) 26, 160.

2   Cheshrow EJ and Kaplitz SE. Anxiety and depression in the geriatric and chronically ill patient. Clin Med (1965) 72, 1281.

3   Janacek J, Schiele BC, Belville T and Anderson R. The effects of withdrawal of trifluoperazine on patients maintained on the combination of tranylcypromine and trifluoperazine. A double blind study. Curr Ther Res (1963) 5, 608.

4   Midwinter RE. Accidental overdose with 'Parstelin'. Br Med J (1962) 2, 1755.

5   Mitchell L. Psychotropic drugs. Br Med J (1968) 1, 381.

6   Mitchell L. (1977) Quoted as a personal communication in 'A Manual of Adverse Drug Interactions' 2nd Edn p 174. Griffin JP and D'Arcy PF. Wright, Bristol (1979).

7   Barsa JA and Saunders JC. A comparative study of tranylcypromine and pargyline. Psychopharmacologia (1964) 6, 295.

8   McQueen EG. New Zealand Committee on Adverse Drug Reactions: 14th Annual Report (1979). NZ Med J (1980) 91, 226.

9   Bucci L. The negative symptoms of schizophrenia and the monoamine oxidase inhibitors. Psychopharmacology (1987) 91, 104–8.

Monoamine oxidase inhibitors + Rauwolfia alkaloids or Tetrabenazine

Abstract/Summary

The use of potentially depressive drugs such as the rauwolfia alkaloids or tetrabenazine is generally contraindicated in patients needing treatment for depression. Central excitation and possibly hypertension can occur if the rauwolfia is given to patients already taking MAOI, but is unlikely if the rauwolfia is given first.

Clinical evidence

A chronically depressed woman treated firstly with nialamide, 100 mg three times a day, and on the third day with reserpine as well, 0.5 mg three times a day, became hypomanic on the following day and almost immediately went into frank mania.[1]

Seven days after stopping 25 mg nialamide daily, a patient was started on tetrabenazine. 6 h later he collapsed and demonstrated epileptiform convulsions, partial unconsciousness, rapid respiration and tachycardia.[2]

Other reports state that the administration of reserpine or tetrabenezine after pretreatment with iproniazid can lead to a temporary (up to three days) disturbance of affect and memory, associated with autonomic excitation, delerious agitation, disorientation and illusions of experience and recognition.[3,4]

A delayed 'reserpine-reversal' was seen in three schizophrenics treated firstly with phenelzine for 12 weeks, then a placebo for 16–33 weeks, and lastly reserpine. Their blood pressures rose slightly and persistently and their psychomotor activity was considerably increased, lasting in two cases throughout the 12-week period of treatment.[5]

Mechanism

Rauwolfia alkaloids such as reserpine cause adrenergic neurones to become depleted of their normal stores of noradrenaline (norepinephrine). In this way they prevent or reduce the normal transmission of impulses at the adrenergic nerve endings of the sympathetic nervous system and thereby act as antihypertensive agents. Since the brain also possesses adrenergic neurones, failure of transmission in the CNS could account for the sedation and depression observed. If these compounds are given to patients already taking MAOI, they can cause the sudden release of large amounts of accumulated noradrenaline (norepinephrine), and in the brain of 5-HT as well, resulting in excessive stimulation of the receptors which is seen as gross central excitation and hypertension. This would account for the case reports cited and the effects seen in animals.[7-9] These stimulant effects are sometime called 'reserpine-reversal' because instead of the expected sedation or depression, excitation or delayed depression is seen. It depends upon the order in which the drugs are given.

Importance and management

The administration of potentially depressive drugs is generally contraindicated in patients needing treatment for depression. However if concurrent use is considered desirable, the MAOI should be given after, and not before, the other drug so that sedation rather than excitation will occur.[6] The documentation of this latter reaction in man is very limited.

References

1 Gradwell BG. Psychotic reactions and phenelzine. Br Med J (1960) 2, 1018.
2 Davies TS. Monoamine oxidase inhibitors and rauwolfia compounds. Br Med J (1960) 2, 739.
3 Voelkel A. Klinische Wirkung von Pharmaka mit Einfluss auf den Monoaminestoffwechsel de Gehirns. Confinia Neurol (1958) 18, 144.
4 Voelkel A. Experiences with MAO inhibitors in psychiatry. Ann NY Acad Sci (1959) 80, 680.
5 Esser AH. Clinical observations on reserpine reversal after prolonged MAO inhibition. Psychiat Neurol Neurochirugica (1967) 70, 59.
6 Natajaran S. Potential dangers of monoamine oxidase inhibitors and alpha-methyldopa. Lancet (1964) i, 1330.
7 Shore PA and Brodie BB. LSD-like effects elicited by reserpine in rabbits pretreated with isoniazid. Proc Soc Exp Biol NY (1957) 94, 433.
8 Chessin M, Kramer R and Scott CC. Modification of the pharmacology of reserpine and serotonin by iproniazid. J Pharmacol exp Ther (1957) 119, 453.
9 von Euler US, Bygoleman S and Persson N-A. Interaction of reserpine and monoamine oxidase inhibitors on adrenergic transmitter release. Biochem Biol Sper (1970) 9, 215.

Monoamine oxidase inhibitors + Sulphonamides

Abstract/Summary

An isolated report describes the development of weakness, ataxia and other adverse effects in a patient on phenelzine when additionally given sulphafurazole (sulfisoxazole).

Clinical evidence, mechanism, importance and management

A woman taking 45 mg phenelzine daily complained of weakness, ataxia, dizziness, tinnitus, muscle pains and parasthesias within seven days of starting to take 4 g of sulphafurazole (sulfisoxazole) daily, which continued until the 10-day sulphonamide course was completed. All the adverse symptoms disappeared when the sulphonamide was withdrawn.[1] The reasons are not understood, but as these adverse effects are a combination of the side-effects of both drugs, it seems possible that a mutual interaction (perhaps saturation of the acetylating mechanisms in the liver) was responsible. Concurrent use need not be avoided, but prescribers should be aware of this case.

Reference

1 Boyer WF and Lake CR. Interaction of phenelzine and sulfisoxazole. Am J Psychiatry (1983) 140, 264–5.

Monoamine oxidase inhibitors + Tricyclic antidepressants

Abstract/Summary

Because of the very toxic and sometimes fatal reactions which have very occasionally taken place in patients taking both MAOI and tricyclic antidepressants, concurrent use came to be regarded as totally contraindicated, but informed opinion now considers that with extremely careful control it is permissible and advantageous for some refractory patients.

Clinical evidence

(a) Toxic reactions due to MAOI/tricyclic antidepressant combinations

The toxic reactions have included (with variations) sweating, flushing, hyperpyrexia, restlessness, excitement, tremor, muscle twitching and rigidity, convulsions and coma. An illustrative example:

A woman with depression who had been taking 20 mg tranylcypromine daily for about three weeks, stopped taking it three days before taking a single tablet of imipramine. Within a few hours she complained of an excruciating headache, and soon afterwards lost consciousness and started to convulse. The toxic reactions manifested were a temperature of 40°C, pulse rate of 120, severe extensor rigidity, carpal spasm, opisthotonos and cyanosis. She was treated with amobarbital and phenytoin, and her temperature was reduced with alcohol-ice-soaked towels. The treatment was effective and she recovered.[11]

Similar reactions have been recorded on a number of other occasions with normal therapeutic doses of iproniazid,[1] isocarboxazid,[1,2] pargyline,[3] or phenelzine[4-9,22] with imipramine; phenelzine with desipramine[13] or clomipramine;[23] and tranylcypromine with clomipramine.[16,24,26] Some other reports are confused by overdosage with one or both drugs, or by the presence of other drugs and diseases. There have been fatalities.[13,16,21] There are far too many reports of these interactions to list them here, but they are extensively reviewed elsewhere.[10,12,20] Three patients with bipolar disorder developed mania when treated with isocarboxazid and amitriptyline.[25]

(b) Advantageous use of MAOI/tricyclic antidepressant combinations

Dr GA Gander of St Thomas's Hospital, London, has stated[14] that 98 out of 149 patients on combined therapy (phenelzine, isocarboxazid or iproniazid with imipramine or amitriptyline) over periods of 1–24 months improved significantly and that the side-effects were '. . .identical in nature and similar in frequency to those seen with a single antidepressant. . . . Side effects were easily controlled by adjusting the dosage. None of the serious side-effects previously reported, such as muscle twitching or loss of consciousness was seen.' He also states that more than 1400 patients having combined antidepressants over a period of four years '. . .tend to confirm these findings described.' Dr William Sargent from the same department has also written[15] that '. . .we have used combined antidepressant drugs for nearly 10 years now on some thousands of patients. We still wait to see any of the rare dangerous complications reported.'

Other reports and reviews describing the beneficial use of MAOI/ tricyclic antidepressant combinations are listed elsewhere.[12,19,20] Moclobemide is reported not to interact with amitriptyline.[24]

Mechanism

Not understood. One idea is that since both types of antidepressant increase the levels of monoamines such as 5-HT and noradrenaline in the brain, each working in concert and reinforcing the effects of the other might raise concentrations so high that a 'spill-over' effect could take place in areas of the brain not concerned with mood elevation, causing the bizarre and serious reactions described. Less likely suggestions are that the MAOI inhibit enzymes concerned with the metabolism of the tricyclic antidepressants, or that active and unusual metabolites of the tricyclic antidepressants are produced.[12]

Importance and management

This interaction when it happens can be serious and life-threatening, but there is no precise information about its incidence. It is probably much lower than was originally thought. No detailed clinical work has been done to find out precisely what sets the scene for a hazardous interaction to occur, but some general empirical guidelines have been suggested so that it can, as far as possible, be avoided when concurrent treatment is thought appropriate:[10,12,18,20,22]

1 Treatment with both types of drug should only be undertaken by those well aware of the problems and can undertake adequate supervision.
2 Only patients refractory to all other types of treatment should be considered.

3 Tranylcypromine, phenelzine, clomipramine and imipramine appear to be high on the list of drugs which have interacted adversely. Amitriptyline, trimipramine and isocarboxazid are possibly safer.
4 Drugs should be given orally, not parenterally.
5 It seems safer to give the tricyclic antidepressants first, or together with the MAOI, than to give the MAOI first. If the patient is already taking an MAOI, it may not be safe to start the tricyclic antidepressant until recovery from MAO-inhibition is complete.
6 Small doses should be given initially, increasing the levels of each drug, one at a time, over a period of 2–3 weeks to levels generally below those used for each one individually.
7 Do not exchange either the MAOI or the tricyclic antidepressant for other members of these drug groups without taking full precautions.

50 mg chlorpromazine given intramuscularly has been used in the treatment of an adverse interaction[24] and one report suggests that patients should carry 300 mg chlorpromazine and take it if a sudden, throbbing, radiating occipital headache occurs, and seek medical help at once.[17]

References

1 Ayd FJ. Toxic somatic and psychopathological reactions to antidepressant drugs. J Neuropsychiat (1961) (Suppl 1), 119.
2 Kane FJ and Freeman D. Non-fatal reaction to imipramine-MAOI inhibitor combination. Amer J Psychiat (1963), 120, 79.
3 McCurdy A and Kane AB. Transient brain syndrome as a non-fatal reaction to combined pargyline-imipramine treatment. Amer J Psychiat (1964), 121, 397.
4 Loeb RH. Quoted in ref 10 below as written communication (1969).
5 Hills NF. Combining the antidepressant drugs. Br Med J (1965) 1, 859.
6 Davies G. Side effects of phenelzine. Br Med J (1960) 2, 1019.
7 Howarth E. Possible synergistic effects of the new thymoleptics in connection with poisoning. J Ment Sci (1961) 107, 1000.
8 Singh H. Atropine-like poisoning due to tranquillizing agents. Amer J Psychiat (1960) 117, 360.
9 Lockett MF and Milner G. Combining the antidepressant drugs. Br Med J (1965) 1, 921.
10 Schukit M, Robins E and Feighner J. Tricyclic antidepressants and monoamine oxidase inhibitors. Combination therapy in the treatment of depression. Arch Gen Psychiat (1971) 24, 509.
11 Brachfield J, Wirtschafter A and Wolfe S. Imipramine-tranylcypromine incompatibility. Near fatal toxic reaction. J Amer Med Ass (1963) 186, 1172.
12 Ponto LB, Perry PJ, Liskow BI and Seaba HH. Drug therapy reviews: tricyclic antidepressant and monoamine oxidase inhibitor combination therapy. Am J Hosp Pharm (1977) 34, 954.
13 Bowen LW. Fatal hyperpyrexia with antidepressant drugs. Br Med J (1964) 2, 1465.
14 Gander GA. In 'Antidepressant Drugs' Proc 1st Int Symp Milan (1966). Int Congr Ser No 122, p 336. Excerpta Medica.
15 Sargent W. Safety of combined antidepressant drugs. Br Med J (1971) 1, 555.
16 Beaumont G. Drug interactions with clomipramine (Anafranil). J Int Med Res (1973) 1, 480.
17 Schildkraut JJ and Klein DF. The classification and treatment of depressive disorders. In 'Manual of Psychiatric Therapeutics' p 61. Shader RI (ed). (1975). Little, Brown, Boston, Mass.
18 Beaumont G. Personal communication (1978).
19 Stockley IH. Tricyclic antidepressants. Part 1. Interaction with drugs affecting adrenergic neurones. In 'Drug Interactions and Their Mechanisms' p 14. (1974) Pharmaceutical Press, London.
20 Anath J and Luchins D. A review of combined tricyclic and MAOI therapy. Compr Psychiatry (1977) 18, 221.
21 Wright SP. Hazards with monoamine oxidase inhibitors: a persistent problem. Lancet (1978) i, 284.

22 Graham PM, Potter JM and Patterson JW. Combination monoamine oxidase inhibitor/tricyclic antidepressant interaction. Lancet (1982) ii, 440.

23 Beeley L and Daly M (eds). Bulletin of the W. Midlands Centre for Adverse Drug Reaction Reporting. (1986) 23, 16.

24 Tackley RM and Tregaskis B. Fatal disseminated intravascular coagulation following a monoamine oxidase inhibitor/tricyclic interaction. Anaesthesia (1987) 42, 760–3.

25 De la Fuente JR, Berlanga C and Leon-Andrade C. Mania induced by tricyclic-MAOI combination therapy in bipolar treatment-resistant disorder. Case reports. J Clin Psychiatry (1986) 47, 40–1.

26 Richards GA, Fritz VU, Pincus P and Reyneke J. Unusual drug interactions between monoamine oxidase inhibitors and tricyclic antidepressants. J Neurol Neurosurg Psychiatry (1987) 50, 1240–1.

Monoamine oxidase inhibitors + L-tryptophan

Abstract/Summary

Although the concurrent use of monoamine oxidase inhibitors and L-tryptophan can be both safe and effective, a few patients may develop both behavioural and neurological signs of toxicity. L-tryptophan has been withdrawn in some countries because of possible toxicity.

Clinical evidence

A man on phenelzine (90 mg daily) developed behavioural and neurological toxicity within 2 h of being given 6 g tryptophan.[1] He showed shivering and diaphoresis, his psychomotor retardation disappeared and he became jocular, fearful and moderately labile. His neurological signs included bilateral Babinski signs, hyperreflexia, rapid horizontal ocular oscillations, shivering of the jaw, trunk and limbs, mild dysmetria and ataxia. The situation resolved on withdrawal of the drugs.

Other reports have described patients who showed hypomania[5] or milder symptoms of toxicity when given both drugs.[2,3,7] Another patient showed toxicity but with transient hyperthermia when the dose of tryptophan was increased.[6] All of the patients appeared to recover fully. Generally concurrent use is said to be both safe and effective,[4] however see the note below.

Mechanism

Not understood.

Importance and management

Information seems to be confined to the reports listed. Concurrent use can be effective in the treatment of depression,[4] but toxicity is possible. The authors of the report detailed here[1] recommend that patients on MAOI should be started on a low dose of L-tryptophan (0.5 g). This should be gradually increased while monitoring the mental status of the patient for mental changes suggesting hypomania, and neurological changes including ocular oscillations and upper motor neurone signs. However it should pointed out that most products containing L-tryptophan for the treatment of depression have been withdrawn in the USA and UK because of a possible association with the development of an eosinophilia-myalgia syndrome.

References

1 Thomas JM and Rubin EH. Case report of a toxic reaction from a combination of tryptophan and phenelzine. Am J Psychiatry (1984) 141, 281–3.

2 Baloh RW, Dietz J and Spooner JW. Myoclonus and ocular oscillations

3 Glassman AH and Platman SR, Potentiation of monoamine oxidase inhibitor by tryptophan. J Psychiatr Res (1969) 7, 83–8.

4 Klein DF, Gittelman R and Quitkin F. Diagnosis and drug treatment of psychiatric disorders: adults and children. Edition 2. Williams and Wilkins Co. (1980) 358.

5 Goff DC. Two cases of hypomania following the addition of L-tryptophan to a Monoamine oxidase inhibitor. Am J Psychiatry (1985) 142, 1487–8.

6 Price WA, Zimmer B and Kucas P. Serotonin syndrome: a case report. J Clin Pharmacol (1986) 26, 77–8.

7 Pare CBM. Potentiation of monoamine oxidase inhibitors by tryptophan. Lancet (1963) 2, 527–8.

19

NEUROLEPTIC, ANXIOLYTIC AND TRANQUILLIZING DRUG INTERACTIONS

The minor tranquillizers include the benzodiazepines, hydroxyzine and other agents used to treat psychoneuroses such as anxiety and tension, and are intended to induce calm without causing drowsiness and sleep. Some of the benzodiazepines and related drugs are also used as anticonvulsants and hypnotics. Table 19.1 contains a list of the benzodiazepines which are referred to in this book.

The major tranquillizers and neuroleptics are represented by chlorpromazine (and other phenothazines), butyrophenones and thioxanthenes. Their major use is in the treatment of psychoses such as schizophrenia and mania. These are listed in Table 19.2. Some of the phenothiazines are also used as antihistamines.

Most of the interactions involving tranquillizers and neuroleptics are listed in this chapter, but there are other synopses elsewhere in this book where the interacting agent is a tranquillizer or neuroleptic. A full listing is given in the Index.

Table 19.1. Benzodiazepines and other minor tranquillizers

Non-proprietary names	Proprietary names
Benzodiazepines	
Alprazolam	Tafil, Trankimazin, Valeans, Xanax
Bromazepam	Bartul, Brozam, Compendium, Durazanil, Gityl, Lectopam, Lexatin, Lexomil, Lexotan, Neo-Opt, Normoc
Brotizolam	Lendormin
Chlordiazepoxide	Ansiacal, A-poxide, Benzodiapin, Binomil, Calmoden Cebrum, Chlotran, Corax, C-tran, Diazebrum, Diazepina, Elenium, Endequil, Equibral, Helogaphen, Huberplex, Karmoplex, Klopoxid, Labican, Liberans, Libritabs, Librium, Lixin, Medilium, Multum, Nack, Normide, Novopoxide, Omnalio, Paliatin, Philcorium, Psicofar, Psicoterina, Relaxil, Reliberan, Reposal, Risachief, Seren, Sintesdan, Smail, Solium, Trilium, Tropium, Viansin, Zeisin
Clobazam	Castilium, Clarmyl, Clopax, Frisin, Frisium, Karadium, Noiafren, Sederlona, Sentil, Urbadan, Urbanol, Urbanyl
Clorazepate	Azene, Belseren, Covengar, Enadine, Justum, Moderane, Nansius, Novoclopate, Tencilan, Transene, Tranxen(e), Tranxilen, Traxilium, Uni-tranxene
Clotiazepam	Clozan, Distensan, Rizen, Tienor, Trecalmo, Veratren
Diazepam	Aliseum, Alupram, Amiprol, Ansiolin, Antenex, Apozepam, Armonil, Atensine, Benzopin, Best, Cuadel, Cyclopam, Diaceplex, Dialar, Diapam, Diaquel, Diatran, Diazemuls, Diazepan, Dipam, Dipezona, Dizam, Domalium, Doval, Drenian, Ducene, E-pam, Eridan, Ethipam, Euphorin, Evacalm, Gubex, Lamra, Lorinon, Mandro-zep, Neo-calme, Neosorex, Neurolitryl, Noan, Notense, Novazam, Paceum,

Table 19.1. *continued*

Non-proprietary names	Proprietary names
	Pax(el), Pidan, Pro-pam, Quetinil, Quievita, Relanium. Relivan X, Rival, Saromet, Scriptopam, Sedapam, Sedaril, Serenack, Solis, Somasedan, Sonacon, Stesolid, Stress-pam, Tensium, Tranquase, Tranquirit, Valoxona, Valium, Valrelease, Vatran, Vivol.
Ketazolam	*Anxon, Contamex, Loftran, Marcen, Sedotime, Solatran, Unakalm*
Loprazolam	*Dormonct, Havlane, Sonin*
Lorazepam	*Almazine, Alzapam, Ativan, Control, Donix, Emotival, Idalprem, Kalmalin, Laubeel, Lorans, Lorax, Lorenin, Orfidal, Piralone, Placidia, Placinoral, Punktyl, Quait, Securit, Sedarkey, Sedatival, Sedicepan, Sidenar, Temesta, Tolid, Tranqil, Tranqipam, Trapaxm, Wypax*
Medazepam	*Anxitol, Azepamid, Benson, Elbrus, Lasazepam, Lerisum, Medacepan, Megasedan, Metonas, Narsis, Navizil, Nivelton, Nobrium, Resmit, Serenium, Siman, Templane*
Oxazepam	*Adumbran, Alepam, Anxiolit, Azutranquil, Aplakil, Benzotran, Durazepam, Enidrel, Isodin, Limbial, Murelax, Nesontil, Neurofren, Noctazepam, Novoxapam, Oxanid, Praxiten, Purata, Quen, Quilibrex, Sedokin, Serenid, Serepax, Seresta, Serpax, Sobile, Wakazepam*
Oxazolam	*Convertal, Hializan, Serenal, Tranquit*
Other drugs	
Buspirone	*Bespar, Buspar*
Hydroxyzine	*Atarax, Atazina, Durrax, Multipax, Neocalma, Orgatrax, Paxistil, Sedaril, Vistaril*

Other benzodiazepines such as flunitrazepam (*Darkene, Flunipam, Rohnipnol*) flurazepam (*Dalmadorm, Dalmane, Dormodor, Felison, Somnol*), lormetazepam (*Loramet, Noctamid, Pronactan*), midazolam (*Dormicum, Hypnovel*), nitrazepam (*Alodorm, Mogadon*), temazepam (*Cerepax, Euhypnos, Lenal, Levanxene, Levanxol, Normison, Planum*) and triazolam (*Halcion, Novodorm*) may be used as sedatives and hypnotics, whereas clonazepam (*Clonopin, Iktorivil, Klonopin, Rivotril*) and diazepam have application as anticonvulsants.

Table 19.2 Phenothiazine, butyrophenone, thioxanthene and related neuroleptics

Non-proprietary names	Proprietary names
Phenothiazines	
Butaperazine	*Randolectil, Repoise*
Chlorpromazine	*Amazin, Ampliactil, Aspersinal, BayClor, Chloractil, Chlorazine, Chlorprom, Chlorpromanyl, Clopratets, Cloracin, Dozine, Hibanil, Klorazin, Klorpromex, Largactil, Megaphen, Novochlorpromazine, Procalm, Promacid, Promapar, Protran, Prozil, Prozin, Repazine*
Fluphenazine	*Anatenazine, Anatensol, Dapotum, Eutimox, Lyogen, Modecate, Moditen, Omca, Pacinol, Permitil, Prolixin, Sevinol*
Mesoridazine	*Imagotan, Serentil*
Methotrimeprazine	*Levonormal, Levoprome, Procrazine, Sinogan, Sofmin, Tisercin, Veractil*
Perphenazine	*Decentan, Fentazin, Trilafon*
Prochlorperazine	*Anti-naus, Buccastem, Compazine, Stemetil, Vertigon*
Promazine	*Calmotal, Neuroplegil, Prazine, Promabec, Promanyl, Protactyl, Sparine, Talofen*
Thioridazine	*Mallorol, Meleril, Mellaril, Melleretten, Melleril*
Trifluoperazine	*Calmazine, Clinazine, Eskazine, Flumatets, Jatroneural, Modalina, Nerolet, Novoflurazine, Pentazine, Solazine, Stelazine, Terfluzin, Triflurin, Tripazine*
Butyrophenones	
Benperidol	*Anquil, Frenactil, Glianimon, Psicoben*
Droperidol	*Dehyrobenperidol, Dridol, Droleptan, Inapsin(e), Sintodian*
Haloperidol	*Bioperidolo, Brotopon, Dozic, Duraperidol, Haldol, Halosten, Linton, Novoperidol, Pacedol, Peluces, Peridol, Serenace, Sigaperidol, Sylador, Tamide*
Thioxanthenes	
Chlorprothixene	*Taractan, Tarasan, Truxal, Truxaletten*
Flupenthixol	*Depixol, Emergil, Fluanxol*
Thiothixene	*Navane*
Other drugs	
Loxapine	*Daxolin, Desconex, Loxapac, Loxitane*
Molindone	*Lidone*
Sulpiride	*Abilit, Aiglonyl, Arminol, Biomaride, Championyl, Confidan, Coolspan, Digton, Dixibon, Dobren, Dogmatil, Dolmatil, Drominetas, Eglonyl, Euquilid, Eusulpid, Guastil, Kalpiride, Lebopride, Lusedan, Meresa, Miradol, Mirbanil, Misulvan, Neogama, Neoride, Omperan, Sato, Sernevin, Sicofrenol, Sulpitil, Tepavil, Vipral*

Benzodiazepines + Antacids

Abstract/Summary

The absorption of chlordiazepoxide and diazepam is slightly delayed by the concurrent use of aluminium and magnesium hydroxide or trisilicate antacids. The absorption of single doses of clorazepate may be reduced, but chronic dosing is unaffected. These interactions appear to be of little or no importance.

Clinical evidence

10 healthy subjects taking 7.5 mg clorazepate nightly were given water, low dose (30 ml) *Maalox* or high dose (120 ml) *Maalox* for 10 days in random sequence. The mean steady-state serum levels of the active metabolite (desmethyldiazepam) were not affected by *Maalox*, although they varied widely between individuals.[1]

This is in line with another report[6] but contrasts with a single-dose study in which the peak plasma concentration of desmethyldiazepam was delayed and reduced about one-third by the use of *Maalox*.[2] The 48-hour AUC (area under the time-concentration curve) was reduced about 10%. Chlordiazepoxide absorption (single dose) is delayed by *Maalox*, though the total amount of drug absorbed is not significantly affected.[3] Similar results have been found with diazepam.[4]

Mechanism

The delay in the absorption of chlordiazepoxide and diazepam is attributed to the effect of the antacid on gastric emptying. Clorazepate on the other hand is a 'pro-drug' which needs acid conditions in the stomach for conversion (hydrolysis and decarboxylation) to its active form. Antacids are presumed to inhibit this conversion by raising the pH of the stomach contents.[5]

Importance and management

Most of the reports describe single dose studies but what is known suggests that no interaction of any clinical importance is likely in patients on long-term treatment with chlordiazepoxide, diazepam or clorazepate. No special precautions seem to be necessary. Whether the delay in absorption (particularly with clorazepate) has an undesirable effect in those who only take benzodiazepines during acute episodes of anxiety and who need rapid relief is uncertain. Information about other benzodiazepines is lacking.

References

1 Shader RI, Ciraulo DA, Greenblatt DJ and Harmatz JS. Steady-state plasma desmethyldiazepam during long-term clorazepate use: effect of antacids. Clin Pharmacol Ther (1982) 31, 180–3.
2 Shader RI, Georgotas A, Greenblatt DJ, Harmatz JS and Allen MD. Impaired absorption of desmethyldiazepam from clorazepate by magnesium aluminium hydroxide. Clin Pharmacol Ther (1978) 24, 308–15.
3 Greenblatt DJ, Shader RI, Harmatz JS, Franke K and Koch-Weser J. Influence of magnesium and aluminium hydroxide mixture on chlordiazepoxide absorption. Clin Pharmacol Ther (1976) 19, 234–9.
4 Greenblatt DJ, Allen DA, MacLaughlin DS, Harmatz JS and Shader RI. Diazepam absorption: effect of antacids and food. Clin Pharmacol Ther (1978) 24, 600–9.
5 Abruzzo CW, Macasieb T, Weinfeld R, Rider JA and Kaplan SA. Changes in the oral absorption characteristics in man of dipotassium clorazepate at normal and elevated gastric pH. J Pharmacokinet Biopharm (1977) 5, 377.
6 Chun AHC, Carrigan PJ, Hoffman DJ, Kershner RP and Stuart JD. Effect of antacids on absorption of clorazepate. Clin Pharmacol Ther (1977) 22, 329.

Benzodiazepines + Atropine or Hyoscine

Abstract/Summary

Atropine and hyoscine do not affect the absorption of diazepam nor its sedative effects.

Clinical evidence, mechanism, importance and management

A study in eight normal subjects given single 10 mg oral doses of diazepam showed that serum diazepam levels were not significantly changed by the concurrent use of 1 mg atropine or 1 mg hyoscine, nor were the sedative effects of the diazepam altered.[1]

Reference

1 Gregoretti SM and Uges DRA. Influence of oral atropine or hyoscine on the absorption of oral diazepam. Br J Anaesth (1982) 54, 1231–4.

Benzodiazepines + Beta-blockers

Abstract/Summary

A small and probably clinically insignificant reduction in the metabolism of diazepam occurs if propranolol or metoprolol are taken concurrently, but more importantly there is some suggestion that patients on diazepam may be more accident-prone while taking metoprolol and possibly other beta-blockers.

Clinical evidence, mechanism, importance and management

The clearance from the body of diazepam in man is reduced 8% by propranolol[1] and 18% by metoprolol,[2] but propranolol has no effect on the clearance of alprazolam or lorazepam.[1] Another study found that the AUC (area under the concentration-time curve) of diazepam was increased 25% by metoprolol, but no statistically significant changes were seen with atenolol or propranolol.[6] These pharmacokinetic changes are small and probably clinically unimportant, however studies of psychomotor performance in man show that those taking diazepam and metoprolol have a reduced kinetic visual acuity (KVA).[3] The significance of this is that low KVA scores are associated with fatigue and accident-proneness in professional drivers.[4] Moreover, choice reaction times at 2 h were also found to be lengthened when taking diazepam and metoprolol, propranolol or atenolol, but at 8 h they only persisted with diazepam and metoprolol.[3,5] Information is very limited indeed, but what is known so far suggests that patients who drive and who are given diazepam and metoprolol in particular should be given some warning. There seems to be no information about other benzodiazepines and beta-blockers. More study is needed.

References

1 Ochs HR, Greenblatt DJ and Verburg-Ochs B. Propranolol interactions with diazepam, lorazepam and alprazolam. Clin Pharmacol Ther (1984) 36, 451–5.
2 Klotz U and Reimann IW. Pharmacokinetic and pharmacodynamic interaction study of diazepam and metoprolol. Eur J Clin Pharmacol(1984) 26, 223–6.
3 Betts TA, Crowe A, Knight R, Raffle A, Parson A, Blake A, Hawksworth G and Petrie JC. Is there a clinically relevant interaction between diazepam and lipophilic beta-blocking drugs? Drugs (1983) 25 (Suppl 2) 279–80.
4 Suzumura A. Visual aptitude tests with the use of the KVS tester. Annual Report of the Research Institute of Environmental Medicine, Nagoya Univerisity, Japan (1969) 17, 59–72.
5 Betts TA, Knight R, Crowe A, Blake A, Harvey P and Mortiboy D. Effect of beta-blockers on the psychomotor performance in normal volunteers. Eur J Clin Pharmacol(1985) 28 (Suppl) 39–49.
6 Hawksworth G, Betts T, Crowe A, Knight R, Nyemitei-Addo I, Parry K, Petrie JC, Raffle JC and Parsons A. Diazepam/beta-adrenoceptor antagonist interactions. Br J clin Pharmac (1984) 17, 69–76S.

Benzodiazepines + Calcium channel blockers

Abstract/Summary

Diltiazem appears not to interact with diazepam.

Clinical evidence, mechanism, importance and management

Single 5 mg doses of diazepam and 60 mg diltiazem were given to six subjects. Plasma levels of each drug were not significantly altered by the presence of the other drug.[1] There seems to be no information about other benzodiazepines and calcium channel blockers.

Reference

1 Etoh A and Kohno K. Studies on the drug interaction of diltiazem. IV. Relationship between first pass metabolism of various drugs and the absorption enhancing effect of diltiazem. Yakugaku Zasshi (1983) 103, 581–8.

Benzodiazepines + Cimetidine, Ranitidine, Famotidine, Nizatidine

Abstract/Summary

Serum levels of alprazolam, chlordiazepoxide, clobazam, clorazepate, diazepam, flurazepam, nitrazepam, triazolam (and probably halazepam and prazepam) are raised by cimetidine but normally this appears to be of little or no clinical importance. Only the occasional patient may experience an increase in the effects. Clotiazepam, lorazepam, oxazepam and temazepam are not affected by cimetidine. Famotidine, nizatidine and ranitidine do not interact with the benzodiazepines except possibly with midazolam which some, but not all studies, suggest is also affected by cimetidine.

Clinical evidence

10 patients showed a combined serum level rise of 75% in diazepam and desmethyldiazepam (the active metabolite) after taking 1200 mg cimetidine daily for a fortnight, but reaction times and other motor and intellectual tests remained unaffected.[1]

Other reports also describe a rise in the serum levels of diazepam[2–4] (associated with increased sedation in one report[19]). Generalized incoordination has also been described in one individual.[22] Rises in serum levels occur with other benzodiazepines: alprazolam,[9,10] chlordiazepoxide,[11] clobazam,[24] clorazepate,[12] flurazepam,[7] nitrazepam,[13] and triazolam.[9,10] Prolonged hypnosis in an elderly woman[21] and CNS toxicity[20] in a woman of 49 have been attributed to a triazolam–cimetidine interaction but this remains unconfirmed. In contrast cimetidine does not interact with lorazepam,[7] oxazepam[7] or temazepam.[8] Ranitidine,[5] nizatidine[26] and famotidine[6] do not interact significantly with diazepam[5,26] nor ranitidine with temazepam.[23] There is some controversy about whether midazolam is or is not affected by cimetidine and ranitidine.[16,17,23,25]

Mechanism

Cimetidine inhibits the liver enzymes concerned with the metabolism (by N-dealkylation plus oxidation or nitro-reduction) of diazepam, alprazolam, chlordiazepoxide, clorazepate, flurazepam, nitrazepam and triazolam. As a result their clearance from the body is reduced and their serum levels rise. However the metabolism of clobazam and clotiazepam seems to be unaffected.[14,15] Lorazepam,[7] oxazepam[7] and temazepam[8] are metabolized by a different metabolic pathway involving glucuronidation which is not affected by cimetidine. Ranitidine, famotidine and nizatidine appear not to inhibit liver microsomal enzymes.

Importance and management

The benzodiazepine–cimetidine interactions are very well documented (not all the references are listed here) but normally they appear to be of little clinical importance, although very occasionally a patient may be adversely affected (increased effects, drowsiness, etc.). Reports of problems are very few indeed, particularly when viewed against the very common use of both drugs. Lorazepam, oxazepam and temazepam are non-interacting alternative benzodiazepines. Ranitidine does not interact with diazepam or temazepam, and neither nizatidine, ranitidine nor famotidine would be expected to interact with other benzodiazepines which are metabolized similarly (see 'Mechanism' above). Midazolam may possibly be an exception: it is claimed that serum levels and sedation are increased by ranitidine and cimetidine[17,25] whereas other reports claim that neither ranitidine nor cimetidine interact.[16,23]

References

1 Greenblatt DJ, Abernethy DR, Morse DS, Harmatz JS and Shader RI. Clinical importance of the interaction of diazepam and cimetidine. Anesth Analg (1986) 65, 176–80.

2 McGowan WAW and Dundee JW. The effect of intravenous cimetidine on the absorption of orally administered diazepam and lorazepam. Br J clin Pharmacol(1982) 14, 207–11.

3 Klotz U and Reimann I. Elevation of steady-state diazepam levels by cimetidine. Clin Pharmacol Ther (1981) 30, 513–7.

4 Gough PA, Curry SH, Aranjo OE, Robinson JD and Dallman JJ. Influence of cimetidine on oral diazepam elimination with measurement of subsequent cognitive change. Br J clin Pharmacol(1982) 14, 739–42.

5 Klotz U, Reimann IW and Ohnhaus EE. Effect of ranitidine on the steady state pharmacokinetics of diazepam. Eur J Clin Pharmacol(1983) 24, 357–60.

6 Locniskar A, Greenblatt DJ, Harmatz JS and Zinny MA. Influence of famotidine and cimetidine on the pharmacokinetic properties of intravenous diazepam. J Clin Pharmacol(1985) 25, 459–50.

7 Greenblatt DJ, Abernethy DR, Koepke HH and Shader RI. Interaction of cimetidine with oxazepam, lorazepam and flurazepam. J Clin Pharmacol(1984) 24, 187–93.

8 Greenblatt DJ, Abernethy DR, Divoll M, Locniskar A, Harmatz JS and Shader RI. Non-interaction of temazepam and cimetidine. J Pharm Sci (1984) 73, 399–401.

9 Pourbaix S, Desager JP, Hulhoven R, Smith RB and Harvengt C. Pharmacokinetic consequences of long-term co-administration of cimetidine and triazolobenzodiazepines, alprazolam and triazolam in healthy subjects. Int J Clin Pharmacol Ther Toxicol (1985) 23, 447–51.

10 Abernethy DR, Greenblatt DJ, Divoll M, Moschitto LJ, Harmatz JS and Shader RI. Interaction of cimetidine with the triazolobenzodiazepines alprazolam and triazolam. Psychopharmacol (1983) 80, 275–8.

11 Desmond PV, Patwardhan RV, Schneker S and Speeg KV. Cimetidine impairs elimination of chlordiazepoxide (Librium) in man. Ann InternMed (1980) 93, 266–8.

12 Divoll M, Abernethy DR and Greenblatt DJ. Cimetidine impairs oxidising capacity in the elderly. Clin Pharmacol Ther (1982) 31, 218.

13 Ochs HR, Greenblatt DJ, Gugler R, Muntefering G, Locniskar A and Abernethy DR. Cimetidine impairs nitrazepam clearance. Clin Pharmacol Ther (1983) 34, 227–30.

14 Grigoleit H-G, Hajdu P, Hundt HK L, Koeppen D, Malerczyk BH, Muller FO and Witte PU. Pharmacokinetic aspects of the interaction between clobazam and cimetidine. Eur J Clin Pharmacol(1983) 25, 139–42.

15 Ochs HR, Greenblatt DJ, Verburg-Ochs B, Harmatz JS and Grehl H. Disposition of clotiazepam: influence of age, sex, oral contraceptives, cimetidine, isoniazid and ethanol. Eur J Clin Pharmacol(1984) 26, 55–9.

16 Greenblatt DJ, Locniskar A, Scavone JM, Blyden GT, Ochs HR, Harmatz JS and Shader RI. Absence of interaction of cimetidine and ranitidine with intravenous and oral midazolam. Anesth Analg (1986) 65, 176–80.

17 Ellwood RJ, Hildebrand PJ, Dundee JW and Collier PS. Ranitidine influences the uptake of oral midazolam. Br J Clin Pharmacol(1983) 15, 743–5.

18 Klotz U and Antilla V-J. Drug interactions with cimetidine: pharmacokinetic studies to evaluate its mechanism. Naunyn-Schmied Arch Pharmacol(1980) 311, R77.

19 Klotz U and Reimann I. Delayed clearance of diazepam due to cimetidine. N Engl J Med (1980) 302, 1012–13.

20 Britton ML and Waller ES. Central nervous system toxicity associated with concurrent use of triazolam and cimetidine. Drug Intell Clin Pharm (1985) 19, 666–8.

21 Parker WA and MacLachlan RA. Prolonged hypnotic response to triazolam-cimetidine combination in an elderly patient. Drug Intell Clin Pharm (1984) 18, 980–1.

22 Anon. Court warns on interaction of drugs. Doctor (1979) 9, 1.

23 Dundee JW, Wilson CM, Robinson FP, Thompson EM and Elliott P. The effect of ranitidine on the hypnotic action of single doses of midazolam, temazepam and zopiclone. Br J clin Pharmac (1984) 20, 553P.

24 Pullar T, Edwards D, Haigh JRM, Peaker S and Feeley MP. The effect of cimetidine on the single dose pharmacokinetics of oral clobazam and N-desmethylclobazam. Br J clin Pharmac (1987) 23, 317–21.

25 Fee JPH, Collier PS, Howard PJ and Dundee JW. Cimetidine and ranitidine increase midazolam bioavailability. Clin Pharmacol Ther (1987) 41, 80–4.

26 Klotz U, Gottlieb W, Keohance PP and Dammann HG. Nocturnal doses of ranitidine and nizatidine do not affect the disposition of diazepam. J Clin Pharmacol(1987) 27, 210–12.

Benzodiazepines + Contraceptives, oral

Abstract/Summary

Pharmacokinetic studies indicate that the oral contraceptives can increase the effects of alprazolam, chlordiazepoxide, diazepam, nitrazepam and triazolam, and reduce the effects of oxazepam, lorazepam and temazepam, but whether in practice there is a need for dosage adjustments has not been determined.

Clinical evidence

(a) Alprazolam, chlordiazepoxide, clotiazepam, diazepam, nitrazepam, triazolam + oral contraceptives

A controlled study in six women showed that the mean half-life of chlordiazepoxide (0.6 mg/kg IV) was virtually doubled while taking oral contraceptives (from 11.6 to 20.6 h) and the total clearance fell by almost two-thirds (from 33.2 to 13.4 ml/min).[1]

Similar but less marked effects were found in other studies with chlordiazepoxide,[2] diazepam,[3,4] alprazolam[8] and to an even lesser extent with triazolam[8] and nitrazepam.[5] No changes were seen with clotiazepam.[7]

(b) Lorazepam, oxazepam, temazepam + oral contraceptives

A controlled study in seven women showed that the mean half-life of lorazepam (2 mg IV) was more than halved while taking oral contraceptives (from 14 to 6 h) and the total clearance increased by a factor of three (from 77.4 to 288.9 ml/min).[1]

A smaller change was seen in other controlled studies with lorazepam,[6,8] and temazepam,[8] and in two other studies both marked[1] and small[6] falls in the half-life of oxazepam of the same order were observed.

Mechanism

Oral contraceptives affect the metabolism of the benzodiazepines by the liver in different ways: oxidative metabolism is reduced (alprazolam, chlordiazepoxide, diazepam, etc.), whereas metabolism by glucuronide conjugation is increased (lorazepam, oxazepam, temazepam, etc.).

Importance and management

Established interactions, but their clinical importance is uncertain. Long-term treatment with benzodiazepines which are highly oxidized (alprazolam, chlordiazepoxide, diazepam, nitrazepam, etc.) in women on the pill should be monitored to ensure that the dosage is not too high. Those taking glucuronidated benzodiazepines (lorazepam, oxazepam, temazepam, etc.) may need a dosage increase. Clotiazepam appears not to interact. Extensive study is needed to determine whether any these interactions is of real importance. No firm conclusions could be drawn from the results of a study which set out to evaluate the importance of this interaction.[9]

References

1 Patwardhan RV, Mitchell MC, Johnson RF and Schenker S. Differential effects of oral contraceptive steroids on the metabolism of benzodiazepines. Hepatology (1983) 3, 248–53.
2 Roberts RK, Desmond PV, Wilkinson GR and Schenker S. Disposition of chlordiazepoxide: sex differences and effects of oral contraceptives. Clin Pharmacol Ther (1979) 25, 826–31.
3 Giles HG, Sellers EM, Naranjo CA, Frecker RC and Greenblatt DJ. Disposition of intravenous diazepam in young men and women. Europ J Clin Pharmacol(1981) 20, 207–13.
4 Abernethy DR, Greenblatt DJ, Divoll M, Arendt R, Ochs HR and Shader RI. Impairment of diazepam metabolism by low-dose estrogen-containing oral contraceptive steroids. N Engl J Med (1982) 306, 791–2.
5 Jochemsen R, Van der Graff M, Boejinga JK and Breimer DD. Influence of sex, menstrual cycles and oral contraception on the disposition of nitrazepam. Br J Clin Pharmacol(1982) 13, 319–24.
6 Abernethy DR, Greenblatt DJ, Ochs HR, Weyers D, Divoll M, Harmatz JS and Shader RI. Lorazepam and oxazepam kinetics in women on low-dose oral contraceptives. Clin Pharmacol Ther (1983) 33, 628–32.
7 Ochs HR, Greenblatt DJ, Verburg-Ochs B, Harmatz JS and Grehl H. Disposition of clotiazepam: influence of age, sex, oral contraceptives, cimetidine, isoniazid and ethanol. Eur J Clin Pharmacol(1984) 26, 55–9.
8 Stoeh GP, Kroboth PD, Juhl RP, Wender DB, Phillips P and Smith RB. Effect of oral contraceptives on triazolam, temazepam, alprazolam and lorazepam kinetics. Clin Pharmacol Ther (1984) 36, 683–90.
9 Kroboth PD, Smith RB, Stoeh GP and Juhl R. Pharmacodynamic evaluation of the benzodiazepine-oral contraceptive interaction. Clin Pharmacol Ther (1985) 38, 525–32.

Benzodiazepines + Dextropropoxyphene

Abstract/Summary

Some evidence suggests that the combined CNS depressant effects of alprazolam and dextropropoxyphene may be greater than with other benzodiazepines because the serum levels of alprazolam may be increased.

Clinical evidence, mechanism, importance and management

A study in 14 normal subjects showed that while taking 65 mg dextropropoxyphene six-hourly the pharmacokinetics of single doses of diazepam and lorazepam were not significantly changed, but the half-life of alprazolam was prolonged from 11.6 to 18.3 h, and its clearance fell from 1.3 to

0.8 ml/min/kg.[1] It would seem that dextropropoxyphene inhibits the metabolism (hydroxylation) of the alprazolam by the liver, thereby reducing its loss from the body, but has little or no effect on the N-demethylation or glucuronidation of the other two benzodiazepines. The clinical importance of this is uncertain, but the inference to be drawn is that the CNS depressant effects of alprazolam will be increased, over and above the simple additive CNS depressant effects likely when other benzodiazepines and dextropropoxyphene are taken together. More study is needed.

Reference

1 Abernethy DR, Greenblatt DJ, Morse DS and Shader RI. Interaction of propoxyphene with diazepam, alprazolam and lorazepam. Br J clin Pharmac (1985) 19, 51–7.

Benzodiazepines + Disulfiram

Abstract/Summary

The serum levels of chlordiazepoxide and diazepam are increased by the use of disulfiram and some patients may possibly experience increased drowsiness. Oxazepam and lorazepam are only minimally affected.

Clinical evidence

After taking 0.5 g disulfiram daily for 14–16 days, the plasma clearances of single doses of chlordiazepoxide and diazepam were reduced by 54 and 41% respectively in alcoholic and normal subjects. The half-lives were increased by 84 and 37% respectively. Serum levels of chlordiazepoxide were approximately doubled. Changes in the pharmacokinetic parameters of oxazepam were minimal.[1]

Another paper by the same workers shows that lorazepam behaves like oxazepam.[2]

Mechanism

Disulfiram inhibits the initial metabolism (N-demethylation and oxidation) of both chlordiazepoxide and diazepam by the liver so that an alternative but slower metabolic pathway is used which results in the accumulation of these benzodiazepines in the body. In contrast, the metabolism (glucuronidation) of oxazepam and lorazepam is minimally affected by disulfiram so that their clearance from the body remains largely unaffected.[1,2]

Importance and management

An established interaction, but the clinical effects are uncertain. Single dose studies are not necessarily reliable predictors of what happens in practice, however it seems probable that some patients will experience increased drowsiness (a) because of this interaction, and (b) because drowsiness is a very common side-effect of disulfiram. Reduce the dosage of the benzodiazepine if necessary. Other benzodiazepines which are metabolized similarly may possibly interact in the same way (clorazepate, prazepam, ketazolam, clobazam, alprazolam, flurazepam, nitrazepam, medazepam, bromazepam, clonazepam, triazolam) but this needs confirmation. Oxazepam and lorazepam appear to be non-interacting alternatives (and possibly temazepam which is also metabolized by glucuronidation).

References

1 MacLoed SM, Sellers EM, Giles HG, Billings BJ, Martin PR, Greenblatt DJ and Marshman JA. Interaction of disulfiram with benzodiazepines. Clin Pharmacol Ther (1978) 24, 583–9.
2 Sellers EM, Giles HG, Greenblatt DJ and Naranjo CA. Differential effects on benzodiazepine disposition by disulfiram and ethanol. Arzneim-Forsch/Drug Res (1980) 30, 882–6.

Benzodiazepines + Ethambutol

Abstract/Summary

Ethambutol appears not to interact with diazepam.

Clinical evidence, mechanism, importance and management

A study on six patients, newly diagnosed as having tuberculosis and treated with ethambutol (25 mg/kg), showed that although some of the pharmacokinetic parameters of diazepam were altered, the changes were not significant.[1] There seems to be nothing in the literature to suggest that ethambutol interacts with other benzodiazepines.

Reference

1 Ochs HR, Greenblatt DJ, Roberts GM and Dengler HJ. Diazepam interaction with antituberculous drugs. Clin Pharmacol Ther (1981) 29, 671.

Benzodiazepines + Indomethacin

Abstract/Summary

Diazepam and indomethacin do not appear to interact adversely, but the feeling of dizziness may be increased.

Clinical evidence, mechanism, importance and management

A study in 119 healthy medical students showed that 10–15 mg diazepam impaired the performance of a number of psychomotor tests (digit symbol substitution, letter cancellation, tracking and flicker fusion). It also caused subjective drowsiness, mental slowness and clumsiness but when 50 or 100 mg indomethacin were given as well, the effects were little different from diazepam alone except that the feeling of dizziness (common to both drugs) was increased.[1]

Reference

1 Nuotto E and Saarialho-Kere U. Actions and interactions of indomethacin and diazepam on performance in healthy volunteers. PharmacolToxicol (1988) 62, 293–7.

Benzodiazepines + Isoniazid

Abstract/Summary

Isoniazid reduces the loss of both diazepam and triazolam from the body. Some increase in their effects would be expected. No interaction occurs with oxazepam or clotiazepam.

Clinical evidence

(a) Diazepam and triazolam

A study in nine normal subjects showed that after three day's treatment with 180 mg isoniazid daily, the half-life of a single dose of diazepam was increased from 34 to 45 h, and the total clearance reduced from 0.54 to 0.40 ml/min.[1] A study in six normal subjects showed that after taking 180 mg isoniazid daily for three days, the half-life of a single dose of triazolam was increased from 2.5 to 3.3 h, the AUC was increased from 26.5 to 38.6 ml^{-1}/h and the clearance was reduced from 6.8 to 3.9 ml/min/kg.[2]

(b) Oxazepam and clotiazepam

A study in nine normal subjects showed that 180 mg isoniazid daily for three days had no effect on the pharmacokinetics of a single 30 mg oral dose of oxazepam.[2] Similarly the pharmacokinetics of clotiazepam were not altered in another study of the effects of isoniazid.[3]

Mechanism

What is known suggests that the isoniazid acts as an enzyme inhibitor, decreasing the metabolism and loss of diazepam and triazolam from the body, thereby increasing and prolonging their effects.

Importance and management

Information is limited but the interactions appear to be established. Their clinical importance is uncertain but be alert for the need to decrease the dosages of diazepam and triazolam if isoniazid is started. There seems to be no direct information about other benzodiazepines, but those undergoing high first-pass extraction and/or liver microsomal metabolism would be expected to interact similarly. Oxazepam and clotiazepam appear not to interact.

References

1 Ochs HR, Greenblatt DJ, Roberts GM and Dengler HJ. Diazepam interaction with antituberculous drugs. Clin Pharmacol Ther (1981) 29, 671.
2 Ochs HR, Greenblatt DJ and Knuchel M. Differential effect of isoniazid on triazolam and oxazepam conjugation. Br J clin Pharmac (1983) 16, 743–46.

3 Ochs HR, Greenblatt DJ, Verburg-Ochs B, Harmatz JS and Grehl H. Disposition of clotiazepam: influence of age, sex, oral contraceptives, cimetidine, isoniazid and ethanol. Eur J Clin Pharmacol(1984) 26, 55–59.

Benzodiazepines + Ketoconazole

Abstract/Summary

Ketoconazole reduces the loss of chlordiazepoxide from the body, but the clinical effects of this seem unlikely to be of great importance.

Clinical evidence, mechanism, importance and management

A study in 12 normal subjects showed that after taking 400 mg ketoconazole daily for five days the clearance of chlordiazepoxide (0.6 mg/kg) was decreased by 38%.[1] It seems unlikely that this will have a marked effect on the treatment of patients, but this needs confirmation. The effects of ketoconazole on other benzodiazepines seems not to have been studied.

Reference

1 Brown MW, Maldonado AL, Meredith CG and Speeg KV. Effect of ketoconazole on hepatic oxidative drug metabolism. Clin Pharmacol Ther (1985) 37, 290–7.

Benzodiazepines + Macrolide antibiotics

Abstract/Summary

Serum levels of triazolam are considerably increased by the concurrent use of erythromycin and triacetyloleandomycin and a marked increase in its effects may occur. The same interaction has been seen in a patient given josamycin. A triazolam dosage reduction may be needed.

Clinical evidence

A study in 16 normal subjects showed that after taking 333 mg erythromycin daily for three days, the clearance of a single 0.5 mg dose of triazolam was reduced by about 50%, the AUC (area under the time-concentration curve) was increased by 106% (from 20.1 to 41.4 ng h/ml) and the maximum serum levels were increased by about one-third (from 2.8 to 4.1 ng/ml)[1]

A study in seven normal subjects showed that after taking 2 g triacetyloleandomycin daily for seven days the peak concentration of triazolam after taking 0.25 mg triazolam was increased by 107%, the AUC between 0 and 8 h was increased by 275%, the half-life was increased from 1.81 to 6.48 h and the apparent oral clearance was reduced by 74%. Marked psychomotor impairment and amnesia was seen.[3] Josamycin and triacetyloleandomycin have been reported to interact similarly in two patients on triazolam, causing an increase in its effects.[2]

Mechanism

The most probable explanation is that these macrolide antibiotics reduce the 'first pass' metabolism of the triazolam by the liver, thereby reducing its loss from the body and raising its serum levels.

Importance and management

Information is limited but the triazolam–erythromycin and triacetyloleandomycin interactions appear to be established. Monitor the effects and anticipate the need to reduce the dosage of the triazolam to avoid excessive effects (drowsiness, memory loss). Some patients are affected much more than others. Much less is known about josamycin but the same precautions should be taken.

References

1 Phillips JP, Antal EJ and Smith RB. A pharmacokinetic interaction between erythromycin and triazolam. J Clin Psychopharmacol (1986) 6, 297–9.
2 Carry PV, Ducluzeau R, Jourdan C, Bourrat C, Vigneou C and Descotes J. De nouvelles interactions avec les macrolides? Lyon Med (1982) 248, 189–90.
3 Warot D, Bergougnan L, Lamiable D, Berlin I, Bensimon G, Danjou P and Puch AJ. Troleandomycin-triazolam interaction in healthy volunteers: pharmacokinetic and psychometric evaluation. Eur J Clin Pharmacol(1987) 32, 389–93.

Benzodiazepines + Metronidazole

Abstract/Summary

Metronidazole does not interact with alprazolam, diazepam or lorazepam.

Clinical evidence, mechanism, importance and management

One study in normal subjects found that 750 mg metronidazole (for an unstated time) had no effect on the pharmacokinetics of lorazepam or alprazolam.[1] Another study found that 800 mg metronidazole daily for five days also had no effect on the pharmacokinetics of a single 0.1 mg/kg intravenous dose of diazepam.[2] Interactions with other benzodiazepines seem unlikely.

References

1 Blyden GT, Greenblatt DJ and Scavone JM. Metronidazole impairs clearance of phenytoin but not of alprazolam or lorazepam. Clin Pharmacol Ther (1986) 39, 181.
2 Jensen JC and Gugler R. Interaction between metronidazole and drugs eliminated by oxidative metabolism. Clin Pharmacol Ther (1985) 37, 407–10.

Benzodiazepines + Omeprazole

Abstract/Summary

Omeprazole can halve the clearance of diazepam from the body. Increased diazepam sedation seems a possibility.

Clinical evidence, mechanism, importance and management

A study in eight normal subjects showed that after taking 40 mg omeprazole daily for a week, the clearance of a single dose of diazepam (0.1 mg/kg IV) was reduced by 54%, due, it is suggested, to inhibition of the liver enzymes concerned with the metabolism of the diazepam.[1] The clinical significance of this is uncertain, but it seems possible that the sedative effects of diazepam during long-term use might be increased. More study is needed.

Reference

1 Gugler R and Jensen JC. Omeprazole inhibits elimination of diazepam. Lancet (1984) i, 1969.

Benzodiazepines + Probenecid

Abstract/Summary

Probenecid markedly reduces the loss of lorazepam from the body. An increase in its sedative effects would be expected.

Clinical evidence, mechanism, importance and management

A study in nine normal subjects showed that while taking 500 mg probenecid six-hourly the clearance of a single 2 mg IV dose of lorazepam was approximately halved (from 80.3 to 44 ml/min) and the elimination half-life was more than doubled (from 14.3 to 33 h). The reason is thought to be that the probenecid inhibits drug clearance by the kidney tubules and also inhibits the metabolism (glucuronidation) of the lorazepam by the liver, the result being that the loss from the body is markedly reduced.[1] The clinical importance of this has not been assessed, but be alert for evidence of an increase in both the therapeutic and toxic effects (sedation, antegrade amnesia). Reduce the dosage as necessary. There seems to be no direct information about other benzodiazepines but those which are metabolized like lorazepam (oxazepam, temazepam) are possible candidates for this interaction. More study is needed.

Reference

1 Abernethy DR, Greenblatt DJ, Ameer B and Shader RI. Probenecid impairment of acetaminophen and lorazepam clearance: direct inhibition of ether glucuronide formation. J PharmacolExp Ther (1985) 234, 345–9.

Benzodiazepines + Rifampicin (Rifampin)

Abstract/Summary

Rifampicin causes a marked increase in the loss of diazepam from the body.

Clinical evidence

A study in seven patients with TB being treated with daily doses of isoniazid (0.5–2.2 g), rifampicin (450–600 mg) and ethambutol (25 mg/kg) showed that the mean half-life of diazepam was reduced to less than a third (from 58 to 14 h) and the clearance increased by more than 300%.[1]

Mechanism

Ethambutol does not interact with diazepam,[1] and isoniazid increases its effects by inhibiting liver microsomal enzymes,[1] so that the increased loss of diazepam is therefore almost certainly due to the rifampicin. It is known to be a potent liver enzyme inducing agent which increases the metabolism (e.g. hydroxylation) of many drugs by the liver, thereby hastening their loss from the body. The effects of the rifampicin clearly dominate the enzyme-inhibiting effects of the isoniazid.

Importance and management

The documentation seems to be limited to this study[1] but it is consistent with the way rifampicin interacts with many other drugs. The clinical importance has not been assessed but it seems likely that the diazepam dosage will need to be raised. Monitor the outcome of concurrent use and alter the dosage accordingly. There seems to be no direct information about other benzodiazepines but if the mechanism suggested for diazepam is true, then those metabolized in a similar way (e.g. chlordiazepoxide, flurazepam) may possibly interact similarly, whereas those which undergo glucuronidation (e.g. lorazepam, oxazepam, temazepam) possibly do not. This needs confirmation. Ethambutol is a non-interacting alternative.

Reference

1 Ochs HR, Greenblatt DJ, Roberts G-M and Dengler HJ. Diazepam interaction with antituberculous drugs. Clin Pharmacol Ther (1981) 29, 671–8.

Benzodiazepines + Theophylline and Caffeine

Abstract/Summary

Aminophylline can be used to antagonize the anaesthesia induced by diazepam or lorazepam, but possibly not midazolam. Caffeine, and to a lesser extent theophylline, may reduce the sedative (and possibly also the anxiolytic) effects of diazepam.

Clinical evidence, mechanism, importance and management

A patient who was unarousable and unresponsive following anaesthesia with diazepam (60 mg over 10 min) and N_2O/O_2 (60%/40%), rapidly returned to consciousness when given 56 mg aminophylline intravenously.[1] Other reports confirm this antagonism by low doses of aminophylline (60 mg IV) of the anaesthesia induced by diazepam[2] or lorazepam,[3] but there is some uncertainty whether it antagonizes midazolam anaesthesia/sedation or not.[4,5] No such interaction occurs if aminophylline is replaced by enprofylline.[2] Caffeine, and to a lesser extent theophylline, counteract the drowsiness and mental slowness induced by diazepam in anxiolytic doses (10–20 mg).[6–9] This may be because they block adenosine receptors.

The aminophylline/benzodiazepine interaction can therefore be used with advantage if reversal of anaesthesia with some benzodiazepines is required. The extent to which theophylline or caffeine (in strong coffee or tea) might reduce the anxiolytic effects of diazepam and other benzodiazepines is uncertain, but it should be borne in mind. Enprofylline might be useful when an antiasthmatic is needed in combination with a benzodiazepine.

References

1 Stirt JA. Aminophylline is a diazepam antagonist. Anesth Analg (1981) 60, 767–8.
2 Nieman D, Martinell S, Arvidsson S, Svedmyr N and Ekstrom-Jodal B. Aminophylline inhibition of diazepam sedation: is adenosine blockade of GABA-receptors the mechanism? Lancet (1984) i, 462–3.
3 Wnagler MA and Kilpatrick DS. Aminophylline is an antagonist of lorazepam. Anesth Analg (1985) 64, 834–6.
4 Kanto J, Aaltonen L, Himberg J-J and Hovi-Viander M. Midazolam as an intravenous induction agent in the elderly: a clinical and pharmacokinetic study. Anesth Analg (1986) 65, 15–20.
5 Sleigh JW. Failure of aminophylline to antagonize midazolam sedation. Anesth Analg (1986) 65, 540.
6 Mattila MJ and Nuotto E. Caffeine and theophylline counteract diazepam effects in man. Med Biol (1983) 61, 337–43.
7 Mattila MJ, Palva E and Savolainen K. Caffeine antagonizes diazepam effects in man. Med Biol (1982) 60, 121–3.
8 Henauer SA, Hollister LE, Gillespie HK and Moore F. Theophylline antagonizes diazepam-induced psychomotor impairment. Eur J Clin Pharmacol (1983) 25, 743–7.
9 Meyer BH, Weis OF and Muller FO. Antagonism of diazepam by aminophylline in healthy volunteers. Anesth Analg (1984) 63, 900–2.

Benzodiazepines + Tobacco smoking

Abstract/Summary

Smokers may need larger doses of the benzodiazepines than non-smokers.

Clinical evidence, mechanism, importance and management

Early studies suggested that smoking did not affect the pharmacokinetics of diazepam[1] or chlordiazepoxide,[2] but a later study found that the clearance of diazepam from the body was increased in smokers.[3] This confirmed the findings of The Boston Collaborative Drug Surveillance Program of a decreased frequency of drowsiness in those on diazepam or chlordiazepoxide who smoked.[4] Smoking has also been found to increase the clearance of alprazolam,[5] lorazepam,[8] oxazepam[6] and clorazepate.[7] The probable reason is that some of the components of tobacco smoke act as enzyme-inducing agents which increase the rate at which the liver metabolizes these benzodiazepines. The inference to be drawn is that smokers may need larger doses than non-smokers to achieve the same therapeutic effects.

References

1 Klotz U, Avant GR, Hoyumpa A, Schenker S and Wilkinson GR. The effects of age and liver disease on the disposition and elimination of diazepam in adult man. J Clin Invest (1975) 55, 347–9.
2 Desmond PV, Roberts RK, Wilkinson GR and Schenker S. No effect of smoking on the metabolism of chlordiazepoxide. N Engl J Med (1979) 300, 199–200.
3 Greenblatt DJ, Allen MD, Harmatz JS and Shader RI. Diazepam disposition determinants. Clin Pharmacol Ther (1980) 27, 301–12.
4 Boston Collaborative Drug Surveillance Program. Clinical depression of the central nervous system due to diazepam and chlordiazepoxide in relation to cigarette smoking and age. N Engl J Med (1973) 288, 277–80.
5 Smith RB, Gwilt PR and Wright CE. Single- and multiple dose pharmacokinetics of oral alprazolam in healthy smoking and non-smoking men. Clin Pharm (1983) 2, 139–43.
6 Greenblatt DJ, Divoll M, Harmatz JS and Shader RI. Oxazepam kinetics: effects of age and sex. J Pharmacol Exp Ther (1980) 215, 86–91.
7 Norman TR, Fulton A, Burrows GD and Maguire KP. Pharmacokinetics of N-desmethyldiazepam after a single oral dose of clorazepate: the effect of smoking. Eur J Clin Pharmacol (1981) 21, 229–33.
8 Greenblatt DJ, Allen MD, Locniskar A, Harmatz JS and Shader RI. Lorazepam kinetics in the elderly. Clin Pharmacol Ther (1979) 26, 103–13.

Buspirone + Cimetidine

Abstract/Summary

Buspirone and cimetidine appear not to interact.

Clinical evidence, mechanism, importance and management

A study in 10 normal subjects found that cimetidine (1 g daily for seven days) had no effect on serum buspirone levels nor on its excretion while taking 45 mg buspirone daily. Some small pharmacokinetic changes were seen, but the performance of three psychomotor function tests remained unaltered and it was concluded that a clinically significant interaction is unlikely.[1]

Reference

1 Gammans RE, Pfeffer M, Wetrick ML, Faulkner HC, Rehm KD and Goodson PJ. Lack of interaction between cimetidine and buspirone. Pharmacotherapy (1987) 7, 72–9.

Buspirone + Fluoxetine

Abstract/Summary

A single case report describes a reduction in the anxiolytic effects of buspirone when fluoxetine was given.

Clinical evidence, mechanism, importance and management

A 35-year-old man with a long history of depression, anxiety and panic was started on 60 mg buspirone daily. His anxiety abated, but worsening depression prompted additional treatment with 200 mg trazodone daily for three weeks which had little effect. He was then additionally given 20 mg fluoxetine daily for persistent dysphoria, but within 48 h his usual symptoms of anxiety had returned and persisted even when the dose was raised to 80 mg daily. Stopping the buspirone did not increase his anxiety.[1] The reasons for this reaction are not understood. Monitor the effects if these drugs are given concurrently. More study is needed.

Reference

1   Bodkin JA and Teicher MH. Fluoxetine may antagonize the anxiolytic action of buspirone. J Clin Psychopharmacol (1989) 9, 150.

Droperidol/Hyoscine + Monoamine oxidase inhibitors (MAOI)

Abstract/Summary

An isolated and unexplained report describes hypotension in a patient given droperidol and hyoscine as premedication, shortly after the withdrawal of phenelzine and perphenazine.

Clinical evidence, mechanism, importance and management

Four days after the withdrawal of phenelzine and perphenazine, a patient was given operative premedication with 20 mg droperidol and 0.4 mg hyoscine. About 2 h later he was observed to be pale, sweating profusely, slightly cyanosed, with a blood pressure of 75/60 mm Hg and a pulse rate of 60. No excitement or changes in respiration were seen. The blood pressure gradually rose to 115/80 mm Hg over the next 45 min, but did not return to normal (160/100 mm Hg) for 36 h. 11 days later, using the same premedication, the operation was successfully undertaken without any hypotensive episodes.[1] The response was attributed to the after-effects of phenelzine treatment, but there is no obvious explanation for this interaction (if indeed it is an interaction).

Reference

1   Penlington GN. Droperidol and monoamine oxidase inhibitors. Br Med J (1966) 1, 483.

Haloperidol + Antituberculars

Abstract/Summary

The serum levels of haloperidol can be reduced by the concurrent use of rifampicin (rifampin).

Clinical evidence, mechanism, importance and management

A study in 18 schizophrenic patients on haloperidol, some of whom were also being treated with a range of antitubercular drugs (ethambutol, isoniazid, rifampicin), showed that those on rifampicin had significantly reduced haloperidol serum levels. The half-life of haloperidol in two patients on rifampicin was 4.8 h compared with 9.4 h in three other patients not taking rifampicin. A likely explanation is that the rifampicin, a recognized enzyme inducing agent, increases the metabolism and loss of the haloperidol from the body. Three of the patients on isoniazid had increased serum haloperidol levels.[1] Information about this interaction is very limited but there is now enough evidence to suggest that the effects of concurrent use should be well monitored. Be alert for any evidence of reduced haloperidol effects. Increase the dosage if necessary. More study is needed.

Reference

1   Takeda M, Nishimura K, Yamasthita S, Matsubayashi T, Tamino S and Nishimura T. Serum haloperidol levels of schizophrenics receiving treatment for tuberculosis. Clin Neuropharmacol (1986) 9, 386.

Haloperidol + Carbamazepine

Abstract/Summary

Serum levels of haloperidol can be more than halved by the concurrent use of carbamazepine. Three reports describe neurotoxicity during concurrent use.

Clinical evidence

(a) Haloperidol serum levels reduced

A cross-over study in nine chronic schizophrenic patients, taking an average of 30 mg haloperidol daily, showed that when they were concurrently treated with carbamazepine (precise dose not stated, but said to be 5–6 tablets daily) over a period of five weeks, their haloperidol serum levels were reduced by 55% (from an average of 45.4 to 21.2 ng/ml). They were also given 10 mg benzhexol daily and 30 mg oxazepam at night whenever necessary. No changes in the serum levels of carbamazepine were seen, nor was the control of the disease changed.[1]

Two other studies similarly showed falls of about 60% in serum haloperidol levels while taking carbamazepine.[2,5] Marked clinical worsening was seen in one of these studies.[5]

(b) Neurotoxicity

A report describes delerium (lethargy, slurred speech, decreased concentration and inattention) in a woman following the replacement of her treatment with thioridazine by haloperidol (15 mg daily) and carbamazepine (400 mg daily). The delerium disappeared within 12 h of withdrawing the medication.[4]

Two other cases of neurotoxicity (drowsiness, slurred speech) during concurrent use have been described.[6,7]

Mechanism

Uncertain. (a) One suggestion is that the carbamazepine may induce the liver enzymes concerned with the metabolism of haloperidol so that it is cleared from the body more quickly.[1,2] (b) The neurotoxicity is not understood.

Importance and management

This combination is not uncommon. One study has shown that there are advantages in adding carbamazepine to haloperidol in treating manic patients, schizoaffective excited patients and others with excited psychoses and schizophrenia.[3] However the studies cited here indicate that concurrent use should be well monitored for any signs of reduced haloperidol effects.

Also be alert for any signs of neurotoxicity.

References

1 Jann MW, Ereshefsky L, Saklad SR, Seidel DR, Davis CM, Burch NR and Bowden CL. Effects of carbamazepine on plasma haloperidol levels. J Clin Psychopharmacol (1985) 5, 106–9.

2 Kidron R, Averbuch I, Klein E and Belmaker RH. Carbamazepine-induced reduction of blood levels of haloperidol in chronic schizophrenics. Biol Psychiatry (1985) 20, 219–22.

3 Klein E, Bental E, Lerer B and Belmaker RH. Combination of carbamazepine and haloperidol versus placebo and haloperidol in excited psychoses: a controlled study. Arch Gen Psychiatry (1984) 41, 165–70.

4 Kanter GL, Yerevanian BI and Ciccone JR. Case report of a possible interaction between neuroleptics and carbamazepine. Am J Psychiatry (1984) 141, 1101–2.

5 Arana GW, Goff DC, Friedman H, Ornstein M, Greenblatt DJ, Black B and Shader RI. Does carbamazepine-induced reduction of plasma haloperidol worsen psychotic symptoms. Am J Psychiatry (1986) 143, 650–1.

6 Brayley J and Yellowlees P. An interaction between haloperidol and carbamazepine in a patient with cerebral palsy. Aust NZ J Psychiatry (1987) 21, 605–7.

7 Yerevanian BI, Hodgeman CH. A haloperidol carbamazepine interaction in a patient with rapid-cycline disorder. Am J Psychiatry (1985) 142, 785–6.

Haloperidol + Fluoxetine

Abstract/Summary

An isolated report describes the development of very severe extrapyramidal symptoms in a woman on haloperidol when additionally given fluoxetine.

Clinical evidence, mechanism, importance and management

A woman who had been on 2–5 mg haloperidol daily for two years with only occasional mild extrapyramidal symptoms, started additionally to take 40 mg fluoxetine twice daily. After five days the haloperidol was stopped but restarted nine days later. Two days later she began to experience severe extrapyramidal symptoms (tongue stiffness, parkinsonism, akathisia) and for three days was virtually incapacitated. Both drugs were stopped and she recovered over a period of a week while treated with benztropine, diphenhydramine and diazepam. She was restarted on perphenazine, later exchanged for 30 mg haloperidol and 6 mg benztropine daily. A slight parkinsonian gait returned but no other extrapyramidal symptoms.[1] The reasons for this severe reaction are not understood. If concurrent use is thought appropriate it should be very well monitored.

Reference

1 Tate JL. Extrapyramidal symptoms in a patient taking haloperidol and fluoxetine. Am J Psychiatry (1989) 146, 399–400.

Haloperidol + Indomethacin

Abstract/Summary

Profound drowsiness and confusion have been described in patients given haloperidol and indomethacin.

Clinical Evidence

A double-blind crossover study on 20 patients to find out the possible advantages of combining haloperidol (5 mg daily) with indomethacin (75 mg daily) in the treatment of pain arising from osteoarthritis of the knee and/or hip was eventually abandoned because 13 patients (11 on haloperidol and two on placebo) failed to complete the trial, six of those on haloperidol being withdrawn because of profound drowsiness or tiredness. The authors of the paper said that the combined treatment '...produced drowsiness and confusion so severe that in some cases the patient's independent existence was in jeopardy; this side-effect was far more intense than anything which might have been expected with haloperidol alone'.[1]

Mechanism

Not understood.

Importance and management

The report cited seems to be the only direct evidence of this interaction, but it appears to be established. The incidence (six out of 11) is high. If concurrent use is thought appropriate, a close watch should be kept to ensure that this severe side-effect does not develop. It might be wiser to avoid concurrent use because the majority of patients requiring this type of treatment are not hospitalized and under the day-to-day scrutiny of the prescriber.

Reference

1   Bird HA, Le Gallez P and Wright V. Drowsiness due to haloperidol/indomethacin combination. Lancet (1983) i, 830–1.

Haloperidol + Tobacco smoking

Abstract/Summary

Those who smoke may need more haloperidol than those who do not.

Clinical evidence

A comparative study showed that steady-state haloperidol levels were lower in a group of 23 cigarette smokers than in another group of 27 non-smokers (16.83 compared with 28.80 ng/ml) and the clearance was increased (1.58 compared with 1.10 l/min).[1] The probable reason is that some of the components of tobacco smoke act as liver enzyme inducers which increase the rate at which the liver metabolizes and clears the haloperidol from the body. It seems likely that smokers will need larger doses of haloperidol than non-smokers, and the dosage of haloperidol may need to be adjusted if patients start or stop smoking.

Reference

1   Jann MW, Sakald SR, Ereshefsky L, Richards AL, Harrington CA and Davis CM. Effects of smoking on haloperidol and reduced haloperidol plasma concentrations and haloperidol clearance. Psychopharmacol (1986) 90, 468–70.

Hydroxyzine + Miscellaneous drugs

Abstract/Summary

Hydroxyzine can cause ECG abnormalities in high doses. It has been suggested that concurrent use with other drugs which can cause cardiac abnormalities might increase the likelihood of dysrhythmias and sudden death.

Clinical evidence, mechanism, importance and management

A study in 25 elderly psychotic patients on 300 mg hydroxyzine over a nine-week period showed that ECG changes were mild except for alteration in T waves which were definite in nine patients and usually observed in leads 1,2 AVL and V_{3-6}. In each case the T-waves were lower in altitude, broadened and flattened and sometimes notched. The QT interval was usually prolonged. A repeat of the study in a few patients, one at least given 400 mg, gave similar results, the most pronounced change being a marked attentuation of the cardiac repolarization. On the basis of these observations the authors suggest that other drugs which cause ECG abnormalities (they mention antiparkinson drugs, atropine, lithium carbonate, phenothiazines, quinidine, procainamide, thioridazine, tricyclic antidepressants), might aggravate and exaggerate these hydroxyzine-induced changes and increase the risk of sudden death.[1] More study is needed to assess the practical importance of these potential interactions.

Reference

1   Hollister LE. Hydroxyzine hydrochloride: possible adverse cardiac interactions. Psychopharmacol Comm (1975) 1, 61.

Neuroleptics (Butyrophenones, Phenothiazines, Thioxanthenes) + Anticholinergics

Abstract/Summary

These drugs are very often given together advantageously and uneventfully, but occasionally serious and even life-threatening interactions occur. These include heat-stroke in hot and humid conditions, severe constipation and adynamic ileus, and atropine-like psychoses. Anticholinergics used to counteract the extrapyramidal side-effects of neuroleptics (e.g. chlorpromazine, haloperidol, etc.) may also reduce or abolish their therapeutic effects. See also 'Phenothiazines + Tricyclic antidepressants'.

Clinical evidence

Concurrent use can result in a generalized low grade but not serious additive increase in the anticholinergic effects of these drugs (blurred vision, dry mouth, constipation, difficulty in urination), however sometimes serious intensification takes place. For the sake of clarity these have been subdivided here into (A) heat stroke, (B) constipation and adynamic ileus, (C) atropine-like psychoses and (D) antagonism of neuroleptic effects.

(A) Heat stroke in hot and humid conditions

Three patients were admitted to hospital in Philadelphia for drug-induced hyperpyrexia during a hot and humid period. In each case their skin and mucous membranes were dry and the pulse fast (120 bpm). The first was taking daily doses of 500 mg chlorpromazine, 200 mg chlorprothixene and 6 mg benztropine; the second was taking 600 mg chlorpromazine, 12 mg trifluoperazine and 2 mg benztropine daily; and the third was on 8 mg haloperidol and 2 mg benztropine daily. There was no evidence of infection.[1]

There are other reports of heat stroke, some of them fatal, in patients taking chlorpromazine, promazine, fluphenazine or other phenothiazines with benztropine or other atropine-like drugs and/or tricyclic antidepressants.[3–5] The danger of heat-stroke in patients or atropine or atropine-compounds was recognized more than half a century ago, and the warning has been repeated many times.[13,14]

Mechanism

Anticholinergic drugs inhibit the parasympathetic nervous system which innervates the sweat glands so that when the ambient temperature rises, the major body heat-losing mechanism can be partially or wholly put out of action.[2] Phenothiazines, thioxanthenes and butyrophenones may also have some anticholinergic effects, but additionally they impair to a varying extent the hypothalamic thermoregulatory mechanisms which control the body's ability to keep a constant temperature when exposed to heat or cold. So, when the ambient temperature rises, the body temperature also rises. The tricyclics can disrupt the temperature control similarly. Thus in very hot and humid conditions when the need to reduce the temperature is great, the additive effects of these drugs can make patients become '...little more able to control their internal responses to heat than are reptiles...'[5] but, unlike poikilothermic animals, they are unable to sustain life once the temperature reaches a certain point.

(B) Constipation and adynamic ileus

Eight cases of adynamic ileus with faecal impaction have been reported in patients treated with phenothiazines (chlorpromazine, levomepromazine, thioridazine, trifluoperazine, perphenazine), imipramine and benztropine or benzhexol, or a combination of two or more of these drugs. Five were treated successfully but three patients died because recognition of the condition was too late.[6]

A number of other cases have been described involving chlorpromazine with nortriptyline,[9] imipramine,[6] benzhexol,[6] trifluoperazine and benztropine,[7] or amitriptyline;[8] mesoridazine with benztropine;[25] trifluoperazine with bentropine or benzhexol;[6,26] imipramine with levomepromazine and benztropine,[6] or with thioridazine and benzhexol.[6] Seven of the cases had a fatal outcome. Severe constipation also occurred in a woman given thioridazine, biperiden and doxepin.[25]

Mechanism

Anticholinergic drugs reduce peristalsis which, in the extreme, can result in total gut stasis. Additive effects can occur if two or more anticholinergic drugs are taken.

(C) Atropine-like psychoses

Three patients taking part in a double-blind study of this interaction and given a phenothiazine and benztropine mesylate for the parkinsonian side-effects, developed an intermittent toxic confusional state (marked disturbance of short-term memory, impaired attention, disorientation, anxiety, visual and auditory hallucinations) with peripheral anticholinergic signs.[12]

Similar reactions occurred in three elderly patients given imipramine or desipramine with benzhexol.[11] A toxic psychosis was seen in a woman on meclozine three days after starting to use a transdermal preparation of hyoscine,[27] and in another man given chlorpromazine, benztropine and doxepin.[25]

Mechanism

These toxic psychoses resemble the CNS effects of atropine or belladonna poisoning and appear to result from the additive effects of the drugs used.

(D) Antagonism of the neuroleptic effects

Studies in psychiatric patients given 300–800 mg chlorpromazine daily showed that when 6–10 mg benzhexol daily was added, the plasma chlorpromazine levels fell from a range of 100–300 ng/ml to less than 30 ng/ml. When the benzhexol was withdrawn the plasma chlorpromazine levels rose again and clinical improvement was seen.[18,21]

Other studied confirm that benzhexol[17,22] and orphenadrine[10] reduce the plasma levels and effects of chlorpromazine. Some of the actions of haloperidol on social avoidance behaviour can be abolished by benztropine, but cognitive integrative function is unaffected.[15,16]

Mechanism

Not understood. Animal studies suggest that the site of interaction is in the gut.[21]

Importance and management

Established and well-documented interactions. While these drugs have been widely used together with apparent advantage and without problems, prescribers should be aware that (i) an unspectacular low-grade anticholinergic toxicity can go undetected in the elderly because the symptoms can be so similar to the general complaints of old people; and (ii) also be aware of the serious problems which can develop, particularly if high doses are used.

(A) Warn patients to minimize outdoor exposure and/or exercise in hot and humid climates, particularly if they are taking high doses of antipsychotic/anticholinergic drugs.

(B) Be alert for severe constipation and for the development of complete gut stasis which can be fatal.

(C) Be aware that the symptoms of central anticholinergic psychosis can be confused with the basic psychotic symptoms of the patient. Withdrawal of one or more of the drugs, or a dosage reduction and/or appropriate symptomatic treatment can be used to control these interactions.

(D) Ensure that the concurrent use of anticholinergics to control the extrapyramidal side-effects of neuroleptics is necessary[19,20] and be aware that the therapeutic effects may possibly be reduced as a result. See also 'Phenothiazines + Tricyclic antidepressants'.

References

1 Westlake RJ and Rastegar A. Hyperpyrexia from drug combinations. J Amer Med Ass (1973) 225, 1250.
2 Kollias J and Bullard RW. The influence of chlorpromazine on the physical and chemical mechanism of temperature regulation in the rat. J Pharmacol Exp Ther (1964) 145, 373.

3 Zelman S and Guillan R. Heat stroke in phenothiazine-treated patients: a report of three fatalities. Am J Psychiat (1970) 126, 1787.

4 Sarnquist F and Larson CP. Drug induced heat stroke. Anesthesiology (1973) 39, 348.

5 Reimer DR, Mohan J and Nagaswami S. Heat dyscontrol syndrome in patients receiving antipsychotic, antidepressant and anti-parkinson drug therapy. J Florida Med Ass (1974) 61, 573.

6 Warnes H, Lehmann HE and Ban TA. Adynamic ileus during psychoactive medication. A report of three fatal and five severe cases. Canad Med Ass J (1976) 96, 1112.

7 Giorano J, Huang A and Canter JW. Fatal paralytic ileus complicating phenothiazine therapy. S Med J (1975) 68, 351.

8 Burkitt EA and Sutcliffe CK. Paralytic ileus after amitriptyline (Tryptizol). Br Med J (1961) 2, 1648.

9 Milner G and Hills NF. Adynamic ileus and nortriptyline. Br Med J (1966) 1, 841.

10 Loga S, Curry S and Lader M. Interactions of orphenadrine and phenobarbitone with chlorpromazine: plasma concentrations and effects in man. Br J clin Pharmac (1975) 2, 197.

11 Roger SC. Imipramine and benzhexol. Br Med J (1967) 1, 500.

12 Davis JM. Psychopharmacology in the aged. Use of psychotropic drugs in geriatric patients. J Geriatric Psychiatry (1974) 7, 145.

13 Wilcox WH. The nature, prevention and treatment of heat hyperpyrexia. Br Med J (1920) 1, 392.

14 Litman RE. Heat sensitivity due to autonomic drugs. J Amer Med Ass (1952) 149, 635.

15 Singh MM and Smith JM. Reversal of some therapeutic effects of an antipsychotic agent by an antiparkinsonian drug. J Nerv Ment Dis (1973) 157, 50.

16 Singh MM and Smith JM. Reversal of some therapeutic effects of haloperidol in schizophrenia by antiparkinson drugs. Pharmacologist (1971) 13, 207.

17 Chan T, Sakalis G and Gershon S. Some aspects of chlorpromazine metabolism in humans. Clin Pharmacol Ther (1973) 14, 133.

18 Rivera-Calimlim L, Castenada L and Lasagna L. Significance of plasma levels of chlorpromazine. Clin Pharmacol Ther (1973) 14, 144.

19 Priest RF. Unpublished surveys from the NIMH collaborative project on drug therapy in chronic schizophrenics and the VA collaborative project on interim drug therapy in chronic schizophrenics. Quoted in Int Drug Ther Newsletter (1974) 9, 29.

20 Klett CJ and Caffey EM. Evaluating the long-term need for antiparkinson drugs by chronic schizophrenics. Arch Gen Psychiatry (1972) 26, 374.

21 Rivera-Calimlim L, Castenada L and Lasagna L. Chlorpromazine and trihexiphenidyl interaction in psychiatric patients. Pharmacologist (1973) 15, 212.

22 Rivera-Calimlim L, Nasrallah H, Strauss J and Lasagna L. Clinical response and plasma levels: effect of dosage schedules and drug interaction on plasma chlorpromazine levels. Am J Psychiat (1976) 133, 647.

23 Wintrobe MM. Harrison's Principles of Internal Medicine, Edn 7. McGraw-Hill (1974) p 1438.

24 Krupp MA and Chatterton MJ. Current Medical Diagnosis and Treatment. Lange Medical Publication, Los Altos (1976) p 354.

25 Ayd FJ. Doxepin with other drugs. S Med J (1973) 66, 465–71.

26 Spiro RK and Kysilewsky RM. Iatrogenic ileus secondary to medication. J Med Soc NJ (1973) 70, 565.

27 Osterholm RK and Camoriano JK. Transdermal scopolamine psychosis. J Amer Med Ass (1982) 247, 3081.

Neuroleptics + Bromocriptine

Abstract/Summary

Concurrent use can be successful but one report describes the re-emergence of schizophrenic symptoms in a patient when bromocriptine was added to molindone and imipramine.

Clinical evidence, mechanism, importance and management

Single low doses of bromocriptine have been found to improve the psychopathology of chronic schizophrenia in patients on neuroleptics[1] and a case report describes the successful concurrent use of bromocriptine and haloperidol.[2] Another report[3] describes a schizoaffective schizophrenic on fluphenazine, benztropine, phenytoin and phenobarbitone whose psychiatric status was unaltered when bromocriptine was given to treat a pituitary adenoma, but the previously normal serum prolactin was reduced to less than detectable levels by the bromocriptine. However a woman with schizoaffective schizophrenia stabilized on 100 mg molindone and 200 mg imipramine daily, relapsed (agitation, delusions, hallucinations) within five days of starting additional treatment with 7.5 mg bromocriptine daily for amenorrhoea-galactorrhoea.[4] Within three days of stopping the bromocriptine these symptoms vanished. The reason suggested by the authors of the report is that the bromocriptine (a dopamine agonist) opposed the actions of the antipsychotic medication (dopamine antagonists) thereby allowing the schizophrenia to re-emerge. If concurrent use is thought appropriate, the outcome should be well monitored.

References

1 Cutler NR, Jeste DV, Kaufmann CA, Karoum F, Schran HF and Wyatt RJ. Low dose bromocriptine: a study of acute effects in chronic medicated schizophrenics. Prog Neuro-Psycho-pharmacol Biol Psychiatry (1984) 8, 277–83.

2 Gattaz WF and Kollisch M. Bromocriptine in the treatment of neuroleptic-resistant schizophrenia. Biol Psychiatry (1986) 21, 519–21.

3 Kellner C, Harris P and Blumhardt C. Concurrent use of bromocriptine and fluphenazine. J Clin Psychiatry (1984) 46, 455.

4 Frye PE, Pariser SF, Kim MH and O'Shaughnessy RW. Bromocriptine associated with symptom exacerbation during neuroleptic treatment of schizoaffective schizophrenia. J Clin Psychiatry (1982) 43, 252–3.

Phenothiazines + Antacids

Abstract/Summary

Antacids containing aluminium hydroxide or magnesium trisilicate can reduce the serum levels of chlorpromazine which would be expected to reduce the therapeutic response.

Clinical evidence

A study in 10 patients taking 600–1200 mg chlorpromazine daily showed that when concurrently treated with 30 ml *Aludrox* (aluminium hydroxide gel) their urinary excretion of chlorpromazine was reduced 10–45%.[3]

A study on six patients, prompted by the observation of one patient on chlorpromazine who relapsed within three days of starting to take an un-named antacid, showed that when 30 ml *Gelusil* (aluminium hydroxide + magnesium trisilicate) was given with a liquid suspension of chlorpromazine, the serum chlorpromazine levels measured 2 h later were reduced by 20% (from 168 to 132 ng/ml).[1,2]

Mechanism

Chlorpromazine becomes bound to the gel structure of these antacids[1,4] which would seem to account for the reduced bioavailability.

Importance and management

Information seems to be limited to the reports cited. Reductions in serum levels of up to 45% would be expected to be clinically important but so far only one case seems to have been reported.[1,2] Separating the dosages as much as possible to avoid admixture in the gut should minimize any effects. An alternative would be to use one of the ionic antacids such as calcium carbonate-glycine or magnesium hydroxide gel which do not seem to affect the gastrointestinal absorption of chlorpromazine to any extent.[4] Nobody appears to have checked on whether other phenothiazines interact similarly.

References

1 Fann WE, Davis JM, Janowsky DS, Sekerke HJ and Schmidt DM. Chlorpromazine: effects of antacids on its gastrointestinal absorption. J Clin Pharmacol (1973) 13, 388.
2 Fann WE, Davis JM, Janowsky DS and Schmidt DM. The effects of antacids on chlorpromazine levels. Ann Pharmacol Ther (1973) 14, 135.
3 Forrest FM and Forrest IS and Serra MT. Modification of chlorpromazine metabolism by some other drugs frequently administered to psychiatric patients. Biol Psychiat (1970) 2, 35.
4 Pinell OC, Fenimore DC, Davis CM and Fann WE. Drug-drug interaction of chlorpromazine and antacid. Clin Pharmacol Ther (1978) 23, 125.

Phenothiazines + Antimalarials

Abstract/Summary

Chloroquine, amodiaquine and Fansidar *(sulphadoxine + pyrimethamine) can markedly increase serum chlorpromazine levels.*

Clinical evidence

15 schizophrenic patients (in three groups of five) given 400 or 500 chlorpromazine daily for at least two weeks were additionally given single doses of either chloroquine sulphate (400 mg), amodiaquine hydrochloride (600 mg) or three tablets of *Fansidar* (25 mg pyrimethamine +500 mg sulphadoxine) an hour before the chlorpromazine. Serum chlorpromazine levels 3 h later were found to be raised approximately threefold by the chloroquine and amodiaquine, and almost fourfold by the *Fansidar*. The plasma levels of one of the major metabolites of chlorpromazine (7-OH-chlorpromazine) were also elevated, but not those of the other (chlorpromazine sulphoxide). Four days later the serum chlorpromazine levels of the patients given chloroquine or *Fansidar* still remained elevated to some extent. There was subjective evidence that the patients were more heavily sedated when given the antimalarials.[1]

Mechanism

Not understood. Both chloroquine and *Fansidar* have relatively long half-lives compared with amodiaquine which may explain the persistence of their effects.

Importance and management

Direct information about this interaction seems to be limited to this study. Its clinical importance is uncertain but it seems possible that these antimalarials could cause chlorpromazine toxicity. Monitor the effects of concurrent use closely and anticipate the need to reduce the chlorpromazine dosage. More study is needed.

References

1 Makanjuola ROA, Dixon PAF and Oforah E. Effects of antimalarial agents on plasma levels of chlorpromazine and its metabolites in schizophrenic patients. Trop Geogr Med (1988) 40, 31–3.

Phenothiazines + Ascorbic acid

Abstract/Summary

A single case report describes a fall in serum fluphenazine levels and deterioration in a patient when given ascorbic acid (vitamin C).

Clinical evidence, mechanism, importance and management

A manic depressive man taking 15 mg fluphenazine daily showed a 25% fall (from 0.93 to 0.705 ng/ml) in his serum drug levels accompanied by a deterioration in behaviour over a 13-day period while taking 1 g ascorbic acid daily.[1] The reason is not understood. There seem to be no other reports of this interaction with fluphenazine or any other phenothiazine.

Reference

1 Dysken MW, Cumming RJ, Channon RA and Davis JM. Drug interaction between ascorbic acid and fluphenazine. J Amer Med Ass (1979) 241, 2008.

Phenothiazines + Attapulgite

Abstract/Summary

An attapulgite-pectin antidiarrhoeal preparation caused a fall in the absorption of promazine in one subject.

Clinical evidence, mechanism, importance and management

A study in a normal subject showed that attapulgite-pectin

reduced the absorption of a single 50 mg dose of promazine by about 25%, possibly due to absorption of the phenothiazine onto the attapulgite.[1] The clinical importance of this and whether other phenothiazines behave similarly appears not to have been studied, but prescribers should be aware of this possible interaction if preparations containing attapulgite-pectin are given. Separating the administration as much as possible to avoid admixture in the gut has been shown with other drugs to minimize the effects of this type of interaction.

Reference

1 Sorby DL and Liu G. Effects of adsorbents on drug absorption. II. Effect of an antidiarrhoea mixture on promazine absorption. J Pharm Sci (1966) 55, 504.

Phenothiazines + Barbiturates

Abstract/Summary

The serum levels of each drug are reduced by the presence of the other, but the clinical importance of these reductions is uncertain. Pentobarbitone, promethazine and scopolamine in combination are said to increase the incidence of operative agitation.

Clinical evidence

(a) Serum phenothiazine levels reduced

A study in 12 schizophrenics on 300 mg chlorpromazine daily showed that when additionally treated with 150 mg phenobarbitone daily, there was a 25–30% fall in serum chlorpromazine levels accompanied by changes in certain physiological measurements which clearly reflected a reduced response. The conclusion was made that there was no advantage to be gained by concurrent use.[1]

In another study on seven patients the serum levels of thioridazine were observed to be reduced by phenobarbitone, the clinical effects of which were uncertain.[2]

(b) Serum phenobarbitone levels reduced

A study in a large number of epileptic patients showed that their serum phenobarbitone levels fell by 29% when treated with phenothiazines including chlorpromazine, thioridazine or mesoridazine, and increased once more when the phenothiazine was withdrawn.[3]

This study confirms another in which 100–200 mg thioridazine daily was found to reduce serum phenobarbitone levels by about 25%.[4] There is also some limited evidence that the concurrent use of pentobarbitone, promethazine and scopolamine increases the incidence of pre-operative, operative and postoperative agitation, and it has been suggested that this triple combination should be avoided.[5]

Mechanisms

Uncertain. The barbiturates are potent liver enzyme inducing agents which, it is presumed, increase the metabolism of the phenothiazines by the liver.

Importance and management

These interactions appear to be established, but the documentation is limited. The importance of both interactions (a and b) is uncertain, but be alert for evidence of reductions in response during concurrent use, and to increased responses if one of the drugs is withdrawn. So far only chlorpromazine, thioridazine, mesoridazine and phenobarbitone are implicated, but it seems possible that other phenothiazines and barbiturates will behave similarly.

References

1 Loga S, Curry S and Lader M. Interactions of orphenadrine and phenobarbitone with chlorpromazine: plasma concentrations and effects in man. Br J clin Pharmac (1975) 2, 197.
2 Ellenor GL, Musa MN and Beuthin FC. Phenobarbital-thioridazine interaction in man. Res Comm Chem Pathol Pharmacol (1978) 21, 185.
3 Haidukewych D and Rodin EA. Effect of phenothiazines on serum antiepileptic drug concentrations in psychiatric patients with seizure disorder. Ther Drug Monitor (1985) 7, 401–4.
4 Gay PE and Madsen JA. Interaction between phenobarbital and thioridazine. Neurology (1983) 33, 1631–2.
5 Macris SG and Levy L. Preanesthetic medication: untoward effects of certain drug combinations. Anesthesiology (1965) 26, 256.

Phenothiazines + Cimetidine

Abstract/Summary

Chlorpromazine serum levels can be reduced by a third if cimetidine is used concurrently.

Clinical evidence

A study in eight patients taking chlorpromazine (75–450 mg daily) showed that when given 1 g cimetidine daily for a week their steady-state serum chlorpromazine levels fell by a third (from 37 to 24 μg/ml). A two-thirds fall was noted in one patient.[1] The reasons are not understood but a decrease in absorption from the gut has been suggested.[1] Information appears to be limited to this report and its clinical importance is uncertain, but be alert for signs of a decreased response to chlorpromazine during concurrent use. An increase in the chlorpromazine dosage would seem to be the logical solution. There seems to be no information about other phenothiazines.

Reference

1 Howes CA, Pullar T, Sourindhrin I, Mistra PC, Capel H, Lawson DH and Tilstone WJ. Reduced steady-state plasma concentrations of indomethacin and chlorpromazine in patients receiving cimetidine. Eur J Clin Pharmacol (1983) 24, 99–102.

Phenothiazines + Disulfiram

Abstract/Summary

A single case report describes a man on perphenazine whose psychotic symptoms re-emerged when he began to take disulfiram.

Clinical evidence, mechanism, importance and management

A psychotic man controlled on 16 mg perphenazine daily by mouth developed marked psychosis soon after starting to take 200 mg disulfiram daily.[1] His serum perphenazine levels had fallen from 2.3 to less than 1 n mol/l. Doubling the dosage of perphenazine had little effect and no substantial clinical improvement or rise in serum levels occurred until the perphenazine was given as the enanthate intramuscularly (50 mg weekly) when the levels rose to about 4 n mol/l. The results of clinical biochemical tests suggested that the disulfiram was acting as a liver enzyme-inducing agent, so that the perphenazine was being metabolized and cleared from the body more rapidly. Disulfiram normally acts as an enzyme inhibitor. Too little is known to assess the general importance of this interaction, but it would seem prudent to be on the alert during concurrent use. There seems to be no information about an interaction with other phenothiazines.

Reference

1 Hansen LB and Larsen N-E. Metabolic interaction between perphenazine and disulfiram. Lancet (1982) ii, 1472.

Phenothiazines + Lithium Carbonate

Abstract/Summary

Serum levels of chlorpromazine can be reduced to non-therapeutic concentrations by the concurrent administration of lithium. Dosage increases may be needed. The development of severe extrapyramidal side-effects or neurotoxicity has been seen in a few patients concurrently treated with lithium and chlorpromazine, thioridazine, thiothixene, flupenthixol, fluphenazine or loxapine. Sleep-walking has been described in some patients taking chlorpromazine-like drugs and lithium.

Clinical evidence

Chlorpromazine + lithium carbonate

(i) Reduced serum chlorpromazine levels

In a double-blind study on psychiatric patients it was found that 400–800 mg daily doses of chlorpromazine (which normally produced serum levels of 100–300 ng/ml) only produced levels of 0–70 ng/ml during the concurrent use of lithium carbonate[1]

Other studies confirm the reduction in serum chlorpromazine

levels by normal therapeutic serum levels of lithium carbonate.[2,3,6] Peak serum chlorpromazine levels in normal subjects were 40% lower and the areas under the time/concentration curves were 26% smaller.[2]

(ii) Toxic reactions

A paranoid schizophrenic maintained on 200–600 mg chlorpromazine daily for five years with no extrapyramidal symptoms developed stiffness of his face, arms and legs, and parkinsonian tremor of both hands within a day of starting to take 900 mg lithium daily. His serum lithium level after three days was 0.5 mEq/l. He was later maintained on daily doses of 1800 mg lithium (serum levels 1.17 mEq/l), 200 mg chlorpromazine and 2 mg benztropine, but he still complained of stiffness and had a persistent hand tremor.[16]

A number of other report describe the emergence of severe extrapyramidal side-effect when chlorpromazine and lithium were used concurrently.[11,13,15]

Other phenothiazines + lithium carbonate

Four patients developed severe neurotoxic complications (seizures, encephalopathy, delerium, abnormal EEG's) while taking high doses of thioridazine (800 mg daily or more) and lithium. Serum lithium levels remained below 1.0 mEq/l. Three of them had used lithium and other phenothiazines uneventfully for extended periods without problems, and the fourth was subsequently successfully treated with lithium and fluphenazine.[4] The sudden emergence of extrapyramidal or other side-effects has been described in patients concurrently treated with lithium and flupenthixol,[5,18] fluphenazine,[12,18] thioridazine,[14] thiothixene[19] or loxapine.[17] Irreversible brain damage has been reported in a patient taking fluphenazine decanoate and lithium.[6] The concurrent use of lithium and chlorpromazine, perphenazine, thioridazine or thiothixene has also been associated with sleep-walking episodes in 9% of a group of patients.[7]

Mechanisms

Not understood. One suggestion to account for the reduced serum levels of chlorpromazine, based on animal studies,[8,9] is that the lithium delays gastric emptying. This exposes the chlorpromazine to the metabolism by the gut wall for a longer time.

Importance and management

Information about the chlorpromazine/lithium interaction which results in reduced serum chlorpromazine levels is limited but it would seem to be established and of clinical importance. Serum chlorpromazine levels below 30 ng/ml have been shown to be ineffective, whereas clinical improvement is associated with levels within the 150–300 ng/ml range or more.[10] Thus a fall in levels to 0–70 ng/ml (study cited above) would be expected to result in a reduced therapeutic response. Monitor the effects and increase the dosage if necessary.

The development of severe neurotoxic and extrapyramidal side-effects with combinations of chlorpromazine or other phenothiazines (thioridazine, flupenthixol, fluphenazine, loxapine) and lithium appears to be very uncommon, but be alert for any evidence of toxicity if lithium is given with any of these drugs. One recommendation is that the onset of neurological manifestations such as excessive drowsiness or movement disorders warrants electroencephalography without delay. Much more study is needed to identify the patients at risk.

References

1 Kerzner B and Rivera-Calimlim L. Lithium and chlorpromazine (CPZ) interaction. Clin Pharmacol Ther (1976) 19, 109.
2 Rivera-Calimlim L, Kerzner B and Karach FE. Effect of lithium on plasma chlorpromazine levels. Clin Pharmacol Ther (1978) 23, 451.
3 Rivera-Calimlim L, Nasrallah H, Strass J and Lasagna L. Clinical response and plasma levels: effect of dose, dosage schedules and drug interactions on plasma chlorpromazine levels. Clin Psychiat (1976) 133, 6.
4 Spring GK. Neurotoxicity with combined use of lithium and thioridazine. J Clin Psychiat (1979) 40, 135.
5 West A. Adverse effects of lithium treatment. Br Med J (1977) 2, 642.
6 Singh SV. Lithium carbonate/fluphemazine decanoate producing irreversible brain damage. Lancet (1982) ii, 278.
7 Charney DS, Kales A, Soldatos CR and Nelson JC. Somnambulistic episodes secondary to combined lithium neuroleptic treatment. Br J Psychiat (1979) 135, 418–24.
8 Sundaresen PR and Rivera-Calimlim L. Distribution of chlorpromazine on the gastrointestinal tract of the rat and its effects on absorptive functions. J Pharmacol Exp Ther (1975) 194, 593.
9 Curry SH, O'Mello A and Mould GP. Destruction of chlorpromazine during absorption in the rat in vivo and in vitro. Br J Pharmacol (1971) 42, 403.
10 Rivera-Calimlim L, Castenada L and Lasogna L. Significance of plasma levels of chlorpromazine. Clin Pharmacol Ther (1973) 14, 978.
11 McGennis AJ. Hazards of lithium and neuroleptics in schizo-affective disorder. Br J Psychiatry (1983)142, 99–100.
12 Sachdev PS. Lithium potentiation of neuroleptic-related extrapyramidal side-effects. Am J Psychiatry (1986) 143, 942.
13 Yassa R. A case of lithium-chlorpromazine interaction. J Clin Psychiatry (1986) 47, 90–1.
14 Bailine SH and Doft M. Neurotoxicity induced by combined lithium-thioridazine treatment. Biol Psychiatry (1986) 21, 834–7.
15 Habib M, Khalil R, Le Pensec-Bertrand, D, Ali-Cherif A, Bongrand MC and Crevat A. Syndrome neurologique persistant apres traitement par les sels de lithium. Rev Neurol(1986) 142, 1, 61–4.
16 Addonizio G. Rapid induction of extrapyramidal side effects with combined use of lithium and neuroleptics. J Clin Psychopharmacol (1985) 5, 296–8.
17 de la Gandara J and Dominguez RA. Lithium and loxapine. A potential interaction. J Clin Psychiatry (1988) 49, 126.
18 Kamlana SH, Kerry RJ and Khan IA. Lithium: some drug interactions. Practitioner (1980) 224, 1291–2.
19 Fetzer J, Kader G and Dahany S. Lithium encephalopathy: a clinical, psychiatric and EEG evaluation. Am J Pschiatry (1981) 138, 1622–3.

Phenothiazines + Naltrexone

Abstract/Summary

Extreme lethargy occurred in two patients on thioridazine when given naltrexone.

Clinical evidence, mechanism, importance and management

Two schizophrenic patients well stabilized on thioridazine (50–200 mg three times daily for 1–7 years) took part in a pilot project to assess the efficacy of naltrexone for the treatment of tardive dyskinesia. Both tolerated the first challenge dose of naloxone (0.8 mg IV) without problems but experienced extreme lethargy and slept almost continuously after the second dose of naltrexone (50–100 mg orally). The severe lethargy cleared up within 12 h of stopping the naltrexone.[1] The reasons for this reaction are not understood. Information seems to be limited to this report but this would seem to be a drug combination to be avoided. There seems to be nothing documented about other phenothiazines.

Reference

1 Maany I, O'Brien CP, Woody G. Interaction between thioridazine and naltrexone. Am J Psychiatry (1987) 144, 966.

Phenothiazines + Phenylpropanolamine

Abstract/Summary

A single case report describes fatal ventricular fibrillation attributed to the concurrent use of thioridazine and phenylpropanolamine.

Clinical evidence, mechanism, importance and management

A 27-year-old schizophrenic woman who was taking regular daily doses of 100 mg thioridazine and 5 mg procyclidine was found dead in bed 2 h after taking a single capsule of *Contac*C* (phenylpropanolamine 50 mg + chlorpheniramine maleate 4 mg). The principal cause of death was aspiration of the stomach contents attributed to ventricular fibrillation.[1] The mechanism is not understood but it is suggested that it may have been due to the combined effects of the thioridazine (known to be cardiotoxic and to cause T-wave abnormalities) and the phenylpropanolamine (possibly able to cause ventricular arrhythmias like adrenaline with anaesthetics).

The general importance of this alleged interaction is uncertain but the authors of the report suggest that ephedrine-like agents such as phenylpropanolamine should not be given to patients on thioridazine or mesoridazine.

Reference

1 Chouinard G, Ghadirian AM and Jones BD. Death attributed to ventricular arrhythmia induced by thioridazine in combination with a single Contac*C capsule. Canada Med Ass J (1978) 119, 729.

Phenothiazines, Butyrophenones or Tricyclic antidepressants + Tea or Coffee

Abstract/Summary

Tea and coffee can cause some drugs to precipitate out of solution, but so far there is no clinical evidence to show that this normally affects the bioavailability of the drugs or that it has a detrimental effect on treatment.

Clinical evidence, mechanism, importance and management

Mikkelson[1] described two patients whose schizophrenia was said to have been exacerbated by an increased consumption of tea and coffee. Subsequent studies[2-5] showed that a number of drugs (chlorpromazine, promethazine, fluphenazine, promazine, prochlorperazine, trifluoperazine, thioridazine, loxapine, haloperidol, droperidol, amitriptyline, imipramine) were precipitated out of solution by tea or coffee due to the formation of a drug-tannin complex which it was thought might possibly lower the absorption of these drugs by the gut. Moreover studies with rats showed that tea abolished the cataleptic effects of chlorpromazine.[6]

However a clinical study[7] of this interaction showed that the serum levels of chlorpromazine, fluphenazine, trifluoperazine and haloperidol in a group of 16 mentally retarded patients were unaffected by the consumption of tea or coffee. Their behaviour also remained unchanged. So at the present time there appears to be little or no direct evidence that this physico-chemical interaction is normally of clinical importance, but more study is needed.

References

1 Mikkelsen EJ. Caffeine and schizophrenia. J Clin Psychiat (1978) 39, 732–5.
2 Kulhanek F, Linde OK and Meisenberg G. Precipitation of antipsychotic drugs in interaction with coffee or tea. Lancet (1979) ii, 1130–1.
3 Hirsch SR. Precipitation of antipsychotic drugs in interaction with tea or coffee. Lancet (1979) ii, 1131.
4 Lasswell WL, Wilkins JM and Weber SS. *In vitro* interaction of selected drugs with coffee, tea and gallotannic acid. Drug-nutrient Interactions (1984) 2, 235–41.
5 Lasswell WL, Weber SS and Wilkins JM. *In vitro* interaction of neuroleptics and tricyclic antidepressants with coffee, tea and gallotannic acid. J Pharm Sci (1984) 73, 1056–8.
6 Cheesman HJ and Neal MJ. Interaction of chlorpromazine with tea and coffee. Br J Clin Pharm (1981) 12, 165–9.
7 Bowen S, Taylor KM and Gibb IAM. Effect of coffee and tea on blood levels and efficacy of antipsychotic drugs. Lancet (1981) i, 1217–18.

Phenothiazines + Tricyclic antidepressants

Abstract/Summary

Concurrent treatment is common but a mutual interaction occurs which results in a rise in the serum levels of both drugs. Although fixed-dose combined preparations are available, it has been suggested that concurrent use might contribute to an increased incidence of tardive dyskinesia. A paradoxical reversal of the therapeutic effects of chlorpromazine after the addition of a tricyclic antidepressant has also been described.

Clinical evidence

Effect of phenothiazines on tricyclic antidepressant serum levels

An extended study of four patients given 12.5 mg fluphenazine decanoate weekly, with 6 mg benztropine mesylate and 300 mg imipramine daily, showed that their mean combined plasma concentrations of imipramine and desipramine were 850 ng/ml compared with only 180 ng/ml in 60 other patients described elsewhere who were taking only 225 mg imipramine daily.[9]

A comparative study[11] of 99 patients taking only amitriptyline or nortriptyline and 60 other patients additionally taking an average of 10 mg perphenazine daily, showed that although the tricyclic antidepressant dosage levels were the same, the plasma tricyclic antidepressant levels of the latter group were up to 70% higher. Similar results were reported in another study on three patients,[3] but minimal or no changes were described in another.[14] Other studies have demonstrated this interaction between imipramine and chlorpromazine,[2,4,13] between amitriptyline,[17] imipramine,[13] desipramine[15] and perphenazine, between desipramine and thioridazine,[16] and between nortriptyline and chlorpromazine.[12] In this last study on seven chronic schizophrenics it was also reported that the addition of full doses of nortriptyline (150 mg daily) to a course of chlorpromazine (300 mg daily) resulted in such a profound worsening of the clinical state, with marked increases in agitation and tension, that the nortriptyline was withdrawn.[12] A temporary reversion to a disruptive behaviour pattern has been seen in other patients on chlorpromazine when given amitriptyline.[10]

Effect of tricyclic antidepressant on phenothiazine serum levels

In a controlled study on eight schizophrenic patients taking 20 mg butaperazine daily, six of them on 150 mg desipramine or more daily showed a rise in serum butaperazine levels of between 50 and 300%.[1]

Mechanism

The rise in the serum levels of both drugs is thought to be due to a mutual inhibition of the liver enzymes concerned with the metabolism of both drugs, resulting in the accumulation of both. The evidence available is consistent with this idea.[1-4,12]

Importance and management

An established interaction, but the advantages and disadvantages of concurrent use are still the subject of debate. These two groups of drugs are widely used together in the treatment of schizophrenic patients who show depression, and for mixed anxiety and depression. A number of fixed-dose combinations have been marketed, e.g. *Triptafen, Etrafon, Triaval* (amitriptyline and perphenazine), *Motival, Motipress* (nortriptyline, and fluphenazine), however the safety of using both drugs together has been questioned.

One of the problems of phenothiazine treatment is the development of tardive dyskinesia, and some evidence suggests that the higher the dosage, the greater the incidence.[6] The symptoms can be transiently masked by increasing the dosage,[7] thus the presence of a tricyclic antidepressant (which increases the levels of the phenothiazine) might not only be a factor causing the tardive dyskinesia to develop, but might also mask the condition and contribute towards its development (or so it has been suggested.)[1,5] Ayd has advised[5] that, until more is known, combined treatment should be the exception rather than the rule. It has also been recommended that the addition of full antidepressant doses of nortriptyline to average antipsychotic doses of chlorpromazine should be avoided because the therapeutic actions of the chlorpromazine may be reversed.[12]

Attention has also been drawn to excessive weight gain associated with several months' use of amitriptyline with thioridazine for the treatment of chronic pain.[8]

References

1 El-Yousef MK and Manier DH. Tricyclic antidepressants and phenothiazines. J Amer Med Ass (1974) 229, 1419.
2 Gram LF and Overo KF. Drug interaction: inhibitory effect of neuroleptics on metabolism of tricyclic antidepressants in man. Br Med J (1972) 1, 463.
3 Gram LF, Overo KF and Kirk L. Influence of neuroleptics and benzodiazepines on metabolism of tricyclic antidepressants in man. Am J Psychiatry (1974) 131, 8.
4 Grammer JL and Rolfe B. Interaction of imipramine and chlorpromazine in man. Psychopharmacologia (1972) 26,(Suppl), 80.
5 Ayd FJ. Pharmacokinetic interaction between tricyclic antidepressants and phenothiazine neuroleptics. Int Drug Ther Newsletter (1974) 9, 31.
6 Crane GE. Persistent dyskinesia. Brit J Psychiatry (1973), 122, 395.
7 Crane GE. Tardive dyskinesia in patients treated with major neuroleptics: a review of the literature. Am J Psychiatry (1968) 124,(Suppl), 40.
8 Pfister AK. Weight gain from combined phenothiazine and tricyclic therapy. J Amer Med Ass (1978) 239, 1959.
9 Siris SG, Cooper TB, Rifkin AE, Brenner R and Lieberman JA. Plasma imipramine concentrations in patients receiving concomitant fluphenazine decanoate. Am J Psychiatry (1982) 193, 104.
10 O'Connor JW. Personal communication 1983.
11 Linnoila M, George L and Guthrie S. Interaction between antidepressants and perphenazine in psychiatric patients. Am J Psychiatry (1982) 139, 1329–31.
12 Loga S, Curry S and Lader M. Interaction of chlorpromazine and nortriptyline in patients with schizophrenia. Clin Pharmacokinetics. (1981) 6, 454–62.
13 Gram LF. Laegemiddelinteraktion: haemmende virkning af neurolepltica pa tricykliske antidepressivas metabolisering. Nord psykiat T. (1971) 25, 357–60.
14 Kragh-Sorensen P,Börga O, Hansen BV, Hansen CE, Hvidberg EF and Larsen N-E. Effect of simultaneous treatment with low doses of perphenazine on plasma and urine concentrations of nortriptyline and

10-hydroxynortriptyline. Europ J clin Pharmacol (1977) 11, 479–483.
15 Nelson JC and Jatlow PI. Neuroleptic effect on desipramine steady-state plasma concentrations. Am J Psychiatry (1980) 137, 1232–34.
16 Hirschowitz J, Bennett JA, Zemlan FP and Garver DL. Thioridazine effect on desipramine plasma levels. J Clin Psychopharmacol (1983) 3, 376–9.
17 Perel JM, Stiller RL and Feldman BL. Therapeutic drug monitoring (TDM) of the amitriptyline (AT)/perphenazine interaction in depressed patients. Clin Chem (1985) 31, 939–40.

Sulpiride + Antacids or Sucralfate

Abstract/Summary

Sucralfate and an aluminium-magnesium hydroxide antacid can reduce the absorption of sulpiride.

Clinical evidence, mechanism, importance and management

A study in six normal subjects showed that the bioavailability of a single 100 mg dose of sulpiride was reduced 40% by 1 g sucralfate and 32% by 30 ml of *Simeco* (an antacid containing 215 mg aluminium hydroxide, 80 mg magnesium hydroxide and 25 mg simethicone in each 5 ml) when taken together, and by 25% when either the sucralfate or the antacid were taken 2 h previously. No change in bioavailability was seen in one subject when the sucralfate was given 2 h after the sulpiride.[1] The mechanisms of these interactions are not understood. Their clinical importance is not established but it would seem reasonable to give the sulpiride 2 h after and not before these other drugs.

Reference

1 Gouda MW, Hikal AH, Babhair SA, ElHofy SA and Mahrous GM. Effect of sucralfate and antacids on the bioavailability of sulpiride in humans. Int J Pharmaceut (1984) 22, 257–63.

Tetrabenazine + Chlorpromazine

Abstract/Summary

An isolated report describes severe Parkinson-like symptoms in a woman with Huntington's Chorea when given tetrabenazine and chlorpromazine.

Clinical evidence, mechanism, importance and management

A woman with Huntington's Chorea, successfully treated with 100 mg tetrabenazine daily for nine years, became motionless, rigid, mute and only able to respond by blinking her eyes within a day of being given two intramuscular injections of 25 mg chlorpromazine. This was diagnosed as severe drug-induced parkinsonism which rapidly responded to withdrawal of both drugs and treatment with bentropine mesylate given intramuscularly and orally.[1] The reason for this reaction is not understood. The authors of this report advise caution if tetrabenazine and other neuroleptics are given.

Reference

1 Moss JH and Stewart DE. Iatrogenic Parkinsonism in Huntington's chorea. Can J Psychiatry (1986) 31, 865–6.

Zolpidem + Miscellaneous drugs

Abstract/Summary

Zolpidem does not interact with warfarin, cimetidine or ranitidine. The sedative effects of chlorpromazine and haloperidol (and probably other sedative drugs) are increased to some extent by zolpidem. Heavy smoking possibly reduces its effects.

Clinical evidence, mechanism, importance and management

A study on the possible interactions of zolpidem[1] (a non-benzodiazepine hypnotic) found that the prothrombin times of eight normal subjects on warfarin were unaffected by four days' treatment with 20 mg zolpidem. The pharmacokinetics of zolpidem in six normal subjects were unaffected by either 1 g cimetidine or 300 mg ranitidine daily for 17 days.

Single 20 mg doses of zolpidem had no effect on the pharmacokinetics of chlorpromazine, imipramine or haloperidol, and neither 50 mg chlorpromazine, 75 mg imipramine nor 2 mg haloperidol had any effect on the pharmacokinetics of zolpidem. Both chlorpromazine and imipramine increased the sedative effects of zolpidem (as indicated by impaired performances of manual dexterity and Stroop's tests) and it seems likely that additive sedation will be seen with other sedative drugs. An anterograde amnesia was seen with zolpidem given with imipramine. There was no evidence that zolpidem could act as either an inducer or an inhibitor of liver microsomal enzymes.

It was also noted in these studies that two heavy smokers had a very high zolpidem clearance and did not experience any sedative effect.[1]

Reference

1 Harvengt C, Hulhoven R, Desager JP, Coupez JM, Guillet Ph, Fuseau E, Lambert D and Warrington SJ. Drug interactions investigated with zolpidem. In 'Imidazopyridines in Sleep Disorders', Sauvanet JP, Langer SZ and Morselli PL (eds.). Raven Press (1988) New York.

20

NEUROMUSCULAR BLOCKER
AND ANAESTHETIC
DRUG INTERACTIONS

This chapter is concerned with the interactions where the effects of neuromuscular blocking drugs and anaesthetics, both general and local, are affected by the presence of other drugs. Where these drugs are responsible for an interaction they are dealt with under the heading of the drug affected. See the index for a full listing.

Nerve impulses originating in the brain and intended to cause the contraction of voluntary muscles achieve the last stage of transmission by the release of acetylcholine from the nerve endings. This neurotransmitter rapidly diffuses across the minute gap which separates the nerve ending from the muscle tissue and attaches itself to the receptors in the specialized area of the muscle called the endplate. At rest this area has negative charges on the outside and positive charges inside, maintained by the energy-using activity of the cells, and is said to be polarized. The arrival of acetylcholine and its attachment to the receptors causes a local disturbance of the endplate, resulting in a reversal of the charges, or depolarization. If this is sufficiently large it sets in motion a much larger electrical disturbance which spreads out almost explosively across the membranes of the muscle fibre and results in its contraction. Almost immediately, within milliseconds, the receptors are cleared of acetylcholine by the activity of a localized enzyme, cholinesterase, in readiness for further stimulation, and the muscle endplate becomes repolarized.

Neuromuscular blockers are of two types. The non-depolarizing or competitive type of blocker (e.g., tubocurarine, gallamine, etc.) competes with acetylcholine for the receptors of the endplate, thereby excluding the acetylcholine and preventing it from acting. A group of drugs called the anticholinesterases, such as neostigmine, can be used as an antidote to this type of blockade because they inhibit the enzymes which destroy acetylcholine so that the concentrations of acetylcholine build up. Thus the competition between the molecules of the blocker and the acetylcholine for occupancy of the receptors swings in favour of the acetylcholine and transmission is restored. The other type of blocker, the depolarizing type, also occupy the receptors on the endplate but they differ in that they act like acetylcholine to cause depolarization. However, they are not immediately removed by cholinesterase so that the depolarization is maintained and the muscle become paralyzed. Anticholinesterase drugs increase the levels of acetylcholine so that they would enhance and prolong this type of blockade. Under some circumstances depolarizing blockade (type I) is converted to the competitive block (type II). The different types of blocker are listed in Table 20.1.

The general and local anaesthetics mentioned in this chapter are listed in Table 20.2. Some of them are also used as antiarrhythmic agents and these are dealt with in the antiarrhythmics chapter.

Table 20.1 Neuromuscular blockers

Non-proprietary names	Proprietary names
Non-depolarizing blockers	
Alcuronium chloride	*Alloferin(e), Aloferin*
Atracurium besylate	*Tacrium*
Fazadinium bromide	*Fazadon*
Gallium triethiodide	*Flaxedil, Miowas G*
Metocurine (dimethyltubocurarine)	*Metubine*
Pancuronium bromide	*Pavulon*
Tubocurarine chloride (curare, d-tubocurarine)	*Curarin(e), Intocostrin(e)-T, Jexin, Tubarine, Tubocuran*
Vecuronium bromide	*Norcuron*
Depolarizing blockers	
Carbolonium bromide(the blockade rapidly changes to non-depolarizing)	*Imbretil*
Decamethonium bromide	*Syncurine*
Decamethonium iodide (C10)	
Suxamethonium bromide/chloride	*Anectine, Brevidil M, Celocurin(e), (succinylcholine), Celocurin-Chloride/Klorid, Curalest, Clysthenon, Midarine, Mioflex, Muscuryl, Myoplegine, Pantolax, Paranoval, Scoline, Succinolin, Succinyl, Sucostrin*
Suxethonium bromide	*Brevidil-E*

Table 20.2 Anaesthetics

Non-proprietary names	Proprietary names
General anaesthetics	
Inhalation:	
Cyclopropane	—
Diethyl ether (ether)	
Enflurane	*Alyrane, Efrane, Ethrane, Inhelthran*
Fluroxene	—
Halothane	*Fluopan, Fluothane, Halovis, Rhodialothan, Somnothane*
Isoflurane	*Aerrane, Forane*
Methoxyflurane	*Penthrane*
Nitrous oxide	*Etonox (N_2O/O_2)*
Trichloroethylene	*Trilene, Triklone*
Parenteral:	
Alphaxalone/Alphadolone	*Alfatesin(e), Alfathesin, Alphadione, Althesin*
Ketamine hydrochloride	*Ketalar, Ketaject, Ketanest, Ketolar*
Thiopentone sodium	*Farmotal, Hypnostan, Intraval Sodium, Leopental, Nesdonal, Pentothal (sodium), Thiobarbityral, Tiobarbital, Trapanal*
Local anaesthetics	
Bupivacaine	
Chloroprocaine	
Lignocaine (lidocaine)	
Mepivacaine	
Procaine	
Propoxycaine	

Anaesthetics + Adrenaline, Noradrenaline and Terbutaline

Abstract/Summary

Patients anaesthetized with volatile anaesthetics (cyclopropane, halothane, enflurane, isoflurane, fluroxene, methoxyflurane, diethyl ether) can develop heart arrhythmias if given adrenaline (epinephrine) or noradrenaline (norepinephrine) unless the dosages are very low. Children appear to be less susceptible. Two patients developed arrhythmias when terbutaline was used with halothane. See also 'Anaesthetics + Phenylephrine'.

Clinical evidence, mechanism, importance and management

(a) Adrenaline and noradrenaline

Oliver and Schaefer were the first to observe in 1895 that an adrenal extract could cause ventricular fibrillation in a dog anaesthetized with chloroform,[1] and it is now very well recognized that similar cardiac dysrhythmias can be caused by adrenaline (epinephrine) and noradrenaline (norepinephrine) in man when anaesthetized with other volatile anaesthetics. A suggested listing of these anaesthetics in order of decreasing sensitivity is as follows: cyclopropane > halothane > enflurane = methoxyflurane > isoflurane = fluroxene > diethyl ether.[2]

The following recommendation has been made if adrenaline is used to reduce surgical bleeding in patients anaesthetized with halothane/nitrous oxide/oxygen: the dosage should not exceed 10 ml of 1:100,000 in any given 10 min period, nor 30 ml per h (i.e. about 100 μg or 1.5 μg/kg/10 min—for a 70 kg person).[3] This dosage guide should also be safe for use with other volatile anaesthetics since halothane and adrenaline are more arrhythmogenic than the others.[2] Solutions containing 0.5% lignocaine (lidocaine) with 1:100,000 also appear to be safe because lignocaine may help to control the potential dysrhythmic effects. For example, a study in 15 adult patients showed that the dose of adrenaline needed to cause three premature ventricular contractions in half the group was 2.11 μg/kg in saline, but 3.69 μg/kg in 0.5% lignocaine (lidocaine).[4] However it should be borne in mind that the arrhythmogenic effects of adrenaline are increased if sympathetic activity is increased, and in hyperthyroidism and hypercapnia.[2]

Children appear to be much less susceptible than adults. A retrospective study of 28 children showed no evidence of dysrhythmia during halothane anaesthesia with adrenaline doses of up to 8.8 μg/kg, and a subsequent study on 83 children (three months to 17 years) found that 10 μg/kg doses were safe.[5]

(b) Terbutaline

Two patients have been described who developed ventricular arrhythmias while anaesthetized with halothane and nitrous oxide/oxygen when given 0.25–0.35 mg terbutaline subcutaneously for wheezing. Both developed unifocal premature ventricular contractions followed by bigeminy which responded to lignocaine.[6] Halothane was also replaced by enflurane in one case. See also 'Anaesthetics + Phenylephrine'.

References

1 Oliver G and Schaefer EA. The physiological effects of extracts of the suprarenal capsules. J Physiol (1895) 18, 230.
2 Wong KC. Sympathomimetic drugs. In 'Drug Interactions in Anesthesia' Smith NT, Miller RD and Corbascio AN (eds). Lea and Febiger, Philadelphia (1981) p 66.
3 Katz RL, Matteo RS and Papper EM. The injection of epinephrine during general anesthesia with halogenated hydrocarbons and cyclopropane in man. 2. Halothane. Anesthesiology (1962) 23, 597–600.
4 Johnston RR, Eger EI and Wilson C. A comparative interaction of epinephrine with enflurane, isoflurane and halothane in man. Anesth Analg (1976) 55, 709–12.
5 Karl HW, Swedlow DB, Leed KW and Downes JJ. Epinephrine-halothane interactions in children. Anesthesiology (1983) 58, 142–5.
6 Thiagarajah S, Grynsztejn M, Lear E and Azar I. Ventricular arrhythmias after terbutaline administration to patients anaesthetized with halothane. Anaesth Analg (1986) 65, 417–8.

Anaesthetics + Alcohol

Abstract/Summary

Those who regularly drink need more thiopentone than those who do not drink.

Clinical evidence, mechanism, importance and management

A study in 532 healthy subjects aged 20–80 showed that those who normally drink alcohol need more thiopentone to achieve anaesthesia than non-drinkers. After adjusting for differences in age and weight distribution, men drinkers (< 40 g alcohol daily) needed 33% more thiopentone for induction than non-drinkers, and women drinkers needed 40% more.

Reference

1 Dundee JW and Milligan KR. Induction dose of thiopentone: the effect of alcohol intake. Br j Clin Pharmac (1989) 27, 693–4P.

Anaesthetics + Anaesthetics

Abstract/Summary

An isolated report describes myoclonic seizures in a man anaesthetized with Alfathesin (alphaxolone-alphadolone) when additionally given enflurane.

Clinical evidence

Anaesthesia was induced uneventfully in a normal man of 23 with 2.5 ml Alfathesin (alphaxolone and alphadolone) given intravenously over 2 min. Anaesthesia was then maintained with 2% enflurane in oxygen through a circle absorber system. After 8 min the patient began to have intermittent myoclonic activity (violent flexion of the extremities and contraction of trunk and facial muscles). The enflurane was stopped and anaesthesia maintained with nitrous oxide and oxygen. The myclonic activity ceased within 3 min. After several minutes the enflurane was restarted and within 3 min the myclonus began again, but it resolved when the enflurane was stopped.[1]

Mechanism

Uncertain. Alfathesin can causes seizures even in normal subjects and enflurane can cause CNS excitation. It seems possible that these effects may be additive, and possibly exacerbated if hypocapnia also occurs.

Importance and management

Direct information seems to be confined to this single report. It has been suggested that concurrent use should be avoided, particularly in patients with known convulsive disorders.[1] Alfathesin has been withdrawn from general use.

Reference

1   Hudson R and Ethans CT. Alfathesin and enflurane: synergistic central nervous system excitation? Canad Anaesth Soc J (1981) 28, 55–60.

Anaesthetics (Methoxyflurane) + Antibiotics and Barbiturates

Abstract/Summary

The nephrotoxic effects of methoxyflurane are increased by the use of barbiturates, tetracyclines and possibly some aminoglycoside antibiotics.

Clinical evidence, mechanism, importance and management

Methoxyflurane has been withdrawn in many countries because it causes kidney damage. This damage can be exacerbated by the concurrent use of some drugs. Five out of seven patients anaesthetized with methoxyflurane who had been given tetracycline before or after surgery showed rises in blood urea nitrogen and creatinine, and three died. Postmortem examination showed pathological changes (oxalosis) in the kidneys.[1] Other reports support this finding.[2–4] Penicillin, streptomycin and chloramphenical appear not to increase the renal toxicity,[1] but gentamicin and kanamycin possibly do so.[5] There is also some evidence that barbiturates can exacerbate the renal toxicity because they alter the metabolism of the methoxyflurane and increase the production of nephrotoxic metabolites.[6,7]

References

1   Kuzucu EY. Methoxyflurane, tetracycline and renal failure. J Amer Med Ass (1970) 211, 1162.

2   Albers DD, Leverett CL and Sandin JH. Renal failure following prostatovesiculectomy related to methoxyflurane anesthesia and tetracycline—complicated by Candida infection. J Urol (1971) 106, 348.
3   Proctor EA and Barton FL. Polyuric acute renal failure after methoxyflurane and tetracycline. Br Med J (1971) 4, 661.
4   Stoelting RK and Gibbs PS. Effect of tetracycline therapy on renal function after methoxyflurane anaesthesia. Anesth Analg (1973) 52, 431.
5   Cousins MJ and Mazze RI. Tetracycline, methoxyflurane anaesthetics and renal dysfunction. Lancet (1972) i, 751.
6   Churchill D, Yacoub JM, Siu KP, Symes A and Gault MH. Toxic nephropathy after low-dose methoxyflurane anesthesia: drug interaction with secobarbital? Canad Med Ass J (1976) 114, 326.
7   Cousins MJ and Mazze RI. Methoxyflurane nephrotoxicity: a study of dose response in man. J Amer Med Ass (1973) 225, 1611.

Anaesthetics + Antihypertensives

Abstract/Summary

Concurrent use normally need not be avoided but it should be recognized that the normal homeostatic responses of the cardiovascular system will be impaired.

Clinical evidence, mechanism, importance and management

The antihypertensive drugs differ in the way they act, but they all interfere with the normal homeostatic mechanisms which control blood pressure and, as a result, the reaction of the cardiovascular system during anaesthesia to fluid and blood losses, body positioning, etc. is impaired to some extent. This instability of the cardiovascular system needs to be recognized and allowed for but it is widely accepted that the antihypertensive treatment should be continued.[1,2] In some cases there is a real risk in stopping, for example a hypertensive rebound can occur if clonidine or the betablockers are suddenly withdrawn. See also 'Clonidine+Betablockers', and 'Anaesthetics+Beta-blockers'. However a warning has been sounded about severe and unexpected hypotension seen during induction in patients on captopril.[3]

References

1   Craig DB and Bose D. Drug interactions in anaesthesia: chronic antihypertensive therapy. Can Anaesth Soc J (1984) 31, 580–8.
2   Foex P, Cutfield GR and Francis CM. Interactions of cardiovascular drugs with inhalation anaesthetics. Anaesthesiol Intensivmed (Berlin) (1982) 150, 109–28.
3   McConachie I and Healy TEJ. ACE inhibitors and anaesthesia. Postgrad Med J (1989) 65, 273–4.

Anaesthetics + Beta-blockers

Abstract/Summary

Anaesthesia in the presence of beta-blockers appears to be safer than withdrawal of the beta-blocker before anaesthesia, provided certain anaesthetics are avoided (methoxyflurane, cyclopropane, diethyl-ether, trichloroethylene) and atropine is used to prevent bradycardia. See also 'Anaesthetics+Timolol', and 'Beta-blockers+Anticholinesterases'.

Clinical evidence and mechanism

It used to be thought that beta-blockers should be withdrawn from patients before surgery because of the risk that their cardiac depressant effects would be additive with those of volatile anaesthetics, reducing cardiac output and lowering blood pressure, but it seems to depend on the anaesthetic used.[1] Lowenstein has drawn up a ranking order of compatibility (from the least to the most compatible) as follows: methoxyflurane, diethyl-ether, cyclopropane, trichloroethylene, enflurane, halothane, narcotics, isoflurane.[1]

(a) Cyclopropane, diethyl-ether, methoxyflurane, trichloroethylene

A risk certainly seems to exist with cyclopropane and diethylether because their depressant effects on the heart are normally counteracted by the release of catecholamines, which would be blocked by the presence of a beta-blocker. There is also evidence (both clinical and animal) that unacceptable cardiac depression may also occur with methoxyflurane and trichloroethylene when a beta-blocker is present.[2,3] For these four anaesthetics it has been stated that an absolute indication for their use should exist before giving them in combination with a beta-blocker.[1]

(b) Enflurane, halothane, isoflurane, narcotics

The situation with enflurane is not clear because it has been widely used with propranolol without apparent difficulties,[1] but a marked reduction in cardiac performance has also been described.[2,3] However beta-blockers and halothane, isoflurane or narcotics appear to be safe.

On the positive side there appear to be considerable benefits to be gained from the continued use of beta-blockers during anaesthesia. Their sudden withdrawal from patients treated for angina or hypertension can result in the development of acute and life-threatening cardiovascular complications (possibly due to the increased sensitivity of the receptors) whether the patient is undergoing surgery or not. In the perioperative period patients benefit from beta-blockade because it can minimize the effects of sympathetic overactivity of the cardiovascular system during anaesthesia and surgery (for example during endotracheal intubation, laryngoscopy, bronchoscopy and various surgical manoeuvres) which can cause heart dysrrhythmias and hypertension.

Importance and management

The consensus of opinion is that beta-blockers should not be withdrawn before anaesthesia and surgery because the advantages of maintaining blockade and the risks accompanying withdrawal are considerable. But it is important to select the safest anaesthetics (isoflurane, halothane, narcotics), to avoid those which appear to be most risky (methoxyflurane, diethylether, chloroform, cyclopropane, trichloroethylene) and to ensure that the patient is protected against bradycardia by atropine (1–2 mg intravenously). See also 'Anaesthetics + Timolol', and 'Beta-blockers + Anticholinesterases'.

References

1 Lowenstein E. Beta-adrenergic blockers. in 'Drug Interactions in Anesthesia.' Smith NT, Miller RD and Corbascio AN (eds). Lea and Febiger, Philadelphia (1981) p 83–101.
2 Foex P, Cutfield GR and Francis CM. Interactions of cardiovascular drugs with inhalation anaesthetics. Anaesthesiol Intensivemed (Berlin) (1982) 150, 109–28.
3 Foex P, Francis CM and Cutfield GR. The interactions between beta-blockers and anaesthetics. Experimental observations. Acta Anaesth scand (1982) Suppl 76, 38–46.

Anaesthetics + Calcium channel blockers

Abstract/Summary

Impaired myocardial conduction has been seen in two patients on diltiazem when anaesthetized with enflurane, but it has been suggested that the concurrent use of anaesthetics and calcium channel blockers is normally without problems.

Clinical evidence, mechanism, importance and management

The author of a review about calcium channel blockers and anaesthetics concludes that concurrent use is normally beneficial except where there are other complicating factors. Thus he warns about possible decreases in ventricular function in patients undergoing open chest surgery given intravenous verapamil or diltiazem.[1] A report describes a patient on diltiazem and atenolol who had impaired AV and sinus node function before anaesthesia which worsened when given enflurane.[2] Another patient also on diltiazem demonstrated severe sinus bradycardia which progressed to asystole when enflurane was used.[2] The authors of this latter report suggest that enflurane and diltiazem can have additive depressant effects on myocardial conduction. Some caution is clearly appropriate.

References

1 Merin RG. Calcium channel blocking drugs and anesthetics: is the drug interaction beneficial or detrimental? Anesthesiology (1987) 66, 111–13.
2 Hantler CB, Wilton N, Learned DM, Hill AEG and Knight PR. Impaired myocardial conduction in patients receiving diltiazem therapy during enflurane anesthesia. Anesthesiology (1987) 67, 94–6.

Anaesthetics + Fenfluramine

Abstract/Summary

An isolated case of fatal cardiac arrest has been attributed to halothane anaesthesia in a woman taking fenfluramine. Animal studies confirm that combined use can cause serious heart arrhythmias and myocardial depression.

Clinical evidence, mechanism, importance and management

A 23-year-old woman, premedicated with diazepam and hyoscine, anaesthetized initially with thiopentone followed by suxamethonium and later halothane with oxygen, became pulseless, cyanosed and showed acute pulmonary oedema within 5 min of induction. She failed to respond to resuscitative measures including cardiac massage. It was later discovered that she had been taking fenfluramine. Later studies in animals showed that during the concurrent use of halothane and fenfluramine, marked ECG changes, sinus bradycardia, heart block, ventricular asystoles, paroxysmal ventricular tachycardia and fibrillation occurred.[1] The reasons are not understood. This is an isolated case and the authors of the report recommend that patients on fenfluramine should not be anaesthetized with halothane,[1] but to keep this alleged interaction in perspective it should be said that the evidence for it has come under heavy fire from at least one author.[2]

References

1 Bennett JA and Eltingham RJ. Possible dangers of anaesthesia in patients receiving fenfluramine. Anesthesia (1977) 32, 8.
2 Winnie AP. Fenfluramine and halothane. Anesthesia (1979) 34, 79.

Anaesthetics + Monoamine oxidase inhibitors

Abstract/Summary

The usual advice is that MAOI should be withdrawn well before anaesthesia, but there is evidence that this is normally unnecessary in most patients, although individual cases of both hypo- and hypertension have been seen. The MAOI can however interact with other drugs sometimes used during surgery.

Clinical evidence and mechanism

The absence of problems during emergency general anaesthesia of two patients on MAOI, prompted further study in six others taking un-named MAOI chronically. All six were premedicated with 10–15 mg diazepam 2 h before surgery. Anaesthesia was induced with thiopentone, intubation facilitated with suxamethonium (succinylcholine), and maintained with nitrous oxide/oxygen and either halothane or isoflurane. Pancuronium was used for muscle relaxation. Morphine was given postoperatively. One patient experienced hypotension which responded to repeated doses of 0.1 mg phenylephrine (IV) without hypertensive reactions. No untoward events occurred either during or after the anaesthesia.[1] A later anaesthetic study on 27 other patients on MAOI (tranylcypromine, phenelzine, isocarboxazid, pargyline) by the same group of workers also found no evidence of adverse reactions.[3] Unexplained hypertension has been described in a patient taking tranylcypromine when etomidate and atracurium were used.[4]

Importance and management

There seems to be little or no documentary evidence that the withdrawal of MAOI before anaesthesia is normally necessary. Scrutiny of reports[2] alleging an adverse reaction usually shows that what happened could be attributed to an interaction between other drugs used during the surgery (e.g. pethidine, sympathomimetics) rather than with the anaesthetics. The authors of the report cited[1,3] here offer the opinion that '...general and regional anesthesia may be provided safely without discontinuation of MAOI therapy, provided proper monitoring, adequate preparation, and prompt treatment of anticipated reactions are utilized.'[1] This implies that the possible interactions between the MAOI and other drugs are fully recognized. Also be alert for the rare unpredictable response.

References

1 El-Ganzouri A, Ivankovich AD, Braverman B and Land PC. Should MAOI be discontinued preoperatively? Anesthesiology (1983) 59, A384.
2 Jenkins LC and Graves HB. Potential hazards of psychoactive drugs in association with anesthesia. Can Anaesth Soc J (1965) 12, 121–8.
3 El-Ganzouri AR, Ivankovitch AD, Braverman B and McCarthy R. Monoamine Oxidase Inhibitors: should they be discontinued preoperatively? Anesth Analg (1985) 64, 592–6.
4 Sides CA. Hypertension during anaesthesia with monoamine oxidase inhibitors. Anaesthesia (1987) 42, 633–5.

Anaesthetics + Neuromuscular blockers

Abstract/Summary

The inhalation anaesthetics (diethyl ether, halothane, enflurane, isoflurane, etc.) increase neuromuscular blockade to differing extents, but nitrous oxide appears not to interact.

Clinical evidence, mechanism, importance and management

Neuromuscular blockade is increased by inhalation anaesthetics, the greater the dosage of the anaesthetic the greater the increase in blockade. In broad terms diethyl ether, enflurane, isoflurane and methoxyflurane have a greater effect than halothane, which is more potent than fluroxene and cyclopropane, whereas nitrous oxide appears not to interact.[1–5] The reasons are not fully understood but the following mechanisms have been suggested: the anaesthetic may have an effect via the CNS, or it may affect the muscle membrane, or possibly that some change in blood flow to the muscle occurs. These anaesthetics do not seem to affect either the release of acetylcholine at neuromuscular junctions or the acetylcholine receptors. The dosage of the neuromuscular blocker may need to be adjusted according to the anaesthetic in use. For example, the dosage of atracurium can be reduced by 25–30% if, instead of balanced anaesthesia (with thiopentone, fentanyl and nitrous oxide/oxygen),[1] enflurane is used, and by about 50% if isoflurane is used.[2] Another study showed that the reversal of blockade by pancuronium with neostigmine was prolonged (roughly doubled) when using enflurane.[6]

References

1 Ramsey FM, White PA, Stullken EH, Allen LL and Roy RC. Enflurane potentiation of neuromuscular blockade by atracurium. Anesthesiology (1982) 57, A255.
2 Sokoll MD, Gergis SD, Mehta M, Ali NM and Lineberry C. Safety and efficacy of atracurium (BW33A) in surgical patients receiving balanced or isoflurane anesthesia. Anesthesiology (1983) 58, 450–5.
3 Schuh FT. Differential increase in potency of neuromuscular blocking agents by enflurane and halothane. Int J Clin Pharmacol Ther Toxicol (1983) 21, 383–6.
4 Fogdall RP and Miller RD. Neuromuscular effects of enflurane alone and in combination with d-tubocurarine, pancuronium and succinylcholine in man. Anesthesiology (1975) 42, 173–8.
5 Miller RD, Way WL, Dolan WM, Stevens WC and Eger EI. Comparative neuromuscular effects of pancuronium, gallamine, and succinylcholine during Forane and halothane anaesthesia in man. Anesthesiology (1971) 35, 509–14.
6 Delisle S and Bevan DR. Impaired neostigmine antagonism of pancuronium during enflurane anaesthesia in man. Br J Anaesth (1982) 54, 441–5.

Anaesthetics + Phenylephrine

Abstract/Summary

Phenylephrine eye drops caused marked cyanosis and bradycardia in a baby anaesthetized with halothane, and hypertension in a woman anaesthetized with isoflurane.

Clinical evidence, mechanism, importance and management

A three-week-old baby anaesthetized with halothane and nitrous oxide/oxygen became cyanosed shortly after the instillation of two drops of 10% phenylephrine solution in one eye. The heart rate decreased from 160 to 60 bpm, S-T segment and T wave changes were seen, and blood pressure measurements were unobtainable. The baby recovered uneventfully when anaesthesia was stopped and oxygen administered. It was suggested that the phenylephrine caused severe peripheral vasodilatation and reflex bradycardia. An adult patient aged 54 anaesthetized with isoflurane developed marked hypertension (a rise from 125/70 to 200/90 mm Hg) shortly after having two drops of 10% phenylephrine in one eye which responded to nasal nitroglycerin and increasing concentrations of isoflurane.[1] The authors of this report say that during anaesthesia the use of phenylephrine should be discouraged, but if necessary use the lowest concentrations of phenylephrine (2.5%). They also point out that the following are effective mydriatics: single drop combinations of 0.5% cyclopentolate and 2.5% phenylephrine or 0.5% tropicamide and 2.5% phenylephrine.

Reference

1 Van der Spek AFL and Hantler CB. Phenylephrine eyedrops and anaesthesia. Anesthesiology (1986) 64, 812–4.

Anaesthetics + Phenytoin or Phenobarbitone

Abstract/Summary

Phenytoin intoxication occurred in a child following halothane anaesthesia, and fatal hepatic necrosis occurred in a woman on phenytoin, phenobarbitone and phenylbutazone after being anaesthetized with fluroxene.

Clinical evidence, mechanism, importance and management

A 10-year-old epileptic girl on long-term treatment with phenytoin (300 mg daily) was admitted to hospital for surgery and was found to have phenytoin serum levels of 25 μg/ml. Three days after anaesthesia with halothane her serum phenytoin levels had risen to 41 μg/ml and she had marked signs of phenytoin intoxication.[1] The probable reason is that the general toxic effects of halothane on the liver slowed the normal rate of phenytoin metabolism so that the serum levels rose. Another epileptic patient controlled on 300 mg phenytoin, 120 mg phenobarbitone and phenylbutazone needed an increase in her phenytoin dosage to 2400 mg daily a week before surgery. She died of massive hepatic necrosis 36 h after anaesthesia with fluroxene.[2]

A suggested explanation is that, just as in animals, pretreatment with phenobarbitone and phenytoin increases the rate of drug metabolism and the hepatotoxicity of halogenated hydrocarbons including chloroform and carbon tetrachlorides.[3] The same may possibly apply to man. No firm conclusions can be drawn from these two cases, but they serve to emphasise the potential hepatotoxicity of these anaesthetics. The authors of the second report[2] suggest that patients with similar drug histories may constitute a high-risk group for liver damage after halogen or vinyl-radical anaesthetics.

References

1 Karline JM and Kutt H. Acute diphenylhydantoin intoxication following halothane anesthesia. J Pediat (1970) 76, 941.
2 Reynolds ES, Brown BR and Vandam LD. Massive hepatic necrosis after fluroxene anesthesia—a case of drug interaction? N Engl J Med (1972) 286, 530.
3 Garner RC and McLean AEM. Increased susceptibility to carbon tetrachloride poisoning in the rat after pretreatment with oral phenobarbitone. Biochem Pharmacol (1969) 18, 645.

Anaesthetics and/or Neuromuscular blockers + Theophylline

Abstract/Summary

Cardiac arrhythmias can develop during the concurrent use of halothane and theophylline but this is possibly less likely with isoflurane. Supraventricular tachycardia occurred in a patient on aminophylline when given pancuronium. Seizures have been attributed to an interaction between ketamine and theophylline.

Clinical evidence, mechanism, importance and management

(a) Development of arrhythmias

A number of reports describe arrhythmias apparently due to an interaction between halothane and theophylline. One describes intraoperative arrhythmias in four out of 67 adult asthmatics given theophylline and halothane (one had supraventricular tachycardia, two had bigeminy and one had multifocal premature ventricular contractions).[9] Nine out of another 45 patients developed heart rates exceeding 145 when given both drugs, whereas no tachycardia occurred in 22 other patients given only halothane.[9] There are other reports of individual adult and child patients who developed ventricular tachycardias[10] attributed to this interaction.[1,8,11,12] One child developed cardiac arrest.[11] The same interaction has been reported in animals.[2,3] Another report describes supraventricular tachycardia in a patient on aminophylline who was anaesthetized with thiopentone and fentanyl, followed by pancuronium. 3 min later his heart rate rose to 180 bpm and the ECG revealed that it was supraventricular in origin.[7] The authors of this report attributed this reaction to an interaction between the pancuronium and the aminophylline. The suggested reason for the interaction with halothane is that the theophylline causes the release of catecholamines (adrenaline—epinephrine, noradrenaline—norepinephrine) from the adrenal medulla which are known to sensitize the myocardium.

The authors of one of the reports advise the avoidance of concurrent use[1] but another says that: '...my own experience with the liberal use of these drugs has convinced me of the efficacy and wide margin of safety associated with their use in combination.'[4] A possibly safer anaesthetic may be isoflurane which in studies with dogs has been shown not to cause cardiac arrhythmias in the presence of aminophylline.[5]

(b) Development of seizures

Tachycardia and extensor-type seizures occurred in four patients initially anaesthetized with ketamine and later with halothane or enflurane.[6] The authors attributed the seizures to an interaction between ketamine and theophylline (aminophylline) and they suggest avoidance of the combination or the use of antiseizure premedication in patients at risk.

(c) Increased neuromuscular blockade

A study in rabbits showed that at therapeutic concentrations the effects of tubocurarine were increased by theophylline, but this does not seem to have been observed in man.[13]

References

1 Roizen MF and Stevens WC. Multiform ventricular tachycardia due to the interaction of aminophylline and halothane. Anesth Analg (1978) 57, 738.
2 Takori M and Loehning RW. Ventricular arrhythmias induced by aminophylline during halothane anaesthesia in dogs. Can Anesth Soc J (1967) 14, 79.
3 Stirt JA, Berger JM, Ricker SM and Sullivan SF. Halothane-induced cardiac arrhythmias following administration of aminophylline in experimental animals. Anesth Analg (1981) 60, 517–20.
4 Zimmerman BL. Arrhythmogenicity of theophylline and halothane used in combination. Anesth Analg (1979) 58, 259.
5 Stirt JA, Berger JM and Sullivan SF. Lack of arrhythmogenicity of isoflurane following administration of aminophylline in dogs. Anesth Analg (1983) 62, 568–71.
6 Hirshman CA, Krieger W, Littlejohn G, Lee R and Julien R. Ketamine-aminophylline-induced decrease in seizure threshold. Anesthesiology (1982) 56, 464–7.
7 Belani KG, Anderson WW and Buckley JJ. Adverse drug interaction involving pancuronium and aminophylline. Anesth Analg (1982) 61, 473–4.
8 Naito Y, Arai T and Miyake C. Severe arrhythmias due to the combined use of halothane and aminophylline in an asthmatic patient. Jpn J Anaesthesiol (1986) 35, 1126–9.
9 Barton MD. Anesthetic problems with aspirin-intolerant patients. Anesth Analg (1975) 54, 376.
10 Roizen MF and Stevens WC. Multiform ventricular tachycardia due to the interaction of aminophylline and halothane. Anesth Analg (1978) 57, 738.
11 Bedger RC, Chang JL and Larson CE. Increased myocardial irritability with halothane and aminophylline. Anesth Prog (1980) 27, 34.
12 Richards W, Thompson J, Lewis G, Levy DS and Church JA. Cardiac arrest associated with halothane anesthesia in a patient receiving theophylline. Ann Allergy (1988) 61, 83–4.
13 Fuke N, Martyn J, Kim C and Basta S. Concentration-dependent interaction of theophylline with d-tubocurarine. J Appl Physiol (1987) 62, 1970–4.

Anaesthetics + Timolol

Abstract/Summary

Marked bradycardia and hypotension occurred in a man using timolol eye-drops when he was anaesthetized.

Clinical evidence, mechanism, importance and management

A 75-year-old man being treated with timolol eye drops for glaucoma developed bradycardia and severe hypotension when anaesthetized (agent not named) which responded poorly to atropine, dextrose-saline infusion and elevation of his feet.[1] It would seem that there was sufficient systemic absorption of the timolol for it to join with the anaesthetic to cause marked depression of cardiac activity. The authors of this report suggest that if patients are to be anaesthetized, low concentrations of timolol should be used (possibly withhold the drops pre-operatively), and that '...induction agents should be used judiciously and beta-blocking antagonists kept readily available.' It is easy to overlook the fact that systemic absorption from eye-drops can be remarkably high. See also 'Anaesthetics + Beta-blockers'.

Reference

1 Mostafa SM. Ocular timolol and induction agents during anaesthesia. Br Med J (1985) 290, 1788.

Anaesthetics + Tricyclic antidepressants

Abstract/Summary

Some very limited evidence suggests that amitriptyline may increase the likelihood of enflurane-induced seizure activity. Tachyarrhythmias have been seen in patients on imipramine when given halothane and pancuronium.

Clinical evidence, mechanism, importance and management

(a) Enflurane + amitriptyline

Two patients taking amitriptyline have been described who showed clonic movements of the leg, arm and hand during surgery while anaesthetized with enflurane and nitrous oxide. The movements stopped when the enflurane was replaced by halothane.[1] A possible reason is that amitriptyline can lower the seizure threshold at which enflurane-induced seizure activity occurs. It is suggested that it may be advisable to avoid enflurane in patients needing tricyclic antidepressants, particularly in those who have a history of seizure or when hyperventilation or high concentrations of enflurane are likely to be used.[1]

(b) Halothane + imipramine and pancuronium

Two patients taking imipramine developed marked tachyarrhthmias when anaesthetized with halothane and given pancuronium.[2] This adverse interaction was subsequently clearly demonstrated in dogs.[2] The authors concluded on the basis of their studies that (i) gallamine should be avoided but tubocurarine would be an acceptable alternative to pancuronium; (ii) caution is appropriate if patients are taking any tricyclic antidepressant and halothane is used; (iii) pancuronium is probably safe in the presence of a tricyclic if enflurane is used. More study is needed.

Reference

1 Sprague DH and Wolf S. Enflurane seizures in patients taking amitriptyline. Anesth Analg (1982) 61, 67–8.
2 Edwards RP, Miller RD, Roizen MF, Ham J, Way WL, Lake CR and Roderick L. Cardiac responses to imipramine and pancuronium during anesthesia with halothane and enflurane. Anesthesiology (1979) 50, 421–5.

Anaesthetics, local + Alcohol and Antirheumatics

Abstract/Summary

The failure rate of spinal anaesthesia with bupivacaine is markedly increased in patients who are receiving anti-rheumatic drugs and who drink.

Clinical evidence, mechanism, importance and management

The observation that regional anaesthetic failures seemed to be particularly high among patients undergoing orthopaedic surgery who were suffering from rheumatic joint diseases, prompted further study of a possible interaction involving antirheumatic drugs and alcohol. It was found that the failure rate of low-dose spinal anaesthesia with bupivacaine (2 ml of 0.5%) increased from 5% in the control group (no alcohol or treatment) to 32–45% in those who had been taking antirheumatic drugs for at least six months or who drank at least 80 g ethanol daily, or both. The percentage of those patients who had a reduced response (i.e. an extended latency period and a reduced duration of action). also increased from 3 to 39–42%. Indomethacin was the specific antirheumatic drug studied in one group.[1]

Reference

1 Sprotte G and Weis KH. Drug interaction with local anaesthetics. Brit J Anaesth (1982) 54, 242P.

Anaesthetics, local + Anaesthetics, local

Abstract/Summary

Mixtures of local anaesthetics are sometimes used to exploit the most useful characteristics of each drug. This normally seems to be safe although it is sometimes claimed that it increases the risk of toxicity. There is a case report of a man who developed toxicity when bupivacaine and mepivacaine were mixed together.

Clinical evidence and mechanism

Local anaesthetics are sometimes mixed together to take advantage of the rapid onset and penetration of one anaesthetic with the prolonged duration of the other.

(a) Evidence of no interaction

A study designed to assess the possibility of adverse interactions in man retrospectively studied the records of 10,538 patients over the 1952–72 period who had been given amethocaine (tetracaine) combined with chloroprocaine, lignocaine (lidocaine), mepivacaine, prilocaine, procaine or propoxycaine for caudal, epidural, brachial plexus, or peripheral nerve block. The incidence of systemic toxic reactions was found to be no greater than when used singly and the conclusion was reached that combined use was advantageous and safe.[1] An animal study using combinations of bupivacaine, lidocaine (lignocaine) and chloroprocaine also found no evidence that the toxicity was greater than if the anaesthetics were used singly.[3] Lignocaine does not affect the pharmacokinetics of bupivacaine in man.[4]

(b) Evidence of a toxic interaction

An animal study showed that if amethocaine (tetracaine) was combined with other local anaesthetics the incidence of systemic toxicity and deaths increased.[1] There is a single case report of a patient given 2% bupivacaine and 0.75% mepivacaine who demonstrated lethargy, dysarthria and mild muscle tremor which the authors of the report correlated with a marked increase in the percentage of unbound (active) bupivacaine. They attributed this to its displacement by the mepivacaine from protein binding sites.[2]

Importance and management

An extensively examined interaction. The overall picture is that combined use does not normally result in increased toxicity although the isolated case report cited above illustrates that the possibility cannot be entirely discounted.

References

1 Moore DC, Bridenbaugh LD, Bridenbaugh PO, Thompson GE and Tucker GT. Does compounding of local anaesthetic agents increase their toxicity in humans? Anesth Analg (1972) 51, 579–85.
2 Hartrick CT, Raj PP, Dirkes WE and Denson DD. Compounding of bupivacaine and mepivacaine for regional anaesthesia. A safe practice? Reg Anaesth (1984) 9, 94–7.
3 De Jong RH and Bonin JD. Mixtures of local anesthetics are no more toxic than the parent drugs. Anesthesiology (1981) 54, 177–81.
4 Freysz M, Beal JL, D'Athis P, Mounie J, Wilkening M and Escousse A. Pharmacokinetics of bupivacaine after axillary brachial plexus block. Int J Clin Pharmacol Ther Tox (1987) 25, 392–5.

Anaesthetics, local + Benzodiazepines

Abstract/Summary

There is conflicting evidence about whether diazepam can increase or decrease serum bupivacaine levels.

Clinical evidence, mechanism, importance and management

21 children aged 2–10 were given single caudal injections of 1 ml/kg of a mixture of 0.5% lignocaine (lidocaine) and 0.125% bupivacaine for regional anaesthesia. Pretreatment with 10 mg diazepam rectally half-an-hour before the surgery had no significant effect on the serum levels of lignocaine, but the AUC and maximal serum bupivacaine levels were increased by 70–75%.[1] This finding conflicts with another in which IV diazepam in adult patients decreased the elimination half-life of epidural bupivacaine.[2]

The diazepam/bupivacaine interaction is not established but anaesthetists should be aware that increased serum levels have been observed. More study is needed.

References

1 Giaufre E, Bruguerolle B, Morisson-Lacombe G and Rousset-Rouviere B. The influence of diazepam on the plasma concentrations of bupivacaine and lignocaine after caudal injection of a mixture of the local anaesthetics in children. Br J clin Pharmac (1988) 26, 116–8.
2 Giasi RM, D'Agostino E and Covino BG. Interaction of diazepam in epidurally administered local anaesthetic agents. Reg Anesth (1980) 5, 8–11.

Anaesthetics, local + Beta-blockers

Abstract/Summary

Propranolol reduces the clearance of bupivacaine and there is the theoretical possibility that the toxicity of bupivacaine may be increased.

Clinical evidence, mechanism, importance and management

A study in six normal subjects showed that the clearance of bupivacaine (30–50 mg IV over 10–15 min) was reduced by 35% (from 0.33 to 0.21 l/min) after taking 40 mg propranolol six-hourly for a day. The reason is thought to be that the propranolol inhibits the activity of the liver microsomal enzymes, thereby reducing the metabolism of the bupivacaine. Changes in blood flow to the liver are unlikely to affect bupivacaine metabolism substantially because it is relatively poorly extracted from the blood. The clinical importance of this interaction is uncertain, but it is suggested that an increase in local anaesthetic toxicity might occur and caution should be exercised if multiple doses of bupivacaine are given.[1] Direct information about other beta-blockers is lacking, but some of them are known to reduce the metabolism of lignocaine (lidocaine). See 'Lignocaine (Lidocaine) + Beta-blockers'.

Reference

1 Bowdle TA, Freund PR and Slattery JT. Propranolol reduces bupivacaine clearance. Anesthesiology (1987) 66, 36–8.

Anaesthetics, local + Cimetidine or Ranitidine

Abstract/Summary

Some studies suggest that both cimetidine and ranitidine can raise bupivacaine levels whereas other evidence suggests that no significant interaction occurs.

Clinical evidence

A controlled study in 36 patients undergoing caesarian section with 0.5% bupivacaine for epidural anaesthesia showed that pretreatment with a single 300 mg dose of cimetidine IM 1–4 h had no effect on the pharmacokinetics of bupivacaine in either mother or foetus, although the unbound bupivacaine levels rose by 22%.[1] Four normal male subjects who were given 400 mg cimetidine at 10.00 pm the previous evening and 8.00 am the following morning, followed by a 50 mg infusion of bupivacaine at 11.0 am, showed a 40% increase in the bupivacaine AUC (area under the curve). 150 mg ranitidine caused a 25% increase but it was not statistically significant.[2] Another study in 16 patients showed that pretreatment with 150 mg ranitidine orally 2 h before bupivacaine for extradural anaesthesia for caesarian section increased the serum levels of bupivacaine at 40 min by about 20%.[3] Similar results by the same group of authors are reported elsewhere.[4] No increased bupivacaine toxicity was reported in any of these reports.

Mechanism

Not understood. A reduction in the metabolism of the bupivacaine by the liver caused by the cimetidine is one suggested explanation. Protein binding displacement is another.

Importance and management

A confusing situation. No clinically important interaction has been established but be alert for any evidence of increased bupivacaine toxicity resulting from raised total serum levels and rises in unbound levels during concurrent use. Cimetidine (but not ranitidine) also raises serum lignocaine (lidocaine) levels when used as an antiarrhythmic agent (see 'Lignocaine + Cimetidine'). More study is needed.

References

1 Kuhnert BR, Zuspan KJ, Kuhnert PM, Syracuse CD, Brashear WT and Brown DE. Lack of influence of cimetidine on bupivacaine levels during parturition. Anesth Analg (1988) 66, 986–90.
2 Noble DW, Smith KJ and Dundas CR. Effects of H-2 antagonists on the elimination of bupivacaine. Br J Anaesth (1987) 59, 735–7.
3 Wilson CM, Moore J, Ghaly RG, McLean E and Dundee JW. Plasma bupivacaine concentrations associated with extradural anaesthesia for Caesarian section: influence of pretreatment with ranitidine. Br J Anaesth (1986) 58, 1330P.
4 Flynn RJ, Moore J, Collier PS and McClean E. Does pretreatment with cimetidine and treatment with cimetidine and ranitidine affect the disposition of bupivacaine? Br J Anaesth (1989) 62, 87–91.

Neuromuscular blockers and/or Anaesthetics + Aminoglycoside antibiotics

Abstract/Summary

The aminoglycoside antibiotics (amikacin, gentamicin, kanamycin, neomycin, streptomycin, tobramycin, etc.) possess neuromuscular blocking activity. Appropriate measures should be taken to accommodate the increased neuromuscular blockade and the prolonged and potentially fatal respiratory depression which can occur if these antibiotics are used with anaesthetics and conventional neuromuscular blocking drugs of any kind.

Clinical evidence

Two examples from many:

(a) Anaesthetic + aminoglycoside antibiotic

A 48-year-old patient anaesthetized with cyclopropane experienced severe respiratory depression after intraperitoneal irrigation with 500 mg 1% neomycin solution. This antibiotic-induced neuromuscular blockade was resistant to treatment with edrophonium but responded to neostigmine.[2]

(b) Anaesthetic + neuromuscular blocker + aminoglycoside antibiotic

A 56-year-old patient, initially anaesthetized with thiopentone followed by nitrous oxide, was given 160 mg gallamine as a muscle relaxant. His respiration was depressed for 18 h following the intraperitoneal administration of 2 g neomycin.[3]

Many other reports confirm that some degree of respiratory embarrassment or paralysis can occur if aminoglycosides are given to anaesthetized patients. When a conventional blocker is also used, the blockade is deepened and recovery prolonged. If the antibiotic is given towards the end of surgery the result can be that a patient who is recovering normally from neuromuscular blockade suddenly develops serious apnoea which can lead on to prolonged and in some cases fatal respiratory depression. Pittinger[1] lists more than a 100 cases in the literature over the 1955–70 period involving tubocurarine with neomycin or streptomycin; gallamine with neomycin, kanamycin or streptomycin; and suxamethonium with neomycin, kanamycin or streptomycin. The routes of antibiotic administration were oral, intraperitoneal, oesophageal, intraluminal, retroperineal, intramuscular, intrapleural, cystic, beneath skin flaps, intradural and intravenous. Later reports involve irrigation of the anterior chamber of the eye with framycetin.[4] Gentamicin given alone[6] or with tubocurarine[7] or pancuronium.[10] Amikacin,[9] tobramycin[8] or ribostamycin[5,14] with tubocurarine or pancuronium,[16] but not ribostamycin with suxamethonium.[5] Pancuronium with streptomcyin[11,15] or neomycin.[14,18] Vecuronium with amikacin/polymyxin,[17] gentamicin (with clindamycin)[13] or tobramycin.[19] Dibekacin causes a small increase in the effects of tubocurarine and suxamethonium,[5,14] but tobramycin seems not to affect alcuronium.[12]

Mechanism

The aminoglycosides appear to reduce or prevent the release of acetylcholine at neuromuscular junctions (related to an impairment of calcium influx) and they may also lower the sensitivity of the postsynaptic membrane, thereby reducing transmission. These effects would be additive with those of conventional neuromuscular blockers which act at the postsynaptic membrane.

Importance and management

Extremely well documented, very long established, clinically important and potentially serious interactions. 10 out of the

111 cases cited by Pittinger[1] were fatal, related directly or indirectly to aminoglycoside-induced respiratory depression. Concurrent use need not be avoided but increased and prolonged neuromuscular blockade should be anticipated with every aminoglycoside and every neuromuscular blocker although the potencies of the aminoglycosides differ. The neuromuscular blocking potencies of the aminoglycosides seem to be in descending order (based on animal studies): gentamicin > streptomycin > amikacin > sisomicin > kanamycin = tobramycin > kanendomycin = dibekacin.[20] The postoperative recovery period should also be closely monitored because of the risk of recurarization if the antibiotic is given during surgery. High risk patients appear to be those with renal disease and hypocalcaemia who may have elevated serum antibiotic levels, and those with pre-existing muscular weakness. Treatment of the increased blockade with anticholinesterases and calcium has met with variable success because the response seems to be inconsistent.

References

1 Pittinger CB, Eryasa Y and Adamson R. Antibiotic-induced paralysis. Anesth Analg (1970) 49, 487.
2 NY State Society of Anesthesiologists Clinical Anesthesia Conference: Postoperative neomycin respiratory depression. NY J Med (1960) 60, 1977.
3 LaPorte J, Mignault J, L'Allier R and Perron P. Un cas d'apnea a la neomycin. Un Med Canada (1959) 88, 149
4 Clark R. Prolonged curarization due to intraocular soframycin. Anesth Int Care (1975) 3, 79.
5 Arai T, Hashimoto Y, Shima Y, Matsukawa S and Iwatsuki K. Neuromuscular blocking properties of tobramycin, dibekacin and ribostamycin in man. Jap J Antibiot (1977) 30, 281.
6 Holtzman JL. Gentamicin and neuromuscular blockade. Ann Int Med (1976) 84, 55.
7 Warner WA and Sanders E. Neuromuscular blockade. J Amer Med Ass (1971) 215, 1157.
8 Waterman PM and Smith RB. Tobramycin-curare interaction. Anesth Analg (1977) 56, 587.
9 Singh YN, Marshall IG and Harvey AL. Some effects of the aminoglycoside antibiotic amikacin on neuromuscular and autonomic transmission. Br J Anaesth (1978) 50, 109.
10 Regan AG and Perumbetti PPV. Pancuronium and gentamicin interaction in patients with renal failure. Anesth Analg (1980) 59, 393.
11 Giala MM and Paradelis AG. Two cases of prolonged respiratory depression due to interaction of pancuronium with colistin and streptomycin. J Antimicrob Chemother (1979) 5, 234.
12 Boliston TA and Ashman R. Tobramycin and neuromuscular blockade. Anesthesia (1978) 33, 552.
13 Jedeikin R, Dolgunski E, Kaplan R and Hoffman S. Prolongation of neuromuscular blocking effect of vecuronium by antibiotics. Anaesthesia (1987) 42, 858–60.
14 Hashimoto T, Shima T, Matsukawa S and Iwatsuki K. Neuromuscular blocking properties of some antibiotics in man. Tohoku J exp Med (1975) 117, 339.
15 Torresi E and Pasotti EM. Su un caso di curarizzazione prolungata da interazione tra pancuronio e streptomicina. Min Anest (1984) 50, 143–5.
16 Monsegur JC, Vidal MM, Beltran J and Felipe MAN. Paralsis neuromuscular prolongada tra administration simultanea de amikacina y pancuronio. Rev Esp Anest Rean (1984) 31, 30–3.
17 Kronenfeld MA, Thomas SJ and Turndorf H. Recurrence of neuromuscular blockade after reversal of vecuronium in a patient receiving polymyxin/amikacin sternal irrigation. Anesthesiol (1986) 65, 93–4.
18 Giala M, Sareyiannis C, Cortsaris N, Paradelis A and Lappas DG. Possible interaction of pancuronium and tubocurarine with oral neomycin. Anaesthesia (1982) 37, 776.
19 Vanacker BF and Van de Walle J. The neuromuscular blocking action of vecuronium in normal patients and in patients with no renal function and interaction vercuronium-tobramycin in renal transplant patients. Acta Anaesth Belg (1986) 37, 95–9.
20 Paradelis AG, Triantaphyllidis C and Giala MM. Neuromuscular blocking activity of aminoglycoside antibiotics. Meth and Find Exptl Clin Pharmacol (1980) 2, 45–51.

Neuromuscular blockers + Aprotinin

Abstract/Summary

Apnoea developed in a number of patients after being given aprotinin (Trasylol) while recovering from neuromuscular blockade with suxamethonium (succinylcholine) with or without tubocurarine.

Clinical evidence

Three patients underwent surgery in which either suxamethonium alone or with tubocurarine was used. At the end of, or shortly after, the operation when spontaneous breathing had recommenced, aprotinin (*Trasylol*) in doses of 2500–5000 kiu was given. In each case respiration rapidly became inadequate and apnoea lasting periods of 7, 30 and 90 min occurred.[1]

Seven other cases have been reported elsewhere.[2]

Mechanism

Not fully understood. Aprotinin is only a very weak inhibitor of serum pseudocholinesterase (100,000 kiu caused a maximal 16% inhibition in man)[3] and on its own would have little effect on the metabolism of suxamethonium. But it might tip the balance in those whose cholinesterase was already very depressed.

Importance and management

The incidence of this interaction is uncertain but probably low. Only a few cases have been reported. It seems probable that it only affects those whose plasma pseudocholinesterase levels are already very low for other reasons. No difficulties should arise in those whose plasma cholinesterase levels are normal.

References

1 Chasapakis G and Dimas C. Possible interaction between muscle relaxants and the kallikrein-trypsin inactivator 'Trasylol'. Br J Anaesth (1966) 38, 838.
2 Marcello B and Porati N. Trasylol e blocco neuromusculare. Minerva anest (Torino) 33, 814.
3 Doenicke A, Gesing H, Krumey I and Schmidinger St. Influence of aprotinin (Trasylol) on the action of suxamethonium. Br J Anaesth (1970) 42, 948–60.

Neuromuscular blockers + Benzodiazepines

Abstract/Summary

Some studies report that diazepam and other benzodiazepines increase the effects of neuromuscular blockers, but others say that they do not. Patients given both drugs should be monitored for possible changes in the depth and duration of neuromuscular blockade.

Clinical evidence

(a) Increased blockade

A comparative study of 10 patients given gallamine and four others given gallamine and diazepam (0.15–0.2 mg/kg) showed that the duration of activity of the blocker was prolonged by a factor of three by the diazepam, and the depression of the twitch response was doubled. Persistent muscle weakness and respiratory depression was seen in two other patients on tubocurarine after premedication with diazepam.[1,2]

Increased neuromuscular blockade has been described with diazepam and tubocurarine,[3,4] suxamethonium[5] and gallamine.[3] Another study found that recovery from 25 to 75% of the twitch height after vecuronium was prolonged 25% by midazolam, and 45% by diazepam.[9] The same study found a 20% prolongation of recovery from the effects of atracurium by midazolam, and 20–35% by diazepam.[9]

(b) Reduced blockade or no effect

The duration of paralysis due to suxamethonium was reduced in one study by 20% when diazepam (0.15 mg/kg) was used and the recovery time was shortened.[2]

In other studies diazepam was found to have no significant effect on the blockade due to tubocurarine,[6] gallamine,[6] decamethonium,[6] pancuronium,[11] fazadinium,[11] alcuronium[11] or suxamethonium.[7,8,11] Lorazepam and lormetazepam have little or no effects on atracurium or vecuronium,[9] and midazolam has no effect on suxamethonium or pancuronium.[10]

Mechanism

Not understood. One suggestion is that where some alteration in response is seen it may be a reflection of a central depressant action rather than a direct effect on the myoneural junction.[6]

Importance and management

There is no obvious explanation for these discordant observations. What is known shows that the benzodiazepines may sometimes unpredictably alter the depth and prolong the recovery period from neuromuscular blockade, but the extent may not be very great and may possibly be little different from the individual variations in the response of patients to neuromuscular blockers. Concurrent use need not be avoided but 'caution and monitoring'[12] has been advised.

References

1 Feldman SA and Crawley BE. Diazepam and muscle relaxants. Br Med J (1970) 1, 691.
2 Feldman SA and Crawley BE. Interaction of diazepam with muscle-relaxant drugs. Br Med J (1970) 2, 336.
3 Vergano F, Zaccagna CA and Zuccaro G. Muscle relaxant properties of diazepam. Minerva Anest (1969) 35, 91.
4 Stovner J and Endresen R. Intravenous anesthesia with diazepam. Acta Anaesth Scand (1965), (Suppl) 24, 223.
5 Jorgensen H. Premedicinering med diazepam. Nord Med (1964) 72, 1395.
6 Dretchen K, Ghoneim MM and Long JP. The interaction of diazepam with myoneural blocking agents. Anesthesiol (1971) 34, 463.
7 Stovner J and Endresen R. Diazepam in intravenous anaesthesia. Lancet (1965) ii, 1298.
8 Hunter AR. Diazepam as a muscle relaxant during general anaesthesia. Br J Anaesth (1967) 39, 633.
9 Driessen JJ, Cruhl JF, Vree TB, van Egmond J and Booij LHDJ. Benzodiazepines and neuromuscular blocking drugs in patients. Acta Anaesthesiol Scand (1986) 30, 642–6.
10 Tassonyi E. Effects of midazolam (Ro 21–3981) on neuromuscular block. Pharmatherapeutica (1984) 3, 678–81.
11 Bradshaw EG and Maddison S. Effect of diazepam at the neuromuscular junction. A clinical study. Br J Anaesth (1979) 51, 955.

Neuromuscular blockers + Beta-blockers

Abstract/Summary

Increases or decreases (often only modest) in the extent of neuromuscular blockade have been seen. The bradycardia and hypotension caused by anaesthetics and beta-blockers may possibly be increased by atracurium.

Clinical evidence

(a) Reduced neuromuscular blockade

A study in 31 patients given 1 mg/kg propranolol IV over a 4 min period during surgery showed that the effects of suxamethonium were slightly reduced. The mean period of apnoea fell from 4.4 min (without propranolol) to 3.6 min. Propranolol was also observed to shorten the recovery from tubocurarine.[1] Other studies describe a shortened recovery period from tubocurarine due to oxprenolol or propranolol, but pindolol affected only a few subjects.[2]

(b) Prolonged neuromuscular blockade

Two patients with thyrotoxicosis showed prolonged neuromuscular blockade with tubocurarine or suxamethonium when given 120 mg propranolol daily.[3]

(c) Bradycardia and hypotension

Eight out of 42 patients on un-named beta-blockers and given atracurium developed bradycardia (less than 50 bpm) and hypotension (systolic pressure less than 80 mm Hg). Most of them had been premedicated with diazepam, induced with methohexitone, and anaesthetized with droperidol, fentanyl and nitrous oxide/oxygen. A further 24 showed bradycardia and eight showed hypotension. All responded promptly to atropine (0.3–0.6 mg IV).[6]

Bradycardia and hypotension have been seen in other patients given alcuronium while using timolol eye drops for glaucoma or atenolol for hypertension.[7,8]

Mechanisms

The changes in the degree of blockade are not understood but it appears to occur at the neuromuscular junction. It has been seen in animal studies.[4,5] The bradycardia and hypotension (c) were probably due to the combined depressant effects on the heart of the anaesthetics, the beta-blocker and atracurium.

Importance and management

Information is limited. Be alert for changes in neuromuscular blockade (increases or decreases) if beta-blockers are used. They seem to be unpredictable and often only modest in extent. The combined cardiac depressant effects of beta-blockade and anaesthesia are well known (see 'Anaesthetics + Beta-blockers') and the possible additional effect of atracurium should also be recognized, but other neuromuscular blockers do not seem to have this effect. It is suggested in one report that it may be wise to avoid atracurium until more is known.[8] See also 'Beta-blockers + Anticholinesterases'.

References

1 Varma Y, Sharma PL and Singh HW. Effect of propranolol hydrochloride on the neuromuscular blocking action of d-tubocurarine and succinylcholine in man. Ind J Med Res (1972) 60, 266.
2 Varma Y, Sharma PL and Singh HW. Comparative effect of propranolol, oxprenolol and pindolol on neuromuscular blocking action of d-tubocurarine in man. Ind J Med Res (1973) 61, 1382.
3 Rozen MS and Whan FM. Prolonged curarization associated with propranolol. Med J Aust (1972) 1, 467.
4 Usubiaga JE. Neuromuscular blocking effects of beta-adrenergic blockers and their interaction with skeletal muscle relaxants. Anesthesiology (1968) 29, 484.
5 Harrah MB, Walter LW and Katzune BC. The interaction of d-tubocurarine with anti-arrhythmic drugs. Anesthesiology (1970) 96, 99.
6 Rowlands DE. Drug interaction? Anaesthesia (1984) 39, 1252.
7 Glynne GL. Drug interaction? Anaesthesia (1984) 39, 293.
8 Yate B and Mostafa SM. Drug interaction? Anaesthesia (1984) 39, 728.

Neuromuscular blockers + Bretylium

Abstract/Summary

In theory there is the possibility of increased and prolonged neuromuscular blockade if bretylium is given with neuromuscular blockers.

Clinical evidence, mechanism, importance and management

Although case reports seem to be lacking, the muscular weakness seen in a few patients given bretylium[1] and the evidence from animal studies which shows that the effects of tubocurarine can be increased and prolonged by bretylium, suggest that an interaction might occur in man.[2] One suggested possibility is that if the bretylium were to be given during surgery to control arrhythmias, its effects (which are delayed) might be additive with the residual effects of the neuromuscular blocker during the recovery period, resulting in apnoea. This needs confirmation.

References

1 Bowman WC. Effects of adrenergic activators and inhibitors on skeletal muscles. In 'Handbook of experimental pharmacology.' Szekeres L (ed). Springer-Verlag (1980) 47–128.
2 Welch GW and Waud BE. Effect of bretylium on neuromuscular transmission. Anesth Analg (1982) 61, 442–4.

Neuromuscular blockers + Calcium channel blockers

Abstract/Summary

Two patients showed increased and prolonged neuromuscular blockade with vecuronium and tubocurarine which was attributed to concurrent treatment with verapamil.

Clinical evidence

A woman of 66, receiving 5 mg verapamil intravenously three times a day for superventricular tachycardia, underwent abdominal surgery during which she was initially anaesthetized with thiopentone and then maintained on nitrous oxide/oxygen with fentanyl. Vecuronium was used as the muscle relaxant. The effects of the vecuronium were increased and prolonged, and at the end of surgery reversal of the blockade using neostigmine was difficult and extended.[1]

Another report similarly describes increased blockade in a patient given tubocurarine which was difficult to reverse with neostigmine but which responded well to edrophonium.[2] Verapamil alone caused respiratory failure in a patient with poor neuromuscular transmission (Duchenne's dystrophy).[3] An increase in the neuromuscular blocking effects of pancuronium, vecuronium, atracurium and suxamethonium by verapamil and nifedipine has been seen in animals.[3,5]

Mechanism

Not fully understood but one suggestion is as follows. Nerve impulses arriving at nerve endings release calcium ions which in turn causes the release of acetylcholine. Verapamil is a calcium channel blocker which reduces the concentration of calcium ions within the nerve so that less acetylcholine is released and this would be additive with the effects of a neuromuscular blocker.[4]

Importance and management

Direct information so far seems to be limited to these two cases cited[1,2] although it is supported by animal studies. The incidence is uncertain but probably small. The authors of one report say that many patients on verapamil do not show a clinically significant increased sensitivity to muscle relaxants[2] but they suggest that as a precaution they should only be given conservative doses of the muscle relaxants. It would be prudent to be alert for this interaction in any patient receiving verapamil or any other calcium channel blocker.

References

1 van Poorten JF, Dhasmana KM, Kuypers RSM and Erdmann W. Verapamil and reversal of vecuronium neuromuscular blockade. Anesth Analg (1984) 63, 155–7.
2 Jones RM, Cashman JN, Casson WR and Broadbent MP. Verapamil potentiation of neuromuscular blockade, Failure of reversal with neostigmine but prompt reversal with edrophonium. Anesth Analg (1985) 64, 1021–5.
3 Durant NN, Nguyen N and Katz RL. Potentiation of neuromuscular blockade by verapamil. Anesthesiology (1984) 60, 298–303.
4 Wali FA. Interactions of nifedipine and diltiazem with muscle relaxants and reversal of neuromuscular blockade with edrophonium and neostigmine. J Pharmacol (1986) 17, 244–53.
5 Bikhazi GB, Leung I and Foldes FF. Interaction of neuromuscular blocking agents with calcium blockers. Anesthesiology (1982) 57, A268.

Neuromuscular blockers + Carbamazepine

Abstract/Summary

Carbamazepine shortens the recovery time from neuromuscular blockade with doxacurium and pancuronium.

Clinical evidence

A study in 18 patients undergoing craniotomy for tumours, seizure foci or cerebrovascular surgery showed that recovery from neuromuscular blockade with pancuronium was on average 65% shorter in those taking carbamazepine.[1] A controlled study in eight patients undergoing surgery showed that those who had been taking carbamazepine for at least a week had recovery times and recovery indices following the use of doxacurium which were about half those of the control group who had not had carbamazepine. For example, the 50% recovery time in those on carbamazepine was 63 min compared with 161 min in the control group.[2]

These findings are consistent with those of another study.[3]

Mechanism

Not understood.

Importance and management

Information is very limited but the interaction appears to be established. Anticipate a decreased response to doxacurium and pancuronium in those taking carbamazepine, and an accelerated recovery.

References

1 Roth S and Ebrahim ZY. Resistance to pancuronium in patients receiving carbamazepine. Anesthesiol (1987) 66, 691–3.
2 Ornstein E, Matteo RS, Halevy JD, Young HL and Abou-Donia M. Accelerated recovery from doxacurium in carbamazepine treated patients. Anesthesiology (1989) 71, A785.
3 Desai P, Hewitt PB and Jones RM. Influence of anticonvulsant therapy on doxacurium and pancuronium-induced paralysis. Anesthesiology (1989) 71, A784.

Neuromuscular blockers + Cimetidine or Ranitidine

Abstract/Summary

One report says that recovery from the neuromuscular blocking effects of suxamethonium (succinylcholine) is prolonged by cimetidine but in fact this may possibly have been due to the presence of metoclopramide. Two others say that no interaction occurs. Ranitidine is also reported not to interact.

Clinical evidence

(a) Evidence of prolonged neuromuscular blockade

A controlled study in 10 patients given 300 mg cimetidine orally at bedtime and another 300 mg 2 h before anaesthesia, showed that while the onset of action of suxamethonium (1.5 mg/kg IV) was unchanged, the time to recover 50% of the twitch height was prolonged 2–2.5 times (from 8.6 to 20.3 min). One patient took 57 min to recover.[1] His serum pseudocholinesterase levels were found to be normal. It was later reported that some patients were also taking metoclopramide which is known to interact in this way.[6]

(b) Evidence of unchanged neuromuscular blockade

A controlled study in 10 patients given 400 mg cimetidine at bedtime and 400 mg 90 min before anaesthesia found no evidence of an effect on the neuromuscular blockade caused by suxamethonium, nor on its duration or recovery period.[5] Another controlled study in patients given 300 mg cimetidine or 150 mg ranitidine the night before and 1–2 h before surgery found no evidence that the duration of action of suxamethonium or the activity of plasma cholinesterase were altered.[6]

Mechanism

Not understood. Studies with human plasma failed to find any evidence that cimetidine in normal serum concentrations inhibits the metabolism of suxamethonium,[3,6] however metoclopramide does. *In vitro* studies with very high cimetidine concentrations found inhibition of pseudocholinesterase activity.[4]

Importance and management

Information seems to be limited to the reports cited. The most likely explanation for the discord between these results is that in the study reporting increased suxamethonium effects[1] some of the patients were also given metoclopramide which can inhibit plasma cholinesterase and prolong the effects of suxamethonium.[6] However until the situation is clarified the possibility of an interaction should be taken into account during concurrent use. A study using a rat phrenic nerve diaphragm preparation found that cimetidine increased the neuromuscular blocking effects of tubocurarine and pancuronium, but there seem to be no reports confirming this in man.[2]

References

1 Kambam JR, Dymond R and Krestow M. Effect of cimetidine on duration of action of succinylcholine. Anesth Analg (1987) 66, 191–2.
2 Galatulas I, Bossa R and Benvenuti C. Cimetidine increases the neuromuscular blocking activity of aminoglycoside antibiotics: antagonism by calcium. Organ-directed toxic: Chem Indices Mech., Proc Symp (1981) 321–5. Pergamon Press, Oxford.
3 Cook DR, Stiller RL, Chakravorti S and Mannenhira T. Cimetidine does not inhibit plasma cholinesterase activity. Anesth Analg (1988) 67, 375–6.
4 Hansen WE and Bertl S. The inhibition of acetylcholinesterase and pseudocholinesterase by cimetidine. Arzneimittelforsch (1983) 33, 161–3.
5 Stirt JA, Sperry RJ and DiFazio CA. Cimetidine and succinylcholine: potential interaction and effect on neuromuscular blockade in man. Anesthesiology (1988) 69, 607–8.
6 Woodworth GE, Sears DH, Grove TM, Ruff RH, Kosek PS and Katz RL. The effect of cimetidine and ranitidine on the duration of action of succinylcholine. Anesth Analg (1989) 68, 295–7.

Neuromuscular blockers + Corticosteroids

Abstract/Summary

Three reports describe antagonism of the neuromuscular blocking effects of pancuronium by prednisone and hydrocortisone in patients with adrenocortical insufficiency, but normally no changes appear to take place.

Clinical evidence

A man undergoing splenectomy and who had been taking 250 mg prednisolone daily had good muscular relaxation in response to 8 mg pancuronium early in the operation, but an hour later began to show signs of inadequate relaxation and continued to do so for the next one-and-a-quarter hours despite being given four additional 2 mg doses of pancuronium.[1]

Another report describes a hypophysectomized man on cortisone and given pancuronium who showed profound paralysis which was rapidly reversed with 100 mg hydrocortisone sodium succinate.[2] Another patient on large doses of hydrocortisone, prenisolone and aminophylline proved to be resistant to the effects of pancuronium.[3]

These reports contrast with another in which 25 patients who had no adrenalcortical dysfunction of histories of corticosteroid therapy who were given pancuronium, metocurine,

tubocurarine or vecuronium. They showed no changes in their neuromuscular blockade when given dexamethasone (0.4 mg/kg) or hydrocortisone (10 mg/kg) intravenously.[4]

Mechanism

Uncertain. One idea, based on animal studies, is that adrenocortical insufficiency causes a defect in neuromuscular transmission (a decrease in the sensitivity of the end-plate) which is reversed by the corticosteroids. Another idea is the effects seen are connected in some way with the steroid nucleus of the pancuronium.

Importance and management

The evidence for an interaction seem to be limited to these reports involving only pancuronium. The evidence from the last study cited[4] suggests that no changes in the neuromuscular blocking effects of non-depolarizing blockers normally takes place if corticosteroids are given.

References

1 Laflin MJ. Interaction of pancuronium and corticosteroids. Anesthesiology (1977) 47, 471.
2 Meyers EF. Partial recovery from neuromuscular blockade following hydrocortisone administration. Anesthesiology (1977) 46, 148.
3 Azar I, Kumar D and Betcher AM. Resistance to pancuronium in an asthmatic patient treated with aminophylline and steroids. Canad Anesth Soc J (1982) 29, 280–2.
4 Schwartz AE, Matteo RS, Ornstein E and Silverberg PA. Acute steroid therapy does not alter non-depolarizing muscle relaxant effects in humans. Anesthesiology (1986) 65, 326–7.

Neuromuscular blockers + Cyclophosphamide

Abstract/Summary

The effects of suxamethonium (succinylcholine) can be increased and prolonged in patients under treatment with cyclophosphamide because their serum pseudocholinesterase levels are depressed. Respiratory insufficiency and prolonged apnoea have been reported.

Clinical evidence

Respiratory insufficiency and prolonged apnoea occurred in a patient on two occasions while receiving cyclophosphamide and undergoing anaesthesia during which suxamethonium and tubocurarine were used. Plasma pseudocholinesterase levels were found to be low. Anaesthesia without the suxamethonium was uneventful. Seven out of eight patients subsequently examined also showed depressed serum pseudocholinesterase levels while taking cyclophosphamide.[1]

Respiratory depression and low serum pseudocholinesterase levels have been described in other reports.[2–4] One report described a 35–70% reduction.[2]

Mechanism

Cyclophosphamide irreversibly inhibits the activity of pseudocholinesterase in the serum, as a result the metabolism of the suxamethonium is reduced and its actions are enhanced and prolonged.[4]

Importance and management

A well-documented and established interaction of clinical importance. Whether all patients are affected to the same extent is uncertain. The depression of the serum pseudocholinesterase levels may last several days, possibly weeks, so that ideally serum pseudocholinesterase levels should be checked before using suxamethonium. It should certainly be used with caution, and the dosage should be reduced.[2] Some have suggested that concurrent use should be avoided.[1] Suxethonium probably interacts similarly, but not other neuromuscular blockers because they are not metabolized by serum pseudocholinesterase.

References

1 Walker IR, Zapf PW and Mackay IR. Cyclophosphamide, cholinesterase and anaesthesia. Aust NZ J Med (1972) 3, 247.
2 Zsigmond EK and Robins G. The effect of a series of anti-cancer drugs on plasma cholinesterase activity. Can Anaesth Soc J (1972) 19, 75.
3 Mone JG and Mathie WE. Qualitative and quantitative effects of pseudocholinesterase activity. Anaesthesia (1967) 22, 55.
4 Wolff H. Die Hemmung der Serumcholinesterase durch Cyclophosphamid (Endoxan). Klin Wsch (1965) 43, 819.

Neuromuscular blockers + Cyclosporin(e)

Abstract/Summary

Two isolated reports describe increases in the effects of vecuronium and pancuronium in patients under treatment with cyclosporin.

Clinical evidence

(a) Pancuronium

A woman with a two-year renal transplant controlled with 100 mg azathioprine, 300 mg cyclosporin and 10 mg prednisone and also taking nifedipine and furosemide for hypertension, underwent surgery during which she was initially anaesthetized with fentanyl and thiopentone, and later nitrous oxide/oxygen and isoflurane. Pancuronium was used as the neuromuscular blocker. She was also infused with cyclosporin before and after surgery. Residual paralysis was seen after surgery and she was re-intubated 20 min later because of increased respiratory distress.

(b) Vecuronium

A girl of 15 on 20 mg cyclosporin IV twice daily and with serum levels of 138 μg.l[-1] was anaesthetized for an endoscopy and bone marrow aspiration using fentanyl, thiopen-

tone and 0.1 mg.kg[-1] vecuronium. Anaesthesia was later maintained with nitrous oxide, oxygen and isoflurane. Attempts were later made to reverse the blockade with edrophonium, atropine and neostigmine but full neuromuscular function was not restored for 3 h and 20 min.[4]

Mechanism

Uncertain. One suggestion is that cremophor (polyoxyl 35 castor oil), a surface-active agent used as a vehicle for the cyclosporin[1] may increase the effective concentration of the pancuronium at the neuromuscular junction. Both compounds have been observed in animal studies to increase vecuronium blockade[2] and cremophor has been seen to decrease the onset time of pancuronium blockade in patients given cremophor-containing anaesthetics.[3]

Importance and management

Direct information seems to be limited to the reports cited. The general importance is uncertain but be alert for an increase in the effects of pancuronium and vecuronium in any patient receiving cyclosporin. The authors suggest that atracurium would be a more suitable blocker in the presence of cyclosporin because any interaction is less pronounced.

References

1 Crosby E and Robblee JA. Cyclosporine-pancuronium interaction in a patient with a renal allograft. Can J Anaesth (1988) 35, 300–2.
2 Gramstad L, Liileaasen P and Misaas B. Onset time for alcuronium and pancuronium after cremophor-containing anaesthetics. Acta Anaesth Scand (1981) 25, 484–6.
3 Viby-Mogensen J. Interaction of other drugs with muscle relaxants. Sem Anaesth (1985) 6, 52.
4 Wodd GG. Cyclosporine-vecuronium interaction. Can J Anaesth (1989) 36 (3 part 1), 358.

Neuromuscular blockers + Dantrolene

Abstract/Summary

The muscle relaxant effects of dantrolene can be additive with those of conventional neuromuscular blockers.

Clinical evidence, mechanism, importance and management

A woman of 60, given a total of 350 mg dantrolene by mouth during the 28 h before surgery to control malignant hyperthermia, showed increased neuromuscular blockade and a slow recovery rate when vecuronium was used subsequently.[1] Dantrolene is a muscle relaxant which acts directly on the muscle by interfering with calcium uptake and release from the sarcoplasmic reticulum. It may also possibly interfere with the release of acetylcholine at the neuromuscular junction. These effects would appear to be additive with those of the neuromuscular blockers. This interaction should be taken into account during concurrent use.

Reference

1 Driessen JJ, Wuis EW and Gielen MJM. Prolonged vecuronium neuro-muscular blockade in a patient receiving orally administered dantrolene. Anesthesiology (1985) 62, 523–4.

Neuromuscular blockers + Dexpanthenol

Abstract/Summary

An increase in the neuromuscular blocking effects of suxamethonium (succinylcholine) has been attributed to the concurrent use of dexpanthenol in one patient, but further studies failed to confirm this interaction.

Clinical evidence, mechanism, importance and management

A patient developed severe respiratory embarrassment following the intramuscular injection of 500 mg dexpanthenol during the recovery period from anaesthesia with nitrous oxide and cyclopropane, and neuromuscular blockade with suxamethonium.[1] However a later study on six patients under general anaesthesia showed that their response to suxamethonium was unaffected by the infusion of 500 mg pantothenic acid.[2]

Several manufacturers of products containing pantothenic acid have issued warnings about this interaction, but they seem to be solely based on the single unconfirmed report cited here,[1] and there seems to be little reason for avoiding concurrent use or for taking particular precautions. However users should be aware of this case.

References

1 Stewart P. Case reports. J Amer Ass Nurse Anesth (1960) 28, 56.
2 Smith RM, Gotthsall SC and Young JA. Succinylcholine-pantothenyl alcohol: a reappraisal. Anesth Analg (1969) 48, 205.

Neuromuscular blockers + Ecothiopate iodide

Abstract/Summary

The neuromuscular blocking effects of suxamethonium (succinylcholine) are markedly increased and prolonged in patients under treatment with ecothiopate iodide. The dosage of suxamethonium should be reduced appropriately.

Clinical evidence

In 1965 Murray McGavi warned that the systemic absorption of ecothiopate iodide from eye drops could lower serum pseudocholinesterase levels to such an extent that '...within a few days of commencing therapy, levels are reached at which protracted apnoea could occur should these patients require general anaesthesia in which muscle relaxation is obtained with suxamethonium.'[1] Cases of apnoea due to this interaction were reported the following year[2,3] and the year after.[5] In one case a woman who had received 200 mg suxamethonium showed apnoea for five and a half hours. Other studies have confirmed that ecothiopate markedly reduces the levels of pseudocholinesterase.[4]

Mechanism

Suxamethonium is metabolized in the body by pseudocholinesterase. In the presence of ecothiopate iodide which is an anticholinesterase, the levels of the enzyme are markedly depressed so that the metabolism of the suxamethonium is reduced and its effects are thereby enhanced and prolonged.[4]

Importance and management

An established, adequately documented and clinically important interaction. Plasma pseudocholinesterase can be rapidly reduced to very low levels (less than 5%) by ecothiopate administered as eye drops, and it can take as long as four weeks to return to approximately normal levels after withdrawal.[6] The dosage of suxamethonium should be reduced appropriately. One report describes the successful use of approximately one fifth of the normal dosage in a patient receiving 0.125% ecothiopate iodide solution, one drop twice a day in both eyes, and with a plasma cholinesterase activity 62% below normal. Recovery from the neuromuscular blockade was rapid and uneventful.[7]

References

1 McGavi DDM. Depressed levels of serum-pseudocholinesterase with ecothiopate-iodide eyedrops. Lancet (1965) ii, 272.
2 Gesztes T. Prolonged apnoea after suxamethonium injection associated with eye drops containing an anticholinesterase agent. Br J Anaesth (1966) 38, 408.
3 Pantuck EJ. Ecothiopate iodide eye drops and prolonged response to suxamethonium. Br J Anaesth (1966) 38, 406.
4 Cavallaro RJ, Krumperman LW and Kugler F. Effect of ecothiopate therapy on the metabolism of succinylcholine in man. Anesth Analg (1974) 47, 570.
5 Mone JG and Mathie WE. Qualitative and quantitative defects of pseudocholinesterase activity. Anaesthesia (1967) 22, 55.
6 de Roetth A, Dettbarn WD, Rosenberg P, Wilensky JG and Wong A. Effect of phopholine iodide on blood cholinesterase levels of normal and glaucoma subjects. Amer J Opthal (1965) 59, 586.
7 Donati F and Bevan DR. Controlled succinylcholine infusion in a patient receiving echothiophate eye drops. Canad Anaesth Soc J (1981) 28, 488.

Neuromuscular blockers + Fentanyl citrate-droperidol (Innovar)

Abstract/Summary

Recovery from the neuromuscular blocking effects of suxamethonium is prolonged by fentanyl citrate-droperidol (Innovar).

Clinical evidence

The observation that patients who had had *Innovar* (fentanyl citrate-droperidol) before anaesthesia appeared to have a prolongation of the effects of suxamethonium, seen as apnoea, prompted further study of this interaction.[1] 19 patients were given suxamethonium and thiopentone during the induction of anaesthesia. The average time from end fasciculation to return of full tetanus was approximately doubled (from 5.83 to 10.45 min) in 10 patients given *Innovar* (2 ml intravenously 10 min before anaesthesia) when compared with nine patients not given *Innovar*.[1]

A much shorter delay in recovery was seen in a later study.[3] Another study[2] showed that the droperidol component of *Innovar* is responsible for this interaction.

Mechanism

Not understood. One suggestion[2] is that droperidol may act as a membrane stabilizer at neuromuscular junctions, and it may also reduce the levels of pseudocholinesterase which is responsible for the metabolism of suxamethonium.

Importance and management.

An established interaction of moderate importance. Delayed recovery should be anticipated in patients on suxamethonium and other neuromuscular blockers if *Innovar* is used.

References

1 Wehner RJ. A case study: The prolongation of Anectine effect by Innovar. AANA Journal (1979) 47, 576–9.
2 Lewis RA. A consideration of prolonged succinylcholine paralysis with Innovar: Is the cause droperidol or fentanyl? AANA Journal (1982) 50, 55–9.
3 Moore GB, Ciresi S and Kallar S. The effect of Innovar versus droperidol or fentanyl on the duration of action of succinylcholine. AANA Journal (1986) 54, 130–6

Neuromuscular blockers + Frusemide (Furosemide)

Abstract/Summary

The effects of the neuromuscular blockers may be increased by low doses of frusemide but opposed by higher doses.

Clinical evidence

(a) Increased neuromuscular blockade

Three patients receiving kidney transplants showed increased neuromuscular blockade with tubocurarine (seen as a pronounced decrease in twitch tension) when given frusemide (40 or 80 mg) and mannitol (12.5 mg) intravenously. One of them showed the same reaction when later given only 40 mg frusemide but no mannitol. The residual blockade was easily antagonized with pyridostigmine (14 mg) or neostigmine (3 mg) with atropine (1.2 mg).[1]

(b) Decreased neuromuscular blockade

10 patients given 1 mg/kg frusemide took 14.7 min to recover from 95 to 50% blockade with pancuronium (as measured by a twitch response) compared with 21.8 min in 10 other patients who had had no frusemide.[3]

Mechanism

Uncertain. Animal studies indicate that what happens probably depends on the dosage of frusemide: 0.1–10 μg/kg increased the blocking effects of tubocurarine and suxamethonium whereas 1–4 mg/kg opposed the blockade.[2] One suggestion is that low doses of frusemide inhibit protein kinase, whereas higher doses cause inhibition of phosphodiesterase.

Importance and management

The documentation is very limited. Be on the alert for changes in the response to any blocker if frusemide is used. Animal studies suggest that increases occur with doses less than 10 μg/kg, but decreases with doses of 1–4 mg/kg. Whether these same changes occur if frusemide is given orally seems not to have been studied.

Reference

1 Miller R, Sohn YJ and Matteo RS. Enhancement of d-tubocurarine neuromuscular blockade by diuretics in man. Anesthesiology (1976) 45, 422.
2 Scappaticci K, Ham JA, Sohn YJ, Miller RD and Dretchen KL. Effects of furosemide on the neuromuscular junction. Anesthesiology (1982) 57, 381–88.
3 Azar I, Cottrell J, Gupta B and Turndorf H. Furosemide facilitates recovery of evoked twitch response after pancuronium. Anesth Analg (1980) 59, 55–7.

Neuromuscular blockers + Immunosuppressants

Abstract/Summary

The neuromuscular blocking effects of tubocurarine are reduced by azathioprine and antilymphocytic globulin. The dosage may need to be increased 2–4-fold.

Clinical evidence, mechanism, importance and management

A retrospective study showed that patients on immunosuppressant drugs following organ transplantation needed an increased dosage of tubocurarine to achieve satisfactory muscle relaxation. A control group of 74 patients needed 0–10 mg tubocurarine; 13 patients on azathioprine needed 12.5–25.0 mg; 11 patients on antilymphocytic globulin needed 10–20 mg and two patients on azathioprine and guanethidine needed 55–90 mg.[1] The reasons are not understood. Since azathioprine is converted within the body to mercaptopurine it is likely that it interacts similarly. Information is very sparse so it is not clear whether this interaction occurs with other neuromuscular blockers. More study is needed.

Reference

1 Vetten KB. Immunosuppressive therapy and anaesthesia. S Afr Med J (1973) 47, 767.

Neuromuscular blockers + Insecticides

Abstract/Summary

Exposure to organophosphate insecticides such as Malathion can markedly prolong the neuromuscular blocking effects of suxamethonium.

Clinical evidence

A man admitted to hospital for an appendectomy became apnoeic during the early part of the operation when given 100 mg suxamethonium to facilitate tracheal intubation, and remained so throughout the 40 min surgery. Spontaneous restoration of neuromuscular activity did not return for 150 min. Later studies showed that he had an extremely low plasma cholinesterase activity (3–10%) although he had a normal phenotype. It subsequently turned out that he had been working with Malathion for 11 weeks, sometimes inside a greenhouse, without any protection.[1]

Mechanism

Malathion, which is an organophosphate insecticide, can inhibit the activity of plasma cholinesterase thereby reducing the metabolism of the suxamethonium and prolonging its effects.

Importance and management

An established and well understood interaction. Particular care should be exercised if suxamethonium is used in individuals known to have been exposed to organophosphate insecticides such as Malathion.

Reference

1 Guillermo FP, Pretel CMM, Royo FT, Macias MJP, Ossorio RA, Gomez JAA, Vidal CJ. Prolonged suxamethonium-induced neuromuscular blockade associated with organophosphate poisoning. Br J Anaesth (1988) 61, 233–6.

Neuromuscular blockers + Lignocaine, Procaine or Procainamide

Abstract/Summary

The neuromuscular blockade due to suxamethonium (succinylcholine) can be increased and prolonged by lignocaine (lidocaine), procaine and possibly procainamide.

Clinical evidence

A patient anaesthetized with fluroxene and nitrous oxide demonstrated 100% blockade with suxamethonium and tubocurarine. About 50 min later when twitch height had fully returned and tidal volume was 0.4 l, she was given 50 mg lignocaine intravenously for premature ventricular contractions. She immediately stopped breathing and the twitch disappeared. About 45 min later the tidal volume was 0.45 l. Later is was found that the patient had a dibucaine number of 23%.[3]

Other studies in man have confirmed that lignocaine and procaine prolong the apnoea following the use of suxamethonium (0.7 mg/kg). A dose-relationship was established. The duration of apnoea was approximately doubled by 7.5 mg/kg of lignocaine or procaine, and tripled by 16.6 mg/kg, although the effects of procaine at higher doses were more marked.[1]

Mechanism

Uncertain. Local anaesthetics appear to act on presynaptic, postsynaptic and muscle membranes. Procaine and lignocaine weakly inhibit pseudocholinesterase[2] which might prolong the activity of suxamethonium. There may additionally be competition between the suxamethonium and the procaine for hydrolysis by pseudocholinesterase which metabolizes them both.[1] Therapeutic serum levels of 4–12 μg/ml procainamide have been found to inhibit cholinesterase activity by 15–30%.[7]

Importance and management

Information is limited but the suxamethonium–lignocaine and lignocaine–procaine interactions appear to be established and of clinical importance. Be alert for signs of increased blockade and/or recurarization with apnoea during the recovery period from suxamethonium blockade if either drug is used. Animal studies indicate that low and otherwise safe doses of lignocaine with other drugs having neuromuscular blocking activity (e.g. polymyxin B, aminoglycoside antibiotics) may possibly be additive with conventional neuromuscular blockers and cause problems.[4]

An increase in the effects of suxamethonium by procainamide has been reported in animals,[5] increased muscle weakness in a myasthenic patient[6] and reductions in serum cholinesterase activity in normal subjects but no marked interaction has yet been reported. Nevertheless be aware that some increase in the neuromuscular blocking effects is possible.

References

1 Usubiaga JE, Wikinski JA, Morales RL and Usubiaga LEJ. Interaction of intravenously administered procaine, lidocaine and succinylcholine in anesthetized subjects. Anesth Analg (1967) 46, 39–45.
2 Reina RA and Cannava N. Interazione di alcuni anestetici locali con la succinilcolina. Act Anaesth Ital (1972) 23, 1–10
3 Miller RD. Neuromuscular blocking agents. In 'Drug Interactions in Anesthesia', Smith NT, Miller RD and Corbascio AN (eds). Lea and Febiger, Philadelphia 1981, p 249.
4 Brueckner J, Thomas KC, Bikhazi GB and Foldes FF. Neuromuscular drug interactions of clinical importance. Anesth Anal (1980) 59, 533–4.
5 Cuthbert MF. The effect of quinidine and procainimide on the neuromuscular blocking action of suxamethonium. Br J Anaesth (1966) 38, 775.
6 Drachman DA and Skom JH. Procainimide—a hazard in myasthenia gravis. Arch Neurol (1965) 13, 316.
7 Kamban JR, Naukam RJ and Sastry BVR. The effect of procainimide on plasma cholinesterase acitivity. Can J Anaesth (1987) 34, 579–81.

Neuromuscular blockers + Lithium carbonate

Abstract/Summary

The concurrent use of neuromuscular blockers and lithium carbonate is normally safe and uneventful, but three patients have been described who experienced prolonged blockade and respiratory difficulties after receiving standard doses of pancuronium and suxamethonium (succinylcholine).

Clinical evidence

A manic depressive woman on lithium carbonate and with a serum lithium concentration of 1.2 mEq/l, underwent surgery and was administered thiopentone, suxamethonium (a total of 310 mg over 2 h) and 0.5 mg pancuronium bromide. Prolonged neuromuscular blockade with apnoea occurred.[1,2]

Two other patients on lithium are described elsewhere who experienced enhanced neuromuscular blockade when given pancuronium alone[3] or with suxamethonium.[10] The authors of the latter report say that '...We have seen potentiation of the neuromuscular blockade produced by succinylcholine in several patients,'[10] but give no further details. In contrast, a study in 17 patients failed to demonstrate any interaction in patients on lithium carbonate when given suxamethonium.[5] A lithium–pancuronium and lithium–suxamethonium interaction has been demonstrated in dogs[1,2,6] and a lithium–d-tubocurarine interaction in cats,[7] but no clear interaction has been demonstrated with any other neuromuscular blocker.[8,9] A case of lithium toxicity has been described in a woman on lithium and suxamethonium, but it is doubtful if it arose because of an interaction.[4]

Mechanism

Uncertain. One suggestion is that, when the interaction occurs, it may be due to changes in the electrolyte balance caused by the lithium which results in a reduction in the release of acetylcholine at the neuromuscular junction.[7]

Importance and management

Information is limited. There are only three definite reports of this interaction in man and evidence that no adverse interaction normally occurs. Concurrent use need not be avoided but it would be prudent to be on the alert for evidence of this interaction in any patient on lithium carbonate who is given any neuromuscular blocker.

References

1 Hill G, Wong KC, Hodges M and Seutker C. Potentiation of succinylcholine neuromuscular blockade by lithium carbonate. Fed Proc (1976) 35, 729.
2 Hill G, Wong KC, and Hodges MR. Potentiation of succinylcholine neuromuscular blockade by lithium carbonate. Anaesthesiol (1976) 44, 439.
3 Borden H, Clark M and Katz H. The use of pancuronium bromide in patients receiving lithium carbonate. Can Anaesth Soc J (1974) 21, 79.
4 Jephcott G and Kerry RJ. Lithium: an anaesthetic risk. Br J Anaesth (1974) 46, 389.
5 Martin BA and Kramer PM. Clinical significance of the interaction between lithium and a neuromuscular blocker. Am J Psychiatry (1982) 139, 1326–8.
6 Reimherr FW, Hodges MR, Hill GE and Wong KC. Prolongation of muscle relaxant effects by lithium carbonate. Am J Psychiatry (1977) 134, 205–6.
7 Basuray BN and Harris CA. Potentiation of d-tubocurarine (d-Tc) neuromuscular blockade in cats by lithium carbonate. Eur J Pharmacol (1977) 45, 79–82.
8 Waud BE, Farrell L and Waud DR. Lithium and neuromuscular transmission. Anesth Analg (1982) 61, 399–402.
9 Hill GE, Wong KC and Hodges MR. Lithium carbonate and neuromuscular blocking agents. Anesthesiol (1977) 46, 122–6.
10 Rosner TM and Rosenberg M. Anesthetic problems in patients taking lithium. J Oral Surgery (1981) 39, 282–5

Neuromuscular blockers + Magnesium salts

Abstract/Summary

The effects of tubocurarine, vecuronium, suxamethonium and possibly other neuromuscular blockers can be increased and prolonged by magnesium sulphate given parenterally.

Clinical evidence

A pregnant 40-year-old with severe pre-eclampsia and receiving magnesium sulphate by infusion, underwent emergency caesarian section during which she was initially anaesthetized with thiopentone, maintained with nitrous oxide/oxygen and enflurane, and given firstly suxamethonium and later vecuronium as muscle relaxants. At the end of surgery the patient rapidly recovered from the anaesthesia but the neuromuscular blockade was very prolonged (an eightfold increase in duration).[1]

Prolonged neuromuscular blockade has been described in two other women with pre-eclampsia given magnesium sulphate and either tubocurarine or suxamethonium.[2] Another study in women undergoing caesarian section showed that those given magnesium sulphate for toxaemia needed less suxamethonium (4.73 compared with 7.39 mg/kg/hr) than other normal patients.[3] Increased blockade has been demonstrated with decamethonium, tubocurarine and suxamethonium in animals.[2,4]

Mechanism

Not fully understood. Magnesium sulphate has direct neuro-muscular blocking activity by inhibiting the normal release of acetylcholine from nerve endings, reducing the sensitivity of the postsynaptic membrane and depressing the excitability of the muscle membranes. These effects are possibly simply additive (or possibly more than additive) with the effects of conventional blockers.

Importance and management

An established interaction but the documentation is limited. Be alert for an increase in the effects of neuromuscular blockers if intravenous magnesium sulphate is used. Intravenous calcium gluconate has been used to assist recovery in one case.[2] No interaction would be expected with magnesium sulphate given orally because its absorption is poor.

References

1 Sinatra RS, Philip BK, Naulty JS and Ostheimer GW. Prolonged neuro-muscular blockade with vecuronium in a patient treated with magnesium sulphate. Anesth Analg (1985) 64, 1220–2.
2 Ghoneim MM and Long JP. The interaction between magnesium and other neuromuscular blocking agents. Anesthesiol (1970) 32, 23.
3 Morris R and Giesecke AH. Potentiation of muscle relaxants by magnesium sulphate in toxemia of pregnancy. South Med J (1968) 61, 25.
4 Giesecke AH, Morris RE, Dalton MD and Stephen CR. Of magnesium, muscle relaxants, toxemic parturients and cats. Anesth Analg (1968) 474, 689.

Neuromuscular blockers + Metoclopramide

Abstract/Summary

The neuromuscular blocking effects of suxamethonium (succinylcholine) can be increased and prolonged in patients taking metoclopramide.

Clinical evidence

A controlled study in 22 patients undergoing elective surgery showed that the recovery from neuromuscular blockade (time from 95% to 25% suppression of the activity of the adductor pollicis muscle) due to suxamethonium was prolonged in those patients who had also been given 10 mg metoclopra-mide IV.[1]

Prolongation of the actions of suxamethonium by metoclopra-mide is also briefly mentioned in another report.[2]

Mechanism

Metoclopramide reduces the activity of plasma cholinesterase which is responsible for the metabolism of suxamethonium. As a result it is metabolized much more slowly and its effects are prolonged.[1,2] One study found that a metoclopramide serum concentration of 0.8 μg/ ml inhibited plasma choli-nesterase activity by 50%. A 10 mg dose of metoclopramide in a 70 kg adult produces serum concentrations of up to 0.14 μg/ml.[2]

Importance and management

An established but not extensively documented interaction of clinical importance. Be alert for enhanced and prolonged neuromuscular blockade during concurrent use. The authors of the first report cited also point out that plasma cholinesterase activity is also reduced in pregnancy and those taking ester-type local anaesthetics, which would be expected to be additive with the effects of metoclopramide.

References

1 Kao YJ and Turner DR. Prolongation of succinylcholine block by metoclopramide. Anesthesiology (1989) 70, 905–8.
2 Kambam JR, Parris WCV, Franks JJ, Sastry BVR, Naukam R and Smith BE. The inhibitory effect of metoclopramide on plasma cholinesterase activity. Can J Anaesth (1988) 35, 476–8.

Neuromuscular blockers + Miscellaneous antibiotics

Abstract/Summary

Colistin, colistin sulphomethate sodium, polymyxins, lincomycin and clindamycin possess neuromuscular blocking activity. Appropriate measures should be taken to accommodate the increased neuromuscular blockade and the prolonged and potentially serious respiratory depression which can occur if these antibiotics are used with anaesthetics and conventional neuromuscular blocking drugs of any kind. In theory amphotericin B might also interact, but the tetracyclines probably not. No interaction is seen with metronidazole, chloramphenicol or penicillin.

Clinical evidence

(a) Amphotericin B

Amphotericin B can induce hypokalaemia resulting in muscle weakness[2,3] which might be expected to enhance the effects of neuromuscular blockers, but there appear to be no reports in the literature confirming that this actually takes place.

(b) Clindamycin or lincomycin

Enhanced blockade has been demonstrated in patients given pancuronium and lincomycin which was reversed by neostigmine.[8] Respiratory paralysis was seen in a man recovering from blockade with tubocurarine[4] and this interaction was confirmed in another report.[5] Other reports describe the same interaction in patients on pancuronium or suxamethonium[12] while treated with clindamycin.

(c) Metronidazole

An increase in the neuromuscular blocking effects of vecuronium has been reported in cats,[13] but a later study in patients failed to find any evidence of an interaction.[14]

(d) Polymyxins

Pittinger in his literature review of antibiotic-neuromuscular blocker interactions found 17 cases over the 1955–70 period in which colistin (polymyxin E) or colistin sulphomethate sodium, with or without conventional neuromuscular blockers, were responsible for the development of increased blockade and respiratory muscle paralysis. Some of the patients had renal disease.[1] A later report describes prolonged respiratory depression in a patient on pancuronium and colistin.[9] Calcium gluconate was found to reverse the blockade.[9] Pittinger also lists five cases of enhanced neuromuscular blockade with polymyxin B. An increase in the blockade due to pancuronium by polymyxin B is described in another report,[11] and prolonged and fatal apnoea occurred in another patient on suxamethonium when his peritoneal cavity was instilled with a solution containing 100 mg polymyxin B and 100,000 U bacitracin.[15]

(e) Tetracyclines, chloramphenicol, penicillins

Pittinger lists four cases of enhanced neuromuscular blockade with rolitetracycline or oxytetracycline in myasthenic patients[1] but there seem to be no reports of interactions in normal patients given neuromuscular blocking drugs. No interaction was seen in the myasthenic patients when given chloramphenicol or penicillin.[6,7]

Mechanisms

Not fully understood but the following sites of action have been suggested.

Antibiotic	Prejunctional	Receptor block	Channel block	Muscle
Polymyxin B	+ +	+ + +		+
Colistin				+
Lincomycin	+ +	+ +	+	+
Tetracyclines				+

After TA Torda, Curr Clin Prac Ser (1983) 11, Clin Exper Norcuron, pp 72–8.

Importance and management

The interactions involving polymyxin B, colistin, colistin sulphomethate sodium, lincomycin and clindamycin are established and clinically important. The incidence is uncertain. Concurrent use need not be avoided, but be alert for increased and prolonged neuromuscular blockade with any neuromuscular blocker. The recovery period should be closely monitored because of the risk of recurarization. No interaction would be expected with the tetracyclines, chloramphenicol, the penicillins or metronidazole.

References

1 Pittinger CB, Eryasa Y and Adamson R. Antibiotic-induced paralysis. Anesth Analg (1970) 49, 487.

2 Holeman CW and Einstein H. The toxic effects of amphotericin B in man. Calif Med (1963) 99, 90.

3 Drutz DJ, Fan JH, Tai TY, Cheng JT and Hsien WC. Hypokalaemic rhabdomylosis and myoglobinuria following amphotericin therapy. J Amer Med Ass (1970) 211. 824.

4 Samuelson RJ, Giesecke AH, Kallus FT and Stanley VF. Lincomycin-curare interaction. Anesth Analg (1975) 54, 103.

5 Hashimoto Y, Iwatsuki N and Shima T. Neuromuscular blocking properties of lincomycin and kanamycin in man. Jap J Anesth (1971) 20, 407.

6 Gibbels E. Further observations on the side-effects of intravenous administration of rolitetracycline in myasthenia gravis pseudoparalytica. Deut Med Wsch (1967) 92, 1153.

7 Wullen F, Kast G and Bruck A. On the side-effects of tetracycline administration in myasthenic patients. Deut Med Wsch (1967) 92, 667.

8 Booij LHD, Miller RD and Crul JF. Neostigmine and 4-aminopyrimidine antagonism of lincomycin-pancuronium neuromuscular blockade in man. Anesth Analg (1978) 57, 316.

9 Giala MM and Paradelis AG. Two cases of prolonged respiratory depression due to interaction of pancuronium with colistin and streptomycin. J Antimicrob Chemother (1979) 5, 234.

10 Crul JF, Booij L, Rutten J, De Groot A, Rutten Ch and Van der Pol F. Interaction of antibiotics and muscle relaxants in abdominal surgery. Proc Symp Intra Abdom Sepsis. Bunge Sci Publ (Utrecht) 1979, p 9.

11 Fogdall RP and Miller RD. Prolongation of pancuronium-induced neuromuscular blockade by polymyxin B. Anesthesiol (1974) 41, 407.

12 Avery D and Finn R. Succinylcholine. Prolonged apnea associated with clindamycin and abonormal liver function tests. Dis Nerv Syst (1977) 38, 473.

13 McIndewar I and Marshall R. Interactions between the neuromuscular blocking drug ORGNC45 and some anaesthetic, analgesic and antimicrobial agents. Br J Anaesth (1981) 53, 785–92.

14 D'Hollander A, Agoston S, Capouet V, Barvais L, Bomblet JP and Esselen M. Failure of metronidazole to alter a vecuronium neuromuscular blockade in humans. Anesthesiology (1985) 63, 99–102.

15 Small GA. Respiratory paralysis after a large dose of intraperitoneal polymyxin B and bacitracin. Anesth Analg (1964) 43, 137–9.

Neuromuscular blockers + Monoamine oxidase inhibitors

Abstract/Summary

Three patients showed an enhancement of the effects of suxamethonium (succinylcholine) during concurrent treatment with phenelzine.

Clinical evidence, mechanism, importance and management

Two patients, one taking phenelzine and the other who had ceased to do so six days previously, developed apnoea following electroconvulsive therapy (ECT) during which suxamethonium was used. Both responded to injections of nikethamide and positive pressure ventilation with oxygen.[1] A later study[2] observed the same response in another patient taking phenelzine. This would appear to be explained by the finding that phenelzine caused a reduction in the levels of serum pseudocholinesterase in four out of 10 patients studied. Since the metabolism of suxamethonium depends on this enzyme, reduced levels of the enzyme would result in a reduced rate of suxamethonium metabolism and in a prolongation of its effects. None of 12 other patients taking tranylcypromine, isocarboxazid or mebanazine showed reduced pseudocholinesterase levels.

It would clearly be prudent to be on the alert for this interaction in patients on phenelzine, but on the basis of limited evidence it seems less likely to occur with the other MAOI's cited.

References

1 Bleaden FA and Czekanska G. New drugs for depression. Br Med J (1960) 1, 200.
2 Bodley PO, Halwax K and Potts L. Low serum pseudocholinesterase levels complicating treatment with phenelzine. Br Med J (1969) 3, 510.

Neuromuscular blockers and Anaesthetics + Morphine

Abstract/Summary

A patient experienced hypertension and tachycardia when given pancuronium bromide after induction of anaesthesia with morphine and nitrous oxide/oxygen. The respiratory depressant effects of ketamine and morphine may be additive.

Clinical evidence, mechanism, importance and management

A woman about to receive a coronary by-pass graft was premedicated with morphine and scopolamine. Morphine (1 mg/kg) was then slowly infused while the patient was ventilated with 50% N_2O/O_2. With the onset of neuromuscular relaxation with pancuronium, the blood pressure rose sharply from 120/60 to 200/110 mm Hg and the pulse rate increased from 54 to 96, persisting for several minutes but restabilizing when 1% halothane was added.[1] The suggested reason is that pancuronium can antagonize the vagal tone (heart slowing) induced by the morphine, thus allowing the blood pressure and heart rate to rise. The authors of the report point out the undesirability of this in those with coronary heart disease. Ketamine is a respiratory depressant like morphine but less potent, and its effects can be additive with morphine.[2]

References

1 Grossman E and Jacobi AM. Hemodynamic interaction between pancuronium and morphine. Anesthesiology (1974) 40, 299.
2 Bourke DL, Malit LA and Smith TC. Respiratory interactions of ketamine and morphine. Anesthesiology (1987) 66, 153–6.

Neuromuscular blockers + Phenytoin

Abstract/Summary

The neuromuscular blocking effects of doxacurium, metocurine, pancuronium and vecuronium are reduced by the concurrent use of phenytoin. Tubocurarine is only minimally affected, and atracurium hardly at all.

Clinical evidence

A comparative study in patients showed that those on phenytoin were resistant to the effects of certain neuromuscular blockers, as measured by the time to recover from 25 to 75% of the response to ulnar nerve stimulation. Compared with the controls, the recovery time for metocurine was reduced by 58%, for pancuronium by 40%, for tubocurarine by 24% and for atracurium by 8% (the last two were deemed not to be statistically significant).[1] Similar results for metocurine are described elsewhere by the same authors.[4] Another study[2] in nine patients on phenytoin showed that on average they needed 80% more pancuronium (0.058 mg/kg/hr) than 18 other patients not taking phenytoin (0.032 mg/kg/hr) while yet another found that in the presence of phenytoin 50% more vecuronium was needed but atracurium was not affected.[6] Only a small reduction in the effects of atracurium by phenytoin was seen in another study.[7] Resistance to pancuronium due to phenytoin has also been described in three other reports,[3,8,9] and a shortening of the recovery period in yet another.[5] Doxacurium seems to be affected even more than pancuronium.[9]

Mechanisms

Not understood. Suggestions include induction of liver enzyme activity which would increase the metabolism of the neuromuscular blocker, and alterations in the myoneural junction response.

Importance and management

Established and clinically important interactions. Anticipate the need to use more doxacurium, pancuronium, metocurine and vecuronium in patients on phenytoin, and expect an accelerated recovery. The effects on tubocurarine appear only to be moderate, and minimal with atracurium.

References

1 Ornstein E, Matteo RS, Silverberg PA, Shwartz AE, Young WL and Diaz J. Chronic phenytoin therapy and non-depolarizing muscular blockade. Anesthesiology (1985) 63, A331.
2 Chen J, Kim YD, Dubois M, Kammerer W and Macnamara TE. The increased requirement of pancuronium in neurosurgical patients receiving Dilantin chronically. Anesthesiology (1983) 59, A288.
3 Callan DL. Development of resistance to pancuronium in adult respiratory distress syndrome. Anesth Analg (1985) 64, 1126-8.
4 Ornstein E, Matteo RS, Young WL and Diaz J. Resistance to metocurine-induced neuromuscular blockade in patients receiving phenytoin. Anesthesiology (1985) 63, 294–8.
5 Messick J, Maass L, Faust R and Cucchiara R. Duration of pancuronium neuromuscular blockade in patients taking anticonvulsant medication. Anesth Analg (1982) 61, 203–4.
6 Ornstein E, Matteo RS, Schwartz AE, Silverberg PA, Young WL and

Diaz J. The effect of phenytoin on the magnitude and duration of neuromuscular block following atracurium or vecuronium. Anesthesiology (1987) 67, 191–6.

7 deBros F, Okutani R, Lai A, Lawrence KW and Basts S. Phenytoin does not interfere with atracurium phamacokinetics and pharmacodynamics. Anesthesiology (1987) 67, A607.
8 Liberan BA, Norman P and Hardy BG. Pancuronium-phenytoin interaction: a case of depressed duration of neuromuscular blockade. Int J Clin Pharmacol Ther Toxicol (1988) 26, 371–4.
9 Desai P, Hewitt PB and Jones RM. Influence of anticonvulsant therapy on doxacurium and pancuronium-induced paralysis. Anesthesiology (1989) 71, A784.

Neuromuscular blockers + Promazine

Abstract/Summary

An isolated report describes prolonged apnoea in a patient given promazine while recovering from neuromuscular blockade with suxamethonium (succinylcholine).

Clinical evidence, mechanism, importance and management

A woman, recovering from surgery during which she had received suxamethonium, was given 25 mg promazine IV for sedation. Within 3 min she had become cyanotic and dyspnoeic, and required assisted respiration for 4 h.[1] The reason is not understood but one suggestion is that promazine possibly depresses pseudocholinesterase levels which would reduce the metabolism of the suxamethonium and thereby prolong recovery. Some caution would seem appropriate if promazine is given to any patient who has had suxamethonium. There seems to be no information about other phenothiazines and other neuromuscular blockers.

Reference

1 Regan AG and Aldrete JA. Prolonged apnea after administration of promazine hydrochloride following succinylcholine infusion. A case report. Anesth Analg (1967) 46, 315.

Neuromuscular blockers + Quinidine

Abstract/Summary

The effects of both depolarizing (e.g. suxamethonium) and non-depolarizing (e.g. tubocurarine) neuromuscular blockers can be increased by quinidine. Recurarization and apnoea have been seen in patients when quinidine was given during the recovery period from neuromuscular blockade.

Clinical evidence

A patient given metocurine (dimethyltubocurarine) during surgery regained her motor functions and was able to talk coherently during the recovery period. Within 15 min of additionally being given 200 mg quinidine sulphate by injection

she developed muscular weakness and respiratory embarrassment. She needed intubation and assisted respiration for a period of two-and-a-half hours. Edrophonium and neostygmine were used to aid recovery.[1]

This interaction has been described in man in reports involving tubocurarine[2] and suxamethonium.[3,4] It has also been seen in animals.[5–8]

Mechanism

Not fully understood. Quinidine appears to have some direct neuromuscular blocking activity of its own which is additive with those of conventional blockers.[5–8]

Importance and management

An established interaction but the documentation in man is limited. The incidence is uncertain but it was seen to a greater or lesser extent in five of six patients studied.[3] It has only been reported in man with metocurine, tubocurarine and suxamethonium, but it occurs in animals with gallamine and decamethonium and it seems possible that it will occur in man with any depolarizing or non-depolarizing neuromuscular blocker. This needs confirmation. Care should clearly be exercised if quinidine is used with any neuromuscular blocking drug.

References

1 Schmidt JL, Vick NA and Sadove MS. The effect of quinidine on the action of muscle relaxants. J Amer Med Ass (1963) 183, 669.
2 Way WL, Katzung BG and Larson CP. Recurarization with quinidine. J Amer Med Ass (1967) 200, 163.
3 Grogono AW. Anesthesia for atrial defibrillation. Effect of quinidine on muscular relaxation. Lancet (1963) ii, 1039.
4 Boere LA. Fehler und Gefahren. Recurarisation nach Chinidinsulfat. Anaesthetist (1964) 13, 368.
5 Miller RD, Way WL and Katzung BG. The neuromuscular effects of quinidine. Proc Soc Exp Biol Med (1968) 129, 215.
6 Miller RD, Way WL and Katzung BG. The potentiation of neuromuscular blocking agents by quinidine. Anesthesiol (1967) 28, 1036.
7 Cuthbert MF. The effect of quinidine and procainamide on the neuromuscular blocking action of suxamethonium. Br J Anaesth (1966) 38, 775.
8 Usubiaga JE. Potentiation of muscle relaxants by quinidine. Anaesthesiol (1968) 29, 1068.

Neuromuscular blockers + Quinine

Abstract/Summary

An isolated report describes recurarization and apnoea in a patient given intravenous quinine after recovering from neuromuscular blockade with suxamethonium and pancuronium.

Clinical evidence

A patient with acute pancreatitis, taking 1800 mg quinine daily, was given penicillin and gentamicin before undergoing surgery during which pancuronium and suxamethonium were used uneventfully. After the surgery the neuromuscular blockade was reversed with neostigmine and atropine, the patient awoke and was breathing well. After an hour and a half an IV infusion of 500 mg quinine in 500 ml isotonic saline (to run over 6 h) was started. Within 10 min (about 15 mg quinine) he became dyspnoeic, his breathing became totally ineffective and he needed re-intubation. Muscle flaccidity persisted for 3 h.[1] The reason for this reaction is not understood. A possible explanation is that it may have been the additive neuromuscular blocking effects of the gentamicin (well recognized as having neuromuscular blocking activity), the quinine (an optical isomer of quinidine which has blocking actions) and the residual effects of the pancuronium and suxamethonium.

There seem to be no other reports of problems in patients on neuromuscular blockers when given quinine, but this isolated case serves to emphasize the importance of being alert for any signs of recurarization in patients concurrently treated with one or more drugs possessing some neuromuscular blocking activity.

Reference

1   Sher MH and Mathews PA. Recurarization with quinine administration after reversal from anaesthesia. Anaesth Intens Care (1983) 11, 241–3.

Neuromuscular blockers + Testosterone

Abstract/Summary

An isolated report describes marked resistance to the effects of suxamethonium and vecuronium, apparently due to the long-term use of testosterone.

Clinical evidence, mechanism, importance and management

A woman transsexual who had been receiving 200 mg testosterone enanthate intramuscularly twice monthly for 10 years was resistant to 100 mg suxamethonium and needed 0.1 mg/kg vecuronium for effective tracheal intubation before surgery. During the surgery it was found necessary to use a total of 22 mg vecuronium over a 50 min period to achieve acceptable relaxation of the abdominal muscles for hysterectomy and salpingo-oophorectomy to be carried out. The reasons are not understood.[1]

Reference

1   Reddy P, Guzman A, Robalino J and Shevde K. Resistance to muscle relaxants in a patient receiving prolonged testosterone therapy. Anesthesiology (1989) 70, 871–3.

Neuromuscular blockers + Thiotepa

Abstract/Summary

An isolated report describes a marked increase in the neuromuscular blocking effects of pancuronium in a myasthenic patient when given thiotepa, but it normally appears not to interact with neuromuscular blocking agents.

Clinical evidence, mechanism, importance and management

A myasthenic patient rapidly developed very prolonged respiratory depression when given thiotepa intraperitoneally after receiving pancuronium.[1] Thiotepa has also been shown to increase the duration of succinylcholine neuromuscular blockade in dogs.[2] However *in vitro* studies show that thiotepa is a poor inhibitor of pseudocholinesterase[3] and in a normal patient it was found not to decrease serum levels significantly.[4] The general silence in the literature would seem to confirm that no special precautions are normally necessary.

References

1   Bennett EJ, Schmidt GB, Patel KP and Grundy EM. Muscle relaxants, myasthenia and mustards? Anesthesiology (1977) 46, 220–1.
2   Cremonesi E and Rodrigues I de J. Interacao de agentes curarizantes com antineoplasico. Rev Bra Anest (1982) 32, 313–15.
3   Zsigmond EK and Robins G. The effects of a series of anti-cancer drugs on plasma cholinesterase activity. Can Anesth Soc J (1972) 19, 75–8.
4   Mone JG and Mathie WE. Qualitative and quantitative defects of pseudocholinesterase activity. Anaesthesia (1967) 22, 55–7.

Neuromuscular blockers + Trimetaphan

Abstract/Summary

Trimet(h)aphan can increase the effects of suxamethonium (succinylcholine) which may result in prolonged apnoea. This may possibly occur with other neuromuscular blocking drugs.

Clinical evidence

A man undergoing neurosurgery was given tubocurarine and suxamethonium. During the recovery period he developed apnoea lasting about two-and-a-half hours attributed to the concurrent use of trimetaphan (4500 mg over a 90 min period). Later when he underwent further surgery using essentially the same anaesthetic techniques and drugs but with a very much smaller dose of trimetaphan (35 mg over a 10 min period) the recovery was normal.[1]

Nine out of 10 patients receiving ECT treatment and given suxamethonium showed an almost 90% prolongation in apnoea (from 142 to 265 s) when 10–20 mg trimetaphan was used instead of 1.2 mg atropine.[2] Prolonged apnoea has been seen in another patient given suxamethonium and trimetaphan.[6] On the basis of an *in vitro* study it was calculated that a typical dose of trimetaphan would double the duration of paralysis due to suxamethonium.[9]

Mechanism

Not fully understood. Trimetaphan can inhibit serum pseudocholinesterase[2] which would reduce the metabolism of the suxamethonium and thereby prolong its activity. Studies in dogs[5] and rats[3,4,8] and case reports in man[7] also indicate that trimetaphan has direct neuromuscular blocking activity. Its effects are additive with the neuromuscular blocking effects of the aminoglycosides.[8]

Importance and management

Information is limited but the interaction appears to be established. If trimetaphan and suxamethonium are used concurrently, be alert for enhanced and prolonged neuromuscular blockade. This has also been seen with non-depolarizing blockers such as tubocurarine in animals[3-5] but not reported so far in man. However respiratory arrest has been seen in man when large doses of trimetaphan were given in the absence of a neuromuscular blocker[7] so that caution is certainly needed. Animal studies also indicate that the blockade is not reversed by neostigmine or calcium chloride.[8]

References

1 Wilson SL, Miller RN, Wright C and Hasse D. Prolonged neuromuscular blockade with trimethaphan: a case report. Anesth Analg (1976) 55, 353.

2 Tewfik GI. Trimethaphan. Its effect on the pseudocholinesterase level of man. Anaesthesia (1957) 12, 326.

3 Pearcy WC and Wittenstein ES. The interactions of trimethaphan (Arfonad), suxamethonium and cholinesterase inhibition in the rat. Br J Anaesth (1960) 32, 156.

4 Deacock AR and Davies TDW. The influence of certain ganglionic blocking agents on the neuromuscular transmission. Br J Anaesth (1958) 30, 217.

5 Randall LD, Peterson WG and Lebmann G. The ganglionic blocking action of thiophan dervatives. J Pharmacol Exp Ther (1949) 97, 48.

6 Poulton TJ, James FM and Lockridge O. Prolonged apnoea following trimethaphan and succinylcholine. Anesthesiology (1979) 50, 54.

7 Dale RC and Schroeder ET. Respiratory paralysis during treatment of hypertension with trimethaphan camsylate. Arch Intern Med (1976) 136, 816.

8 Paradelis AG, Crassaris LG, Karachalios DN and Triantaphyllidis CJ. Aminoglycoside antibiotics: interaction with trimethaphan at the neuromuscular junctions. Drugs Exptl Clin Res (1987) 8, 233–6.

9 Sklar GS and Lanks KW. Effects of trimethaphan and sodium nitroprusside on hydrolysis of succinylcholine *in vitro*. Anesthesiology (1977) 47, 31–3.

21
SYMPATHOMIMETIC DRUG INTERACTIONS

Noradrenaline (norepinephrine, levarterenol) is the principal neurotransmitter involved in the final link between nerve endings of the sympathetic nervous system and the adrenergic receptors of the organs or tissues innervated. The effects of stimulation of this system can be reproduced or mimicked by noradrenaline itself and by a number of other drugs which can also cause stimulation of these receptors. The drugs which can behave in this way are described as 'sympathomimetics' and act either directly on the adrenergic receptors like noradrenaline itself or indirectly by releasing stored noradrenaline from the nerve endings. Some of them do both. This is very simply illustrated in Figure 21.1.

We now know that the adrenergic receptors of the sympathetic system are not identical but can be subdivided into at least four main types, α_1, α_2, β_1 and β_2, and it is now possible broadly to categorize the sympathomimetics into groups according to their activity. The value of this categorization is that individual sympathomimetic drugs can be selected for their stimulant actions on articular organs or tissues. For example, salbutamol and terbutaline are so-called β-agonists which selectively stimulate the β_2 receptors in bronchi causing bronchodilation. This represents a significant improvement on isoprenaline (isoproterenol) which also stimulates β_1 receptors in the heart, and on ephedrine, which stimulates α receptors as well. Although the sympathomimetics are categorized together in this chapter, it is important to appreciate that they have a very wide range of actions and uses. One should not, therefore, extrapolate the interactions seen with one drug to any other without fully taking into account their differences and similarities. The Index should be consulted for a full listing of all interactions involving drugs with sympathomimetic activity.

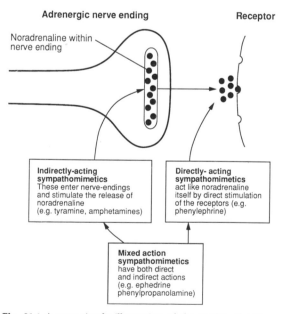

Fig. 21.1 A very simple illustration of the modes of action indirectly-acting, directly-acting and mixed action sympathomimetics at adrenergic neurones.

Table 21.1 A categorization of some sympathomimetic drugs.

Drug	Receptors stimulated
Direct stimulators of α and β receptors	
Adrenaline (epinephrine)	β more marked than α
Mainly direct stimulators of α receptors	
Phenylephrine	Predominantly α
Methoxamine	Premoninantly α
Metaraminol	Predominantly α
Noradrenaline (norepinephrine)	Predominantly α
Mainly direct stimulators of β$_1$ receptors	
Dopamine	Predominantly β$_1$, some α
Dobutamine	Predominantly β$_1$, some β$_2$ and α
Direct stimulators of β$_1$ and β$_2$ receptors	
Fenoterol	Predominantly β$_2$
Isoetharine	Predominantly β$_2$
Isoprenaline (Isoproterenol)	β$_1$ and β$_2$
Orciprenaline	Predominantly β$_2$
Ritodrine	Predominantly β$_2$
Salbutamol	Predominantly β$_2$
Terbutaline	Predominantly β$_2$
Direct and indirect stimulators of α and β receptors	
Ephedrine	α and β
Etefedrine	α and β
Phenylpropanolamine	α and β
Pseudoephedrine	α and β
Mainly indirect stimulators of α and β receptors	
Amphetamine	α and β ⎫
Mephentermine	α and β ⎬ also central stimulants
Methylphenidate	α and β ⎭
Tyramine	α and β

Amphetamines and Related drugs + Chlorpromazine

Abstract/Summary

The appetite suppressant and other effects of amphetamines, chlorphentermine and phenmetrazine are opposed by chlorpromazine. The antipsychotic effects of chlorpromazine can be opposed by amphetamine.

Clinical evidence

(a) Dextroamphetamine + phenothiazines

A study in 20 obese schizophrenic patients being treated with phenothiazines and other drugs (including chlorpromazine, thioridazine, imipramine and chlordiazepoxide) showed that they not only failed to respond to concurrent treatment with dextroamphetamine for obesity, but the expected sleep disturbance was not seen.[3] Antagonism of the effects of amphetamines by chlorpromazine has been described in other reports.[2,4]

A study in a very large number of patients taking 200–600 mg chlorpromazine daily indicated that the addition of 10–40 mg amphetamine had a detrimental effect on the control of their schizophrenic symptoms.[1]

(b) Chlorphentermine or phenmetrazine + chlorpromazine

A double-blind controlled study in patients taking chlorpromazine showed the effect of phenmetrazine in reducing weight was diminished.[5] Another study in which phenmetrazine or chlorphentermine were being used similarly showed that their effects on the control of obesity were inhibited by chlorpromazine.[6]

Mechanism

Not understood. However it is known that phenothiazines such as chlorpromazine are able to inhibit the uptake mechanism by which the amphetamines enter neurones. If this occurs at peripheral adrenergic neurones and centrally at both adrenergic and dopaminergic neurones, some part of the antagonism of the amphetamines can be explained.

Importance and management

Established interactions. These reports amply demonstrate that it is not desirable to attempt to treat patients with chlorpromazine and amphetamines, phenmetrazine or chlorphentermine concurrently. It is not clear whether this interaction takes place with phenothiazines other than chlorpromazine, but it seems possible.

This interaction has been deliberately exploited, and with success, in the treatment of 22 children poisoned with various amphetamines (dexamphetamine, methamphetamine, phenmetrazine).[2] They were given 1 mg/kg chlorpromazine intramuscularly initially, followed by further doses as necessary.

References

1 Casey JF, Hollister LE, Klett CJ, Lasky JJ and Caffrey EM. Combined drug therapy of chronic schizophrenics. Controlled evaluation of placebo, dextroamphetamine, imipramine, isocarboxazid and trifluoperazine added to maintenance doses of chlorpromazine. Am J Psychiat (1961) 117, 997.
2 Espelin DE and Done AK. Amphetamine poisoning: effectiveness of chlorpromazine. N Engl J Med (1968) 278, 1361.
3 Modell W and Hussar AE. Failure of dextroamphetamine sulphate to influence eating and sleeping patterns in obese schizophrenic patients: clinical and pharmacological significance. J Amer Med Ass (1965) 193, 275.
4 Jonsson LE. Pharmacological blockade of amphetamine effects in amphetamine-dependent subjects. Eur J Clin Pharmacol (1972) 4, 206.
5 Reid AA. Pharmacological antagonism between chlorpromazine and phenmetrazine in mental hospital patients. Med J Aust (1964) 1, 187.
6 Sletten IW, Orgnjanov V, Menendez S, Sunderland D and El-Toumi A. Weight reduction with chlorphentermine and phenmetrazine in obese psychiatric patients during chlorpromazine therapy. Curr Ther Res (1967) 9, 570.

Amphetamines + Lithium carbonate

Abstract/Summary

The effects of the amphetamines can be opposed by lithium carbonate.

Clinical evidence, mechanism, importance and management

Two depressed patients spontaneously abandoned abusing amphetamines (methamphetamine with cannabis and phenmetrazine) because, while taking lithium carbonate, they were unable to get 'high'. Another patient complained of not feeling any effects from amphetamines taken for weight reduction until lithium carbonate was withdrawn.[1] Another report confirmed these findings.[2] The reasons for these reactions is not known, but one suggestion is that amphetamines and lithium seem to have mutually opposing pharmacological actions on noradrenaline uptake at adrenergic neurones.[1] Information is very limited, but what is known indicates that a reduction in the effects of amphetamine may occur if lithium carbonate is given concurrently.

References

1 Flemenbaum A. Does lithium block the effects of amphetamine? A report of three cases. Am J Psychiatry (1974) 131, 820.
2 Van Kammen DP and Murphy D. Attentuation of the euphoriant and activating effects of d- and l-amphetamine by lithium carbonate treatment. Psychopharmacologia (1975) 44, 215.

Amphetamines + Nasal decongestants

Abstract/Summary

An isolated report describes the antagonism of l-amphetamine in a hyperactive child by nasal decongestants containing phenylpropanolamine and chlorpheniramine.

Clinical evidence

Maintenance therapy with 42 mg levoamphetamine succinate daily in a 12-year-old hyperactive boy was found to be ineffective on two occasions when he was concurrently treated with *Contac* and *Allerest* for colds. Both of these proprietary nasal decongestants contain phenylpropanolamine and chlorpheniramine.[1] The reason is not understood. There is too little information to make any statement about the general importance of this reaction.

Reference

1 Heustis RD and Arnold LE. Possible antagonism of amphetamine by decongestant-antihistamine compounds. J Pediatrics (1974) 85, 579.

Amphetamines + Urinary acidifiers or Alkalinizers

Abstract/Summary

The loss of amphetamine in the urine is increased by urinary acidifiers, and reduced by urinary alkalinizers.

Clinical evidence

A study in six normal subjects given 10–15 mg amphetamine by mouth showed that when the urine was made alkaline (approximately pH 8) by giving sodium bicarbonate, only 3% of the original dose of amphetamine was excreted over a 16 h period compared with 54% when the urine was made acid (approximately pH 5) by taking ammonium chloride.[1]

Similar results have been reported elswhere.[3] Psychoses resulting from amphetamine retention in patients with alkaline urine have been described.[2]

Mechanism

Amphetamine is a base which is excreted by the kidneys. In alkaline solution most of it exists in the un-ionized form which is readily reabsorbed by the kidney tubules so that little is lost in the urine. In acid solution, little of the drug is in the un-ionized form so that little can be reabsorbed and much is lost in the urine. A more detailed and illustrated account of this interaction mechanism is given in the introductory chapter.

Importance and management

A well-established interaction. It can be usefully exploited to clear amphetamine from the body more rapidly in cases of overdosage by acidifying the urine with ammonium chloride. Conversely it can represent an undesirable interaction if therapeutic doses of amphetamine are excreted too rapidly. Care is also needed to ensure that amphetamine intoxication does not develop if the urine is made alkaline with, for example, sodium bicarbonate or acetazolamide.

References

1 Beckett AH, Rowland M and Turner P. Influence of urinary pH on excretion of amphetamine. Lancet (1965) i, 303.
2 Anggard E, Jonsson L-E, Hogmark A-L and Gunne L-M. Amphetamine metabolism in amphetamine psychosis. Clin Pharmacol Ther (1973) 14, 870.
3 Rowland M and Beckett AH. The amphetamines: clinical and pharmacokinetic implications of recent studies of an assay procedure and urinary excretion in man. Arzneim-Forsch (1966) 16, 1369.

Directly-acting sympathomimetics + Beta-blockers

Abstract/Summary

(i) Effects on blood pressure. The pressor effects of adrenaline (epinephrine) can be markedly increased in patients taking non-selective beta-blockers such as propranolol: a severe and potentially life-threatening hypertensive reaction with bradycardia can develop. An isolated report describes a fatal hypertensive reaction with propranolol and phenylephrine but concurrent use normally seems to be uneventful. (ii) Effects on bronchi. No adverse interaction normally occurs during the concurrent use of sympathomimetic brochodilators (e.g. isoprenaline, isoproterenol) and cardio-selective beta-blockers (e.g. metoprolol). Non-selective beta-blockers (e.g. propranolol) should not be used in asthmatic subjects because they can cause serious bronchoconstriction. (iii) Anaphalaxis. The incidence of anaphylaxis is possibly increased by the beta-blockers and patients may be resistant to treatment with adrenaline (epinephrine) and other sympathomimetics.

Clinical evidence

(i) Effects on blood pressure

(a) Propranolol + adrenaline (epinephrine) or levonordefrin

Five normal subjects and four patients with hyperthyroidism showed a small increase in heart rate but little change in blood pressure after the subcutaneous injection of 0.4 mg adrenaline. After pre-treatment with 40 mg propranolol the same dose of adrenaline caused a 20–40 mm Hg rise in blood pressure and a fall in heart rate of 23–36 beats per minute.[1]

Six patients on 20–80 mg propranolol daily and undergoing plastic surgery experienced marked hypertensive reactions (blood pressures in the range 190/110 to 260/150 mm Hg) and bradycardia when their eyelids and/or faces were infiltrated with 8–40 ml of local anaesthetic solutions of lignocaine (lidocaine) containing 1:100,000 or 1:200,000 adrenaline (epinephrine). Cardiac arrest occurred in one patient.[7]

Similar marked increases in blood pressure,[2–5,10,11,20,22] associated in some instances with severe bradycardia, have been described in other reports involving propranolol. Only a small blood pressure rise was seen in a comparative study with metoprolol.[4] This was confirmed in another study in which patients given identical infusions of adrenaline (epinephrine) developed a hypertensive-bradycardial reaction while taking propranolol but not while taking metoprolol.[8] A hypertensive reaction has also been seen in a patient on propranolol when given an injection of 2% mepivacaine with 1:20,000 levonordefrin.[21]

(b) Propranolol + phenylephrine

A woman with hypertension, well controlled with propranolol (30 mg four times a day), was given one drop of a 10% phenylephrine hydrochloride solution in each eye during an ophthalmic examination. 45 min later she complained of a sudden and sharp bi-temporal pain and shortly afterwards became unconscious. She later died of an intracerebral haemorrhage due to the rupture of a berry aneurysm.[9] She had had a similar dose of phenylephrine on a previous occasion in the absence of propranolol without any problems. No change in blood pressure was seen in another study in subjects taking metoprolol who were administered 0.5–4.0 mg doses of phenylephrine intranasally[6] or in 12 hypertensive patients on propranolol or metoprolol when given intravenous infusions of phenylephrine.[11]

Mechanism

Adrenaline stimulates alpha- and beta-receptors of the cardiovascular system, the former resulting in vasoconstriction and the latter in both vasodilatation and stimulation of the heart. The net result is usually a modest increase in heart rate and a small rise in blood pressure. If however the beta-receptors are blocked, the unopposed alpha vasoconstriction causes a marked rise in blood pressure, followed by bradycardia due to the unopposed increase in reflex vagal tone. Cardioselective beta-blockers have a much smaller effect on the beta-2 receptors in the blood vessels and therefore the effects of any interaction is relatively small. Phenylephrine is largely an alpha-stimulator.

Importance and management

The propranolol–adrenaline (epinephrine) interaction is established. It may be serious and potentially life-threatening, depending on the dosage of adrenaline (epinephrine) used. Marked and serious rises have occurred in patients given 300–400 μg adrenaline subcutaneously[1,9] or 80–400 μg by infiltration of skin and eyelids during plastic surgery. Patients on non-selective beta-blockers such as propranolol should only be administered adrenaline in very reduced dosages because of the marked bradycardia and hypertension which can occur. A less marked effect is likely with the selective beta-blockers such as metoprolol.[4] A list of the different types of beta-blockers is given in the introduction to Chapter

10. Local anaesthetics used in dental surgery usually contain very low concentrations (e.g. 5–20 μg/ ml, i.e. 1 in 200,000—1 in 50,000) and only small volumes are usually given, so that an undesirable interaction is unlikely.

No interaction between phenylephrine and the beta-blockers would be expected. Apart from the single unexplained case cited above,[9] the literature would appear to be silent. Concurrent use normally appears to be clinically unimportant,[6,11] particularly bearing in mind the widespread use of the beta-blockers and the ready availability of phenylephrine in the form of over-the-counter cough-and-cold remedies and nasal decongestants.

Acute hypertensive episodes can be controlled with chlorpromazine given in 1 mg increments, or phentolamine, both of which are alpha-blockers. Intravenous hydralazine, 20mg in 250 ml saline, administered at 40 drops per min for 10–20 min has been used successfully[7]. Nifedipine has also been used.[20]

(ii) Effects on bronchi

(a) Cardio-selective beta-blockers

Normally the cardio-selective beta-blockers do not affect the beta-receptors in the bronchi although there a few cases on record of brocho-spasm following their use by asthmatics. No adverse interaction occurs between beta-agonist sympathomimetic bronchodilators and these beta-blockers. A study in 29 patients with chronic bronchial asthma taking 200 mg practolol daily, showed that the effects of terbutaline, 15 mg daily, were unaltered and no subjective or objective worsening of the asthmatic symptoms was seen.[14] Similar results have been described in other studies with metoprolol[12,13] or practolol[12] with isoprenaline (isoproterenol); and atenolol or metoprolol with terbutaline.[17]

(b) Non-selective beta-blockers

Non-selective beta-blockers, such as propranolol, are contraindicated in asthmatic subjects because they can precipitate an asthmatic attack by blocking the normal dilation of the bronchi which is under the control of the sympathetic nervous system.[12,13] Even eye drops containing the non-selective beta-blocker timolol have been reported to precipitate an asthmatic attack.[15]

Mechanism

Non-selective beta-blockers, intended for their actions on the heart, also block the beta-receptors in the bronchi so that the normal brochodilation which is under the control of the sympathetic nervous system is reduced or abolished. As a result the brochoconstriction of asthma is made worse. Cardioselective beta-blockers, on the other hand, preferentially block beta-1 receptors in the heart, leaving the beta-2 receptors largely unaffected, so that beta-2 stimulating bronchodilators such as isoprenaline, terbutaline, etc. continue to have their bronchodilator effects.

Importance and management

Non-selective beta-blockers should be avoided in asthmatic subjects, whether given orally or in eye-drops. The cardioselective beta-blockers are very much safer for patients with chronic obstructive airway disease, and the evidence indicates that no adverse interaction is likely with the beta-agonist bronchodilator sympathomimetics (isoprenaline, terbutaline, salbutamol).

(iii) Anaphylaxis: resistance to treatment

Clinical evidence, mechanism, importance and management

A patient who suffered an anaphylactic reaction after receiving an allergy injection was resistant to the bronchodilatory effects of adrenaline (epinephrine) because she was taking propranolol.[15] Resistance to treatment in patients on beta-blockers has been described in a number of reports.[16] There is some suggestion that the incidence of anaphylactic reactions may also be increased.[18,19] The reasons are not well understood but it seems possible that the adrenoceptors concerned with suppressing the release of the mediators of anaphylaxis may be blocked by either beta-1 or beta-2 antagonists.[18]

It may be necessary to use much larger doses of adrenaline (epinephrine) or other sympathomimetics to overcome the resistance. An 80-fold increase in the IV dose of isoprenaline (isoproterenol) has even been suggested.[18]

References

1 Varma DR, Sharma KK and Arora RC. Response to adrenaline and propranolol in hyperthyroidism. Lancet (1976), 1, 260.
2 Kram J, Bourne HR, Melmon KL and Malbach H. Propranolol. Ann Int Med (1974) 80, 282.
3 Harris WS, Schoenfeld CD, Brooks RH and Weissler AM. Effect of beta adrenergic blockade on the hemodynamic responses to epinephrine. Amer J Cardiol (1966) 17, 484.
4 van Herwaarden CLA. Effects of adrenaline during treatment with propranolol and metoprolol. Br Med J (1977) 2, 1029.
5 Berchtold P and Bessman AN. Propranolol. Ann Int Med (1974) 80, 119.
6 Myers MG and Iazetta JJ. Intranasally administered phenylephrine and blood pressure. Can Med Ass J (1982) 127, 365–8.
7 Foster CA and Aston SJ. Propranolol-epinephrine interaction: a potential disaster. Plastic Surg and Reconstr Surg (1983) July, 74–8.
8 Houben H, Thien T and Laor VA. Effect of low-dose epinephrine infusion on hemodynamics after selective and non-selective beta-blockade in hypertension. Clin Pharmacol Ther (1982) 31, 685.
9 Cass E, Kadar D, and Stein HA. Hazards of phenylephrine topical medication in persons taking propranolol. Can Med Ass J (1979) 120, 1261–2.
10 Hansbrough JF and Near A. Propranolol-epinephrine antagonism with hypertension and stroke. Ann InternMed (1980) 92, 717.
11 Myers MG. Beta-adrenoceptor antagonism and pressor response to phenylephrine. Clin Pharmacol Ther (1984) 36, 57–63.
12 Thringer G and Svedmyr N. Interaction of orally administered metoprolol, practolol and propranolol with isoprenaline in asthmatics. Eur J Clin Pharmacol(1976) 10, 163.
13 Johnsson G, Svedmyr N and Thurnier G. Effects of intravenous propranolol and metoprolol and their interaction with isoprenaline on pulmonary function, heart rate and blood pressure in asthmatics. Eur J Clin Pharmacol(1975) 8, 175.
14 Fromgren H and Eriksson NE. Effects of practolol in combination with terbutaline in the treatment of hypertension and arrhythmias in asthmatic patients. Scand J Resp Dis (1975) 56, 217.

15 Charan NB amd Lakshminarayan S. Pulmonary effects of topical timolol. Arch InternMed (1980) 120, 843.
16 Newman BR and Schultz LK. Epinephrine-resistant anaphylaxis in a patient taking propranolol hydrochloride. Ann Allergy (1981) 47, 35.
17 Lofdahl C-G and Svedmyr N. Cardioselectivity of atenolol and metoprolol. A study in asthmatic patients. Eur J Resp Dis (1981) 62, 396–404.
18 Toogood JH. Beta-blocker therapy and the risk of anaphylaxis. Canad Med Ass J (1987) 136, 929–33.
19 Berkelman RL, Finton RJ and Elsea W. Beta-adrenergic antagonists and fatal anaphylactic reactions to oral penicillin. Ann InternMed (1986) 104, 143.
20 Whelan TV. Propranolol, epinephrine and accelerated hypertension during hemodialysis. Ann InternMed (1987) 106, 327.
21 Mito RS and Yagiela JA. Hypertensive response to levonordefrin in a patient receiving propranolol: report of a case. J Am Dent Ass (1988) 116, 55–7.
22 Gandy W. Severe epinephrine-propranolol interaction. Ann Emerg Med (1989) 18, 98–9.

Directly and Indirectly-acting sympathomimetic amines + Furazolidone

Abstract/Summary

After 5–10 days' use furazolidone has MAO-inhibitory activity approximately equivalent to the antidepressant and antihypertensive MAOI's. The concurrent use of sympathomimetic amines with indirect activity (amphetamines, phenylpropanolamine, ephedrine, etc.) or tyramine-rich foods and drinks may be expected to result in a potentially serious rise in blood pressure, although direct evidence of accidental adverse reactions of this kind seem not to have been reported. The pressor effects of noradrenaline (norepinephrine) are unchanged.

Clinical evidence

A study in four hypertensive patients showed that after six days' treatment with 400 mg furazolidone daily, the pressor responses to tyramine or dexamphetamine had increased two- to threefold, and after 13 days about tenfold. These responses were approximately the same as those found in two other patients on pargyline.[1] The MAO-inhibitory activity of furazolidone was confirmed by measurements taken on jejunal specimens. The pressor effects of noradrenaline were unchanged.[1]

Mechanism

The MAO-inhibitory activity of furazolidone is not immediate and may in fact be due to a metabolite of furazolidone[4]. It develops gradually so that, after 5–10 days use, indirectly-acting sympathomimetics will interact with furazolidone in the same way as they do in the presence of other MAOI's. More details of the mechanisms of this interaction are to be found elsewhere (see 'Tyramine-rich foods + MAOI', 'Indirectly-acting sympathomimetics + MAOI').

Importance and management

The MAO-inhibitory activity of furazolidone after 5–10 days' use is established, but reports of hypertensive crises either with sympathomimetics or tyramine-containing foods or drinks appear to be lacking. Notwithstanding, it would seem prudent to warn patients given furazolidone not to take any of the drugs, foods or drinks which are prohibited to those on antidepressant or antihypertensive MAOI (e.g. cough, cold and influenza remedies containing phenylpropanolamine, phenylephrine, pseudoephedrine, etc., appetite-suppressants containing sympathomimetics, or tyramine-rich foods or drinks). See the appropriate synopses for more detailed lists of these drugs, foods and drinks ('Tyramine-rich foods+MAOI', 'Tyramine-rich alcoholic drinks+MAOI'). No adverse interaction would be expected with noradrenaline (norepinephrine).

References

1 Pettinger WA and Oates JA. Supersensitivity to tyramine during monoamine oxidase inhibition in man. Mechanism at the level of the adrenergic neurone. Clin Pharmacol Ther (1968) 9, 341.
2 Pettinger WA, Soyangco FG and Oates JA. Monoamine oxidase inhibition by furazolidone in man. Clin Res (1966) 14, 258.
3 Pettinger WA, Soyangco F and Oates JA. Inhibition of monoamine oxidase in man by furazolidone. Clin Pharmacol Ther (1968) 9, 442.
4 Stern IJ, Hollifield RD, Wilk S and Buzard JA. The anti-monoamine oxidase effects of furazolidone. J PharmacolExp Ther (1967) 156, 492–9.

Directly-acting sympathomimetics + Guanethidine and Related drugs

Abstract/Summary

The pressor effects of noradrenaline (norepinephrine, levarterenol), phenylephrine, metaraminol and similar drugs can be increased two- to fourfold in the presence of guanethidine and related drugs (bethanidine, debrisoquine, guanadrel, etc.). The mydriatic effects are similarly enhanced and prolonged.

Clinical evidence

(a) Pressor responses

A study in six normal subjects, given 200 mg guanethidine on the first day of study and 100 mg daily for the next two days, showed that their pressor responses (one third pulse pressure + diastolic pressure) when infused with noradrenaline in a range of doses were enhanced two-and-a-half to four times. Moreover cardiac arrhythmias appeared at lower doses of noradrenaline and with greater frequency than in the absence of guanethidine, and were more serious in nature.[1]

There are reports of this enhanced pressor response involving debrisoquine with phenylephrine,[3,4] (even when given orally[9]), with bretylium and noradrenaline,[5] and guanethidine with metaraminol.[2] In the latter instance, 10 mg metaraminol given intravenously rapidly caused a blood pressure rise to 220/130 mm Hg accompanied by severe headache and extreme angina. An increased blood pressure (from 165/92 to 210/120 mm Hg) was also seen in a patient on guanethidine who, prior to surgery, was treated with phenylephrine eye drops.[10]

(b) Mydriatic responses

The mydriasis due to phenylephrine administered as a 10% eyedrop solution was observed to be prolonged for up to 10 h in a patient concurrently receiving guanethidine for hypertension.[6] This enhanced mydriatic response has been described in other studies involving guanethidine with adrenaline, phenylephrine or methoxamine;[7] and debrisoquine with phenylephrine[9] or ephedrine.[7]

Mechanism

If sympathetic nerves are cut surgically, the receptors which they normally stimulate become hypersensitive. By preventing the release of noradrenaline (norepinephrine) from adrenergic neurones, guanethidine and other adrenergic neurone blockers cause a temporary 'drug-induced sympathectomy' which is also accompanied by hypersensitivity of the receptors. Hence the increased response to the stimulation of the receptors by directly acting sympathomimetics.

Importance and management

An established, well-documented and potentially serious interaction. Since the pressor effects are grossly exaggerated, dosages of directly-acting sympathomimetics (alpha-agonists) should be reduced appropriately. The pressor effects of noradrenaline (levarterenol) are increased two- to fourfold, and of phenylephrine twofold. In addition it should be remembered that the incidence and severity of heart arrhythmias is increased.[1,4] Considerable care is required. Direct evidence seems to be limited to noradrenaline, phenylephrine and metaraminol, but dopamine and methoxamine possess direct sympathomimetic activity and may be expected to interact similarly. No interaction would be expected with the beta-agonist drugs used for the treatment of asthma (such as terbutaline, salbutamol). Bethanidine and other guanethidine-like drugs (guanoclor, guanoxan, guanadrel, etc.) are also expected to behave like guanethidine. If as a result of this interaction the blood pressure becomes grossly elevated, it can be controlled by the administration of an alpha-adrenergic blocker such as phentolamine.[3,9]

Phenylephrine is contained in a number of over-the-counter cough and cold preparations, a few of which contain up to 10 mg in a dose. This dose is only likely to cause a moderate blood pressure rise, compared with the marked rise seen in subjects on debrisoquine given 0.75 mg/kg (roughly 45 mg in a 10-stone individual).[4,8] However this requires confirmation.

An exaggerated pressor response is clearly much more potentially serious than enhanced and prolonged mydriasis, but the latter is also possible and undesirable. It can occur whether or not the guanethidine-like drug has been given systemically or topically. The same precautions apply about using smaller amounts of the sympathomimetic drugs.

References

1 Mulheims GH, Entrup RW, Palewonsky D and Mierzwiak DS. Increased sensitivity of the heart to catecholamine-induced arrhythmias following guanethidine. Clin Pharmacol Ther (1965) 6, 757.
2 Stevens FRT. A danger of sympathomimetic drugs. Med J Aust (1966) 2, 576.
3 Aminu J, D'Mello A and Vere DW. Interaction between debrisoquine and phenylephrine. Lancet (1970) ii, 935.
4 Allum W, Aminu J, Bloomfield TH, Davies C, Scales AH and Vere DW. Interaction between debrisoquine and phenylephrine in man. Brit J Pharmacol(1973) 47, 675P.
5 Laurence DR and Nagle RE. The interaction of bretylium with pressor agents. Lancet (1961) i, 593.
6 Cooper B. Neo-synephrine (10%) eye drops. Med J Aust (1968) 55, 420.
7 Sneddon JM and Turner P. The interactions of local guanethidine: tolerance and effects on adrenergic nerve function and response to sympathomimetic amines. Brit J Pharmac(1962) 19, 13.
8 Boura ALA and Green AF. Comparison of bretylium and guanethidine; tolerance and effects on adrenergic nerve function and responses to sympathomimetic amines. Br J Pharmac (1962) 19, 3.
9 Allum W, Aminu J, Bloomfield TH, Davies C, Scales AH and Vere DW. Interaction between debrisoquine and phenylephrine in man. Br J clin Pharmac (1974) 1, 51.
10 Kim JM, Stevenson CE and Matthewson HS. Hypertensive reactions to phenylephrine eyedrops in patients with sympathetic denervation. Am J Ophthalmol (1978) 85, 862–8.

ministration of indirectly-acting sympathomimetics such as phenypropranolamine in cough and cold remedies, need to be imposed. However the isolated report cited indicates that the occasional patient may possibly experience unpleasant adverse effects.

References

1 Ghose K, Coppen A and Turner P. Autonomic actions and interactions of mianserin hydrochloride (Org GB94) and amitriptyline in patients with depressive illness. Psychopharmacology (1976) 49, 201.
2 Coppen A, Ghose K, Swade C and Wood K. Effect of mianserin hydrochloride on peripheral uptake mechanisms for noradrenaline and 5-hydroxytryptamine in man. Br J clin Pharmac (1978) 5, 13s.
3 Ghose K. Studies on the interaction between mianserin and noradrenaline in patients suffering with depressive illness. J clin Pharmacol(1977) 4, 712.
4 Coppen AJ and Ghose K. Clinical and pharmacological effects of treatment with a new antidepressant. Arzneim-Forsch/Drug Res (1976) 26, 1166.
5 Larochelle P, Hamet P, Enjalbert M. Responses to tyramine and norepinephrine after imipramine and trazodone. Clin Pharmacol Ther (1979) 26, 24.
6 Weddige RL. Possible trazodone-pseudoephedrine toxicity: a case report. Neurobehav toxicol teratol (1985) 7, 201

Directly-acting sympathomimetics + Mianserin or Trazodone

Abstract/Summary

No adverse interaction would be expected in patients on mianserin or trazodone who are treated with sympathomimetic amines, however a single report describes toxicity in a woman on trazodone when she took pseudoephedrine.

Clinical evidence, mechanism, importance and management

Studies in depressed patients have shown that the pressor (increased blood pressure) responses to tyramine and noradrenaline (norepinephrine) remain virtually unchanged after 14 days treatment with 60 mg mianserin daily.[1-4] Other studies on normal subjects given 50 mg trazodone three times a day found that the pressor response to tyramine remained unchanged whereas the response to noradrenaline was reduced.[5] However an isolated report describes a woman who had been taking 250 mg trazodone daily for two years who took two doses of an over-the-counter medicine containing pseudoephedrine. Within 6 h she experienced dread, anxiety, panic, confusion, depersonalization and the sensation that parts of her body were separating. None of these symptoms had been experienced in the past on either preparation alone.[6] The reasons for this reaction are not understood.

The practical importance of these observations is that, unlike the tricyclic antidepressants, no special precautions would normally seem necessary if patients on mianserin or trazodone are given noradrenaline or other directly-acting sympathomimetics. Similarly none of the dietary precautions against eating tyramine-rich foods or drinks, or the ad-

Directly-acting sympathomimetic amines + Monoamine oxidase inhibitors (MAOI)

Abstract/Summary

The pressor effects of adrenaline (epinephrine, levarterenol), isoprenaline (isoproterenol) and methoxamine may be unchanged or only moderately increased in patients taking MAOI. The increase may possibly be more marked in those who show a significant hypotensive response to the MAOI. An isolated case of tachycardia and apprehension has also been described in an asthmatic on phenelzine after taking salbutamol, and hypomania in another asthmatic after taking isoetharine.

Clinical evidence

(a) Effects in normal subjects

Two subjects given 45 mg phenelzine daily, and another given 30 mg tranylcypromine daily, for seven days showed no significant changes in their pressor responses to either adrenaline (epinephrine) or isoprenaline (isoproterenol). Another subject on tranylcypromine, similarly treated, showed a twofold increase in the pressor response in the mid-range of noradrenaline (norepinephrine) concentrations infused, but not in the upper or low ranges.[1]

These results confirm those found in two other studies, one with noradrenaline and phenelzine[2] and the other with noradrenaline and methoxamine in patients taking nialamide.[3] However yet another study in three volunteers on tranylcypromine found that the effects of noradrenaline were slightly increased and while with adrenaline a two- to fourfold increase in the effects on heart rate and diastolic pressure took place, but a less marked increase in systolic pressure. Isoprenaline behaved very much like adrenaline, but there was no enhancement of systolic pressure.[4] Tachycardia and apprehension in a man on phenelzine after taking salbutamol has also been described,[5] and hypomania in a man on phenelzine while taking isoetharine.[6]

(b) Effects in patients with MAOI-induced hypotension

In a study in seven hypertensive patients who showed postural hypotension after being given either pheniprazine or tranylcypromine, it was demonstrated that the doses of noradrenaline required to produce a 25 mm Hg rise in systolic pressure were reduced to 13–38% and of methoxamine to 30–39%.[3] However another study found no significant change when noradrenaline was given to two patients treated with pargyline.[7]

Mechanism

These sympathomimetic amines act directly on the receptors at the nerve endings which innervate arterial blood vessels, so that the presence of the MAOI-induced accumulation of noradrenaline within these nerve endings would not be expected to alter the extent of direct stimulation. The enhancement seen in those patients whose blood pressure was lowered by the MAOI might possibly be due to an increased sensitivity of the receptors which is seen if the nerves are cut, and is also seen during temporary 'pharmacological severance'. The reactions of the two patients given beta-adrenergic agonists (salbutamol, isoetherine) is not understood.

Importance and management

The evidence is limited, but the overall picture is that some slight to moderate enhancement of the effects of noradrenaline (levarterenol) and adrenaline (epinephrine) may occur, but the authors of two of the reports cited[1,4] are in general agreement that the extent is normally not likely to be hazardous. Some caution is, however, appropriate. Direct evidence about methoxamine is even more limited but it seems to behave similarly. None of the studies demonstrated any marked changes in the effects of isoprenaline (isoproterenol).

The situation in patients who show a reduced blood pressure due to the use of an MAOI (this would seem to apply principally to pargyline) is less clear. One study found a very marked increase in the pressor efforts of noradrenaline and methoxamine[3] in hypertensive patients on pheniprazine or tranylcypromine, whereas another[7] found no changes in the pressor effects of noradrenaline in patients on pargyline. Some caution is clearly needed.

The cases involving salbutamol and isoetharine are isolated and possibly not of general importance. This needs confirmation. The interaction between phenylephrine and the MAOI is dealt with separately elsewhere.

References

1 Boakes AJ, Laurence DR, Teoh PC, Barar FSK, Benedikter L and Prichard BNC. Interactions between sympathomimetic amines and antidepressant agents in man. Br Med J (1973) 1, 311.
2 Elis J, Laurence DR, Mattie H and Prichard BNC. Modification by monoamine oxidase inhibitors of the effect of some sympathomimetics on blood pressure. Br Med J (1967) 2, 75.
3 Horwitz D, Goldberg LI and Sjoerdsma A. Increased blood pressure responses to dopamine and norepinephrine produced by monoamine oxidase inhibitors in man. J Lab Clin Med (1960) 56, 747.
4 Cuthbert MF and Vere DW. Potentiation of the cardiovascular effects of some catecholamines by a monoamine oxidase inhibitor. Brit J Pharmacol(1971) 43, 471P.
5 Shader RI and Greenblatt DJ. MAOI's and drug interactions—a proposal for a clearing house. J Clin Psychopharmacol (1985) 5, A17.
6 Goldman LS and Tiller JA. Hypomania related to phenelzine and isoetharine interaction in one patient. J Clin Psychiatry (1987) 48, 170.
7 Pettinger WA, Oates JA. Supersensitivity to tyramine during monoamine oxidase inhibition in man. Clin Pharmacol Ther (1968) 9, 341–4.

Directly- and indirectly-acting sympathomimetics + Rauwolfia alkaloids

Abstract/Summary

The pressor and other effects of directly acting sympathomimetics (adrenaline, noradrenaline, phenylephrine, etc.) are slightly increased in the presence of the rauwolfia alkaloids. The effects of indirectly acting sympathomimetics or those with mixed activity (amphetamines, mephentermine, ephedrine, phenylpropanolamine, etc.) may be reduced or abolished.

Clinical evidence

A study in seven normal subjects showed that after taking 0.25–1.0 mg reserpine daily for two weeks their pressor responses to noradrenaline (levarterenol) were slightly increased (20–40%) but their responses to tyramine (an indirectly acting amine) were reduced about 75%.[9] A man on reserpine who became hypotensive while undergoing surgery failed to respond to an intravenous injection of ephedrine, but did so after 30 min treatment with noradrenaline (levarterenol), presumably because the stores of noradrenaline at adrenergic neurones had become replenished.[1] A child who had accidentally taken reserpine (thought to be about 6.5 mg) also failed to respond to an intramuscular injection of ephedrine (16 mg).[3] The mydriatic effects of ephedrine in man were shown to be antagonized by pretreatment with reserpine,[2] but a number of patients on reserpine were found to have increased blood pressures (+30/+13 mm Hg) during surgery if pretreated with phenylephrine eyedrops.[10]

Experiments with dogs have demonstrated that adrenaline (epinephrine), noradrenaline (norepinephrine) and phenylephrine—all with direct actions—remain effective vasopressors after treatment with reserpine and their actions are enhanced to some extent, whereas the vasopressor actions of ephedrine, amphetamine, methamphetamine, tyramine and mephentermine—all with indirect actions—are reduced or abolished by reserpine.[5-7]

Mechanism

The rauwolfia alkaloids cause adrenergic neurones to lose their stores of noradrenaline (norepinephrine), so that they can no longer stimulate adrenergic receptors and transmission ceases. Indirectly acting sympathomimetics (which depend on their ability to stimulate the release of stored noradrenaline) may therefore be expected to become ineffective, whereas the effects of directly acting sympathomimetics should remain unchanged or possibly even enhanced because of the supersensitivity of the receptors which occurs when they are deprived of stimulation by noradrenaline for any length of time. Drugs with mixed direct and indirect actions, such as ephedrine, should fall somewhere between the two, although the reports cited seem to indicate that ephedrine has predominantly indirect activity in man.[1-3]

Importance and management

These are established interactions, but the paucity of clinical information suggests that in practice these interactions have not presented many problems. If a pressor drug is required, a directly acting drug such as noradrenaline (levarterenol) or phenylephrine may be expected to be effective. Metaraminol has also been successfully used as a pressor drug in reserpine-treated patients.[8] The receptors may show some supersensitivity so that a dosage reduction may be required. Somewhat surprisingly in the light of the other evidence, one report claims that 25 mg ephedrine given orally or intramuscularly, once or twice a day, proved to be an effective treatment for reserpine-induced hypotension and bradycardia in schizophrenic patients.[4]

References

1 Ziegler CH and Lovette JB. Operative complications after therapy with reserpine and reserpine compounds. J Amer Med Ass (1961) 176, 916.
2 Sneddon JM and Turner P. Ephedrine mydriasis in hypotension and the response to treatment. Clin Pharmacol Ther (1969) 10, 64.
3 Phillips T. Overdose of reserpine. Br Med J (1955) 2, 969.
4 Noce RH, Williams DB and Rapaport W. Reserpine (Serpasil) in the management of the mentally ill. J Amer Med Ass (1955) 158, 11–15.
5 Stone CA, Ross AC, Wenger HC, Ludden CT, Blessing JA, Totaro JA and Porter CC. Effect of alpha-methyl-3,4-dihydroxyphenylalanine (methyldopa), reserpine, and related agents on some vascular responses in the dog. J PharmacolExp Ther (1962) 136, 80.
6 Eger EI and Hamilton WK. The effect of reserpine on the action of various vasopressors. Anaesthesiology (1959) 20, 641.
7 Moore JI and Moran NC. Cardiac contractile force responses to ephedrine and other sympathomimetic amines in dogs after pretreatment with reserpine. J PharmacolExp Ther (1962) 136, 89.
8 Smessaert AA and Hicks RG. Problems caused by rauwolfia drugs during anaesthesia and surgery. NY State J Med (1961) 61, 2399.
9 Abboud FM and Ekstein JW. Effects of small oral doses of reserpine on vascular responses to tyramine and norepinephrine in man. Circulation (1964) 29, 219–23.
10 Kim JM, Stevenson CE and Matthewson HS. Hypertensive reactions to phenylephrine eyedrops in patients with sympathetic denervation. Am J Ophthalmol (1978) 85, 862–8.

Directly-acting sympathomimetic amines + Tricyclic antidepressants

Abstract/Summary

Patients being treated with tricyclic antidepressants show a grossly exaggerated response (hypertension, cardiac arrhythmias, etc.) to injections of noradrenaline (norepinephrine, levarterenol), adrenaline (epinephrine) or, to a lesser extent, to phenylephrine. Local anaesthetics containing these vasoconstrictors and levonordefrin should not be used, but felypressin is a safe alternative. Doxepin and maprotiline appear not to interact to the same extent as most tricyclic antidepressants.

Clinical evidence

The effects of intravenous infusions of noradrenaline were increased approximately ninefold, and of adrenaline approximately sixfold, in six healthy subjects who had been taking 60 mg protriptyline daily for four days.[1,2]

The effects of intravenous infusions of noradrenaline were increased 4-8-fold, of adrenaline 2-4-fold, and to phenylephrine 2-3-fold in four healthy subjects who had been taking 75 mg imipramine daily for five days. There were no noticeable or consistent changes in their response to isoprenaline (isoproterenol).[5]

Five patients taking nortriptyline, desipramine or other unnamed tricyclic antidepressants experienced adverse reactions, some of them severe (throbbing headache, chest pain) following the injection of *Xylestin* (lignocaine with 1:25,000 noradrenaline) during dental treatment.[4] Several episodes of marked increases in blood pressure, dilated pupils, intense malaise, violent but transitory tremor and palpitations have been reported in patients taking un-named tricyclic antidepressants when they were given local anaesthetics containing adrenaline or noradrenaline for dental treatment.[3]

There are other reports describing this interaction of noradrenaline with imipramine,[6,9] desipramine,[9,10] nortriptyline,[8] protriptyline[10] and amitriptyline;[9,10] of adrenaline with amitriptyline,[7] and of levonordefrin with desipramine (in dogs).[19]

Mechanism

The tricyclics and some related antidepressants block or inhibit the uptake of noradrenaline into adrenergic neurones. Thus the most important means by which noradrenaline is removed from the adreno-receptor area is inactivated and the concentration of noradrenaline outside the neurone can rise. If therefore more noradrenaline (or one of the other directly acting alpha or alpha/beta agonists) is infused into the body, the adreno-receptors of the cardiovascular system concerned with raising blood pressure become grossly stimulated by this superabundance of amines, and the normal response is accordingly exaggerated.

Importance and management

A well-documented, well-established and potentially serious interaction. The parenteral administration of noradrenaline (norepinephrine, levarterenol), adrenaline (epinephrine), phenylephrine or any other sympathomimetic amine with predominantly direct activity should be avoided in patients under treatment with tricyclic antidepressants. If these sympathomimetics must be used, the rate and amount injected must be very much reduced to accommodate the exaggerated responses which will occur. Local anaesthetics containing conventional vasoconstrictors (noradrenaline, adrenaline, levonordefrin) should not be given to patients taking tricyclic antidepressants, but felypressin has been shown to be a safe alternative.[11,12,16] If an adverse interaction occurs it can be controlled by the use of an alpha-receptor blocking agent such as phentolamine.

Doxepine in doses of less than 200 mg daily blocks neuronal uptake much less than other tricyclic antidepressants and so is unlikely to show this interaction to the same degree, but in larger doses it will interact like other tricyclics.[13,15] Maprotiline (a tetracyclic antidepressant) also blocks uptake much less than most of the tricyclics and in normal therapeutic doses in one study on three subjects was shown not to increase the pressor response to noradrenaline.[14] The pressor response to noradrenaline is also not significantly increased in the presence of mianserin (see 'Noradrenaline + Mianserin) or iprindole,[18] and is reported to be reduced in the presence of trazodone.[17] It does not seem to have been established whether the response to oral doses of phenylephrine is enhanced.

References

1 Svedmyr N. The influence of a tricyclic antidepressive agent (protripytline) on some circulatory effects of noradrenaline and adrenaline in man. Life Sci (1968) 7, 77.

2 Svedmyr N. Potentieringsvisker vid tillforsel au katekolaminer till patienter som behandlas med trickyliska antidepressiva medel. Svenska Lak Tidn (1968) 65, 72.

3 Dam WH. Personal communication cited by Kristoffersen MB. Antidepressivas potensering af Katekolaminvirkning. Ugeskr Laeg (1969) 131, 1013.

4 Boakes AJ, Laurence DR, Lovel KW, O'Neil R and Verrill PJ. Adverse reactions to local anaesthetic/vasoconstrictor preparations. A study of the cardiovascular responses to Xylestin and hostacain-with-adrenaline. Brit Dent J (1972) 133, 137.

5 Boakes AJ, Laurence DR, Teoh PC, Barar FSK, Benedikter LT and Prichard BNC. Interactions between sympathomimetic amines and antidepressant agents in man. Br Med J (1973) 1, 311.

6 Gershon S, Holmberg G, Mattsson E. Mattsson N and Marshall A. Imipramine hydrochloride. Its effects on clinical, autonomic and psychological functions. Arch Gen Psychiat (1962) 6, 96.

7 Siemkowicz E. Hjertestop efter amitriptylin og adrenalin. Ugeskrift Laeg (1975) 137, 1403.

8 Persson G and Siwers B. The risk of potentiating effect of local anaesthesia with adrenalin in patients treated with tricyclic antidepressants. Sven Tanlak Tiskr (1975) 68, 9.

9 Fischbach R, Harrer G and Harrer H. Verstarkung der Noradrenalinwirkung durch Psychopharmaka beim Menschen. Arzneim-Forsch (1966) 16, 263.

10 Mitchell JR, Cavanaugh JH, Arias L and Oates JA. Guanethidine and related agents. III. Antagonism by drugs which inhibit the norepinephrine pump in man. J Clin Invest (1970) 49, 1596.

11 Aelig WH, Laurence DR, O'Neil R and Verrill PJ. Cardiac effects of adrenaline and felypressin as vasoconstrictors in local anaesthesia for oral surgery under diazepam sedation. Br J Anaesth (1970) 42, 174.

12 Goldman V, Astrom A and Evers H. The effects of a tricyclic antidepressant on the cardiovascular effects of local anaesthetic solutions containing different vasoconstrictors. Anesthesia (1971) 26, 91.

13 Fann WE, Cavanaugh JH, Kaufmann JS, Griffith JD, Davis JM, Janowsky DS and Oates JA. Doxepin: effects on transport of biogenic amines in man. Psychopharmacologia (1971) 22, 111.

14 Briant RH and George CF. The assessment of potential drug interactions with a new tricyclic antidepressant drug. Br J clin Pharmacol(1974) 1, 113.

15 Oates JA, Fann WE and Cavanaugh JH. Effect of doxepin on the norepinephrine pump. Psychosomatics (1969) 10 (Suppl) 12.

16 Perovic J, Terzic M and Todorovic L. Safety of local anaesthesia induced by prilocaine with felypressin in patients on tricyclic antidepressants. Bull Group Int Rech Sci Stomatol Odontol (1979) 22, 57.

17 Larochelle P, Hamet P and Enjalbert M. Responses to tyramine and norepinephrine after imipramine and trazodone. Clin Pharmacol Ther (1979) 26, 24.

18 Fann WE, Davis JM, Janowsky DS, Kaufmann JS, Griffith JD and Oates JA. Effect of iprindole on amine uptake in man. Arch Gen Psychiatry (1972) 26, 158–62.

19 Dreyer AC and Offermeier J. The influence of desipramine on the blood pressure elevation and heart rate stimulation of levonordefrin and felypressin alone and in the presence of local anaesthetics. J Dent Ass SA (1986) 41, 615–18.

Dopamine + Ergometrine

Abstract/Summary

A single report attributes the development of gangrene in a patient to the infusion of dopamine after ergometrine.

Clinical evidence, mechanism, importance and management

Gangrene of the extremities has been described in a patient who was given an infusion of dopamine following the administration of ergometrine.[1] This would seem to have resulted from the additive peripheral vasoconstrictor effects of both drugs which reduced the circulation to such an extent that infection became unchecked. It would seem prudent to avoid concurrent use.

Reference

1 Buchanan N, Cane RD and Miller M. Symmetrical gangrene of the extremities associated with the use of dopamine subsequent to ergometrine administration. Intens Care Med (1977) 3, 55.

Dopamine + Phenytoin

Abstract/Summary

There is evidence that patients needing dopamine to support their blood pressure can become severely hypotensive if phenytoin is added to their treatment.

Clinical evidence, mechanism, importance and management

Five critically ill patients with a variety of conditions and under treatment with a number of different drugs, were given dopamine hydrochloride to maintain an adequate blood pressure. When seizures developed they were additionally given phenytoin. Coincidentally their hitherto stable blood pressures fell rapidly and one patient died from cardiorespiratory arrest. A similar reaction was demonstrated in dogs made hypovolemic and hypotensive by bleeding.[1] The reason for this reaction is not understood, but one suggestion is that the phenytoin may have a greater myocardial depressant effect during dopamine-induced catecholamine depletion.

The documentation is limited to this single report. This suspected interaction is not fully established, but there is enough evidence to indicate that phenytoin should only be used with great caution, or not at all, in those requiring dopamine to maintain their blood pressure.

Reference

1 Bivins BA, Rapp RP, Griffin WO, Bloudin R and Bustrack J. Dopamine-phenytoin interaction. A cause of hypotension in the critically ill. Arch Surg (1978) 113, 245.

Indirectly-acting sympathomimetic amines + Methyldopa

Abstract/Summary

Indirectly-acting sympathomimetics might be expected to cause a blood pressure rise in patients taking methyldopa, and an isolated case report describes a hypertensive reaction in a patient taking methyldopa and oxprenolol when he took a decongestant containing phenylpropanolamine, but in practice this interaction seems to be of little or no general practical importance. The mydriatic effects of ephedrine are reported to be depressed by methyldopa.

Clinical evidence, mechanism, importance and management

Studies in man have shown that after taking 2–3 g methyldopa daily, the pressor (rise in blood pressure) effects of tyramine were doubled.[1] In another study the pressor rise was 50/16 mm Hg compared with 18/10 before methyldopa treatment.[2] A man with renal hypertension, whose blood pressure was well controlled with 500 mg methyldopa and 480 mg oxprenolol daily, showed a rise in blood pressure from about 120–140/70–80 mm Hg to 200/150 mm Hg within two days of starting to take two tablets of *Triogesic* (phenylpropanolamine 12.5 mg and paracetamol 500 mg) three times a day. His blood pressure fell when the *Triogesic* was withdrawn.[4] The reason for this is uncertain. One suggestion is that the methyldopa causes the replacement of noradrenaline (epinephrine) at adrenergic nerve endings by methyl-noradrenaline which has weaker pressor (alpha) ac-

tivity but greater vasodilator (beta) activity. With the vasodilator activity blocked by the oxprenolol, the vasoconstrictor activity (pressor) of the phenylpropanolamine would be unopposed and exaggerated.

Despite the information derived from the studies outlined above[1,2] and the single report cited, there seems to be nothing else in the literature to suggest that indirectly-acting sympathomimetics normally cause an adverse reaction (rise in blood pressure) with methyldopa. More study is needed. One report states that the normal mydriatic effects of ephedrine are depressed by methyldopa.[3]

References

1 Pettinger W, Horwitz D, Spector S and Sjoerdsma A. Enhancement by methyldopa of tyramine sensitivity in man. Nature (1963) 200, 1107.
2 Dollery CT, Harrington M and Hodge JV. Haemodynamic studies with methyldopa: effect on cardiac output and response to pressor amines. Br Heart J (1963) 25, 670.
3 Sneddon JM and Turner P. Ephedrine mydriasis in hypertension and the response to treatment. Clin Pharmacol Ther (1969) 10, 64.
4 McLaren EH. Severe hypertension produced by interaction of phenylpropanolamine with methyldopa and oxprenolol. Br Med J (1976) 3, 283.

Indirectly-acting sympathomimetic amines + Monoamine oxidase inhibitors (MAOI)

Abstract/Summary

The concurrent use of sympathomimetic amines with indirect activity (amphetamines, phenylpropanolamine, ephedrine, pseudoephedrine, metaraminol, etc.) and MAOI can result in a potentially fatal hypertensive crisis. These amines are found in many proprietary cough, cold and influenza preparations, or are used as appetite suppressants. (See also 'Tyramine-rich foods + MAOI').

Clinical evidence

The interaction can result in a rapid and serious rise in blood pressure accompanied by tachycardia, chest pains and severe occipital headache. Neck stiffness, flushing, sweating, nausea, vomiting, hypertonicity of the limbs and sometimes epileptiform convulsions can occur. Fatal intracranial haemorrhage, cardiac arrhythmias and cardiac arrest may result. Two examples from many:

A woman who, unknown to her doctors, was taking pargyline, was given phenylpropanolamine for nasal decongestion on the eve of surgery which promptly caused a hypertensive reaction. Her blood pressure rose rapidly from 130/80 to 220/160 mm Hg and she complained of occipital headache, photophobia and nausea. She also exhibited sweating and vomited. Two intravenous injections of 5 mg phentolamine partially controlled her blood pressure.[1]

A 30-year-old depressed woman who was taking 45 mg

phenelzine daily and 2 mg trifluoperazine at night, acquired some dexamphetamine tablets from a friend and took 20 mg. Within 15 min she complained of severe headache which she described as if 'her head was bursting'. An hour later her blood pressure was 150/100 mm Hg. Later she became comatose and died. A postmortem examination revealed a haemorrhage in the left cerebral hemisphere, disrupting the internal capsule and adjacent areas of the corpus striatum.[2]

This interaction has been reported with amphetamine sulphate,[3] d-l amphetamine,[4] metaraminol,[11] methylamphetamine,[5–8] mephentermine,[19] ephedrine,[9,10] phenylpropanolamine,[12–15] pseudoephedrine,[18,22] and methylphenidate,[19] in patients on tranylcypromine,[3,5,6,9,10,13] phenelzine,[2,4–9,12,14,15,20] isocarboxazid,[6] iproniazid,[22] mebanazine,[12] and pargyline.[11] There are other reports and studies of this interaction not listed here. Extreme hyperpyrexia, apparently without hypertension, has with described with tranylcypromine and amphetamines.[16,17]

Mechanism

The symptoms of the interaction can be attributed to overstimulation of the adrenergic receptors of the cardiovascular system.[21] During treatment with MAOI, large amounts of noradrenaline (norepinephrine) accumulate at adrenergic nerve endings not only in the brain, but also within the sympathetic nerve endings which innervate arterial blood vessels. Stimulation of these nerve endings by sympathomimetic amines with indirect actions causes the release of the accumulated noradrenaline and in the massive stimulation of the receptors. Consequently an exaggerated blood vessel constriction occurs and the blood pressure rise is proportionately excessive. Intracranial haemorrhage can occur if the pressure is so high that a blood vessel ruptures.[2]

Importance and management

An extremely well-documented, serious, and potentially fatal interaction. Patients taking any of the older MAOI, whether for depression or hypertension, should not take any sympathomimetic amine with indirect activity. These include the amphetamines (dexamphetamine, hydroxyamphetamine, methylamphetamine), mephentermine, phenylpropanolamine, ephedrine, pseudoephedrine and metaraminol. Cyclopentamine, methylephedrine and pholedrine also have indirect sympathomimetic activity and may be expected to interact similarly. Direct evidence implicating benzphetamine, chlorphentermine, diethylpropion, mazindol,[23] phendimetrazine and phenmetrazine seems not to have been documented, but on the basis of their known pharmacology the manufacturers warn about their concurrent administration with the MAOI.

Many of these sympathomimetic amines occur in a considerable number of over-the-counter cough, cold and influenza preparations, and as proprietary appetite suppressants. Patients should be strongly cautioned about not taking any of these without first seeking informed advice. If a hypertensive reaction occurs, it can be controlled with alpha-adrenoreceptor blockers such as phentolamine, 5 mg given intravenously and repeated as necessary, or failing that intramuscular injections of 50 mg chlorpromazine.

References

1 Jenkins LC and Graves HB. Potential hazards of psychoactive drugs in association with anaesthesia. Can Anaes Soc J (1965) 12, 121.
2 Lloyd JT and Walker DRH. Death after combined dexamphetamine and phenelzine. Br Med J (1965) 2, 168.
3 Zeck P. The dangers of some antidepressant drugs. Med J Aust (1961) 2, 607.
4 Tonks CM and Livingstone D. MAOI. Lancet (1963) i, 1323.
5 MacDonald R. Tranylcypromine. Lancet (1963) i, 269.
6 Mason A. Fatal reaction associated with tranylcypromine and methylamphetamine. Lancet (1962) i, 1073.
7 Dally PJ. Fatal reaction associated with tranylcypromine and methylamphetamine. Lancet (1962) i, 1235.
8 Nymark M and Nielsen IM. Reactions due to the combination of MAOI's with thymoleptics, pethidine or methylamphetamine. Lancet (1963) ii, 524.
9 Ellis J, Laurence DR, Mattie H and Prichard BNC. Modification by monoamine oxidase inhibitors of the effects of some sympathomimetics on blood pressure. Br Med J (1967) 2, 75.
10 Low-Beer GA and Tidmarsh D. Collapse after Parstelin. Br Med J (1963) 2, 683.
11 Horler AR and Wynne NA. Hypertensive crisis due to pargyline and metaraminol. Br Med J (1965) 2, 460.
12 Tonks CM and Lloyd AT. Hazards with monoamine oxidase inhibitors. Br Med J (1965) 1, 589.
13 Cuthbert MF, Greenberg MP and Morley SW. Cough and cold remedies: potential danger to patients on monoamine oxidase inhibitors. Br Med J (1969) 1, 404.
14 Mason AMS and Buckle RM. 'Cold' cures and monoamine oxidase inhibitors. Br Med J (1969) 1, 845.
15 Humberstone PM. Hypertension from cold remedies. Br Med J (1969) 1, 846.
16 Lewis E. Hyperpyrexia with antidepressant drugs. Br Med J (1965) 1, 1671.
17 Krisko I, Lewis E and Johnson JE. Severe hyperpyrexia due to tranylcypromine and amphetamine toxicity. Ann InternMed (1969) 70, 559.
18 Wright SP. Hazards with monoamine oxidase inhibitors: a persistent problem. Lancet (1978) i, 284.
19 Sherman M, Hauser GC and Glover BH. Toxic reactions to tranylcypromine. Ann J Psychiat (1964) 120, 1019.
20 Stark DCC. Effects of giving vasopressors to patients on monoamine oxidase inhibitors. Lancet (1962) i, 1405.
21 Simpson LL. Mechanism of the adverse interaction between monoamine oxidase inhibitors and amphetamine. J Pharm Exp Ther (1978) 205, 392.
22 Davies R. Patient medication records. Pharm J (1982) 287, 652.
23 Magrath SM (Sandoz Products Ltd). Personal communication (1987).

Indirectly-acting sympathomimetic amines + Tricyclic antidepressants

Abstract/Summary

The effects of indirectly acting sympathomimetics (amphetamines, phenylpropanolamine, etc.) would be expected to be reduced by the tricyclic antidepressants, but so far only one case involving ephedrine and amitriptyline seems to have been reported.

Clinical evidence, mechanism, importance and management

Indirectly-acting sympathomimetic amines like tyramine exert their effects by causing the release of noradrenaline (norepinephrine) from adrenergic neurones rather than by a direct stimulant action on the receptors. In the presence of a tricyclic antidepressant, the entry of these amines into adrenergic neurones is partially or totally prevented and the noradrenaline-releasing effects are therefore blocked. The reduction in the pressor response to tyramine has been used to monitor the efficacy of treatment with the tricyclic antidepressants.[1] However tyramine itself is only used as a research tool, or as a model of the behaviour of the indirectly acting sympathomimetics. The activity of other similar sympathomimetics might be expected to be blocked by the tricyclics in the same way, but only one case seems to have been reported. An elderly woman on 75 mg amitriptyline daily developed hypotension (70 mm Hg systolic) during subarachnoid anaesthesia. Her blood pressure rose only minimally when given IV boluses of ephedrine (a mixed action sympathomimetic) totalling 90 mg but she responded normally when given adrenaline (a directly-acting sympathomimetic).[2]

References

1 Mulgirigama LD, Pare CMB, Turner P, Wadsworth J and Witts DJ. Tyramine pressor responses and plasma levels during tricyclic antidepressant therapy. Postgrad Med J (1977) 53 (Suppl 4) 30.
2 Serle DG. Amitriptyline and ephedrine in subarachnoid anesthesia. Anaesth Int Care (1985) 13, 214

Isoprenaline + Tricyclic antidepressants

Abstract/Summary

Although isoprenaline (isoproterenol) and amitriptyline have been used together safely and with advantage in the treatment of asthma, an isolated case has been reported of death arising from their current use (or abuse?).

Clinical evidence, mechanism, importance and management

Amitriptyline alone[2,3] and with isoprenaline[4] is beneficial in the treatment of asthma, and in a study of possible adverse interactions between the two, no abnormalities of heart rhythm were seen, although one out of the four patients studied showed tachycardia.[5] However a woman taking *Tedral* (theophylline, ephedrine and phenobarbitone), twice daily, died as a result of aspiration of vomit in response to cardiac arrhythmias induced by the use of amitriptyline and isoprenaline.[1] It was estimated that she had taken forty 125 μg doses of isoprenaline daily for several days prior to her death. Amitriptyline, isoprenaline, ephedrine and the fluorocarbon inhaler propellant appear to have had additive cardiotoxic effects, but just why cardiac arrhythmias should cause vomiting is not understood. This fatal interaction would seem to be due to the abuse rather than the responsible use of these drugs. However the case serves to emphasize the risk attached to the over-use of isoprenaline inhalers if cardiotoxic drugs such as the tricyclic antidepressants are being used concurrently.

References

1 Kadar D. Amitriptyline and isoproterenol: a fatal combination. Can Med Ass J (1975) 112, 556.
2 Ananth J. Antiasthmatic effect of amitriptyline. Can Med Ass J (1974) 110, 1131.
3 Meares RA, Mills JE and Horvath TB. Amitriptyline and asthma. Med J Aust (1971) 2, 25.
4 Matilla MJ and Muittari A. Modification by imipramine of the bronchodilator response to isoprenaline in asthmatic patients. Ann Med Int Fenn (1968) 57, 185.
5 Boakes AJ, Laurence DR, Teoh PC, Barar FSK, Benedikter LT and Prichard BNC. Interactions between sympathomimetic amine and antidepressant agents in man. Br Med J (1973) 1, 311.

3,4-methylene-dioxy-methamphetamine (MDMA) + Monoamine oxidase inhibitors (MAOI)

Abstract/Summary

A man experienced a marked hypertensive reaction with diaphoresis, altered mental status and hypertonicity after taking MDMA and phenelzine.

Clinical evidence, mechanism, importance and management

A man on phenelzine took a pill containing MDMA (3,4-methylene-dioxy methamphetamine) and 1 h later his usual 15 mg dose of phenelzine. During the next hour he experienced palpitations, uneasiness, difficulty in controlling his movements and in speaking. This progressed into slow, sustained, forceful twisting and arching movements. When hospitalized 3 h later he was sweating, his blood pressure was found to be raised (208/80 mm Hg), heart rate 64 bpm, respiration 28/min and temperature 36.9°. He failed to respond to 50 mg diphenhydramine IV and was given 50 g activated charcoal and 30 g magnesium sulphate by nasogastric tube. He recovered rapidly over the next 3 h.[1]

Many of these symptoms are consistent with those seen when indirectly-acting sympathomimetic amines such as amphetamines and MAOI interact (see 'Indirectly-acting sympathomimetics + MAOI). Direct information seems to be limited to this case report but on the basis of what is known about other sympathomimetic/MAOI interactions, patients taking any MAOI should be strongly warned against taking MDMA. The authors of this report advise standard treatment where indicated for hypertensive crisis (phentolamine, nitroprusside), hyperpyrexia (cooling measures, dantrolene, pancuronium), seizures (diazepam, phenytoin), and rhabdomyolysis (hydration, mannitol). MDMA is prescribed by some psychiatrists in dosages of 75–125 mg, but it is also 'street-available' as a recreational drug in doses of 50–100 mg. Its alternative names include AKA, ecstasy, XTC, MDM, Adam, doctor, M and M's.

Reference

1 Smilkstein MJ, Smolinske SC, Rumack BH. A case of MAO inhibitor/MDMA interaction: agony after ecstasy. Clin Toxicol (1987) 25, 149–59.

Phenylpropanolamine + Indomethacin

Abstract/Summary

An isolated case report describes a patient on phenylpropanolamine who developed serious hypertension after taking a single dose of indomethacin.

Clinical evidence, mechanism, importance and management

A woman who had been taking one *Trimolet* (85 mg D-phenylpropanolamine) daily for several months as an appetite suppressant, developed a severe bifrontal headache within 15 min of taking 25 mg indomethacin. 30 min later her systolic blood pressure was 210 mm Hg and the diastolic was unrecordable. A later study confirmed that neither drug on its own caused this response, but when taken together the blood pressure rose to a maximum of 200/150 mm Hg within half an hour of taking the indomethacin, and was associated with bradycardia. The blood pressure was rapidly reduced by phentolamine.[1] A possible explanation is that the indomethacin suppressed the synthesis of the vasodilator prostaglandins which are normally produced by the kidney. As a result the vasoconstrictor effects of the phenylpropanolamine became unopposed, leading to a sharp rise in blood pressure which in its turn lead to bradycardia induced reflexly by the stimulation of the arterial baroreceptors.

The general importance of this interaction is uncertain, but bearing in mind the increasing body of evidence showing that phenylpropanolamine, even on its own, can sometimes cause severe hypertension,[2-4] it might be prudent to avoid this combination of drugs.

References

1 Lee KY, Bellin LJ and Vandongen R. Severe hypertension after ingestion of an appetite suppressant (phenylpropanolamine) with indomethacin. Lancet (1979) i, 1110.
2 Livingstone PH. Transient hypertension and phenylpropanolamine. J Am Med Ass (1966) 196, 1159.
3 Duvernoy WFC. Positive phentolamine test in hypertension induced by a nasal decongestant. N Engl J Med (1969) 280, 877.
4 Shapiro SR. Hypertension due to anorectic agent. N Engl J Med (1969) 280, 1363.

Phenylephrine + Monoamine oxidase inhibitors (MAOI)

Abstract/Summary

The concurrent use of phenylephrine, taken orally, and the MAOI can result in a potentially life-threatening hypertensive crisis. Phenylephrine is a common ingredient of many proprietary cough, cold and influenza preparations. The effects of phenylephrine given parenterally may be approximately doubled.

Clinical evidence

A study in four normal subjects, given either 45 mg phenelzine or 30 mg tranylcypromine daily for seven days, showed that the pressor response (blood pressure rise) to phenylephrine given orally was grossly enhanced. In three experiments in which 45 mg was given orally, the rise in blood pressure became potentially disastrous and had to be stopped with phentolamine. The enhancement was about 13 times in the only experiment which was not stopped, and 6–35 times in the two which were curtailed. The rise in blood pressure was accompanied by a severe headache. An approximately twofold increase was seen following parenteral administration.[2]

Another study describes a 2–2.5 times increase in the effects of phenylephrine given parenterally,[2] and an exaggerated pressor response is described in a case report.[3]

Mechanism

Phenylephrine is given in large doses by mouth because a very large proportion is destroyed by the MAO in the gut and liver, and only a small amount gets into general circulation. If the MAO is inhibited, most of the oral dose escapes destruction and passes freely into circulation as an overdose. Hence the gross enhancement of the pressor effects. Phenylephrine has mainly direct sympathomimetic activity, but it may also have some minor indirect activity as well which would be expected to result in the release of some of the MAOI-accumulated noradrenaline (norepinephrine) at adrenergic nerve endings. This might account for the increased response to phenylephrine given parenterally.

Importance and management

By no means as extensively documented as some of the other sympathomimetic–MAOI interactions, but just as serious and potentially life-threatening. Patients on any MAOI, whether for depression or hypertension, should not take phenylephrine in normal oral doses. Phenylephrine is a common ingredient of oral over-the-counter cough, cold and influenza preparations and patients should be strongly warned against them. Whether the effects of nose drops and nasal sprays are also enhanced is uncertain, but it would be prudent to avoid them until they have been shown to be safe. The response to parenteral administration is also approximately doubled so that an appropriate dosage reduction is necessary.

If a hypertensive reaction occurs, it can be controlled with an alpha-adrenoreceptor blocker such as phentolamine, 5 mg, given intravenously, or failing that an intramuscular injection of 50 mg chlorpromazine. There is some indirect evidence that no interaction occurs between phenylephrine and moclobemide.[4] This requires confirmation.

References

1 Boakes AJ, Laurence DR, Teoh PC, Barar FSK, Benedikter L and Prichard BNC. Interactions between sympathomimetic amines and antidepressant agents in man. Br Med J (1973) 1, 311.
2 Elis J, Laurence DR, Mattie H and Prichard BNC. Modification by monoamine oxidase inhibitors of the effect of some sympathomimetics on blood pressure. Br Med J (1967) 2, 75.
3 Jenkins LC and Graves HB. Potential hazards of psychoactive drugs in association with anaesthesia. Can Anaes Soc J (1965) 12, 121.
4 Korn A, Eichler HG and Gasic S. Moclobemide, a new specific MAO-inhibitor does not interact with direct adrenergic agonists. The Second Amine Oxidase Workshop, Uppsala. August 1986. Pharmacology and Toxicology (1987) 60, Suppl I, 31.

Phenylpropanolamine + Caffeine

Abstract/Summary

Phenylpropanolamine can raise blood pressure and this may be further increased by caffeine. This may result in a hypertensive crisis in few particularly susceptible individuals and increase the risk of intercranial haemorrhage.

Clinical evidence, mechanism, importance and management

A study in 16 normal subjects found that after taking a placebo their mean blood pressures over the following 5 h were 137/85 mm Hg. After taking 75 mg phenylpropanolamine or 400 mg caffeine alone, or both together, their blood pressures rose to 148/97 mm Hg. After 150 mg phenylpropanolamine alone they rose to 173/103 mm Hg. One of the subjects had a hypertensive crisis after 150 mg phenylpropanolamine and again 2 h after 400 mg caffeine which needed antihypertensive treatment.[1] This illustrates the potential hazards of these drugs, even in normal healthy individuals. The authors of this report advise that likely users (those with allergies, or overweight, or postpartum women) and those particularly vulnerable (elderly or hypertensive) should be warned about taking more than the recommended doses, and of taking caffeine at the same time, because of the risk of intracranial haemorrhage.

Reference

1 Lake CR, Zaloga G, Bray J, Rosenberg D and Chernow B. Transient hypertension after two phenylpropanolamine diet aids and the effects of caffeine: a placebo-controlled follow-up study. Am J Med (1989) 86, 427–32.

Ritodrine + Glycopyrrolate

Abstract/Summary

Supraventricular tachycardia developed in a woman on ritodrine when given glycopyrronium.

Clinical evidence, mechanism, importance and management

Premature labour in a 39-year-old who was 28 weeks pregnant was arrested with an IV infusion of ritodrine hydrochloride. Two weeks later while on the maximum dose of ritodrine (0.3 mg.min⁻¹) uterine contractions began again and she was scheduled for emergency caesarian section. It was noted in the operating room that she had copious oral secretions so she was given 100% oxygen by mask and 0.2 mg glycopyrronium intravenously. Shortly afterwards she developed superventricular tachycardia (a rise from 80 to 170–180 bpm) which was converted to sinus tachycardia (130 bpm) with 0.5 mg propranolol IV in divided doses.[1] The reason for this reaction is not understood. Ritodrine alone has been responsible for tachyarrhythmias and a possible explanation is that the effects of these two drugs were additive. Two other cases of tachyarrhythmia have been described in patients premedicated with atropine who were given ritodrine as a single IV bolus.[2]

Information is very limited and the interaction is not well established but some caution is clearly appropriate if both drugs are used. The authors of the first report advise avoidance.

References

1 Simpson JI and Giffin JP. A glycopyrrolate-ritodrine drug-drug interaction. Can J Anaesth (1988) 35, 187–9.
2 Sheybany S, Murphy JF, Evans D, Newcombe RG and Pearson JF. Ritodrine in the management of fetal distress. Br J Obstet Gynaecol (1982) 89, 723–6.

Tyramine-rich foods + Cimetidine

Abstract/Summary

A woman on cimetidine experienced a severe headache with hypertension when she drank Bovril and ate some cheese.

Clinical importance, mechanism, importance and management

A woman of 77 with hiatus hernia who had been treated for three years with 400 mg cimetidine four times daily, experienced a severe frontal headache and hypertension which appeared to be related to the ingestion of a cup of *Bovril* and some English cheddar cheese, both of which can contain substantial amounts of tyramine.[1] The authors point out the similarity between this reaction and that which is seen in patients on MAOI who eat tyramine-rich foods (see

Table 21.2 The tyramine-content of some drinks.

Drink	Tyramine content (mg/L)	Ref	Drink	Tyramine content	Ref.
Ale (Canada)	8.8	1	Wine (from different regions in France)	5.17–3.70	6
Beer (Canada)	6.4, 11.1, 11.2	2			
Beer (UK)	1.34	7	Wine, red (Canada, France, Italy, Spain, USA)	3.51–8.64 (mean 5.18)	2,6
Beer (USA)	1.8, 2.3, 4.4	1			
Champagne (Canada)	0.2, 0.6	2			
Chianti (Italy)	0,1.48,1.76,12.2,10.36,25.4	1–3,7	Wine, red (unstated origin)	1.36	7
Port	0.2	1			
Reisling	0.6	1	Wine, white (Germany, Italy, Portugal, Spain)	1.26–5.87 (mean 4.41)	2,6
Sauterne	0.4	1			
Sherry (USA)	3.6	1	Wine, white (Germany, Jugoslavia)	1.22	
Sherry (Canada)	0.2	2			

'Tyramine-rich foods+MAOI'), but there is no satisfactory explanation for what occurred. This is an isolated report and there is no reason why patients in general on cimetidine should avoid tyramine-rich foods.

Reference

1 Griffin MJJ and Morris JS. MAOI-like reaction associated with cimetidine. Drug Intell Clin Pharm (1987) 21, 219.

Tyramine-rich alcoholic drinks + Monoamine oxidase inhibitors (MAOI)

Abstract/Summary

(a) Patients taking the older MAOI (tranylcypromine, phenelzine, nialamide, pargyline, etc.) may suffer a serious hypertensive reaction if they drink tyramine-rich drinks such as beer or wine. (b) The hypotensive side-effects of the MAOI may be exaggerated in a few patients by alcohol and they may experience dizziness and faintness after drinking relatively modest amounts.

Interaction, mechanism, importance and management

(a) Hypertensive reactions

A severe and potentially life-threatening hypertensive reaction can occur in patients on MAOI if they have alcoholic drinks containing significant amounts of tyramine. The details of this reaction, its mechanism, the names of the older MAOI which interact and the newer ones which are unlikely to do so are described in the synopsis 'Tyramine-rich foods + Monoamine oxidase inhibitors'. A dose of 10–25 mg tyramine is required before a serious rise in blood pressure takes place. Calculations made from the figures in Table 21.2 show that a litre (a little under two pints) of the samples of Canadian ale or beer, and about 400 ml of one sample of Italian Chianti wine, contain enough tyramine to reach the 10–25 mg threshold dosage, and would represent a hazard to patients on MAOI. But some drinks contain too little tyramine to matter. The problem is that there is no way of knowing the probable tyramine-content without a detailed analysis.

The table can be used as broad general guide when advising patients, but it cannot be an absolute guide because all alcoholic drinks are the end-product of a biological fermentation process and no two batches are ever absolutely identical. There may be a 50-fold difference even between wines from the same grape stock.[7] It is claimed by the Chianti producers[4] that the new methods which have replaced the ancient 'governo' process result in negligible amounts of tyramine in today's Chianti. This seems to be borne out by the results of recent analyses[3,7] one of which found a tyramine-content of only 1.48 mg/l. Whiskey, brandy, gin or other spirits seem unlikely to contain significant amounts of tyramine because they are distilled and the volumes drunk are relatively small. On the other hand alcohol-free beer may not be safe. Its tyramine-content is similar to ordinary beer[8] and one patient on tranylcypromine suffered an acute cerebral haemorrhage after drinking a de-alcoholised Irish beer.[7]

(b) Hypotensive reactions

Some degree of hypotension can occur in patients on MAOI (therapeutically exploited in the case of pargyline). This may be exaggerated by the vasodilation and reduced cardiac output caused by alcohol, and patients should be warned of the possibility of orthostatic hypotension and syncope if they drink.[5] They should be advised not to stand up too quickly, and to remain sitting or lying if they feel faint or begin to 'black out'.

References

1 Horwitz D, Lovenberg W, Engelman K and Sjoerdsma A. Monoamine oxidase inhibitors, tyramine and cheese. J Amer Med Ass (1964) 188, 1108.

2 Sen NP. Analysis and significance of tyramine in foods. J Food Sci (1969) 34, 127.

3 Korn A, Eichler HG, Fischbach R and Gasic S. Moclobemide, a new reversible MAO inhibitor—interaction with tyramine and tricyclic anti-

depressants in healthy volunteers and depressive patients. Psycho-pharmacology (1986) 88, 153–7.

4 Anon. Statement from the Consorzio Vino Chianti Classico, London. Undated (circa 1984).

5 Anon. MAOI's—a patient's tale. Pulse (1981) December 5th, p 69.

6 Zee JA, Simard RE, L'Heureux L and Tremblay J. Biogenic amines in wines. Am J Enol Vitic (1983) 34, 6–9.

7 Hannah P, Glover V and Sandler M. Tyramine in wine and beer. Lancet (1988) i, 879.

8 Murray JA, Walker JF and Doyle JS. Tyramine in alcohol-free beer. Lancet (1988) i, 1167–8.

Tyramine-rich foods + Monoamine oxidase inhibitors (MAOI)

Abstract/Summary

The concurrent use of the older MAOI (nialamide, pargyline, phenelzine, tranylcypromine, etc.) and tyramine-rich foods can result in a potentially life-threatening hypertensive crisis. Deaths from intracranial haemorrhage have occurred. Significant amounts of tyramine occur in cheese, yeast extracts (e.g. Marmite) and some types of salami. Caviar, pickled herrings, chicken and beef livers, and avacados have been implicated in this interaction. Some of the newer MAOI (amiflamine, moclobemide, selegiline, toloxatone) do not interact at all or only minimally, and there is less likelihood of an interaction with cimoxatone or brofaromine.

Clinical evidence

A rapid, serious, and potentially fatal rise in blood pressure can occur in patients on MAOI who ingest tyramine-rich foods or drinks. A violent occipital headache, pounding heart, neck stiffness, flushing, sweating, nausea and vomiting may be experienced. Two illustrative examples: the first being one of the earliest recorded observations by Rowe, a pharmacist, in a letter after seeing the reaction in his wife who was taking *Parstelin* (tranylcypromine with trifluoperazine).

'After cheese on toast; within a few minutes face flushed, felt very ill; head and heart pounded most violently, and perspiration was running down her neck. She vomited several times, and her condition looked so severe that I dashed over the road to consult her GP. He diagnosed 'palpitations' and agreed to call if the symptoms had not subsided in an hour. In fact the severity diminished and after about 3 h she was normal, other than a severe headache—but 'not of the throbbing kind'. She described the early part of the attack 'as though her head must burst'.'[1]

A man on pargyline who, despite eating Sweitzer cheese uneventfully on a number of previous occasions, experienced severe substernal chest pain and palpitations within 15 min of eating the cheese. His blood pressure was found to have risen to 200/114 mm Hg. Two other patients experienced headache after eating aged cheese. One of them had a severe nose-bleed and was found to have a blood pressure of 240/140 mm Hg.[2]

Table 21.3. The tyramine-content of some foods

Food	Tyramine (μg/g)	Ref.
Avocado	23,0	15,32
Banana pulp	7,0	15,32
Banana (whole)	65	15
Caviar (Iranian)	680	13
Cheese—see Table 21.4		
Country cured ham	not detectable	14
Farmer salami sausage	314	14
Genoa salami sausage	0–1237 (average 534)	14
Hard salami	0–392 (average 210)	14
Herring (pickled)	3030	16
Lebanon bologna	0–333 (average 224)	14
Liver—chicken	94-113	17
Liver—beef	0–274	18
Orange pulp	10	15
Pepperoni sausage	0-195 (average 39)	14
Plum, red	6	15
Smoked landjaeger sausage	396	14
Summer sausage	184	14
Tomato	4,0	15,32
Thuringer cervelat	0-162	14
Yeast extracts		
Barmene	157	5
Befit	419	5
Bovril	200–500	23
Bovril beef cubes	200–500	23
Bovril chicken cubes	50–200	23
Marmite	500–3000	23,32
Oxo chicken cubes	130	24
Red Oxo cubes	250	24
Yeastrel	101	5
Yex	506	5
Yoghurt	0.2, 3–4	19,32

There are too many reports of this interaction to list them here individually, but they are reviewed extensively elsewhere.[1,9] Blackwell and his colleagues list[5] a total of 110 instances caused by tyramine-rich foods which came to their attention during the 1963–66 period. There have been many since. Tranylcypromine, phenelzine, mebanazine or pargyline have been implicated in this interaction with cheese, yeast extracts, protein diet supplements, pickled herrings, chicken livers, caviar, soy sauce, avocados, New Zealand prickly spinach, beef livers and chianti wine. Many patients recovered fully, but Blackwell lists 26 cases of intracranial haemorrhage and nine deaths.[1] Another review lists 38 cases of haemorrhage and 21 deaths.[8]

Mechanism

Tyramine is formed in foods such as cheese by the bacterial degradation of milk and other proteins, firstly to tyrosine and other amino acids, and the subsequent decarboxylation of the

Table 21.4. The tyramine-content of some cheeses. This table should not be used to predict the probable tyramine-content of a cheese. It is only intended to show the extent and the variation which can occur.

Variety of cheese	Tyramine content (μg/g)	Ref.
American processed	50	3
Argenti	188	11
Blue	49,203,266	10.11
Boursault	1116	10
Brick	194	11
Brie	180	3
Brie type (Danish)	0	10
Camembert	86,125,	3, 11
Cheddar		
Australian	226	5
Canadian	120,136,192,251,535 1000, 1530	5,10
English	0,72,182,281,332,480,953	5
Farmhouse	284	5
Kraft	214	5
New York State	1416	5
New Zealand	416, 580	5
Cream cheese	<0.2	3
Cottage cheese	<0.2	3
Danish Blue (Gorgonzola type)	31,93,256	10
d'Oka	100,310	11
Edam	100,214	11
Emmental	225	11
Gouda	54,95	11
Gouda type (Canadian)	20	10
Gourmandise	216	10
Gruyere	64 (mean of seven samples) 514	12
Kashar	44 (mean of seven samples)	12
Liederkrantz	1226,1683	11
Limburger	204	11
Mozzarela	410	10
Munster	110	11
Mycelia	1340	11
Parmesan	65	10
Parmesan type (USA)	4,5,290	10
Provolone	38	10
Romano	197,238	10,11
Roquefort	27,48,520,267	10,11
Stilton	466,2170	10
Swiss	50,434	11
Tulum	208 (mean of eight samples)	12
White (Turkish)	17.5	12

tyramine to tyrosine. This interaction is therefore not associated with fresh foods, but with those which have been allowed to 'mature' in some way. (Note that tyramine was first isolated from cheese in 1903 and is named after the Greek word for cheese: tyros).[21] Tyramine is an indirectly-acting sympathomimetic amine, one of its actions being to release noradrenaline (norepinephrine) from the adrenergic neurones associated with blood vessels which causes a rise in blood pressure by stimulating their constriction. Normally any ingested tyramine is rapidly metabolized before it escapes into general circulation because both the intestinal wall and the liver, to which the blood first flows, contain the enzyme monoamine oxidase (MAO). However, if the activity of the enzyme at these sites is inhibited (by the presence of an MAOI), any tyramine passes freely into circulation to cause not just a rise in blood pressure, but a highly exaggerated rise due to the release from the adrenergic neurones of the large amounts of noradrenaline which accumulate there during inhibition of the MAO. This final step in the interaction is identical with that which occurs with any other indirectly-acting sympathomimetic amine in the presence of an MAOI (see synopsis 'Indirectly-acting sympathomimetics + MAOI'). The violent headache seems to occur when the blood pressure reaches about 200 mm Hg. There is also some evidence that other amines such as tryptamine and phenylethylamine may play a part in this interaction.

Importance and management

An extremely well-documented, well-established, serious and potentially fatal interaction. The incidence is uncertain but estimates range from 1–20%.[6,7] Patients taking any of the older MAOI (isocarboxazid, nialamide, phenelzine, pargyline, tranycypromine, etc.) should not eat foods which contain substantial amounts of tyramine (see Tables 21.3, 21.4). As little as 6 mg can raise the blood pressure[3] and 10–25 mg would be expected to cause a serious interaction.[3] Because tyramine levels vary so much it is impossible to guess the amount present in any food or drink. An old and mature cheese may contain trivial amounts of tyramine compared with one which is innocuous looking and even mild-tasting. The tyramine-content can even differ significantly within a single cheese between the centre and the rind.[4] There is no guarantee that patients who have risked eating these hazardous foodstuffs on many occasions uneventfully may not eventually experience a full-scale hypertensive crisis if all the many variables conspire together.[2]

A total prohibition should be imposed on the following: cheese and yeast extracts such as *Marmite* (tyramine content up to 3 mg/g), possibly *Bovril* (0.5 mg/g) and pickled herrings (3 mg/g) (see Table 21.3). Hypertensive reactions have been seen with chicken livers[17] and beef livers,[18] caviar,[13] pickled herrings,[16] avocados,[21] soy sauce,[28] a powdered protein diet supplement (*Ever-so-slim*)[31] and New Zealand prickly spinach (*tetragonia tetragonides*).[22] This is not a true spinach as found in the USA or Europe. A number of other foods should also be viewed with great suspicion such as fermented bolognas and salamis, pepperoni and summer sausage because some of them may contain significant amounts of tyramine (see Table 21.3). However the following are often viewed with unjustifiable suspicion: yoghourt, cream and possibly chocolate. It also seems very doubtful if either cream cheese or cottage cheese represent a hazard. *Whole* green bananas contain up to 65 μg/g, but the pulp contains relatively small amounts.

It is usual practice to recommend avoidance of the prohibited foods for 2–3 weeks after withdrawal of the MAOI to allow full recovery of the enzymes. If a hypertensive reaction occurs it can be controlled with an alpha-blocker such as phentolamine (5 mg IV) or phenoxybenzamine, or failing that an IM injection of 50 mg chlorpromazine. 20 mg labetolol given intravenously over 5 min has also proved to be successful.[28]

Selegiline[20] and toloxatone[26] have been shown not to interact with tyramine because they selectively inhibit MAO B, leaving MAO A in the gut wall unaffected,[20] Moclobemide, brofaromine and cimoxatone selectively inhibit MAO A, but the moclobemide-tyramine interaction is minimal with food present,[27,29,31] and the likelihood of a hypertensive reaction with cimoxatone or brofaromine[33] is less than with the older non-selective MAOI. It has been calculated that patients taking 20 mg cimoxatone daily would need to ingest 57 g *Marmite*, 120 g average cheddar cheese or three litres of Chianti wine to reach the critical tyramine dosage level.[25,26] The risk of an interaction is also very much reduced with amiflamine.[30]

References

1 Blackwell B, Marley E, Price J and Taylor D. Hypertensive interactions between monoamine oxidase inhibitors and foodstuffs. Br J Psychiat (1967) 113, 349.

2 Hutchison JC. Toxic effects of monoamine oxidase inhibitors. Lancet (1964) ii, 150.

3 Horwitz D, Lovenberg W, Engelman K and Sjoerdsma A. Monoamine oxidase inhibitors, tyramine and cheese. J Amer Med Ass (1964) 188, 1108.

4 Price K and Smith SE. Cheese reaction and tyramine. Lancet (1971) i, 130.

5 Blackwell B and Marley E. Hypertensive interactions between MAOI and foodstuffs. In Neuropsychopharmacology. Proc 5th Int Congr Coll Int Neuro-psycho-pharmacologium. Brill H, Cole JO, Deniker P, Hippius H and Bradley PB (Eds). Int Congr Series no 129, Washington, March 1966. Excerpta Medica Foundation (1967).

6 Anon. Hypertensive reactions to monoamine oxidase inhibitors. Brit Med J (1964) i, 578.

7 Cooper AJ, Magnus RV and Rose MJ. A hypertensive syndrome with tranylcypromine medication. Lancet (1964) i, 527.

8 Sadusk JF. The physician and the Food and Drug Administration. J Amer Med Ass (1964) 190, 907.

9 Stockley IH. Drug Interactions and their Mechanisms. Pharmaceutical Press, London, (1974) p. 5.

10 Sen NP. Analysis and significance of tyramine in foods. J Food Sci (1969) 34, 127.

11 Kosikowsky FV and Dahlberg AC. The tyramine content of cheese. J Diary Sci (1948) 31, 293.

12 Kayaalp SO, Renda N, Kaymarkcalan S and Ozer A. Tyramine content of some cheeses. Toxicol appl Pharmacol(1970) 16, 459.

13 Isaac P, Mitchell B and Grahame-Smith DG. Monoamine oxidase inhibitors and caviar. Lancet (1977) ii, 816.

14 Rice S, Eitenmiller RR and Koehler PE. Histamine and tyramine content of meat products. J Milk Food Technol (1975) 38, 256.

15 Udenfriend S, Lovenberg W and Sjoerdsma A. Physiologically active amines in common fruits and vegetables. Arch Biochem (1959) 85, 487.

16 Nuessle WF, Norman FC and Miller HE. Pickled herring and tranylcypromine reaction. J Amer Med Ass (1965) 192, 726.

17 Heberg DL, Gordon MW and Glueck BC. Six cases of hypertensive crisis in patients on tranylcypromine after eating chicken livers. Amer J Psychiatry (1966) 122, 933.

18 Boulton AA, Cookson B and Paulton R. Hypertensive crisis in a patient on MAOI antidepressants following a meal of beef liver. Can Med Ass J (1970) 102, 1394.

19 van Slyke L and Hart B. Conditions affecting the proportions of fat and proteins in cows milk. Amer Chem J (1903) 30, 8.

20 Elsworth JD, Glover V, Reynolds GP, Sandler M, Lees AJ, Phuapradit P, Shaw KM, Stern GM and Kumar P. Deprenyl administration in man: a selective monoamine oxidase B inhibitor without the cheese effect. Psychopharmacol (1978) 57, 33.

21 Generali JA, Hogan LC, McFarland M, Schwab S and Hartman CR. Hypertensive crisis resulting from avocados and a MAO inhibitor. Drug Intell Clin Pharm (1981) 15, 904–6.

22 Comfort A. Hypertensive reaction to New Zealand prickly spinach in a woman taking phenelzine. Lancet (1981) ii, 472.

23 Clarke A. (Bovril Ltd). Personal communication (1987).

24 Oxo Ltd. Personal communication (1987).

25 Dollery CT, Brown MJ, Davies DS, Lewis PJ and Strolin-Benedetti M. Oral absorption and concentration-effect relationship of tyramine with and without cimoxatone, a type-A specific inhibitor of monoamine oxidase. Clin Pharmacol Ther (1983) 34, 651–63.

26 Dollery CT, Brown MJ, Davies DS and Strolin Benedetti M. Pressor amines and monoamine oxidase inhibitors. In Monoamine Oxidase and Disease. Proc Conf Paris, Oct 1983. Tipton KF, Dostert P and Strolin Benedetti M. (Eds) Academic Press (1984) p 429–41.

27 Korn A, Eichler HG, Fischbach R and Gasic S. Moclobemide, a new reversible MAO inhibitor—interaction with tyramine and tricyclic antidepressants in healthy volunteers and depressive patients. Psychopharmacology (1986) 88, 153–7.

28 Abrams JH, Schulman P and White WB. Successful treatment of a monoamine oxidase inhibitor-tyramine hypertensive emergency with intravenous labetolol. N Engl J Med (1985) 313, 52.

29 Korn A, Da Prada M, Raffesberg W, Gasic S and Eichler HG. Tyramine absorption and pressure response after MAO-inhibition with moclobemide. The Second Amine Oxidase Workshop, Uppsala, August 1986. Pharmacology and Toxicology (1987) 60, 30

30 Grind M, Alvan G, Graffner A, Gustavsson L, Helleday J, Lindgren JE, Selander H and Siwers B. Clinical investigation of the interaction between amiflamine and oral tyramine in man. In Monoamine Oxidase and Disease, p 497–503, Academic Press, London 1984.

31 Zetin M, Plon L and De Antonio M. MAOI reaction with powdered protein diet supplement. J Clin Psychiatry (1987) 48, 499.

32 Da Prada M, Zurcher G, Wuthrich I and Haefely WE. On tyramine, food, beverages and the reversible MAO inhibitor moclobemide. J Neural Transm (1988) (Suppl) 26, 31–56.

33 Bieck PR, Firkusny L, Schick C, Antonin K-H, Nilsson E, Schulz R, Schwenk M, Wollman H. Monoamine oxidase inhibition by phenelzine and brofaromine in healthy volunteers. Clin Pharmacol Ther (1989) 45, 260–9.

22
THEOPHYLLINE AND
RELATED XANTHINE
DRUG INTERACTIONS

The main xanthines used in medicine are theophylline and aminophylline, the latter being used when greater water solubility is needed. They are of particular value in the treatment of asthma because they relax the bronchial smooth muscle. In an attempt to overcome the gastrointestinal irritation caused by theophylline, various formulations have been devised and different derivatives have been made such as diprophylline and enprofylline which do not liberate theophylline in the body. Within the context of interactions aminophylline would be expected to behave like theophylline because it is a complex of theophylline with ethylenediamine, but derivatives of theophylline seem to act differently and it should not be assumed that they all share common interactions.

Caffeine is also a xanthine and it is principally used because it stimulates the central nervous system, increasing wakefulness, mental and physical activity. There are hundreds of over-the-counter preparations containing caffeine with other ingredients such as aspirin, codeine and paracetamol, but caffeine is most commonly taken in the form of tea, coffee, cola drinks and cocoa.

Table 22.1 Caffeine-containing herbs and caffeine-containing drinks[1]

Source	Caffeine-content	Caffeine-content of drink
Coffee beans	1–2%	up to 100 mg/100 ml decaffeinated about 3 mg/100 ml
Kola	1.5–2.5%	up to 20 mg/100 ml in 'Coke' drinks
Mate	0.2–2.0%	
Tea	1–4%	up to 60 mg/100 ml

[1] Martindale. The Extra Pharmacopoeia. Edn 29 (1989) p1535.

Table 22.2 Theophylline and related xanthines

Non-proprietary names	Proprietary names
Aminophylline	Afonilum, Aminocont, Aminodur, Aminomal, Aminophyl(lin), Androphyllin, Cardophyl(l)in, Carine, Corophyllin, Corophyllamin, Duraphyllin, Escophyllin, Eufilina, Euphyllin(a), Fergupina, Lixaminoil, Mini-lix, Paralon, Peterphyllin, Phyldrox, Phyllocontin, Phyllotemp, Planophylline, Tefamin, Teofylamin, Variaphylline, Vernaphyllin.
Diprophylline (diphylline)	Aerophylline, Airet, Asthmolysin, Astmamasitt, Brosema, (dyphylline), Dicoryllin, Difilina, Difillin, Dilin, Dilor, Droxine, Dyflex, Emfabid, Glyfillin, Katasma, Lancephylline, Lufylin, Neophyllin, Neothylline, Neo-vasophylline, Neothylline, Neutralfillina, Neutraphylline, Prophyllen, Protophylline, Silbephylline, Synthophylline, Thylline
Enprofylline	
Theophylline	Accurbron, Aerobin, Aerolate, Afonilum, Aminomal, Aminomed, Aquaphyllin, Armophylline, Asmafil, Aspertal-t, Asthmophylline, Bilordyl, Biophylline, Bronchoparat, Bronchoretard, Brokodyl, Cetraphylline, Cronasma, Diffumal, Dilatrane, Duraphyl(llin), Elexicon, Elexomin, Elixophyllin, Englate, Euphylline, Godafilin, Inophyline, Labid, Labophylline, Lasma, Lodrane, Neulin, Oxyphyllin, Physpan, Pro-vent, Pulmidur, Pulmophylline, Respid, Rona-phyllin, Slo-phyllin, Sodiphylline, Solosin, Somophyllin, Sustaire, Synophylate, Tagilen, Techniphylline, Tefamin, Teoclasma, Teolix, Teonova, Theobid, Theocap, Theoclear, Theocontin, Theocot, Theo-dur, Theofrenon, Theograd, Theolair, Teolixir, Theospan, Theovent, Unifyl, Uniphyl(llin), Unixan, Xantivent

Caffeine + Calcium channel blockers

Abstract/Summary

A small and relatively unimportant increase in the effects of caffeine may occur in patients given verapamil.

Clinical evidence, mechanism, importance and management

A study in six normal subjects given single 200 mg doses of caffeine showed that the concurrent use of verapamil (80 mg three times daily for two days) decreased the total clearance of caffeine by 25% (from 4.6 to 5.8 h).[1] These changes are not large and unlikely to be of much importance in most patients. In excess the caffeine from tea, coffee and 'Coke' can cause jitteriness and insomnia.

Reference

1 Nawoot S, Wong D, Mays DC and Gerber N. Inhibition of caffeine elimination by verapamil. Clin Pharmacol Ther (1988) 43, 148.

Caffeine + Cimetidine

Abstract/Summary

The stimulant effects of caffeine may be increased to some extent by cimetidine.

Clinical evidence, mechanism, importance and management

After giving 1 g cimetidine daily to five subjects for six days, it was found that the half-life of caffeine was increased about 70% and the average plasma levels were estimated as being about 1.7 times higher.[1] Another study confirmed that the caffeine half-life is increased by cimetidine.[2] The probable reason is that the cimetidine inhibits the metabolism of the caffeine by the liver, resulting in its accumulation in the body. Such an increase is unlikely to be of much importance in most patients, but it might have a part to play in exaggerating the undesirable effects of caffeine-containing drinks (tea, coffee, Coca-Cola) in a few patients who have insomnia or anxiety.

References

1 Broughton LJ and Rogers HJ. Decreased systemic clearance of caffeine due to cimetidine. Br J clin Pharmacol (1981) 12, 155–9.
2 Beach CA, Gerber N, Ross J and Bianchine JR. Inhibition of elimination of caffeine by cimetidine. Clin Res (1982) 30, 438A.

Caffeine + Oral contraceptives

Abstract/Summary

The stimulant effects of caffeine may be increased to some extent in women taking combined oral contraceptives.

Clinical evidence, mechanism, importance and management

A study over three months in nine women showed that, while using low dose combined oral contraceptives, the clearance of caffeine (single 162 mg doses) was reduced, the half-life prolonged (from 5.4 to 7.9 h) and the serum levels raised.[1] This confirmed the results of another study.[2] The probable mechanism of this interaction is that the contraceptives inhibit the metabolism of caffeine by the liver resulting in its accumulation in the body. Women on the pill who drink caffeine-containing drinks (tea, coffee, Coca-Cola, etc.) may find the stimulant effects of caffeine increased. In excess caffeine can cause jitteriness and insomnia.

References

1 Abernethy DR and Todd EL. Impairment of caffeine clearance by chronic use of low-dose oestrogen-containing oral contraceptives. Eur J Clin Pharmacol (1985) 28, 425–8.
2 Patwardhan RV, Desmond PV, Johnson RF, Schenker S. Impaired elimination of caffeine by oral contraceptive steroids. J Lab Clin Med (1980) 95, 603–8.

Caffeine + Disulfiram

Abstract/Summary

Disulfiram reduces the loss of caffeine from the body which may complicate the withdrawal from alcohol, particularly in a few individuals.

Clinical evidence, mechanism, importance and management

A study in normal subjects and recovering alcoholics showed that disulfiram treatment (250 mg maintenance dose) reduced the clearance of caffeine by about 30%, but a few of the alcoholics had a more than 50% reduction.[1] As a result the levels of caffeine in the body increase. Raised levels of caffeine can cause irritability, insomnia and anxiety, and as coffee consumption is often particularly high among recovering alcoholics, there is the risk that they may turn to alcohol to calm them down. To avoid this possible complication it might be wise for recovering alcoholics not to drink too much tea or coffee. De-caffeinated coffee and tea are widely available.

Reference

1 Beach CA, Mays DC, Guiler RC, Jacober CH and Gerber N. Inhibition of elimination of caffeine by disulfiram in normal subjects and recovering alcoholics. Clin Pharmacol Ther (1986) 39, 265–70.

Caffeine + Idrocilamide

Abstract/Summary

Idrocilamide causes the marked retention in the body of caffeine from tea, coffee and other drinks. This can lead to caffeine intoxication (insomnia, extreme nervousness, jitteriness, anxious agitation).

Clinical evidence

The possibility that caffeine ingestion might have some part to play in the development of psychiatric disorders seen in patients on idrocilamide, prompted a pharmacokinetic study in four normal subjects. It was found that while taking 400 mg idrocilamide three times a day, the half-life of caffeine from a cup of coffee containing about 150–200 mg caffeine was prolonged by a factor of nine (from about 7 to 59 h). The overall clearance of caffeine was decreased about 90%.[1,2]

Mechanism

The experimental evidence indicates that idrocilamide causes marked inhibition of the metabolism and clearance of caffeine from the body, leading to its accumulation.

Importance and management

Evidence is limited but the interaction appears to be established. Patients on idrocilamide should avoid caffeine-containing drinks (tea, coffee, Coca-Cola, etc.) or only take very small amounts otherwise caffeine intoxication may develop. Decaffeinated teas and coffee are widely available.

References

1 Brazier JL, Descotes J, Lery N, Ollagnier M and Evreux J-Cl. Inhibition by idrocilamide of the disposition of caffeine. Eur J Clin Pharmacol (1980) 17, 37.
2 Evreux JC, Bayere JJ, Descotes J, Lery N, Ollagnier M and Brazier JL. Les accidents neuropsychiques de l'idrocilamide: consequences d'une inhibition due metabolisme de la cafeine? Lyon Medical (1979) 241, 89.

Caffeine + Methoxsalen

Abstract/Summary

Methoxsalen markedly reduces the loss of caffeine from the body. Caffeine intoxication seems to be a possibility.

Clinical evidence, mechanism, importance and management

A study in five normal subjects with psoriasis showed that a single 1.2 mg/kg oral dose of methoxsalen given 1 h before a single 200 mg oral dose of caffeine reduced the clearance of the caffeine by 69% (from 110 to 34 ml/min). The elimination half-life of caffeine over the period 2–16 h after taking the methoxsalen increased tenfold (from 5.6 to 57 h).[1] The reason is believed to be that the methoxsalen acts as a potent inhibitor of the metabolism of the caffeine by the liver, thereby markedly reducing its loss from the body. The practical consequences of this interaction are as yet uncertain, but it seems possible that the toxic effects of caffeine will be increased. In excess the caffeine from tea, coffee and Coca-Cola can cause jitteriness, headache and insomnia. More study is needed.

Reference

1 Mays DC, Camisa C, Cheney P, Pacula CM, Nawoot S and Gerber N. Methoxsalen is a potent inhibitor of the metabolism of caffeine in humans. Clin Pharmacol Ther (1987) 42, 621–6.

Caffeine + Mexiletine

Abstract/Summary

The clearance of caffeine from the body is reduced 30–60% by the concurrent use of mexiletine. Whether this might result in caffeine toxicity is uncertain.

Clinical evidence

A study in five normal subjects showed that the clearance of a single 366 mg dose of caffeine was reduced by 57% (from 126 to 54 ml/min) by a single 200 mg dose of mexiletine. The elimination half-life rose from 246 to 419 min. Seven patients with cardiac arrhythmias showed a 48% reduction in caffeine clearance when given long-term treatment with 600 mg mexiletine daily.[1] In a similar study by the same authors the caffeine clearance was reduced 30% (from 77 to 54 ml/min) in seven normal subjects by 200 mg mexiletine, and by 48% (from 71 to 37 ml/min) in five patients taking 600 mg mexiletine daily. Fasting caffeine levels were almost sixfold higher during than after mexiletine treatment (1.99 compared with 0.35 μg/ml).[2] 200 mg lignocaine (lidocaine), 100 mg flecainide or 500 mg tocainide had no effect on the caffeine clearance.[2]

Mechanism

Not understood. The pharmacokinetics of the mexiletine were unaffected by the caffeine.

Importance and management

The interaction appears to be established but its clinical importance is uncertain. The authors of these reports point out that caffeine-consumption is very common (in tea, coffee, Coca-Cola) and some of the side-effects of mexiletine treatment might be partially due to caffeine-retention. In excess caffeine can cause jitteriness, tremor and insomnia. They also suggest that the caffeine test for liver function might also be impaired by mexiletine.

References

1 Joeres R, Klinker H, Heusler H, Epping J and Richter E. Influence of mexiletine on caffeine elimination. Pharmac Ther (1987) 33, 163–9.
2 Joeres R, Richter E. Mexiletine and caffeine elimination. N Engl J Med (1987) 317, 117.

Caffeine + Quinolone antibiotics

Abstract/Summary

Enoxacin and pipemidic acid can markedly increase the blood levels of caffeine. The side-effects of caffeine (restlessness, insomnia, jitteriness, etc.) derived from drinks such as tea, coffee or 'Coke' would be expected to be increased. Ciprofloxacin and nofloxacin interact to a lesser extent and ofloxacin not at all.

Clinical evidence

(a) Ciprofloxacin

A study in which 12 normal subjects were given 500 mg ciprofloxacin for five days showed that the AUC (area under the concentration-time curve) of caffeine was increased about 60% by ciprofloxacin.[1]

Another study found that the AUC of caffeine increased by 16.8, 57.1 and 57.8% respectively when given 100 mg, 250 mg and 500 mg ciprofloxacin twice daily for four days.[3]

(b) Enoxacin

A study in 12 normal subjects found that the AUC of a single 230 mg dose of caffeine increased by 138%, 176% and 346% respectively when given 100 mg, 200 mg or 400 mg twice daily for three days.[3]

(c) Pipemidic acid

A study in six normal subjects found that after taking 800 mg pipemidic acid twice daily for a day the clearance of 350 mg caffeine was reduced two-thirds (from 9.7 to 3.56 l/h). The steady-state caffeine levels after repeated doses in two of the subjects rose about threefold.[2]

Another study found that 400 mg pipemidic acid twice daily for three days increased the AUC (area under the concentration-time curve) of a single 230 mg dose by 179%.[3]

(d) Norfloxacin

A study in six normal subjects found that after taking 800 mg norfloxacin twice daily for a day the clearance of 350 mg caffeine was reduced about one third (from 9.7 to 3.56 l/h).[2] Another study found no statistically significant change in the AUC of caffeine in subjects given 400 mg nofloxacin daily for three days.[3]

(e) Ofloxacin

A study in 12 subjects given 400 mg ofloxacin daily for five days showed that it had no significant effects on the pharmacokinetics of a single dose of caffeine.[1] This was confirmed in another study.[3]

Mechanism.

It would seem that the metabolism (N-demethylation) of caffeine is markedly reduced by some quinolones (pipemidic acid, enoxacin) but to a lesser extent by the others.[4]

Importance and management

An established interaction. Patients taking enoxacin or pipemidic acid may possibly experience an increase in the side-effects of caffeine (headache, jitteriness, restlessness, insomnia) if they continue to drink normal amounts of caffeine-containing drinks (tea, coffee, 'Coke', etc.). They should be warned to cut out or reduce their intake of caffeine. The authors of one report[1] suggest that patients with hepatic disorders, cardiac arrhythmias or latent epilepsy should avoid caffeine if they take enoxacin for a week or more. The effects of ciprofloxacin and norfloxacin are likely to be smaller than those of enoxacin and of lesser importance. Ofloxacin seems to be a non-interacting alternative.

References

1 Staib AH, Stille W, Dietlin G, Shah PM, Harder S, Mieke S and Beer C. Interaction between quinolones and caffeine. Drugs (1987) 34 (Suppl 1) 170–4.
2 li Carbo M, Segura J, De la Torre R, Badenas JM and Cami J. Effect of quinolones on caffeine disposition. Clin Pharmacol Ther (1989) 45, 234–40.
3 Harder S, Staib AH, Beer C, Papenburg A, Stille W and Shah PM. 4-quinolones inhibit biotransformation of caffeine. Eur J Clin Pharmacol (1988) 35, 651–6.
4 Still W, Harder S, Mieke S, Beer C, Shah PM, Frech K and Staib AH. Decrease of caffeine elimination in many patients during co-administration of 4-quinolones. J Antimicrob Chemother (1987) 20, 729–34.

Theophylline + Allopurinol

Abstract/Summary

Some limited evidence indicates that the effects of theophylline may be increased by the concurrent use of allopurinol.

Clinical evidence

A study in 12 normal subjects showed that the concurrent use of allopurinol (600 mg daily) for 14 days, increased the half-life of theophylline given orally (5 mg/kg) by 25% and increased the area under the curve by 27%.[1] Two other studies with 300 mg allopurinol daily given for only a week failed to show any effect on the pharmacokinetics of theophylline,[2,3] possibly because the dosage was smaller and the trial lasted only a week.

Mechanism

Uncertain. One suggestion is that the allopurinol inhibits the metabolism of the theophylline by the liver.

Importance and management

Evidence appears to be limited to the studies cited which were on normal healthy subjects. The clinical importance of this interaction is uncertain, but it would now seem prudent to check for any signs of theophylline overdosage during concurrent use, particularly in patients whose disease condition may result in a reduction in the metabolism of the theophylline.

References

1 Manfredi RL and Vessell ES. Inhibition of theophylline metabolism by long-term allopurinol administration. Clin Pharmacol Ther (1981) 29, 224.
2 Vozeh S, Powell RJ, Cupit GC, Riegelman S and Sheiner LB. Influence of allopurinol on theophylline disposition in adults. Clin Pharmacol Ther (1980) 27, 194.
3 Grygiel JJ, Wing LMH, Farkas J and Birkett DJ. Effects of allopurinol on theophylline metabolism and clearance. Clin Pharmacol Ther (1979) 26, 660.

Theophylline + Aminoglutethimide

Abstract/Summary

The loss of theophylline from the body is increased by the concurrent use of aminoglutethimide and some reduction in its serum levels and therapeutic effects seems probable.

Clinical evidence

A study in three patients taking a sustained release theophylline preparation (200 mg twice daily) showed that the concurrent use of aminoglutethimide (250 mg four times a day) increased the theophylline clearance by 32%.[1]

Mechanism

Aminoglutethimide is a known enzyme inducing agent which increases the metabolism of some drugs by the liver, thereby increasing their loss from the body. It seems likely that it affects theophylline in this way.

Importance and management

Direct information is limited to this study. Its clinical importance is uncertain, but the effects of theophylline would be expected to be reduced to some extent by the addition of aminoglutethimide. Monitor the effects and increase the dosage if necessary.

Reference

1 Lonning PE, Kvinnsland S and Bakke OM. Effect of aminoglutethimide on antipyrine, theophylline and digitoxin disposition in breast cancer. Clin Pharmacol Ther (1984) 36, 796–802.

Theophylline + Albendazole and Mebendazole

Abstract/Summary

Neither albendazole nor mebendazole appear to interact with theophylline.

Clinical evidence, mechanism, importance and management

Studies in 12 and six normal subjects showed that the pharmacokinetics of theophylline were unaffected by 100 mg mebendazole twice daily for three days or a single 400 mg dose of albendazole respectively. No special precautions would seem to be needed if either of these anthelmintics is given to patients taking theophylline.

Reference

1 Adebayo GI and Mabadeje AFB. Theophylline disposition—effects of cimetidine, mebendazole and albendazole. Aliment Pharmacol Ther (1988) 2, 341–6.

Theophylline + Ampicillin or Amoxycillin

Abstract/Summary

Neither ampicillin nor amoxycillin interacts adversely with theophylline, nor amoxycillin with enprofylline.

Clinical evidence, mechanism, importance and management

A study[1] on 11 asthmatic children aged three months to six years showed that the mean half-life of theophylline was unchanged by the concurrent use of ampicillin. Another study[2,3] on nine normal adults similarly showed that the concurrent use of amoxycillin (750 mg daily for nine days) did not affect the pharmacokinetics of theophylline. Amoxycillin causes a small but not statistically significant reduction in the renal clearance of enprofylline.[4] No special precautions would seem to be necessary during concurrent use.

References

1 Kadlec GJ, Ha Le Thanh, Jarboe CH, Richard D and Karibo JM. Effect of ampicillin on theophylline half-life in infants and young children. South Med J (1978) 71, 1584.
2 Jonkman JHG, van der Boon WJV, Schoenmaker R, Holtkamp A and Hempenius J. Lack of effect of amoxycillin on theophylline pharmacokinetics. Br J clin Pharmac (1985) 19, 99–101.
3 Jonkman JHG, van der Boon WJV, Schoenmaker R, Holtkamp AH and Hempenius J. Clinical pharmacokinetics of amoxycillin and theophylline during cotreatment with both medicaments. Chemotherapy (1985) 31, 329–35.
4 Sitar DS, Aoki FY, Hoban DJ, Hidinger K-G, Montgomery PR and Mitenko PA. Enprofylline disposition in the presence and absence of amoxycillin and erythromycin. Br J clin Pharmac (1987) 24, 57–61.

Theophylline + Antacids

Abstract/Summary

The absorption of theophylline from the gut does not normally appear to be significantly affected by the concurrent use of aluminium or magnesium hydroxide antacids such as **Maalox, Mylanta** *or* **Amphojel,** *but a significant rise in theophylline levels has been described with one sustained-release theophylline preparation* (**Nuelin Depot**).

Clinical evidence, mechanism, importance and management

A study[1] in 12 normal subjects showed that the absorption of aminophylline (200 mg) was slightly reduced by the concurrent use of 30 ml *Maalox* (magnesium-aluminium hydroxide gel) but the extent was considered to be clinically unimportant. Another three-day study[2] on nine asthmatic patients showed that neither 30 ml *Mylanta* nor 60 ml *Amphojel* had a predictable or significant effect on the steady-state serum levels of theophylline when administered as aminophylline or as a sustained-release preparation of theophylline. The absence of a significant interaction was confirmed in another study using an aluminium-magnesium hydroxide antacid and a sustained release theophylline preparation (un-named).[3] No changes were seen in the pharmacokinetics of *K1-b Riker*, a sustained-release preparation, in another study using an un-named antacid.[5] In contrast, in another study[4] it was found that serum theophylline levels from a sustained-release formulation (*Nuelin Depot*) but not from *Theo-dur* were raised when an antacid (*Novalucid*—magnesium and aluminium hydroxides, and magnesium carbonate) was given concurrently. In this last instance the side-effects of theophylline might be increased in those with serum levels at the top end of the range, but generally speaking no special precautions seem to be necessary during the concurrent use of theophylline and antacids.

References

1 Arnold LA, Spurbeck GH, Shelver WH and Henderson WM. Effect of an antacid on gastrointestinal absorption of theophylline. Am J Hosp Pharm (1979) 36, 1059–62.
2 Reed RC and Schwartz HJ. Lack of influence of an intensive antacid regimen on theophylline bioavailability. J Pharmacokinetic Biopharm (1984) 12, 315–331.
3 Darzentas LJ, Stewart RB, Curry SH and Yost RL. Effect of antacid on bioavailability of a sustained-release theophylline tablet preparation. Drug Intell Clin Pharm (1982) 16, 4714
4 Myhre KI and Walstad RA. The influence of antacid on the absorption of two different sustained-release formulations of theophylline. Br J clin Pharmac (1983) 15, 683–7.
5 Moreland TA, McMurdo MET and McEwen J. The effect of food and antacid on the pharmacokinetics of a sustained release theophylline preparation. Br J clin Pharmac (1987) 24, 275–6.

Theophylline + Antihistamines and Related drugs

Abstract/Summary

Terfenadine, temelastine and ketotifen appear not to interact adversely with theophylline.

Clinical evidence, mechanism, importance and management

Three studies in normal subjects showed that the pharmacokinetics of theophylline were unchanged by the concurrent use of 200 mg temelastine daily[1] or 60 mg terfenadine.[2,5] Another two studies showed that ketotifen does not affect the pharmacokinetics of theophylline.[3,4] No adverse effects were seen and the symptom score was improved.[4]

References

1 Charles BG, Schneider JJ, Norris RLG and Ravenscroft PJ. Temelastine does not affect theophylline pharmacokinetics in normal subjects. Br J clin Pharmac (1987) 24, 673–5.
2 Luskin AT, Fitzsimmons WE, Luskin S and MacLeod CM. Single dose study of the effect of terfenadine on theophylline absorption and disposition. Ann Allergy (1987) 60, 184.
3 Garty M, Scolnik D, Danziger Y, Volovitz B, Ilfeld DN and Varsano I. Non-interaction of ketotifen and theophylline in children with asthma—an acute study. Eur J Clin Pharmacol (1987) 32, 187–9.
4 Hendy MS, Burge PS and Stableforth DE. Effects of ketotifen on the bronchodilating action of aminophylline. Respiration (1986) 49, 296–9.
5 Brion N, Naline E, Beaumont D, Pays M and Advenier C. Lack of effect of terfenadine on theophylline pharmacokinetics and metabolism in normal subjects. Br J clin Pharmac (1989) 27, 391–5.

Theophylline + Barbiturates

Abstract/Summary

Theophylline serum levels can be reduced by the concurrent use of phenobarbitone (phenobarbital). Single reports involving quinalbarbitone (secobarbital) and pentobarbitone show that sometimes the serum theophylline levels may be considerably reduced.

Clinical evidence

A study in seven asthmatic children (6–12 years old) showed that after taking phenobarbitone (2 mg/kg daily) for 19 days their mean steady-state serum theophylline levels were reduced by 30%, and the clearance was increased 35% (range 12–71%).[1]

Increases in theophylline clearance of up to 34% and decreases in half-life have been seen in other studies in normal subjects given phenobarbitone for periods of 2–4 weeks.[2–4] Premature babies are reported to need more theophylline if treated with phenobarbitone.[8] A single case report describes a man who showed a 95% rise in the clearance of theophylline when treated with high dose pentobarbitone(-al)[6], and another report describes a 337% increase in the clearance of theophylline over a four-week period in a child treated with quinalbarbitone (secobarbital).[7]

Mechanism

Barbiturates are potent liver enzyme inducing agents which increase the metabolism of theophylline by the liver, thereby hastening its removal from the body. This has been seen in animal studies[5] and is also likely to be true for man.

Importance and management

A moderately well documented, established and clinically important interaction. Patients treated with phenobarbitone may need above-average doses of theophylline to achieve and maintain adequate serum levels. Concurrent use should be monitored and appropriate dosage increases made. All of the barbiturates can cause enzyme induction and may, to a greater or lesser extent, be expected to behave similarly. This is illustrated by the single reports cited involving pentobarbitone and quinalbarbitone.

References

1 Saccar CL, Danish M, Ragni MG, Rocci ML, Greene J, Yaffe SJ and Mansmann HC. The effects of phenobarbital on theophylline disposition in children with asthma. J Allergy Clin Immunol (1985) 75, 716–9.
2 Landay RA, Gonzalez MA and Taylor JC. Effect of phenobarbital on theophylline disposition. J Allergy Clin Immunol (1978) 62, 27.
3 Piafsky KM, Sitar DS and Ogilvie RI. Effect of phenobarbital on the disposition of intravenous theophylline. Clin Pharmacol Ther (1977) 22, 336.
4 Jacobs MH and Senior R. Personal communication (1978) cited by Ogilvie RI in Clin Pharmacokinetics (1978) 3, 267–93.
5 Williams JF and Szentivanyi A. Implications of hepatic metabolising activity in the therapy of bronchial asthma. J Allergy Clin Immunol (1975) 55, 125.
6 Gibson GA, Blouin RA, Bauer LA, Rapp RP and Tibbs PA. Influence of high dose pentobarbital on theophylline pharmacokinetics: a case report. Ther Drug Monit (1985) 7, 181–4.
7 Paladino JA, Blumer NA and Maddox RR. Effect of secobarbital on theophylline clearance. Ther Drug Monit (1983) 5, 133–9.
8 Yazdani M, Kissling GE, Tran TH, Gottschalk SK and Schuth CR. Phenobarbital increases the theophylline requirements of premature infants being treated for apnea. Am J Dis Child (1987) 141, 97–9.

Theophylline + BCG vaccine

Abstract/Summary

There is evidence that BCG vaccine can cause a small increase in the serum levels of theophylline but the clinical importance of this is uncertain.

Clinical evidence, mechanism, importance and management

A study on 12 normal subjects showed that a fortnight after receiving BCG vaccination (0.1 ml *Tubersol*, equivalent to five TU of tuberculin PPD), the clearance of single doses of theophylline was reduced by 21% and the theophylline half-life was prolonged by 14% (range 4 to 47%).[1] It seems possible therefore that the occasional patient may develop some signs of theophylline toxicity, particularly if their serum levels are already towards the top end of the therapeutic range. More study is needed to determine the clinical importance of this interaction.

Reference

1 Gray JD, Renton KW and Hung OR. Depression of theophylline elimination following BCG vaccination. Br J clin Pharmac (1983) 16, 735–7.

Theophylline + Beta-agonist bronchodilators

Abstract/Summary

The concurrent use of theophylline and beta-agonist bronchodilators is common and usually advantageous but some adverse reactions can occur. The side-effects of ephedrine may be increased and the risk of hypokalaemia may be increased if salbutamol or terbutaline are given intravenously. Some patients may show a clinically significant fall in serum theophylline levels if given salbutamol or isoprenaline (isoproterenol). Orciprenaline is reported not to alter serum theophylline levels.

Clinical evidence, mechanism, importance and management

(a) Theophylline + ephedrine

A double-blind randomized study of theophylline, ephedrine and hydroxyzine given separately and together (conventional ephedrine/theophylline ratios of 25:130) to 23 children showed that given singly none of the drugs caused a significant number of adverse reactions, but ephedrine/theophylline in combination was associated with insomnia (14 patients), nervousness (13 patients) and gastrointestinal complaints (18 patients) including vomiting (12 patients). This combination was also no more effective than theophylline alone.[1,2] A previous study in 12 asthmatic children produced essentially similar results,[3] however a later study suggested that no adverse effects occurred if lower doses of ephedrine were used.[14]

(b) Theophylline + isoprenaline (isoproterenol)

A study in six asthmatic children with status asthmaticus and respiratory failure showed that the infusion of isoprenaline increased the clearance of theophylline (given as IV aminophylline) by 19%.[13]

(c) Theophylline + orciprenaline (metaproterenol)

A study on six normal subjects showed that orciprenaline given orally (20 mg eight-hourly) or by inhalation (1.95 mg six-hourly) had no effect on the clearance of theophylline.[11] This confirms a previous finding in asthmatic children in whom it was shown that orciprenaline does not alter serum theophylline levels.[12]

(d) Theophylline + salbutamol

A study in normal subjects showed that the presence of theophylline significantly increased the hypokalaemia and tachycardia caused by infusions of salbutamol and may cause profound hypokalaemia in a few individuals. Concurrent use in acutely ill hypoxic patients could increase the risk of cardiac arrhythmias arising from the hypokalaemia.[5] A case report describes a marked increase in the clearance of theophylline in a child aged 19 months when given intravenous salbutamol and theophylline. The theophylline dosage had to be increased threefold to achieve adequate serum concentrations.[6] Other reports describe reduced theophylline levels, worsened peak flow rates, and increased tachycardia in patients taking theophylline and salbutamol orally.[8,9] No changes in the pharmacokinetics of theophylline were found in another study in normal subjects.[10]

(e) Theophylline + terbutaline

A study in seven normal subjects with therapeutic serum levels of theophylline showed that the unwanted side-effects of intravenous terbutaline (6 μg/kg in 100 ml normal saline over 1 h) were increased, namely, a fall in serum potassium levels and rises in serum glucose levels, pulse rates and systolic blood pressures. The authors suggest that these unwanted effects should be monitored, in particular the serum potassium levels of those already at risk for hypokalaemia.[4] Another study in adult asthmatics found that terbutaline decreased serum theophylline levels by about 10% by increasing its clearance, but the control of the asthma was improved.[7]

References

1 Weinberger M and Bronsky E. Interaction of ephedrine and theophylline. Clin Pharmacol Ther (1974) 15, 223.
2 Weinberger M, Bronsky E, Bensch GW, Brock GN and Yeckles JJ. Interaction of ephedrine and theophylline. Clin Pharmacol Ther (1975) 17, 585.
3 Weinberger M and Bronsky EA. Evaluation of oral bronchodilator therapy in asthmatic children. J Pediat (1974) 84, 421.
4 Smith SR and Kendall MJ. Potentiation of the adverse effects of intravenous terbutaline by oral theophylline. Br J clin Pharmac (1986) 21, 451–3.
5 Whyte KF, Reid C, Addis GJ, Whitesmith R and Reid JL. Salbutamol induced hypokalaemia: the effect of theophylline alone and in combination with adrenaline. Br J clin Pharmac (1988) 25, 571–8.
6 Amirav I, Amitai Y, Avital A and Godfrey S. Enhancement of theophylline clearance by intravenous albuterol. Chest (1988) 94, 444–5.
7 Garty MS, Keslin LS, Ilfeld DN, Mazar A, Spitzer S and Rosenfeld JB. Increased theophylline clearance by terbutaline in asthmatic adults. Clin Pharmacol Ther (1988) 43, 150.
8 Danziger Y, Garty M, Volwitz B, Ilfeld D, Versano I and Rosenfeld JB. Reduction of serum theophylline levels by terbutaline in children with asthma. Clin Pharmacol Ther (1985) 37, 469–71.
9 Dawson KP and Fergusson DM. Effects of oral theophylline and oral salbutamol in the treatment of asthma. Arch Dis Child (1982) 57, 674–6.
10 McCann JP, McElnay JC, Nicholls DP, Scott MG and Stanford CF. Oral salbutamol does not affect theophylline kinetics. Br J Pharmac (1986) 89 (Proc Suppl) 715P.
11 Conrad KA and Woodworth JR. Orciprenaline does not alter theophylline elimination. Br J clin Pharmac (1981) 12, 756–7.
12 Rachelefsky GS, Katz RM, Mickey MR and Siegel SC. Metaproterenol and theophylline in asthmatic children. Ann Allergy (1980) 45, 207–12.
13 Hemstreet MP, Miles MV and Rutland RO. Effect of intravenous isoproterenol on theophylline kinetics. J Allerg Clin Immunol (1982) 69, 360–4.
14 Tinkelman DG and Avener SE. Ephedrine therapy in asthmatic children. J Amer Med Ass (1977) 237, 553.

Theophylline + Beta-blockers

Abstract/Summary

Non-selective beta-blockers such as propranolol should not be given to asthmatic patients because they can cause bronchospasm. The concurrent use of theophylline and selective beta-blockers such as metoprolol is not contraindicated, but some caution is still appropriate.

Clinical evidence, mechanism, importance and management

A study in nine normal subjects (six of whom smoked 10–30 cigarettes daily) showed that the clearance of theophylline was reduced 37% by propranolol (40 mg six-hourly) but not in the group as a whole by metoprolol (50 mg six-hourly), although the smokers did show some reduction in clearance.[1] However non-selective beta-blockers such as propranolol are contraindicated in asthmatic patients because they can cause bronchospasm. The clinical importance of a possible interaction between theophylline and selective beta-blockers such as metoprolol in those who smoke awaits assessment. Some caution would seem appropriate because metoprolol can block the inotropic effects of theophylline,[2] and also because the safety of the selective (beta-1 selective) beta-blockers in all asthmatic patients is not absolutely certain. More study is needed.

References

1 Conrad KA and Nyman DW. Effects of metoprolol and propranolol on theophylline elimination. Clin Pharmacol Ther (1980) 28, 463.
2 Conrad KA and Prosnitz EH. Cardiovascular effects of theophylline. Partial attenuation by beta-blockade. Eur J Clin Pharmacol (1981) 21, 109.

Theophylline and Related drugs + Caffeine

Abstract/Summary

Caffeine raises serum theophylline levels, but the clinical importance of this is uncertain. Furafylline, a new xanthine, causes a very marked rise in caffeine levels accompanied by toxicity.

Clinical evidence, mechanism, importance and management

A study in six normal subjects showed that when given 8 or 18 mg caffeine daily for six days the clearance of theophylline was decreased by 18–27% and the half-life was prolonged by 21% and 44% (depending on the dosage of the caffeine).[1] The extent to which the ingestion of caffeine in coffee or tea raises the serum levels of theophylline and affects its therapeutic use appears not to have been studied. In another study on furafylline, a new theophylline-like xanthine compound, it was found that it causes caffeine (ingested in coffee) to accumulate in the body to a very marked extent, (a 5–10-fold rise), accompanied by a number of unacceptable side-effects.[2] The probable reason is that the furaylline inhibits the metabolism and clearance of caffeine from the body. The authors of this report point out that the toxic side-effects of some other new drugs may be related to caffeine-intoxication.

References

1 Loi CM, Jue SG, Bush ED, Crowley JJ and Vestal RE. Effect of caffeine dose on theophylline metabolism. Clin Res (1987) 35, 377A.
2 Tarrus E, Cami J, Roberts DJ, Spickett RGW, Celdran E and Segura J. Accumulation of caffeine in healthy volunteers treated with furafylline. Br J clin Pharmac (1987) 23, 9–18.

Theophylline + Calcium channel blockers

Abstract/Summary

Diltiazem and verapamil normally cause a small increase or no change in the serum theophylline levels of asthmatic patients and normal subjects. Nifedipine may cause a decrease or no change, and felodipine causes a small decrease. The control of asthma seems not to be adversely affected. However there are individual case reports describing unexplained intoxication in two patients when given nifedipine and one patient when given verapamil.

Clinical evidence

(a) Theophylline + diltiazem

A study in nine normal subjects (four smokers and five non-smokers) showed that after taking 90 mg diltiazem twice daily for 10 days the clearance of theophylline (given as aminophylline) fell by 21% (from 51 to 64.6 ml/min/1.73 m²) and its half-life increased from 6.1 to 7.5 h.[8]

A 12% fall in clearance was seen in another study[9] whereas another study found no significant change in the half-life of theophylline when diltiazem was given.[5]

(b) Theophylline + felodipine

A study in 10 normal subjects showed that 5 mg felodipine eight-hourly for four days reduced the plasma AUC of theophylline by 18.3% (from 270 to 220 μmol.h.l^{-1}).[13]

(c) Theophylline + nifedipine

A study in eight asthmatic patients on theophylline showed that 20 mg nifedipine twice daily in a slow-release form

caused their serum theophylline levels to fall by 30% (from 9.7 to 6.8 μg/ml); they were below the therapeutic range (<4 μg/ml) in three of the patients, but no changes in the control of the asthma was seen as measured by peak flow determinations and symptom scores.[4]

No changes in the pharmacokinetics of theophylline were seen in other studies of asthmatic patients given nifedipine[6,10] and the control of asthma was unchanged.[6] Another study in normal subjects found that the nifedipine deceased the clearance of theophylline by 9%,[2] whereas another found no changes in the theophylline pharmacokinetics.[7] However there are two case reports of patients who developed theophylline intoxication apparently due to the addition of nifedipine.[11,12]

(d) Theophylline + verapamil

A study in five asthmatic subjects given 200 mg aminophylline six-hourly showed that the concurrent use of 80 mg verapamil six-hourly for two days had no effect on the pharmacokinetics of theophylline, and no effects on the spirometric measurements made (FVC, FEV1, FEF25–7).[1] Reductions of 14%, 18% and 23% in theophylline clearance were found in three pharmacokinetic studies in normal subjects.[2,5,9] There is an isolated report of a woman on digoxin and theophylline who developed signs of toxicity (tachycardia, nausea, vomiting) which was attributed to the concurrent use of verapamil.[3] Her theophylline serum levels doubled over a six-day period.

Mechanism

It is believed that diltiazem, nifedipine and verapamil alter (increase or decrease) the metabolism of theophylline by the liver, as a result its loss from the body is changed. Felodipine possibly reduces theophylline absorption.

Importance and management

Adequately but not extensively documented. The results are not entirely consistent but the overall picture is that concurrent use is normally safe. Despite the small decreases in the clearance or absorption of theophylline seen with diltiazem, felodipine and verapamil, and the quite large reductions in serum levels seen in one study with nifedipine, no adverse changes in the control of the asthma were seen in any of the studies. However very occasionally and unpredictably theophylline levels have risen causing intoxication in patients given nifedipine (two patients) or verapamil (one patient) so it would be prudent to monitor the effects. There seems to be no information about other calcium channel blockers.

References

1 Gotz VP and Russell WL. Effect of verapamil on theophylline disposition. Chest (1987) 92, 75S.
2 Robson RA, Miners JO and Birkett DJ. Selective inhibitory effects of nifedipine and verapamil on oxidative metabolism: effects on theophylline. Br J clin Pharmac (1988) 25, 397–400.
3 Burnakis TG, Seldon M and Czaplicki AD. Increased serum theophylline concentrations secondary to oral verapamil. Clin Pharm (1983) 2, 458–61.
4 Smith SR, Wiggins J, Stableforth DE, Skinner C and Kendall MJ. Effect

of nifedipine on serum theophylline concentrations and asthma control. Thorax (1987) 42, 794–6.

5   Abernethy DR, Egan JM, Dickinson TH and Carrum G. Substrate-selective inhibition by verapamil and diltiazem: differential disposition of antipyrine and theophylline in humans. J Pharmacol Exp Ther (1988) 244, 994–9.
6   Garty M, Cohen E, Mazar A, Ilfeld DN, Spitzer S and Rosenfeld JB. Effect of nifedipine and theophylline in asthma. Clin Pharmacol Ther (1986) 40, 195–8.
7   Jackson SHD, Shah K, Debbas NMG, Johnston A, Peverel-Cooper CA and Turner P. The interaction between IV theophylline and chronic oral dosing with slow release nifedipine in volunteers. Br J clin Pharmac (1986) 21, 389–92.
8   Nafziger AN, May JJ and Bertino JS. Inhibition of theophylline elimination by diltiazem therapy. J Clin Pharmacol (1987) 27, 862–5.
9   Sirmans A, Pieper JA, Lalonde RL, Self TH and Smith D. Effect of calcium channel antagonists on theophylline disposition. Drug Intell Clin Pharm (1987) 21, 16A.
10 Christopher MA, Harman E, Bell JA and Hendeles L. Measurement of steady-state theophylline concentrations before and during concurrent therapy with diltiazem or nifedipine. Drug Intell Clin Pharm (1987) 21, 4A.
11 Parrillo SJ and Venditto SJ. Elevated theophylline blood levels from institution of nifedipine therapy. Ann Emerg Med (1984) 43, 216–17.
12 Harrod CS. Theophylline toxicity and nifedipine. Ann Intern Med (1987) 106, 480.
13 Bratel T, Billing B and Dahlqvist R. Felodipine reduces the absorption of theophylline in man. Eur J Clin Pharmacol (1989) 36, 481–5.

Theophylline + Carbamazepine

Abstract/Summary

Two case reports describe a marked fall in serum theophylline levels during the concurrent use of carbamazepine. Another single case report describes a fall in serum carbamazepine levels when theophylline was given.

Clinical evidence

An asthmatic girl of 11 was well controlled for two months with theophylline until the phenobarbitone she was taking was replaced by carbamazepine.[1] The asthma worsened, theophylline serum levels fell to subtherapeutic levels and the half-life of the theophylline halved (from 5.25 to 2.75 h). Asthmatic control was restored when the carbamazepine was replaced by ethotoin. The clearance of theophylline in another patient was halved when carbamazepine (600 mg daily) was withdrawn.[3]

A girl of 10 showed a fall in serum carbamazepine levels (trough concentrations roughly halved) when she was treated with theophylline, and experienced grand mal convulsions.[2] Her serum theophylline levels were also unusually high (142 μmol/l) for the dosage taken (5 mg/kg six-hourly), so it may be that the convulsions were as much due to this as to the fall in carbamazepine levels.

Mechanism

The mechanisms of these reactions is not understood but it has been suggested that each drug possibly increases the liver metabolism and clearance of the other drug, resulting in a reduction in their effects.[1,2]

Importance and management

Information seems to be limited to the reports cited so that their general importance is uncertain. Concurrent use need not be avoided, but it would be prudent to check that the serum concentrations of each drug (and their effects) are not reduced to subtherapeutic levels.

References

1   Rosenberry KR, Defusco CJ, Mansmann HC and McGeady SJ. Reduced theophylline half-life induced by carbamazepine therapy. J Ped (1983) 102, 472–4.
2   Mitchell EA, Dower JC and Green RJ. Interaction between carbamazepine and theophylline. NZ Med J (1986) 99, 69–70.
3   Reed RC and Schwartz HJ. Phenytoin-theophylline-quinidine interaction. N Engl J Med (1983) 308, 724–5.

Theophylline + Cimetidine, Etintidine, Famotidine or Ranitidine

Abstract/Summary

Theophylline serum levels are raised by cimetidine and toxicity may develop if appropriate reductions (one third to a half) are not made in the theophylline dosage. Ranitidine would not be expected to interact but has been reported to do so in a few patients. So far famotidine appears not to interact but etintidine behaves like cimetidine.

Clinical evidence

(a) Cimetidine

The theophylline serum levels of an asthmatic 15-year-old rose threefold (from 13 to 37 μg/ml) within a fortnight of starting to take cimetidine (dosage not stated). Theophylline levels fell once again when the cimetidine was withdrawn.[1] This appears to be a particularly exaggerated response to the interaction.

Other case reports describe the development of toxic theophylline serum levels caused by the use of cimetidine.[7,8,11] A number of well-controlled pharmacokinetic studies on groups of healthy subjects[2,4–6,9,21] and in patients[3,4,10,13] have all clearly demonstrated that cimetidine (1000–1200 mg daily) prolongs the theophylline half-life by about 60% and reduces the clearance by 30–40%. Trough serum levels are raised about one-third.[13] The extent of the interaction does not depend on the dosage of cimetidine (within the 1200–2400 mg daily range).[9]

(b) Etintidine

A study in 10 normal subjects showed that 800 mg etintidine daily for four days almost tripled the half-life of theophylline (from 6 to 16.8 h) and reduced the clearance by about 65% (from 0.0564 to 0.02 l/h/kg).[28]

(c) Famotidine

A study on 10 healthy subjects showed that 40 mg famotidine twice daily for five days had no effect on the pharmacokinetics of theophylline.[23]

(d) Ranitidine

A number of pharmacokinetic studies on considerable numbers of subjects clearly show that ranitidine does not affect the pharmacokinetics of theophylline,[8,12,14,16,24] even in daily doses up to 4200 mg daily.[22] However five reports describe a total of six patients who developed theophylline toxicity when given ranitidine.[19,20,26,27,29]

Mechanism

Cimetidine is a well-recognised enzyme inhibitor which depresses the metabolism of theophylline by the liver, thereby prolonging its stay in the body and raising its serum levels. It has also been suggested that a theophylline-cimetidine complex may be formed in the body which is less easily metabolized than theophylline.[17] Etintidine behaves similarly. Famotidine appears not to have enzyme inhibiting effects but just why ranitidine interacts sometimes is not clear.

Importance and management

The theophylline-cimetidine interaction is very well documented (not all the references being listed here), very well established and clinically important. Theophylline serum levels should be monitored if cimetidine is given concurrently and suitable dosage adjustments made to ensure that theophylline toxicity does not develop. Levels normally rise by about one-third, but much greater increases have been seen in individual patients. Initial dosage reductions of 30–50% have been suggested to accommodate the rise.[8] There is some disagreement about whether smokers do or do not need a greater reduction.[15,25] The extent of the interaction seems to be the same in both young and old.[18] Etintidine appears to behave like cimetidine. The situation with ranitidine is not clear; it would not be expected to interact but it does so occasionally and unpredictably. Monitor concurrent use closely and be alert for any evidence of toxicity. Famotidine would also not be expected to interact but, as with ranitidine, the effects should be monitored.

References

1 Weinberger MM, Smith G, Milavetz G and Hendeles L. Decreased theophylline clearance due to cimetidine. N Engl J Med (1981) 304, 672.
2 Jackson JE, Powell JR, Wandell M, Bentley J and Dorr R. Cimetidine-theophylline interaction. Pharmacologist (1980) 22, 231.
3 Campbell MA, Platetka JR, Jackson JE, Moon JF and Finley PR. Cimetidine decreases theophylline clearance. Ann Intern Med (1981) 95, 68.
4 Wood L, Grice J, Petroff V, McGuffie C and Roberts RK. Effect of cimetidine on the disposition of theophylline. Aust NZ J Med (1980) 10, 586.
5 Roberts RK, Grice J, Wood L, Petroff V and McGuffie C. Cimetidine impairs the elimination of theophylline and antipyrine. Gastroenterol (1981) 81, 19.
6 Reitberg DP, Bernhard H and Schentag JJ. Alteration of theophylline clearance and half-life by cimetidine. An Intern Med (1981) 95, 582.
7 Lofgren RP and Gilbertson A. Cimetidine and theophylline. Ann Intern Med (1982) 96, 378.
8 Bauman JH, Kimelblatt BJ, Carracio DR, Silverman HM, Simon GI and Beck GJ. Cimetidine-theophylline interaction. Report of four patients. Ann Allergy (1982) 48, 100–2.
9 Powell JR, Rogers JF, Wargin WA, Cross RE and Eshelman FN. The influence of cimetidine vs ranitidine on theophylline pharmacokinetics. J Pharmacol Ther (1982) 31, 261.
10 Fenje PC, Isles AF, Baltodan A, Macleod SM and Soldin S. Interaction of cimetidine and theophylline in two infants. Can Med Ass J (1982) 126, 1178.
11 Uzzan D, Uzzan B, Bernard N and Caubarrere I. Interaction medicamenteuse de la cimetidine et de la theophylline. Nouv Presse Med (1982) 11, 1950.
12 Ruff F. Interferences medicamenteuses de la theophylline. Absence d'interaction theophylline-ranitidine. Nouv Presse Med (1982) 11, 3512,
13 Vestal RE, Thummel KE, Musser B and Mercer GD. Cimetidine inhibits theophylline clearance in patients with chronic obstructive pulmonary disease. A study using stable isotope methodology during multiple oral dose administration. Br J clin Pharmacol (1983) 15, 411–18.
14 Powell JR, Rogers JF, Wargin WA, Cross RE and Eshelman FN. Inhibition of theophylline clearance by cimetidine but not ranitidine. Arch Intern Med (1984) 144, 484–6.
15 Grygiel JJ, Miners JO, Drew R and Birkett DJ. Differential effects of cimetidine on theophylline metabolic pathways. Eur J Clin Pharmacol (1984) 26, 335–40.
16 Ferrari M, Angelini GP, Barozzi E, Olivieri M, Penna S and Accardi R. A comparative study of ranitidine and cimetidine effects on theophylline metabolism. Giornale Italiano Malattie del Torace (1984) 38, 31–4.
17 Ritschel WA, Alcorn GJ, Streng WH and Zoglio MA. Cimetidine-theophylline complex formation. Meth Find Exptl Clin Pharmacol (1983) 5, 55–8.
18 Cohen IA, Johnson CE, Berardi RR, Hyneck ML and Achem SR. Cimetidine-theophylline interaction: effects of age and cimetidine dose. Ther Drug Monit (1985) 7, 426–34.
19 Fernandes E and Melewicz FM. Ranitidine and theophylline. Ann Intern Med (1984) 100, 459.
20 Gardner ME and Sikorski GW. Ranitidine and theophylline. Ann Intern Med (1985) 102, 559.
21 Mulkey PM, Murphy JE and Shleifer NH. Steady-state theophylline pharmacokinetics during and after short-term cimetidine administration. Clin Pharm (1983) 2, 439–41.
22 Kelly HW, Powell JR and Donohue JF. Ranitidine at very large doses does not inhibit theophylline elimination. Clin Pharmacol Ther (1986) 39, 577–81.
23 Chremos AN, Lin JH, Yeh KC, Chiou WF, Bayne WF, Lipschutz K and Williams P.L. Famotidine does not interfere with the disposition of theophylline in man. Comparison with cimetidine. Clin Pharmacol Ther (1986) 39, 187.
24 Seggev JS, Barzilay M and Schey G. No evidence for interaction between ranitidine and theophylline. Arch Intern Med (1987) 147, 179–80.
25 Cusack BJ, Dawson GW, Mercer GD and Vestal RE. Cigarette smoking and theophylline metabolism: effects of cimetidine. Clin Pharmacol Ther (1985) 37, 330–6.
26 Roy AK, Cuda MP and Levine RA. Theophylline toxicity induced by ranitidine. Gastroenterol (1988) 94, A389.
27 Dietemann-Molard A, Popin E, Oswald-Mammosser M, Colas des Francs V and Pauli G. Intoxication a la theolphylline par interaction avec la ranitidine a dose elevee. La Presse Med (1988) 17, 280.
28 Huang S-M, Weintraub HS, Marriott TB, Marinan B, Abels R and Leese PT. Etintidine-theophylline interaction study in humans. Biopharm and Drug Disp (1987) 8, 561–9.
29 Skinner MH, Lenert L and Blaschke TT. Theophylline toxicity subsequent to ranitidine administration: a possible drug-drug interaction. Am J Med (1989) 86, 129–32.

Theophylline + Contraceptives (oral)

Abstract/Summary

Serum theophylline levels are raised to some extent in women taking oral contraceptives, but no toxicity has been reported.

Clinical evidence

A controlled study[1] in eight women on oral contraceptives showed that their total plasma clearance of a single oral dose of aminophylline (4 ml/kg) was about 30% lower than in eight other women not on oral contraceptives (35.1 compared with 53.1 ml/h/kg).[1] The theophylline half-life was also prolonged by about 30% (from 7.34 to 9.79 h).

These findings are confirmed by other studies[2-4,7] which also showed that the plasma clearance of theophylline is decreased about 30% by the use of oral contraceptives. In contrast, no significant changes were seen in 10 adolescent women (16–18 years).[6]

Mechanism

Uncertain, but it seems possible that the oestrogenic component (rather than the progestogen[5]) may inhibit the metabolism of the theophylline by the liver microsomal enzymes, thereby reducing its clearance.

Importance and management

An established interaction but there seem to be no reports of theophylline toxicity resulting from concurrent use. Women (possibly not adolescents) on oral contraceptives may need less theophylline than those not taking oral contraceptives. There is a small risk that patients with serum theophylline at the top end of the range may show some toxicity.

References

1 Tornatore KM, Kanarkowski R, McCarthy TL, Gardner MJ, Yurchak AM and Jusko WJ. Effect of chronic oral contraceptive steroids on theophylline disposition. Eur J Clin Pharmacol (1982) 23, 129–34.
2 Jusko WJ, Gardner MJ, Mangione A, Schentag JJ, Koup JR, and Vance JW. Factors affecting theophylline clearances: age, tobacco, marijuana, cirrhosis, congestive heart failure, obesity, oral contraceptives, benzodiazepines, barbiturates and ethanol. J Pharm Sci (1979) 68, 1358–66.
3 Roberts RK, Grice J, McGuffie C and Heilbron L. Oral contraceptive steroids impair the elimination of theophylline. J Lab Clin Med (1983) 101, 821–5.
4 Gardner MJ, Tornatore KM, Jusko WJ, Karnankowski R. Effects of tobacco smoking and oral contraceptive use on theophylline disposition. Br J clin Pharmacol (1983) 16, 271–80.
5 Gotz VP, Dolly FR and Block AJ. Influence of medroxyprogesterone on theophylline disposition. J Clin Pharmacol (1983) 23, 281–4.
6 MacLeod S, Koren G, Chin T, Correia J and Tesoro A. Theophylline pharmacokinetics in adolescent females following coadministration of oral contraceptives. Clin Pharmacol Ther (1985) 37, 209.
7 Long DR, Roberts EA, Brill-Edwards M, Quaggin S, Correia J, Koren G and MacLeod SM. The effect of the oral contraceptive Ortho 7/7/7 on theophylline clearance in non-smoking women aged 18–22. Clin Invest Med (1987) 10 (4 Suppl B) B59.

Theophylline + Corticosteroids

Abstract/Summary

Concurrent use is not uncommon but increases in serum theophylline levels (sometimes associated with toxicity), decreases and no changes have been described during concurrent use. The general clinical importance of these interactions is uncertain.

Clinical evidence

(a) Increased serum theophylline levels

Six patients in status asthmaticus with stable serum concentrations of theophylline (by infusion) were given an intravenous 500 mg bolus of hydrocortisone followed 6 h later by three two-hourly doses of 200 mg. In each case the serum theophylline levels rapidly climbed from about 20 to between 30 and 50 μg/ml. At least two of the patients complained of nausea and headache.[1] Another study on 10 children (aged 2–6) with status asthmaticus showed that methylprednisolone increased the half-life of theophylline.[4] Another study using an un-named corticosteroid also reported a prolonged theophylline half-life (from 4.98 to 6.18 h) and a clearance reduced by about one-third.[6]

(b) Reduced serum theophylline levels

Seven normal subjects stabilized on theophylline given intravenous methylprednisolone (1.6 mg/kg) and hydrocortisone (33 mg/kg) separately showed a 21% increase in clearance when the results of the two were combined.[2] Another study[3] on six normal subjects showed that prednisone (20 mg) caused a small but clinically trivial reduction in the serum levels of theophylline. An increase in the clearance of theophylline was seen in a normal subject given methylprednisolone but no changes in the kinetics of theophylline were seen in two subjects given methylprednisolone.[5]

Mechanism

Not understood.

Importance and management

The interactions of theophylline with the various corticosteroids is poorly documented and their clinical importance is difficult to assess because both increases, small decreases and no changes in the serum levels of theophylline have been reported. It is also questionable whether the results of studies in normal healthy subjects can validly be extrapolated to patients with status asthmaticus. There is no good reason for avoiding concurrent use, but the effects and/or serum theophylline levels should be checked.

References

1 Buchanan N, Hurwitz S and Butler P. Asthma—a possible interaction between hydrocortisone and theophylline. S Afr Med J (1979) 56, 1147.
2 Leavengood DC, Bunker-Soler AL and Nelson HS. The effect of

corticosteroids on theophylline metabolism. Ann Allergy (1983) 50, 249.

3 Anderson JL, Ayres JW and Hall CA. Potential pharmacokinetic interaction between theophylline and prednisone. Clin Pharm (1984) 3, 187–8.
4 De La Morena E, Borges MT, Rebollar CG and Escorihuela R. Efecto de la metil-prednisolona sobre los niveles sericos de teofilina. Rev Clin Esp (1982) 167, 297–300.
5 Squire EN and Nelson HS. Corticosteroids and theophylline clearance. NER Allergy Proc (1987) 8, 113–15.
6 Elvey SM, Saccar CL, Rocci ML, Mansmann HC, Martynec DM and Kester MB. The effect of corticosteroids on theophylline metabolism in asthmatic children. Ann Allergy (1986) 56, 520.

Theophylline + Co-trimoxazole

Abstract/Summary

Co-trimoxazole does not interact with theophylline.

Clinical evidence, mechanism, importance and management

A cross-over study on six normal subjects showed that eight day's treatment with co-trimoxazole (960 mg twice daily) had no effect on the pharmacokinetics of theophylline given intravenously.[1] Another study found that co-trimoxazole (960 mg twice daily) for five days had no effect on the pharmacokinetics of theophylline given orally.[2] No special precautions would seem necessary if these two drugs are given concurrently.

Reference

1 Jonkman JHG, van der Boon WJV, Schoenmaker R, Holtkamp AH and Hempenius J. Lack of influence of co-trimoxazole on theophylline pharmacokinetics. J Pharm Sci (1985) 74, 1103–4.
2 Lo KF, Nation RL and Sansom LN. Lack of effect of co-trimoxazole on the pharmacokinetics of orally administered theophylline. Biopharm Drug Disp (1989) 10, 573–80.

Theophylline + Dextropropoxyphene

Abstract/Summary

Dextropropoxyphene does not interact significantly with theophylline.

Clinical evidence, mechanism, importance and management

A study in six normal subjects showed that the concurrent use of 65 mg dextropropoxyphene eight-hourly for five days did not significantly change the plasma clearance of theophylline (125 mg eight-hourly).[1] There would seem to be no need to avoid concurrent use or to take particular precautions.

Reference

1 Robson RA, Miners JO, Whitehead AG and Birkett DJ. Specificity of the inhibitory effect of dextropropoxyphene on oxidative drug metabolism in man: effects on theophylline and tolbutamide disposition. Br J clin Pharmac (1987) 23, 772–5.

Theophylline + Disulfiram

Abstract/Summary

Blood theophylline levels are increased by disulfiram. The theophylline dosage may need to be reduced to avoid the development of toxicity.

Clinical evidence

A study in 20 recovering alcoholics showed that after taking 250 mg disulfiram daily for a week the clearance of theophylline (5 mg/kg infused IV) was decreased by 21% (from 105.7 to 83.1 ml/kg/h). Those taking 500 mg disulfiram daily showed a decrease of 32.5% (from 94.3 to 65.4 ml/kg/h).[1,2] Smoking appeared to have no important effects on the extent of this interaction.

Mechanism

Disulfiram inhibits the liver enzymes concerned with the metabolism of the theophylline, thereby reducing its clearance from the body.

Importance and management

Information appears to be limited to this study but it would seem to be an established and clinically important interaction. Monitor the serum levels of theophylline and its effects if disulfiram is added, anticipating the need to reduce the theophylline dosage, bearing in mind that the extent of this interaction depends upon the dosage of disulfiram used. Some patients on 500 mg disulfiram showed a 50% reduction in clearance.

References

1 Loi C-M, Day JD, Jue SG, Costello P and Vestal RE. The effect of disulfiram on theophylline disposition. Clin Pharmacol Ther (1987) 41, 165.
2 Loi C-M, Day JD, Jue SG, Bush ED, Costello P, Dewey LV and Vestal RE. Dose-dependent inhibition of theophylline metabolism by disulfiram in recovering alcoholics. Clin Pharmacol Ther (1989) 45, 476–86.

Theophylline + Enprostil

Abstract/Summary

Enprostil does not interact with theophylline.

Clinical evidence, mechanism, importance and management

A double-blind cross-over study[1] in 10 asthmatic patients showed that the concurrent use of enprostil (70 μg daily) for five days had no effect on serum theophylline levels, vital capacity or FEV₁. It would seem that concurrent use is safe.

Reference

1 Gross G and Bynum L. Use of enprostil in asthmatics taking theophylline. Gastroenterol (1985) 88, 1407.

Theophylline + Erythromycin

Abstract/Summary

Theophylline serum levels can be increased by the concurrent use of erythromycin and intoxication may develop in those patients whose serum levels are already high unless the dosage is reduced. At the same time erythromycin levels may possibly fall to subtherapeutic concentrations.

Clinical evidence

(a) Theophylline serum levels increased

A cross-over pharmacokinetic study on 12 patients with chronic bronchitis given aminophylline (4 mg/kg/day) showed that peak serum theophylline levels were raised 28% when concurrently treated with erythromycin stearate (500 mg six-hourly) and the clearance was reduced 22%.[1]

Rises in serum theophylline levels of up to 40% as a result of this interaction have been described in numerous studies[2-10,16] some of which report the development of theophylline toxicity. Not all patients show this interaction. One report states that it occurred in only three of the nine subjects studied[11] and two other studies[12,13,15] involving eight and 13 subjects failed to demonstrate this interaction.

(b) Erythromycin serum levels reduced

A study on six normal subjects taking 500 mg erythromycin eight-hourly showed that when given a single 250 mg dose of theophylline intravenously their peak serum erythromycin levels were almost halved. Over an 8 h period the area under the serum concentration/time curve was reduced 38%.[14]

Another pharmacokinetic study found that serum erythromycin levels fell by more than 30% when theophylline was given concurrently,[18] whereas an earlier study found no changes apart from a marked increase in renal clearance.[16]

Mechanisms

Not fully understood. It seems most likely that erythromycin inhibits the metabolism of theophylline by the liver resulting in a reduction in its clearance from the body and in a rise in its serum levels. It also seems possible that theophylline can affect both the absorption and the elimination of erythromycin.[17,18]

Importance and management

The effects of erythromycin on theophylline (a) are established (but still debated) and well documented. Not all the reports are referenced here. It does not seem to matter which erythromycin salt is used. Monitor concurrent use closely and anticipate the need to reduce the theophylline dosage to avoid toxicity. Not all will show this interaction but it may take several days to manifest itself. Those particularly at risk are patients with already high serum theophylline levels and/or taking high dosages (20 mg/kg body weight or more). A 25% reduction has been recommended for those in the 15–20 μg/ml range,[1,5] but little dosage adjustment is probably needed for those at the lower end of the range (8–15 μg/ml) unless toxic symptoms appear.[1,9] Enprofylline appears not to interact with erythromycin and is a possible alternative.[19] The fall in erythromycin levels caused by theophylline (b) is not well documented but what is known suggests that it may be clinically important. Be alert for any evidence of an inadequate response to the erythromycin and increase the dosage if necessary. More study is needed.

References

1 Reisz G, Pingleton SK, Melethil S and Ryan P. The effect of erythromycin on theophylline pharmacokinetics in chronic bronchitis. Am Rev Resp Dis (1983) 127, 581–4.
2 Cummins LH, Kozak PP and Gillman SA. Erythromycin's effects on theophylline blood levels. Pediatric (1977) 59, 144.
3 Cummins LH, Kozak PP and Gillman SA. Theophylline determinations. Ann Allergy (1976) 37, 450.
4 Anderson RJ. Review of antimicrobial drug interactions. Clin Med (1978) 85, 13.
5 Prince RA, Wing DS, Weinberger MM, Hendeles LS and Riegleman S. Effect of erythromycin on theophylline kinetics. J Allergy Clin Immunol (1981) 68, 427–31.
6 May DC, Jarboe CH, Ellenberg DT, Roe EJ and Karibo J. The effects of erythromycin on theophylline elimination in normal males. J Clin Pharmacol (1982) 22, 125–30.
7 Branigan TA, Robbins RA, Cady WJ, Nickols JG and Ueda CT. The effects of erythromycin on the absorption and disposition kinetics of theophylline. Eur J clin Pharmac (1981) 21, 115–20.
8 Green JA and Clementi WA. Decrease in theophylline clearance after the administration of erythromycin to a patient with obstructive lung disease. Drug Intell Clin Pharm (1983) 17, 370–2.
9 Zarowitz BJM, Szefler SJ and Lasezkay GM. Effect of erythromycin base on theophylline kinetics. Clin Pharmacol Ther (1981) 29, 601–5.
10 Richer C, Matthieu M, Bah H, Thuillez C, Duroux P and Guidicelli J-F. Theophylline kinetics and ventilatory flow in bronchial asthma and chronic airflow obstruction: influence of erythromycin. Clin Pharmacol Ther (1982) 31, 579–86.
11 Pfeifer HJ, Greenblatt DJ and Friedman P. Effects of three antibiotics on theophylline kinetics. Clin Pharmacol Ther (1979) 26, 36.
12 Kelly SJ, Pingleton SK, Ryan PB and Sri M. The lack of influence of erythromycin on plasma theophylline serum levels. Chest (1980) 78, 523.
13 Maddux M, Organek H, Hasegawa G, Leeds N and Bauman J. Erythromycin alteration of theophylline pharmacokinetics. Lack of effect at steady-state. Am Rev Resp Dis (1981) 123, 60.
14 Iliopoulou A, Aldhous ME, Johnston A and Turner P. Pharmacokinetic interaction between theophylline and erythromycin. Br J clin Pharmac (1982) 14, 495–9.
15 Maddux MS, Leeds NH, Organek HW, Hasegawa GR and Bauman JL. The effect of erythromycin on theophylline pharmacokinetics at steady-state. Chest (1982) 81, 563–5.
16 LaForce CF, Miller MF and Chai H. Effect of erythromycin on

theophylline clearance in asthmatic children. J Ped (1981) 99, 153–6.

17 Hildebrandt R, Moller H and Gundert-Remy U. Influence of theophylline on the renal clearance of erythromycin. Int J Clin Pharmacol Ther Tox (1987) 25, 601–4.

18 Paulsen O, Hoglund P, Nilsson L-G and Bengtsson H-I. The interaction of erythromycin with theophylline. Eur J Clin Pharmacol (1987) 32, 493–8.

19 Sitar DS, Aoki FY, Hoban DJ, Hidinger K-G, Montgomery PR and Mitenko PA. Enprofylline disposition in the presence and absence of amoxycylline and erythromycin. Br J clin Pharmac (1987) 24, 57–61.

Theophylline + Food

Abstract/Summary

The bioavailability of theophylline from a number of sustained-release formulations can be increased or decreased by food and by the type of food eaten (high protein diets increase the loss of theophylline from the body, whereas high carbohydrate diets reduce the loss). Changes in the bioavailability of theophylline can also occur in patients fed by nasogastric tube or intravenously.

Clinical evidence

(a) Theophylline and food given orally

A study in seven normal subjects showed that the absorption of theophylline from a controlled release tablet (*Theograd*) increased from 65 to 87% when taken after a meal.[1] Another showed that food did not affect the bioavailability of theophylline in *Theolin Retard*[4] but increased it from 53 to 96% with *Uniphyl*.[6] The area under the concentration-time curve for theophylline given as *Nuelin SA* increased by 33% in eight patients with airways obstruction after eating a high carbohydrate/low protein diet for a week when compared with a high protein/low carbohydrate diet.[2] Another study on 18 normal subjects indicated that carbohydrate delayed the absorption of theophylline from *Teovent*.[3] Food is reported to increase the absorption of theophylline from *Theo-24*[5] but reduce (by 53%) the bioavailability of *Theo-Dur Sprinkle*.[6] A patient with chronic obstructive pulmonary disease showed a two-thirds fall in his serum theophylline levels accompanied by bronchospasm when he was fed through a nasogastric tube with *Osmolite*. The interaction occurred with both theophylline tablets (*Theo-Dur*) and liquid theophylline, but not when the theophylline was given intravenously as aminophylline.[7] Food was found to alter the absorption pattern of *Uniphylline* in children but not adults. 'Dose dumping' and toxic serum theophylline levels occurred in some children and it was concluded that children should not take this sustained release preparation in large doses with food.[11] Only slight and clinically unimportant changes in absorption were seen in studies of *Theostat 300*, *Uniphyl* and *Teonova* in normal adults when given with food.[12–15]

(b) Theophylline and food given parenterally

An isolated report describes an elderly woman treated with aminophylline by intravenous infusion who showed a marked fall in her serum theophylline levels (from 16.3 to 6.3 mg/l) when the amino acid concentration of her parenteral nutrition regimen was increased from 4.25 to 7%.[8]

Mechanism

Not fully understood. One suggestion is that high protein diets stimulate liver enzymes (the cytochrome P-450 mono-oxygenase system) thereby increasing the metabolism of the theophylline and hastening its loss from the body. High carbohydrate diets have the opposite effect.[9,10]

Importance and management

The theophylline-food interactions have been thoroughly studied but there seems to be no consistent pattern in the way the absorption of different theophylline preparations is affected. Be alert for any evidence of an inadequate response which can be related to food intake, and monitor the effects if one preparation is exchanged for another. Encourage patients to take their theophylline consistently in relation to meals, and not to make major changes in their diet without consulting the prescriber.

References

1 Lagas M and Jonkman JHG. Influence of food on the rate and extent of absorption of theophylline after a single dose oral administration of a controlled release tablet. Int J Clin Pharmacol Ther Tox (1985) 23, 424–6.

2 Thompson PJ, Skypala I, Dawson S, McAllister WAC and Warwick MT. The effect of diet upon serum concentrations of theophylline. Br J clin Pharmac (1983) 16, 267–70.

3 Johansson O, Lindberg T, Melander A and Whalin-Boll E. Different effects of different nutrients on theophylline absorption in man. Drug-Nutr Interactions (1985) 3, 205–11.

4 Sips AP, Edelbroek PM, Kulstad S, de Wolff FA and Dijkman JH. Food does not effect bioavailability of theophylline from *Theolin Retard*. Eur J Clin Pharmacol (1984) 26, 405–7.

5 Vaughan L, Milavetz G, Hill M, Weinberger M and Hendeles L. Food-induced dose-dumping of *Theo-24*, a 'once-daily' slow release theophylline product. Drug Intell Clin Pharm (1984) 18, 510.

6 Karim A, Burns T, Wearley L, Streicher J and Palmer M. Food-induced changes in theophylline absorption from controlled release formulations. Part I. Substantial increased and decreased absorption with *Uniphyl* tablets and *Theo-Dur Sprinkle*. Clin Pharmacol Ther (1985) 38, 77–83.

7 Gal P and Layson R. Interference with oral theophylline absorption by continuous nasogastric feedings. Ther Drug Monitor (1986) 8, 421–3.

8 Ziegenbein RC. Theophylline clearance increase from increased amino acid in a CPN regimen. Drug Intell Clin Pharm (1987) 21, 220–1.

9 Kappas A, Anderson KE, Conney AH and Alvares AP. Influences of dietary protein and carbohydrate on antipyrine and theophylline metabolism in man. Clin Pharmacol Ther (1976) 20, 643–53.

10 Feldman CH, Hutchinson VE, Pippenger CE, Blumenfeld TA, Feldman BR and Davis WJ. Effect of dietary protein and carbohydrate on theophylline metabolism in children. Pediatrics (1980) 66, 956–62.

11 Steffensen G and Pedersen S. Food induced changes in theophylline absorption from a once-a-day theophylline product. Br J clin Pharmac (1986) 22, 571–7.

12 Thebault JJ, Aiache JM, Mazoyer F and Cardot JM. The influence of food on the bioavailability of a slow release theophylline preparation. Clin Pharmacokinet (1987) 13, 267–72.

13 Schulz H-U, Karlsson S, Sahner-Ahrens I, Steinijans VW and Beier W. Effect of drug intake prior to or after meals on serum theophylline concentrations: single-dose studes with Euphylong. Int J Clin Pharmacol Ther Toxicol (1987) 25, 222–8.

14 Boner AL, Setter L, Messori A, Plebani M, Vallone G and Martini N.

Effect of food on the bioavailability of a slow-release theophylline formulation. J Clin Pharm Ther (1988) 13, 77–81.

15 Arkinstall WW, Hopkinson M, Rivington RN and Stewart JH. The clinical significance of food induced changes in the pharmacokinetics of theophylline with *Uniphyl*. Am Rev Resp Dis (1988) 137, 33.

Theophylline + Frusemide

Abstract/Summary

The outcome of concurrent use is uncertain. Frusemide is reported to increase, decrease or to have no effect on serum theophylline levels.

Clinical evidence

Eight patients with chronic stable asthma were given 300 mg of a sustained-release theophylline preparation. When given 25 mg frusemide concurrently their mean serum theophylline levels measured at 1 and 6 h were reduced by 41% (from 12.14 to 7.16 μg/ml).[1] Four premature neonates, two given theophylline and frusemide orally and the other two intravenously, showed a fall in steady-state serum theophylline levels from 8 to 2–3 μg/ml when the frusemide was given within 30 min of the theophylline.[2] 10 patients with asthma, chronic bronchitis or emphysema on continuous maintenance infusion with aminophylline showed a 21% rise in their serum theophylline levels (from 13.7 to 16.6 μg/ml) 4 h after being given a 40 mg dose of frusemide (intravenously over 2 min).[3]

A study in 12 normal subjects given theophylline failed to find any change in serum theophylline levels when given 40 mg frusemide orally.[4]

Mechanism

Not understood.

Importance and management

Information is limited and the outcome of concurrent use is inconsistent and uncertain. If both drugs are used the serum theophylline levels should be monitored and appropriate dosage adjustments made as necessary.

References

1 Carpentiere G, Marino S and Castello F. Furosemide and theophylline. Ann Intern Med (1985) 103, 957.
2 Toback JW and Gilman ME. Theophylline-furosemide inactivation? Pediatrics (1983) 71, 140–1.
3 Conlon PF, Grambau GR, Johnson CE and Weg JR. Effect of intravenous furosemide on serum theophylline concentration. Am J Hosp Pharm (1981) 38, 1345–7.
4 Janicke U-A and Gundert-Remy U. Failure to detect a clinically significant interaction between theophylline and furosemide. Naunyn-Schmied Arch Pharmacol (1986) 332, R100.

Theophylline + Idrocilamide

Abstract/Summary

Idrocilamide can increase serum theophylline levels. A reduction in the theophylline dosage may be needed to avoid intoxication.

Clinical evidence, mechanism, importance and management

A study in six normal subjects showed that the concurrent use of idrocilamide (600 mg daily for seven days) increased the half-life of a single dose of theophylline by 2.5 (from 8.5 to 21.6 h) due, so it is suggested, to a reduction in the liver metabolism caused by the idrocilamide.[1] Information is very limited but it indicates that concurrent use should be closely monitored. The need to reduce the theophylline dosage should be anticipated.

Reference

1 Lacroix C, Nouveau J, Hubscher Ph, Tardif D, Ray M and Goulle JP. Influence de l'idrocilamide sur le metabolisme de la theophylline. Rev Pneumol Clin (1986) 42, 164–6.

Theophylline + Influenza vaccines

Abstract/Summary

Normally none of the influenza vaccines (whole virus, split virus and purified subunit) interact with theophylline, but there are three reports describing rises in serum theophylline levels in a few patients attributed to the use of an influenza vaccine, accompanied by toxicity in some instances.

Clinical evidence

(a) Evidence of no interaction

No evidence of a rise in serum theophylline levels was seen in 12 patients given influenza vaccine, trivalent, Types A and B[9] or in 119 elderly people given an un-named influenza vaccine.[4] No evidence of an interaction was found in a number of other studies involving 23 normal subjects (split virus vaccine),[5] seven subjects and five patients (purified subunit vaccine),[6] 12 patients (trivalent vaccine—*Fluzone*),[7] 11 patients and 12 normal subjects (trivalent vaccine—*Fluogen*),[8] 16 normal subjects (whole virus vaccine),[10] and 16 patients (trivalent vaccine—*Fluzone*),[11] or 49 asthmatic children (trivalent subvirion influenza V).[12]

(b) Evidence of an interaction

Three patients taking 200 mg oxytriphylline (equivalent to 128 mg theophylline) orally six-hourly for at least seven days showed a rise in their serum theophylline levels of 219, 89 and 85% respectively within 12–24 h of receiving 0.5 ml trivalent influenza vaccine (*Fluogen*—Parke Davis). Two of them showed signs of theophylline toxicity. A subsequent study on four normal subjects showed that the same dose of vaccine more than doubled the half-life of theophylline (from 3.3 to 7.3 h) and halved its clearance (from 52 to 25 mg/kg/h).[1]

A girl of 15 showed a transient rise in theophylline levels (no sign of toxicity) when given a split-virus vaccine,[3] and a woman showed a rise accompanied by headaches and palpitations.[7] Theophylline intoxication has been seen in children during an influenza epidemic accompanied by changes in serum theophylline levels.[2]

Mechanism

Uncertain. It is thought that if the interaction occurs it is due to inhibition by the vaccine of the activity of the liver enzymes concerned with the metabolism of theophylline, resulting in its accumulation in the body.[1] One suggestion is that vaccine contaminants rather than the vaccine itself may be responsible so that no interaction would seem likely with highly purified subunit vaccines.[13]

Importance and management

A very thoroughly investigated interaction, the weight of evidence indicating that no adverse interaction normally occurs with any type of influenza vaccine in children, adults or the elderly. Even so, bearing in mind the occasional and unexplained reports of interaction,[1,3,7] it would seem prudent to monitor the effects of concurrent use although problems are very unlikely to arise now that purer vaccines are available (see 'Mechanism').

References

1 Renton KW, Gray JD and Hall RI. Decreased elimination of theophylline after influenza vaccination. Can Med Ass J (1980) 123, 288.
2 Kraemer MJ, Furukawa CT, Koup JR, Shapiro GG, Pierson WE and Bierman CW. Altered theophylline clearance during an influenza B outbreak. Paediatrics (1982) 69, 476–80.
3 Walker S, Schreiber L and Middelkamp JN. Serum theophylline levels after influenza vaccination. Can Med Ass J (1981) 125, 243–4.
4 Patriarca PA, Kendal AP, Stricof RL, Weber JA, Meissner MK and Dateno B. Influenza vaccination and warfarin or theophylline toxicity in nursing home residents. N Engl J Med (1983) 308, 1601–2.
5 Grabowski N, May JJ, Pratt DS, Richtmeier WJ, Bertino JS and Sorge KF. The effect of split virus influenza vaccination on theophylline pharmacokinetics. Am Rev Resp Dis (1985) 131, 934–8.
6 Winstanley PA, Tjia J, Back DJ, Hobson D and Breckenridge AM. Lack of effect of highly purified subunit influenza vaccination on theophylline metabolism. Br J clin Pharmac (1985) 20, 47–53.
7 Fischer R, Booth B, Mitchell D and Kibbe A. Influence of trivalent influenza vaccine on serum theophylline levels. Can Med Ass J (1982) 126, 1312–13.
8 Bukowskyj M, Munt P, Wigle R and Nakatou K. Theophylline clearance: lack of effect of influenza vaccination and ascorbic acid. Am Rev Resp Dis (1984) 129, 672–5.
9 Gomolin IH, Chapron DJ and Luhan PA. Effects of influenza virus vaccine on theophylline and warfarin clearance in institutionalised elderly. J Amer Ger Soc (1984) 32, Suppl S21.
10 Hannan SE, May JJ, Pratt DS, Richtsmeier WJ and Bertino JS. Lack of effect of whole virus influenza vaccine on theophylline pharmacokinetics. Am Rev Resp Dis (1986) 133, A61.
11 Goldstein RS, Cheung OT, Seguin R, Lobley G and Johnson AC. Decreased elimination of theophylline after influenza vaccination. Can Med Ass J (1981) 126, 470.
12 Feldman CH, Rabinowitz A, Levison M, Klein R, Feldman BR and Davis WJ. Effects of influenza vaccine on theophylline metabolism in children with asthma. Am Rev Respir Dis (1985) 131 (4 Suppl) A9.
13 Winstanley PA, Back DJ and Breckenridge AM. Inhibition of theophylline metabolism by interferon. Lancet (1987) ii, 1340.

Theophylline + Interferon

Abstract/Summary

The clearance of theophylline from the body is reduced (on average halved) by interferon. Theophylline intoxication is likely if the dosage is not reduced appropriately.

Clinical evidence

A study in five patients with stable chronic active hepatitis B and four healthy subjects showed that 20 h after being given a single 9 or 18 mega unit IM injection of interferon (recombinant alpha A, Hoffman La Roche), the theophylline clearance of eight patients was approximately halved (from 0.7 to 0.36 ml/kg/min) with a range of 33–81%. The mean theophylline elimination half-life was increased from 6.3 to 10.7 h (1.5 to 6-fold increases). One healthy subject showed no change. Four weeks after the study the theophylline clearances were noted to have returned to their former values.[1]

Mechanism

Interferon inhibits the liver enzymes[2] concerned with the metabolism of some drugs, including theophylline, so that it is cleared from the body more slowly and accumulates.[1]

Importance and management

Direct information appears to be limited to this report[1] but the interaction appears to be established. So far there are no reports of toxicity but it would be expected to occur if the theophylline dosage is not reduced. Concurrent use should be closely monitored. What is known suggests that on average the dosage should be roughly halved, but individual patients who normally have increased rates of theophylline clearance (e.g. smokers) may need even greater dosage reductions.[1]

References

1 Williams SJ, Baird-Lambert JA and Farrell GC. Inhibition of theophylline metabolism by interferon. Lancet (1987) ii, 939–41.
2 Williams SJ and Farrell GC. Inhibition of antipyrine metabolism by interferon. Br J Clin Pharmacol (1986) 22, 610–12.

Theophylline + Isoniazid

Abstract/Summary

One study found that theophylline serum levels were increased by the concurrent use of isoniazid whereas another found that the clearance of theophylline was increased.

Clinical evidence, mechanism, importance and management

A study in seven normal subjects showed that after taking 10 mg/kg isoniazid daily for the 10 days, the half-life and AUC (area under the curve) of theophylline were increased by 15% (from 152 to 175 min) and 31% (from 439–620 μmol/h/l) respectively. The theophylline was given as an IV infusion and the serum levels after 6 h were 22% higher (58 μmol/l compared with 48.5 μmol/l). Five subjects also showed an increase in isoniazid half-life and AUC but they were not statistically significant.[1] In contrast another study on four normal subjects, given 300 mg isoniazid daily for six days, found that the clearance of theophylline given orally was increased by 16%, but no consistent changes were seen in any of the other pharmacokinetic parameters measured.[2] The reason for these inconsistent results is not understood. The outcome of concurrent use is uncertain but it would clearly be prudent to monitor the effects.

References

1 Hoglund P, Nilsson L-G and Paulsen O. Interaction between isoniazid and theophylline. Eur J Resp Dis (1987) 70, 110–6.
2 Thompson JR, Burckart GJ, Self TH, Brown RE and Straughn AB. Isoniazid-induced alterations in theophylline pharmacokinetics. Curr Ther Res (1982) 32, 921–5.

Theophylline + Ketoconazole

Abstract/Summary

Although ketoconazole normally appears not to interact with theophylline in normal subjects, one report says that it can reduce theophylline levels in asthmatics.

Clinical evidence, mechanism, importance and management

No changes in the pharmacokinetics of theophylline (3 mg/kg IV) were seen in 12 normal subjects after taking 400 mg ketoconazole daily for five days.[1] Similar results were found in another study in 10 normal subjects.[2] However a case report describes a man whose serum theophylline levels fell sharply from about 16.5 to 9 mg/l (a subtherapeutic level) over the 2 h immediately after taking 200 mg ketoconazole. A less striking fall was seen in two other patients.[3] The reasons for these discordant results are not understood but it would now seem prudent to monitor the effects of concurrent use closely to confirm that the theophylline continues to be effective. More study is needed.

References

1 Brown MW, Maldonado AL, Meredith CG and Speeg KV. Effect of ketoconazole on hepatic oxidative drug metabolism. Clin Pharmacol Ther (1985) 37, 290–7.
2 Heusner JJ, Dukes GE, Rollins DE, Tolman KG and Galinsky RE. Effect of chronically administered ketoconazole on the elimination of theophylline in man. Drug Intell Clin Pharm (1987) 21, 514–7.
3 Murphy E, Hannon D and Callaghan B. Ketoconazole-theophylline interaction. Irish Med J (1987) 80, 123–4.

Theophylline + Macrolide antibiotics

Abstract/Summary

Theophylline serum levels can rise during concurrent treatment with triacetyloleandomycin (troleandomycin) and theophylline toxicity may develop if the dosage is not reduced appropriately. Josamycin may cause a fall in serum theophylline levels or not interact at all. Midecamycin, miocamycin, ponsinomycin, rokitamycin, roxithromycin and spiramycin do not interact significantly. See also 'Theophylline + Erythromycin'.

Clinical evidence

(a) Josamycin

No significant changes in the serum theophylline levels were seen in three studies in adult and child patients given josamycin concurrently.[4–6] Another study[8] reported a fall of 23% in five patients with particularly severe respiratory impairment, but no significant effect in five other patients with less severe disease. No interaction was seen in another study using josamycin.[7]

(c) Midecamycin, miocamycin, ponsinomycin, rokitamycin, roxithromycin and spiramycin

18 asthmatic children showed a slight decrease in serum theophylline levels when given midecamycin (40 mg/kg/day) for 10 days for a bronchopulmonary infection, but no changes were seen in a pharmacokinetic study in five normal adults.[9] No significant changes in serum theophylline levels were seen in 20 patients on slow-release theophylline (*Theo-dur*), 600 mg daily, or four mg/kg intravenous theophylline, three times daily, when concurrently treated with 1200 mg miocamycin daily for 10 days.[10] A study in five chronic asthmatic children and another in 25 other patients confirmed the absence of an interaction between theophylline and miocamycin.[12,16] A human study showed that 800 mg ponsinomycin twice daily for five days had little effect on steady-state serum theophylline levels, although renal clearance was slightly increased.[15] 11 elderly patients on theophylline showed no significant changes in serum theophylline levels when given 600 mg rokitamycin daily for a week.[13] 12 normal subjects showed only small changes in the pharmacokinetics of theophylline when given 300 mg roxithromycin daily for four days.[14] A study in 15 asthmatic patients on theophylline showed that the concurrent use of 1 g spiramycin for at least five days had no significant effect on their steady-state serum theophylline levels.[11]

(c) Triacetyloleandomycin

Eight patients with severe chronic asthma showed a 50% reduction in their clearance of theophylline when treated with triacetyloleandomycin (250 mg four times daily). One of them had a theophylline-induced seizure after 10 days and was found to have a serum theophylline level of 40 μg/ml (normal range 10–20 μg/ml). The theophylline half-life in this patient had increased from 4.6 to 11.3 h.[1–3]

Mechanism

It is believed that triacetyloleandomycin forms inactive cytochrome P-450-metabolite complexes within the liver cells, the effect of which is to reduce the metabolism of theophylline, thereby reducing its loss from the body. Josamycin, midecamycin, miocamycin, rokitamycin and spiramycin have different molecular structures which apparently do not behave like triacetyloleandomycin.[11]

Importance and management

The theophylline–triacetyloleandomycin interaction is established. Increases in serum theophylline levels should be expected during concurrent use. This may have a beneficial effect on the control of asthma, but it may also lead to toxicity if the levels rise too high. Concurrent use should be monitored and the theophylline dosage reduced as necessary. Josamycin would seem to be an alternative antibiotic which appears only to interact (a fall in serum theophylline levels) in those with particularly severe respiratory impairment. Other effectively non-interacting macrolide antibiotics are midecamycin, miocamycin, ponsinomycin, rokitamycin, roxithromycin and spiramycin.

References

1. Weinburger M, Hudgel D, Spector S and Chidsey C. Troleandomycin (TAO): an inhibitor of theophylline metabolism. J Allergy Clin Immunol (1976) 57, 262.
2. Weinburger M, Hudgel D, Spector S and Chidsey C. Effect of triacetyloleandomycin (TAO) on the metabolism of theophylline. Clin Pharmacol Ther (1976) 19, 118.
3. Weinburger M, Hudgel D, Spector S and Chidsey C. Inhibition of theophylline clearance by troleandomycin. J Allergy Clin Immunol (1977) 59, 228.
4. Ruff F, Prosper M and Pujet JC. Theophylline et antibiotiques. Absence d'interaction avec la josamycine. Therapie (1984) 39, 1–6.
5. Baos RJ, de Frias EC, Cadorniga R and Moreno M. Estudio de posibles interaccinones entre josamicina y teofilina en ninos. Rev Farmacol Clin Exp (1985) 2, 345–8.
6. Ruff F, Santais MC, Chastagnol D, Huchon G and Durieux P. Macrolide et theophylline: absence d'interaction josamycine-theophylline. Nouv Presse Med (1981) 10, 175.
7. Brazier JL, Kofman J, Faucon G, Perrin-Fayolle M, Lepape A and Lanove R. Retard d'elimination de la theophylline du a la troleandomycine. Absence d'effet de la josamycine. Therapie (1980) 35, 545.
8. Bartolucci L, Gradoli C, Vincenzi V, Iapadre M and Valori C. Macrolide antibiotics and serum theophylline levels in relation to the severity of the respiratory impairment: a comparison between the effects of erythromycin and josamycin. Chemioterapia (1984) 3, 286–90.
9. Lavarenne J, Paire M and Talon O. Influence d'un nouveau macrolide, la mydecamycine, sur les taux sanguins de theophylline. Therapie (1981) 36, 451–6.
10. Rimoldi R, Babdera M, Fioretti M and Giorcelli R. Miocamycin and theophylline blood levels. Chemioterapia (1986) 5, 213–6.
11. Debruyne D, Jehan A, Bigot M-C, Lechevalier B, Prevost J-N and Moulin M. Spiramycin has no effect on serum theophylline in asthmatic patients. Eur J Clin Pharmacol (1986) 30, 505–7.
12. Principi N, Onorato J, Giuliani MG and Vigano A. Effect of miocamycin on theophylline kinetics in children. Eur J Clin Pharmacol (1987) 31, 701–4.
13. Ishioka T. Effect of a new macrolide antibiotic, 3'-O-propionyl-leucomycin A5 (Rokitamycin), on serum concentrations of theophylline and digoxin in the elderly. Acta Therapeutica (1987) 13, 17–23.
14. Saint-Salvi B, Tremblay D, Surjust A and Lefebvre MA. A study of the interaction of roxithromycin with theophylline and carbmazepine. J Antimicrob Chemother (1987) 20, Suppl B, 121–9.
15. Couet W, Ingrand I, Reigner B, Girault J, Bizouard J and Fourtillan JB.

Lack of effect of ponsinomycin on the plasma pharmacokinetics of theophylline. Eur J Clin Pharmacol (1989) 37, 101–4.
16. Dal Negro R, Turco P, Pomari C and de Conti F. Miocamycin doesn't affect theophylline serum levels in COPD patients. Int J Clin Pharmacol Ther Tox (1988) 26, 27–9.

Theophylline + Metronidazole

Abstract/Summary

No interaction of clinical importance takes place if metronidazole is given to patients taking theophylline.

Clinical evidence, mechanism, importance and management

A study in five women showed that while taking metronidazole (250 mg three times a day) for trichmoniasis the pharmacokinetics of theophylline were slightly but not significantly changed.[1] Another study in five normal subjects confirmed this finding.[2] Although the evidence is limited, no special precautions would seem to be necessary during concurrent use.

Reference

1. Reitberg DP, Klarnet JP, Carlson JK and Schentag JJ. Effect of metronidazole on theophylline pharmacokinetics. Clin Pharm (1983) 2, 441–4.
2. Adebayo GI. Lack of inhibitory effect of metronidazole on theophylline disposition in healthy subjects. Br J clin Pharmacol (1987) 24, 110–13.

Theophylline + Mexiletine

Abstract/Summary

Two isolated reports describe increased serum theophylline levels and evidence of toxicity in two patients when given mexiletine.

Clinical evidence, mechanism, importance and management

A man with coronary heart disease and chronic obstructive lung disease developed nausea, vomiting and loss of appetite within a few days of starting to take 200 mg mexiletine three times daily. His serum theophylline levels had risen from 15.3 to 25 μg/ ml. The symptoms disappeared when the theophylline dosage was reduced from 600 mg to 200 mg daily, and his serum theophylline levels fell to 14.2 μg/ml.[1] The serum theophylline levels of another patient approximately doubled when he started to take mexiletine. He experienced significant nausea and gastric upset. The reason for this response is not known, but changes in the metabolism of the theophylline by the liver have been suggested.[1,2] The effects of concurrent use should be well monitored for signs of theophylline toxicity.

References

1 Katz A, Buskila D and Sukenik S. Oral mexiletine-theophylline interaction. Int J Cardiol (1987) 17, 227–8.
2 Stanley R, Comer T, Taylor JL and Saliba D. Mexiletine-theophylline interaction. Amer J Med (1989) 86, 733–4.

Theophylline + Pirenzepine

Abstract/Summary

Pirenzepine does not interact with theophylline.

Clinical evidence, mechanism, importance and management

A pharmacokinetic study in five normal subjects showed that 50 mg pirenzepine daily for five days had no effect on the pharmacokinetics of theophylline (given as aminophylline, 6.5 mg/kg body weight, intravenously).[1] This would suggest that concurrent use need not be avoided.

Reference

1 Sertl K, Rameis H and Meryn S. Pirenzepin does not alter the pharmacokinetics of theophylline. Int J Clin Pharmacol Ther Toxicol (1987) 25, 15–17.

Theophylline + Piroxicam

Abstract/Summary

Piroxicam does not interact with theophylline.

Clinical evidence, mechanism, importance and management

A study in six normal subjects showed that seven days' treatment with 20 mg piroxicam daily had no effect on the pharmacokinetics of theophylline, given as aminophylline 6 mg/kg intravenously.[1] No special precautions would seem to be necessary during concurrent use.

Reference

1 Maponga C, Barlow JC and Schentag JJ. Lack of effect of piroxicam on theophylline clearance in healthy volunteers. DICP Ann Pharmacotherapy (1990) 24, 123–6.

Theophylline + Pneumococcal vaccine

Abstract/Summary

Pneumococcal vaccination does not affect theophylline.

Clinical evidence, mechanism, importance and management

A study in six normal subjects showed that the pharmacokinetics of theophylline (250 mg given orally three times daily for 10 days) were unaltered the day after receiving 0.5 ml of a pneumococcal vaccine, and week later.[1] These findings need confirmation in patients, but what is known suggests that no special precautions are needed during concurrent use.

Reference

1 Cupit GC, Self TH, Pieper JA and Bekemayer WB. Effect of pneumococcal vaccine (PV) on theophylline (T) disposition. Clin Pharmacol Ther (1987) 41, 199.

Theophylline and Related drugs + Probenecid

Abstract/Summary

Serum levels of theophylline are unaffected by the concurrent use of probenecid, but serum diprophylline (dyphylline) and enprofylline levels can be raised.

Clinical evidence, mechanism, importance and management

A study in 12 subjects showed that the half-life of dyphylline (dihydroxypropyl theophylline) (20 mg/kg) was doubled (from 2.6 to 4.9 h) and the clearance halved (from 173 to 95 ml/h/kg) by the concurrent use of 1 g probenecid resulting in raised serum dyphylline levels.[1] In another study in six normal subjects the total body clearance of enprofylline was halved (from 21 to 9.8 l/h) by the concurrent use of 1 g probenecid.[3] In contrast, a study in seven normal subjects showed that 1 g probenecid given 30 min before an oral dose of aminophylline (5.6 mg/kg) had no significant effect on the pharmacokinetics of theophylline.[2] The probable reason for the difference is that theophylline is largely cleared from the body by liver metabolism, whereas dyphylline and enprofylline are mostly lost in the urine which is where probenecid is most likely to interfere.

These are single doses studies and the outcome of chronic concurrent use is therefore uncertain, but it would seem to be prudent to monitor serum dyphylline and enprofylline levels if probenecid is started or stopped.

References

1 May DC and Jarboe CH. Inhibition of clearance of dyphylline by probenecid. N Engl J Med (1981) 304, 791.
2 Chen TWD and Patton TF. Effect of probenecid on the pharmacokinetics of aminophylline. Drug Intell Clin Pharm (1983) 17, 465–6.
3 Borga O, Parsson R and Lunell E. Effects of probenecid on enprofylline kinetics in man. Eur J Clin Pharmacol (1986) 30, 221–3.

Theophylline + Pyrantel

Abstract/Summary

A single case report describes increased serum theophylline levels in a child when given pyrantel embonate (pyrantel pamoate).

Clinical evidence

A boy of eight with status asthmaticus was treated firstly with aminophylline and then switched to oral theophylline on day three. On day four he was additionally given a single 160 mg dose of pyrantel embonate at the same time as his second theophylline dose for an *Ascaris Lumbricoides* infection. About 2.5 h later his serum theophylline level had risen from 15 to 24 μg/ml. The theophylline was stopped. 1.5 h later it had risen to 30 μg/ml. No theophylline toxicity occurred and the patient was discharged later in the day without theophylline.[1]

Mechanism

Not understood. One suggestion is that the pyrantel inhibited the liver enzymes concerned with the metabolism of the theophylline, thereby reducing its loss from the body. Another is that it increased drug release from the sustained-release theophylline preparation.

Importance and management

Information is limited to this single case report. No general conclusions can be based on such slim evidence but concurrent use should be well monitored because in this case the serum theophylline concentration increase was very rapid. More study is needed.

Reference

1 Hecht L and Murray WE. Theophylline-pyrantel pamoate interaction. DICP Ann Pharmacotherapy (1989) 23, 258.

Theophylline + Quinolone antimicrobials

Abstract/Summary

Theophylline serum levels can be markedly increased in some patients (two–threefold) by the concurrent use of enoxacin or ciprofloxacin. The theophylline dosage may need to be approximately halved if toxicity is to be avoided. Norfloxacin, lomefloxacin, ofloxacin and pefloxacin cause a much smaller rise in theophylline levels, or even no rise at all, and no theophylline dosage adjustment may be needed.

Clinical evidence

(a) Theophylline + ciprofloxacin

A study in 33 patients on theophylline showed that when given ciprofloxacin, 750 mg twice daily, their serum theophylline levels doubled (from 7.8 to 14.6 μg/ml). Seven of the older patients showed symptoms of theophylline toxicity.[1]

A two- to threefold increase in serum theophylline levels was seen in another study in patients given 500 mg ciprofloxacin twice daily.[8] The clearance of theophylline (6 mg/kg IV over 30 min) was decreased by 17.8% in eight normal subjects given ciprofloxacin, 750 mg twice daily for 6–8 days. Three of the subjects showed a 42–113% decrease.[2] The CSM in the UK has eight reports of clinically important toxic interactions between these two drugs.[3] One elderly woman taking 440 mg theophylline daily died with toxic serum levels shortly after starting to take ciprofloxacin.[3] In contrast another report said that no increases in theophylline levels and no toxicity occurred in 20 patients given 500–750 mg ciprofloxacin twice daily.[4]

(b) Theophylline + enoxacin

An interaction study was made when unexpectedly high serum theophylline levels (accompanied by toxicity) were seen in patients concurrently treated with enoxacin. 14 patients showed a two-threefold rise (mean 8.5 to 21.7 μg/ml) in serum theophylline levels after taking 800–1200 mg enoxacin for 3–5 days. Nine of them complained of nausea and vomiting which disappeared when the theophylline dosage was reduced. Six patients subsequently given aminophylline intravenously showed a doubling of their serum theophylline concentrations within three days.[5,6]

Signs of theophylline toxicity have been described elsewhere in patients on theophylline when given enoxacin.[7] In one study serum theophylline levels were seen to double when 800 mg enoxacin daily were taken,[11] and in another a threefold rise was seen.[18]

(c) Theophylline + lomefloxacin

A study in 25 normal subjects found that 400 mg lomefloxacin daily for seven days had little or no effect on the pharmacokinetics of theophylline although the half-life was slightly increased (from 6.72 to 7.02 h).[17]

(d) Theophylline + norfloxacin

A study in 10 normal subjects taking 600 mg aminophylline daily showed that while taking 800 mg norfloxacin concurrently for four days no significant changes in serum theophylline levels occurred.[12]

Norfloxacin was found not to affect theophylline in two other studies[13,14] but some changes were found in another. 800 mg norfloxacin daily for six days increased the half-life of aminophylline given IV from 8.3 to 9.6 h, increased the AUC from 96.1 to 112.0 mg/h/l, and decreased the clearance from 0.74 to 0.63 ml/kg/min.[15] The greatest individual change in clearance was −29%.[15]

(e) Theophylline + ofloxacin

A study in 15 normal subjects showed that when given 400 mg ofloxacin twice daily for eight days, their steady-state theophylline levels rose by 10.3% and the AUC by 9.9%.[10] In another study an 11% decrease in clearance was seen,[2] and no changes were seen in two other studies.[11,13,19]

(f) Theophylline + pefloxacin

A study in eight patients taking 600–1200 mg theophylline daily showed that when treated with 800 mg pefloxacin daily for five-and-a-half days, their serum pefloxacin levels rose by 19.6% and the clearance fell by 29.4%.[9,11] No changes were seen in another study.[13]

Mechanism

These quinolone antibiotics appear to inhibit the metabolism of theophylline by liver to different extents, so that it is cleared from the body more slowly and its serum levels rise. The renal clearance may also be reduced.[16]

Importance and management

The theophylline–enoxacin and –ciprofloxacin interactions are well documented, well established and of clinical importance. The incidence is uncertain but it does not cause problems in all patients.[7] The risk seems greatest in the elderly[1] and those with theophylline levels already towards the top end of the therapeutic range. Toxicity may develop rapidly (within 2–3 days) unless the dosage of theophylline is reduced. Avoid concurrent use unless the theophylline levels can be monitored and appropriate dosage reductions made where necessary. Halving the dose has been suggested.[6,11] One study found that new steady-state serum theophylline levels were achieved within about three days of starting and stopping enoxacin.[20]

Keep a check on the effects if norfloxacin, ofloxacin or pefloxacin are used because theophylline serum levels may rise to a small extent (10–20%[10,11]), but these antibiotics appear to be much safer and there seem to be no reports of adverse interactions. Lomefloxacin appears not to interact.

References

1 Raoof S, Wollschlager C and Khan FA. Ciprofloxacin increases serum levels of theophylline. Am J Med (1987) 82 (Suppl 4A) 115–18.
2 Nix DE, DeVito JM, Whitbread MA and Schentag JJ. Effect of multiple dose oral ciprofloxacin on the pharmacokinetics of theophylline and indocyanine green. J Antimicrob Chemother (1987) 19, 263–9.
3 Bem JL and Mann RD. Danger of interaction between ciprofloxacin and theophylline. Br Med J (1988) 296, 1131.
4 Maesen FPV, Teengs JP, Bauer C and Davies BI. Quinolones and raised concentrations of theophylline. Lancet (1984) ii, 530.
5 Wijnands WJA, van Herwaarden CLA and Vree TB. Enoxacin raises plasma theophylline concentrations. Lancet (1984) ii, 108.
6 Wijnands WJA, Vree TB and van Herwaarden CLA. Enoxacin decreases the clearance of theophylline in man. Br J clin Pharmac (1985) 20, 583–8.
7 Davies BI, Maessen FP and Teengs JP. Serum and sputum concentrations of enoxacin after oral single dosing in a clinical and bacteriological study. J Antimicr Chemother (1984) 14 (Suppl C), 83–9.
8 Thomsen AH, Thompson GD, Hepburn M and Whiting BA. Clinically significant interaction between ciprofloxacin and theophylline. Eur J Pharmacol (1987) 33, 435–6.
9 Wijnands WJA, Vree TB and van Herwaarden CLA. Comment: potential theophylline toxicity with enoxacin. Drug Intell Clin Pharm (1987) 21, 383.
10 Gregoire SL, Grasela TH, Freer JP, Tack KJ and Schentag JJ. Inhibition of theophylline clearance by coadministered ofloxacin without alteration of theophylline effects. Antimicrob Ag Chemother (1987) 31, 375–8.
11 Wijnands WJA, Vree TB and van Herwaarden CLA. The influence of quinolone derivatives on theophylline clearance. Br J clin Pharmac (1986) 22, 677–83.
12 Bowles SK, Popovski Z, Rybak MJ, Beckman H and Edwards DJ. Effect of norfloxacin on theophylline pharmacokinetics. Clin Pharmacol Ther (1988) 43, 156.
13 Niki Y, Soejima R, Kawane H, Sumi M and Umeki S. New synthetic quinolone antibacterial agents and serum concentration of theophylline. Chest (1987) 92, 663–9.
14 Sano M, Yamamoto I, Ueda J, Yoshikawa E, Yamashinia H and Goto M. Comparative pharmacokinetics of theophylline following two fluoroquinolones co-administration. Eur J Clin Pharmacol (1987) 32, 431–2.
15 Tierney MG, Ho G and Dales RE. Effect of norfloxacin on theophylline pharmacokinetics. Clin Pharmacol Ther (1988) 43, 156.
16 Beckmann J, Elsasser W, Gundert-Remy U and Hertrampf R. Enoxacin—a potent inhibitor of theophylline metabolism. Eur J Clin Pharmacol (1987) 33, 227–30.
17 Nix DE, Norman A and Schentag JJ. Effect of lomefloxacin on theophylline pharmacokinetics. Antimicrob Ag Chemother (1989) 33, 1006–8.
18 Takagi K, Hasegawa T, Yamaki K, Suzuki R, Watanabe T and Satake T. Interaction between theophylline and enoxacin. Int J Clin Pharmacol Ther Tox (1988) 26, 288–92.
19 Al-Turk WA, Shaheen OM, Othman S, Khalaf RM and Awidi AS. Effect of ofloxacin on the pharmacokinetics of a single intravenous theophylline dose. Ther Drug Monit (1988) 10, 160–3.
20 Rogge MC, Solomon WR, Sedman AJ, Welling PG, Koup JR and Wagner JG. The theophylline-enoxacin interaction: II. Changes in the disposition of theophylline and its metabolites during intermittent administration of enoxacin. Clin Pharmacol Ther (1989) 46, 420–8.

Theophylline + Repirinast

Abstract/Summary

Repirinast appears not to interact adversely with theophylline.

Clinical evidence, mechanism, importance and management

A study in seven adult asthmatics given 400–800 mg theophylline twice daily showed that the concurrent use of repirinast (dosage not clearly stated but by implication 150 mg twice daily) for three weeks had no effect on the pharmacokinetics of the theophylline.[1] No special precautions would seem necessary if both drugs are given.

Reference

1 Tagaki K, Kuzuya T, Horiuchi T, Nadai M, Apichartpichean R, Ogura Y and Hasegawa T. Lack of effect of repirinast on the pharmacokinetics of theophylline in asthmatic patients. Eur J Clin Pharmacol (1989) 37, 301–3.

Theophylline + Ribavirin

Abstract/Summary

Ribavirin does not interact with theophylline.

Clinical evidence, mechanism, importance and management

A study in 13 normal subjects given aminophylline, and six children with influenza superimposed on bronchial asthma or an asthmatic syndrome treated with theophylline, showed that 200 mg ribavirin six-hourly had no effect on the serum levels of theophylline.[1]

Reference

1 Fraschini F, Scaglione F, Maierna G, Cogo R, Furcolo F, Gattei R, Borghu C and Palazzini E. Ribavirin influence on theophylline plasma levels in adults and children. Int J Clin Pharmacol Ther Toxicol (1988) 26, 30–2.

Theophylline + Rifampicin (Rifampin)

Abstract/Summary

Serum theophylline levels can be reduced by the concurrent use of rifampicin. An increase in the theophylline dosage may be necessary.

Clinical evidence

A study in seven normal subjects showed that after taking 600 mg rifampicin daily for a week, the area under the concentration-time curve following 450 mg of a sustained-release aminophylline preparation was reduced by 18%. A parallel study with eight normal subjects showed that the metabolic clearance of intravenous aminophylline was increased by 45%.[1]

Other studies in normal subjects given 600 mg rifampicin daily for 1–2 weeks showed that rises in theophylline clearance of 25–82% occurred.[2–7] A 61% fall in serum theophylline levels occurred in a 15-month-old boy when given rifampicin.[8]

Mechanism

Rifampicin is a potent liver enzyme inducing agent which increases the metabolism of the theophylline, thereby speeding up its clearance from the body resulting in reduced serum levels.[4]

Importance and management

An established interaction. Serum theophylline levels and its therapeutic effects may be expected to be reduced during concurrent treatment with rifampicin. It can occur within 36 h.[8] The wide range of increases in clearance which have been reported (25–82%) makes it difficult to predict the increase in theophylline dosage required, but in some instances it may possibly need to be doubled.[4]

References

1 Powell-Jackson PR, Jamieson AP, Gray BJ, Moxham J and Williams R. Effect of rifampicin administration on theophylline pharmacokinetics in humans. Am Rev Resp Dis (1985) 131, 939–40.
2 Boyce EG, Dukes GE, Rollins DE and Sudds TW. The effect of rifampin on theophylline kinetics. Clin Pharmacol Ther (1985) 37, 183.
3 Straughn AB, Henderson RP, Lieverman PL and Self TH. Effect of rifampin on theophylline disposition. Ther Drug Monit (1984) 6, 153–6.
4 Robson RA, Miners JO, Wing LMH and Birkett DJ. Theophylline-rifampicin interaction: non-selective induction of theophylline metabolic pathways. Br J clin Pharmac (1984) 18, 445–8.
5 Lofdahl CG, Mellstrad T and Svedmyr N. Increased metabolism of theophylline by rifampicin. Respiration (1984) 46 (Suppl 1), 104.
6 Hauser AR, Lee C, Teague RB and Mullins C. The effect of rifampin on theophylline disposition. Clin Pharmacol Ther (1983) 33, 254.
7 Boyce EG, Dukes GE, Rollins DE and Sudds TW. The effect of rifampin on theophylline kinetics. J Clin Pharmacol (1986) 26, 696–9.
8 Brocks DR, Lee KC, Weppler CP and Tam YK. Theophylline-rifampin in a pediatric patient. Clin Pharm (1986) 5, 602–4.

Theophylline + Sucralfate

Abstract/Summary

One study indicates that no interaction occurs. Another suggests that the absorption of sustained-release theophylline is reduced by sucralfate.

Clinical evidence, mechanism, importance and management

A study in normal subjects showed that while taking 1 g sucralfate four times daily, no clinically important changes occurred in the absorption of a single 5 mg/kg dose of an oral non-sustained release theophylline preparation (*Slo-Phyllin*, WH Storer).[1] In contrast, another group of workers found that when 1 g sucralfate was given 30 min before a 350 mg sustained-release theophylline preparation, the theophylline absorption was reduced by 40%.[2] The reasons are not understood. As many patients are given sustained-release preparations and neither of these studies clearly show what is likely to happen in clinical practice, be alert for any evidence of a reduced response to theophylline. Increase the dosage if necessary.

Reference

1 Cantral KA, Schaaf LJ, Jungnickel PW and Monsour HP. Effect of sucralfate on theophylline absorption in healthy volunteers. Clin Pharm (1988) 7, 58–61.
2 Fleischmann R, Bozler G and Boekstegers P. Bioverfugbarkeit von Theophylline unter Ulkustherapeutika. Verh Dtsch Ges Inn Med (1984) 90 (II), 1876–9.

Theophylline + Sulphinpyrazone

Abstract/Summary

Sulphinpyrazone can cause a small reduction in serum theophylline levels.

Clinical evidence, mechanism, importance and management

A study in six normal subjects given 125 mg theophylline every 8 h for four days showed that while taking 800 mg sulphinpyrazone daily the total clearance of theophylline was increased by 22% (range 8.5 to 42%).[1] This appears to be the sum of an increase in the metabolism of the theophylline by the liver, and a decrease in its renal clearance.

Information seems to be limited to this study. The fall in serum theophylline levels in most patients is unlikely to be very significant, but it may possibly affect a few. Concurrent use should be monitored.

Reference

1 Birkett DJ, Miners JO and Attwood J. Evidence for a dual action of sulphinpyrazone on drug metabolism in man: theophylline-sulphinpyrazone interaction. Br J clin Pharmac (1983) 15, 567–9.

Theophylline + Tetracyclines or Cephalosporins

Abstract/Summary

The effects of theophylline are not normally significantly altered or only minimally raised by the concurrent use of tetracycline, doxycycline, cephalexin or cefaclor but the occasional patient may possibly be adversely affected if serum theophylline levels are already high.

Clinical evidence, mechanism, importance and management

A trial[1] on nine healthy adults given single doses of aminophylline (5 mg/kg IV) showed that the concurrent use of tetracycline or cephalexin, 250 mg six-hourly for 48 h, had no significant effect on the kinetics of theophylline. Five non-smoking patients with chronic obstructive airway disease showed an average 14% rise in serum theophylline levels after five days' treatment with 1000 mg tetracycline daily, but

when a sixth patient was included (a smoker) the results were deemed not to be statistically significant.[4] Another study[2] on 10 asthmatic subjects given doxycycline (100 mg twice daily on day one and then 100 mg four times daily for three days) showed that on average their serum theophylline levels were not significantly altered, although four of them showed rises of more than 20%. The failure of doxycycline to interact significantly with theophylline is confirmed by another study in nine normal subjects.[3] A single case report suggested that cefaclor might have been responsible for the development of theophylline toxicity in a child[7] but a single dose and a steady-state study found that 750 mg cefaclor daily for eight and nine days respectively had no effect on the pharmacokinetics of theophylline,[5,6] and this was confirmed in another study.[7] The concurrent use of any of these antibiotics should be monitored.

References

1 Pfeifer HJ, Greenblatt DJ and Friedman P. Effects of three antibiotics on theophylline kinetics. Clin Pharmacol Ther (1979) 26, 36.
2 Seggev JS, Shefi M, Schey G and Farfel Z. Serum theophylline concentrations are not affected by coadministration of doxycycline. Ann Allergy (1986) 56, 156–7.
3 Jonkman JHG, van der Boom WJV, Schoenmaker R, Holtkamp A and Hempenius J. No influence of doxycycline on theophylline pharmacokinetics. Ther Drug Monit (1985) 7, 92–4.
4 Gotz VP and Ryerson GG. Evaluation of tetracycline on theophylline disposition in patients with chronic obstructive airways disease. Drug Intell Clin Pharm (1986) 20, 694–7.
5 Bachmann K, Schwartz J, Forney RB and Jauregui L. Impact of cefaclor on the pharmacokinetics of theophylline. Ther Drug Monit (1986) 8, 151–4.
6 Jonkman JHG, van der Boon WJV, Schoenmaker R, Holtkamp A and Hempenius J. Clinical pharmacokinetics of theophylline during cotreatment with cefaclor. Int J Clin Pharmacol Ther Toxicol (1986) 24, 88–92.
7 Jauregui L, Bachmann K, Forney R, Bischoff M and Schwartz J. The impact of cefaclor on the pharmacokinetics of theophylline. Recent Adv Chemother., Proc Int Congr Chemother 14th Antimicrob Section 1 (1985) 694–5.

Theophylline + Thiabendazole

Abstract/Summary

Theophylline serum levels can be markedly increased by the concurrent use of thiabendazole. Toxicity may develop if the theophylline dosage is not reduced appropriately. A 50% reduction has been suggested.

Clinical evidence

An elderly man on prednisone, frusemide, terbutaline, orciprenaline and theophylline was additionally given theophylline by infusion (40–50 mg/h). When he was additionally given 4 g thiabendazole daily for five days for a *strongloides* infestation he developed theophylline toxicity and his serum levels were found to have more than doubled (from 19.2 to 46 μg/ml), although he had previously been treated with 3 g thiabendazole daily for three days uneventfully (and unsuccessfully).[1]

Another report describes an increase in the serum theophylline levels, despite a reduction in the theophylline dosage, when a man was started on 1.8 g thiabendazole twice daily. Theophylline levels fell when the thiabendazole was stopped.[2] A study in six normal subjects clearly showed that 1.5 mg thiabendazole twice daily for three days markedly affected the pharmacokinetics of aminophylline; the half-life increased (from 6.72 to 18.60 h), the clearance fell (from 0.067 to 0.023 l/h/kg) and the elimination rate constant also decreased (from 0.11 to 0.039 h⁻¹). Two of the subjects experienced severe nausea, vomiting and dizziness.[3]

Mechanism

Uncertain. It is suggested that the thiabendazole inhibits the metabolism of the theophylline by the liver thereby prolonging its stay in the body and raising its serum levels. The nausea and vomiting may have been due to both the theophylline and the thiabendazole.

Importance and management

An established interaction of clinical importance. Monitor the effects of concurrent use and reduce the theophylline dosage accordingly. The authors of the second report suggest a 50% theophylline dosage reduction.

References

1 Sugar AM, Kearns PJ, Haulk AA and Rushing JL. Possible thiabendazole-induced theophylline toxicity? Amer Rev Resp Dis (1980) 122, 501.
2 Lew G, Murray WE, Lane JR and Haeger E. Theophylline-thiabendazole drug interaction. Clin Pharm (1989) 8, 225–7.
3 Schneider D, Gannon R, Sweeney K and Shore E. Theophylline and antiparasitic drug interactions. A case report and a study of the influence of thiabendazole and mebendazole on theophylline kinetics in adults. Chest (1990) 97, 84–7.

Theophylline + Thyroid and Antithyroid compounds

Abstract/Summary

The serum levels of theophylline can increase and toxicity may develop if hyperthyroidic patients are treated with antithyroid compounds without reducing the theophylline dosage. An increase in the theophylline requirements may occur if thyroid hormones are given to hypothyroidic patients.

Clinical evidence

The clearance of theophylline is much greater in hyperthyroidic patients (0.155 h⁻¹) than in euthyroidic (0.107 h⁻¹) or hypothyroidic patients (0.60 h⁻¹).[1] Drug-induced changes in the thyroid status will therefore alter the amount of theophylline which is needed to maintain therapeutic levels.

(a) Theophylline + antithyroid compounds

The serum theophylline levels of an asthmatic patient doubled (from 16.8 to 30.9 µg/ml) accompanied by toxicity, following treatment for hyperthyroidism with radioactive iodine (I¹³¹).[2] Five hyperthyroidic patients showed a reduction in their clearance of theophylline from 3.98 to 3.17 l/h, and a rise in the theophylline half-life from 4.6 to 5.9 h when treated with carbimazole.[3]

(b) Theophylline + thyroid hormones

A patient taking 1 g theophylline daily and who was hypothyroidic (serum thyroxine 1.4 µg/100 ml) developed severe theophylline intoxication (serum levels 34.7 µg/ml) accompanied by life-threatening cardiac arrhythmia. Two months later after treatment with thyroid hormones which increased his serum levels to 4.3 µg/100 ml, his serum theophylline levels had fallen to 13.5 µg/ml while continuing to take the same theophylline dosage (1 g daily).[4]

Mechanism

The thyroid status affects the rate at which theophylline is metabolized. In hyperthyroidism it is increased, whereas in hypothyroidism it is decreased.

Importance and management

It is well established that changes in thyroid status affect how the body handles theophylline. Monitor the effects and anticipate the need to reduce the theophylline dosage if treatment for hyperthyroidism is started (e.g. with radioactive iodine, carbimazole, etc.). Similarly anticipate the need to increase the theophylline dosage if treatment is started for hypothyroidism (e.g. with levothyroxine).

References

1 Pokrajac M, Simic D and Varagic VM. Pharmacokinetics of theophylline in hyperthyroid and hypothyroid patients with chronic obstructive pulmonary disease. Eur J Clin Pharmacol (1987) 33, 483–6.
2 Johnson CE and Cohen IA. Theophylline toxicity after iodine 131 treatment for hyperthyroidism. Clin Pharm (1988) 7, 620–2.
3 Vozeh S, Otten M, Staub J-J and Follath F. Influence of thyroid function on theophylline kinetics. Clin Pharmacol Ther (1984) 36, 634–40.
4 Aderka D, Shavit G, Garfinkel D, Santo M, Gitter S and Pinkhas J. Life-threatening theophylline intoxication in a hypothyroidic patient. Respiration (1983) 44, 77–80.

Theophylline + Ticlopidine

Abstract/Summary

Ticlopidine reduces the clearance of theophylline from the body.

Clinical evidence, mechanism, importance and management

A study in 10 normal subjects showed that after taking

250 mg ticlopidine twice daily for 10 days, the clearance of a single 5 mg/kg oral dose of theophylline was reduced by 37% (from 0.682 to 0.431 ml/kg/min) and the half-life was reduced by 30% (from 731 to 514 min).[1] The reason is not understood but it seems possible that the ticlopidine inhibits the metabolism of the theophylline by the liver. Information is very limited, but it would now seem prudent to monitor the effects of concurrent use. It may be necessary to reduce the dosage of the theophylline.

Reference

1 Colli A, Buccino G, Cocciolo M, Parravicini R, Elli GM and Scaltrini G. Ticlopidine-theophylline interaction. Clin Pharmacol Ther (1987) 41, 358–62.

Theophylline + Tobacco smoking

Abstract/Summary

Smokers and non-smokers heavily exposed to tobacco smoke may need more theophylline than non-smokers to achieve the same therapeutic benefits because the theophylline is cleared from the body more quickly. An increased dosage may also be needed by those who chew tobacco or take snuff but not if they chew nicotine gum.

Clinical evidence

A comparative study in man showed that the mean half-life of theophylline in a group of smokers was 4.3 h compared with 7 h in a group of non-smokers.[1] Almost identical results were found in another study,[2] and a number of other studies confirm these findings.[3–5] The same increased clearance has been seen in a patient who chewed tobacco (1.11 compared with the more usual 0.59 ml/kg/min).[8] The theophylline half-life in passive smokers (non-smokers regularly exposed to tobacco smoke in the air they breathe) was also found in one study to be shorter than in non-smokers (6.93 compared with 8.69 h).[10]

Mechanism

Tobacco smoke contains polycyclic hydrocarbons which act as liver enzyme inducing agents, and this results in a more rapid clearance of theophylline from the body.[6]

Importance and management

An established interaction of moderate clinical importance. It is noteworthy (and explicable) that smokers experience fewer theophylline side-effects than non-smokers,[7] nevertheless patients needing theophylline should be strongly encouraged not to smoke. It has been estimated that those who smoke heavily (20–40 cigarettes daily) may need daily doses of theophylline which are about twice those of non-smokers, and the need to use an increased dosage seems likely in those who regularly chew tobacco or take it as snuff. Nicotine chewing gum is reported not to affect theophylline clearance.[8] One report says that within a week of stopping smoking the clearance of theophylline falls by almost 40% so that a dosage reduction may be needed,[9] whereas another says that recovery takes many months.[1]

Investigators of the possible interactions of theophylline with other drugs should take into account the theophylline-tobacco smoke interaction in both smokers and passive smokers when selecting their subjects.[10]

References

1 Hunt SN, Jusko WJ and Yurchak AM. Effect of smoking on theophylline disposition. Clin Pharmacol Ther (1976) 19, 546.
2 Jenne J, Nagasawa H, McHugh R, Macdonald F and Wyse E. Decreased theophylline half-life in cigarette smokers. Life Sci (1975) 17, 195.
3 Powell JR, Thiercelin J-F, Vozeh S, Sansom L and Riegelman S. The influence of cigarette smoking and sex on theophylline disposition. Am Rev Resp Dis (1977) 116, 17–23.
4 Cusack B, Kelly JG, Lavan J, Noel J and O'Malley K. Theophylline kinetics in relation to age; the importance of smoking. Br J clin Pharmac (1980) 10, 109–14.
5 Jusko WJ, Schentag JJ, Clark JH, Garndern M, and Yurchak AM. Enhanced biotransformation of theophylline in marihuana and tobacco smokers. Clin Pharmacol Ther (1978) 24, 406–10.
6 Grygiel J and Birkett DJ. Cigarette smoking and theophylline clearance and metabolism. Clin Pharmacol Ther (1981) 30, 491–6.
7 Pfeifer HJ and Greenblatt DJ. Clinical toxicity of theophylline in relation to cigarette smoking. Chest (1978) 73, 455–9.
8 Rockwood R and Henann N. Smokeless tobacco and theophylline clearance. Drug Intell Clin Pharm (1986) 20, 624–5.
9 Lee BL, Benowitz NL and Jacob P. Cigarette abstinence, nicotine gum and theophylline metabolism. Clin Pharmacol Ther (1987) 41, 245.
10 Matsunga SK, Plezia PM, Karol MD, Katz MD, Camilli AE and Benowitz NL. Effects of passive smoking on theophylline clearance. Clin Pharmacol Ther (1989) 46, 399–407.

Theophylline + Vidarabine

Abstract/Summary

A single case report describes a woman who showed a rise in serum theophylline levels when concurrently treated with vidarabine.

Clinical evidence, mechanism, importance and management

A woman under treatment with several drugs (ampicillin, gentamicin, clindamycin, digoxin and aminophylline for congestive heart failure, chronic pulmonary disease and suspected abdominal sepsis) developed elevated serum theophylline levels four days after starting to take vidarabine (400 mg daily) for herpes.[1] The suggestion is that the vidarabine inhibited the metabolism of the theophylline. Whether this is, in fact, an interaction is uncertain, but it would now seem prudent to be on the alert for a rise in serum theophylline levels if vidarabine is given concurrently.

Reference

1 Gannon R, Sullman S, Levy RM and Grober J. Possible interaction between vidarabine and theophylline. Ann Intern Med (1984) 101, 148.

Theophylline + Viloxazine

Abstract/Summary

Viloxazine increases serum theophylline levels and intoxication may occur unless the theophylline dosage is reduced.

Clinical evidence

A study in eight normal subjects given a single 200 mg dose of theophylline showed that the concurrent use of 300 mg viloxazine daily increased the 24-h AUC (area under the concentration-time curve) of the theophylline by 47%, increased the maximal serum concentration and reduced its clearance.[3]

An elderly woman on theophylline developed acute intoxication (a grand mal seizure) two days after starting to take 200 mg viloxazine daily. Her serum theophylline levels had increased threefold (from about 10 to 28 mg/l) and fell again when the viloxazine was withdrawn.[1] Nausea and vomiting, associated with raised serum theophylline levels, occurred in another patient when treated with viloxazine.[2] The theophylline fell to subtherapeutic levels when the viloxazine was eventually stopped.

Mechanism

The suggestion is that the viloxazine competitively antagonizes the metabolism of the theophylline by the liver, thereby reducing its loss from the body and resulting in an increase in its serum levels.

Importance and management

Information seems to be limited to these reports but it would seem to be a clinically important interaction. Theophylline serum levels should be monitored if viloxazine is added, anticipating the need to reduce the dosage.

References

1 Laaban JP, Dupeyron JP, Lafay M, Sofeir M, Rochemaure J and Fabiani P. Theophylline intoxication following viloxazine induced decrease in clearance. Eur J Clin Pharmacol (1986) 30, 351–3.
2 Thompson AH, Addis GJ, McGovern EM and McDonald NJ. Theophylline toxicity following coadministration of viloxazine. Ther Drug Monitor (1988) 10, 359–60.
3 Perault MC, Griesemann E, Bouquet S, Lavoisy J, Vandel B. A study of the interaction of viloxazine with theophylline. Ther Drug Monit (1989) 11, 520–2.

23

TRICYCLIC ANTIDEPRESSANT AND RELATED DRUG INTERACTIONS

The development of the tricyclic antidepressants arose out of work carried out on phenothiazine compounds related to chlorpromazine. The earlier ones possessed two benzene rings joined by a third ring of carbon atoms, with sometimes a nitrogen, and of having antidepressant activity (hence their name), however some of the later ones have one, two or even four rings. Table 23.1 lists the common tricyclic antidepressants and a number of other compounds which are also used for depression.

The antidepressant activity of the tricyclic antidepressants

The arrival of a nerve impulse at the end of a nerve causes the release of a small amount of chemical transmitter which, after diffusing to the receptors of the next nerve or organ, stimulates a response. In the case of neurones which used noradrenaline (norepinephrine) as the transmitting substance, the receptors are 'cleared' for further stimulation by the return of the chemical transmitter into the nerve endings, although a small proportion is destroyed by the enzyme catechol-O-methyl transferase (COMT). The noradrenaline re-enters the nerve ending by means of an uptake or 'pump' mechanism.

The tricyclic antidepressants appear to act by inhibiting the activity of this uptake mechanism and in this way they raise the concentrations of the chemical transmitter in the receptor area. If depression represents some inadequacy in transmission between the nerves in the brain, increasing amounts of transmitter may go some way towards reversing this inadequacy by improving transmission. Neurones which used 5-HT (serotonin) instead of noradrenaline appear to respond to the tricyclics in a similar way.

Other properties of the tricyclic antidepressants

The tricyclics also possess other characterstics which are responsible for their side-effects. They have anticholinergic (atropine-like) activity and can cause dry mouth, blurred vision, constipation, urine retention and an increase in ocular tension. Postural hypotension occurs sometimes and there are also cardiotoxic effects. Among the central side effects are sedation, the precipitation of seizures in certain individuals, and extrapyramidal reactions.

Other interactions involving the tricyclic and other antidepressants but not discussed in this chapter are categorized elsewhere. Consult the Index for a full listing.

Table 23.1 Tricyclic and other antidepressants

Non-proprietary names	Proprietary names
Amitriptyline	Adepril, Amival, Amilent, Amiline, Amilit, Amitid, Amitril, Amitrip(tol), Annolytin, Deprestat, Deprex, Domical, Elavil, Endep, Equilibrin, Laroxyl, Lentizol, Levate, Miketorin, Novotryptin, Redomox, Saroten, Sarotex, Teperin, Trepiline, Triptizol, Tryptanol, Tryptizol
Amoxapine	Asendin, Demolox, Omnipress
Butriptyline	Centrolyse, Evadene, Evadyne
Clomipramine	Anafranil
Desipramine	Nebril, Norpramin, Nortimil, Pertofran(a), Pertofrin, Sertofren
Dibenzepin	Deprex, Ecatril, Noveril
Dothiepin	Adapin, Aponal, Co-Dox, Novoxapin, Quitaxon, Sin(e)quan, Sinquane, Spectra, Toruan, Triadapin
Femoxetine	Malexil
Fluoxetine	Prozac
Fluvoxamine	Faverin, Fevarin, Floxyfal
Imipramine	Antipress, Berkomine, Chimoreptin, Dimipressin, Dynaprin, Efuranol, Ethipramine, Imavate, Imidol, Imiprin, Iramil, Janimine, Medipramine, Melipramine, Norpramine, Novopramine, Oppanyl, Panpramine, Praminil, Presamine, Prodepress, Somipra, Tizipramine, Tofranil
Iprindole	Prondol
Lofepramine	Amplit, Deftan, Deprimil, Didalen-70, Gamanil, Gamonil, Tymelyt
Maprotiline	Ludiomil
Melitracen	Dixeran, Melixeran, Trausabun
Mianserin	Athimil, Athymil, Bolvidon, Lantanon, Lerivon, Norval, Tetramide, Tolvin, Tolvon
Nomifensine	(withdrawn 1986)
Nortriptyline	Allegron, Altilev, Ateben, Aventyl, Kareon, Martimil, Noritren, Nortab, Nortrilen, Pamelor, Paxtibi, Psychostyl, Sensaval, Sensival, Vividyl
Protriptyline	Concordin, Maximed, Triptil
Trazodone	Deprax, Desyrel, Manegan, Molipaxin, Pragmarel, Thomban, Tramensan, Trittico
Trimipramine	Stangyl, Surmontil, Tydamine
Viloxazine	Vicilan, Vivalan
Zimeldine	(withdrawn 1983)

Femoxetine + Cimetidine

Abstract/Summary

Femoxetine serum levels are increased by cimetidine.

Clinical evidence, mechanism, importance and management

A study in six normal subjects on 600 mg femoxetine daily showed that the concurrent use of 1 g cimetidine daily for seven days raised the steady-state trough serum levels of femoxetine by 140% (from 10 to 24 ng/ml). The AUC (area under the curve) was increased but not significantly.[1] The probable reason for this interaction is that the cimetidine inhibits the oxidative metabolism of the femoxetine by the liver, reducing its loss from the body and thereby raising the serum levels. The authors of the paper recommend that the initial femoxetine dosage should be reduced from 600 to 400 mg daily.

Reference

1 Schmidt J, Sorensen AS, Gjerris A, Rafaelsen OJ and Mengel H. Femoxetine and cimetidine: interaction in healthy volunteers. Eur J Clin Pharmacol(1986) 31, 299–302.

Fluoxetine + Miscellaneous drugs

Abstract/Summary

Fluoxetine does not interact with diazepam, chlorothiazide, tolbutamide or warfarin.

Clinical evidence, mechanism, importance and management

Fluoxetine given as a single dose or in multiple doses over eight days had no effect on the pharmacokinetics of 10 mg diazepam, 500 mg chlorothiazide, 1 g tolbutamide or 20 mg warfarin, nor were the pharmacokinetics of fluoxetine changed. The hypoglycaemic effects of tolbutamide and the anticoagulant effects of the tolbutamide and warfarin respectively also remained unchanged.[1]

Reference

1 Lemberger L, Bergstrom RF, Wolen RL, Farid NA, Enas GG and Aronoff GR. Fluoxetine: clinical pharmacology and physiologic disposition. J Clin Psychiatry (1985) 46, 3 (Sec 2), 14–19.

Fluoxetine + Monoamine oxidase inhibitors (MAOI)

Abstract/Summary

A serious and possibly fatal toxic reaction can occur if fluoxetine is stopped and an MAOI started without leaving sufficient time in between.

Clinical evidence

A report describes a patient who took 20 mg fluoxetine for a fortnight, replaced two days later by 10 mg tranylcypromine daily. Four days later within 2–3 h of taking a 20 mg dose of tranylcypromine the patient began to experience such uncontrollable shivering that her teeth could be heard chattering. She was alert and orientated but she had double vision, nausea, confusion and anxiety. These all resolved within a day of stopping the tranylcypromine, and did not recur when fluoxetine was tried again six weeks later.[1] Dista Products, the manufacturers of fluoxetine, have on record three unpublished reports of fatal toxic reactions attributed to the use of an MAOI after fluoxetine was stopped.[1]

Mechanism

Not understood. The symptoms were not typical of an MAOI-tyramine reaction (no headache, chest pain or a raised blood pressure) and more closely resembled the serotonin-syndrome which is typified by CNS irritability, increased muscle tone, shivering, altered consciousness and mycolonus. Toxicity of this kind has been seen in patients on fluoxetine within a few days of starting additional treatment with L-tryptophan which is a precursor of serotonin (see 'Fluoxetine + L-tryptophan'). A not dissimilar reaction has been seen with phenelzine and tryptophan (see 'MAOI + Tryptophan').

Importance and management

Not well established nor well documented, but the seriousness of the reaction indicates that concurrent use should be avoided and sequential use undertaken with great care. Dista, the manufacturers of fluoxetine, recommend that (a) five weeks should elapse between stopping the fluoxetine and starting the MAOI because the effects of fluoxetine are very persistent, and (b) two weeks between stopping an MAOI and starting fluoxetine.[2]

References

1 Sternbach H. Danger of MAOI therapy after fluoxetine withdrawal. Lancet (1988) ii, 850–1.
2 Doyle MJ (Dista Products). Personal communication (1988).

Fluoxetine + L-tryptophan

Abstract/Summary

Central and peripheral toxicity developed in five patients on fluoxetine when given L-tryptophan.

Clinical evidence, mechanism, importance and management

Five patients who had been on fluoxetine (50–100 mg daily) for at least three months developed a number of reactions including central toxicity (agitation, restlessness, aggressivity, worsening of obsessive-compulsive disorders) and peripheral toxicity (abdominal cramps, nausea, diarrhoea) within a few days of starting 1–4 g L-tryptophan daily. These symptoms disappeared when the tryptophan was stopped. Some of the patients had had tryptophan before without problems. The reason for this reaction is not understood but the authors point out that the symptoms resemble the 'serotonin syndrome' seen in animals when serotonin levels are increased, and warn against the concurrent use of tryptophan with fluoxetine or other serotonin re-uptake inhibitors.[1] Most products containing L-tryptophan for the treatment of depression have been withdrawn in the USA and UK because of a possible association with the development of an eosinophilia-myalgia syndrome.

Reference

1 Steiner W and Fontaine R. Toxic reaction following the combined administration of fluoxetine and L-tryptophan: five case reports. Biol Psychiatry (1986) 21, 1067–71.

Fluvoxamine + Miscellaneous drugs

Abstract/Summary

Serum warfarin levels are increased by fluvoxamine and bleeding can occur if the anticoagulant dosage is not reduced. Adverse reactions have been reported when fluvoxamine and lithium were used concurrently. On theoretical grounds an adverse reaction is possible with the MAOI or tryptophan. No clinically important interaction appears to occur if fluvoxamine is used with propranolol, atenolol, chloral hydrate or the benzodiazepines.

Clinical evidence, mechanism, importance and management

The concurrent use of fluvoxamine can increase serum warfarin levels by 65% and a few cases of bleeding have been described.[1,4] Concurrent use need not be avoided but the need to decrease the anticoagulant dosage should be anticipated. The Committee on the Safety of Medicines (CSM) in the UK has warned of possible adverse reactions if fluvoxamine is given with other antidepressants such as the MAOI, lithium and tryptophan. 19 reports have been received of adverse reactions when fluvoxamine was given with lithium (five reports of convulsions and one of hyperpyrexia).[3] The warning about the MAOI and tryptophan appears to be an extrapolation from the reactions (a serotonin-syndrome) which have been seen with fluoxetine, another serotonin re-uptake inhibitor (see 'Fluoxetine+MAOI', and 'Fluoxetine+Tryptophan'). Most products containing L-tryptophan for the treatment of depression have been withdrawn in the USA and UK because of a possible association with the development of an eosinophilia-myalgia syndrome.

100 mg fluvoxamine daily raised the serum levels of propranolol (160 mg) 5-fold in normal subjects, but the heart-slowing effects were only slightly increased (3 beats/min). The diastolic pressure following exercise was slightly reduced but the general hypotensive effects remained unaltered. No changes in plasma levels of atenolol were seen but the heart-slowing effects were slightly increased and the hypotensive effects slightly decreased.[1] Fluvoxamine has also been found not to interact adversely with either chloral hydrate or benzodiazepines.[2]

References

1 Duphar files, quoted by Benfield P and Ward A. Fluvoxamine, a review of its pharmacodynamic and pharmocokinetic properties and therapeutic efficacy in depressive illness. Drugs (1986) 32, 313–34.
2 Wagner W, Cimander K, Schnitker J and Koch HF. Influence of concomitant psychotropic medication on the efficacy and tolerance of fluvoxamine. Adv Pharmacotherapy (1986) 2, 34–56.
3 Committee on the Safety of Medicines. Current Problems, May 1989, 26, 3.
4 Ashford G (Duphar). Personal communication(s) 1989.

Mianserin or Nomifensine + Anticonvulsants

Abstract/Summary

There is evidence that the serum levels of both mianserin and nomifensine can be markedly reduced by the concurrent use of phenytoin, phenobarbitone or carbamazepine. Nomifensine has been withdrawn.

Clinical evidence, mechanism, importance and management

A comparative study in six epileptics and six normal subjects showed that phenytoin with either phenobarbitone or carbamazepine markedly reduced the serum levels of single doses of mianserin and nomifensine. The mean half-life of mianserin was reduced by 75% (from 16.9 to 4.8 h) and the area under the time-concentration curve (AUC) by 86%. The half-life of nomifensine was not significantly altered, despite the fact that the AUC was reduced by almost 50%.[1,2] The reasons are not known, but it seems possible that these anticonvulsants may have increased the metabolism of mianserin and nomifensine by the liver. The clinical importance of these interactions is still uncertain, but it would be prudent to be alert for a reduction in the antidepressant response in patients. More study is needed. Nomifensine was withdrawn world-wide in January 1986 by the manufacturers because it has been associated with acute immune haemolytic anaemia and intravascular haemolysis

References

1 Nawishy S, Hathaway N and Turner P. Interactions of anticonvulsant drugs with mianserin and nomifensine. Lancet (1981) ii, 871.
2 Richens A, Nawishy S and Trimble M. Antidepressant drugs, convulsions and epilepsy. Br J clin Pharmac (1983) 15, 295–8S.

Tetracyclic antidepressants + Beta-blockers

Abstract/Summary

Maprotiline toxicity attributed to the concurrent use of propranolol has been described in three patients.

Clinical evidence

A patient experienced maprotiline toxicity (dizziness, hypotension, dry mouth, blurred vision, etc.) after taking 120 mg propranolol daily for two weeks. His trough serum maprotiline levels had risen by 40%. The serum levels fell and the side-effects disappeared when the propranolol was withdrawn.[2] A man on 120 mg propranolol daily began to experience visual hallucinations and psychomotor agitation with a few days of starting to take 200 mg maprotiline daily.[3] Another man on haloperidol, benztropine, triamterene, hydrochlorothiazide and propranolol became disorientated, agitated and uncooperative with visual hallucinations and incoherent speech within a week of starting to take 150 mg maprotiline daily. These symptoms disappeared when all the drugs were withdrawn. Reintroduction of the antihypertensive drugs with haloperidol and desipramine proved effective and uneventful.[1]

Mechanism

Not understood. A suggested reason is that the propranolol reduces the blood flow to the liver so that the metabolism of the maprotiline is reduced, leading to its accumulation in the body.

Importance and management

Information seems to be limited to the cases cited. The general importance of this interaction is uncertain, but if concurrent use it thought appropriate the outcome should be very well monitored. The authors of one of the reports[3] say that simultaneous use is inadvisable. Another tetracyclic antidepressant, mianserin, appears not to interact with propranolol. See Index.

References

1 Malkek-Ahmadi P and Tran T. Propranolol and maprotiline toxic interaction. Neurobehav Toxicol Teratol (1985) 7, 203–9.
2 Tollefson G and Lesar T. Effect of propranolol on maprotiline clearance. Am J Psychiatry (1984) 141, 148–9.

3 Saiz-Ruiz J and Moral L. Delerium induced by association of propranolol and maprotiline. J Clin Psychopharmacol (1988) 8, 77–8.

Tetracyclic Antidepressants + Oral contraceptives or Tobacco smoking

Abstract/Summary

Neither tobacco smoking nor the oral contraceptives affect maprotiline.

Clinical evidence, mechanism, importance and management

A study in women showed that, over a 28-day period, the use of oral contraceptives did not significantly affect the steady-state serum levels of maprotiline (75 mg nightly), nor was its therapeutic effectiveness changed.[1] Smoking also has no effect on maprotiline serum levels nor on its effectiveness.[1,2]

References

1 Luscombe DK. Interaction studies: the influence of age, cigarette smoking and the oral contraceptive on blood concentrations of maprotiline. In 'Depressive Illness—Far Horizons?' McIntyre JNM (ed), Cambridge Med Publ, Northampton 1982, p 62–3.
2 Holman RM. Maprotiline and cigarette smoking: an interaction study: clinical findings. In 'Depressive Illness—Far Horizons?' McIntyre JNM (ed), Cambridge Med Publ, Northampton 1982, p 66–7.

Trazodone + Phenothiazines

Abstract/Summary

Undesirable hypotension occurred in two patients on chlorpromazine or trifluoperazine when given trazodone.

Clinical evidence, mechanism, importance and management

A depressed patient on chlorpromazine began to complain of dizziness and unstable gait within two weeks of starting to take 100 mg trazodone daily. When his blood pressure was checked it was found to be between 92/58 and 126/72 mm Hg. Within two days of stopping the trazodone his blood pressure had restabilized.[1] Another patient on trifluoperazine was given 100 mg trazodone daily and within two days she complained of dizziness and was found to have a blood pressure of 86/52 mm Hg. Within a day of withdrawing the trazodone her blood pressure was back to 100/65 mm Hg.[1] It would seem that the hypotensive side-effects of the two drugs can be additive. Patients given both groups of drugs should be monitored for signs of hypotension.

Reference

1 Asayesh K. Combination of trazodone and phenothiazines: a possible additive hypotensive effect. Can J Psychiatry (1986) 31, 857–8.

Tricyclic antidepressants + Baclofen

Abstract/Summary

An isolated report describes a patient with multiple sclerosis on baclofen who was unable to stand within a few days of starting to take nortriptyline, and later imipramine.

Clinical evidence, mechanism, importance and management

A man with multiple sclerosis who was taking 10 mg baclofen four times a day to relieve spasticity, complained of leg weakness and was unable to stand within six days of starting to take 50 mg nortriptyline at bedtime. 48 h after stopping the nortriptyline his muscle tone returned. Two weeks later he was given 75 mg imipramine daily and once again his muscle tone was lost.[1] The reason is not understood. Prescribers should be aware of this report if the concurrent use of baclofen and any tricyclic antidepressant is being considered.

Reference

1 Silverglat MJ. Baclofen and tricyclic antidepressants: possible interaction. J Am Med Ass (1981) 246, 1659.

Tricyclic antidepressants + Barbiturates

Abstract/Summary

The serum levels of amitriptyline, desipramine and nortriptyline are reduced by the concurrent use of barbiturates. A reduced therapeutic response would be expected.

Clinical evidence

A comparative study in five pairs of twins given nortriptyline showed that the twins concurrently treated with un-named barbiturates developed steady-state serum nortriptyline levels which were reduced by 14–60%.[2]

Similar observations have been made in patients and normal subjects taking nortriptyline with amylobarbitone[3,5] and protriptyline with sodium amylobarbitone.[4] A patient showed a 50% reduction in serum desipramine levels when given 100 mg phenobarbitone each night as a hypnotic.[1]

Mechanism

The barbiturates are potent liver enzyme inducing agents which increase the metabolism and clearance of the tricyclic antidepressants from the body, thereby reducing their serum levels.

Importance and management

An established interaction although the documentation is limited. Its clinical importance is uncertain but if concurrent use is thought appropriate, be on the alert for a reduced antidepressant response. As all the barbiturates are potent liver enzyme inducing agents, this interaction may possibly occur between any barbiturate and any tricyclic antidepressant. This needs confirmation. Toxic overdosage with the tricyclics can cause convulsions and other effects including respiratory depression which may be increased by the use of a barbiturate. It is thought that diazepam[6] may be a better choice of anticonvulsant in this situation, although sodium amylobarbitone[7,8] and paraldehyde[9] have been used successfully.

References

1 Hammer W, Idestrom CM and Sjoqvist F. In 'Antidepressant Drugs' p 301, Garattini S and Dukes MNG (eds) Proc 1st Int Symp, Milan (1966). Int Congr Series no 122, Excerpta Medica.
2 Alexanderson A, Evans DAP and Sjoqvist F. Steady state plasma levels of nortriptyline in twins: influence of genetic factors and drug therapy. Br Med J (1969) 4, 764.
3 Burrows GD and Davies B. Antidepressants and barbiturates. Br Med J (1971) 4, 113.
4 Moody JP, Whyte SF, MacDonald AJ and Naylor GJ. Pharmacokinetic aspects of protriptyline plasma levels. Eur J Clin Pharmacol(1977) 11, 51.
5 Silverman G and Braithwaite R. Interaction of benzodiazepines and tricyclic antidepressants. Br Med J (1972) 4, 111.
6 Crocker J and Morton B. Tricyclic (antidepressant) drug toxicity. Clin Toxicol (1969) 2, 397.
7 Arneson GAA. A near fatal case of imipramine overdosage. Am J Psychiat (1961) 177, 934.
8 Luby ED and Domino EF. Toxicity from large doses of imipramine and MAO inhibitor in suicidal intent. J Am Med Ass (1961) 117, 68.
9 Connelly JF and Venables AA. A case of poisoning with 'Tofranil'. Med J Aust (1961) 1, 108.

Tricyclic antidepressants + Benzodiazepines

Abstract/Summary

Concurrent use is not uncommon and normally appears to be uneventful. Roche markets a combined amitriptyline-chlordiazepoxide preparation (Limibitrol) but its advantages have been questioned. However three patients have been described who became drowsy, forgetful and appeared uncoordinated and drunk while taking amitriptyline and chlordiazepoxide, and four others have been described who showed toxic effects while taking Limibitrol.

Clinical evidence, mechanism, importance and management

Clinical trials on large numbers of patients have shown that the incidence of adverse reactions while taking amitriptyline and chlordiazepoxide was no greater than might have been expected with either of the drugs used singly,[3,4] but a few adverse reports have been documented. A depressed patient on 150 mg amitriptyline and 40 mg chlordiazepoxide daily became confused, forgetful and uncoordinated. He acted as though he was drunk.[1] Two other patients taking amitriptyline and chlordiazepoxide experienced drowsiness, memory impairment, slurring of the speech and an inability to concentrate. Both were unable to work and one described himself as feeling drunk.[2] Four patients on *Limibitrol* are reported to have experienced some manifestations of toxicity (delusions, confusion, agitation, disorientation, dry mouth, blurred vision).[8] Some of these effects seem to arise from increased CNS depression (possibly additive) and/or an increase in the anticholinergic side-effects of the tricyclic.

Studies on the effects of nitrazepam, diazepam, oxazepam and chlordiazepoxide on steady-state plasma levels of nortriptyline and amitriptyline,[5] and of diazepam and chlordiazepoxide on nortriptyline[6] failed to find any interaction. Another study demonstrated an increase in amitriptyline levels when diazepam was given.[7] An isolated report describes a patient whose serum desipramine levels (300 mg daily) were halved when he was given 3 mg clonazepam daily and rose again when it was withdrawn.[9]

There seems to be no reason for avoiding concurrent use although the advantages and disadvantages remain the subject of debate. Other tricyclic antidepressant/benzodiazepine combinations would not be expected to behave differently from those described here. There is the theoretical possibility that during during the first few days patients may experience increased drowsiness with the more sedative antidepressants such as amitriptyline.

References

1 Kane FJ and Taylor TW. A toxic reaction to combined Elavil-Librium therapy. Am J Psychiat (1963) 119, 1179.
2 Abdon FA. Elavil-Librium combination. Am J Psychiat (1964) 120, 1204.
3 Haider IA. A comparative trial of RO-4–6270 and amitriptyline in depressive illness. Br J Psychiat (1967) 113, 993.
4 General Practitioner Clinical Trials. Chlordiazepoxide with amitriptyline in neurotic depression. Practitioner (1969) 202, 437.
5 Silverman G and Braithwaite R. Benzodiazepines and tricyclic antidepressant plasma levels. Br Med J (1973) 2, 18.
6 Gram LF, Overo KF and Kirk L. Influence of neuroleptics and benzodiazepines on metabolism of tricyclic antidepressants in man. Am J Psychiat (1974) 131, 863.
7 Dugal R, Caille G, Albert J-M and Cooper SF. Apparent pharmacokinetic interaction of diazepam and amitriptyline in psychiatric patients: a pilot study. Curr Ther Res (1975) 18, 679.
8 Beresford TP, Feinsilver DL and Hall RCW. Adverse reactions to a benzodiazepine-tricyclic antidepressant compound. J Clin Psychopharmacol (1981) 1, 392.
9 Deicken RF. Clonazepam-induced reduction in serum desipramine concentrations. J Clin Psychopharmacol (1988) 8, 71–2.

Tricyclic antidepressants + Cannabis

Abstract/Summary

Marked tachycardia has been described in two patients, one taking imipramine and the other nortriptyline, when they smoked cannabis.

Clinical evidence, mechanism, importance and management

A 21-year-old student who had had no problems with either nortriptyline or cannabis separately, experienced marked tachycardia (160 bpm) when used together.[1] It was controlled with propranolol.[1] A man of 25 complained of restlessness, dizziness and tachycardia (120 bpm) after smoking cannabis while taking 50 mg imipramine daily.[2] Increased heart rates are well-documented side-effects of both the tricyclic antidepressants and cannabis, and what occurred was probably due to the additive beta-adrenergic and the anticholinergic effects of the tricyclic antidepressants, and the beta-adrenergic effect of the marijuana. Direct information is limited but it has been suggested that concurrent use should be avoided.[1]

References

1 Hillard JR and Vieweg WVR. Marked sinus tachycardia resulting from the synergistic effects of marijuana and nortriptyline. Am J Psychiatry (1983) 140, 626–7.
2 Kizer KW. Possible interaction of TCA and marijuana. Ann Emerg Med (1980) 19, 444.

Tricyclic antidepressants + Carbamazepine

Abstract/Summary

Serum imipramine levels can be halved by the concurrent use of carbamazepine. An isolated report describes carbamazepine toxicity in a patient shortly after starting to take desipramine.

Clinical evidence

(a) Serum imipramine levels reduced

A study in 30 children (aged 6–16) with attention-deficit disorder being treated with imipramine showed that those concurrently treated with carbamazepine for 1–6 months had total serum antidepressant levels which were approximately half those found in the children not taking carbamazepine, necessitating a doubling of the imipramine dosage.[1]

(b) Serum carbamazepine levels increased

A woman on long-term treatment with carbamazepine developed intoxication (nausea, vomiting, blurred vision, slurred speech, ataxia) within six days of starting to take

150 mg desipramine daily. Her serum carbamazepine levels were found to have doubled (from 7.7 to 15 µg/ml).[2]

Mechanism

It seems likely that the carbamazepine (a recognized enzyme-inducing agent) increases the metabolism and loss of the imipramine from the body, thereby reducing the serum levels. The reason for the increased serum carbamazepine levels is not understood.

Importance and management

Information seems to be limited to these two reports. Monitor the effects if carbamazepine is combined with imipramine or any other tricyclic antidepressant and be alert for a reduction in the effects of the tricyclic. An increased dosage may be needed. Also be alert for any evidence of carbamazepine toxicity if desipramine or any other tricyclic is added to established treatment with carbamazepine.

References

1 Brown CS, Wells BG, Self TH and Jabbour JT. Influence of carbamazepine on plasma imipramine concentration in children with attention-deficit hyperactivity disorder. Pharmacotherapy (1988) 8, 135.
2 Lesser I. Carbamazepine and desipramine: a toxic reaction. J Clin Psychiatry (1984) 45, 360.

Tricyclic antidepressants + Cholestyramine

Abstract/Summary

A single case report describes a marked reduction in the serum levels and antidepressant effectiveness of doxepin caused by the concurrent use of cholestyramine.

Clinical evidence

A man whose depression was controlled with doxepin relapsed within a week of starting to take 6 g cholestyramine twice daily. Within three weeks of increasing the dosage separation of the doxepin and cholestyramine from 4 to 6 h his combined serum antidepressant (i.e. doxepin plus n-desmethyldoxepin) levels had risen from 39 to 81 ng/ml and his depression had improved. Reducing the cholestyramine dosage to a single 6 g dose daily, separated from the doxepin by 15 h, resulted in a further rise in his serum antidepressant levels to 117 ng/ml accompanied by relief of his depression.[1]

Mechanism

The most likely explanation is that the doxepin became bound to the cholestyramine within the gut, thereby reducing its absorption.

Importance and management

Direct information seems to be limited to this single report. As the authors point out, it is difficult to generalize from this case because the patient had an abnormal gastrointestinal tract (hemigastrectomy with pyloroplasty and chronic diarrhoea), nevertheless be alert for reduced antidepressant levels and reduced effects in patients treated with any tricyclic antidepressant and cholestyramine. A 6-h dosage separation may only be partially effective.

Reference

1 Geeze DS, Wise MG and Stigelman WH. Doxepin-cholestyramine interaction. Psychosomatics (1988) 29, 233–5.

Tricyclic antidepressants + Cimetidine or Ranitidine

Abstract/Summary

The concurrent use of cimetidine can raise the serum levels of amitriptyline, desipramine, doxepin, imipramine and nortriptyline. Toxicity may develop if the dosage of the tricyclic antidepressant is not reduced appropriately. Other tricyclic antidepressants are expected to interact similarly. Ranitidine does not interact.

Clinical evidence

(a) Amitriptyline + cimetidine or ranitidine

A double-blind cross-over study in normal subjects showed that, after taking 1200 mg cimetidine daily for two days, peak serum levels and the AUC (area under the concentration-time curve) of amitriptyline following a single 25 mg dose were raised by 37% and 80% respectively.[1]

Another study by the same authors found that ranitidine does not interact with amitriptyline.[12]

(b) Desipramine + cimetidine

A study in eight depressed patients taking 100–250 mg desipramine daily showed that after taking 1200 mg cimetidine daily for four days their serum desipramine levels were raised by 51% and its hydroxylated metabolite (2-hydroxydesipramine) by 46%.[2]

Another study showed that this interaction only occurs in those individuals who are 'rapid' hydroxylators.[3]

(c) Doxepin + cimetidine or ranitidine

A study in 10 normal subjects showed that 12 h after starting to take 300 mg cimetidine daily, peak serum levels and the AUC of doxepin after a single 100 mg oral dose were raised by 28% and 31% respectively.[4]

In another study 1200 mg cimetidine daily was found to

double the steady-state serum levels of doxepin (50 mg daily) whereas 300 mg ranitidine daily had no effect.[13] A patient being treated with doxepin complained that the normally mild side-effects (urinary hesitancy, dry mouth and decreased visual acuity) became incapacitating when additionally treated with cimetidine. His serum doxepin levels were found to be elevated.[5]

(d) Imipramine + cimetidine or ranitidine

A study in 12 normal subjects showed that after taking 1200 mg cimetidine daily for three days, peak serum levels and the AUC of imipramine after a single 100 mg dose were raised by 65% and 172% respectively. After taking 300 mg ranitidine daily for three days the pharmacokinetics of imipramine were unaltered.[6]

These findings with cimetidine confirm those of a previous study.[9] There are case reports of patients taking imipramine who developed severe anticholinergic side-effects (dry mouth, urine retention, blurred vision) associated with very marked rises in serum imipramine levels when concurrently treated with cimetidine.[7,8]

(e) Nortriptyline + cimetidine

A study in six healthy subjects showed that after taking 1200 mg cimetidine daily for two days, peak serum nortriptyline levels were not significantly raised but the AUC was increased by 20%.[9]

A case report describes a patient whose serum nortriptyline levels were raised about one-third while taking cimetidine.[10] Another patient complained of abdominal pain and distention (but no other anticholinergic side-effects) when treated with nortriptyline and cimetidine.[11]

Mechanism

Cimetidine is a potent liver enzyme inhibitor which reduces the metabolic clearance of the tricyclic antidepressants from the body. This results in a rise in their serum levels. Ranitidine does not interact because it is not an enzyme inhibitor.

Importance and management

The interactions with cimetidine are well established, well documented and of clinical importance. The incidence is uncertain but a study with desipramine[3] showed that only 'rapid' hydroxylators demonstrate this interaction so that not all patients will be affected. Those taking amitriptyline, desipramine, doxepin, imipramine or nortriptyline who are given cimetidine should be monitored for evidence of increased toxicity (an excessive increase in mouth dryness, urine retention, blurred vision, constipation, tachycardia, postural hypotension). Other tricyclic antidepressants would be expected to be similarly affected. Ideally the antidepressant serum levels should be monitored. Reduce the dosage of the antidepressant by 33–50% where necessary or replace the cimetidine with ranitidine which, because it is not an enzyme inhibitor, does not interact with amitriptyline, doxepin or imipramine and would not be expected to interact with other tricyclic antidepressants. Other H_2-blockers which do not cause enzyme inhibition include famotidine and nizatidine.

References

1 Curry SH, CL De Vane and Wolfe MM. Cimetidine interaction with amitriptyline. Eur J Clin Pharmacol(1985) 29, 429–33.
2 Amsterdam JD, Brunswick DJ, Potter L and Kaplan MJ. Cimetidine-induced alterations in desipramine plasma concentrations. Psychopharmacology (1984) 83, 373–5.
3 Steiner E and Spina E. Differences in the inhibitory effect of cimetidine on desipramine metabolism betwen rapid and slow debrisoquin hydroxylators. Clin Pharmacol Ther (1987) 42, 278–82.
4 Abernethy DR and Todd EL. Doxepin-cimetidine interaction: increased bioavailability during cimetidine treatment. J Clin Psychopharmacol (1986) 6, 8–12.
5 Brown MA, Haight KR and McKay G. Cimetidine-doxepin interaction. J Clin Psychopharmacol (1985) 5, 245–7.
6 Wells BG, Pieper JA, Self TH, Stewart CF, Waldon SL, Bobo L and Warner C. The effect of ranitidine and cimetidine on imipramine disposition. Eur J Clin Pharmacol(1986) 31, 285–90.
7 Shapiro PA. Cimetidine-imipramine interaction: case report and comments. Am J Psychiatry (1984) 141, 152.
8 Miller DD and Macklin M. Cimetidine-imipramine interaction: a case report. Am J Psychiatry (1983) 140, 351.
9 Henauer SA and Hollister LE. Cimetidine interaction with imipramine and nortriptyline. Clin Pharmacol Ther (1984) 35, 183–7.
10 Miller DD and Macklin M. Cimetidine-imipramine interaction: case report and comments. Am J Psychiatry (1984) 141, 153.
11 Lerro FA. Abdominal distention syndrome in a patient receiving cimetidine-nortriptyline therapy. J Med Soc New Jersey (1983) 80, 631–2.
12 Curry SH, DeVane CL and Wolfe MM. Lack of interaction of ranitidine with amitriptyline. Eur J Clin Pharmacol(1987) 32, 317–20.
13 Sutherland DL, Remillard AJ, Haight KR, Brown MA and Old L. The influence of cimetidine versus ranitidine on doxepin pharmacokinetics. Eur J Clin Pharmacol(1987) 32, 159–64.

Tricyclic and related antidepressants + Co-trimoxazole

Abstract/Summary

Four patients on tricyclics and one on viloxazine relapsed when given cotrimoxazole.

Clinical evidence, mechanism, importance and management

A report describes four patients taking tricyclic antidepressants (imipramine, clomipramine, dibenzepine) and one taking viloxazine who relapsed into depression when they were concurrently treated with co-trimoxazole (trimethoprim + sulphamethoxazole) for 2–9 days.[1] The reasons are not known. This seems to be the first and only report of a possible interaction between these very commonly prescribed drugs so that its general importance is very uncertain, but it would now seem prudent to monitor the outcome of concurrent use.

Reference

1 Brion S, Orssaud E, Chevalier JF, Plas J and Waroquaux O. Interaction entre le cotrimoxazole et les antidepresseurs. L'Encephale (1987) 8, 123–6.

Tricyclic antidepressants + Dextropropoxyphene

Abstract/Summary

An elderly patient on doxepin experienced increased lethargy and daytime sedation when additionally given dextropropoxyphene.

Interaction, mechanism, importance and management

An elderly man taking 150 mg doxepin daily, was noted to have increased lethargy and daytime sedation when he started to take 65 mg dextropropoxyphene every 6 h. His plasma doxepin levels were found to be raised by almost 150% (from 20 to 48.5 ng/ml). Desmethyldoxepin levels were similarly increased (from 8.8 to 20.7 ng/ml). A study subsequently carried out on 10 young normal subjects, using antipyrine as a marker of drug inhibition, showed that the same dose of dextropropoxyphene reduced the metabolism of the antipyrine by 16%.[1]

The general clinical significance of this interaction is uncertain. The patient cited was elderly and his liver function possibly may not have been good. Concurrent use need not be avoided, but it would seem prudent to check that the dosage of the tricyclic antidepressant is not excessive, particularly in those known or suspected to have poor liver function.

Reference

1 Abernethy DR, Greenblatt DJ and Steel K. Propoxyphene inhibition of doxepin and antipyrine metabolism. Clin Pharmacol Ther (1982) 31, 199.

Tricyclic antidepressants + Disulfiram

Abstract/Summary

Disulfiram reduces the clearance of imipramine and desipramine from the body. The concurrent use of amitriptyline and disulfiram is reported to cause a therapeutically useful increase in the effects of disulfiram but organic brain syndrome has been seen in two patients.

Clinical evidence, mechanism, importance and management

Amitriptyline is reported to have been successfully used to increase the effects of both disulfiram and citrated calcium carbimide without any increase in side effects.[1,2] However there is evidence that an adverse interaction can occur. A study in two men showed that while taking 500 mg disulfiram daily, the AUC (area under the curve) of imipramine given intravenously increased by 32.5 and 26.7%, and in one subject given desipramine, by 32.3%.[1] Peak serum levels were also increased. The suggested reason is that the disulfiram inhibits the metabolism of the antidepressants by the

liver. There is also a report of a man taking disulfiram who, when given amitriptyline, complained of dizziness, visual and auditory hallucinations, and who became disorientated to person, place and time. A not dissimilar reaction was seen in another patient.[2] Concurrent use should be monitored for any evidence of toxicity.

References

1 MacCallum WAG. Drug interactions in alcoholism treatment. Lancet (1969) i, 313.
2 Pullar-Strecker H. Drug interactions in alcoholism treatment. Lancet (1969) i, 735.
3 Ciraulo DA, Barnhill J and Boxenbaum H. Pharmacokinetic interaction of disulfiram and antidepressants. Am J Psychiatry (1985) 142, 1373–4.
4 Maany I, Hayashida M and Pfeffer SL. Possible toxic interaction between disulfiram and amitriptyline. Arch Gen Psychiatry (1982) 39, 743–4.

Tricyclic antidepressants + Ethchlorvynol

Abstract/Summary

Transient delerium has been attributed to the concurrent use of amitriptyline and ethchlorvynol.

Clinical evidence, mechanism, importance and management

A report claims that transient delerium has been seen when amitriptyline and ethchlorvynol were used concurrently,[1] but no details are given and there appear to be no other reports confirming this alleged interaction.

Reference

1 Hussar DA. Tabular compilation of drug interactions. Am J Pharm (1969) 141, 109.

Tricyclic antidepressants + Fenfluramine

Abstract/Summary

A confusing situation: some say that concurrent use is safe and effective while others say that fenfluramine can cause depression and should not be used in patients with depression.

Clinical evidence, mechanism, importance and management

Depression has been seen in some patients given fenfluramine[2] and several cases of withdrawal depression have been observed in patients on amitriptyline and fenfluramine, following episodes of severe depression.[3] The manufacturers say that fenfluramine should not be used in patients with a history of depression or while being treated with antidepressants.[1] On the other hand it has also been claimed that depression is not a serious problem in most patients taking fenfluramine[6] and that it can be used safely and effectively with tricyclic antidepressants.[5-7] One report describes a rise in the serum levels of amitriptyline when 60 mg fenfluramine was given to patients on 150 mg amitripytline daily for depression.[4]

References

1 ABPI Data Sheet Compendium, 1985–6 p 1400. Datapharm publications, London.

2 Gaind R. Fenfluramine (Ponderax) in the treatment of obese psychiatric outpatients. Br J Psychiatry (1969) 115, 963.

3 Harding T. Fenfluramine dependence. Br Med J (1971) 3, 305.

4 Gunne LM, Antonijevic S and Jonsson J. Effect of fenfluramine on steady state plasma levels of amitriptyline. Postgrad Med J (1975) 51 (Suppl 1) 113.

5 Pinder RM, Brogden RN, Sawyer PR, Speight TM and Avery GS. Fenfluramine: a review of its pharmacological properties and therapeutic efficacy in obesity. Drugs (1975) 10, 241.

6 Poire R, Rombach F and Crance JP. Obesite et fenfluramine (768 S). Experiences de trois ans d'utilisation prolongee et controlee du medicament en milieu psychiatrique hospitalies. Ann Medicopsychologiques (1966) 1, 26.

7 Mason EC. Servier Laboratories Ltd. Personal Communication (1976).

Tricyclic and related antidepressants + Fluoxetine

Abstract/Summary

The serum levels of desipramine, imipramine, nortriptyline and trazodone can be markedly increased by the concurrent use to fluoxetine. Toxicity may occur.

Clinical evidence

(a) Desipramine, nortriptyline and imipramine

Four patients taking either 250 mg desipramine daily, 150 mg imipramine daily or 100 mg nortriptyline daily showed 2–4-fold increases in serum tricyclic antidepressant levels within 1–2 weeks of additionally taking 50–400 mg fluoxetine daily. Two of them developed typical tricyclic antidepressant anticholinergic side-effects (constipation, urinary hesitancy).[1]

Another patient on 300 mg desipramine daily and tryptophan developed marked lethargy, fatigue and worsening depression within five days of starting 20–40 mg fluoxetine daily. Her serum desipramine levels doubled after five days and tripled after 12 days concurrent use. She recovered when the fluoxetine was stopped.[2] The serum imipramine and desipramine levels of another patient on imipramine approximately doubled after taking 20 mg fluoxetine twice daily for 12 days.[3] Markedly raised serum desipramine levels during fluoxetine treatment have been described in another patient.[4] A marked increase in serum nortriptyline levels occurred in two other patients when given fluoxetine.[5,6]

(b) Trazodone

A patient on trazodone showed a 31% increase in the antidepressant/dose ratio when given 40 mg fluoxetine daily. She experienced sedation and an unstable gait.[1]

Mechanism

Unknown. A likely explanation is that the fluoxetine inhibits the metabolism of these antidepressants by the liver, resulting in a reduction in their loss from the body.

Importance and management

Information is limited to these reports but the interaction seems to be established. Monitor the effects of concurrent use and be alert for any evidence of antidepressant toxicity. Reduce the dosage if necessary. More study is needed.

References

1 Aranow RB, Hudson JI, Pope HG, Grady TA, Laage TA, Bell IR and Cole JD. Elevated antidepressant plasma levels after addition of fluoxetine. Am J Psychiatry (1989) 146, 911–13.

2 Bell IR and Cole JD. Fuoretine induces elevation of desipramine and exacerbation of geriatric non-psychotic symptoms. J Clin Psychopharmacol (1988) B, 447–8.

3 Faynor SM and Espina V. Fluoxetine inhibition of imipramine metabolism. Clin Chem (1989) 35, 1180.

4 Goodrick PJ. Influence of fluoxetine on plasma levels of desipramine. Am J Psychiatry (1989) 146, 552.

5 Kahn DG. Increased plasma nortriptyline concentration in a patient cotreated with fluoxetine. J Clin Psychiatry (1990) 51, 36.

6 Vaughan DA. Interaction of fluoxetine with tricyclic antidepressants. Am J Psychiatry (1989) 145, 1478.

Tricyclic antidepressants + Food

Abstract/Summary

Food does not affect the absorption of imipramine from the gut.

Clinical evidence, mechanism, importance and management

A study in 12 healthy subjects showed that the ingestion of food (breakfast) had no effect on the bioavailability of imipramine, the peak serum concentrations or the time to peak concentrations following a 50 mg oral dose.[1]

Reference

1 Abernethy DR, Divoll M, Greenblatt DJ and Shader RI. Imipramine pharmacokinetics and absolute bioavailability. Clin Res (1983) 31, 626A.

Tricyclic antidepressants + Furazolidone

Abstract/Summary

A report describes the development of toxic psychosis, hyperactivity, sweating and hot and cold flushes in a woman on amitriptyline when given furazolidone with diphenoxylate and atropine.

Clinical evidence, mechanism, importance and management

A depressed woman taking daily doses of 1.25 mg conjugated oestrogen substances and 75 mg amitriptyline, was additionally given 300 mg furazolidone and diphenoxylate with atropine sulphate. Three days later she began to experience blurred vision, profuse perspiration followed by alternate chills and hot flushes, restlessness, motor activity, persecutory delusions, auditory hallucinations and visual illusions. The symptoms cleared within a day of stopping the furazolidone.[1] The reasons are not understood but the authors point out that furazolidone has MAO-inhibitory properties and that the symptoms were similar to those seen when the tricyclic antidepressants and MAOI interact. However the MAO-inhibitory activity of furazolidone normally takes about five days to develop. Whether the concurrent use of atropine and amitriptyline (both of which have anticholinergic activity) had some part to play in the reaction is uncertain. No firm conclusions can be drawn from this slim evidence, but prescribers should be aware of this case when considering the concurrent use of tricyclic antidepressants and furazolidone.

Reference

1   Aderhold RM and Munitz CE. Acute psychosis with amitriptyline and furazolidone. J Am Med Ass (1970) 213, 2080.

Tricyclic antidepressants + Haloperidol

Abstract/Summary

Serum tricyclic antidepressant levels can be considerably increased in a few patients by the concurrent use of haloperidol. This was apparently the cause of a grand mal seizure in one case but toxic reactions appear to be uncommon.

Clinical evidence

A comparative study in 30 patients on similar doses of desipramine (2.5–2.55 mg/kg) showed that two of them concurrently treated with haloperidol had steady-state serum desipramine levels which were more than double those of 15 others not taking haloperidol (255 compared with 110 ng/ml).[3]

A case report describes a patient who had a grand mal seizure when concurrently treated with desipramine and haloperidol. Her serum desipramine levels were unusually high (610 ng/ml).[4]

Mechanism

Haloperidol reduces the metabolism of the tricyclic antidepressants, thereby reducing their loss from the body and resulting in a rise in their serum levels. For example, the urinary excretion of a test dose of C^{14}-imipramine given to two schizophrenic patients was reduced 35–40% while taking 12–20 mg haloperidol daily.[1] In a similar study on another schizophrenic patient given C^{14}-nortriptyline it was found that the urinary excretion and plasma metabolite levels of nortriptyline fell while taking 16 mg haloperidol daily, while plasma levels of unchanged nortriptyline rose.[2]

Importance and management

An established interaction though its documentation is small. Concurrent use is common and adverse reactions are uncommon but be aware that the serum tricyclic levels will be elevated. This was apparently the cause of a grand mal seizure in the case cited.[4]

References

1   Gram LF and Overo KF. Drug interaction: inhibitory effect of neuroleptics on metabolism of tricyclic antidepressants in man. Br Med J (1972) 1, 463.
2   Gram LF, Overo KF and Kirk L. Influence of neuroleptics and benzodiazepines on metabolism of tricyclic antidepressants in man. Am J Psychiatry (1974) 131, 8.
3   Nelson JC and Jatlow I. Neuroleptic effect on desipramine on steady-state plasma concentrations. Am J Psychiatry (1980) 137, 1232–4.
4   Mahr GC, Berchon R and Balon R. A grand mal seizure associated with desipramine and haloperidol. Can J Psychiatry (1987) 32, 463–4.

Tricyclic antidepressants + Methadone

Abstract/Summary

Methadone can double serum desipramine levels.

Clinical evidence

A study on five men, stabilized on 2.5 mg/kg desipramine daily, showed that after taking 0.5 mg/kg methadone daily for two weeks their mean serum desipramine levels had risen by 108%. Previous observations on patients given both drugs had shown that desipramine levels were higher than expected and desipramine side-effects developed at relatively low doses.[1]

Mechanism

Not understood.

Importance and management

Information seems to be limited to this study but the interaction would seem to be established. Monitor the effects of concurrent use and anticipate the need to reduce the desipramine dosage. There seems to be nothing reported about the effects of methadone on other tricyclic antidepressants.

References

1 Maany I, Dhopesh V, Arndt IO, Burke W, Woody G and O'Brien CP. Increase in desipramine serum levels associated with methadone treatment. Am J Psychiatry (1989) 146, 1611–13.

References

1 Dayton PG, Perel JM, Israili ZH, Faraj BA, Rodewig K, Black N and Goldberg LI. Studies with methylphenidate: drug interactions and metabolism. In 'Clinical Pharmacology of Psychoactive Drugs', Sellers EM (ed). Alcoholism and Drug Addiction Reseach Foundation. Toronto (1975) p 183.
2 Cooper TB and Simpson GM. Concomitant imipramine and methylphenidate administration: a case report. Am J Psychiat (1973) 130, 721.
3 Wharton RN, Perel JM, Dayton PG and Malitz S. A potential use for the interaction of methylphenidate with tricyclic antidepressants. Am J Psychiat (1971) 127, 1619.
4 Grob CS and Coyle JT. Suspected adverse methylphenidate-imipramine interactions in children. J Dev Behav Pediatrics (1986) 7, 265–7.

Tricyclic antidepressants + Methylphenidate

Abstract/Summary

Methylphenidate can cause a marked increase in the blood levels of imipramine resulting in clinical improvement. Whether levels can rise to toxic concentrations appears not to be documented but two adolescents have been described who experienced severe mood deterioration while taking both drugs.

Clinical evidence

A study in '... several patients...' demonstrated a dramatic increase in the blood levels of desipramine and imipramine during concurrent treatment with imipramine and methylphenidate. In one patient taking 150 mg imipramine daily it was observed that 20 mg methylphenidate a day increased the blood levels of the imipramine from 100 to 700 μg/l and of desipramine from 200 to 850 μg/l over a period of 16 days.[1]

Similar effects have been described in other reports.[2,3] A 9-year-old and a 15-year-old exhibited severe behavioural problems until the imipramine and methylphenidate they were taking were stopped.[4]

Mechanism

In-vitro experiments with human liver slices indicate that methylphenidate inhibits the metabolism of imipramine, resulting in its accumulation, and this is reflected in raised blood levels.[3]

Importance and management

Information is limited. Some therapeutic improvement is seen because of the very marked rise in the blood levels of the antidepressant, but whether this also can lead to tricyclic antidepressant toxicity is uncertain. It does not seem to have been reported, but the possibility should be considered. Information about other tricyclic antidepressants is lacking. It has been suggested that concurrent use in children and adolescents may be undesirable.[3]

Tricyclic Antidepressants + Oestrogens (estrogens)/Oral contraceptives

Abstract/Summary

There is evidence that oestrogens can sometimes paradoxically reduce the effects of imipramine yet at the same time cause imipramine toxicity. The general clinical importance of this interaction has yet to be evaluated.

Clinical evidence

A study in 10 women taking 150 mg imipramine daily for primary depression found that those given 50 μg ethinyloestradiol daily for a week showed less improvement than other women given only 25 μg or a placebo. Four out of the 10 developed signs of imipramine toxicity which was dealt with by halving the imipramine dose.[1] Long-standing imipramine toxicity was also relieved in a woman taking 100 mg daily when her dosage of conjugated oestrogen was reduced to a quarter.[2] In contrast, several studies which showed that serum clomipramine levels were raised or remained unaffected by the concurrent use of oestrogen-containing contraceptives, failed to confirm that tricyclic antidepressant toxicity occurs more often in those on the pill than those who are not.[5-8] Akathisia in three patients has been attributed to an interaction betwen conjugated oestrogens and amitriptyline or chlorimipramine.[9]

Mechanism

Among the possible reasons for these effects are that the oestrogens increase the bioavailability of imipramine,[3] or inhibit its metabolism.[4]

Importance and management

This interaction is inadequately established. There is no obvious reason for avoiding concurrent use, but it would seem reasonable to be alert for any evidence of toxicity and/or lack of response to tricyclic antidepressant treatment. More study is needed.

References

1 Prange AJ, Wilson JC and Alltop A. Estrogen may well affect response to antidepressant. J Amer Med Ass (1972) 219, 143.
2 Khurana RC. Estrogen-imipramine interaction. J Amer Med Ass (1972) 222, 702.
3 Abernethy DR, Greenblatt DJ and Shader RI. Imipramine disposition in users of oral contraceptives. Clin Pharmacol Ther (1984) 35, 792.
4 Somani SM and Khurana RC. Mechanism of estrogen-imipramine interaction. J Amer Med Ass (1973) 223, 560.
5 Beaumont G. Drug interactions with clomipramine (Anafranil). J Int Med Res (1973) 1, 480.
6 Gringras M, Beaumont G and Grieve A. Clomipramine and oral contraceptives: an interaction study—clinical findings. J Int Med Res (1980) 8, (Suppl 3), 76.
7 Luscombe DK and Jones RB. Effects of concomitantly administered drugs on plasma levels of clomipramine and desmethyl-clomipramine in depressive patients receiving clomipramine therapy. Postgrad Med J (1977) 53 (Suppl 4), 77.
8 John VA, Luscombe DK and Kemp H. Effects of age, cigarette smoking and oral contraceptives on the pharmacokinetics of clomipramine and its desmethyl metabolite during chronic dosing. J Int Med Res (1980) 8,(Suppl 3), 88.
9 Krishnan KRR, France RD and Ellmwood EH. Tricyclic-induced akathisia in patients taking conjugated estrogens. Am J Psychiatry (1984) 141, 696–7.

Tricyclic antidepressants + Quinidine

Abstract/Summary

There is some evidence that quinidine can markedly reduce the loss of nortriptyline from the body.

Clinical evidence, mechanism, importance and management

A study[1] in five normal subjects showed that 50 mg quinidine given 1 h before a single 50 mg dose of nortriptyline increased the AUC (area under the concentration-time curve) of the nortriptyline fourfold (from 0.6 to 2.8 mg l^{-1} h) and the half-life threefold (from 14.2 to 44.7 h). The clearance fell from 5.4 to 1.9 ml min^{-1}. A possible explanation is that the quinidine reduces the metabolism of the nortriptyline. The clinical importance of this interaction awaits assessment, but be alert for evidence of an increase in the effects, and possibly the toxicity, of nortriptyline. More study is needed.

Reference

1 Ayesh R, Dawling S, Widdop B, Idle JR and Smith RL. Influence of quinidine on the pharmacokinetics of nortriptyline and desipramine. Br J clin Pharmac (1988) 25, 140–1P.

Tricyclic antidepressants + Sucralfate

Abstract/Summary

Sucralfate causes a marked reduction in the absorption of amitriptyline.

Clinical evidence, mechanism, importance and management

A single-blind cross-over study in six normal subjects showed that when a single 75 mg dose of amitriptyline was taken with a single 1 g dose of sucralfate, the AUC (area under the concentration-time curve) of the amitriptyline was reduced by 50% (from 680 to 320 ng h/ml).[1] Concurrent use should be monitored to confirm that the therapeutic effects of the antidepressant are not lost. An increase in the dosage may be needed. Information about other tricyclic antidepressants seems to be lacking.

Reference

1 Ryan R, Carlson J and Farris F. Effect of sucralfate on the absorption and disposition of amitriptyline in humans. Fed Proc (1986) 45, 205.

Tricyclic antidepressants + Thioxanthenes

Abstract/Summary, Clinical evidence, mechanism, importance and management

A study using C^{14}-imipramine showed that, unlike the situation between the tricyclic antidepressants and phenothiazines, no interaction occurred with flupenthixol.[1]

Reference

1 Gram LF and Overo KF. Drug interaction: inhibitory effect of neuroleptics on metabolism of tricyclic antidepressants in man. Br Med J (1972) 1, 463.

Tricyclic antidepressants + Thyroid preparations

Abstract/Summary

The antidepressant response to imipramine, amitriptyline and possibly other tricyclics can be accelerated by the use of thyroid preparations. An isolated case of paroxysmal atrial tachycardia, another of thyrotoxicosis and yet another of hypothyroidism due to concurrent therapy have been described.

Clinical evidence, mechanism, importance and management

Normally an advantageous interaction. The addition of 25 μg tri-iodothyronine daily was found to increase the speed and efficacy of imipramine in relieving depression.[1] Similar results have been described in other studies with imipramine, desipramine[2] and amitriptyline[3] but the reasons are not understood. However adverse reactions have also been seen. A patient being treated for both hypothyroidism and depression with 60 mg thyroid and 150 mg imipramine daily complained of dizziness and nausea. She was found to have developed paroxysmal atrial tachycardia.[4] A 10-year-old girl with congenital hypothyroidism, well controlled on 150 mg desiccated thyroid daily, developed severe thyrotoxicosis after taking 25 mg imipramine daily for five months for enuresis. The problem disappeared when the imipramine was withdrawn.[5] In another patient the effect of thyroxine was lost and hypothyroidism developed when given dothiepin.[6] These apparent interactions remain unexplained.

References

1 Wilson IC, Prange AJ, McLane TK, Rabon AM and Lipton MA. Thyroid-hormone enhancement of imipramine in non-retarded depressions. N Engl J Med (1970) 282, 1063.

2 Extein I. Case reports of L-triiodothyronine potentiation. Am J Psychiatry (1982) 139, 966–7.

3 Wheatley D. Potentiation of amitriptyline by thyroid hormone. Arch Gen Psychiatr (1972) 26, 229.

4 Prange AJ. Paroxysmal auricular tachycardia apparently resulting from combined thyroid-imipramine treatment. Am J Psychiatry (1963) 119, 994.

5 Colantonio LA and Orson JM. Triiodothyronine thyrotoxicosis. Induction by desiccated thyroid and imipramine. Am J Dis Child (1974) 128, 396.

6 Beeley L, Beadle F and Lawrence R. Bull West Midl Centre for Adverse Drug Reaction Reporting (1984) 19, 11.

Tricyclic antidepressants + Tobacco smoking

Abstract/Summary

Smoking reduces the serum levels of amitriptyline, clomipramine, desipramine, imipramine and nortriptyline, but the concentration of the free and unbound antidepressant rises which appears to offset the effects of this interaction.

Clinical evidence, mechanism, importance and management

Two studies failed to find any difference between the steady-state nortriptyline serum levels of smokers and non-smokers,[1,2] but others have found that smoking lowers the serum levels of amitriptyline, clomipramine,[5] desipramine, imipramine[4] and nortriptyline.[3] For example a 25% reduction in serum nortriptyline levels was found in one study,[3] and a 45% reduction in imipramine/desipramine levels.[4] The probable reason is that some of the components of tobacco smoke are enzyme inducing agents which increase the metabolism of these depressants by the liver. However it might wrongly be concluded from these figures that smokers need larger doses to control their depression. Preliminary data shows that the serum concentrations of free (and pharmacologically active) nortriptyline are greater in smokers than non-smokers (10.2 compared with 7.4%) which probably offsets the fall in total serum levels.[3] Thus the lower serum levels in smokers may be as therapeutically effective as the higher levels in non-smokers and there is probably no need to raise the dosage to accommodate this interaction.

References

1 Norman TR, Burrows GD, Maguire KP, Rubinstein G, Scoggins BA and Davies B. Cigarette smoking and plasma nortriptyline levels. Clin Pharmacol Ther (1977) 21, 453–6.

2 Alexander B, Price-Evans and Sjoqvist F. Steady-state plasma levels of nortriptyline in twins: influence of genetic factors and drug therapy. Br Med J (1969) 4, 764–8.

3 Perry PJ, Browne JL, Prince RA, Alexander B and Tsuang MT. Effects of smoking on nortriptyline plasma concentrations in depressed patients. Ther Drug Monit (1986) 8, 279–84.

4 Perel JM, Hurwie MJ and Kanzler MB. Pharmacodynamics of imipramine in depressed patients. Psychopharmacol Bull (1975) 11, 16–18.

5 John VA, Luscombe DK and Kemp H. Effects of age, cigarette smoking and the oral contraceptive on the pharmacokinetics of clomipramine and its desmethyl metabolite during chronic dosing. J Int Med Res (1980) eight (Suppl 3) 88–95.

Tricyclic antidepressants + Urinary alkalinizers or Acidifiers

Abstract/Summary

Blood levels of desipramine, nortriptyline and other tricyclic antidepressants are not significantly affected by agents which alter urinary pH.

Clinical evidence, mechanism, importance and management

Because the tricyclics are bases it might be expected that changes in the urinary pH would have an effect on their excretion, but in fact the excretion of unchanged drug is small (less than 5% with nortriptyline and desipramine) compared with the amounts metabolized by the liver.[1] No significant changes in blood levels occur with agents such as acetazolamide or ammonium chloride which can have a marked effects on the pH of the urine.[1] Even in cases of poisoning '...vigorous procedures such as forced diuresis, peritoneal dialysis, or haemodialysis can therefore not be expected to markedly accelerate the elimination of these drugs.'[1] Only in the case of hepatic dysfunction is simple urinary clearance likely to take on a more important role.

Reference

1 Sjoqvist F, Berglund F, Borga O, Hammer W, Andersson S and Thorstrad C. The pH-dependent excretion of monomethylated tricyclic antidepressants. Clin Pharmacol Ther (1969) 10, 826.

24
MISCELLANEOUS
DRUG INTERACTIONS

Acipimox + Cholestyramine

Abstract/Summary

Acipimox does not interact significantly with cholestyramine

Clinical evidence, mechanism, importance and management

A randomized cross-over study in seven normal subjects given 150 mg of acipimox with 4 g cholestyramine, followed by two additional 4 g doses of cholestyramine 8 and 16 h later showed that the pharmacokinetics of acipimox were slightly but not significantly altered by the cholestyramine.[1] There would seem to be no good reason for avoiding concurrent use.

Reference

1 De Paolis C, Farina R, Pianezzola E, Valzelli G, Celotti F and Pontiroli AE. Lack of pharmacokinetic interaction between cholestyramine and acipimox, a new lipid lowering agent. Br J clin Pharmac (1986) 22, 496–7.

Allopurinol + Antacids

Abstract/Summary

Three patients showed a marked reduction in the effects of allopurinol while concurrently taking an aluminium hydroxide antacid. Separating the dosages by 3 h reduced the effects of this interaction.

Clinical evidence, mechanism, importance and management

Three patients on chronic haemodialysis, taking 5.7 g aluminium hydroxide daily and 300 mg allopurinol daily for high uric acid and phosphate levels, failed to show any fall in their hyperuricaemia until the antacid was given 3 h before the allopurinol. When this was done their uric acid levels fell by 40–65%. One of them started once again to take both preparations together whereupon his uric acid levels began to climb. It would appear that the aluminium hydroxide considerably reduces the absorption of allopurinol from the gut by some as yet unknown mechanism.

Information seems to be limited to this report. Advise patients to separate the administration of these two drugs by 3 h or more to avoid admixture in the gut and monitor the outcome. Follow the same precautions with any other antacid until more information becomes available.

Reference

1 Weissman I and Krivoy N. Interaction of aluminium hydroxide and allopurinol in patients on chronic haemodialysis. Ann Intern Med (1987) 107, 787.

Allopurinol + Iron

Abstract/Summary

No adverse interaction occurs if iron and allopurinol are given concurrently.

Clinical evidence, mechanism, importance and management

Some early animal studies suggested that allopurinol might have an inhibitory effect on the metabolism of iron. This led the manufacturers of allopurinol in some countries to issue a warning about their concurrent use,[1,2] however it would now seem that no special precautions are necessary if they are administered concurrently.[3]

References

1 Emmerson BT. Effects of allopurinol on iron metabolism in man. Ann Rheum Dis (1966) 25, 700.
2 Davis PS and Deller DJ. Effect of a xanthine oxidase inhibitor (allopurinol) on radio-iron absorption in man. Lancet (1966) ii, 470.
3 Ascione FJ. Allopurinol and iron. J Amer Med Ass (1975) 232, 1010.

Allopurinol + Probenecid

Abstract/Summary

The theoretical possibility of an adverse interaction between allopurinol and probenecid which could lead to uric acid precipitation in the kidneys appears not to be realized in practice.

Clinical evidence, mechanism, importance and management

Probenecid appears to increase the renal excretion of allopurinol or its active metabolite (oxipurinol, or alloxanthine),[1] while allopurinol is thought to inhibit the metabolism of probenecid. It certainly increases the half-life of probenecid.[2] It has been suggested that the outcome might be an increase in the excretion of uric acid which could result in the precipitation of uric acid in the kidneys. However the clinical importance of these mutual interactions seems to be minimal. No problems were seen in a study in patients given 200–600 mg allopurinol and 500–1000 mg probenecid daily, although the half-life of the probenecid was increased by about 50%.[3]

References

1 Elion GB, Yu T-F, Gutman AB and Hitchings GH. Renal clearance of oxipurinol, the chief metabolite of allopurinol. Amer J Med (1968) 45, 69.
2 Horwitz D, Thorgeirsson SS and Mitchell JR. The influence of allopurinol and size of dose on the metabolism of phenylbutazone in patients with gout. Eur J clin Pharmacol(1977) 12, 133.
3 Yu T-F and Gutman AB. Effect of allopurinol (4-hydroxypyrazolo(3,4-dl) pyrimidine on serum and urinary uric acid in primary and secondary gout. Amer J Med (1964) 37, 885.

Allopurinol + Tamoxifen

Abstract/Summary

A single case report describes a marked exacerbation of allopurinol hepatotoxicity in a man when given tamoxifen

Clinical evidence, mechanism, importance and management

An elderly man who had been taking 300 mg allopurinol daily for 12 years and who had mild chronic allopurinol hepatotoxicity, developed fever and marked increases in his serum levels of lactic dehydrogenase and alkaline phosphatase within a day of starting to take 10 mg tamoxifen twice daily.[1] This was interpreted as an exacerbation of the heptatotoxicity. He rapidly recovered when the allopurinol was stopped. The reasons for the reaction are not understood. It would now seem prudent to monitor the effects of concurrent use, but the general importance of this interaction is not known.

Reference

1 Shad KA, Levin J, Rosen N, Greenwald E and Zumoff B. Allopurinol hepatotoxicity potentiated by tamoxifen. NY State J Med (1982) 82, 1745–6.

Allopurinol + Thiazides

Abstract/Summary

Severe allergic reactions to allopurinol have been seen in a few patients, tentatively attributed to renal failure and the use of thiazide diuretics.

Clinical evidence, mechanism, importance and management

Most patients tolerate allopurinol very well, but life-threatening hypersensitivity reactions (rash, vasculitis, hepatitis, eosinophilia, progressive renal insufficiency, etc.) develop very occasionally even with standard doses of 200–400 mg. Most of the reported cases are associated with renal insufficiency and about half were taking thiazide diuretics.[4] For example, four patients developed a hypersensitivity vasculitis while taking allopurinol and hydrochlorothiazide.[1] Renal failure impairs the loss of oxipurinol (the major metabolite of allopurinol) but a study in normal subjects failed to find any alteration in its clearance by thiazides which might provide a pharmacokinetic link between thiazide use and allopurinol toxicity.[3] Other studies have shown that the effects of allopurinol on pyrimidine metabolism are enhanced by the use of thiazides.[2] Some caution is therefore appropriate if both drugs are used, particularly if renal function is abnormal, but more study is needed to confirm this possible interaction.

References

1 Young JL, Boswell RB and Nies AS. Severe allopurinol sensitivity. Association with thiazides and prior renal compromise. Arch InternMed (1974) 134, 553.
2 Wood MH, O'Sullivan WJ, Wilson M and Tiller DJ. Potentiation of an effect of allopurinol on pyrimidine metabolism by chlorothiazide in man. Clin Exp PharmacolPhysiol (1974) 1, 53.
3 Hande KR. Evaluation of a thiazide-allopurinol drug interaction. Am J Med Sci (1986) 292, 213–16.
4 Hande KR, Noon RM and Stone WJ. Severe allopurinol toxicity: description and guidelines for prevention in patients with renal insufficiency. Am J Med (1984) 76, 47–56.

Anistreplase (APSAC) + Streptokinase

Abstract/Summary

The effects of streptokinase are likely to be reduced or abolished if given within 6 months of streptokinase or anistreplase because the persistently high levels of streptokinase antibodies reduce or prevent its activation.

Clinical evidence

A study in 25 patients who had been given streptokinase for the treatment of acute myocardial infarction found that 12 weeks later they still had enough anti-streptokinase antibodies in circulation to neutralize an entire 1.5 million unit dose. At 4–8 months 18 out of 20 still had enough to neutralize half of a 1.5 million unit dose, and after 8 months the neutralization ranged from 0.4 to two million units.[1]

Mechanism

The administration of streptokinase causes the production of anti-streptokinase antibodies. These antibodies persist in the circulation so that the clot-dissolving effects of another dose of streptokinase given many months later may be ineffective or less effective because it becomes bound and neutralised by these antibodies before it can activate the plasmin which dissolves the fibrin of the clot. Many people already have a very low titre of antibodies against streptokinase even before they are given a first dose because they have become sensitized by a previous streptococcal infection, yet the incidence of allergic and anaphylactic reactions to anistreplase and streptokinase seems to be low (3% or less). At risk patients can be identified by means of a skin test.[3]

Importance and management

An established and clinically important interaction. One author says that 'the real practical reason why therapy is not repeated within a year is that it simply would not work.'[2] On the other hand the authors of the report cited[1] suggest that the streptokinase neutralization titres should be measured before giving a second dose within a year so that an effective dosage can be calculated.

References

1 Jalihal S and Morris GK. Antistreptokinase titres after intravenous streptokinase. Lancet (1990) i, 184–5.
2 Moriarty AJ. Anaphylaxis and streptokinase. Hosp Update (1987) 13, 342.
3 Dykewicz MS, McGrath KG, Davison R, Kaplan KJ and Patterson R. Identification of patients at risk for anaphylaxis due to streptokinase. Arch InternMed (1986) 146, 305–7.

Anticholinesterases + Miscellaneous drugs

Abstract/Summary

Diuretic doses of acetazolamide can oppose the actions of anticholinesterases used in the treatment of myasthenia gravis. Dipyridamole, procainamide and quinidine also oppose the activity of drugs used to treat myasthenia.

Clinical evidence, mechanism, importance and management

Acetazolamide (500 mg intravenously) given as a diuretic has been observed to worsen the muscular weakness of patients with myasthenic gravis who are taking anticholinesterase drugs.[1] This was confirmed in an electromyographic study in patients taking edrophonium and in an isolated animal nerve-muscle preparation.[1] A patient well maintained on distigmine bromide experienced an aggravation of his myasthenic symptoms on two occasions when additionally given 75 mg dipyridamole three times daily.[4] The mechanisms of these interactions are not understood. Both procainamide and quinidine also increase the muscular weakness of patients with myasthenia gravis and should therefore be avoided.[2,3]

References

1 Carmignani M, Scoppetta C, Ranelletti FO and Tonali P. Adverse interaction between acetazolamide and anticholinesterase drugs at the normal and myasthenic neuromuscular junction. Int J Clin Pharmacol Ther Toxicol (1984) 22, 140–4.
2 Drachman DA and Skom JH. Procainamide—a hazard in myasthenia gravis. Arch Neurol(1965) 13, 316.
3 Aviado DM and Salem H. Drug action, reaction and interaction. I. Quinidine for cardiac arrhythmias. J Clin Pharmacol(1975) 15, 477.
4 Haddad M, Zelikovski A and Reiss R. Dipyridamole counteracting distigmine in a myasthenic patient. IRCS Med Sci (1986) 14, 297.

Antihistamines + Contraceptives, oral

Abstract/Summary

The effects of doxylamine and diphenhydramine appear not to be affected by the concurrent use of oral contraceptives.

Clinical evidence, mechanism, importance and management

A controlled study in two groups of women (13 and 10) found that the pharmacokinetics of 25 mg doxylamine and 50 mg diphenhydramine were unaltered by the use of low dose oestrogen-containing contraceptives.[1] No particular precautions would seem to be necessary during concurrent use.

Reference

1 Luna BG, Scavone JM and Greenblatt DJ. Doxylamine and diphenhydramine pharmacokinetics in women on low-dose estrogen oral contraceptives. J Clin Pharmacol(1989) 29, 257–60.

Baclofen + Ibuprofen

Abstract/Summary

A man developed baclofen toxicity when given ibuprofen.

Clinical evidence, mechanism, importance and management

An isolated report describes a man taking 20 mg baclofen

three times a day without problems who developed baclofen toxicity (confusion, disorientation, bradycardia, blurred vision, hypotension and hypothermia) after taking eight 600 mg doses of ibuprofen (600 mg ibuprofen three times daily). It appeared that the toxicity was caused by baclofen accumulation arising from acute renal insufficiency caused by the ibuprofen.[1] The general importance of this interaction is likely to be small, but concurrent use should be monitored.

Reference

1 Dahlin PA and George J. Baclofen toxicity associated with declining renal clearance after ibuprofen. Drug Intell Clin Pharm (1984) 18, 805–8.

References

1 Masbernard A. Quoted as personal communication (1977) by Heel RC, Brogden RN, Speight TM and Avery GS. Benzbromarone: a review of its pharmacological properties and their use in gout and hyperuricaemia. Drugs (1977) 14, 349–66.
2 Sinclair DS and Fox IH. The pharmacology of hypouricaemic effect of benzbromarone. J Rheumatol (1975) 2, 437.
3 Sorensen LB and Levinson DJ. Clinical evaluation of benzbromarone. Arth Rheum (1976) 19, 183.
4 Lee IK. Mead Johnson Research Centre. A clinical study of benzbromarone, unpublished data 1977. Quoted by Heel et al (reference 1).
5 Gross A and Giraud V. Uber die Wirkung von Benzbromaron auf Urikamie und Urikosurie. Med Welt (1972) 23, 133–6.
6 Kropp A. Uricosuric action of benzbromarone upon pyrazinamide-induced hyperuricaemia. Med Welt (1970) 65, 1448.

Benzbromarone + Miscellaneous drugs

Abstract/Summary

It is uncertain whether benzbromarone interacts with the oral anticoagulants but aspirin antagonizes its uricosuric effects. It is also not clear whether benzbromarone remains effective in the presence of pyrazinamide, but it is not affected by chlorothiazide.

Clinical evidence, mechanism, importance and management

Although there seems to be no direct evidence that benzbromarone interacts with the oral anticoagulants, concurrent use should be monitored because increased anticoagulant effects occur when other benzofuran derivatives are given (e.g. benziodarone, amiodarone). However it is claimed that no increases in the anticoagulant effects of nicoumalone, ethylbiscoumacetate or phenindione were seen in a few patients given benzbromarone.[1]

A study in six gouty subjects found that a single 600 mg dose of aspirin reduced the peak ratio of urate to creatinine clearance with 160 mg benzbromarone by a half (23 compared with 12%).[2] 2600 mg aspirin daily given to 29 normal subjects on 40–80 mg benzbromarone daily reduced the urate lowering effects by 20–40%.[3] Aspirin should be avoided by patients taking benzbromarone.

It is not clear whether benzbromarone remains effective in patients taking pyrazinamide. One report claims that when 50 mg benzbromarone was given to 10 patients taking 35 mg/kg pyrazinamide daily, uric acid levels were reduced in all of them (averaging 24.3%) and were normal in 4 of the 10.[6] However another report says that 160 mg benzbromarone daily had no uricosuric effect on 5 patients taking 3 g pyrazinamide daily,[2] and other authors also refer to this failure to reduce uric acid levels.[3]

The uricosuric effects of benzbromarone appear to be unaffected by the concurrent use of chlorothiazide.[4,5]

Bismuth subcitrate + Miscellaneous drugs

Abstract/Summary

Antacids, food and large amounts of milk can reduce the effects of bismuth subcitrate. It is as yet uncertain whether other drugs which raise gastric pH can reduce the ulcer-healing effects.

Clinical evidence, mechanism, importance and management

Bismuth subcitrate (bismuth chelate, tripotassium dicitratobismuthate, TDB) is believed to act by precipitating in gastric juice within the stomach where it coats and binds to the ulcerated site, thereby blocking the irritant actions of stomach acid. If the pH of the stomach rises above 3.5 precipitation does not occur to any great extent[1] and the ulcer-healing properties could be reduced or lost. Bismuth subcitrate can also bind to antacids and for these reasons the manufacturers suggest that antacids should not be taken half-an-hour before or after bismuth subcitrate. On theoretical grounds H_2-blockers (e.g. cimetidine, ranitidine) or proton pump inhibitors (e.g. omeprazole) which can raise gastric pH should also be avoided but there seems as yet to be no direct evidence confirming this.[4] The manufacturers also suggest that large amounts of milk should not be taken with bismuth subcitrate but small amounts on breakfast cereals, or in tea or coffee do not matter.[3] One recommendation is that the bismuth subcitrate should be taken half-an-hour before food, and any antacid half-an-hour after food to minimize any interactions.[2] Bismuth subcitrate would also be expected to interact with tetracyclines given orally (see 'Tetracyclines + Antacids').

References

1 Lee SP. A potential mechanism of action of colloidal bismuth subcitrate: diffusion barrier to hydrochloric acid. Scand J Gastroenterol (1982) 17 (Suppl 80) 17–21.
2 Baguley J. Ranitidine interactions. Pharm J (1990) 244, 5.
3 Data Sheet Compendium 1989–90. Datapharm Publications (1989).
4 Baxter GF. Ranitidine interactions. Pharm J (1990) 244,117.

Calcium and Vitamin D + Diuretics

Abstract/Summary

Excessive serum calcium levels can develop in patients given calcium and vitamin D if they are additionally treated with diuretics such as the thiazides which can reduce the urinary excretion of calcium.

Clinical evidence

An elderly woman treated with hydrochlorothiazide 25 mg and triamterene 50 mg daily for hypertension, and 5000 U vitamin D_2 with 1.5 g calcium daily for osteoporosis, became confused, disorientated and dehydrated. She was found to have a serum calcium level of 13.9 mg/dl (normal 8.2–10.5 mg/dl).[1]

Another elderly woman with normal kidney function on hydrochlorothiazide, 50 mg daily, and 2.5–7.5 mg calcium daily also developed hypercalcaemia.[2] A young woman with osteoporosis taking 120,000 IU vitamin D_2 and 2 g calcium daily became hypercalcaemic when given chlorothiazide.[3] 5 out of 12 patients under treatment for hypoparathyroidism with vitamin D became hypercalcaemic when treated with thiazides.[4]

Mechanism

The thiazide diuretics (and triamterene) can cause calcium-retention by reducing the urinary excretion. This, added to the increased intake of calcium, resulted in excessive calcium levels.

Importance and management

An established interaction. The incidence is unknown. Concurrent use need not be avoided but the serum calcium levels should be regularly monitored to ensure that they do not become excessive.

References

1 Drinka PJ and Nolten WE. Hazards of treating osteoporosis and hypertension concurrently with calcium, vitamin D and distal diuretics. J Am Geriat Soc (1984) 32, 405–7.
2 Hakim R, Tolis G, Golzman D et al. Severe hypercalcemia associated with hydrochlorothiazide and calcium carbonate therapy. Can Med Ass J (1979) 121, 591.
3 Parfitt AM. Chlorothiazide-induced hypercalcaemia in juvenile osteoporosis and hyperparathyroidism. N Engl J Med (1969) 281, 55.
4 Parfitt AM. Thiazide-induced hypercalcaemia in vitamin D-treated hypoparathyroidism. Ann InternMed (1972) 77, 557.

Cannabis + Disulfiram

Abstract/Summary

An isolated case report describes a hypomanic-like reaction in a man on disulfiram when he used cannabis.

Clinical evidence, mechanism, importance and management

A man with a 10-year history of drug abuse (alcohol, amphetamines, cocaine, cannabis) experienced a hypomanic-like reaction (euphoria, hyperactivity, insomnia, irritability) on two occasions while being treated with 250 mg disulfiram daily which was attributed to the concurrent use of cannabis. The patient said that he felt as though he had been taking amphetamine.[1] The reason for this reaction is not understood.

Reference

1 Lacoursiere RB and Swatek R. Adverse interaction between disulfiram and marijuana: a case report. Am J Psychiatry (1983) 140, 242–4.

Carbenoxolone + Antacids

Abstract/Summary

There is some evidence that antacids may possibly reduce the effects of carbenoxolone.

Clinical evidence, mechanism, importance and management

The bioavailability of carbenoxolone combined with magnesium and aluminium hydroxide antacids in a liquid formulation was found to be approximately half that of carbenoxolone in granular and capsule formulations.[1] The extent to which antacids might reduce the ulcer-healing effects of carbenoxolone given in other formulations seems not to have been assessed but the possibility should be borne in mind.

Reference

1 Crema F, Parini J, Visconti M and Perucca E. Effetto degli antiacidi sulla biodisponibilita del carbenoxolone. Il Farmaco (1987) 42, 357–64.

Carbenoxolone + Antihypertensives and Diuretics

Abstract/Summary

Carbenoxolone causes fluid retention and raises the blood pressure in some patients. This may be expected to oppose the effects of antihypertensive drugs. Thiazides can be used to treat the adverse side-effects of carbenoxolone, but not spironolactone or amiloride which oppose its ulcer-healing effects. The potassium-losing effects of the thiazides and carbenoxolone can be additive so that a potassium supplement may be needed to prevent hypokalaemia.

Clinical evidence, mechanism, importance and management

(a) Antihypertensives + carbenoxolone

Carbenoxolone can raise the blood pressure. Five out of 10 patients on 300 mg carbenoxolone daily, and two out of 10 taking 150 mg daily, showed a rise in diastolic blood pressure of 20 mm Hg or more.[1] Other reports[2-8] confirm that fluid retention and hypertension commonly occur, the incidence of the latter being variously reported as being as low as 4%[10] or as high as 50%,[8] and fluid retention as absent[2] or affecting 46%.[8] The reason for the blood pressure rise is that carbenoxolone has mineralocorticoid-like activity. There appear to be few direct reports of adverse interactions between antihypertensive drugs and carbenoxolone, but any patient on carbenoxolone should have regular checks on their weight and blood pressure, whether taking an antihypertensive agent or not. An increase in the dosage of the antihypertensive agent may be necessary.

(b) Carbenoxolone + diuretics

Thiazide diuretics can be used to control the oedema and hypertension caused by carbenoxolone, but not spironolactone (an aldosterone-antagonist) or amiloride[11] because they oppose its ulcer-healing effects.[4] Deglycyrrhizinated liquorice which is an analogue of carbenoxolone has reduced mineralocorticoid activity and fewer side-effects.[8,9] If thiazides are used it should be remembered the potassium-losing effects of the carbenoxolone and the diuretic will be additive so that a potassium supplement may be needed to prevent hypokalaemia. Alternative drugs for the treatment of ulcers are the H_2-blockers, ranitidine being one which interacts with very few other drugs.

References

1 Turpie AGG and Thomson TJ. Carbenoxolone sodium in the treatment of gastric ulcer with special reference to side-effects. Gut (1965) 6, 591.
2 Bank S and Marks IN. Maintenance carbenoxolone sodium in the treatment of gastric ulcer recurrence. In 'Carbenoxolone Sodium', Baron A and Sullivan (eds), Butterworths, London (1970) p.103.
3 Doll R, Langman MJS and Shawdon HH. Effect of different doses of carbenoxolone and different diuretics. In 'A Symposium on Carbenoxolone Sodium', Robson A and Sullivan S (eds), Butterworths, London (1968) p 51.
4 Doll R, Langman MJS and Shawdon HH. Treatment of gastric ulcer with carbenoloxone: antagonistic effect of spironolactone. Gut (1968) 9, 42.
5 Montgomery RD and Cookson JB. Comparative trial of carbenoxolone and a deglycyrrhizinated liquorice preparation (Cavid-S). Clin Trials J (1972) 9, 33.
6 Langman MJS, Knapp DR and Wakley EJ. Treatment of chronic gastric ulcer with carbenoxolone and gefarnate; a comparative trial. Br Med J (1973) 3, 84.
7 Horwich L and Galloway R. Treatment of gastric ulcer with carbenoxolone sodium. Clinical and radiological evaluation. Br Med J (1965) 2, 1272.
8 Fraser PM, Doll R, Langman MJS, Misiewicz JJ and Shawdon HH. Clinical trial of a new carbenoxolone analogue BX-24, zinc sulphate and vitamin A in the treatment of gastric ulcer. Gut (1972) 13, 459.
9 Brogden RN, Speight TM and Avery GS. Deglycyrrhizinized liquorice: a report of its pharmacological properties and therapeutic efficacy in peptic ulcer. Drugs (1974) 8, 330.
10 Montgomery RD. Side-effects of carbenoxolone sodium: a study of ambulant therapy of gastric ulcer. Gut (1967) 8, 148.
11 Reed PI, Lewis SI, Vincent-Brown A, Holdstock DJ, Gribble RJN, Murgatroyd RE and Baron JH. The influence of amiloride on the therapeutic and metabolic effects of carbenoxolone in patients with gastric ulcer. Scand J Gastroenterol (1980) 15, Suppl 65, 51.

Carbenoxolone + Chlorpropamide, Tolbutamide, Phenytoin, Warfarin

Abstract/Summary

Of these drugs, only chlorpropamide appears to have an effect on the pharmacokinetics of carbenoxolone, causing a small reduction in serum levels.

Clinical evidence, mechanism, importance and management

A study on four normal subjects showed that single doses of 500 mg tolbutamide, 100 mg phenytoin or 10 mg warfarin had no significant effect on the half-life of single 100 mg doses of carbenoxolone. A single 250 mg dose of chlorpropamide delayed the absorption of carbenoxolone and this was confirmed in six patients with benign gastric ulcers taking 300 mg carbenoxolone daily who showed a depression in their serum levels (about 20%). Some delay in absorption also occurred.[1] The clinical importance of this is uncertain. More study is needed.

Reference

1 Thornton PC, Papouchado M and Reed PI. Carbenoxolone interactions in man—preliminary report. Scand J Gastroenterol (1980) 15, Suppl 65, 35.

Charcoal + Other drugs

Abstract/Summary

Charcoal adsorbs drugs onto its surface and can markedly reduce their availability for absorption by the gut. Separating their administration as much as possible would be expected to reduce this interaction.

Clinical evidence, mechanism, importance and management

Activated charcoal can adsorb gases, toxins and drugs onto its surface. Most of the reports in the literature are concerned with the treatment of cases of poisoning and overdosage where these adsorptive properties are exploited, but charcoal in doses intended to adsorb intestinal gas or for the treatment of diarrhoea and dysentery can also adsorb drugs given in normal therapeutic doses. For example, in one human study it was found that 98% of 0.5 mg digoxin and 500 mg phenytoin, and 70% of 1 g aspirin were adsorbed by 50 g activated charcoal in water.[1] Similar levels of adsorption would be expected with many other drugs. For this reason the administration of charcoal and drugs should be separated as much as possible to avoid their admixture in the gut, although it should be said that as yet there is little or no documentation to confirm that this is effective.

Reference

1 Neuvonen PJ, Elfving SM and Elonen E. Reduction of absorption of digoxin, phenytoin and aspirin by activated charcoal in man. Eur J Clin Pharmacol(1978) 13, 213.

Chlormethiazole (Clomethiazole) + Cimetidine or Ranitidine

Abstract/Summary

The sedative and hypnotic effects of chlormethiazole are markedly increased by cimetidine, but ranitidine does not interact.

Clinical evidence

A study in eight normal subjects showed that after one week's treatment with 1 g cimetidine daily the clearance of a single 1 g oral dose of chlormethiazole (the normal hypnotic dose) was reduced by 69%, and the elimination half-life and AUC (area under the curve) were increased by 60 and 55% respectively. Without the cimetidine the subjects slept for 30–60 min after taking the chlormethiazole, whereas after the cimetidine treatment most of them slept for at least 2 h.[1,2]

Subsequent studies showed that 300 mg ranitidine daily does not interact significantly with chlormethiazole.[3,4]

Mechanism

Cimetidine not only inhibits the liver enzymes concerned with the metabolism of the chlormethiazole but it also reduces the flow of blood through the liver, both of which results in a reduction in the rate at which the chlormethiazole is removed from the body. Ranitidine does not inhibit liver enzymes.

Importance and management

Information about cimetidine appears to be limited to this study, but it is consistent with the way it increases and prolongs the activity of other drugs. The authors emphasize that the risks of over-sedation and respiratory depression are likely to be greatest in the elderly and those with liver disease. The dosage of chlormethiazole should be reduced to accommodate this interaction (probably approximately halved) or the cimetidine replaced by ranitidine or another H$_2$-blocker which lacks enzyme inhibitory activity.

References

1 Shaw G, Bury RW, Mashford ML, Breen KJ and Desmond PV. Cimetidine impairs the elimination of chlormethiazole. Eur J Clin Pharmacol(1981) 21, 83.
2 Desmond PV, Shaw RG, Bury RW, Mashford ML and Breen KJ. Cimetidine impairs the clearance of an orally administered high clearance drug, chlormethiazole. Gastroenterol (1981) 80, 21.
3 Desmond PV, Breen KJ, Harman P, Mashford ML and Morphett B. No effect of ranitidine on the disposition or elimination of clormethiazole or indocyanin green (ICG). Scand J Gastroenterol (1982) 17, Suppl 78, A50.
4 Mashford ML, Harman PJ, Morphett BJ, Breen KJ and Desmond PV. Ranitidine does not affect chlormethiazole or indocyanine green disposition. Clin Pharmacol Ther (1983) 34, 231–3.

Cholestyramine + Spironolactone

Abstract/Summary

Hyperchloraemic metabolic acidosis has been seen in two patients associated with the use of cholestyramine and spironolactone.

Clinical evidence, mechanism, importance and management

Two case reports describe the development of hyperchloraemic metabolic acidosis in two elderly patients with hepatic cirrhosis treated with cholestyramine (up to four sachets daily) who were concurrently receiving spironolactone. Other predisposing factors included mild renal impairment and upper respiratory tract infection.[1,2] This adverse reaction appears to be rare, but electrolyte monitoring during concurrent use has been advised.[1]

References

1 Eaves ER and Korman MG. Cholestyramine induced hyperchloremic metabolic acidosis. Aust NZ J Med (1984) 14, 670–1.
2 Clouston WM and LLoyd HM. Cholestyramine induced hyperchloremic metabolic acidosis. Aust NZ J Med (1985) 15, 271.

Cisapride + Miscellaneous drugs

Abstract/Summary

Cisapride increases the rate of absorption of diazepam and alcohol. No clinically important interactions are apparent with cimetidine, ranitidine, antacids or propranolol.

Clinical evidence, mechanism, importance and management

Cisapride speeds up gastrointestinal motility. This would be expected to accelerate drug transit through the gut, to increase the absorption rate of drugs, and it may to some extent reduce the extent of absorption. For this reason the manufacturers of cisapride suggest[10] that for drugs which need careful individual titration (e.g. anticonvulsants) it may be useful to measure their plasma concentrations, however there seems to be no direct evidence that a clinically important interaction actually occurs. Cisapride does not cause sedation but it accelerates the absorption of diazepam[3] and alcohol so that their sedative effects occur more quickly and may possibly be transiently increased.[4] Cisapride was found not to affect serum propranolol levels nor the blood pressure control of 10 mildly hypertensive patients given a sustained-release propranolol preparation.[9] The concurrent use of anticholinergic drugs would be expected to oppose the effects of cisapride.

Peak serum cisapride levels are increased 22% by cimetidine (possibly by enzyme inhibition) whereas the bioavailability of cimetidine is reduced (17%).[1,5] Cisapride enhances the absorption rate of ranitidine but reduces its absorption (AUC reduced 26%).[6,8] The increase in the bioavailability of cisapride by ranitidine[6] was not confirmed in one study.[8] The concurrent use of aluminium oxide and magnesium hydroxide was found in another study not to affect the absorption of cisapride.[7] It seems doubtful if the concurrent use of any of these drugs is likely to result in a clinically important adverse interaction.

15 normal subjects were given 30 mg cisapride daily for 28 days to find out if it induces or inhibits liver microsomal enzymes, using antipyrine as a marker or index drug. No changes in metabolism were found.[2]

References

1 Kirsch W, Rose I and Ohnhaus EE. Cispride and cimetidine. Both drugs alter the pharmacokinetics of each other. Clin Pharmacol Ther (1986) 39, 202.
2 Davies DS, Mills FJ and Welburn PJ. Cisapride has no effect on antipyrine clearance. Br J clin Pharmac (1988) 26, 808–9.
3 Bateman DN. The action of cisapride on gastric emptying and the pharmacodynamics and pharmacokinetics of oral diazepam. Eur J Clin Pharmacol (1986) 30, 205–8.
4 Idzikowski C and Welburn P. An evaluation of possible interactions between ethanol and cisapride. Unpublished report N 49087 on file, Janssen Pharmaceuticals (1986).
5 Kirch W, Janisch HD, Ohnhaus EE and Van Peer A. Cisapride-cimetidine interaction: enhanced cisapride bioavailability and accelerated cimetidine absorption. Ther Drug Monit (1989) 11, 411–14.
6 Castelli G, van Peer A, Gasparini R, Woestenborghs R, Heykants J, Verlinden M and Capozzi C. Cisapride-ranitidine interaction. Unpublished report N49638 on file, Janssen Pharmaceuticals (1986).
7 Verlinden M, Van Peer A, Gasparini R, Woestenborghs R, Heykants J and Reyntjens A. Unaltered oral absorption of cisapride on coadministration of antacids. Unpublished report N49374 on file, Janssen Pharmaceuticals (1986).
8 Milligan KA, McHugh P and Rowbotham DJ. Effects of concomitant administration of cisapride and ranitidine on plasma concentrations in volunteers. Br J Anaesth (1989) 63, 628P.
9 Van der Kleijn E and Van Mameren C. Effect of cisapride on the plasma concentrations of a delayed formulation of propranolol and on its clinical effects on blood pressure in mildly hypertensive patients. Unpublished report N46957 on file, Janssen Pharmaceuticals (1986).
10 PREPULSID (cisapride). Data sheet Janssen Pharmaceuticals (1989).

Clofibrate + Cholestyramine

Abstract/Summary

No significant interaction occurs between clofibrate and cholestyramine.

Clinical evidence, mechanism, importance and management

A study in 15 patients taking 1 g clofibrate twice daily showed that 16 g cholestyramine daily had no effect on the fasting plasma levels, urinary and faecal excretion, or the half-life of clofibrate.[1]

Reference

1 Sedaghat A and Ahrens EH. Lack of effect of cholestyramine on the pharmacokinetics of clofibrate in man. Eur J Clin Invest (1975) 5, 177.

Clofibrate + Contraceptives, oral

Abstract/Summary

Serum cholesterol and triglyceride levels can be increased by the oral contraceptives, and in two cases this is reported to have opposed the cholesterol-lowering effects of clofibrate.

Clinical evidence, mechanism, importance and management

A woman with hypercholesterolaemia, taking clofibrate, showed a rise in her serum cholesterol levels on two occasions when concurrently using an oral contraceptive.[1] Another patient with type IV hyperlipoproteinaemia reacted similarly.[2] Rises in serum levels of cholesterol and triglycerides in women taking oral contraceptives are well recognized.[3,4] It is questionable therefore whether oral contraceptives are suitable for women needing treatment with clofibrate. More study is needed.

References

1 Smith RBW and Prior IAM. Oral contraceptive opposition to hypercholesterolaemic action of clofibrate. Lancet (1968) i, 750.
2 Robertson-Rintoul J. Raised serum-lipids and oral contraceptives. Lancet (1972) ii, 1320.
3 Wynn V, Doar JWH, Mills GL and Stokes T. Fasting serum triglyceride, cholesterol and lipoprotein levels during oral contraceptive therapy. Lancet (1969) ii, 756.
4 Stokes T and Wynn V. Serum lipids in women on oral contraceptives. Lancet (1971) ii, 677.

Clofibrate + Probenecid

Abstract/Summary

Serum clofibrate levels can be approximately doubled by probenecid.

Clinical evidence, mechanism, importance and management

A pharmacokinetic study in four normal subjects taking 500 mg clofibrate 12-hourly showed that 500 mg probenecid six-hourly almost doubled steady-state clofibric acid levels (from 72 to 129 mg/l) and raised free clofibric acid levels from 2.5 to 9.1 mg/l. The suggested reasons is that the probenecid reduces the renal and metabolic clearance of the clofibrate by inhibiting its conjugation with glucuronic acid.[1] The clinical importance of this interaction is uncertain. It appears not to have been assessed.

Reference

1 Veenendaal JR, Brooks PM and Meffin PJ. Probenecid-clofibrate interaction. Clin Pharmacol Ther (1981) 29, 351.

CNS depressants + CNS depressants

Abstract/Summary

The concurrent use of two or more drugs which depress the central nervous system may be expected to result in increased depression. This may have undesirable and even life-threatening consequences.

Clinical evidence, mechanism, importance and management

The primary effect of some drugs and the unwanted, secondary or side-effect of many other drugs is depression of the activity of the central nervous system. If taken together their effects may be additive. It is not uncommon for patients, particularly the elderly, to be taking half-a-dozen drugs or more (and alcohol as well) and for the cumulative CNS-depressant effects to range from mild drowsiness through to a befuddled stupor which can make the performance of the simplest everyday task more difficult or even impossible. The importance of this will depend on the context: at home and at bedtime it may even be advantageous, whereas in the kitchen, at work, in a busy street, driving a car or handling other potentially dangerous machinery where alertness is at a premium, it may considerably increase the risk of accident. An example of the lethal effects of combining an antihistamine, a benzodiazepine tranquillizer and alcohol is briefly mentioned in the synopsis 'Alcohol+Antihistamines'. A less spectacular but socially distressing example is that of a woman accused of shop-lifting while in a confused state arising from the combined sedative effects of *Actifed*, a *Beechams Powder* and *Dolobid* (containing triprolidine, salicylamide and diflunisal respectively).[1]

Few if any well-controlled studies have been made on the cumulative or additive detrimental effects of CNS depressants (except with alcohol), but the following is a list of some of the drugs which to a greater or lesser extent possess CNS depressant activity and which may be expected to interact in this way: alcohol, analgesics, antibiotics, anticonvulsants, antidepressants, antihistamines, antinauseants, antipsychotics, cough and cold preparations, hypnotics, narcotics, sedatives and tranquillizers. Some of the interactions of alcohol with these drugs are dealt with in individual synopses. The Index should be consulted.

Reference

1 Herxheimer A and Haffner BD. Prosecution for alleged shoplifting: successful pharmacological defence. Lancet (1982) i, 634.

Colestipol + Clofibrate or Fenofibrate

Abstract/summary, clinical evidence, mechanism, importance and management

Studies in normal subjects showed that over a six-day period no adverse interaction occurred when given daily doses of 10–15 g colestipol with either 500 mg clofibrate or 300 mg fenofibrate.[1,2]

References

1 Harvengt C and Desager JP. Lack of pharmacokinetic interaction of colestipol and fenofibrate in volunteers. Eur J Clin Pharmacol(1980) 17, 459.
2 DeSante KA, Disanto AR, Albert KS, Weber DJ, Welch RD and Vecchio TJ. The effect of colestipol hydrochloride on the bioavailability and pharmacokinetics of clofibrate. J Clin Pharmacol(1979) 11–12, 721.

Colestipol + Miscellaneous drugs

Abstract/Summary

Colestipol is reported not to interact significantly with aspirin or methyldopa. A report suggests that colestipol is active in insulin-treated diabetics but may be ineffective in those treated with phenformin and sulphonylureas.

Clinical evidence, mechanism, importance and management

Although colestipol can undoubtedly bind to a number of drugs in the gut, the effects on the bioavailability of most of them is usually small and clinically unimportant. The rate of absorption of aspirin is increased by 10 g colestipol but the extent is unaltered and no particular precautions seem to be necessary.[3] Colestipol is also reported to have no important effect on the absorption of methyldopa.[1]

A long-term double-blind trial in 12 diabetics with elevated serum cholesterol levels showed that the concurrent use of phenformin and a sulphonylurea (chlorpropamide, tolbutamide or tolazamide) inhibited the normal hypocholesterolaemic effects of the colestipol. No such antagonism was seen in two maturity-onset diabetics treated with insulin. The control of diabetes was not affected by the colestipol.[2] This suggests that colestipol may not be suitable for lowering the blood cholesterol levels of diabetics treated with these oral hypoglycaemic agents. More study is needed to confirm these findings.

References

1 Hunningshake DB and King S. Effect of cholestyramine and colestipol on the absorption of methyldopa and hydrochlorothiazide. Pharmacologist (1978) 20, 220.
2 Bandisole MS and Boshell BR. Hypocholesterolemic activity of colestipol in diabetics. Curr Ther Res (1975) 18, 276.
3 Hunningshake DB and Pollack E. Effect of bile acid sequestering agents on the absorption of aspirin, tolbutamide and warfarin. Fed Proc (1977) 36, 996.

Desferrioxamine + Miscellaneous drugs

Abstract/Summary

Vitamin C may cause cardiac disorders in some patients treated with desferrioxamine. Prochlorperazine caused unconsciousness in two patients being treated with desferrioxamine.

Clinical evidence, mechanism, importance and management

(a) Desferrioxamine + vitamin C (ascorbic acid)

Sometimes vitamin C is given to increase the excretion of iron when desferrioxamine is being used, however some patients given 500 mg vitamin C daily have shown a striking, but often transitory, deterioration in left ventricular function. For this reason it has been suggested that extreme caution should be used in patients with excess tissue iron.[1,2] The need for the use of the vitamin needs to be clearly established. Patients with advanced primary or secondary hemochromatosis, particularly those with overt cardiac disease, should reduce their vitamin C intake to a minimum. It has also been stated that the use of orange juice as a source of potassium in those receiving diuretic therapy is most injudicious.[2] The need for the use of vitamin C needs to be clearly established, however under very well controlled conditions concurrent use can be undertaken.[3]

(b) Desferrioxamine + prochlorperazine

Two out of seven patients treated for rheumatoid arthritis with desferrioxamine lost consciousness for 48–72 h when given prochlorperazine, the presumed reason being that this drug combination removes essential iron from the nervous system.[4] It has also been suggested that desferrioxamine-induced damage of the retina may be more likely in the presence of phenothiazines.[5] The concurrent use of desferrioxamine and prochlorperazine should be avoided, but there seems to be no direct evidence of adverse interactions with any of the other phenothiazines.

References

1 Henry W. Echocardioagraphic evaluation of the heart in thalassaemia major. In Nienhaus AW, moderator. Thalassaemia major: molecular and clinical aspects. Ann Intern Med (1979) 91, 892–4.
2 Nienhaus A W. Vitamin C and iron. N Engl J Med (1981) 304. 170–1.
3 Cohen A, Cohen IJ and Schwartz E. Scurvy and altered iron stores in Thalassaemia major. N Engl J Med (1981) 304, 150–60.

4 Blake DR, Winyard P, Lunec A, Williams A, Good PA, Crewers S J, Gutteridge J, Rowley D, Halliwell B, Cornish A and Hidor RC. Cerebral and ocular toxicity induced by desferrioxamine. Quart J Med (1985) 56, 345–55.
5 Pall H, Blake DR, Good PA and Wynyard AC. Copper chelation and the neuro-ophthalmic toxicity of desferrioxamine. Lancet (1986) ii, 1279.

Dimethicone + Cimetidine or Doxycycline

Abstract/Summary

The bioavailabilities of cimetidine and doxycycline are not affected by dimethicone.

Clinical evidence, mechanism, importance and management

The pharmacokinetics of a 200 mg dose of cimetidine were not significantly changed by 2.25 g dimethicone in 11 normal subjects.[1] Another study in eight subjects found that 2.25 g dimethicone did not alter the bioavailability of doxycycline.[2]

References

1 Boismare F, Flipo JL, Moore N and Chanteclair G. Etude de l'effet du dimticone sur la disponibilite de la cimetidine. Therapie (1987) 42, 9–11.
2 Bistue C, Perez P, Becquart D, Vincon G and Albin H. Effet du dimeticone sur la biodisponibilite de la doxycycline. Therapie (1987) 42, 13–16.

Dinoprostone (Prostaglandin E2) + Oxytocin

Abstract/Summary

Concurrent use may result in uterine hypertonus.

Clinical evidence, mechanism, importance and management

The makers of *Propess*, a slow-release pessary containing dinoprostone for the initiation or continuation of cervical ripening in patients at term (38–40 weeks gestation), say that concurrent or close sequential use of these drugs should only be undertaken under exceptional circumstances because it is known that the prostaglandins potentiate the uterotonic effects of oxytocics. Uterine activity should be monitored for evidence of hypertonus. Normally the pessary is removed when labour is established.[1] *Propess* was withdrawn in the UK in July 1990 because of an unacceptable incidence of hypertonus and foetal distress.

Reference

1 Propress data sheet (1989), Rousell Labs.
2 CSM current problems series, no 29, Aug 1990.

Enteral tube feeding + Antacids

Abstract/Summary

Aluminium-containing antacids can interact with high protein liquid enteral feeds within the oesophagus to produce an obstructive plug.

Clinical evidence, mechanism, importance and management

Three patients who were being fed with a liquid high protein nutrient (*Fresubin* liquid) through an enteral tube developed an obstructing protein-aluminium complex oesophageal plug when intermittently given an aluminium/magnesium hydroxide antacid (*Alucol-Gel*). The authors of the report advise that high molecular protein solutions should not be mixed with antacids or followed by antacids, and if an antacid is needed it should be given some time after the nutrients and the tube should be vigorously flushed beforehand.[1]

Reference

1 Valli C, Schulthess H-K, Asper R, Escher F and Hacki WH. Interaction of nutrients with antacids: a complication during enteral tube feeding. Lancet (1986) i, 747.

Ergot + Glyceryl trinitrate (GTN)

Abstract/Summary

The ergot alkaloids such as dihydroergotamine would be expected to oppose the anti-anginal effects of glyceryl trinitrate (nitroglycerin).

Clinical evidence, mechanism, importance and management

There seem to be no clinical reports of adverse interactions between these drugs but since ergot causes vasoconstriction and can provoke angina, it would be expected to oppose the effects of glyceryl trinitrate used as a vasodilator in the treatment of angina. Glyceryl trinitrate has also been shown to increase the bioavailability of dihydroergotamine in hypotensive subjects[1] which would increase its vasoconstrictor effects.

Reference

1 Bobik A, Jennings G, Skews H, Esler M and McLean A. Low oral bioavailability of dihydroergotamine and first-pass extraction in patients with orthostatic hypotension. Clin Pharmacol Ther (1981) 30, 673–9.

Ergot + Macrolide antibiotics

Abstract/Summary

Ergot toxicity can develop rapidly if patients on ergotamine or dihydroergotamine are concurrently treated with erythromycin or triacetyloleandomycin. A single case has occurred with josamycin but none appear to have been described with midecamycin or spiramycin and none would be expected.

Clinical evidence

(a) Ergot + erythromycin

A woman who had regularly and uneventfully taken *Migral* (ergotamine tartrate 2 mg, cyclizine hydrochloride 50 mg, caffeine 100 mg) on a number of previous occasions, took one tablet during a course of treatment with erythromycin (250 mg every six hours). Within two days she developed severe ischaemic pain in her arms and legs during exercise, with a burning sensation in her feet and hands. When admitted to hospital 10 days later her extremities were cool and cyanosed. Her pulse could not be detected in the lower limbs.[3]

Five other cases of acute ergotism are reported elsewhere[1,2,4–6] involving ergotamine tartrate or dihydroergotamine with erythromycin. The reaction developed within a few hours[5] or days.[2] The spasm of the blood vessels was moderate or severe, and prolonged.

(b) Ergot + josamycin

An isolated report describes a woman of 33 who developed severe ischaemia of the legs within three days of starting to take 2 g josamycin daily and capsules containing 0.3 mg ergotamine tartrate. Her legs and feet were cold, white and painful, and most of her peripheral pulses were impalpable.[16]

(c) Ergot + triacetyloleandomycin

A woman of 40 who had been taking dihydroergotamine, 90 drops daily, for three years without problems, developed cramp in her legs within a few hours of starting to take triacetyloleandomycin (250 mg four times a day). Five days later she was admitted to hospital as an emergency with severe ischaemia of her arms and legs. Her limbs were cold and all her peripheral pulses were impalpable[1].

There are reports[2–12,17] of 10 other patients taking normal doses of ergotamine tartrate or dihydroergotamine for months or years without problems who developed severe ergotism within hours or days of starting to take normal doses of triacetyloleandomycin.

Mechanism

Erythromycin and triacetyloleandomycin form metabolites in the liver which make stable complexes with the iron of cytochrome P-450 so that the normal metabolizing activity of the liver enzymes is reduced.[15] The ergot is poorly metabolized as a result so that it accumulates in the body and its vasoconstrictive effects are increased. Spiramycin, midecamycin and josamycin do not form these complexes.[15]

Importance and management

The interactions of ergot with erythromycin and triacetyloleandomycin are well documented, well established and clinically important. Concurrent use should be avoided because the outcome can be serious. Some of the cases cited were effectively treated with sodium nitroprusside or naftidrofuryl oxalate.[2,5,13] Spiramycin, midecamycin and josamycin would not be expected to interact because they do not form cytochrome P-450 complexes (see 'Mechanism'), however there is one unexplained and unconfirmed report of an interaction with josamycin (cited above[17]).

References

1 Lagier G, Castot A, Riboulet G and Bosesh C. Un cas d'ergotisme mineur semblant en rapport avec une potentialisation de l'ergotamine par l'ethylsuccinate d'erythromcyine. Therapie (1979) 34, 515.

2 Neveux E, Lesgourgues B, Luton J-P, Guilhaume B, Bertagna A and Picard J. Ergotisme aigu par association propionate d'erythromycine-dihydroergotamine. Nouv Presse med (1981) 10, 2830.

3 Francis H, Tyndall A and Webb J. Severe vascular spasm due to erythromycin-ergotamine interaction. Clin Rheumatol (1984) 3, 243–6.

4 Collet AM, Moncharmont D, San Marco JL, Eissinger F. Pinot JJ and Laselve L. Ergotisme iatrogene: role de l'association tartrate d'ergotamine-propionate d'erythromycine. Semm Hop Paris (1982) 58, 1624–6.

5 Boucharlat J, Franco A, Carpentier P, Charignon Y, Denis B and Hommel M. Ergotisme en milieu psychiatrique par association DHE propionate d'erythromycine. Ann Med Psychol(1980) 138, 292–6.

6 Leroy F, Asseman P, Pruvost P, Adnet P, Lacroix D and Thery C. Dihydroergotamine-erythromycin-induced ergotism. Ann InternMed (1988) 109, 249.

7 Franco A, Bourland P, Massot C, Lecoeur J, Guidicelli H and Bessard G. Ergotisme aigu par association dihyroergotamine-triacetyloleandomycine. Nouv Presse med (1978) 7, 205.

8 Lesca H, Ossard D, and Reynier Ph. Les risques de l'association triacetyl oleandomycine et tartrate d'ergotamine. Nouv Presse med (1976) 5, 1832.

9 Hayton AC. Precipitation of acute ergotism by triacetyloleandomycin. NZ Med J (1969) 69, 42.

10 Dupuy JC, Lardy Ph, Seaulau P, Kervoelen O and Paulet J. Spasmes arteriels systemiques. Tartrate d'ergotamine. Arch Mal Coeur (1979) 72, 86.

11 Bigorie B, Aimez P, Soria RJ, Samama F di Maria G, Guy-Grand B and Bour H. L'association triacetyl oleandomycin-tartrate d'ergotamine. Est-elle dangereuse? Nouv Presse med (1975) 4, 2723.

12 Vayssairat M, Fiessinger J-N, Becquemin M-H and Housset E. Association dihydroergotamine et triacetyloleandomycine. Role dans une necrose digitale iatrogene. Nouv Presse med (1978) 7, 2077.

13 Matthews NT, and Havill JH. Ergotism with therapeutic doses of ergotamine tartrate. NZ Med J.(1979) 89, 476–7.

14 Meunier P, Courpron P and Vignon G. Ergotisme iatrogene aigu par association medicamenteuse diagnostique par exploration non invasive (velocimetrie a effet Doppler). Nouv Presse med (1978) 7, 2478.

15 Pessayre D, Larrey D, Funck-Brentano C and Benhamou JP. Drug interactions and hepatitis produced by some macrolide antibiotics. J Antimicrob Chemother (1985) 16, Suppl A, 181–94.

16 Grolleau JY, Martin M, De la Guerrande B, Barrier J and Peltier P. Ergotism aigu lors d'une association josamycine/tartrate d'ergotamine. Therapie (1981) 36, 319–21.

17 Bacourt F and Couffinhal J-C. Ischemie des membres par association dihydroergotamine-triacetyloleandomycine. Nouvelle observation. Nouv Presse Med (1978) 7, 1561.

Ergot + Tetracyclines

Abstract/Summary

Five patients taking ergotamine or dihydroergotamine have been reported who developed ergotism when they were additionally treated with doxycycline or tetracycline.

Clinical evidence

A woman who had previously taken ergotamine tartrate succesfully and uneventfully for 16 years, was treated with doxycycline and dihydroergotamine methane sulfonate (DHE—Sandoz), 30 drops three times a day. Five days later her hands and feet became cold and reddened, and she was diagnosed as having developed a mild form of ergotism.[1]

Other cases of ergotism, some of them more severe, have been described in patients taking ergotamine tartrate and doxycycline (one patient) or tetracycline-trypsin-alpha chymotrypsin (three patients).[2–4]

Mechanism

Unknown. One suggestion[1] is that these antibiotics may have inhibited the activity of the liver enzymes concerned with the metabolism and clearance of the ergotamine, thereby prolonging its stay in the body and enhancing its activity. One of the patients had a history of alcoholism[2] and two of them were in their eighties[4] so that their liver function may have already been reduced.

Importance and management

Information is very limited indeed. The general importance of this interaction is uncertain, but it would clearly be prudent to be on the alert for any signs of ergotism in patients given ergot derivatives and any of the tetracyclines. Impairment of liver function may possibly be a contributory factor.

References

1 Amblard P, Reymond JL, Franco A, Beani JC, Carpentier P, Lemonnier D and Bessard G. Ergotism. Forme mineure par association dihydroergotamine-chlorhydrate de doxycycline, etude capillaroscopique. Nouv Presse Med. (1978) 7, 4148.

2 Dupuy JC, Lardy Ph, Seaulau P, Kervoelen P and Paulet J. Spasmes arteriels systemiques. Tartrate d'ergotamine. Arch Mal Coeur (1978) 72, 86.

3 L'Yvonnet M, Boillot A, Jacquet AM, Barale F, Grandmottet P, Zurlinden B and Gillet JY. A propos d'un cas exceptionnel d'intoxication aigue par un derive de l'ergot de seigle. Gynecologie (1974) 30, 541.

4 Sibertin-Blanc M. Les dangers de l'ergotisme a propos de deux observations. Arch Med Ouest (1977) 9, 265.

Ethylene dibromide + Disulfiram

Abstract/Summary

The very high incidence of malignant tumours in rats exposed to both ethylene dibromide and disulfiram is the basis of the recommendation that concurrent exposure of man to these compounds should be avoided.

Clinical evidence, mechanism, importance and management

The incidence of malignant tumours in rats exposed to 20 ppm ethylene dibromide (6 h daily, five days weekly) while receiving 0.05% disulfiram is very high indeed.[1] The reasons are not understood. In addition to the precautions needed to protect workers from the toxic effects of ethylene dibromide, it has been strongly recommended that disulfiram should not be given to those who may be exposed to this compound.[2,3]

References

1 Plotnick HB. Carcinogenesis in rats of combined ethylene dibromide and disulfiram. J Amer Med Ass (1978) 239, 1609.
2 Anon. Ethylene dibromide and disulfiram toxic interaction. NIOSH Current Intelligence Bulletin (1978) 23, Apr 11. US Department of Health, Education and Welfare Publication No 78–145.
3 Yodaiken RE. Ethylene dibromide and disulfiram—a lethal combination. J Am Med Ass (1978) 239, 2783.

Famotidine, Nizatidine and Roxatidine + Other drugs

Abstract/Summary

Famotidine, nizatidine and roxatidine do not inhibit liver microsomal enzymes and what is known so far suggests that, in the context of drug interactions, they are likely to behave more like ranitidine than cimetidine.

Clinical evidence, mechanism, importance and management

Cimetidine interacts with a wide range of other drugs because it is a potent liver enzyme inhibiting agent, the effect of which is to reduce the metabolism and clearance from the body of drugs taken concurrently, thereby raising their serum levels, sometimes into the toxic range. Ranitidine on the other hand does not inhibit liver microsomal enzymes so that it interacts with far fewer drugs. Studies using antipyrine as an indicator of changes in liver enzyme activity have shown that famotidine, nizatidine and roxatidine are more like ranitidine in not inhibiting the liver microsomal enzymes (cytochrome P-450 mixed function oxidase system) which are affected by cimetidine.

For example, cimetidine increases serum theophylline levels by inhibiting its metabolism by the liver whereas famotidine and roxatidine do not.[1,6] Cimetidine also interacts with diazepam in the same way whereas famotidine, nizatidine and roxatidine do not.[2–6] Roxatidine also does not interact with propranolol.[6]

Thus in the absence of direct information about the outcome of giving famotidine, nizatidine or roxatidine with other drugs which are known to interact with cimetidine because their metabolism by the liver is reduced, the behaviour of ranitidine rather than cimetidine is likely to be the better guide.

References

1 Chremos AN, Lin JH, Yeh KC, Chiou WF, Bayne WF, Lipschutz K and Williams RL. Famotidine does not interfere with the disposition of theophylline in man: comparision with cimetidine. Clin Pharmacol Ther (1986) 39, 187.
2 Sambol NC, Upton RA, Chremos AN, Lin E, Gee W and Williams RL. Influence of famotidine and cimetidine on the disposition of phenytoin and indocyanine green. Clin Pharmacol Ther (1986) 39, 225.
3 Locniskar A, Greenblatt DJ, Harmatz JS, Zinny MA and Shader RI. Interaction of diazepam with famotidine and cimetidine, two H_2-receptor antagonists. J Clin Pharmacol(1986) 26, 299–303.
4 Klotz U, Arvela P and Rosenkranz B. Famotidine, a new H_2-receptor antagonist, does not affect hepatic elimination of diazepam or tubular secretion of procainamide. Eur J Clin Pharmacol(1985) 28, 671–5.
5 Klotz U. Lack of effect of nizatidine on drug metabolism. Scand J Gastroenterol (1987) 22 (Suppl 136) 18-23
6 Labs RA. Interaction of roxatidine acetate with antacids, food or other drugs. Drugs (1988) 35 (Suppl 3) 82–9.

Fenfluramine + Mazindol

Abstract/Summary

There is an isolated case of cardiomyopathy attributed to the use of fenfluramine and mazindol.

Clinical evidence, mechanism, importance and management

A woman of 36 developed acute cardiomyopathy while taking 40 mg fenfluramine and 1 mg mazindol daily for obesity. The problem resolved within a week of stopping both drugs and appropriate cardiac treatment with digoxin, frusemide and hydralazine.[1]

Reference

1 Gillis D, Wengrower D, Witztum E and Leitersdorf E. Fenfluramine and mazindol: acute reversible cardiomyopathy associated with their use. Int J Psychiatry Med (1985–6) 15, 197–200.

Folic acid + Sulphasalazine

Abstract/Summary

Sulphasalazine can reduce the absorption of folic acid.

Clinical evidence, mechanism, importance and management

A study in patients with ulcerative colitis and granulomatous colitis showed that their absorption of folic acid was reduced about a third (from 65.0% to 44.4%) by the inflammatory bowel disease when compared with normal subjects, and even further reduced (down to 32.0%) while taking sulphasalazine.[1] The clinical importance of this is uncertain, but it should be borne in mind when both compounds are given together.

Reference

1 Franklin JL and Rosenberg IH. Impaired folic acid absorption in inflammatory disease: effects of salicylazosulfapyridine (Azulfidine). Gastroenterology (1973) 64, 517.

Gemfibrozil + Colestipol

Abstract/Summary

Colestipol can reduce the absorption of gemfibrozil if given at the same time.

Clinical evidence

A study in 10 patients with raised serum cholesterol and triglyceride levels found that if 600 mg gemfibrozil was given alone or 2 h before or 2 h after 5 g colestipol, the serum gemfibrozil concentration curves were similar. However when given at the same time, the AUC (area under the concentration/time curve) was reduced about 30% (from 62.6 to 43.6 mg/h/l).[1]

Mechanism

Not understood. It seems probable that the colestipol binds with the gemfibrozil in the gut, thereby reducing its absorption.

Importance and management

Information is very limited and the clinical importance of this reduction in bioavailability is uncertain. However the interaction can be avoided by separating the administration of the two drugs by at least 2 h. More study is needed.

Reference

1 Forland SC, Feng Y and Cutler RE. Apparent reduced absorption of gemfibrozil when given with colestipol. J Clin Pharmacol (1990) 30, 29–32.

Gemfibrozil + Ispaghula (Psyllium)

Abstract/Summary

Psyllium causes a small, but almost certainly clinically unimportant, reduction in the absorption of gemfibrozil.

Clinical evidence, mechanism, importance and management

A study in 10 normal subjects found that when 600 mg gemfibrozil was taken together with 3 g psyllium in 240 ml water or 2 h after the psyllium, the AUC (area under the concentration/time curve) was reduced about 10%. This small change in bioavailability is almost certainly too small to matter. No special precautions would seem to be necessary.

Reference

1 Forland SC and Cutler RE. The effect of psyllium on the pharmacokinetics of gemfibrozil. Clin Res (1990) 38, 94A.

Gemfibrozil + Rifampicin

Abstract/Summary

Rifampicin appears not to interact with gemfibrozil.

Clinical evidence, mechanism, importance and management

A study in which 10 normal subjects were given 600 mg gemfibrozil before and after taking 600 mg rifampicin daily for six days showed that the pharmacokinetics of the gemfibrozil were not significantly changed by the rifampicin.[1]

Reference

1 Forland SC, Feng Y and Cutler RE. The effect of rifampin on the pharmacokinetics of gemfibrozil. J Clin Pharmacol(1988) 28, 908–959.

Glucagon + Beta-blockers

Abstract/Summary

The hyperglycaemic effects of glucagon may be reduced by propranolol.

Clinical evidence, mechanism, importance and management

A study in five normal subjects showed that the hyperglycaemic activity of glucagon was reduced to some extent in the presence of propranolol. The reason is uncertain, but one suggestion is that the propranolol inhibits the effects of the catecholamines which are released by glucagon. A similar response would be expected in patients under treatment with propranolol. Whether this is also true for other beta-blockers awaits confirmation.

Reference

1 Messerli FH, Kuchel O and Tolis G. Effects of beta-adrenergic blockage on plasma cyclic AMP and blood sugar responses to glucagon and isoproterenol in man. Int J Clin Pharmacol(1976) 14, 189.

Glyceryl trinitrate (GTN) + Anticholinergics

Abstract/Summary, clinical evidence, mechanism, importance and management

Drugs with anticholinergic effects such as the tricyclic antidepressants and disopyramide depress salivation and most patients complain of having a dry mouth. In theory sublingual glyceryl trinitrate will dissolve less readily under the tongue in these patients, thereby reducing its absorption and its effects. However no formal studies to confirm this seem to have been carried out.

Glyceryl trinitrate (GTN) + Aspirin

Abstract/Summary

Some limited evidence suggests that analgesic doses of aspirin can increase the serum levels of glyceryl trinitrate, possibly resulting in an increase in its side-effects such as hypotension and headaches.

Clinical evidence

A study in seven normal subjects found that when 0.8 mg glyceryl trinitrate (GTN, nitroglycerin) was given as a sublingual spray an hour after taking 1 g aspirin, the mean plasma GTN levels half-an-hour later were increased by 54% (from 0.24 to 0.37 ng.ml^{-1}). The haemodynamic effects of the GTN (reduced diastolic blood pressure, end-diastolic diameter and end-systolic diameter) were enhanced. Some changes were seen when 500 mg aspirin was given every two days (described as an antiaggregant dose) but the effects were not statistically significant.[1]

Mechanism

Although prostaglandin-synthetase inhibitors such as aspirin can suppress the vasodilator effects of GTN to some extent by blocking prostaglandin release, it seems that a much greater pharmacodynamic interaction also occurs in which aspirin reduces the flow of blood through the liver so that the metabolism of the glyceryl trinitrate is reduced, thus increasing its effects.

Importance and management

Information is very limited but it seems possible that patients taking GTN may experience an exaggeration of its side-effects such as hypotension and headaches if they are taking analgesic doses of aspirin. More study is needed to find out if this is of any practical importance.

Reference

1 Weber S, Rey E, Pipeau C, Lutfalla G, Richard M-O, Daoud-El-Assaf H, Olive G and Degeorges M. Influence of aspirin on the hemodynamic effects of sublingual nitroglycerin. J Cardiovasc Pharmacol(1983) 5, 874–7.

H$_2$-blockers + Antacids

Abstract/Summary

The absorption of cimetidine, ranitidine and famotidine may possibly be reduced to some extent by antacids but whether this reduces their ulcer-healing effects is uncertain. Separate the dosages by at least an hour to reduce the possibility.

Clinical evidence

(a) Cimetidine

A study in which 12 normal subjects were given 300 mg cimetidine orally four times a day, with and without 30 ml *Mylanta II*, indicated that the absorption of cimetidine was unaffected.[10]

The serum levels and urinary excretion of cimetidine were unaffected in six healthy subjects when given either 20 ml *Aludrox SA* (4.75 ml aluminium hydroxide gel + 100 mg magnesium hydroxide in every 5 ml) or two *Rennies* (80 mg light magnesium carbonate + 680 mg chalk per tablet).[1] No interaction was found in another study with an aluminium phosphate antacid.[5,12]

In contrast, a number of other single dose studies indicated that antacids reduce absorption: 30 ml *Novalucol* (6 g aluminium hydroxide + 2.5 g magnesium hydroxide in every 100 ml) reduced serum cimetidine levels by 22% (range 3–48%)[2]; *Maalox* and *Mylanta* were found to reduce peak serum cimetidine levels 40–50% and the 4 h AUC (area under the curves) were similarly reduced.[3] Reductions have been found in other studies.[4,6]

(b) Famotidine

A study in 17 normal subjects showed that *Mylanta II* reduced the absorption of famotidine to some extent.[11]

(c) Ranitidine

A study in six subjects showed that the concurrent use of 30 ml *Mylanta II* (aluminium/magnesium hydroxide mixture) reduced the peak ranitidine serum levels and the AUC (area under the curve) after a single 150 mg dose by one-third.[7]

A reduction was found in another study.[9] Another study showed that aluminium phosphate reduced the bioavailability of ranitidine by 30%.[13]

Mechanism

Not fully understood. Changes in gastric pH caused by the antacid and retarded gastric motility have been suggested.

Importance and management

A reduction in the bioavailability of famotidine and ranitidine can occur with some antacids, but none of these interactions is well established and evidence that the ulcer-healing effects are reduced to a significant extent seems to be lacking. It may prove not be necessary to take any special precautions. However until the absence of an interaction is confirmed it might be prudent to follow the general recommendation that the antacid should be given 1 h before or after the H$_2$-blocker if fasting, or 1 h after if the blocker is taken with food, in which case no significant reduction in absorption should occur.[3,8,9,11]

References

1 Burland WL, Darkin DW and Mills MW. Effect of antacids on absorption of cimetidine. Lancet (1976) ii, 965.
2 Bodemar G, Norland B and Walan A. Diminished absorption of cimetidine caused by antacids. Lancet (1979) i, 444.
3 Steinberg WM, Lewis JH and Katz DM. Antacids inhibit absorption of cimetidine. N Engl J Med (1982) 307, 400–4.
4 Russell WL, Lopez LM, Normann SA, Doering PL and Guild RT. Effect of antacids on predicted steady-state cimetidine concentrations. Dig Dis Sci (1984) 29, 385–9.
5 Albin H, Vincon G, Pehoucq F and Dangoumau J. Influence d'un antacide sur la biodisponibilite de la cimetidine. Therapie (1982) 37, 563–6.
6 Gugler R, Brand M and Somogyi A. Impaired cimetidine absorption due to antacids and metoclopramide. Eur J Clin Pharmacol(1981) 20, 225–8.
7 Mihaly GW, Marino AT, Webster LK, Jones DB, Louis WJ and Smallwood RA. High dose of antacid (*Mylanta II*) reduces the bioavailability of ranitidine. Br Med J (1982) 285, 998–9.
8 Frislid K and Berstad A. High dose antacid reduced bioavailability of ranitidine. Br Med J (1983) 286, 1358.
9 Desmond PV, Harman PJ, Gannoulis N, Kamm M and Mashford ML. The effect of antacids and food on the absorption of cimetidine and ranitidine. Gastroenterology (1986) 90, 1393.
10 Shelly DW, Doering PL, Russell WL, Guild RT, Lopez LM and Perrin J. Effect of concomitant antacid administration on plasma cimetidine concentrations during repetitive dosing. Drug Intell Clin Pharm (1986) 20, 792–5.
11 Tupy-Visich MA, Tarzian SK, Schwartz S, Lin JH, Hessey GA, Kanovsky SM and Chremos AN. Bioavailability of oral famotidine when administered with antacid or food. J Clin Pharmacol(1986) 26, 541–60.
12 Albin H, Vincon G, Demotes-Mainard F, Begaud B and Bedjaoui A. Effect of aluminium phosphate on the bioavailability of cimetidine and prednisolone. Eur J Clin Pharmacol(1984) 26, 271–3.
13 Albin H, Vincon G, Begaud B, Bistue C and Perez P. Effect of aluminium phosphate on the bioavailability of ranitidine. Eur J Clin Pharmacol(1987) 32, 97–99.

H$_2$-blockers + Sucralfate

Abstract/Summary

Sucralfate normally appears not to affect the bioavailability of cimetidine or ranitidine and there is some preliminary evidence that the healing rate may possibly be increased.

Clinical evidence, mechanism, importance and management

Most *in vitro* and human studies show that sucralfate does not affect the absorption of either cimetidine or ranitidine,[1–5] but one study found a 30% reduction in ranitidine bioavailability.[6] There is no clear reason (apart from cost) for avoiding concurrent use and there is some indication that it may possibly be valuable: sucralfate and cimetidine were not different in the rate at which they healed duodenal ulcers in eight patients and there was some evidence of a possible trend towards more rapid healing if given together.[7] More confirmatory study of this is needed.

References

1 Mullersman G, Gotz VP, Russell WL and Derendorf H. Lack of clinically significant *in vitro* and *in vivo* interactions between ranitidine and sucralfate. J Pharm Sci (1986) 75, 995–8.
2 Mullersman G, Gotz VP, Russell WL and Derendorf H. *In vitro* and *in vivo* interactions between ranitidine and sucralfate. Drug Intell Clin Pharm (1986) 20, 452.
3 Albin H, Vincon G, Lalague MC, Couzigou P and Amouretti M. Effect of sucralfate on the bioavailability of cimetidine. Eur J Clin Pharmacol(1986) 30, 493–4.
4 D'Angio R, Mayersohn M, Conrad KA and Bliss M. Cimetidine absorption in humans during sucralfate coadministration. Br J clin Pharmac (1986) 21, 515–20.
5 Beck CL, Dietz AJ, Carlson JD and Letendre PW. Evaluation of potential cimetidine sucralfate interaction. Clin Pharmacol Ther (1987) 41, 168.
6 Maconochie JG, Thomas M, Michael MF, Jenner WR and Tannger WR. Ranitidine sucralfate interaction study. Clin Pharmacol Ther (1987) 41, 205.
7 Van Deventer G, Schneidman D, Olson C and Walsh J. Comparison of sucralfate and cimetidine taken alone and in combination for treatment of active duodenal ulcers. Gastroenterology (1984) 86, 1287.

H$_2$-blockers + Tobacco smoking

Abstract/Summary

Duodenal ulcers treated with H$_2$-blockers heal less easily in smokers and are more likely to recur when treatment is over if smoking continues.

Clinical evidence, mechanism, importance and management

There is ample evidence that the healing of duodenal ulcers in those given gastric antisecretory drugs (H$_2$-blockers such as cimetidine, ranitidine, etc.) is slower than in non-smokers and recurrence is more common.[1–3] One of the reasons appears to be that smoking reduces the serum levels of these drugs although peak levels occur sooner and are higher.[4] It seems that the rate of gastric emptying is increased by smoking which has an effect on drug absorption.[4] Patients treated for ulcers should be encouraged to stop smoking, but if persuasion fails it may be necessary to increase the drug dosage.

References

1 Korman MG, Hansky J, Eaves ER and Schmidt GT. Cigarette smoking and the healing of duodenal ulcer. Gastroenterology (1982) 82, 1104.
2 Korman MG, Hetzel DJ, Hansky J, Shearman DJC, Eaves ER, Schmidt GT, Hecker R and Fitch R. Oxmetidine or cimetidine in duodenal ulcer: healing rate and effect of smoking. Gastroenterology (1982) 82, 1104.
3 Boyd EJS, Wilson JA and Wormsely KG. Smoking inhibits therapeutic gastric inhibition. Lancet (1983) i, 95.
4 Boyd EJS, Johnston DA, Wormsley KG, Jenner WN and Salanson X. The effects of cigarette smoking on plasma concentrations of gastric antisecretory drugs. Aliment Pharmacol Ther (1987) 1, 57–65.

Iron preparations + Antacids

Abstract/Summary

The absorption of iron and an expected haematological response can be reduced by the concurrent use of antacids. Separate their administration as much as possible.

Clinical evidence

(a) Magnesium trisilicate

When oral iron failed to cause an expected rise in haemoglobin levels, a study was undertaken in nine patients who were given 5 g of isotopically labelled ferrous sulphate. 35 g magnesium trisilicate reduced the absorption from an average of 30 to 12%. The reduction was small in some patients, but one individual showed a fall from 67 to 5%.[1]

(b) Aluminium and magnesium hydroxides, sodium bicarbonate and calcium carbonate

A study in 22 healthy subjects who were mildly iron deficient (due to blood donation or menstruation) showed that one teaspoonful of *Mylanta II* had little effect on the absorption at 2 h of 10 or 20 mg ferrous sulphate, whereas 1 g sodium bicarbonate almost halved the absorption and 500 mg calcium carbonate reduced it by two-thirds. Iron absorption from a multivitamin-mineral preparation was little affected by calcium carbonate.[5]

Another study found that an antacid containing aluminium and magnesium hydroxides and magnesium carbonate reduced the absorption of 15 mg ferrous sulphate and ferrous fumarate in healthy iron-replete subjects by 38 and 31% respectively.[6] Poor absorption of iron during treatment with sodium bicarbonate and aluminium hydroxide has been described elsewhere.[2,3]

Mechanism

Uncertain. One suggestion is that magnesium sulphate changes ferrous sulphate into less easily absorbed salts, or increases its polymerization.[1] Carbonates possibly cause the formation of poorly soluble iron complexes.[2] Aluminium hydroxide is believed to precipitate iron as the hydroxide and ferric ions can become intercalated into the aluminum hydroxide lattice.[4]

Importance and management

Information is limited and difficult to assess because of the many variables (different dosages, different subjects and patients), however a 'blanket precaution' to achieve maximal absorption would be to separate the administration of iron preparations and antacids as much as possible to avoid admixture in the gut. This may prove not to be necessary with some preparations.

References

1 Hall GJL and Davis AE. Inhibition of iron absorption by magnesium trisilicate. Med J Aust (1969) 2, 95.
2 Benjamin IB, Cortell S and Conrad ME. Bicarbonate-induced iron complexes and iron absorption. Gastroenterology (1967) 35, 389.
3 Rastogi SP, Padilla F and Boyd CM. Effect of aluminium hydroxide on iron absorption. Am Soc Neph (1975) 8, 21.
4 Coste JF, De Bari VA, Keil LB and Needle MA. *In vitro* interactions of oral haematinics and antacid preparations. Curr Ther Res (1977) 22, 205.
5 O'Neil-Cutting MA and Crosby WH. The effect of antacids on the absorption of simultaneously ingested iron. J Am Med Ass (1986) 255, 1468–70.
6 Ekenved G, Halvorsen L and Solvell L. Influence of a liquid antacid on the absorption of different iron salts. Scand J Haematol (1976) Suppl 28, 65–77.

Iron preparations or Vitamin B$_{12}$ + Chloramphenicol

Abstract/Summary

In addition to the serious and potentially fatal bone marrow depression which can occur with chloramphenicol, it may also cause a milder, reversible depression which can oppose the treatment of anaemia with iron or vitamin B$_{12}$.

Clinical evidence

10 out of 20 patients on iron-dextran for iron-deficiency anaemia given chloramphenicol failed to show the expected haematological response, and all four patients on vitamin B$_{12}$ for pernicious anaemia were similarly refractory until the chloramphenicol was withdrawn.[4]

Mechanism

Chloramphenicol can cause two forms of bone marrow depression. One is serious and irreversible and can result in fatal aplastic anaemia, whereas the other is probably unrelated, milder and reversible, and appears to occur at serum levels of 25 μg/ml or more. The reason is that chloramphenicol can inhibit protein synthesis, the first sign of which is a fall in the reticulocyte count which reflects inadequate red cell maturation. This response has been seen in animals,[1] normal individuals,[2] normal individuals receiving vitamin B_{12} and folic acid,[3] and in anaemic patients being treated with iron-dextran or vitamin B_{12}.[4]

Importance and management

An established interaction of clinical importance. The authors of one study recommend that dosages of 25–30 mg/kg are usually adequate for treating infections without running the risk of elevating serum chloramphenicol levels to 25 μg/ml or more when marrow depression occurs.[5] A preferable alternative would be to use a safer antibiotic. It has been claimed that the optic neuritis which sometimes occurs with chloramphenicol can be reversed with large doses of vitamins B_6 and B_{12}.[6]

References

1 Rigdon RH, Crass G and Martin A. Anemia produced by chloramphenicol (chloromycetin) in the duck. AMA Arch Pathol (1954) 58, 85.
2 McCurdy PR. Chloramphenicol bone marrow toxicity. J Amer Med Ass (1961) 176, 588.
3 Jiji RM, Gangarosa EJ and de la Marcorra F. Chloramphenicol and its sulfamoyl analogue. Report of reversible erythropoietic toxicity in healthy volunteers. Arch InternMed (1963) 111, 70.
4 Saidi P, Wallerstein RO and Aggeler PM. Effect of chloramphenicol on erythropoiesis. J Lab Clin Med (1961) 57, 247.
5 Scott JL, Finegold SM, Belkin GA and Lawrence IS. Chloramphenicol and bone marrow depression. N Engl J Med (1965) 272, 1137.
6 Cocke JC. Chloramphenicol optic neuritis. Amer J Dis Child (1967) 114, 424.

Iron preparations + Cholestyramine

Abstract/Summary

Cholestyramine binds with ferrous sulphate in the gut, thereby reducing its absorption, but the clinical importance of this is uncertain.

Clinical evidence, mechanism, importance and management

A single case report briefly describes the development of iron-deficiency anaemia in a patient with erythropoietic protoporphyria treated with cholestyramine.[1] Subsequent studies showed that cholestyramine binds with iron (as it does with many other drugs), and in rats this was found to halve the absorption from the gut of a single 100 μg dose of ferrous sulphate.[2] But nobody seems to have checked on the general clinical importance of this in patients. Until more is known it would seem prudent to separate the dosages of the iron and cholestyramine to avoid mixing in the gut, thereby minimizing the effects of this possible interaction.

References

1 Kuffin JC, Noyes WD and Porter S. Iron and cholestyramine in erythropoietic protoporphyria. Clin Res (1970) 18, 38.
2 Thomas FB, McCullough F and Greenberger NJ. Inhibition of the intestinal absorption of inorganic and hemoglobin iron by cholestyramine. J Lab Clin Med (1971) 78, 70–80.

Iron preparations + Tea

Abstract/Summary

Tea does not affect the absorption of iron given by mouth.

Clinical evidence, mechanism, importance and management

A single dose study in 10 iron-deficient anaemic children taking 2–15.8 mg/kg daily doses of iron found that tea did not affect its absorption.[1]

Reference

1 Koren G, Bolchis H and Keren G. Effects of tea on the absorption of pharmacological doses of an oral iron preparation. Isr J Med Sci (1982) 18, 547.

Liquorice + Other drugs

Abstract/Summary

Very large amounts of liquorice can cause pseudoaldosteronism which may adversely affect the treatment of cardiac failure and hypertension, and the control of body potassium levels.

Clinical evidence, mechanism, importance and management

The serum potassium levels of 11 out of 14 normal subjects fell by over 0.3 mmol/l after eating 100–200 g liquorice daily for four weeks. Four withdrew from the study because of hypokalaemia. Mild or uncomfortable oedema of the face, hands and ankles occurred in six and some of them gained weight.[1] Another previously healthy patient developed fulminant congestive heart failure after eating large amounts of liquorice for a week.[2] The reason is that liquorice contains glycyrrhizic acid which has potent mineralocorticoid properties. The conclusion to be drawn is that patients under treatment for hypertension or cardiac failure, or taking drugs which lower body potassium levels, should avoid large amounts of liquorice.

References

1 Epstein MT, Espiner EA, Donald RA and Hughes H. Effects of eating liquorice on the renin-angiotensin-aldosterone axis in normal subjects. Br Med J (1977) 1, 488.

2   Chamberlain TJ. Licorice poisoning, pseudoaldosteronism, and heart failure. J Amer Med Ass (1970) 213, 1343.

Loperamide + Cholestyramine

Abstract/Summary

An isolated report, supported by an in vitro study, indicates that the effects of loperamide can be reduced by cholestyramine. Separate the dosages as much as possible.

Clinical evidence

A man who had had extensive surgery of the gastrointestinal tract with the creation of an ileostomy needed treatment for excessive fluid loss. His fluid loss was observed to be 'substantially less' (not precisely quantified) when given loperamide alone (2 mg six-hourly) than when given in combination with cholestyramine (2 g every 4 h).[1]

Mechanism

The probable reason is that the cholestyramine, which is an ion-exchange resin, binds with the loperamide in the gut, thereby reducing its activity. An *in vitro* study using 50 ml simulated gastric fluid showed that 64% of a 5.5 mg dose of loperamide was bound by 4 g of cholestyramine.[1]

Importance and management

Direct information is limited to this report but what occurred is consistent with the way cholestyramine interacts with other drugs. It has been suggested that the two drugs should be separated as much as possible to prevent mixing in the gut, or the loperamide dosage should be increased.[1]

Reference

1   Ti TY, Giles HG and Sellers EM. Probable interaction of loperamide and cholestyramine. Can Med Ass J (1978) 119, 607.

Methoxsalen + Phenytoin

Abstract/Summary

The serum levels of methoxsalen can be markedly reduced by the concurrent use of phenytoin.

Clinical evidence

A patient with epilepsy failed to respond to treatment for psoriasis with PUVA (12 treatments of 30 mg 8-methoxypsoralen given orally and ultraviolet A irradiation) while taking 250 mg phenytoin daily. Methoxsalen serum levels were normal in the absence of phenytoin but abnormally low while taking phenytoin,[1] due, it is suggested, to the enzyme inducing effects of the phenytoin. This interaction could lead to serious erythema and blistering because the stimulant effects of the methoxsalen on the melanin pigmentation of the skin is reduced. Concurrent use should be avoided or very closely monitored.

Reference

1   Stasberg B and Hueg B. Interaction between 8-methoxpsoralen and phenytoin. Acta Derm Venereol (1985) 65, 552–3.

Metyrapone + Phenytoin

Abstract/Summary

The results of the metyrapone hypothalamic-hypophyseal function test are unreliable in patients taking phenytoin. Doubling the dose of metyrapone gives results which are close to normal.

Clinical evidence, mechanism, importance and management

A study in five normal subjects and three patients taking 300 mg phenytoin showed that their serum metyrapone levels 4 h after taking a regular 750 mg dose were very low indeed compared with a control group (6.5 compared with 48 μg/100 ml). Their response to metyrapone was proportionately lower.[1] Other reports confirm that the urinary steroid response is subnormal in patients taking phenytoin.[3,4] The reason is that phenytoin is a potent liver enzyme inducing agent which increases the metabolism of the metyrapone, thereby reducing its biological activity,[1,2] as a result of which the results of the metyrapone test for hypothalamic-hypophyseal function are invalid. Doubling the dose of metyrapone from 750 mg four-hourly to two-hourly has been shown to give results similar to those in subjects not taking phenytoin.[1]

References

1   Meikle AW, Jubiz W, Matsukura S, West CD and Tyler FH. Effect of diphenylhydantoin on the metabolism of metyrapone and release of ACTH in man. J Clin Endocrinol Metab(1969) 29, 1553.
2   Jubiz W, Levinson RA, Meikle AW, West CD and Tyler FH. Absorption and conjugation of metyrapone during diphenylhydantoin therapy: mechanism of the abnormal response to oral metyrapone. Endocrinology (1970) 86, 328.
3   Krieger DT. Effect of diphenylhydantoin on pituitary-adrenal interrelations. J Clin Endocrinol (1962) 22, 490.
4   Werk EE, Thrasher K, Choi Y and Sholiton LJ. Failure of metyrapone to inhibit 11-hydroxylation of 11-deoxycortisol during drug therapy. J Clin Endocrinol (1967) 27, 1358.

Oxygen (hyperbaric) + Acetazolamide, Barbiturates, Narcotics

Abstract/Summary, clinical evidence, mechanism, importance and management

It has been suggested, but not confirmed, that because increased levels of carbon dioxide in the tissues can increase the sensitivity to oxygen-induced convulsions, drugs such as acetazolamide which are carbonic anhydrase-inhibitors are contraindicated in those given hyperbaric oxygen. Nor should oxygen be given during narcotic or barbiturate withdrawal because the convulsive threshold of such patients is already low.[1]

Reference

1 P G. HBO can interact with pre-existing patient conditions. J Amer Med Ass (1981) 246, 1177–8.

Paraldehyde + Disulfiram

Abstract/Summary

Concurrent use should be avoided because toxic reactions seem likely.

Clinical evidence, mechanism, importance and management

It is thought that paraldehyde is depolymerized in the liver to acetaldehyde, and then oxidized by acetaldehyde dehydrogenase.[1] Since disulfiram inhibits this enzyme, concurrent use would be expected to result in the accumulation of acetaldehyde and in a modified 'antabuse' reaction,[2] but so far there appear to be no reports of this in man. In addition, alcoholics with impaired liver function are said to be sensitive to the toxic effects of paraldehyde and may show restlessness rather than sedation. These are all good reasons for avoiding concurrent use.

References

1 Hitchcock P and Nelson EE. The metabolism of paraldehyde: II. J Pharmac Exp Ther (1943) 79. 286.
2 Keplinger ML and Wells JA. Effect of antabuse on the action of paraldehyde in mice and dogs. Fed Proc (1956) 15, 445.

Piperine + Miscellaneous drugs

Abstract/Summary

Piperine can increase the bioavailability of phenytoin and other drugs.

Clinical evidence, mechanism, importance and management

A study in five normal subjects found that piperine (20 mg for seven days) increased the absorption of a single 300 mg oral dose of phenytoin (AUC + 50%) and raised the peak serum levels.[1] The significance of this is that piperine is a major alkaloid of black and long peppers (*Piper nigrum* and *longum*) both of which are used in Ayurvedic formulations, the presumption being that these plant products are empirically included to increase the bioavailability of other constituents, thereby increasing their efficacy. This report also quotes other studies showing that the piperine increases blood levels of rifampicin, sulphadiazine and tetracycline.[1] It might therefore be possible to exploit this interaction in cases where it is difficult to achieve therapeutic levels with conventional drug doses. No cases of adverse interactions seem to have been reported.

Reference

1 Bano G, Amla V, Raina RK, Zutshi U and Chopra CL. The effect of piperine on pharmacokinetics of phenytoin in healthy volunteers. Planta Medica (1987) 53, 568–9.

Pirenzepine + Cimetidine

Abstract/Summary, clinical evidence, mechanism, importance and management

The pharmacokinetics of pirenzepine and cimetidine are not affected by the presence of the other drug, but pirenzepine increases the cimetidine-induced reduction in gastric acid secretion. An apparently advantageous interaction.[1]

Reference

1 Jamali F, Mahachai V, Reilly PA and Thomson AB R. Lack of pharmacokinetic interaction between cimetidine and pirenzepine. Clin Pharmacol Ther (1985) 38, 325–30.

Pravastatin + Miscellaneous drugs

Abstract/Summary

Cholestyramine and colestipol markedly reduce the bioavailability of pravastatin if given together, but not if the dosages are well separated. No clinically significant interactions have been seen when aspirin, cimetidine, gemfibrozil, Maalox, nicotinic acid or probucol were given concurrently. Pravastatin does not interact with warfarin.

Clinical evidence, mechanism, importance and management

(a) Pravastatin + antipyrine

Antipyrine is used as a model or marker drug to find out if drugs are likely to affect the metabolism of others. A study in 24 type II hypercholesterolaemic patients given 5, 10 or 20 mg pravastatin twice daily for four weeks found that antipyrine saliva samples showed no changes in either its elimination half-life or its clearance.[1] Thus pravastatin appears not to induce or inhibit liver microsomal enzymes (cytochrome P450 system) and would not be expected to interact with other drugs commonly affected in this way (e.g. phenytoin, warfarin).

(b) Pravastatin + cholestyramine and colestipol

A study in 24 subjects found that cholestyramine reduced the bioavailability of the pravastatin by about 40% when given together, but when the pravastatin was given 1 h before or 4 h after the cholestyramine only a small and clinically insignificant reduction occurred. Similarly, colestipol in 18 subjects reduced the bioavailability of pravastatin by about 50%, but not when given 1 h before or with food.[3] It would seem that these bile acid binding resins can bind with pravastatin if they are allowed to mix together in the gut, thereby reducing its absorption. Separate the dosages of these drugs appropriately.

(c) Pravastatin + miscellaneous drugs

No clinically significant changes in the bioavailability of single 20 mg doses of pravastatin were seen in studies on the concurrent use of 600 mg gemfibrozil or 500 mg probucol in 20 normal subjects.[4] The concurrent use of *Maalox TC* (15 ml four times daily) or cimetidine (300 mg four times daily)— both given 1 h previously—was found to reduce the bioavailability of single 20 mg doses of pravastatin by 52 and 68% respectively, however the manufacturers say that it is unlikely that these changes will affect the clinical efficacy of pravastatin.[5,6] Other studies found that neither aspirin (324 mg) nor nicotinic acid (1 g) affected the bioavailability of pravastatin.[7] The manufacturers also say that during clinical trials of pravastatin no noticeable drug interactions were seen in patients taking diuretics, antihypertensives, digitalis, ACE-inhibitors, calcium channel blockers, beta-blockers or nitroglycerins.[6]

(d) Pravastatin + warfarin

10 normal subjects were given 20 mg pravastatin alone twice daily for three and a half days, 5 mg warfarin alone twice daily for six days, and then both pravastatin and warfarin together for six days. The warfarin did not alter the pharmacokinetics of pravastatin, and the anticoagulant effects of the warfarin were not significantly changed.[2]

References

1 Pan HY, Swanson BN, DeVault AR, Willard DA and Brescia D. Antipyrine elimination is not affected by chronic administration of pravastatin (SQ31,000). A tissue-selective HMG CoA reductase inhibitor. Clin Res (1988) 36, 368A.
2 Light RT, Pan HY, Glaess SR and Bakry D. A report on the pharmacokinetic and pharmacodynamic interaction of pravastatin and warfarin in healthy male volunteers. Unpublished report on file of ER Squibb. Protocol No 27, 201–59 (1988).
3 Pan HY, DeVault AR, Ivashkiv E, Whigan D, Brennan JJ and Willard DA. Pharmacokinetic interaction studies of pravastatin with bile-acid-binding resins. 8th Int Symp Atherosclerosis, October 9–13, Rome (1988), 711.
4 Pan HY, Glaess SR, Kassalow LM, Meehan RL and Martynowicz H. A report on the bioavailability of pravastatin in the presence and absence of gemfibrozil or probucol in healthy male subjects. Unpublished report on file of ER Squibb. Protocol No. 277, 201–18 (1988).
5 Marino MR, Pan HY, Bakry D, Glaess SR and Martyniwicz H. A report on the comparative pharmacokinetics of pravastatin in the presence and absence of cimetidine or antacids in healthy male subjects. Unpublished report on file of ER Squibb. Protocol No 27, 201–43 (1988).
6 Lipostat (Pravastatin) datasheet, ER Squibb (1990).
7 Pan HY, DeVault AR and Waclawski AP. A report on the effect of nicotinic acid alone and in the presence of aspirin on the bioavailability of SQ 31,000 in healthy male subjects. Unpublished report on file of ER Squibb. Protocol No 27, 201–6 (1987).

Retinoids + Tetracyclines, Vitamin A

Abstract/Summary

The development of 'pseudotumour cerebri' has been associated with the concurrent use of isotretinoin and tetracyclines. A condition similar to vitamin A overdosage may occur if isotretinoin and vitamin A are given concurrently.

Clinical evidence, mechanism, importance and management

(a) Retinoids + tetracyclines

The concurrent use of isotretinoin and a tetracycline has resulted in the development of 'pseudotumour cerebri' (i.e. a clinical picture of cranial hypertension with headache, dizziness and dysopia). By 1983 the FDA had received reports of 10 patients with pseudotumour cerebri and/or papilloedema associated with the use of isotretinoin. Four had retinal haemorrhages. Five of the 10 were also being treated with a tetracycline.[2] The manufacturers (Hoffman La Roche) also have similar reports on file of three patients given isotretinoin and either minocycline or tetracycline.[3] The same reaction has been seen in two patients given etretinate with minocycline or prednisolone.[4] A possible reason for this reaction is that the two drugs have an additive effect in increasing intracranial pressure. Be alert for the development of this adverse response if these drugs are used.

(b) Retinoids + vitamin A

Combined treatment may result in a condition similar to overdosage with vitamin A, for which reason concurrent use should be avoided or very closely monitored because changes in bone structure can occur, including premature fusion of the epiphyseal disc in children.[1]

References

1 Milstone LM, McGuire J and Ablow RC. Premature epiphyseal closure in a child receiving oral 13-cis-retinoic acid. J Am Acad Dermatol (1982) 7, 663–6.
2 Adverse effects with isotretinoin. FDA Drug Bull (1983) 13, 21–3. Quoted verbatim in J Amer Acad Dermatol (1984) 10, 519–20.
3 Hoffmann La Roche, data on file. Quoted by Shalita AR, Cunningham WJ, Leyden JJ, Pochi PE and Strauss JS. Isotretinoin treatment of acne and related disorders; an update. J Amer Acad Dermatol (1983) 9, 629–38.
4 Viraben R, Matthieu C and Fonton B. Benign intracranial hypertension during etretinate therapy for mycosis fungoides. J Amer Acad Dermatol (1985) 13, 515–17.

Roxatidine + Antacids and Food

Abstract/Summary

Neither food nor Maalox interacts to an important extent with roxatidine.

Clinical evidence, mechanism, importance and management

A study in 10 normal subjects given 150 mg roxatidine found that food slightly delayed but increased the peak serum levels, but the extent of the absorption (bioavailability) was unchanged.[1] Another study in 24 normal subjects found that two tablespoons of *Maalox* (aluminium and magnesium hydroxides) four times daily had no clinically important effects on the absorption of 150 mg roxatidine.[1]

References

1 Labs RA. Interaction of roxatidine acetate with antacids, food and other drugs. Drugs (1988) 35 (Suppl 3) 82–9.

Simvastatin + Miscellaneous drugs

Abstract/Summary

Simvastatin causes a small but probably clinically unimportant increase in the serum levels of digoxin. It appears not to interact with beta-blockers, calcium antagonists, diuretics or NSAID's.

Clinical evidence, mechanism, importance and management

A study found that the serum digoxin levels were slightly raised (+0.3 ng/ml) by simvastatin. This appears to be of little or no clinical importance. In clinical studies no interaction was seen with propranolol or other beta-blockers, calcium antagonists, diuretics or non-steroidal anti-inflammatory drugs. Simvastatin also has little effect on the pharmacokinetics of antipyrine in hypercholesterolaemic patients which suggests that simvastatin is unlikely to interact with other drugs which use the same metabolic pathway in the liver.[1,2]

References

1 ZOCOR (simvastatin) data sheet (MSD). February 1989.
2 ZOCOR information booklet (MSD) 1989.

Sodium polystyrene sulphonate + Antacids

Abstract/Summary

The concurrent use of antacids with sodium polystyrene sulphonate can result in metabolic alkalosis.

Clinical evidence, mechanism, importance and management

A man with metabolic acidosis developed metabolic alkalosis when given 90 g sodium polystyrene sulphonate with 90 ml magnesium hydroxide mixture.[1] Alkalosis has also been described in a study on a number of patients given this cation exchange resin with *Maalox* (magnesium-aluminium hydroxides) and calcium carbonate.[2] The suggested reason is that the sodium polystyrene sulphonate and magnesium react together within the gut to form magnesium polystyrene sulphonate and sodium chloride. As a result the normal neutralization of the bicarbonate ions by the gastric juice and the resin within the gut fails to occur, resulting in the absorption of the bicarbonate leading to metabolic alkalosis. This interaction appears to be established. Concurrent use should be undertaken with caution and serum electrolytes should be closely monitored. Administration of the resin rectally as an enema can avoid the problem.

References

1 Fernandez PC and Kovnat PJ. Metabolic acidosis reversed by the combination of magnesium and a cation-exchange resin. N Engl J Med (1972) 286, 23.
2 Schroeder ET. Alkalosis resulting from combined administration of a 'non-systemic' antacid and a cation-exchage resin. Gastroenterology (1969) 56, 868.

Sodium polystyrene sulphonate + Sorbitol

Abstract/Summary

Potentially fatal colonic necrosis may occur if sodium polystyrene sulphonate is given as an enema with sorbitol.

Clinical evidence

Five patients with uraemia developed severe colonic necrosis after being given enemas containing sodium polystyrene sulphonate and sorbitol. Four of the five died as a result. Associated studies in rats made uraemic found that all of them died over a two-day period after being given enemas of sodium polystyrene sulphonate with sorbitol, but none died after enemas without sorbitol. Extensive haemorrhage and transmural necrosis developed.[1]

Mechanism

Not understood.

Importance and management

Information is very limited and the interaction is not firmly established, nevertheless its seriousness suggests that sodium polystyrene sulphonate should not be given as an enema in aqueous vehicles containing sorbitol. More study is needed.

Reference

1 Lillemore KD, Romolo JI, Hamiltion SR, Pennington LR, Burdick JF and Williams GM. Intestinal necrosis due to sodium polystyrene (Kayexalate) in sorbitol enemas: clinical and experimental support for the hypothesis. Surgery (1987) 101, 266.

Somatropin (human growth hormone) + Miscellaneous hormones

Abstract/Summary

The glucocorticoid corticosteroids can oppose the effects of somatropin. Somatropin opposes the hypoglycaemic effects of insulin and may also reduce thyroid function.

Clinical evidence, mechanism, importance and management

Large doses of glucocorticoid corticosteroids can inhibit the growth stimulating effects of somatropin. Close monitoring of concurrent use is needed.[1] Somatropin raises blood sugar levels. The control of blood sugar levels in diabetic children will therefore need to be closely monitored if somatotropin and insulin are used concurrently.[1] Somatropin can cause the development of hypothyroidism which can reduce the growth stimulating effects of somatotropin. Monitor the thyroid function and administer thyroid hormone if necessary.[1]

Reference

1 Humatrope (somatotropin). Data sheet, Lilley (1989).

Sulphinpyrazone + Flufenamic, Meclofenamic or Mefenamic acid

Abstract/Summary, clinical evidence, mechanism, importance and management

The uricosuric effects of sulphinpyrazone are not opposed by the concurrent use of flufenamic acid, meclofenamic acid or mefenamic acid.[1,2]

References

1 Latham BA, Radcliff F and Robinson RG. The effect of mefenamic acid and flufenamic acid on plasma uric acid levels. Ann Phys Med (1966) 8, 242.
2 Robinson RG and Radcliff FJ. The effect of meclofenamic acid on plasma uric acid levels. Med J Aust (1972) 1, 1079–80.

Sulphinpyrazone + Probenecid

Abstract/Summary

Probenecid reduces the loss of sulphinpyrazone in the urine, but the uricosuria remains unaltered.

Clinical evidence, mechanism, importance and management

A study in eight gouty patients showed that while probenecid was able to inhibit the renal tubular excretion of sulphinpyrazone, reducing it by about 75%, the maximal uric acid clearance seen with each drug alone remained unchanged. There would therefore seem to be no advantage in using these drugs together. Whether the toxic effects of sulphinpyrazone are increased seems not to have been studied.

Reference

1 Perel JM, Dayton PG, McMillan PG, Snell M, Yu TF and Gutman AB. Studies of interactions among drugs in man at the renal level: probenecid and sulphinpyrazone. Clin Pharmacol Ther (1969) 10, 834.

Thyroid hormones + Anticonvulsants

Abstract/Summary

An isolated report describes a reduction in the effects of thyroxine when phenytoin was given. Both carbamazepine and phenytoin can reduce serum thyroid hormone levels but clinical hypothyroidism seems to be rare.

Clinical evidence

A patient with hypothyroidism, successfully treated with 0.15 mg thyroxine daily for four years, became hypothyroidic again when given 300 mg phenytoin daily. Doubling the thyroxine dosage proved to be effective. A later study in this patient during which the phenytoin was withdrawn and then restarted confirmed this interaction.[1]

A number of other reports describe very significant reductions in serum thyroid hormone levels in considerable numbers of subjects and patients when treated with phenytoin or carbamazepine,[3–6] but there seem to be only two cases in which hypothyroidism (reversible) has been seen, one with carbamazepine and phenytoin and the other with carbamazepine alone.[2]

There is also a report attributing arrhythmia to the use of phenytoin in a hypothyroidic patient with rheumatic heart disease,[7] but this report was later criticized by others as being inaccurate and misleading.[8,9]

Mechanism

Both phenytoin and carbamazepine can increase the metabolism of the thyroid hormones, thereby reducing their serum levels.

Importance and management

Despite very clear evidence that both carbamazepine and phenytoin can cause a marked reduction in serum thyroid hormone levels, the development of clinical hypothyroidism seems to be very rare and there seems to be only one case on record (cited above). There seems to be little reason for avoiding the concurrent use of thyroid hormones and either phenytoin or carbamazepine, but the outcome should be monitored. Increase the thyroid dosage if necessary. See also 'Thyroid hormones + Barbiturates'.

References

1 Blackshear JL, Schultz AL, Napier JS and Stuart DD. Thyroxine replacement requirements in hypothyroid patients receiving phenytoin. Ann InternMed (1983) 99, 341.
2 Aanderud S and Strandjord RE. Hypothyroidism induced by anti-epileptic therapy. Acta NeurolScand (1980) 61, 330–2.
3 Hansen JM, Skovsted L, Lauridsen UB, Kirkegaard C and Siersbaek-Nielsen K. The effect of diphenylhydantoin on thyroid function. J Clin Endocrinol Metab(1974) 39, 785.
4 Oppenheimer JH, Fisher LV, Nelson KM and Jailer JW. Depression of the serum protein-bound iodine level by diphenylhydantoin. J Clin Endocrinol Metab(1961) 21, 252–62.
5 Rootwelt K, Ganes T and Johannessen SI. Effect of carbamazepine phenytoin and phenobarbitone on serum levels of thyroid hormones and thyrotropin in humans. Scand J Clin Lab Invest (1978) 38, 731–6.
6 Connell JMC, Rapeport WG, Gordon S and Brodie MJ. Changes in circulating thyroid hormones during short-term hepatic enzyme induction with carbamazepine. Eur J Clin Pharmacol(1984) 26, 453–6.
7 Fulop M, Widrow DR, Colmes RA and Epstein EJ. Possible diphenylhydantoin-induced arrhythmia in hypothyroidism. J Amer Med Ass (1966) 196, 454–7.
8 Farzan S. Diphenylhydantoin and arrhythmia. J Amer Med Ass (1966) 197, 63.
9 Gaspar HL. Diphenylhydantoin and arrhythmia. J Amer Med Ass (1966) 197, 63.

Thyroid Hormones + Barbiturates

Abstract/Summary

An isolated report describes a reduction in the response of a woman to thyroxine when treated with a barbiturate hypnotic.

Clinical evidence, mechanism, importance and management

An elderly woman on 0.3 mg L-thyroxine daily for hypothyroidism complained of severe breathlessness within a week of reducing her nightly dose of *Tuinal* (quinalbarbitone sodium 199 mg + amylobarbitone sodium 100 mg) from two capsules to one. She was subsequently found to be thyrotoxic. She became symptom-free once again when the dosage of the thyroxine was halved.[1] The reason is not understood, but an animal study showed that barbiturates increase the turnover of thyroxine by increasing its hepatocellular binding.[2] The general importance of this interaction is uncertain, but be alert for any evidence of changes in thyroid status if barbiturates are added or withdrawn from patients being treated for hypothyroidism.

References

1 Hoffbrand BI. Barbiturate/thyroid-hormone interaction. Lancet (1970) ii, 903.
2 Oppenheimer JH, Bernstein G and Surks MI. Increased thyroxine turnover and thyroidal function after stimulation of hepatocellular binding of thyroxine by phenobarbital. J Clin Invest (1968) 47, 1399.

Thyroid hormones + Cholestyramine

Abstract/Summary

The absorption of thyroid extract, levothyroxine and tri-iodothyronine from the gut is reduced by the concurrent use of cholestyramine. Separate the dosages by 4–5 h.

Clinical evidence

Prompted by the observation of a hypothyroidic patient under treatment with thyroxine whose basal metabolic rate fell when given cholestyramine, a further study was made on two similar patients taking 60 mg thyroid extract or 100 μg levothyroxine sodium daily, and on five normal subjects. When they were given 4 g cholestyramine four times daily their absorption of thyroxine[131] was reduced and the amount remaining in the faeces was roughly doubled. One of the patients showed a worsening of her hypothyroidism. Separating the dosages by 4–5 h reduced the interaction to a minimum.[1]

Mechanism

Cholestyramine binds to thyroxine in the gut, thereby reducings its absorption. Since thyroxine probably also takes part in the entero-hepatic shunt (after absorption it is resecreted in the bile), continued contact with the cholestyramine is possible.

Importance and management

An established interaction (although the documentation is very limited) and of clinical importance. *In vitro* tests show that tri-iodothyronine interacts similarly.[1] The effects can be minimized by separating the dosages by 4–5 h, even so the outcome should be monitored so that any necessary thyroid hormone dosage adjustments can be made.

Reference

1 Northcutt RC, Stiel JN, Hollifield JW and Stant EG. The influence of cholestyramine on thyroxine absorption. J Amer Med Ass (1969) 208, 1857.

Thyroid hormones + Lovastatin

Abstract/Summary

An isolated report describes raised serum thyroid hormone levels and evidence of thyrotoxicosis in a patient on levothyroxine when given lovastatin.

Clinical evidence, mechanism, importance and management

A 54-year-old diabetic taking 20 mg levothyroxine daily and a number of other drugs (gemfibrozil, clofibrate, propranolol, diltiazem, quinidine, aspirin, dipyridamole, insulin) was started on 20 mg lovastatin daily. Weakness and muscle aches developed within 2–3 days and over a 27-day period he lost 10% of his body weight. His serum thyroxine levels rose from 11.3 to 27.2 μg/dl. The reasons are not understood but the author of the report postulated that the lovastatin may have displaced the thyroid hormones from their binding sites, thereby causing this thyrotoxic state.[1]

The general importance of this interaction is uncertain, but the thyroid status should be monitored if lovastatin is added or discontinued in any patient receiving thyroid hormone treatment.

Reference

1 Lustgarten BP. Catabolic response to lovastatin therapy. Ann InternMed (1988) 109, 171–2.

Thyroid hormones + Rifampicin (Rifampin)

Abstract/Summary

A case report suggests the possibility that rifampicin might reduce the effects of the thyroid hormones.

Clinical evidence, mechanism, importance and management

A woman with Turner syndrome who had had total thyroidectomy and who was being treated with 0.1 mg L-thyroxine daily, showed a marked fall in serum thyroxine levels and free thyroxine index with a dramatic rise in serum thyrotropin levels when given rifampicin. However no symptoms of clinical hypothyroidism developed.[1] A possible reason for the changes seen is that rifampicin is a potent enzyme inducing agent which can markedly increase the metabolism of many drugs, thereby increasing their loss from the body and reducing their effects. Rifampicin given to normal subjects also reduces endogenous serum thyroxine levels. There seem to be no reports of adverse effects in patients given both drugs but it would seem prudent to monitor the effects of concurrent use.

Reference

1 Isley WL. Effect of rifampicin therapy on thyroid function tests in a hypothyroidic patient on replacement L-thyroxine. Ann InternMed (1987) 107, 517–18.

Total parenteral nutrition + Potassium-sparing diuretics

Abstract/Summary

Metabolic acidosis occurred in two patients receiving total parenteral nutrition which was attributed to the use of triamterene or amiloride.

Clinical evidence, mechanism, importance and management

A report describes the development of metabolic acidosis in two patients receiving total parenteral nutrition associated with the concurrent use of triamterene and amiloride. The cases were complicated by a number of pathological and other factors, but the suggestion is that the major reason for the acidosis was because these diuretics prevented the kidneys from responding normally to the acid load. Caution is advised during concurrent use.[1]

Reference

1 Kushner RF and Sitrin MD. Metabolic acidosis. Development in two patients receiving a potassium-sparing diuretic and total parenteral nutrition. Arch InternMed (1986) 146, 343–5.

Trimoprostil + Antacids

Abstract/Summary, clinical evidence, mechanism, importance and management

The bioavailability of trimoprostil is not affected by **Mylanta I, Di-Gel** *or food.*[1]

Reference

1 Wills RJ, Rees MMC, Rubio F, Gibson DM, Givens S, Parsonnet M and Gallo-Torres HE. Influence of antacids on the bioavailability of trimoprostil. Eur J Clin Pharmacol(1984) 27, 251–2.

Vitamin A + Aminoglycoside antibiotics

Abstract/Summary

Neomycin can markedly reduce the absorption of vitamin A from the gut.

Clinical evidence, mechanism, importance and management

A study in five normal subjects showed that 2 g neomycin markedly reduced the absorption of a test dose of vitamin A (retinyl palmitate) due, it is suggested, to a direct chemical interference between the neomycin and bile and fatty acids in the gut which disrupts the absorption of fats and fat-soluble vitamins.[1] The extent to which chronic treatment with neomycin (or other aminoglycosides) would impair the treatment of vitamin A deficiency has not been determined.

Reference

1 Barrowman JA, D'Mello A amd Herxheimer A. A single dose of neomycin impairs absorption of vitamin A (Retinol) in man. Eur J clin Pharmacol(1973) 5, 199.

Vitamin C (Ascorbic acid) + Aspirin

Abstract/Summary

Aspirin reduces the absorption of ascorbic acid by about a third.

Clinical evidence, mechanism, importance and management

Studies in guinea pigs and man have shown that 900 mg aspirin reduces the absorption of ascorbic acid (single 500 mg doses) from the gut by about a third, and reduces the urinary excretion by about a half.[1] The clinical importance of this is uncertain, but in view of the increased ascorbic acid requirements in conditions such as rheumatoid arthritis and the common cold, both of which are often treated with aspirin, there may be a case for increasing the intake of ascorbic acid. One suggestion is an increase from the normal physiological requirement of 30–60 mg to 100–200 mg daily. More study is needed. Studies in man have shown that ascorbic acid does not significantly affect serum salicylate levels.[2]

References

1 Basu TK. Vitamin C—aspirin interactions. Int J Vitam Nutr Res (1982) Suppl 23, 83–90.
2 Hansten PD and Hayton WL. Effect of antacids and ascorbic acid on serum salicylate concentration. J Clin Pharmacol(1980) 24, 326.

Vitamin D + Phenytoin

Abstract/Summary

The long-term use of phenytoin and other anticonvulsants can disturb vitamin D and calcium metabolism which may result in osteomalacia. There are a few reports of patients taking vitamin D supplements who responded poorly while taking phenytoin. Serum phenytoin levels are not altered.

Clinical evidence

(a) Effect of phenytoin on vitamin D

A 16-year-old with grand mal epilepsy and under treatment for idiopathic hypoparathyroidism failed to respond adequately to daily doses of 10 μg 1-alpha-hydroxycholecalciferol and 6–12 g calcium, apparently due to the concurrent use of 200 mg phenytoin and 500 mg primidone daily. Replacement with 0.6–2.4 mg dihydrotachysterol daily produced a satisfactory response.[1]

Two other reports describe patients whose response to vitamin D was poor because of concurrent anticonvulsant treatment with phenytoin.[2,5] Other reports clearly show that while taking phenytoin the serum levels of vitamin D are reduced.[6–8]

(b) Effect of vitamin D on phenytoin

A controlled trial on 151 epileptic patients on phenytoin and calcium showed that the addition of 2000 IU vitamin D2 daily over a three-month period had no significant effect on serum phenytoin levels.[4]

Mechanism

The well-recognized enzyme-inducing effects of phenytoin and other anticonvulsants increase the metabolism of the vitamin D, thereby reducing its effects and disturbing the calcium metabolism.[3] In addition the phenytoin may possibly reduce the absorption of the calcium from the gut.[1]

Importance and management

The disturbance of calcium metabolism by phenytoin and other anticonvulsants is very well established but there are only a few reports describing a poor response to vitamin D. The effects of concurrent treatment should be well monitored. Those who need vitamin D supplements may probably need greater than usual doses.

References

1 Rubinger D, Korn-Lubetzki I, Feldman S and Popovtzer MM. Delayed response to 1-alpha-cholecalciferol therapy in a case of hypo-parathyroidism during anticonvulsant therapy. Isr J Med Sci (1980) 16, 772.
2 Asherov J, Weinberger A and Pinkhas H. Lack of response to vitamin D therapy in a patient with hypoparathyroidism under anticonvulsant drugs. Helv Pediatr Acta (1977) 32, 369.
3 Chan JCM, Oldham SB, Holick MF and DeLuca HF. One alpha-hydroxyvitamin D3 in chronic renal failure. A potent analogue

of the kidney hormone 1,25-dihydroxycholecalciferol. J Amer Med Ass (1975) 234, 47.

4 Christiansen D and Redbro P. Effect of vitamin D2 on serum phenytoin. A controlled therapeutic trial. Acta NeurolScand (1974) 50, 661.

5 McLaren N and Lifschitz F. Vitamin D-dependency rickets in institutionalized, mentally retarded children on long-term anticonvulsant therapy. III. The response to 25-hydroxycholecalciferol and to vitamin D2. Pediatr Res (1973) 7, 914–22.

6 Mosekilde L and Melsen F. Anticonvulsant osteomalacia determined by quantitative analyses of bone changes. Population study and possible risk factors. Acta Med Scand (1976) 199, 349–55.

7 Hahn TJ and Avioli LV. Anticonvulsant osteomalacia. Arch InternMed (1975) 135, 997–1000.

8 Hunter J, Maxwell JD, Stewart DA, Parson V and Williams R. Altered calcium metabolism in epileptic children on anticonvulsants. Br Med J (1971) 4, 202–4.

Vitamin K + Gentamicin and Clindamycin

Abstract/Summary

Seven patients in intensive care failed to respond to intravenous vitamin K for hypoprothrombinaemia while receiving gentamicin and clindamycin.

Clinical evidence, mechanism, importance and management

Some patients, particularly those in intensive care[1,2] who are not eating, can quite rapidly develop acute vitamin K deficiency which leads to prolonged prothrombin times and possibly bleeding. This can normally be controlled by giving vitamin K parenterally. However one report[2] describes seven such patients, all with normal liver function, who unexpectedly failed to respond to vitamin K. Examination of their records showed that all were receiving gentamicin/clindamycin. Just why these antibiotics oppose the effects of vitamin K is not understood, but it would seem prudent to avoid the use of these particular antibiotics wherever possible in patients within this category. More study is needed.

References

1 Ham JM. Hypoprothrombinaemia in patients undergoing prolonged intensive care. Med J Aust (1971) 2, 716.

2 Rodriguez-Erdmann F, Hoff JV and Carmody G. Interaction of antibiotics with vitamin K. J Amer Med Ass (1981) 246, 937.

X-ray contrast media + Calcium channel blockers

Abstract/Summary

The hypotensive effects of intravenous bolus doses of ionic X-ray contrast media are increased by the presence of calcium channel blockers (diltiazem, nifedipine, verapamil, etc.). No interaction or only a small interaction appears to occur with non-ionic contrast media. A case report describes serious ventricular tachycardia in a patient on prenylamine when given sodium iothalamate.

Clinical evidence, mechanism, importance and management

(a) Hypotensive effects increased

It is well recognized that ionic X-ray contrast media used for ventriculography reduce the systemic blood pressure due to peripheral vasodilation. They also have a direct depressant effect on the heart muscle. A comparative study of the haemodynamic response of 65 patients showed that the hypotensive effect of a bolus dose of an ionic agent (0.5 ml/kg diatrizoate meglumine and diatrizoate sodium with edetate sodium or disodium) was increased by the concurrent use of nifedipine or diltiazem: it occurred earlier (3.1 s instead of 12.9 s), was more profound (a fall in systolic pressure of 48.4 instead of 36.9 mm Hg) and more prolonged (62 s instead of 36 s).[1] A similar interaction was seen in dogs given verapamil.[2] No interaction or only a minimal interaction was seen in the patients and dogs when non-ionic contrast media (iopamidol or iohexol) were used instead.[1,2]

(b) Ventricular arrhythmia precipitated

An elderly man who had been taking 60 mg prenylamine and 10 mg nifedipine three times a day for two years experienced cardiorespiratory arrest a few seconds after a bolus intravenous injection of 80 ml sodium iothalamate 70% (*Conray 420*), and a further arrest 90 seconds later. On the second occasion the rhythm was identified as ventricular tachycardia, converted to sinus rhythm by a 100 Joule DC shock.[3] The reason is thought to be the additive effects of the prenylamine and sodium iothalamate both of which can prolong the QTC (corrected QT interval of the heart) which predisposes the development of serious ventricular arrhythmias. Concurrent use should be avoided. The manufacturers of sodium iothalamate also advise the avoidance of hypokalaemia and of drugs such as procainamide and quinidine which also tend to prolong the QTC interval.

References

1 Morris DL, Wisneski JA, Gertz EW, Wexman M, Axelrod R and Langberg JJ. Potentiation by nifedipine and diltiazem of the hypotensive response after contrast angiography. J Am Coll Cardiol (1985) 6, 785–91.

2 Higgins CB, Kuber M and Slutsky RA. Interaction between verapamil and contrast media in coronary arteriography: comparison of standard ionic and new non-ionic media. Circulation (1983) 68. 628–35.

3 Duncan JS and Ramsay LE. Ventricular tachycardia precipitated by sodium iothalamate (Contray 420) injection during prenylamine treatment: a predictable adverse drug interaction. Postgrad Med J (1985) 61, 415–7.

X-ray contrast media + Cholestyramine

Abstract/Summary

A single report describes poor radiographic visualization of the gall bladder in a man due to an interaction between iopanoic acid and cholestyramine within the gut.

Clinical evidence, mechanism, importance and management

A cholecystogram of a man on cholestyramine with postgastrectomy syndrome who was given oral iopanoic acid as an X-ray contrast medium, suggested that he had an abnormal and apparently collapsed gall bladder. A week after stopping the cholestyramine a repeat cholecystogram gave excellent visualization of a gall bladder of normal appearance.[1] The same effects have been observed experimentally in dogs.[2] The reason seems to be that the cholestyramine binds with the iopanoic acid in the gut so that little is absorbed and little is available for secretion in the bile. Hence the poor visualization of the gall bladder.

On the basis of reports about other drugs which similarly bind to cholestyramine, it seems probable that this interaction could be avoided if the administration of the iopanoic acid and the cholestyramine were to be separated as much as possible. Whether other oral acidic X-ray contrast media such as iobenzamic acid, ioglycamic acid, iophenoxic acid, iothalamic acid and others bind in a similar way to cholestyramine is uncertain, but this possibility should be considered.

References

1 Nelson JA. Effect of cholestyramine on teleopaque oral cholecystography. Am J Roentgenol Radium Ther Nucl (1974) 122, 333.
2 Berk RN. Cited as a personal communication in ref 1.

X-ray contrast media + Phenothiazines

Abstract/Summary

Two isolated case reports describe epileptiform reactions in two patients when metrizamide was used in the presence of chlorpromazine and dixyrazine.

Clinical evidence, mechanism, importance and management

A patient on chronic treatment with 75 mg chlorpromazine daily had grand mal seizures three and a half hours after being given metrizamide (16 ml of 170 mg iodine per ml) by the lumbar route. 5 h later he had another seizure.[1] One out of 34 other patients demonstrated epileptogenic activity on the EEG when given metrizamide for lumbar myelography. He was taking 10 mg dixyrazine three times daily.[2] A clinical study of 77 patients given levomepromazine for the relief of lumbago-sciatic pain found no evidence of an increased risk of epilepsy after receiving metrizamide.[3]

References

1 Hindmarsh T, Grepe A and Widen L. Metrizamide-phenothiazine interaction. Report of a case with seizures following myelography. Acta Radiol Diag (1975) 16, 129.
2 Hindmarsh T. Lumbar myelography with meglumine locarinate and metrizamide. A double-blind investigation. Acta Radiol Diag (1975) 16, 24.
3 Standnes B, Oftedal S-I and Weber H. Effect of levopromazine on EEG and on clinical side-effects after lumbar myelography with metrizamide. Acta Radiol Diag (1982) 23, 111–14.

INDEX

This index lists all of the pairs of drugs discussed in the text of this book which are known to interact in man, or not to interact, but not those where the interactions are speculative or based solely on the results of experiments in animals. The only exception to this being the possible interactions of some of the cytotoxic drugs. Double check the index by looking up the names of both drugs in which you are interested, and possibly their group names as well.

You can possibly get a lead on the way an unlisted pair of drugs behaves if you look up the group names of the drugs or one of their related drugs, but you should bear in mind that even closely related drugs are not identical and therefore any conclusion reached should only be tentative.

In order to keep the index to a manageable size, most brand names have been avoided except for some compound preparations which are printed in italics. Tables of international brand names/generic names are included in the introductory sections of most chapters. You can find these tables by looking up the group names of the drugs in question (e.g. Anticoagulants, Anticonvulsants etc).

Antilymphocytic globulin
+Tubocurarine 529
Antimalarials, *see also* individual drugs
+Antacids 110
+Antidiarrhoeals 110
+Contraceptives, oral 335
+Hypoglycaemic agents 428
+Kaolin 110
+Magnesium trisilicate 110
+Phenothiazines 504
Antimicrobials, *see* individual drugs
Antineoplastics, *see* Cytotoxics and individual drugs
Antiparkinson drugs, *see also* individual drugs
Generic and brand names 290, 291
+Betel nuts 292
Antipsychotics, *see* individual drugs
+Encainide 79
Antipyrine, *see* Phenazone
Antirheumatic agents, *see* individual drugs
Generic and brand names 39, 40
Antischistosomals
+Contraceptives, oral 335
Antituberculars, *see* individual drugs
Apomorphine
+Clonidine 268
Appetite suppressants, *see also* individual drugs
+Monoamine oxidase inhibitors 549
Aprindine
+Amiodarone 76
Aprobarbitone
+Dicoumarol 164
Aprotinin
+Neuromuscular blockers 522
+Suxamethonium 522
Ascorbic acid, *see* Vitamin C
Aspartame
+Anticonvulsants 215
+Phenytoin 215
+Warfarin 183
Asparaginase, *see* Colaspase
Aspirin (acetylsalicylic acid)
+Acetazolamide 42
+Alcohol 17
+Aluminium hydroxide 41
+Aminosalicylic acid (PAS) 108
+Antacids 41
+Anticoagulants 163
+Atenolol 314
+Benzbromarone 603
+Benzylpenicillin 134
+Betamethasone 43
+Calcium channel blockers 325
+Captopril 263
+Carbonic anhydrase inhibitors 42
+Charcoal 605
+Chlorpropamide 429
+Cimetidine 42
+Colestipol 608
+Corticosteroids 43, 443
+Dexamethasone 43
+Dichlorphenamide 42
+Dicoumarol 163

+Diflunisal 47
+Digoxin 376
+Food 43
+Glyceryl trinitrate (GTN) 614
+H2-blockers 42
+Heparin 211
+Indomethacin 50
+Insulin 429
+Interferon 122
+Isoxicam 52
+IUD's 341
+Levamisole 43
+Lithium carbonate 469
+*Maalox* 42
+Magnesium hydroxide 41
+Meclofenamic acid 53
+Methotrexate 362
+Methylprednisolone 43
+Misoprostol 44
+Nabumetone 57
+Naproxen 57
+Nefopam 59
+Nicoumalone (acenocoumarol) 163
+Phenylbutazone 44
+Phenytoin 236
+Pindolol 314
+Pravastatin 619
+Prednisone 43
+Probenecid 44
+Propranolol 314
+Prostaglandins 44
+Pyrazinamide 137
+Quinidine 93
+Ranitidine 42
+Sodium bicarbonate 41
+Sodium valproate 257
+Spironolactone 285
+Sucralfate 60
+Sulphinpyrazone 45
+Triamcinolone 43
+Verapamil 325
+Vitamin C (ascorbic acid) 625
+Warfarin 163
+Zidovudine 154
Astemizole
+Alcohol 16
Atenolol, *see also* Beta-blockers
+Alcohol 305
+Allopurinol 305
+Aluminium hydroxide 305
+Amiodarone 74
+Aspirin 314
+Caffeine 321
+Calcium carbonate 305
+Calcium gluconate 305
+Cimetidine 308
+Clonidine 267
+Diazepam 491
+Disopyramide 77
+Fluvoxamine 588
+Food 313
+Imidazole salicylate 314
+Indomethacin 314
+Insulin 413
+Ketanserin 280
+Lignocaine (lidocaine) 82
+Magnesium carbonate 305
+Magnesium hydroxide 305
+Neostigmine 306

+Nicoumalone (acenocoumarol) 167
+Nifedipine 316
+Penicillins 317
+Phenprocoumon 167
+Prazosin 283
+Prenylamine 328
+Ranitidine 319
+Terbutaline 541
+Tobacco smoking 321
+Verapamil 322
+Warfarin 167
Atracurium, *see also* Neuromuscular blockers
+Beta-blockers 523
+Diazepam 523
+Enflurane 516
+Isoflurane 516
+Lorazepam 523
+Lormetazepam 523
+Midazolam 523
+Nitrous oxide 516
+Phenytoin 534
Atropine
+Alcohol 16
+Diazepam 491
+Ritrodrine 553
Attapulgite-pectin
+Phenothiazines 504
+Promazine 504
Azapropazone
+Antacids 45
+Anthraquinone laxatives 45
+Anticoagulants 164
+Bisacodyl 45
+Chloroquine 45
+Digitoxin 376
+Dihydroxyaluminium sodium carbonate 45
+Frusemide (furosemide) 273
+Hypoglycaemic agents 412
+Magnesium aluminium silicate 45
+Methotrexate 362
+Phenytoin 237
+Tolbutamide 412
+Warfarin 164
Azathioprine, *see also* Mercaptopurine
+Allopurinol 345
+ACE inhibitors 261
+Captopril 261
+Cotrimoxazole 346
+Cyclosporin 450
+Doxorubicin (adriamycin) 346
+Trimethoprim 346
+Tubocurarine 529
Azathioprine/guanethidine
+Tubocurarine 529
Azlocillin
+Gentamicin 104
+Netilmicin 104
+Tobramycin 104

Bacampicillin
+Chloroquine 133
Baclofen
+Ibuprofen 602
+Lithium carbonate 463
+Tricyclic antidepressants 590

Bactericides, *see* individual drugs
+bacteriostatics 100
Barbiturates, *see also* individual drugs
+Alcohol 18
+Anaesthetics, general 514
+Anticoagulants 164
+Beta-blockers 306
+Calcium channel blockers 215
+Cimetidine 224
+Corticosteroids 438
+Cyclophosphamide 351
+Disopyramide 78
+Doxorubicin (adriamycin) 355
+Hypoglycaemic agents 413
+Lignocaine (lidocaine) 82
+Methoxyflurane 514
+Metronidazole 130
+Miconazole 224
+Monoamine oxidase inhibitors 478
+Oxygen 619
+Phenothiazines 505
+Phenytoin 237
+Primidone 255
+Quinidine 92
+Rifampicin (rifampin) 224
+Sulphonamides 145
+Theophylline 563
+Thyroid hormones 623
+Tricyclic antidepressants 590
BCG vaccine
+Theophylline 564
BCNU, *see* Carmustine
Beer, *see also* Alcohol
Alcohol content 15
+Monoamine oxidase inhibitors 554
+Tranylcypromine 554
+Tyramine content 554
Beer-shampoo
+Disulfiram 26
Bemetizide
+Indomethacin 287
Benazepril
+Nicoumalone (acenocoumarol) 157
+Warfarin 157
Bendrofluazide, *see also* Thiazides
+Aminoglutethimide 345
+Diazoxide 270
+Ibuprofen 287
+Indomethacin 287
+Lithium carbonate 474
Benfluorex
+Anticoagulants 165
+Phenprocoumon 165
Benoxaprofen
+Digoxin 377
Benzbromarone
+Anticoagulants 603
+Aspirin 603
+Chlorothiazide 603
+Ethylbiscoumacetate 603
+Nicoumalone (acenocoumarol) 603
+Phenindione 603
+Pyrazinamide 603
Benzhexol (trihexyphenidyl), *see also* Anticholinergics
+Chlorpromazine 501

+Desipramine 501
+Imipramine 501
+Levodopa 294
+Perphenazine 501
+Thioridazine 501
+Tricyclic antidepressants 501
+Trifluoperazine 501
Benziodarone
+Anticoagulants 166
+Clorindione 166
+Dicoumarol 166
+Diphenadione 166
+Ethylbiscoumacetate 166
+Nicoumalone (acenocoumarol) 166
+Phenindione 166
+Phenprocoumon 166
+Warfarin 166
Benznidazole
+Alcohol 33
Benzodiazepines, *see also* individual drugs
Generic and brand names 488, 489
+Alcohol 18
+Aminophylline 497
+Anaesthetics, local 520
+Antacids 491
+Anticholinergics 491
+Anticoagulants 166
+Beta-blockers 491
+Caffeine 497
+Calcium channel blockers 492
+Contraceptives, oral 493
+Cyclophosphamide 351
+Dextropropoxyphene 494
+Digoxin 377
+Disulfiram 494
+Ethambutol 495
+Fluvoxamine 588
+H2-blockers 492
+Hypoglycaemic agents 413
+Indomethacin 495
+Isoniazid 495
+Ketoconazole 496
+Levodopa 294
+Macrolide antibiotics 496
+Metronidazole 496
+Monoamine oxidase inhibitors 478
+Narcotic analgesics 59
+Neuromuscular blockers 523
+Omeprazole 497
+Phenytoin 238
+Probenecid 497
+Rifampicin (rifampin) 497
+Sodium valproate 258
+Theophylline 497
+Tobacco smoking 498
+Tricyclic antidepressants 590
Benztropine, *see also* Anticholinergics
+Chlorpromazine 501
+Chlorprothixene 501
+Fluphenazine 501
+Haloperidol 501
+Mesoridazine 501
+Methotrimeprazine 501
+Perphenazine 501
+Promazine 501
+Thioridazine 501

+Trifluoperazine 501
Benzydamine
+Anticoagulants 167
+Phenprocoumon 167
Benzylpenicillin, *see also* other penicillins
+Aspirin 134
+Chloramphenicol 113
+Chlorothiazide 134
+Chlortetracycline 135
+Cimetidine 110
+Contraceptives, oral 338
+Indomethacin 134
+Methoxyflurane 514
+Oxytetracycline 135
+Phenylbutazone 134
+Sulphamethizole 134
+Sulphamethoxypyridazine 134
+Sulphaphenazole 134
+Sulphinpyrazone 134
+Warfarin 197
Benzylprocaine penicillin
+Chloramphenicol 113
Bepridil
+Digoxin 378
+Food 327
Beta-acetyl digoxin, *see* Acetyl digoxin
Beta-blockers, *see also* individual drugs
Classification 303
Generic and brand names 304–5
+Alcohol 265, 305
+Amiodarone 74
+Anaesthetics, general 514, 518
+Anaesthetics, local 520
+Antacids 305
+Antiasthmatics 541
+Anticholinesterases 306
+Anticoagulants 167
+Atracurium 523
+Barbiturates 306
+Benzodiazepines 491
+Caffeine 321
+Calcium channel blockers 307, 316, 322
+Chloroform 514
+Cimetidine 308
+Cimetidine/phenylephrine 309
+Clonidine 267
+Contraceptives, oral 310
+Cyclopropane 514
+Dextromoramide 310
+Dextropropoxyphene 310
+Digoxin 377
+Diltiazem 310
+Disopyramide 77
+Encainide 79
+Enflurane 514
+Ergot alkaloids 311
+Ergotamine 311
+Erythromycin 312
+Etintidine 312
+Ether 514
+Fenfluramine 265
+Flecainide 312
+Fluvoxamine 588
+Food 313
+Glucagon 613
+H2-blockers 319
+Halofenate 313

637

Carbenoxolone
+ Aluminium hydroxide 604
+ Amiloride 604
+ Antacids 604
+ Antihypertensives 604
+ Chlorpropamide 601
+ Digitoxin 380
+ Digoxin 380
+ Diuretics 604
+ Magnesium hydroxide 604
+ Phenytoin 605
+ Spironolactone 604
+ Thiazides 604
+ Tolbutamide 605
+ Warfarin 605
Carbimazole
+ Corticosteroids 440
+ Prednisolone 440
+ Theophylline 582
Carbon tetrachloride
+ Anticoagulants 168
+ Dicoumarol 168
Carbonic anhydrase inhibitors, see
  also individual drugs
+ Aspirin 42
Carbutamide
+ Cyclophosphamide 420
+ Phenylbutazone 427
Cardiac glycosides, see Digitalis
  glycosides and individual drugs
Cardioselective beta-blockers, see
  Beta-blockers and individual
  drugs
Carmofur
+ Alcohol 348
Carmustine (BCNU)
+ Cimetidine 348
+ Digoxin 383
+ Phenytoin 217
CCNU, see Lomustine
Cefaclor
+ Probenecid 112
+ Theophylline 581
Cefadroxil
+ Cholestyramine 111
+ Diclofenac 47
Cefazeflur
+ Alcohol 21
Cefazolin
+ Methyldopa 281
Cefmenoxime
+ Alcohol 21
Cefmetazole
+ Alcohol 21
+ Probenecid 112
Cefonicid
+ Alcohol 21
Cefoperazone
+ Alcohol 21
+ Anticoagulants 169
Ceforanide
+ Alcohol 21
+ Probenecid 112
Cefotaxime
+ Mezlocillin 112
+ Tobramycin 102
Cefotetan
+ Alcohol 21
Cefotiam
+ Alcohol 21

Cefoxitin
+ Alcohol 21
+ Frusemide (furosemide) 111
+ Probenecid 112
Cefpiramide
+ Alcohol 21
Cefsoludin
+ Alcohol 21
Ceftazidime
+ Chloramphenicol 113
+ Cyclosporin 446
Ceftizoxime
+ Alcohol 21
+ Probenecid 112
Ceftriaxone
+ Frusemide (furosemide) 111
+ Probenecid 112
Cefuroxime
+ Tobramycin 102
Central Nervous System
  depressants, see CNS
  depressants
Cephacetrile
+ Frusemide (furosemide) 111
+ Probenecid 112
Cephalexin
+ Cholestyramine 111
+ Gentamicin 102
+ Probenecid 112
+ Theophylline 581
Cephalexin/clindamycin
+ Contraceptives, oral 332
Cephaloglycin
+ Probenecid 112
Cephaloridine
+ Frusemide (furosemide) 111
+ Probenecid 112
Cephalosporins, see also individual
  drugs
+ Alcohol 21
+ Aminoglycoside antibiotics 102
+ Anticoagulants 169
+ Cholestyramine 111
+ Frusemide (furosemide) 111
+ Methyldopa 281
+ Penicillins 112
+ Probenecid 112
+ Theophylline 581
Cephalothin
+ Alcohol 21
+ Anticoagulants 169
+ Colistin sulphomethate
  sodium 113
+ Frusemide (furosemide) 111
+ Gentamicin 102
+ Methotrexate 360
+ Probenecid 112
+ Tobramycin 102
Cephamandole
+ Alcohol 21
+ Probenecid 112
+ Warfarin 169
Cephazolin
+ Alcohol 21
+ Anticoagulants 169
+ Digoxin 387
+ Probenecid 112
Cephradine
+ Alcohol 21
+ Frusemide (furosemide) 111
+ Methyldopa 281

+ Probenecid 112
CHAP-V
+ Anticonvulsants 217
Charcoal
+ Aspirin 605
+ Digoxin 605
+ Phenytoin 605
Cheese
Cheese reaction 555
Tyramine content 556
+ Cimetidine 553
+ Debrisoquine 279
+ Demeclocycline 150
+ Isocarboxazid 555
+ Isoniazid 123
+ Mebanazine 555
+ Monoamine oxidase
  inhibitors 555
+ Nialamide 555
+ Pargyline 555
+ Procarbazine 368
+ Tetracyclines 150
+ Tranylcypromine 555
Chianti
Tyramine content 554
+ Monoamine oxidase
  inhibitors 554
Chloral betaine
+ Alcohol 23
Chloral hydrate
+ Alcohol 23
+ Anticoagulants 170
+ Dicoumarol 170
+ Fluvoxamine 588
+ Frusemide (furosemide) 271
+ Monoamine oxidase
  inhibitors 479
+ Phenelzine 479
+ Warfarin 170
Chloramphenicol
+ Acetaminophen (paracetamol)
  113
+ Ampicillin 113
+ Anticoagulants 170
+ Benzylpenicillin 113
+ Benzylprocaine penicillin 113
+ Ceftazidime 113
+ Chlorpropamide 416
+ Contraceptives, oral 332
+ Cyclophosphamide 352
+ Dicoumarol 170
+ Ethylbiscoumacetate 170
+ Hypoglycaemic agents 416
+ Iron preparations 616
+ Iron-dextran 616
+ Methicillin 113
+ Methotrexate 360
+ Methoxyflurane 514
+ Nicoumalone (acenocoumarol)
  170
+ Paracetamol (acetaminophen)
  113
+ Penicillins 113
+ Phenobarbitone 114
+ Phenytoin 240
+ Procaine penicillin 113
+ Rifampicin (rifampin) 115
+ Streptomycin 113
+ Tolbutamide 416
+ Vitamin B12 (cyanocobalamin)
  616

Chlordiazepoxide, *see also*
Benzodiazepines
+Alcohol 18
+Aluminium hydroxide 491
+Amitriptyline 590
+Cimetidine 492
+Contraceptives, oral 493
+Disulfiram 494
+Ethylbiscoumacetate 166
+Insulin 413
+Iproclozide 478
+Isocarboxazid 478
+Ketoconazole 496
+Levodopa 294
+Magnesium hydroxide 491
+Nortriptyline 590
+Phenelzine 478
+Phenobarbitone 226
+Phenytoin 238
+Tobacco smoking 498
+Tolbutamide 413
+Warfarin 166
Chlorinated pesticides, *see*
Pesticides
Chlormerodrin
+Lithium carbonate 463
Chlormethiazole
+Cimetidine 606
+H2-blockers 606
+Ranitidine 606
Chloroform
+Adrenaline (epinephrine) 513
+Beta-blockers 514
+Epinephrine (adrenaline) 513
Chloroprocaine
+Amethocaine (tetracaine) 519
Chloroquine
+Antacids 110
+Antidiarrhoeals 110
+Ampicillin 133
+Azapropazone 45
+Bacampicillin 133
+Chlorpromazine 504
+Cimetidine 115
+Contraceptives, oral 335
+Digoxin 389
+Hypoglycaemic agents 428
+Kaolin 110
+Magnesium trisilicate 110
+Metronidazole 131
+Penicillins 133
+Ranitidine 115
Chlorothiazide, *see also* other
Thiazides
+Acetohexamide 433
+Allopurinol 601
+Benzbromarone 603
+Benzylpenicillin 134
+Calcium carbonate 286
+Calcium/vitamin D 604
+Chlorpropamide 433
+Colestipol 286
+Cyclosporin 452
+Fluoxetine 587
+Insulin 433
+Lithium carbonate 474
+Phenformin 433
+Tolbutamide 433
+Warfarin 179
Chlorotrianisene
+Hydrocortisone 440

+Prednisone 440
Chlorozotocin
+Mitomycin 367
Chlorpheniramine
+Alcohol 16
+Dexamphetamine
(amphetamine) 541
+Phenytoin 241
Chlorphentermine
+Chlorpromazine 540
Chlorpromazine, *see also*
Phenothiazines
+Alcohol 34
+Aluminium hydroxide 503
+Amitriptyline 508
+Amodiaquine 504
+Benzhexol 501
+Benztropine 501
+Calcium carbonate 503
+Chloroquine 504
+Chlorphentermine 540
+Cimetidine 505
+Clonidine 266
+Coffee 508
+Dexamphetamine
(amphetamine) 540
+Diazoxide 270
+Guanethidine 277
+Hypoglycaemic agents 416
+Imipramine 508
+Levodopa 299
+Lithium carbonate 506
+Magnesium hydroxide 503
+Magnesium trisilicate 503
+Meperidine (pethidine) 66
+Methylamphetamine 540
+Metrizamide 627
+Nicoumalone (acenocoumarol)
198
+Nortriptyline 508
+Orphenadrine 501
+Pethidine (meperidine) 66
+Phenmetrazine 540
+Phenobarbitone 505
+Phenytoin 248
+Piperazine 135
+Propranolol 319
+Sodium valproate 258
+Sotalol 319
+Sulphadoxine/pyrimethamine
504
+Tea 508
+Tetrabenazine 509
+Tranylcypromine 484
+Trazodone 589
+Tricyclic antidepressants 501
+Zolpidem 510
Chlorpropamide, *see also*
Hypoglycaemic agents
+Alcohol 407
+Allopurinol 409
+Ammonium chloride 435
+Aspirin 429
+Carbenoxolone 601
+Chloramphenicol 416
+Chlorothiazide 433
+Cimetidine 417
+Clofibrate 418
+Colestipol 608
+Cortisone 420
+Cotrimoxazole 431

+Demeclocycline 432
+Diazepam 413
+Dicoumarol 411
+Fenclofenac 426
+Flurbiprofen 426
+Gemfibrozil 422
+Halofenate 423
+Hydrochlorothiazide 433
+Ibuprofen 426
+Indomethacin 426
+Mebanazine 425
+*Moduretic* 433
+Nicoumalone (acenocoumarol)
411
+Nifedipine 415
+Nortriptyline 434
+Phenylbutazone 427
+Probenecid 428
+Propranolol 413
+Rifampicin (rifampin) 429
+Sodium bicarbonate 435
+Sodium salicylate 429
+Sucralfate 430
+Sulphafurazole 431
+Sulphamethizole 431
+Trichlormethiazide 433
Chlorprothixene
+Benztropine 501
Chlortetracycline, *see also*
Tetracyclines
+Aluminium hydroxide 147
+Benzylpenicillin 135
+Carbamazepine 148
+Phenobarbitone 148
+Phenytoin 148
Chlorthalidone
+Captopril 261
+Clorindione 179
+Digoxin 386
+Lithium carbonate 474
+Nicoumalone (acenocoumarol)
179
+Phenprocoumon 179
+Warfarin 179
Cholestyramine
+Acetaminophen (paracetamol)
62
+Acipimox 600
+Amiodarone 75
+Anticoagulants 171
+Cefadroxil 111
+Cephalexin 111
+Cephalosporins 111
+Clofibrate 607
+Cyclosporin 450
+Digitoxin 380
+Digoxin 380
+Doxepin 592
+Ferrous sulphate 617
+Flecainide 81
+Flufenamic acid 49
+Fusidic acid 144
+Hydrochlorothiazide 286
+Iopanoic acid 627
+Iron preparations 617
+Loperamide 618
+Medigoxin 380
+Mefenamic acid 49
+Methotrexate 360
+Metronidazole 130
+Naproxen 58

646

Ferrous - *see* individual drugs and
Iron
Ferrous fumarate
+Aluminium hydroxide 616
+Magnesium hydroxide 616
Ferrous gluconate
+Methyldopa 282
Ferrous sulphate
+Aluminium hydroxide 616
+Calcium carbonate 616
+Cholestyramine 617
+Ciprofloxacin 140
+Doxycycline 149
+Levodopa 296
+Magnesium carbonate 616
+Magnesium hydroxide 616
+Magnesium trisilicate 616
+Methacycline 149
+Methyldopa 282
+*Mylanta* 616
+Oxytetracycline 149
+Penicillamine 64
+Sodium bicarbonate 616
+Sulphasalazine 144
+Tetracycline 149
Fibre (bran)
+Amoxycillin 133
+Digoxin 384
Fish
+Isoniazid 123
Flecainide
+Aluminium hydroxide 81
+Amiodarone 80
+Antacids 81
+Beta-blockers 312
+Caffeine 560
+Cholestyramine 81
+Cimetidine 81
+Digoxin 388
+Food 81
+Milk 81
+Propranolol 312
+Quinine 81
+Tobacco smoking 82
Floctafenine
+Anticoagulants 182
+Nicoumalone (acenocoumarol)
182
+Phenprocoumon 182
Flucloxacillin, *see also* other
penicillins
+Contraceptives, oral 338
+Warfarin 197
Fluconazole
+Contraceptives, oral 337
+Cyclosporin 452
+Phenytoin 243
Flucytosine
+Aluminium hydroxide 120
+Amphotericin 120
+Antacids 120
+Cytarabine 120
+Magnesium hydroxide 120
+Procarbazine 120
Fludrocortisone, *see also*
Corticosteroids
+Ethambutol 445
+Phenytoin 443
+Rifampicin (rifampin) 445
Flufenamic acid
+Cholestyramine 49

+Sulphinpyrazone 622
Fluindione, *see also* Anticoagulants
+Miconazole 192
Flunitrazepam, *see also*
Benzodiazepines
+Alcohol 18
Fluocortolone
+Contraceptives, oral 440
Fluorouracil (5FU)
+Aminoglycoside antibiotics 356
+Cimetidine 356
+Methotrexate 362
+Neomycin 356
+Warfarin 175
Fluoxetine
+Alcohol 27
+Buspirone 499
+Chlorothiazide 587
+Desipramine 595
+Diazepam 587
+Haloperidol 500
+Imipramine 595
+Lithium carbonate 466
+Monoamine oxidase
inhibitors 587
+Nortriptyline 595
+Tolbutamide 587
+Tranylcypromine 587
+Trazodone 595
+Tricyclic antidepressants 595
+Tryptophan 588
+Warfarin 587
Flupenthixol
+Alcohol 34
+Betel nuts 292
+Imipramine 598
+Lithium carbonate 506
Fluphenazine, *see also*
Phenothiazines
+Alcohol 34
+Benztropine 501
+Betel nuts 292
+Clonidine 266
+Coffee 508
+Imipramine 508
+Lithium carbonate 506
+Tea 508
+Vitamin C (ascorbic acid) 504
Flurazepam
+Alcohol 18
+Cimetidine 492
+Levodopa 294
+Warfarin 166
Flurbiprofen
+Chlorpropamide 426
+Cimetidine 49
+Frusemide (furosemide) 273
+H2-blockers 49
+Metformin 426
+Nicoumalone (acenocoumarol)
193
+Phenprocoumon 193
+Ranitidine 49
+Warfarin 193
Flurithromycin
+Carbamazepine 229
Fluroxene
+Adrenaline (epinephrine) 513
+Epinephrine (adrenaline) 513
+Neuromuscular blockers 516
+Noradrenaline (norepinephrine)

513
+Norepinephrine (noradrenaline)
513
+Phenobarbitone 517
+Phenytoin 517
Flutamide
+Anticoagulants 183
+Warfarin 183
Fluvoxamine
+Alcohol 28
+Anticoagulants 588
+Atenolol 588
+Benzodiazepines 588
+Beta-blockers 588
+Chloral hydrate 588
+Digoxin 382
+Lithium carbonate 588
+Propranolol 588
+Tryptophan 588
+Warfarin 588
Folic acid
+Anticonvulsants 219
+Contraceptives, oral 341
+Cotrimoxazole 116
+Phenobarbitone 219
+Phenytoin 219
+Primidone 219
+Sulphasalazine 612
Food, *see also* individual foods
Tyramine content 555
Vitamin K content 210
+Anticoagulants 183, 210
+Antihypertensives 266
+Aspirin 43
+Atenolol 313
+Bepridil 327
+Beta-blockers 313
+Bismuth subcitrate 603
+Calcium channel blockers 327
+Captopril 266
+Clindamycin 129
+Cyclosporin 450
+Dextropropoxyphene 46
+Dicoumarol 183
+Enalapril 266
+Etoposide 354
+Flecainide 81
+Frusemide (furosemide) 272
+Imipramine 595
+Indomethacin 51
+Isoniazid 125
+Isoniazid 123
+Itraconazole 127
+Ketoconazole 127
+Labetalol 313
+Levodopa 296
+Lincomycin 129
+Melphalan 354
+Mercaptopurine 358
+Methotrexate 354
+Metoprolol 313
+Monoamine oxidase
inhibitors 555
+Morphine 56
+Nabumetone 57
+Nifedipine 327
+Oxprenolol 313
+Penicillamine 64
+Pentopril 266
+Phenytoin 243
+Pindolol 313

Hypoglycaemic agents (cont.)
+ Urinary alkalinizers 435
Hypokalaemic agents
+ Liquorice 617

Ibuprofen
+ Alcohol 17
+ Aluminium hydroxide 49
+ Antacids 49
+ Baclofen 602
+ Bendrofluazide 287
+ Captopril 263
+ Chlorpropamide 426
+ Cimetidine 49
+ Digoxin 389
+ Frusemide (furosemide) 273
+ H2-blockers 49
+ Hydrochlorothiazide 287
+ Lithium carbonate 469
+ Magnesium hydroxide 49
+ Methotrexate 362
+ Metoprolol 314
+ Nizatidine 49
+ Phenprocoumon 193
+ Phenytoin 245
+ Pindolol 314
+ Propranolol 314
+ Ranitidine 49
+ Sucralfate 60
+ Tolbutamide 426
+ Warfarin 193
Ice-cream
+ Warfarin 183
Idrocilamide
+ Caffeine 560
+ Theophylline 573
Ifosfamide
+ Cisplatin 357
+ Phenobarbitone 357
Imidazole salicylate
+ Atenolol 314
Imipenem
+ Aminoglycoside antibiotics 122
Imipenem/cilastin
+ Cyclosporin 455
Imipramine, *see also* Tricyclic
antidepressants
+ Adrenaline (epinephrine) 547
+ Benzhexol 501
+ Bethanidine 278
+ Bromocriptine 503
+ Cannabis 591
+ Carbamazepine 591
+ Chlorpromazine 508
+ Cimetidine 592
+ Clonidine 269
+ Co-trimoxazole 593
+ Disulfiram 594
+ Epinephrine (adrenaline) 547
+ Estrogens 597
+ Ethinyloestradiol 597
+ Fluoxetine 595
+ Flupenthixol 598
+ Fluphenazine 508
+ Food 595
+ Guanethidine 278
+ Haloperidol 596
+ Halothane 519
+ Hexamethylmelamine 356
+ Iproniazid 485

+ Isocarboxazid 485
+ Isoprenaline (isoproterenol) 547
+ Isoproterenol (isoprenaline) 547
+ Levodopa 302
+ Methylphenidate 597
+ Noradrenaline (norepinephrine)
547
+ Norepinephrine
(noradrenaline) 547
+ Oestrogens 597
+ Pancuronium 519
+ Pargyline 485
+ Perphenazine 508
+ Phenelzine 485
+ Phenylephrine 547
+ Phenytoin 255
+ Ranitidine 592
+ Reserpine 284
+ Thyroid hormones 598
+ Tobacco smoking 599
+ Tranylcypromine 485
+ Tricyclic antidepressants 590
+ Zolpidem 510
Immunosuppressants, *see*
individual drugs and
Cytotoxics
Generic and brand names 436
Indanedione anticoagulants, *see*
Anticoagulants
Indigestion remedies, *see* Antacids
and individual drugs
Indirectly-acting
sympathomimetics, *see*
Sympathomimetics
Indobufen
+ Glipizide 426
Indomethacin
+ Alcohol 29
+ Allopurinol 50
+ Aluminium hydroxide 50
+ Amikacin 106
+ Aminoglycoside antibiotics 106
+ Anaesthetics, general 519
+ Antacids 50
+ Anticoagulants 187
+ Aspirin 50
+ Atenolol 314
+ Bemetizide 287
+ Bendrofluazide 287
+ Benzodiazepines 495
+ Benzylpenicillin 134
+ Beta-blockers 314
+ Bumetanide 273
+ Bupivacaine 519
+ Calcium channel blockers 327
+ Captopril 263
+ Chlorpropamide 426
+ Cimetidine 51
+ Clorindione 187
+ Diazepam 495
+ Diflunisal 47
+ Digoxin 390
+ Enalapril 263
+ Felodipine 327
+ Food 51
+ Frusemide (furosemide) 273
+ Gentamicin 106
+ H2-blockers 51
+ Haloperidol 500
+ Hydralazine 280
+ Hydrochlorothiazide 287

+ Lisinopril 263
+ Lithium carbonate 469
+ Magnesium carbonate 50
+ Magnesium hydroxide 50
+ Mazindol 41
+ Metformin 426
+ Methotrexate 362
+ Nefopam 59
+ Nifedipine 327
+ Oxprenolol 314
+ Pentopril 263
+ Phenprocoumon 187
+ Phenylbutazone 70
+ Phenylpropanolamine 552
+ Pindolol 314
+ Prednisolone 443
+ Prednisone 443
+ Probenecid 51
+ Propranolol 314
+ Sucralfate 60
+ Triamterene 288
+ Vaccines 52
+ Warfarin 187
Indoprofen
+ Glipizide 426
+ Tolbutamide 426
+ Warfarin 193
Indoramin
+ Alcohol 280
Influenza vaccine
+ Acetaminophen (paracetamol)
122
+ Alprazolam 122
+ Anticoagulants 187
+ Anticonvulsants 220
+ Carbamazepine 220
+ Cyclosporin 460
+ Lorazepam 122
+ Paracetamol (acetaminophen)
122
+ Phenobarbitone 220
+ Phenytoin 245
+ Theophylline 573
+ Warfarin 187
Innovar (fentanyl/droperidol)
+ Neuromusculard blockers 528
+ Suxamethonium 528
Insecticides, *see* Pesticides
Insulin, *see also* Hypoglycaemic
agents
+ Acebutolol 413
+ Alcohol 407
+ Alprenolol 413
+ Aspirin 429
+ Atenolol 413
+ Captopril 407
+ Chlordiazepoxide 413
+ Chlorothiazide 433
+ Clonidine 419
+ Colestipol 608
+ Contraceptives, oral 419
+ Corticosteroids 420
+ Cyclophosphamide 420
+ Debrisoquine 422
+ Dicoumarol 411
+ Diltiazem 415
+ Doxycycline 432
+ Droperidol 410
+ Enalapril 407
+ Encainide 79
+ Ether 410

Insulin (cont.)
+ Ethyloestrenol 410
+ Gemfibrozil 422
+ Guanethidine 422
+ Halofenate 423
+ Halothane 410
+ Isoniazid 424
+ Mebanazine 425
+ Methandienone 410
+ Methoxyflurane 410
+ Metoprolol 413
+ Nandrolone 410
+ Nitrous oxide 410
+ Oxprenolol 413
+ Oxytetracycline 432
+ Penbutolol 413
+ Phenprocoumon 411
+ Phenylephrine 428
+ Phenytoin 244
+ Pindolol 413
+ Propranolol 413
+ Somatropin 622
+ Stanozolol 410
+ Sulphinpyrazone 431
+ Testosterone 410
+ Thiopentone 410
+ Timolol 413
+ Tobacco smoking 434
+ Trichlormethiazide 433
+ Warfarin 411
Interferon
+ Acetaminophen (paracetamol) 122
+ Aspirin 122
+ Paracetamol (acetaminophen) 122
+ Prednisone 122
+ Theophylline 574
Intrauterine Contraceptive Devices, *see* IUD's
Iodine preparations
+ Lithium carbonate 468
Iodine-131
+ Theophylline 582
Iohexol, *see also* X-ray contrast media
+ Calcium channel blockers 330
Iopamidol, *see also* X-ray contrast media
+ Calcium channel blockers 330
Iopanoic acid, *see also* X-ray contrast media
+ Cholestyramine 627
Iothalamate, *see also* X-ray contrast media
+ Calcium channel blockers 330
Iprindole
+ Noradrenaline (norepinephrine) 547
+ Norepinephrine (noradrenaline) 547
Iproclozide
+ Chlordiazepoxide 478
Iproniazid
+ Imipramine 485
+ Meperidine (pethidine) 67
+ Morphine 483
+ Pethidine (meperidine) 67
+ Pseudoephedrine 549
+ Reserpine 484
+ Tetrabenazine 484

Iron preparations, *see also* Ferrous salts
+ Allopurinol 600
+ Antacids 616
+ Chloramphenicol 616
+ Cholestyramine 617
+ Ciprofloxacin 140
+ Levodopa 296
+ Methyldopa 282
+ Ofloxacin 140
+ Penicillamine 64
+ Quinolone antibiotics 140
+ Sulphasalazine 144
+ Tea 617
+ Tetracyclines 149
Iron-dextran
+ Chloramphenicol 616
Iron-glycine-sulphate
+ Ciprofloxacin 140
+ Ofloxacin 140
Isocarboxazid, *see also* Monoamine Oxidase Inhibitors
+ Amitriptyline 485
+ Anaesthetics, general 516
+ Cheese 555
+ Chlordiazepoxide 478
+ Dextromethorphan 479
+ Food 555
+ Imipramine 485
+ Levodopa 298
+ Methylamphetamine 549
+ Morphine 483
+ Sympathomimetics 549
+ Tranylcypromine 482
+ Tyramine-rich foods 555
Isoetharine
+ Phenelzine 545
Isoflurane, *see also* Anaesthetics, general
+ Adrenaline (epinephrine) 513
+ Aminophylline 517
+ Amiodarone 74
+ Atracurium 516
+ Beta-blockers 514
+ Epinephrine (adrenaline) 513
+ Monoamine oxidase inhibitors 516
+ Neuromuscular blockers 516
+ Noradrenaline (norepinephrine) 513
+ Norepinephrine (noradrenaline) 513
+ Phenylephrine 517
Isoniazid
+ Alcohol 30
+ Aluminium hydroxide 123
+ Aminosalicylic acid (PAS) 123
+ Antacids 123
+ Anticoagulants 159
+ Benzodiazepines 495
+ Carbamazepine 228
+ Cheese 123
+ Cimetidine 124
+ Clotiazepam 495
+ Contraceptives, oral 332
+ Cycloserine 117
+ Cyclosporin 458
+ Diazepam 495
+ Disulfiram 124
+ Ethambutol 125
+ Ethosuximide 232

+ Fish 123
+ Food 123, 125
+ Haloperidol 499
+ Hypoglycaemic agents 424
+ Insulin 424
+ Ketoconazole 128
+ Levodopa 125
+ Magaldrate 123
+ Meperidine (pethidine) 126
+ Oxazepam 495
+ Pethidine (meperidine) 126
+ Phenytoin 246
+ Primidone 256
+ Propranolol 126
+ Ranitidine 124
+ Rifampicin (rifampin) 126
+ Theophylline 574
+ Tolbutamide 424
+ Triazolam 495
+ Warfarin 159
Isoniazid/aminosalicylic acid
+ Warfarin 159
Isoniazid/pyridoxine
+ Vincristine 369
Isoprenaline (isoproterenol)
+ Amitriptyline 551
+ Imipramine 547
+ Metoprolol 541
+ Phenelzine 545
+ Practolol 541
+ Theophylline 564
+ Tranylcypromine 545
Isopropamide iodide
+ Lithium carbonate 468
Isoproterenol, (isoprenaline)
+ Amitriptyline 551
+ Imipramine 547
+ Metoprolol 541
+ Phenelzine 545
+ Practolol 541
+ Theophylline 564
+ Tranylcypromine 545
Isotretinoin
+ Contraceptives, oral 338
+ Minocycline 620
+ Tetracycline 620
Isoxicam
+ Acetyldigoxin 390
+ Anticoagulants 188
+ Aspirin 52
+ Cimetidine 52
+ Phenytoin 52
+ Propranolol 314
+ Warfarin 188
Ispaghula, *see* Psyllium
Isradipine
+ Digoxin 378
Itraconazole
+ Cyclosporin 452
+ Food 127
Ivoqualine (viqualine)
+ Alcohol 38
IUD's (Intrauterine Contraceptive Devices)
+ Aspirin 341
+ Corticosteroids 341
+ Mefenamic acid 341

654

+ Flucytosine 120
+ Ibuprofen 49
+ Indomethacin 50
+ Ketoconazole 127
+ Levodopa 294
+ Lithium carbonate 472
+ Mefenamic acid 48
+ Naproxen 57
+ Norfloxacin 139
+ Ofloxacin 139
+ Pefloxacin 139
+ Penicillamine 64
+ Phenoperidine 69
+ Phenytoin 234
+ Prednisone 437
+ Quinidine 98
+ Ranitidine 614
+ Roxatidine 621
+ Sodium polystyrene
   sulphonate 621
+ Sodium valproate 257
+ Sulpiride 509
+ Suprofen 60
+ Tetracycline 147
+ Theophylline 563
+ Tolfenamic acid 48
+ Tolmetin 60
+ Trimoprostil 624
+ Warfarin 162
+ Zomepirac 60

Magnesium oxide *see also* Antacids
+ Naproxen 57
+ Phenytoin 234

Magnesium sulphate
+ Aminoglycoside antibiotics 106
+ Calcium channel blockers 328
+ Gentamicin 106
+ Neuromuscular blockers 531
+ Nifedipine 328
+ Suxamethonium 531
+ Tetracycline 147
+ Tubocurarine 531
+ Vecuronium 531

Magnesium trisilicate *see also*
   Antacids
+ Antimalarials 110
+ Chloroquine 110
+ Chlorpromazine 503
+ Contraceptives, oral 332
+ Dexamethasone 437
+ Digoxin 375
+ Ferrous sulphate 616
+ Mexiletine 86
+ Nitrofurantoin 132
+ Phenytoin 234
+ Prednisolone 437
+ Prednisone 437
+ Rifampicin (rifampin) 142
+ Sodium valproate 257
+ Trimethoprim 153
+ Warfarin 162

Malathion
+ Suxamethonium 530

MAOI, *see* Monoamine Oxidase
   Inhibitors

Mandrax
+ Alcohol 31

Mannitol
+ Cyclosporin 452

Maprotiline
+ Alcohol 30

+ Clonidine 265
+ Contraceptives, oral 589
+ Nicoumalone (acenocoumarol)
   207
+ Noradrenaline (norepinephrine)
   547
+ Norepinephrine (noradrenaline)
   547
+ Propranolol 589
+ Tobacco smoking 589

Marmite (yeast extract)
+ Monoamine oxidase
   inhibitors 555

Mazindol
+ Bethanidine 276
+ Debrisoquine 276
+ Fenfluramine 612
+ Indomethacin 41
+ Lithium carbonate 468
+ Monoamine oxidase
   inhibitors 481
+ NSAID's 41
+ Phenelzine 481
+ Prednisone 41
+ Sodium salicylate 41

M-BACOD
+ Bleomycin 348

MDMA (3,4-methylene-dioxy-
   methamphetamine)
+ Monoamine oxidase
   inhibitors 551
+ Phenelzine 551

Mebanazine, *see also* Monoamine
   Oxidase Inhibitors
+ Butobarbitone 478
+ Cheese 555
+ Chlorpropamide 425
+ Insulin 425
+ Meperidine (pethidine) 67
+ Pethidine (meperidine) 67
+ Phenylpropanolamine 549
+ Propranolol 482
+ Quinalbarbitone 478
+ Tolbutamide 425
+ Tyramine-rich foods 555

Mebendazole
+ Anticonvulsants 130
+ Carbamazepine 130
+ Cimetidine 130
+ Phenytoin 130
+ Sodium valproate 130
+ Theophylline 562

Mebhydrolin
+ Alcohol 16

Meclofenamic acid
+ Anticoagulants 190
+ Aspirin 53
+ Sulphinpyrazone 622
+ Warfarin 190

Meclozine
+ Hyoscine 501

Medazepam
+ Alcohol 18

Medigoxin, *see also* other Digitalis
   glycosides
+ Cholestyramine 380
+ Diltiazem 384
+ Pinaverium 396

Medroxyprogesterone
+ Aminoglutethimide 342

Mefenamic acid
+ Anticoagulants 190
+ Cholestyramine 49
+ IUD's 341
+ Lithium carbonate 469
+ Magnesium hydroxide 48
+ Sulphinpyrazone 622
+ Warfarin 190

Mefloquine
+ Contraceptives, oral 335
+ Hypoglycaemic agents 428

Meglumine diatrizoate
+ Diltiazem 330
+ Nadolol 323
+ Nifedipine 330
+ Propranolol 323

Melphalan
+ Cimetidine 358
+ Cyclosporin 455
+ Digoxin 383
+ Food 354
+ Warfarin 175

Menadiol, *see* Vitamin K
Menaphthone, *see* Vitamin K
Mepacrine (quinacrine)
+ Pamaquine 136
+ Primaquine 136

Meperidine (pethidine)
+ Acetaminophen (paracetamol)
   63
+ Acyclovir 65
+ Chlorpromazine 66
+ Cimetidine 67
+ Cyclophosphamide 353
+ Furazolidone 67
+ H2-blockers 67
+ Iproniazid 67
+ Isoniazid 126
+ Mebanazine 67
+ Monoamine oxidase inhibitors
   67, 483
+ Mustine 353
+ Paracetamol (acetaminophen) 63
+ Pargyline 67
+ *Parstelin* 483
+ Phenelzine 67
+ Phenobarbitone 66
+ Phenothiazines 66
+ Phenytoin 68
+ Prochlorperazine 66
+ Promethazine 59
+ Propiomazine 66
+ Ranitidine 67
+ Thioridazine 66
+ Tranylcypromine 67

Mephentermine
+ Monoamine oxidase
   inhibitors 549
+ Phenelzine 549
+ Tranylcypromine 549

Mepivacaine
+ Amethocaine (tetracaine) 519
+ Bupivacaine 519

Meprobamate
+ Alcohol 31
+ Anticoagulants 190
+ Warfarin 190

Meptazinol
+ Anticoagulants 190
+ Warfarin 190

657

Mercaptopurine
+ Allopurinol 345
+ Co-trimoxazole 346
+ Doxorubicin (adriamycin) 346
+ Food 358
+ Trimethoprim 346
+ Vaccines 354
+ Warfarin 175
Mesoridazine
+ Benztropine 501
+ Phenobarbitone 505
Metaclazepam
+ Alcohol 18
Metaproterenol, *see* Orciprenaline
Metaraminol
+ Guanethidine 544
+ Monoamine oxidase
inhibitors 549
+ Pargyline 549
+ Reserpine 546
Metformin, *see also* Hypoglycaemic
agents
+ Alcohol 407
+ Captopril 407
+ Cimetidine 417
+ Fenclofenac 426
+ Flurbiprofen 426
+ Indomethacin 426
+ Nicardipine 415
+ Nifedipine 415
+ Phenprocoumon 411
Methacycline, *see also* Tetracyclines
+ Carbamazepine 148
+ Ferrous sulphate 149
+ Milk 150
+ Phenobarbitone 148
+ Phenytoin 148
Methadone
+ Anticonvulsants 53
+ Carbamazepine 53
+ Cimetidine 54
+ Desipramine 596
+ Diazepam 59
+ Disulfiram 54
+ Monoamine oxidase
inhibitors 483
+ Phenobarbitone 53
+ Phenytoin 53
+ Rifampicin (rifampin) 54
+ Tranylcypromine 483
+ Tricyclic antidepressants 596
+ Urinary acidifiers 55
+ Urinary alkalinizers 55
Methandienone
+ Bromindione 161
+ Insulin 410
+ Oxyphenbutazone 61
+ Phenylbutazone 61
+ Warfarin 161
Methaqualone
+ Alcohol 31
+ Anticoagulants 191
+ Diazepam 31
+ Warfarin 191
Methenamine, *see* Hexamine
Methchlorethamine, *see* Mustine
Methicillin, *see also* other Penicillins
+ Chloramphenicol 113
+ Gentamicin 102
+ Tobramycin 102

Methimazole
+ Corticosteroids 440
+ Prednisolone 440
+ Warfarin 209
Methionine
+ Levodopa 297
Methotrexate
+ Alcohol 358
+ Aminoglycoside antibiotics 359
+ Amiodarone 359
+ Aspirin 362
+ Azapropazone 362
+ Bleomycin 348
+ Carbenicillin 364
+ Cephalothin 360
+ Chloramphenicol 360
+ Cholestyramine 360
+ Cisplatin 350
+ Corticosteroids 360
+ Co-trimoxazole 361
+ Diclofenac 362
+ Dicloxacillin 364
+ Digoxin 383
+ Diuretics 361
+ Etoposide 354
+ Etretinate 365
+ Fluorouracil (5FU) 362
+ Food 354
+ Frusemide (furosemide) 361
+ Hydrocortisone 360
+ Hydroflumethiazide 361
+ Ibuprofen 362
+ Indomethacin 362
+ Kanamycin 359
+ Ketoprofen 362
+ Naproxen 362
+ Neomycin 359
+ Nitrous oxide 362
+ NSAID's 362
+ Paromomycin 359
+ Penicillin 364
+ Penicillins 364
+ Phenobarbitone 359
+ Phenylbutazone 362
+ Phenytoin 217
+ Piperacillin 364
+ Prednisone 360
+ Probenecid 364
+ Smallpox vaccine 354
+ Sodium bicarbonate 366
+ Sodium salicylate 362
+ Tetracycline 365
+ Thiazides 361
+ Ticarcillin 364
+ Tolbutamide 360
+ Trimethoprim 361
+ Urinary alkalinizers 366
+ Vaccines 354
+ Vitamin C (ascorbic acid) 359
+ Warfarin 175
Methotrimeprazine
+ Benztropine 501
+ Metrizamide 627
+ Pargyline 484
+ Tranylcypromine 484
Methoxamine
+ Guanethidine 544
+ Nialamide 545
+ Pheniprazine 545
+ Tranylcypromine 545

Methoxsalen
+ Caffeine 560
+ Phenytoin 618
Methoxyflurane, *see also*
Anaesthetics, general
+ Adrenaline (epinephrine) 513
+ Aminoglycoside antibiotics 514
+ Barbiturates 514
+ Benzylpenicillin 514
+ Beta-blockers 514
+ Chloramphenicol 514
+ Epinephrine (adrenaline) 513
+ Gentamicin 514
+ Insulin 410
+ Kanamycin 514
+ Neuromuscular blockers 516
+ Noradrenaline (norepinephrine)
513
+ Norepinephrine (noradrenaline)
513
+ Quinalbarbitone 514
+ Streptomycin 514
+ Tetracycline 514
Methylamphetamine
(Methamphetamine)
+ Chlorpromazine 540
+ Guanethidine 276
+ Isocarboxazid 549
+ Monoamine oxidase
inhibitors 549
+ Phenelzine 549
+ Tranylcypromine 549
Methyldopa
+ Alcohol 265
+ Amitriptyline 283
+ Cefazolin 281
+ Cephalosporins 281
+ Cephradine 281
+ Colestipol 608
+ Contraceptives, oral 335
+ Desipramine 283
+ Digoxin 391
+ Disulfiram 282
+ Ephedrine 549
+ Fenfluramine 265
+ Ferrous gluconate 282
+ Ferrous sulphate 282
+ Haloperidol 282
+ Iron preparations 282
+ Levodopa 297
+ Lithium carbonate 469
+ Mianserin 265
+ Monoamine oxidase
inhibitors 481
+ Pargyline 481
+ Phenobarbitone 281
+ Phenoxybenzamine 282
+ Phenylpropanolamine 549
+ Salbutamol 267
+ Sympathomimetics 549, 267
+ Tricyclic antidepressants 283
+ Trifluoperazine 266
+ Tyramine 549
Methylphenidate
+ Anticoagulants 191
+ Ethylbiscoumacetate 191
+ Guanethidine 276
+ Imipramine 597
+ Phenylbutazone 70
+ Phenytoin 247
+ Primidone 247

+ Tranylcypromine 549
+ Tricyclic antidepressants 597
Methylphenobarbitone
+ Ethosuximide 232
Methylprednisolone, *see also*
Corticosteroids
+ Aspirin 43
+ Carbamazepine 439
+ Cyclosporin 451
+ Erythromycin 442
+ Ketoconazole 442
+ Phenobarbitone 438
+ Phenytoin 443
+ Rifampicin (rifampin) 445
+ Theophylline 569
+ Triacetyloleandomycin (TAO)
442
Methylsalicylate
+ Warfarin 163
Methyltestosterone, *see also*
Anabolic steroids
+ Cyclosporin 459
+ Phenprocoumon 161
Methysergide
+ Hypoglycaemic agents 424
+ Propranolol 311
+ Tolbutamide 424
Metoclopramide
+ Alcohol 32
+ Cyclosporin 455
+ Digoxin 392
+ Levodopa 298
+ Misonidazole 366
+ Morphine 56
+ Neuromuscular blockers 532
+ Quinidine 97
+ Suxamethonium 532
Metocurine (Dimethyltubocurarine)
+ Phenytoin 534
+ Quinidine 535
Metolazone
+ Captopril 261
+ Cyclosporin 452
Metoprolol, *see also* Beta-blockers
+ Adrenaline (epinephrine) 541
+ Alcohol 305
+ Aluminium hydroxide 305
+ Amiodarone 74
+ Antacids 305
+ Caffeine 321
+ Cimetidine 308
+ Contraceptives, oral 310
+ Dextropropoxyphene 310
+ Diazepam 491
+ Epinephrine (adrenaline) 541
+ Felodipine 307
+ Food 313
+ Hydralazine 314
+ Ibuprofen 314
+ Insulin 413
+ Isoprenaline (isoproterenol) 541
+ Isoproterenol (isoprenaline) 541
+ Lignocaine (lidocaine) 82
+ Magnesium carbonate 305
+ Nicoumalone (acenocoumarol)
167
+ Nifedipine 316
+ Pentobarbitone 306
+ Phenelzine 482
+ Phenprocoumon 167
+ Phenylephrine 541

+ Procainamide 89
+ Propafenone 319
+ Ranitidine 319
+ Rifampicin (rifampin) 320
+ Terbutaline 541
+ Theophylline 565
+ Tolbutamide 413
+ Verapamil 322
+ Warfarin 167
Metriphonate
+ Contraceptives, oral 335
Metrizamide, *see also* X-ray contrast
media
+ Chlorpromazine 627
+ Dixyrazine 627
+ Methotrimeprazine 627
Metronidazole
+ Alcohol 32
+ Alprazolam 496
+ Aluminium hydroxide 130
+ Anticoagulants 191
+ Barbiturates 130
+ Benzodiazepines 496
+ Chloroquine 131
+ Cholestyramine 130
+ Cimetidine 131
+ Contraceptives, oral 332
+ Cyclosporin 450
+ Diazepam 496
+ Disulfiram 131
+ Kaolin-pectin 130
+ Lithium carbonate 469
+ Lorazepam 496
+ Phenobarbitone 130
+ Phenprocoumon 191
+ Phenytoin 247
+ Prednisone 131
+ Sulphadoxine/pyrimethamine
131
+ Sulphasalazine 145
+ Theophylline 576
+ Vecuronium 532
+ Warfarin 191
Metronidazole/cimetidine
+ Cyclosporin 450
Metyrapone
+ Phenytoin 618
Mexiletine
+ Aluminium hydroxide 86
+ Amiodarone 76
+ Antacids 86
+ Anticonvulsants 88
+ Caffeine 560
+ Cimetidine 87
+ Diamorphine 87
+ Digoxin 392
+ H2-blockers 87
+ Magnesium trisilicate 86
+ Morphine 87
+ Phenytoin 88
+ Propranolol 87
+ Quinidine 87
+ Ranitidine 87
+ Rifampicin (rifampin) 88
+ Theophylline 576
+ Urinary acidifiers 86
+ Urinary alkalinizers 86
Mezlocillin
+ Cefotaxime 112
+ Gentamicin 104
+ Netilmicin 104

+ Tobramycin 104
Mianserin
+ Alcohol 35
+ Anticonvulsants 588
+ Bethanidine 265
+ Carbamazepine 588
+ Clonidine 265
+ Guanethidine 265
+ Hydralazine 265
+ Hypoglycaemic agents 425
+ Methyldopa 265
+ Noradrenaline (norepinephrine)
545
+ Norepinephrine (noradrenaline)
545
+ Phenobarbitone 588
+ Phenprocoumon 207
+ Phenytoin 588
+ Propranolol 265
+ Sympathomimetics 545
+ Tyramine 545
+ Warfarin 207
Miconazole
+ Amphotericin 109
+ Anticoagulants 192
+ Barbiturates 224
+ Carbamazepine 229
+ Ethylbiscoumacetate 192
+ Fluindione 192
+ Glibenclamide 425
+ Gliclazide 425
+ Hypoglycaemic agents 425
+ Nicoumalone (acenocoumarol)
192
+ Pentobarbitone 224
+ Phenindione 192
+ Phenprocoumon 192
+ Phenytoin 248
+ Tioclomarol 192
+ Tobramycin 107
+ Tolbutamide 425
+ Warfarin 192
Midazolam
+ Alcohol 18
+ Aminophylline 497
+ Atracurium 523
+ Cimetidine 492
+ Pancuronium 523
+ Ranitidine 492
+ Suxamethonium 523
+ Vecuronium 523
Midecamycin
+ Theophylline 575
Milk and Milk Products
+ Alcohol 33
+ Bismuth subcitrate 603
+ Cyclosporin 450
+ Demeclocycline 150
+ Doxycycline 150
+ Flecainide 81
+ Methacycline 150
+ Minocycline 150
+ Nabumetone 57
+ Oxytetracycline 150
+ Tetracycline 150
+ Tetracyclines 150
Mineral oil, *see* Liquid Paraffin
Minocycline, *see also* Tetracyclines
+ Contraceptives, oral 332
+ Etretinate 620
+ Isotretinoin 620

661

Pargyline (cont.)
+ Imipramine 485
+ Levodopa 298
+ Meperidine (pethidine) 67
+ Metaraminol 549
+ Methotrimeprazine 484
+ Methyldopa 481
+ Noradrenaline (norepinephrine) 545
+ Norepinephrine (noradrenaline) 545
+ Pethidine (meperidine) 67
+ Phenylpropanolamine 549
+ Sympathomimetics 545, 549
+ Tyramine-rich foods 555
Paromomycin, *see also* Aminoglycoside antibiotics
+ Dicoumarol 159
+ Methotrexate 359
Parstelin
(tranylcypromine + trifluoperazi-ne), *see also* Tranylcypromine and Monoamine Oxidase Inhibitors
+ Meperidine (pethidine) 483
+ Morphine 483
+ Pethidine (meperidine) 483
PAS, *see* Aminosalicylic acid
Pefloxacin, *see also* Quinolone antibiotics
+ Aluminium hydroxide 139
+ Antacids 139
+ Cimetidine 140
+ Magnesium hydroxide 139
+ Nicoumalone (acenocoumarol) 202
+ Theophylline 578
Penbutolol, *see also* Beta-blockers
+ Cimetidine 308
+ Insulin 413
+ Lignocaine (lidocaine) 82
Penicillamine
+ Aluminium hydroxide 64
+ Antacids 64
+ Digoxin 394
+ Ferrous sulphate 64
+ Food 64
+ Iron preparations 64
+ *Maalox* 64
+ Magnesium hydroxide 64
Penicillin, *see also* Penicillins
+ Digoxin 387
+ Erythromycin 118
+ Methotrexate 364
+ Probenecid 134
Penicillin V *see also* Penicillins (phenoxymethylpenicillin)
+ Alcohol 110
+ Contraceptives, oral 338
+ Neomycin 107
Penicillins, *see also* individual drugs
+ Allopurinol 109
+ Aminoglycoside antibiotics 104, 107
+ Anticoagulants 197
+ Atenolol 317
+ Cephalosporins 112
+ Chloramphenicol 113
+ Chloroquine 133
+ Contraceptives, oral 338
+ Methotrexate 364

+ Probenecid 134
+ Tetracyclines 135
Pentazocine
+ Nefopam 59
+ Polluted air 65
+ Promethazine 59
+ Tobacco smoking 65
Pentobarbitone, *see also* other Barbiturates
+ Alprenolol 306
+ Caffeine 223
+ Cimetidine 224
+ Ethylbiscoumacetate 164
+ Metoprolol 306
+ Miconazole 224
+ Promethazine/hyoscine 505
+ Quinidine 92
+ Theophylline 563
Pentopril, *see also* ACE inhibitors
+ Cimetidine 262
+ Food 266
+ Indomethacin 263
Perphenazine
+ Alcohol 34
+ Amitriptyline 508
+ Benzhexol 501
+ Benztropine 501
+ Desipramine 508
+ Disulfiram 506
+ Imipramine 508
+ Lithium carbonate 506
+ Minocycline 151
+ Nortriptyline 508
Pesticides
+ Anticoagulants 188
+ Neuromuscular blockers 530
+ Phenylbutazone 70
+ Warfarin 188
Pethidine (meperidine)
+ Acetaminophen (paracetamol) 63
+ Acyclovir 65
+ Chlorpromazine 66
+ Cimetidine 67
+ Cyclophosphamide 353
+ Furazolidone 67
+ H2-blockers 67
+ Iproniazid 67
+ Isoniazid 126
+ Mebanazine 67
+ Monoamine oxidase inhibitors 67, 483
+ Mustine 353
+ Paracetamol (acetaminophen) 63
+ Pargyline 67
+ *Parstelin* 483
+ Phenelzine 67
+ Phenobarbitone 66
+ Phenothiazines 66
+ Phenytoin 68
+ Prochlorperazine 66
+ Promethazine 59
+ Propiomazine 66
+ Ranitidine 67
+ Thioridazine 66
+ Tranylcypromine 67
Petrichloral
+ Anticoagulants 170
Pharmacodynamic interactions 10–12

Pharmacokinetic interactions 3–10
Phenazone (antipyrine)
+ Amylobarbitone 69
+ Anticoagulants 198
+ H2-blockers 612
+ Pravastatin 619
+ Simvastatin 621
+ Warfarin 198
Phenelzine, *see also* Monoamine Oxidase Inhibitors
+ Adrenaline (epinephrine) 545
+ Amantadine 478
+ Anaesthetics, general 516
+ Broad beans 298
+ Chloral hydrate 479
+ Chlordiazepoxide 478
+ Clomipramine 485
+ Cyproheptadine 479
+ Desipramine 485
+ Dexamphetamine (amphetamine) 549
+ Dextromethorphan 479
+ Dextropropoxyphene 480
+ Droperidol/hyoscine 499
+ Epinephrine (adrenaline) 545
+ Ephedrine 549
+ Fenfluramine 480
+ Ginseng 480
+ Guaiphenesin 483
+ Hexamethylmelamine 356
+ Imipramine 485
+ Isoetharine 545
+ Isoprenaline (isoproterenol) 545
+ Isoproterenol 545
+ Levodopa 298
+ Lithium carbonate 481
+ Mazindol 481
+ MDMA 551
+ Meperidine (pethidine) 67
+ Mephentermine 549
+ Methylamphetamine 549
+ Metoprolol 482
+ Morphine 483
+ Nadolol 482
+ Nitrazepam 478
+ Noradrenaline (norepinephrine) 545
+ Norepinephrine (noradrenaline) 545
+ Oxtriphylline 483
+ Pethidine (meperidine) 67
+ Phenylephrine 552
+ Phenylpropanolamine 549
+ Reserpine 484
+ Salbutamol 545
+ Sulphafurazole 485
+ Suxamethonium 533
+ Sympathomimetics 545, 549
+ Tranylcypromine 482
+ Tryptophan 487
+ Tyramine-rich drinks 554
+ Tyramine-rich foods 555
Pheneturide
+ Phenytoin 248
Phenformin, *see also* Hypoglycaemic agents
+ Alcohol 407
+ Chlorothiazide 433
+ Colestipol 608
+ Halofenate 423
+ Tetracycline 432

664

665

Prednisolone, *see also*
Corticosteroids
+ Aloxiprin 43
+ Aluminium hydroxide 437
+ Aluminium phosphate 437
+ Carbamazepine 439
+ Carbimazole 440
+ Cimetidine 440
+ Contraceptives, oral 440
+ Cyclosporin 451
+ Etretinate 620
+ Indomethacin 443
+ Ketoconazole 442
+ Magnesium trisilicate 437
+ Methimazole 440
+ Naproxen 443
+ Pancuronium 526
+ Phenobarbitone 438
+ Phenytoin 443
+ Rifampicin (rifampin) 445
+ Triacetyloleandomycin (TAO) 442
Prednisone, *see also* Corticosteroids
+ Aluminium hydroxide 437
+ Aspirin 43
+ Chlorotrianisene 440
+ Choline salicylate 43
+ Cimetidine 440
+ Cyclophosphamide 352
+ Dicoumarol 175
+ Gastrogel 437
+ Hexestrol 440
+ Indomethacin 443
+ Interferon 122
+ Ketoconazole 442
+ Magnesium hydroxide 437
+ Magnesium trisilicate 437
+ Mazindol 41
+ Methotrexate 360
+ Metronidazole 131
+ Oxyphenbutazone 61
+ Phenobarbitone 438
+ Phenytoin 443
+ Ranitidine 440
+ Rifampicin (rifampin) 445
+ Smallpox vaccine 446
+ Sucralfate 446
+ Theophylline 569
+ Tolbutamide 420
+ Vaccines 446
Prenylamine
+ Amiodarone 328
+ Atenolol 328
+ Beta-blockers 328
+ Lignocaine (lidocaine) 328
+ Oxprenolol 328
+ Phenprocoumon 168
+ Procainamide 328
+ Propranolol 328
+ Quinidine 328
+ Sodium iothalamate 330
+ Sotalol 328
Prilocaine
+ Amethocaine (tetracaine) 519
Prilocaine-lignocaine
+ Co-trimoxazole 116
Primaquine
+ Contraceptives, oral 335
+ Mepacrine (quinacrine) 136
Primidolol
+ Prazosin 283

Primidone
+ Acetazolamide 215
+ Barbiturates 255
+ Carbamazepine 230
+ Carbamazepine 255
+ Clonazepam 255
+ Clorazepate 255
+ Contraceptives, oral 333
+ Corticosteroids 445
+ Denzimol 217
+ Dexamethasone 445
+ Ethosuximide 232
+ Folic acid 219
+ Isoniazid 256
+ Methylphenidate 247
+ Phenobarbitone 255
+ Phenytoin 256
+ Quinidine 92
+ Sodium valproate 256
+ Vitamin D 625
+ Vitamin D/calcium 625
Pristinamycin
+ Cyclosporin 454
Probenecid
+ Allopurinol 601
+ Aminophylline 577
+ Aminosalicylic acid (PAS) 108
+ Amoxycillin 134
+ Ampicillin 134
+ Aspirin 44
+ Benzodiazepines 497
+ Bumetanide 275
+ Captopril 262
+ Cefaclor 112
+ Cefmetazole 112
+ Ceforanide 112
+ Cefoxitin 112
+ Ceftizoxime 112
+ Ceftriaxone 112
+ Cephacetrile 112
+ Cephalexin 112
+ Cephaloglycin 112
+ Cephaloridine 112
+ Cephalosporins 112
+ Cephalothin 112
+ Cephamandole 112
+ Cephazolin 112
+ Cephradine 112
+ Chlorpropamide 428
+ Cisplatin 350
+ Clofibrate 607
+ Dapsone 117
+ Digoxin 396
+ Diprophylline 577
+ Enprofylline 577
+ Frusemide (furosemide) 275
+ Heparin 213
+ Hypoglycaemic agents 428
+ Indomethacin 51
+ Ketoprofen 53
+ Lorazepam 497
+ Methotrexate 364
+ Nafcillin 134
+ Nalidixic acid 132
+ Naproxen 58
+ Penicillins 134
+ Pyrazinamide 137
+ Rifampicin (rifampin) 143
+ Sodium salicylate 44
+ Sulphinpyrazone 622
+ Theophylline 577

+ Tolbutamide 428
+ Zidovudine 154
Probucol
+ Cyclosporin 457
+ Pravastatin 619
Procainamide
+ Anticholinesterases 602
+ Aluminium phosphate 76
+ Aminobenzoic acid (PABA) 90
+ Amiodarone 89
+ Antacids 76
+ Beta-blockers 89
+ Captopril 262
+ Cimetidine 89
+ Co-trimoxazole 91
+ Digoxin 385
+ H2-blockers 89
+ Hydroxyzine 501
+ Lignocaine (lidocaine) 85
+ Metoprolol 89
+ Prenylamine 328
+ Propranolol 89
+ Quinidine 90
+ Ranitidine 89
+ Suxamethonium 530
+ Trimethoprim 91
Procaine
+ Sulphadiazine 145
+ Suxamethonium 530
Procaine penicillin
+ Chloramphenicol 113
Procarbazine
+ Acetyldigoxin 383
+ Alcohol 35
+ Antihypertensives 367
+ Cheese 368
+ CNS depressants 367
+ Digitoxin 383
+ Etoposide 354
+ Flucytosine 120
+ Food 368
+ Mustine 367
+ Sympathomimetics 368
+ Tyramine-rich foods 368
+ Vaccines 354
+ Verapamil 353
+ Warfarin 175
Procetofene, *see* Fenofibrate
Prochlorperazine
+ Desferrioxamine 609
+ Levodopa 299
+ Meperidine (pethidine) 66
+ Pethidine (meperidine) 66
+ Phenytoin 248
Procyclidine
+ Betel nuts 292
Progabide
+ Anticonvulsants 221
+ Carbamazepine 221
+ Clonazepam 221
+ Phenobarbitone 221
+ Phenytoin 221
+ Sodium valproate 221
Progestogens, *see* Contraceptives, oral
Prolintane
+ Anticoagulants 200
+ Ethylbiscoumacetate 200
PROMACE-MOPP
+ Warfarin 175

671

673

675

Tuinal
(amylobarbitone
+quinalbarbitone)
+Thyroid hormones 623
Tyramine, *see also* Tyramine rich
foods and drinks
+Furazolidone 543
+Methyldopa 549
+Mianserin 545
+Monoamine Oxidase
Inhibitors 555
+Reserpine 546
+Trazodone 545
Tyramine-rich drinks
Tyramine content 554
+Monoamine oxidase
inhibitors 554
Tyramine-rich foods
Tyramine content 555
+Cimetidine 553
+Debrisoquine 279
+Furazolidone 543
+Isocarboxazid 555
+Mebanazine 555
+Monoamine oxidase
inhibitors 555
+MOPP 368
+Nialamide 555
+Pargyline 555
+Phenelzine 555
+Procarbazine 368
+Tranylcypromine 555

Urinary acidifiers, *see also*
individual drugs
+Amphetamines 541
+Erythromycin 119
+Hexamine 121
+Hypoglycaemic agents 435
+Methadone 55
+Mexiletine 86
+Quinine 138
+Sulphonamides 121
+Tricyclic antidepressants 599
Urinary alkalinizers, *see also*
individual drugs
+Amphetamines 541
+Erythromycin 119
+Hexamine 121
+Hypoglycaemic agents 435
+Lithium carbonate 472
+Methadone 55
+Methotrexate 366
+Mexiletine 86
+Quinidine 98
+Quinine 138
+Tocainide 98
+Tricyclic antidepressants 599

VAC
+Verapamil 353
Vaccines, *see also* individual
vaccines
+Acetaminophen (paracetamol)
122
+Actinomycin 354
+Alprazolam 122
+Anticoagulants 187
+Anticonvulsants 220

+Bleomycin 354
+Carbamazepine 220
+Corticosteroids 446
+Cortisone 446
+Cyclophosphamide 354
+Cyclosporin 460
+Cytotoxics 354
+Indomethacin 52
+Lorazepam 122
+Mercaptopurine 354
+Methotrexate 354
+Mustine 354
+Paracetamol (acetaminophen)
122
+Phenobarbitone 220
+Phenytoin 245
+Prednisone 446
+Procarbazine 354
+Theophylline 564, 573, 577
+Vinblastine 354
+Vincristine 354
+Warfarin 187
Valproic acid, *see* Sodium valproate
Valpromide
+Carbamazepine 231
Vancomycin
+Aminoglycoside antibiotics 107
+Nifedipine 330
+Warfarin 169
Vasodilators, *see* individual drugs
Vecuronium *see also* Neuromuscular
blockers
+Amikacin/polymyxin 521
+Cyclosporin 527
+Dantrolene 527
+Diazepam 523
+Gentamicin 521
+Lorazepam 523
+Lormetazepam 523
+Magnesium sulphate 531
+Metronidazole 532
+Midazolam 523
+Phenytoin 534
+Testosterone 536
+Tobramycin 521
+Verapamil 524
Vegetables
Vitamin K content 211
+Anticoagulants 210
Verapamil, *see also* Calcium channel
blockers
+Alcohol 21, 265
+Aminophylline 566
+Aspirin 325
+Atenolol 322
+Barbiturates 215
+Beta-blockers 322
+Bupivacaine 328
+Caffeine 559
+Calcium/vitamin D 325
+Carbamazepine 215
+Cimetidine 325
+Cisplatin 353
+COPP 353
+Cyclophosphamide 353
+Cyclosporin 449
+Dantrolene 327
+Digitoxin 403
+Digoxin 403
+Doxorubicin (adriamycin) 353
+Ethambutol 329

+Glibenclamide 415
+Lignocaine (lidocaine) 328
+Lithium carbonate 464
+Metoprolol 322
+Phenobarbitone 215
+Pindolol 322
+Practolol 322
+Prazosin 284
+Procarbazine 353
+Propranolol 322
+Quinidine 94
+Rifampicin (rifampin) 329
+Sulphinpyrazone 329
+Theophylline 566
+Tubocurarine 524
+VAC 353
+Vecuronium 524
+Vincristine 353
+Vindesine 353
+Vitamin D/calcium 325
Vidarabine
+Aminophylline 583
+Allopurinol 153
+Theophylline 583
Vigabatrin
+Anticonvulsants 222
+Carbamazepine 222
+Phenobarbitone 222
+Phenytoin 222
Viloxazine
+Anticonvulsants 223
+Carbamazepine 223
+Co-trimoxazole 593
+Phenytoin 223
+Theophylline 584
Vinbarbitone
+Dicoumarol 164
Vinblastine
+Bleomycin/cisplatin 368
+Mitomycin 369
+Phenytoin 217
+Vaccines 354
Vinca alkaloids, *see* individual
drugs
Vincristine
+Acetyldigoxin 383
+Bleomycin 348
+Colaspase 369
+Digitoxin 383
+Isoniazid/pyridoxine 369
+Vaccines 354
+Verapamil 353
+Warfarin 175
Vindesine
+Mitomycin 369
+Verapamil 353
+Warfarin 175
Vitamin A
+Aminoglycoside antibiotics 625
+Contraceptives, oral 341
+Neomycin 625
+Retinoids 620
Vitamin B12 (cyanocobalamin)
+Chloramphenicol 616
+Contraceptives, oral 341
Vitamin B6 (pyridoxine)
+Anticonvulsants 221
+Contraceptives, oral 341
+Levodopa 300
+Phenobarbitone 221
+Phenytoin 221